Radiologic Oncology of the Abdomen and Pelvis

An Atlas and Text

Radiologic Oncology of the Abdomen and Pelvis

An Atlas and Text

ALI SHIRKHODA, M.D.

Professor of Radiology
University of Texas System Cancer Center
Radiologist and Director of Computed Tomography
M. D. Anderson Hospital and Tumor Institute
Houston, Texas

YEAR BOOK MEDICAL PUBLISHERS, INC.
CHICAGO • LONDON • BOCA RATON

1   2   3   4   5   6   7   8   9   0   KC   92   91   90   89   88

Library of Congress Cataloging-in-Publication Data
Shirkhoda, Ali.
    Radiologic oncology of the abdomen and pelvis: an atlas and text
    Ali Shirkhoda.
       p.   cm.
    Includes bibliographies and index.
    ISBN 0-8151-7652-X
    1. Abdomen—Cancer—Diagnosis.   2. Pelvis—Cancer—Diagnosis.
    3. Diagnostic imaging.   4. Abdomen—Imaging.
    5. Pelvis—Imaging.
    I. Title.
       [DNLM: 1. Abdominal Neoplasms—radionuclide—atlases.   2. Pelvic
Neoplasms—radionuclide—atlases.   WI 17 S558r]
RC280.A2S55 1988   88-5515
616.99′4950757—dc19   CIP
DNLM/DLC
for Library of Congress

Sponsoring Editor: James D. Ryan, Jr.
Associate Director, Manuscript Services: Frances M. Perveiler
Production Project Manager: Gayle Paprocki
Proofroom Supervisor: Shirley E. Taylor

To my Wife,
Shahrzad
And my Daughters,
Layla and
Roxana

Contributors

James L. Buck, L.C.D.R., M.C., U.S.N.R.
Chief, Section of Gastrointestinal Radiology Pathology
Armed Forces Institute of Pathology, Washington D.C.
Assistant Professor of Radiology
Uniformed Services University of the Health Sciences
Bethesda, Maryland

Chusilp Charnsangavej, M.D.
Radiologist and Professor of Radiology
Chief of Interventional and Cardiovascular Radiology
The University of Texas M. D. Anderson Hospital and
    Tumor Institute at Houston
Houston, Texas

Marvin H. Chasen, M.D.
Formerly Associate Radiologist and Associate Professor of
    Clinical Radiology
The University of Texas M. D. Anderson Hospital and
    Tumor Institute at Houston
Houston, Texas
Currently Associate Professor of Clinical Radiology
Baylor College of Medicine
Houston, Texas

Ronelle DuBrow, M.D.
Assistant Radiologist and Assistant Professor of
    Radiology
The University of Texas M. D. Anderson Hospital and
    Tumor Institute at Houston
Houston, Texas

Farzin Eftekhari, M.D.
Associate Radiologist and Associate Professor of
    Radiology
The University of Texas M. D. Anderson Hospital and
    Tumor Institute at Houston
Houston, Texas

Thomas W. Koonce, M.D.
Formerly Fellow in Sectional Body Imaging and
    Interventional Radiology
The University of Texas M. D. Anderson Hospital and
    Tumor Institute at Houston
Houston, Texas
Currently Radiologist
The Radiology Consultant
Little Rock, Arkansas

Lamk M. Lamki, M.D., F.R.C.P.(C.)
Associate Internist and Associate Professor of Medicine
    (Nuclear Medicine)
The University of Texas M. D. Anderson Hospital and
    Tumor Institute at Houston
Houston, Texas

Errol Lewis, M.D.
Formerly Associate Radiologist and Associate Professor of
    Radiology
The University of Texas M. D. Anderson Hospital and
    Tumor Institute at Houston
Houston, Texas
Currently Radiologist
Baptist Hospital
Memphis, Tennessee

Anthony R. Lupetin, M.D.
Senior Attending Radiologist
Allegheny General Hospital
Pittsburgh, Pennsylvania

John E. Madewell, M.D.
Formerly Professor and Vice Chairman
Department of Radiology
Director of Radiologic Education
Baylor College of Medicine
Houston, Texas
Currently Professor and Chairman
Department of Radiology
Pennsylvania State University
Hershey, Pennsylvania

Luceil B. North, M.D.
Radiologist and Associate Professor of Radiology
The University of Texas M. D. Anderson Hospital and
    Tumor Institute at Houston
Houston, Texas

Golden Pan, M.D.
Senior Resident in Diagnostic Radiology
The University of Texas Health Science Center
Houston, Texas

Donald A. Podoloff, M.D.
Associate Radiologist and Associate Professor of Nuclear
    Medicine and Radiology
Deputy Chairman, Department of Nuclear Medicine
The University of Texas M. D. Anderson Hospital and
    Tumor Institute at Houston
Houston, Texas

Pablo R. Ros, M.D.
Formerly Chief, Section of Gastrointestinal Radiology
    Pathology
Armed Forces Institute of Pathology
Washington, D.C.
Assistant Professor of Radiology and Nuclear Medicine
Uniformed Services University of the Health Sciences
Bethesda, Maryland
Currently Associate Professor of Radiology
Director of Abdominal Imaging Services
University of Florida School of Medicine
Gainesville, Florida

Ali Shirkhoda, M.D.
Radiologist and Professor of Radiology
Director of Computed Tomography
The University of Texas M. D. Anderson Hospital and
    Tumor Institute at Houston
Houston, Texas

Anita J. Thomas, M.D.
Formerly Assistant Radiologist and Assistant Professor of
    Radiology
The University of Texas M. D. Anderson Hospital and
    Tumor Institute at Houston
Houston, Texas
Currently Radiologist
Erlanger Hospital
Chattanooga, Tennessee

Foreword

The identification and staging of tumors represent a large portion of the practice of diagnostic radiology. Unfortunately, the pertinent literature is widely scattered, and frequently only the typical manifestations of a given neoplasm are described. While most tumors are readily recognized, there is less appreciation of their early appearances and limited recognition of the roles of diagnostic imaging in staging and treatment. All aspects are essential if cancer survival rates are to be improved.

To obtain the most detailed information, a variety of imaging procedures must be employed. These range from conventional radiography to sectional imaging techniques such as ultrasound, computed tomography, and magnetic resonance imaging. Although reasonably well-defined indications for each exist, their number and complexity can cause confusion, particularly for the referring physician. The newer modalities have proved to be most helpful, making possible the visualization of certain organs and tissues that formerly required the use of contrast material or radionuclides. In addition, the multiplanar capabilities of sectional examinations permit use of a third dimension in the localization and definition of tumors. Such information may be used for the guidance of percutaneous biopsy needles and in treatment planning. Also, the ability of computed tomography to determine the relative densities of imaged structures has proved useful in the pretreatment calculation of the scattering effects of various tissues on high-energy particles.

While the newer techniques have considerably broadened the capabilities of diagnostic radiologists, the gradual evolution and refinement of conventional imaging procedures have also made a significant contribution to the diagnosis and staging of tumors. The earlier recognition of disease by radiologic means has improved survival rates in certain tumors. Undoubtedly, this trend will continue as the value of early detection becomes more apparent through such studies as the breast screening program of the Health Insurance Plan of New York.

The University of Texas M. D. Anderson Hospital and Tumor Institute is a referral center dedicated to the treatment of neoplastic diseases. The concentration of pathology that occurs in a categorical institution has permitted the authors to cover most neoplasms in detail. Three fourths of this book's contributors are members of the M. D. Anderson staff, and over 90% of its material has been derived from the M. D. Anderson files. Where deficits were encountered, detailed contributions were made by collaborators from other institutions.

The material selected by Dr. Shirkhoda and his associates emphasizes an integrated approach to the use of the various imaging modalities and illustrates the capabilities of each. Both common and uncommon neoplasms are included, and the book is heavily pictorial, affording an opportunity for the reader to become familiar with the nuances of individual neoplasms. The legends function as additional text, illustrating the relative importance of specific diagnostic modalities.

Technical advances aside, the skill of the radiologist remains pivotal in the amount of information that can be obtained from an imaging procedure. The hard-won experience of the authors should prove of value to all radiologists and oncologists and provide a sound approach to the use of imaging techniques in the cancer patient.

Gerald D. Dodd, M.D.
Professor and Head
Division of Diagnostic Imaging
The University of Texas System Cancer Center
M. D. Anderson Hospital and Tumor Institute
Houston, Texas

Preface

Over the past decade, there has been a revolution in the understanding of cancer, mostly as a result of developments in molecular biology. The mechanisms of carcinogenesis are gradually unfolding. During the same period there has been another revolution. Advances in imaging technology and interventional radiologic procedures have had a profound impact on the practice of radiology in general and on radiologic oncology in particular. The first of these advances was the development of computed tomography and its application in the head and body. This major step allowed the radiologist to look at anatomy and pathology from a cross-sectional rather than the conventional view. Next, high-resolution ultrasound was discovered and most recently, magnetic resonance imaging was introduced. These noninvasive, sectional imaging modalities have proved to be of significant value not only in permitting the recognition of neoplasia in early stages and providing means for staging, but also in their increased specificity, with even pathognomonic findings in many conditions. These improvements should be heightened in the near future with further progression in spectroscopy and in imaging utilizing monoclonal antibodies.

This text and atlas has been designed not only to bring together data from these radiologic advances but also to discuss other conventional techniques where applicable and to provide the reader with a wide spectrum of oncologic material. The text is deliberately brief. It avoids details of technical procedures: these will change rapidly over time. But each subject is presented from a comprehensive perspective. It is hoped that the reader will be able to study this book in a short time and come away with the fundamental information necessary to confidently recognize radiologic manifestations of abdominal and pelvic oncologic conditions. The role of this book is indeed complementary to other textbooks written in this field.

The book is in fact in two parts. The first seven chapters are organ or system oriented, and the last seven cover oncologic conditions related to a broader spectrum of anatomic structures or focus on selected imaging modalities. The cases presented comprise both common and uncommon and occasionally unusual or exotic lesions. The latest references related to each subject are provided.

Despite my efforts and those of my colleagues, the book is certainly not without imperfections. This is not surprising considering that an ambitious task has been undertaken that requires a greater breadth of knowledge than we could master and a luxury of time none but the idle could afford.

I am indebted to many individuals for the success of this book. Most important, I thank my colleagues who gave time and effort to share their expertise with me in order to bring depth and completeness to the book. A special note of gratitude goes to Suzanne Simpson, my editor at the Department of Scientific Publications of the University of Texas System Cancer Center. With her special devotion, she has spent countless numbers of hours working on each chapter. My appreciation is extended to my secretary, Sharon Williams, who spent many hours collecting references and typing the manuscript. I also thank Gene Swarzc and Robert Czimny from the photography section of Diagnostic Radiology for their careful preparation of the images used for this book. And finally my special appreciation goes to my wife, Shahrzad, and my daughters, Layla and Roxana, who accepted patiently the inconvenience of my long preoccupation with this work.

Ali Shirkhoda

Contents

1

Gastrointestinal Neoplasms

Ronelle DuBrow, M.D.

Patients with primary gastrointestinal malignancies often present with symptoms referable to the site of disease. Thus, dysphagia is seen in patients with esophageal and esophagogastric junction tumors, constipation or rectal bleeding with colorectal tumors, small bowel obstruction with small bowel tumors, and epigastric pain and early satiety with gastric lesions. Less frequently, systemic symptoms such as anorexia, weight loss, or anemia will predominate. The first step in the diagnostic workup at this initial stage is to examine the appropriate portion of the gastrointestinal tract. This can be done with endoscopy or with barium studies. The major advantage of endoscopy is the opportunity to detect and to perform a biopsy on a tumor at the same time. The advantages of barium studies would include the generally lower cost, the production of a permanent record, and the ability to examine parts of the bowel not reached by the endoscope, mainly the small bowel, but occasionally the right colon or colon proximal to a partially obstructing tumor. The sensitivity of the two modalities for the detection of tumors is probably comparable. In some cases they can be complementary. The barium examination gives a better appreciation of the overall extent of the tumor. Except in very large exophytic tumors where percutaneous biopsy might be performed, endoscopy is essential for histologic diagnosis.

Once a tumor is detected and histologic diagnosis is made, staging becomes the next concern. Computed tomography (CT) is the most accurate and comprehensive imaging tool for this purpose. The tumor itself can usually be imaged, and extension beyond the gastric or intestinal wall and invasion of adjacent structures can often be detected. Nodal and hepatic metastases are also detectable in a large percentage of cases. The limitations of CT include the inability to detect subtle, often microscopic extension of tumor through the wall and serosa, the inability to diagnose tumor in normal-sized lymph nodes, and the inability to image peritoneal metastases when the metastatic deposits are small. It can be argued that staging should be done at the time of surgery because patients will need at least palliative surgery in most cases to circumvent obstructing or bleeding lesions. Computed tomography is primarily useful in following patients after resection or staging (or both), in looking for recurrence and metastasis, and in monitoring the effects of treatment on metastases or unresectable tumors.

Adenocarcinomas make up the overwhelming majority of tumors affecting the stomach, small bowel, and colorectum. In the following chapter, more specific information regarding adenocarcinomas in each particular site and many examples will be presented. In addition, a brief discussion and examples of rarer tumors, including sarcomas, lymphoma, and carcinoid tumors, in each site will be presented. Finally, metastatic disease to the gastrointestinal tract will be discussed and illustrated.

ESOPHAGOGASTRIC JUNCTION

Although most primary malignant tumors of the esophagus are squamous cell carcinomas, malignant lesions involving the esophagogastric junction are usually adenocarcinomas (Fig 1–1). The latter typically arise from the cardia of the stomach, although tumors arising in a distal columnar-lined (Barrett's) esophagus, or arising in the mucous glands of the esophagus, or in heterotopic gastric mucosa, are occasionally seen.[1] In 1976, 30% of all gastric carcinomas arose at the cardia compared with 7% in 1930.[2] Thus, despite the falling incidence of gastric cancer in the United States, the incidence of adenocarcinoma of the esophagogastric junction is rising, and there may be evidence that the latter tumors are increasingly occurring in young patients.[3]

Primary malignant esophageal tumors other than adenocarcinoma and squamous cell carcinoma are extremely rare. They include leiomyosarcoma (Fig 1–2) and other sarcomas, small cell tumor (i.e., carcinoid or oat cell), melanoma, lymphoma, and tumors resembling salivary gland primaries (mucoepidermoid and adenoid cystic carcinomas). Carcinosarcoma, pseudosarcoma, and spindle cell carcinoma are all variants of squamous cell carcinoma that show sarcomatous elements histologically; although these tumors are rare, their differentiation is important because they may have a better prognosis than the usual squamous cell carcinoma.[4, 5] They tend to present as bulky intraluminal masses in the middle or distal esophagus, sometimes mimicking a large food bolus (Fig 1–3).[4–6]

The hallmark of the clinical presentation of tumors of the esophagogastric junction is dysphagia. Initial evaluation is usually by a barium swallow or upper gastrointestinal (UGI) series. Both adenocarcinomas and squamous cell carcinomas can be infiltrating, ulcerating, or predominantly polypoid. Very small tumors sometimes mimic benign intramural masses. Multinodular circumferential tumors sometimes mimic varices, although there will be no change in the filling defects on different films, and the lumen will not be distensible as in the case of varices. Ulcerating or infiltrating tumors are sometimes difficult to differentiate from peptic esophagitis or stricture, and smooth submucosal tumor extension from the cardia can mimic achalasia radiographically (Fig 1–4) and manometrically.[7] Radiologic features to differentiate this pseudoachalasia from true primary achalasia have been described.[8, 9] The double-contrast examination with its better distension of the gastric fundus and detailed en face visualization of the mucosa at the cardia may be particularly helpful in this regard. Amyl nitrate may be used to relax the esophagogastric junction to aid in differentiation.[10] In these cases, one must have a high index of suspicion, especially in older patients presenting with a relatively short history of symptoms. Persistent endoscopic efforts must be made to obtain adequate biopsy specimens and brushings for cytological analysis.

Computed tomography has little to add in the initial diagnosis of tumors of the esophagogastric junction. This is a confusing area on CT, and a soft tissue pseudomass is present in as many as 38% of normal patients.[11, 12] With meticulous attention to gastric distension and patient positioning, the question of real mass vs. pseudomass can usually be resolved. However, barium studies are far more sensitive and certainly cheaper for initial evaluation.

Computed tomography has potential for use in the preoperative staging of known esophagogastric junction malignancy.[9, 13] Unfortunately, periesophageal invasion into the mediastinum is not reliably identified. Because the esophagus has no serosa, this invasion is a frequent and early event. Both false positive and false-negative diagnoses of mediastinal spread are predominantly encountered. Metastases to the celiac axis and left gastric nodes and to the liver, adrenals, and retroperitoneum can often be detected. However, metastases within normal-sized lymph nodes will be missed. Between two reported studies, CT's sensitivity for periesophageal invasion was 67%, and its sensitivity for regional lymph node involvement was 59%.[13, 14]

In the follow-up of patients who have undergone resection for tumors of the esophagogastric junction, CT can be an important tool in detecting regional recurrence and distant metastases (Fig 1–5). Barium swallow and endoscopy are important in assessing for anastomotic recurrence as well.

STOMACH

Adenocarcinoma

In the United States, cancer of the stomach (Figs 1–6 to 1–11), despite its falling incidence, still ranks eighth in cancer-related deaths, with 24,600 new cases estimated for 1987.[15] The overall five-year survival remains at 10% to 30%.[16] Early gastric cancer, that is, carcinoma with invasion no deeper than submucosa, carries a much better prognosis: five-year survival rates are as high as 95% in Japan.[17] There, where stomach cancer is six to eight times more prevalent than in the United States, mass screening programs have been effective in raising the rate of diagnosis of early cancer from 5% to 35% of all stomach cancers.[17] In the United States, mass screening is unlikely to be undertaken because of the lower prevalence of disease, so that diagnosis will continue to be made in patients with symptoms. The overwhelming number of patients with gastric carcinoma will have advanced disease at presentation.

Patients often present with vague abdominal complaints or with epigastric pain that mimics peptic ulcer disease. The UGI series is the best imaging means for finding and describing the primary tumor. The lesions can be polypoid, ulcerating, or diffusely infiltrating. The last type of tumor usually reduces gastric volume and obliterates the normal folds, giving the so-called leather-bottle appearance (Fig 1–8). However, some diffusely infiltrating tumors do not reduce gastric volume and may be seen as thickened folds alone (Figs 1–9 and 1–10).[18] Endoscopic biopsies of infiltrating lesions may yield normal results, because these tumors are predominantly submucosal. A high index of suspicion on the basis of radiographic findings is important in encouraging deeper biopsies or even surgery.

The differential diagnosis includes other malignancies that involve the stomach—commonly, lymphoma and leiomyosarcoma. Metastasis from breast carcinoma is at times indistinguishable from the linitis plastica form of primary gastric cancer. Benign entities that can mimic carcinoma include peptic ulcer disease, hypertrophic pyloric stenosis, and gastritis, especially that due to syphilis, tuberculosis, or corrosive agents.

Once a diagnosis has been made, CT scanning may be of help in staging the disease.[14, 19–21] The primary tumor often appears as generalized or focal wall thickening (wall thickness > 1 cm) or as a polypoid mass. Distension with contrast or air is essential for adequate evaluation. In most cases, local lymph node involvement cannot be separated from the primary tumor mass. Similarly, tumor in normal-sized distant lymph nodes cannot be diagnosed.However, enlarged nodes in the gastrohepatic ligament, celiac axis, or mesentery can often be detected. Computed tomography can also suggest that there is local invasion of adjacent structures such as the spleen and pancreas (Fig 1–9). Metastases to the liver or to an ovary (Krukenberg's tumor) (Fig 1–10)

can be diagnosed with this modality.[22, 23] In patients who have undergone resection, CT can be helpful in follow-up to detect local recurrence and distant metastases.[24]

Leiomyoma and Leiomyosarcoma

Leiomyosarcoma is a rare tumor, accounting for only 1% to 3% of all gastric malignancies. The tumor arises from smooth muscle fibers in the wall of the stomach and may reach quite a large size before it is clinically apparent.[25] A leiomyoma is a benign smooth muscle tumor that is sometimes difficult to differentiate from the malignant variety both radiologically and pathologically.[26] Malignant smooth muscle tumors tend to be larger, but that generalization may not help in an individual case.

Patients with leiomyoma or leiomyosarcoma most often present with gastrointestinal bleeding, abdominal fullness or pain, or all of these. A mass is often palpated. Radiographically, the tumor is classically seen as an intramural mass, often with a central area of ulceration (Figs 1–12 and 1–13). These tumors frequently grow exogastrically to a great size, and they sometimes produce a predominantly extrinsic mass effect on the stomach and adjacent organs (Fig 1–14).[27] A smaller intramural component or ulceration may be the clue to the site of origin of the tumor. The tumors frequently ulcerate and may on occasion excavate. When they grow predominantly intraluminally, especially if the surface is ulcerated or lobulated, they may be difficult to differentiate from adenocarcinoma or even lymphoma. The large exogastric variety may be mistaken for retroperitoneal tumor or even abscess.

When a mass is found, an appropriate next step would be a CT scan of the abdomen. The extent of disease, including invasion into adjacent organs and presence of hepatic or nodal metastases, can be assessed. Leiomyosarcomas tend to be large, irregular masses that contain areas of low attenuation or necrosis.[28–30] Leiomyomas are usually sharply outlined masses of homogeneous density.[28] Unless the lesion is ulcerated, and occasionally even when it is, endoscopic biopsies can be nondiagnostic, demonstrating only the normal overlying gastric mucosa. If a mass is seen on the CT scan and endoscopic biopsies are normal, percutaneous aspiration biopsy may establish the diagnosis prior to surgery.

Once the tumor has been excised, CT has an important role in documenting local recurrence and metastasis. Recurrent tumor in the peritoneum or in the liver has the same CT appearance as primary lesions, namely, soft tissue masses with necrotic or cystic components.

Lymphoma

Gastric lymphoma accounts for less than 5% of all gastric malignancies.[31] Stomach involvement is much more common in the non-Hodgkin's lymphomas than in Hodgkin's disease. The stomach is the most common site of involvement in the gastrointestinal tract: 50% of patients with gastrointestinal lymphoma have disease in the stomach.[32] At times, the stomach will be involved in patients with widespread nodal and extranodal disease. At other times, the stomach is the principal site of involvement.

Because the stomach is in some cases the only site of involvement, the clinical and radiographic presentation of gastric lymphoma may closely mimic that of gastric adenocarcinoma (Fig 1–15). Epigastric discomfort, bleeding, and weight loss are common presenting symptoms. On UGI studies, the findings of each entity overlap. However, there are some features that favor a diagnosis of lymphoma,[31–36] most importantly: (1) infiltration of the wall, that is, thickened, often bizarre folds, without loss of distensibility (Fig 1–16); (2) multiple ulcerated lesions separated by intervening normal mucosa; and (3) a large (> 10-cm) intraluminal mass (Fig 1–17).

It has long been said that lymphoma crosses the pylorus and involves the duodenum more frequently than does carcinoma. This may not be so, however; at least one study failed to find duodenal involvement in any of the 72 patients examined.[33] In other studies, extension to the duodenal bulb was observed in 20% to 33% of patients with gastric lymphoma and in only 5% to 6% of patients with gastric adenocarcinoma.[35–37] Even if these findings are verified, since 95% of all malignant tumors are adenocarcinomas, the overwhelming majority of disease extending to the duodenal bulb would be expected to be due to carcinoma.

Abdominal CT is particularly helpful in patients who have gastric lymphoma because of its ability to evaluate the abdominal and pelvic nodal areas, the liver and spleen, and the structures contiguous to the stomach.[38, 39] Invasion of contiguous structures is less common in lymphoma than in adenocarcinoma, but it does occur. The gastric involvement is frequently seen on CT as thickening of the gastric wall to a diameter greater than 1 cm. The stomach must be adequately distended with contrast or air for application of this measurement.

Although surgery may still be performed for primary gastric lymphoma, it has been shown that chemotherapy combined with local radiation therapy, without resection, may also be effective. In addition, when the gastric lesion is part of a more diffuse process, the treatment will not involve resection. The response of the gastric lesions can be followed by repeated UGI series.[40 41] Besides shrinkage of the tumor mass (or masses), some overall or focal volume loss has been observed after treatment, particularly when radiation is employed. The most involved area on pretreatment studies shows the most marked constriction after treatment (Fig 1–17). Other response patterns include (1) an accentuation or new development of ulceration or even frank perforation as the tumor recedes and (2) healing to benign-appearing ulcer or ulcer scar.

SMALL INTESTINE

Adenocarcinoma

Despite the fact that the small intestine makes up 75% of the length of the entire gastrointestinal tract, small intestinal cancers constitute less than 1% of all gastrointestinal tract malignancies.[42] Metastasis is often present at diagnosis, and the prognosis is generally poor. Distribution of adenocarcinomas tends to be proximal. Forty percent occur in the duodenum and 35% in the jejunum, three fourths of those being within 100 cm of the ligament of Treitz. Symptoms most often include upper abdominal pain, obstruction, weight loss, and evidence of bleeding. Duodenal tumors are less likely than more distal cancers to obstruct the lumen. Patients with periampullary tumors frequently present with jaundice.

The UGI series and small bowel examination are the procedures of choice in diagnosing small bowel cancers (Figs 1–18 to 1–21). Like adenocarcinomas of the rest of the gastrointestinal tract, they tend to be seen as infiltrating circumferential tumor masses with mucosal destruction and ulceration, often with proximal dilatation of the small bowel. Tumors in the duodenum are sometimes polypoid.

The main value of CT in small bowel carcinoma is in the detection of metastatic disease to nodes and liver as well as the demonstration of the extent of disease outside of the bowel wall. A recent study of duodenal neoplasms notes that the intrinsic nature of the tumor can often be identified on CT, so that this tumor is clearly differentiated from a locally advanced pancreatic, colon, or renal primary invading the duodenum (Fig 1–20).[43]

Carcinoid Tumor

Carcinoid tumors are the most common primaries of the small bowel. However, many are asymptomatic and found incidentally at autopsy or at abdominal surgery for other causes. They are much more common in the ileum than in the jejunum or duodenum. They arise from argentaffin cells in the mucosa deep in the intestinal crypts and grow initially as intramural nodules. If detected at this stage, the tumor is seen radiographically as a small (usually < 1.5-cm) submucosal mass, most often in the distal ileum. Approximately 30% of cases have multiple submucosal masses.[44, 45] As the tumor grows, it causes smooth muscle hypertrophy, which may thicken the bowel wall and contribute to obstructive symptoms. Obstruction may also occur because of intussusception or annular tumor growth, the latter resulting in an apple core appearance that mimics adenocarcinoma. As the tumor invades the serosa and then the mesentery, it incites an intense desmoplastic reaction in the mesentery, producing areas of fixation, kinking, and tethering of small bowel loops (Fig 1–22). This appearance can be seen as well in mesenteric fibrosis from other causes, including regional enteritis, radiation, and postoperative adhesions. It is at this stage that small bowel obstruction is most common.

The angiographic findings in carcinoid tumor have been described[46] and consist of a tumor stain corresponding to the primary tumor, kinking and encasement of mesenteric arteries and veins associated with the mesenteric fibrosis, and hypervascular liver metastases.

The carcinoid syndrome is due to the production of serotonin and other substances by metastatic tumor in the liver. It develops in a small proportion of patients with small bowel carcinoids; however, most patients with this syndrome have primary tumors arising in the small bowel.[47] Even with hepatic disease, the course may be somewhat indolent. Intraarterial embolization plus chemotherapy shows promise as a means of controlling symptoms of the carcinoid syndrome and perhaps in prolonging survival.[48]

Sarcoma

Sarcomas account for approximately 20% to 25% of all malignant primary small bowel tumors.[42] The overwhelming majority are of smooth muscle origin.

They are most common in the ileum, of moderate incidence in the jejunum, and relatively uncommon in the duodenum (about 10% occur in the duodenum). They arise in the muscularis propria and often grow predominantly toward the serosa, usually presenting as large, extrinsic masses. Small bowel sarcomas are likely to become necrotic and may ulcerate or excavate. Common clinical symptoms include pain, chronic blood loss, weight loss, and a palpable abdominal mass.

Small bowel series may show evidence of the site of origin. Occasionally, the bowel will be extensively involved (Fig 1–23). At other times, traction at one point on the bowel wall or ulceration into the mass from a single point (Fig 1–24) will be the only clue as to the site of origin. The differential diagnosis includes extrinsic tumor secondarily involving the bowel or, occasionally, abscess.

Computed tomography can document the extent of disease more completely than can barium study.[28–30] The CT scan is also useful in assessing for hepatic metastases. The tumors tend to be large, nonhomogeneous masses, often with large areas of low attenuation compatible with necrosis. Barium can occasionally be seen within the mass. If a tissue diagnosis is needed, percutaneous biopsy is easily performed with CT or ultrasound guidance. Local recurrence after resection is not uncommon, and CT is useful in the follow-up of these patients to document the recurrences or metastases.

Lymphoma

Approximately one third of patients with gastrointestinal lymphoma have involvement of the small bowel.[32] As with gastric lymphoma, the involvement is seen almost exclusively in the non-Hodgkin's lymphomas and may represent the primary site of disease or be a manifestation of a diffuse lymphomatous process. Radiologically, there is no difference in the small bowel manifestations if the involvement is primary or secondary. The distribution of lymphoma in the small bowel roughly approximates the distribution of normal lymphoid tissue, both being more common in the ileum, particularly in the terminal ileum. Involvement of the duodenum is uncommon.

The lymphoma arises in the lymphoid tissue of the submucosa and may infiltrate the wall diffusely or grow predominantly into the mesentery, where it may excavate. Thus, two common radiographic appearances are (1) segmental narrowing with effacement of the mucosa (Fig 1–25,A), representing a diffusely infiltrating tumor; and (2) a mass containing an amorphous collection of barium communicating with an abnormal loop of bowel (Fig 1–25,B), representing the endoexoenteric form. Other forms include diffuse nodules (Fig 1–25,C)[49]; scattered nodules, often with ulceration; diffuse fold thickening (Fig 1–25,D); and aneurysmal dilatation, this last probably due to infiltration of the autonomic plexus and destruction of the muscularis propria. A sprue-like malabsorption pattern has been described, probably due to mesenteric infiltration with lymphatic obstruction. True sprue may precede the development of lymphoma. Typically, small bowel lymphoma does not cause complete obstruction unless associated with intussusception of a submucosal nodule.[31] This contrasts with small bowel carcinoma. However, the patterns are relatively nonspecific, and carcinoma, metastasis, and mesenchymal tumors have to be considered in the differential, as well as, occasionally, Crohn's disease.

In *Mediterranean lymphoma*, a subgroup of intestinal lymphoma that affects young adults in Mediterranean countries, the radiographic appearances are characteristic and differ from those previously mentioned.[50,51] The involvement is usually proximal and diffuse, including the duodenum and jejunum, and is characterized by marked fold thickening, often with nodules. Pathologic examination of the bowel demonstrates diffuse infiltration of the lamina propria by plasma cells.

In lymphoma, CT scanning is always helpful in evaluating the abdomen for adenopathy and for liver and spleen involvement.[38] The extent of the small bowel abnormality can be seen to best advantage as well, especially when the small bowel involvement is the manifestation of even larger mesenteric disease.

LARGE INTESTINE

Adenocarcinoma

Carcinoma of the colon and rectum is the second most common malignancy in the United States, with close to 145,000 cases estimated for 1987.[15] Overall five-year survival is less than 50% and has not changed significantly in the last two decades.[52] It is generally believed that survival could be substantially increased if cancers could be found at earlier stages. In theory, it is possible that the overall incidence of colorectal cancer could also be decreased by the detection and removal of benign adenomas. Because the population at risk for the development of colon cancer is so large, that is, people age 40 or more, it is unlikely that mass screening is possible. In the individual case, however, the goal should always be the detection of small polyps and cancers. This may mean the more widespread use of good double-contrast radiography of the large bowel.

The radiographic detection of small cancers of the colon and rectum is basically a matter of finding small polyps (Fig 1–26).[53] It is not possible in most cases to determine whether the polyp is benign or malignant. The most reliable criterion is size: polyps less than 1 cm harbor carcinoma approximately 1% of the time, polyps 1 to 2 cm have a 10% incidence of malignancy, and those larger than 2 cm are malignant 33% to 46% of the time.[53] Other features are unreliable, particularly for small lesions. As cancers grow, they assume the more classic appearance of fungating, infiltrating, or ulcerating masses, usually of moderate size (Fig 1–27). They may grow around the circumference of the bowel, ultimately producing the so-called apple core appearance. Although they are usually obvious, large masses on double-contrast enema examination can at times be quite subtle in appearance (Fig 1–28). Occasionally, tumors grow as flat, carpetlike lesions, often with a reticular or villous surface pattern (Fig 1–29).[54] A rare manifestation of colorectal cancer is the linitis plastica appearance, in which there is a long, narrowed segment without ulceration and with tapered rather than overhanging margins.[55, 56] This is seen more frequently in patients with long-standing ulcerative colitis.

There is about a 5% incidence of synchronous cancer and a 23% incidence of synchronous benign polyps associated with a known primary lesion.[52] In patients with ulcerative colitis, the rate of synchronous cancers is higher (Fig 1–30). In all cases, it is extremely important that the whole large intestine be well examined when a primary lesion is discovered. If the primary cancer obstructs the lumen, a complete evaluation must be performed soon after resection. The malignant nature of the obstruction can often be diagnosed by the detection on barium enema of shouldering and mucosal destruction at the distal margin of the obstructing lesion (Fig 1–31). Peritoneal spread of tumor can occasionally be documented on the enema when the tumor is far advanced (Fig 1–32). Occasionally, carcinomas will perforate, and the inflammatory reaction in adjacent normal bowel may simulate diverticulitis (Fig 1–33). In rare instances, bladder symptoms are the presenting complaint, when the inflammation has spread to involve this organ (Fig 1–34). The differential diagnosis in malignant-appearing lesions of the colon and rectum would have to include lymphoma, carcinoid and other rare tumors, and amebomas and other masses produced by uncommon infestations.

Computed tomography has been disappointing in the pretherapy staging of patients with colorectal cancer because of its inability to accurately assess the depth of bowel wall invasion and the presence or absence of tumor in normal-sized lymph nodes.[57–59] These are crucial factors in determining stage and, hence, prognosis. The overall accuracy of CT has been shown to be only 50% to 70%, and generally this modality is not recommended for routine preoperative screening.[60]

For the follow-up of patients after initial resection, there is some basis for routine CT scanning.[58–63] Local recurrence of rectosigmoid cancer is common, seen in between 30% and 50% of patients.[52] Frequently, recurrent tumor at the anastomosis will grow extramurally and may be difficult to detect on barium studies (Fig 1–35). Computed tomography is an excellent way to look at extension beyond the bowel wall (Fig 1–36). In patients who have had abdominoperineal resection, CT is the only way to examine the pelvis, although magnetic resonance imaging may soon become an important modality for this purpose. It is important that a baseline CT study be performed after surgery, because the presence of mass in the presacral space on any one study is not definitive evidence of local recurrence.[64, 65] Such a mass may represent postoperative fibrosis, which can be presumed if the mass is seen to stay the same size or diminish in size and become better defined over time. If this is not the case, or if a baseline study for comparison is not available, CT-guided percutaneous biopsy should be performed to determine if recurrence is present.[66] Computed tomography is also helpful in detecting metastasis to the liver and occasionally in documenting peritoneal metastases (Fig 1–37). The overall accuracy of this modality in detecting recurrent or metastatic colorectal carcinoma was reported to be close to 90% in two studies.[58, 59]

Epithelial Tumors of the Anal Canal

Cancer of the anal canal accounts for between 2% and 4% of malignant tumors of the large intestine.[67] Patients typically present with local signs and symptoms such as bleeding, pain on defecation, or sensation of a mass, and the initial clinical impression may be of benign disease such as hemorrhoids or anal fissures. Two main histologic subsets exist:

squamous cell carcinoma arising from squamous epithelium below the pectinate line, and basaloid or cloacogenic carcinoma arising from transitional epithelium around the pectinate line. They are generally treated together as one disease because the stage of disease is far more important in determining therapy and prognosis than the histology.

Initial diagnosis is in most cases by physical examination and anoscopy or proctoscopy. When a barium enema examination is performed, the tumor may appear as a submucosal, eccentric mass, occasionally with ulceration (Figs 1–38 to 1–40). Small nodular or plaque-like masses are also seen. The differential diagnosis would include distal adenocarcinoma of the rectum and other, more rare tumors, as well as hemorrhoids and perirectal abscesses.[68]

A CT scan may be of help in pretreatment staging.[69] Lymphatic spread is common, occurring in up to 40% of patients; CT may document pelvic, mesenteric, or paraaortic nodal disease, as well as inguinal metastases, which would be clinically apparent. Hematogenous spread, predominantly to liver and lungs, is uncommon, occurring in less than 6% of patients.[67] Disease recurs in about 40% of patients treated with abdominoperineal resection. Radiation therapy is being used more frequently now, both with and without surgery, yielding lower, although still significant, recurrence rates.

Computed tomography is important in following these patients to look for local recurrence and nodal spread. As after abdominoperineal resection for adenocarcinoma, a baseline CT two to four months after completion of therapy may be a sound policy to ensure that recurrences will be differentiated from postoperative or postirradiation change.

Lymphoma

Less than 1% of all malignant tumors of the large intestine are lymphomas, and only 10% of patients with lymphoma of the gastrointestinal tract have colorectal involvement.[31] Like all gastrointestinal sites, non-Hodgkin's lymphoma is much more common than Hodgkin's disease; either may be primary or secondary in the bowel. In primary lymphoma of the large intestine, the cecum is most commonly involved, followed by the rectum.

Radiologically, lesions are frequently large (5- to 10-cm) intramural or intraluminal masses (Fig 1–41). Circumferential infiltration of the wall occasionally produces a focal stricture. The major differential diagnosis in both cases is carcinoma. Small nodules account for about 45% of cases and may be confused with metastases, polyposis syndromes, or inflammatory processes such as Crohn's disease or pseudomembranous colitis. If the nodules are very small (2–3 mm), lymphoid hyperplasia would have to be considered. If the tumor involves the mesentery, large extrinsic masses may occur.

Carcinoid Tumor

Carcinoid tumors are rare in the large bowel. They usually arise in the rectum and radiographically appear most often as smooth, submucosal-appearing masses less than 2 cm in diameter (Fig 1–42); they are typically found incidentally at proctoscopy.[70] Only 10% of rectal carcinoids metastasize.[45] On the contrary, carcinoids in the colon, exclusive of the appendix, are aggressive and malignant lesions; more than 50% have metastasized at presentation.[45] Most are in the ascending colon and radiographically may be indistinguishable from adenocarcinoma of the colon, appearing as fungating masses or infiltrating apple core lesions with destruction of the mucosa. Carcinoid syndrome is rare.

Leiomyosarcoma

Leiomyosarcomas are the most common mesenchymal malignancy affecting the colon but, again, are rare in this location. They have a predilection for the rectum. They arise in the wall, usually in the muscularis propria, and often grow extramurally, frequently not producing symptoms until a large mass is present (Fig 1–43). As in other parts of the alimentary tract, the tumors tend to become necrotic and excavate. Thus, the radiologic findings are usually those of a large mass displacing the bowel with evidence of irregular ulceration into the mass.

TUMOR SPREAD TO THE GASTROINTESTINAL TRACT

It is helpful to think of secondary neoplastic involvement of the gastrointestinal tract (Figs 1–44 to 1–58) in terms of the mechanism of tumor spread. Meyers and McSweeney classified this spread as occurring by direct invasion, peritoneal seeding, or embolic, hematogenous dissemination.[72]

Tumors that spread by direct invasion do so either directly by contiguity or indirectly via fascial planes. Examples of the former are the spread of cancer of the prostate, ovaries, or uterus to the rectosigmoid or of renal cancer to the ascending or descending colon. The latter is exemplified by the spread of gastric or pancreatic cancer to the transverse colon via the gastrocolic ligament or transverse mesocolon, respectively. Direct spread to the bowel may also occur from nodal masses in the mesentery or omentum.

Tumors that spread by peritoneal seeding include, most commonly, ovarian, gastric, colon, and pancreatic neoplasms. Malignant cells may be deposited anywhere but tend to lodge and grow in the pouch of Douglas, the root of the mesentery in the right lower quadrant, and the right paracolic gutter.

Hematogenous or embolic metastases are deposited submucosally anywhere in the bowel but most frequently in the small bowel, probably because of the greater proportion of blood flow to the small bowel. The tumors that most commonly metastasize in this way to the bowel are melanoma, Kaposi's sarcoma, and breast and lung cancer.

Barium studies are the most appropriate radiologic examinations for looking for metastatic disease to the bowel.[73–82] The radiographic appearance depends on the type of spread as well as on the amount of growth of tumor that has occurred before the bowel is examined. Thus, hematogenous metastases might be seen as small submucosal masses, as masses with central ulceration (the so-called bull's eye lesion), as large excavated masses, or as circumferential infiltrating lesions, depending on the type and extent of growth. Breast cancer metastatic to the bowel may be seen as submucosal nodules but more commonly infiltrates the submucosa and incites a desmoplastic reponse, giving rise to a linitis plastica appearance of the involved bowel (Fig 1–58). Serosal disease may be manifested as small masses, as masses with tethering of the overlying mucosa, as fixation and kinking of the bowel if the mesentery is infiltrated, or as circumferential or intraluminal or excavated masses if the tumor is advanced. With direct spread of tumor, there is usually focal mass effect with traction change or ulceration of the mucosa and occasionally bulky intraluminal mass when invasion is extensive. Obstruction may result from circumferential tumor, intraluminal mass, or intussusception of a submucosal mass. When the involvement is advanced, it is difficult to tell what the original mode of spread was.

Differential diagnosis in metastatic disease of the bowel is not usually a problem, because in most cases there is a known primary lesion. With mesenteric fibrosis, the differentiation between fibrosis due to radiation therapy, postoperative adhesions, and tumors may be difficult. With focal lesions, a second primary might have to be considered in the differential.

Computed tomography is not the primary modality for detecting metastases to the bowel but may be useful in documenting the extent of disease outside of the lumen. In addition, because CT is used for following patients with metastatic tumor, the first demonstration of bowel involvement may be on the CT scan. This means that the bowel must be well opacified and that attention should be paid to the thickness of the bowel wall and the contiguity of bowel to tumor masses. Intussusception may give a very characteristic appearance on CT (Fig 1–53).[83–85] The radiologist should be familiar with and look for such abnormalities.

REFERENCES

1. Faintuch J., Shepard K.V., Levin B.: Adenocarcinoma and other unusual variants of esophageal cancer. *Semin. Oncol.* 11:192–202, 1984.
2. Cady B., Ramsden D.A., Stein A., et al.: Gastric cancer: contemporary aspects. *Am. J. Surg.* 133:423–428, 1977.
3. Levine M.S., Laufer I., Thompson J.J.: Carcinoma of the gastric cardia in young people. *AJR* 140:69–72, 1983.
4. DeMeester T.R., Skinner D.B.: Polypoid sarcomas of the esophagus: a rare but potentially curable neoplasm. *Ann. Thorac. Surg.* 20:405–417, 1975.
5. Olmsted W.W., Lichtenstein J.E., Hyams V.J.: Polypoid epithelial malignancies of the esophagus. *AJR* 140:921–925, 1983.
6. Agha F., Keren D.F.: Spindle-cell squamous carcinoma of the esophagus: a tumor with biphasic morphology. *AJR* 145:541–545, 1985.
7. Lawson T.L., Dodds W.J.: Infiltrating carcinoma simulating achalasia. *Gastrointest. Radiol.* 1:245–248, 1976.
8. Marshak R.H., Eliasoph J.: Cardiospasm or carcinoma? The roentgen findings. *American Journal of Digestive Diseases* 2:11–25, 1957.
9. Freeny P.C., Marks W.M.: Adenocarcinoma of the gastroesophageal junction: barium and CT examination. *AJR* 138:1077–1084, 1982.
10. Dodds W.J., Steward E.T., Kishk S.M., et al.: Radiologic amyl nitrite test for distinguishing pseudoachalasia from idiopathic achalasia. *AJR* 146:21–23, 1986.
11. Marks W.M., Callen P.W., Moss A.A.: Gastroesophageal region: source of confusion on CT. *AJR* 136:359–362, 1981.
12. Thompson W.M., Halvorsen R.A., Williford M.E., et al.: Computed tomography of the gastroesophageal junction. *RadioGraphics* 2:179–193, 1982.
13. Thompson W.M., Halvorsen R.A., Foster W.L., et al.: Computed tomography for staging esophageal and gastroesophageal cancer: reevaluation. *AJR* 141:951–958, 1983.
14. Halvorsen R.A., Thompson W.M.: Computed tomographic staging of gastrointestinal tract malignancies: I. Esophagus and stomach. *Invest. Radiol.* 22:2–16, 1987.
15. Silverberg E., Lubera J.: Cancer statistics. *CA* 37:2–19, 1987.
16. Adashek K., Sanger J., Longmire W.P.: Cancer of the stomach: review of consecutive 10 year intervals. *Ann. Surg.* 189:6–10, 1979.
17. White, R.M., Levine M.S., Enterline H.T., et al.: Early gastric cancer: recent experience. *Radiology* 155:27–57, 1985.
18. Balthazar E.J., Davidian M.M.: Hyperrugosity in gastric carcinoma: radiographic, endoscopic, and pathologic features. *AJR* 136:531–535, 1981.
19. Lee K.R., Levine E., Moffat R.E., et al.: Computed tomographic staging of malignant gastric neoplasms. *Radiology* 133:151–155, 1979.
20. Moss A.A., Schnyder P., Marks W., et al.: Gastric adenocarcinoma: a comparison of the accuracy and economics of staging by computed tomography and surgery. *Gastroenterology* 80:45–50, 1981.
21. Balfe D.M., Koehler R.E., Karstaedt N., et al.: Computed tomography of gastric neoplasms. *Radiology* 140:431–436, 1981.
22. Cho K.C., Gold B.M.: Computed tomography of Krukenberg tumors. *AJR* 145:285–288, 1985.
23. Megibow A.J., Julnick D.H., Bosniak M.A., et al.: Ovarian metastases: computed tomographic appearances. *Radiology* 156:161–164, 1985.
24. Mullin D., Shirkhoda A.: Computed tomography after gastrectomy in primary gastric carcinoma. *J. Comput. Assist. Tomogr.* 9:30–33, 1985.
25. Shiu M.H., Farr G.H., Papachristou D.N., et al.: Myosarcomas of the stomach: natural history, prognostic factors and management. *Cancer* 49:177–187, 1982.
26. Helinger H.: The recognition of exogastric tumours: report of six cases. *Br. J. Radiol.* 39:25–36, 1966.
27. Nauert T.C., Zornoza J., Ordonez N.: Gastric leiomyosarcoma. *AJR* 139:291–297, 1982.
28. Megibow A.J., Balthazar E.J., Hulnick D.H., et al.: CT evaluation of gastrointestinal leiomyomas and leiomyosarcomas. *AJR* 144:727–731, 1985.
29. McLeod A.J., Zornoza J., Shirkhoda A.: Leiomyosarcoma: computed tomographic findings. *Radiology* 152:133–136, 1984.
30. Clark R.A., Alexander E.S.: Computed tomography of gastrointestinal leiomyosarcoma. *Gastrointest. Radiol.* 7:127–129, 1982.
31. Zornoza J., Dodd G.D.: Lymphoma of the gastrointestinal tract. *Semin. Roentgenol.* 15:272–287, 1980.
32. Brady L.W., Asbell S.O.: Malignant lymphoma of the gastrointestinal tract. *Radiology* 137:291–298, 1980.
33. Sherrick D.W., Hodgson J.R., Dockerty M.B.: The

roentgenologic diagnosis of primary gastric lymphoma. *Radiology* 84:925–932, 1965.

34. Privett J.T.J., Davies E.R., Roylance J.: The radiological features of gastric lymphoma. *Clin. Radiol.* 28:457–463, 1977.

35. Menuck L.S.: Gastric lymphoma: a radiologic diagnosis. *Gastrointest. Radiol.* 1:157–161, 1976.

36. Sato T., Sakai Y., Ishiguro S., et al.: Radiologic manifestations of early gastric lymphoma. *AJR* 146:513–517, 1986.

37. Hricak H., Thoeni R.F., Margulis A.R., et al.: Extension of gastric lymphoma into the esophagus and duodenum. *Radiology* 135:309–312, 1980.

38. Burgener F.A., Hamlin D.J.: Histiocytic lymphoma of the abdomen: radiographic spectrum. *AJR* 137:337–342, 1981.

39. Buy J.N., Moss A.A.: Computed tomography of gastric lymphoma. *AJR* 138:859–865, 1982.

40. Fox E.R., Laufer I., Levine M.S.: Response of gastric lymphoma to chemotherapy: radiologic appearance. *AJR* 142:711–714, 1984.

41. Libshitz H.I., Lindell M.M., Maor M.H., et al.: Appearance of the intact lymphomatous stomach following radiotherapy and chemotherapy. *Gastrointest. Radiol.* 10:25–29, 1985.

42. Sindelar W.: Cancer of the small intestine, in DeVita V.T. Jr., Hellman S., Rosenberg S.A. (eds.): *Cancer: Principles and Practice of Oncology*, ed. 2. Philadelphia, J.B. Lippincott Co., 1985, pp. 771–794.

43. Farah M.C., Jafri S.Z.H., Schwab R.E., et al.: Duodenal neoplasms: role of CT. *Radiology* 162:839–843, 1987.

44. Bancks N.H., Goldstein H.M., Dodd G.D.: The roentgenologic spectrum of small intestinal carcinoid tumors. *AJR* 123:274–280, 1975.

45. Balthazar E.J.: Carcinoid tumors of the alimentary tract: I. Radiographic diagnosis. *Gastrointest. Radiol.* 3:47–56, 1978.

46. Kinkhabwala M., Balthazar E.J.: Carcinoid tumors of the alimentary tract: II. Angiographic diagnosis of small intestinal and colonic lesions. *Gastrointest. Radiol.* 3:57–61, 1978.

47. Moertel C.G., Sauer W.G., Dockerty M.B., et al.: Life history of the carcinoid tumor of the small intestine. *Cancer* 14:901–912, 1961.

48. Carrasco C.H., Charnsangavej C., Ajani J., et al.: The carcinoid syndrome: palliation by hepatic artery embolization. *AJR* 147:149–154, 1986.

49. Fernandez B.J., Amato D., Goldfinger M.: Diffuse lymphomatous polyposis of the gastrointestinal tract: a case report with immunohistochemical studies. *Gastroenterology* 88:1267–1270, 1985.

50. Ramos L., Marcos J., Illanas M., et al.: Radiological characteristics of primary intestinal lymphoma of the Mediterranean type: observations on twelve cases. *Radiology* 126:379–385, 1978.

51. Nasr K., Haghighi P., Bakhshandeh K., et al.: Primary upper small intestinal lymphoma: a report of 40 cases. *American Journal of Digestive Diseases* 21:313–322, 1976.

52. Sugarbaker P.H., Gunderson L.L., Wittes R.E.: Colorectal cancer, in DeVita V.T. Jr., Hellman S., Rosenberg S.A. (eds.): *Cancer: Principles and Practice of Oncology*, ed. 2. Philadelphia, J.B. Lippincott Co., 1985, pp. 795–884.

53. Skucas J., Spataro R.F., Cannucciari D.P.: The radiographic features of small colon cancers. *Radiology* 143:335–340, 1982.

54. Rubesin S.E., Saul S.H., Laufer I., et al.: Carpet lesions of the colon. *RadioGraphics* 5:537–552, 1985.

55. Raskin M.M., Viamonte M., Viamonte M. Jr.: Primary linitis plastica carcinoma of the colon. *Radiology* 113:17–22, 1974.

56. Oliver T.W. Jr., Somogyi J., Gaffney E.F.: Primary linitis plastica of the rectum. *AJR* 140:79–80, 1983.

57. Butch R.J., Stark D.D., Wittenberg J., et al.: Staging rectal cancer by MR and CT. *AJR* 146:1155–1160, 1986.

58. Thompson W.M., Halvorsen R.A., Foster W.L. Jr., et al.: Preoperative and postoperative CT staging of rectosigmoid carcinoma. *AJR* 146:703–710, 1986.

59. Freeny P.C., Marks W.M., Ryan J.A., et al.: Colorectal carcinoma evaluation with CT: preoperative staging and direction of postoperative recurrence. *Radiology* 158:347–353, 1986.

60. Thompson W.M., Halvorsen R.A.: Computed tomographic staging of gastrointestinal malignancies: II. The small bowel, colon and rectum. *Invest. Radiol.* 22:96–105, 1987.

61. McCarthy S.M., Barnes D., Deveney K., et al.: Detection of recurrent rectosigmoid carcinoma: prospective evaluation of CT and clinical factors. *AJR* 144:577–579, 1985.

62. Grabbe E., Winkler R.: Local recurrence after sphincter-saving resection for rectal and rectosigmoid carcinoma. *Radiology* 155:305–310, 1985.

63. Husband J.E., Hodson N.J., Parsons C.A.: The use of computed tomography in recurrent rectal tumors. *Radiology* 134:677–682, 1980.

64. Kelvin F.M., Korobkin M., Heaston D.K., et al.: The pelvis after surgery for rectal carcinoma: serial CT observations with emphasis on nonneoplastic features. *AJR* 141:959–964, 1983.

65. Reynak R.H., White F.E., Young J.W.R., et al.: The appearance on computed tomography after abdomino-perineal resection for carcinoma of the rectum: a comparison between the normal appearances and those of recurrence. *Br. J. Radiol.* 56:237–240, 1983.

66. Butch R.J., Wittenberg J., Mueller P.R., et al.: Presacral masses after abdominoperineal resection for colorectal carcinoma: the need for needle biopsy. *AJR* 144:309–312, 1985.

67. Sugarbaker P.H., Gunderson L.L., Wittes R.E.: Cancer of the anal region, in DeVita V.T. Jr., Hellman S., Rosenberg S.A. (eds.): *Cancer: Principles and Practice of Oncology*, ed. 2. Philadelphia, J.B. Lippincott Co., 1985, pp. 885–894.

68. Thoeni R.F., Venbrux A.C.: Work in progress. The anal canal: distinction of internal hemorrhoids from small cancers by double-contrast barium enema examination. *Radiology* 145:17–19, 1982.

69. Cohan R.H., Silverman P.M., Thompson W.M., et al.: Computed tomography of epithelial neoplasms of the anal canal. *AJR* 145:569–573, 1985.

70. Sato T., Sakai Y., Sonoyama A., et al.: Radiologic spectrum of rectal carcinoid tumors. *Gastrointest. Radiol.* 9:23–26, 1984.

71. Chait M.M., Kurty R.C., Hajdu S.I.: Gastrointestinal tract metastasis in patients with germ-cell tumor of the testis. *Dig. Dis. Sci.* 23:925, 1978.

72. Meyers M.A., McSweeney J.: Secondary neoplasms of the bowel. *Radiology* 105:1–11, 1972.

73. Libshitz H.I., Lindell M.M., Dodd G.D.: Metastases to the hollow viscera. *Radiol. Clin. North Am.* 20:487–499, 1982.

74. Zornoza J., Goldstein H.M.: Cavitating metastases of the small intestine. *AJR* 129:613–615, 1977.

75. Chang S.F., Burrell M.I., Brand M.H., et al.: The protean gastrointestinal manifestations of metastatic breast carcinoma. *Radiology* 126:611–617, 1978.

76. Smith S.J., Carlson H.C., Gisvold J.J.: Secondary neoplasms of the small bowel. *Radiology* 125:29–33, 1977.

77. Kidd, R., Freeny P.C.: Radiographic manifestations of extrinsic processes involving the bowel. *Gastrointest. Radiol.* 7:21–28, 1982.

78. Goldstein H.M., Beydoun M.T., Dodd G.D.: Radiologic spectrum of melanoma metastatic to the gastrointestinal tract. *AJR* 129:605–612, 1977.

79. Rose H.S., Balthazar E.J., Megibow A.J., et al.: Alimentary tract involvement in Kaposi sarcoma: radiographic and endoscopic findings in 25 homosexual men. *AJR* 139:661–666, 1982.

80. Yuhasz M., Laufer I., Sutton G., et al.: Radiography of the small bowel in patients with gynecologic malignancies. *AJR* 144:303–307, 1985.

81. Rubesin S.E., Levine M.S.: Omental cakes: colonic involvement by omental metastases. *Radiology* 154:593–596, 1985.

82. Ginaldi S., Lindell M.M., Zornoza J.: The striped colon: a new radiographic observation in metastatic serosal implants. *AJR* 134:453–455, 1980.

83. Parienty R.A., Lepreux J.F., Gruson B.: Sonographic and CT features of ileocolic intussusception. *AJR* 136:608–610, 1981.

84. Curcio C.M., Feinstein R.S., Humphrey R.L., et al.: Computed tomography of entero-enteric intussusception. *J. Comput. Assist. Tomogr.* 6:969–974, 1982.

85. Merine D., Fishman E.K., Jones B., et al.: Enteroenteric intussusception: CT findings in nine patients. *AJR* 148:1129–1132, 1987.

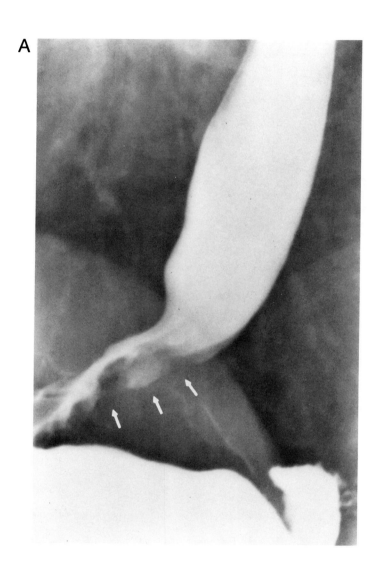

FIG 1–1.

Adenocarcinoma of the esophagogastric junction. This 54-year-old man experienced epigastric pain for six months. The results of the UGI series and endoscopy were initially normal at the onset of symptoms. The patient lost 6 kg (13 lb) over the six-month period and noted one episode of hematemesis.

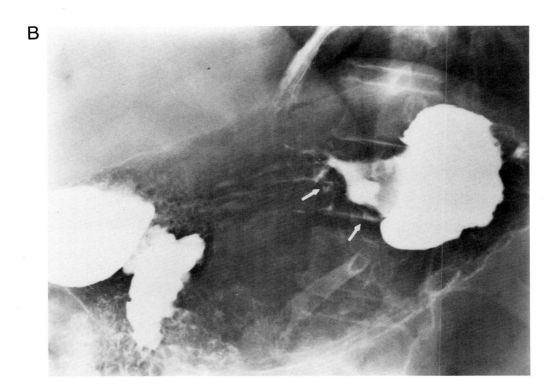

A and **B,** repeat UGI examination reveals a small submucosal ulcerated mass *(arrows)* at the esophagogastric junction. Biopsy and resection confirmed the diagnosis of adenocarcinoma.

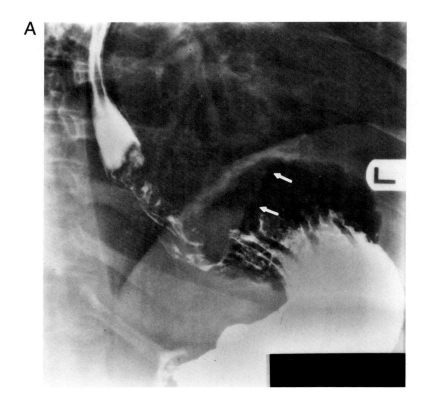

FIG 1–2.

Leiomyosarcoma of the distal esophagus. This 40-year-old man had a three-year history of progressive dysphagia with two prior "normal" UGI series. At this presentation, he had no other symptoms, including no complaints of anorexia and no significant weight loss.

A, a UGI film at this presentation reveals a long, infiltrating tumor of the distal esophagus, with an abrupt upper margin and mass extension into the gastric fundus *(arrows).*

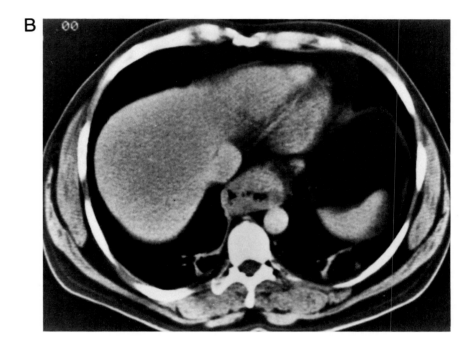

B, a CT scan confirms the circumferential thickening of the esophageal wall and eccentric distortion of the lumen.

The tumor was completely excised. Pathologic examination revealed a 7 by 3.5 cm mass, which on microscopic examination proved to be a high-grade leiomyosarcoma.

This was an unusual tumor, but there was nothing specific about the radiographic findings in this case that would have allowed differentiation from a squamous cell carcinoma or adenocarcinoma involving the distal esophagus.

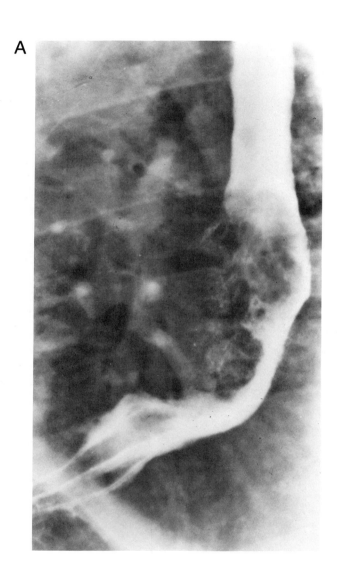

FIG 1–3.
Carcinosarcoma of the distal esophagus. This 71-year-old man presented because of progressive dysphagia to solid food.

A, a barium swallow film reveals a bulky tumor in the distal esophagus. The tumor is expanding the lumen.

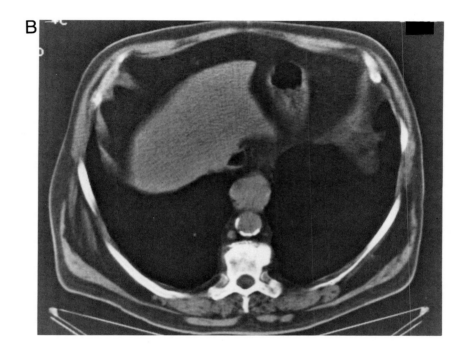

B, a CT scan demonstrates the bulky distal esophagus with clear fat planes separating it from surrounding structures.

The surgical specimen revealed squamous cell carcinoma with spindle cell elements. There was no invasion of the muscularis propria.

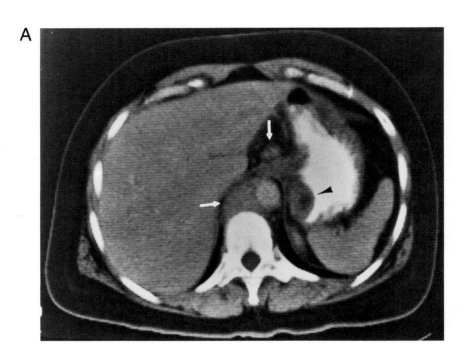

FIG 1–4.
Pseudoachalasia in gastric adenocarcinoma. This 43-year-old woman was initially treated at the age of 32 for mediastinal and axillary Hodgkin's disease, nodular sclerosing type. Four years later, the disease recurred in the abdomen and was treated with systemic chemotherapy and abdominal radiation therapy. The patient remained disease free for one year and was then lost to follow-up. When she presented six years later for routine follow-up, a CT scan was obtained.

A, the CT scan shows retrocrural and gastrohepatic ligament adenopathy *(arrows),* which was considered by the clinicians to represent treated Hodgkin's disease. The mass in the gastric fundus *(arrowhead)* was not appreciated by the radiologists at that time. Over the next six months, the patient developed weight loss and dysphagia.

B

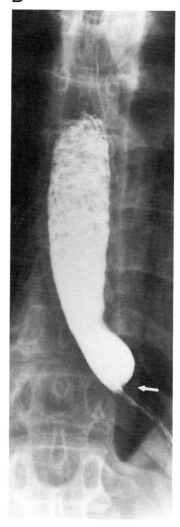

C

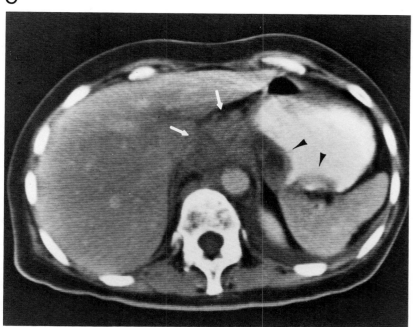

B, a film from a barium swallow demonstrates narrowing of the distal esophagus with stasis of barium and food. Fluoroscopically, there was absence of ordered peristalsis, consistent with achalasia. The narrowing is not classically tapered, however, and should be interpreted as shouldered on one side *(arrow),* raising the possibility of pseudoachalasia.

C, a repeat CT scan reveals enlargement of the gastrohepatic ligament adenopathy *(arrows)* and extension of the gastric mass *(arrowheads).*

Endoscopic biopsies confirmed adenocarcinoma of the stomach.

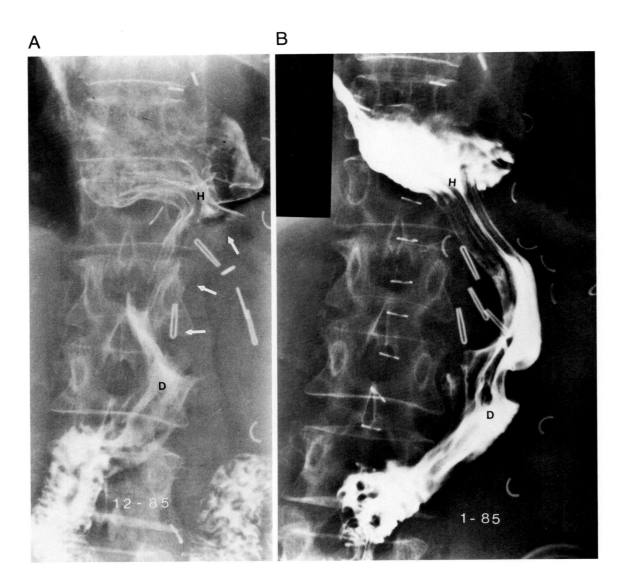

FIG 1–5.
Recurrent squamous cell carcinoma of the esophagus. This 63-year-old woman originally complained of dysphagia for four months. She was found by UGI series and endoscopic biopsy to have a squamous cell carcinoma of the esophagogastric junction. Resection with esophagogastrostomy was performed. The tumor was 4 cm in its maximum dimension and the margins were clear, but there was involvement of one of five perigastric lymph nodes. The patient did well for 11 months, when she began to experience early satiety.

A, a barium swallow film demonstrates extrinsic mass effect on the distal stomach *(arrows).* (**D**, duodenum; **H**, hiatus).

B, it can particularly be appreciated in comparison with the appearance on an initial postoperative swallow (*D,* duodenum; *H,* hiatus). Endoscopy revealed no mucosal disease.

C, a CT scan demonstrates a large necrotic mass in the epigastrium. This mass corresponds to the area of extrinsic compression.

D, percutaneous biopsy was performed with CT guidance. Analysis of the material from this biopsy confirmed the diagnosis of recurrent squamous cell carcinoma.

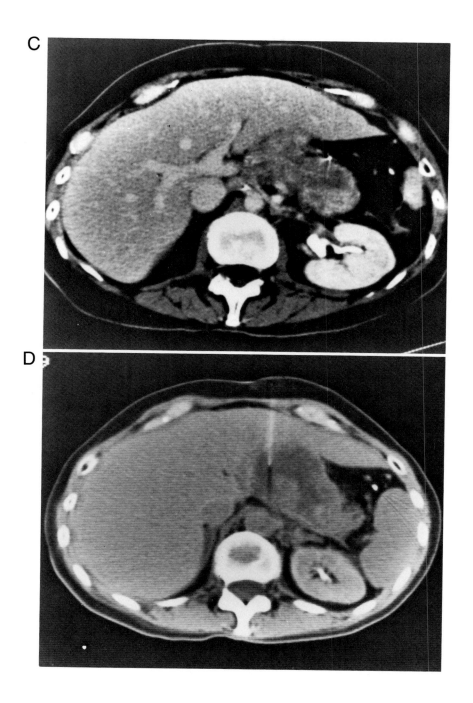

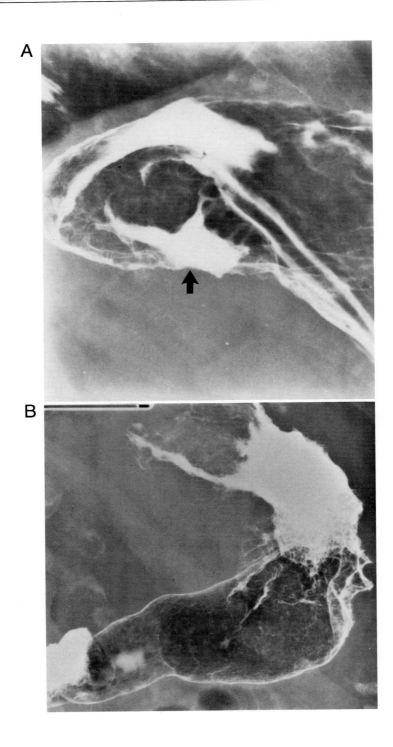

FIG 1–6.
Typical appearances of gastric carcinoma.
     A, polypoid mass with large, stellate, central ulceration *(arrow).*

B, lobular mass in the fundus with extensive infiltration of the mucosa to the distal body, manifested by decreased distensibility, distorted folds, and mucosal destruction.

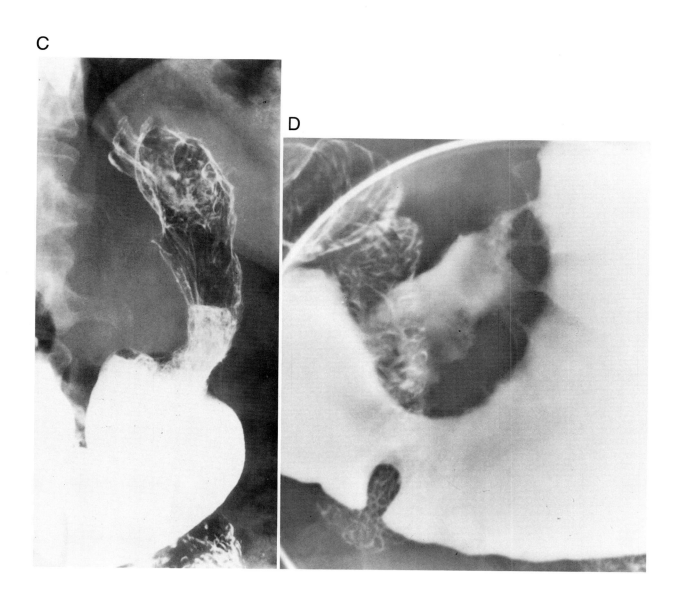

C, decreased distensibility of the proximal half of the stomach, without definite mucosal destruction.

D, Carman-Kirklin complex: shallow ulcer with rolled tumor border seen folded, in tangent, as an ulcer that is convex toward the lumen.

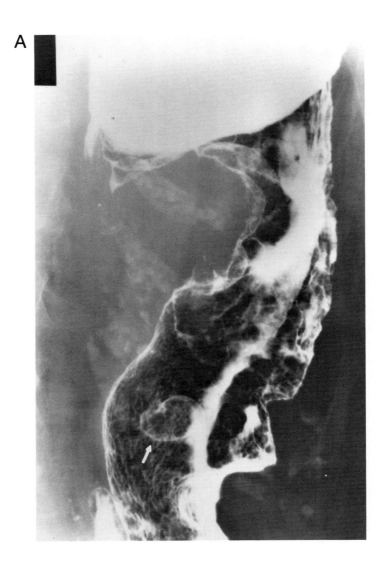

FIG 1–7.

Adenocarcinoma of the stomach and benign polyps. This 71-year-old woman presented with gradual-onset fatigue, anorexia, and weight loss. She was found to have an iron deficiency anemia.

A and **B,** a UGI series was performed. The films reveal a large lobulated mass involving the posterior wall and lesser curvature of the upper body. In addition, there are multiple polyps ranging from 0.5 to 2.0 cm in the distal body *(arrows).* The stomach is unusually vertical because of a prior thoracoplasty for tuberculosis with subsequent elevation of the left hemidiaphragm.

C, the CT scan illustrates the predominantly intraluminal extension of this mass.

Endoscopy confirmed the UGI findings. Biopsies and subsequent gastrectomy revealed moderately well differentiated invasive adenocarcinoma with adjacent intestinal metaplasia. There were multiple benign adenomatous and hyperplastic polyps.

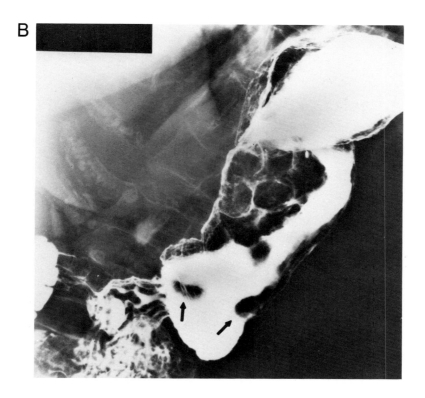

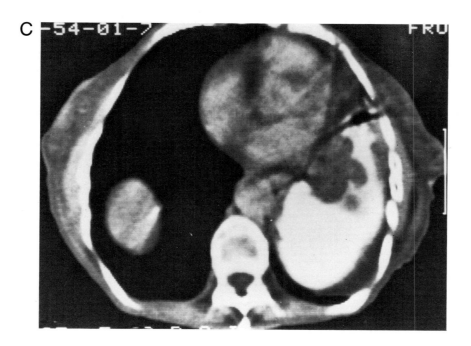

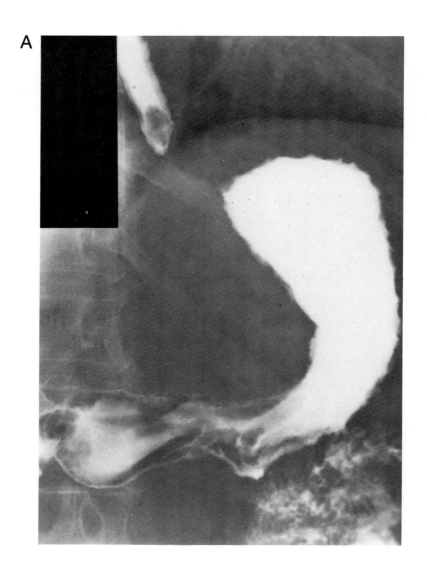

FIG 1–8.
Adenocarcinoma of the stomach, linitis plastica type. This 59-year-old woman had a two-month history of early satiety and epigastric pain.

A, the UGI series reveals diffuse narrowing of the stomach, with the exception of the prepyloric antrum. There is mucosal irregularity but no ulceration. The stomach maintained a fixed, unchanging appearance on all radiographs. This is compatible with the linitis plastica appearance, which is usually due to scirrhous carcinoma of the stomach.

B

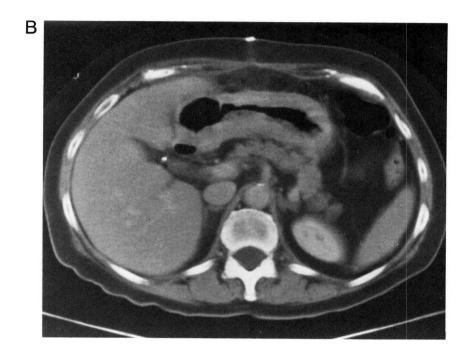

B, the CT scan confirms the diffuse wall thickening.

Results of the endoscopic biopsies, including a snare biopsy, were normal on three separate occasions. At exploratory laparotomy, there was locally advanced tumor involving the stomach and extending into the lesser omentum and distal esophagus. The pathology was signet ring adenocarcinoma of the stomach.

A

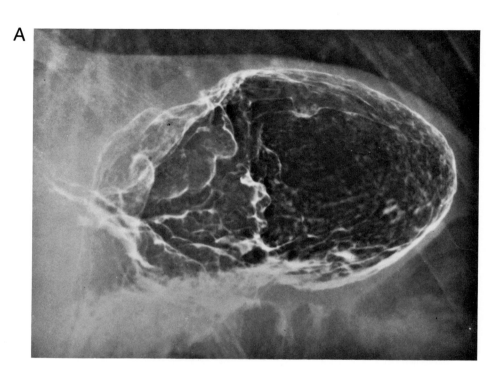

FIG 1–9.
Adenocarcinoma of the stomach. This 38-year-old man had a history of dysphagia for one year. Results of prior UGI series at the onset of symptoms were reported to be normal.

A, a UGI film at this presentation reveals thickening and rigidity of the folds in the fundus around the cardia, compatible with submucosal infiltration.

B, the CT scan confirms the focal gastric wall thickening posteriorly, which is more than can be accounted for by the pseudotumor effect of the oblique orientation of the esophagogastric junction.

C, on a lower CT slice, there is suggestion of splenic invasion.

Endoscopy revealed thickened folds, and biopsy results were normal. At operation, the patient was seen to have extensive adenocarcinoma of the stomach invading the left hemidiaphragm and spleen. Although submucosal infiltration of gastric folds without luminal compromise is often seen in lymphoma, it should be emphasized that this pattern is not infrequently encountered in gastric carcinoma as well (see Fig 1–10 also).

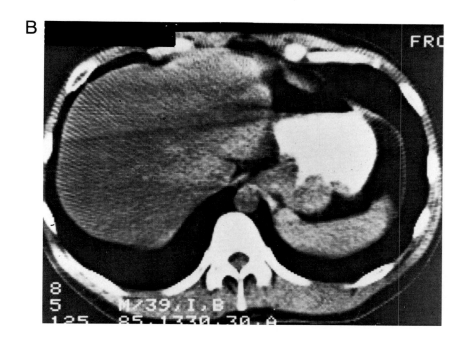

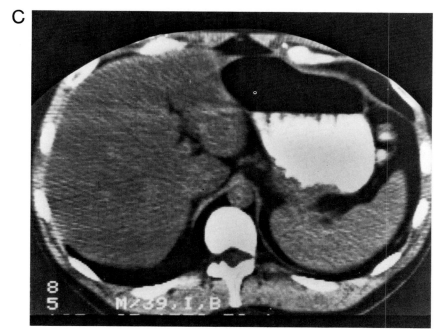

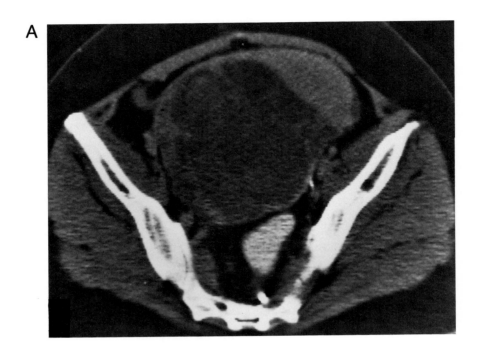

FIG 1–10.
Krukenberg's tumor: adenocarcinoma of stomach metastatic to ovary. This 22-year-old woman presented originally in February 1982 because of abdominal pain. Endoscopy revealed a posterior wall gastric ulcer; biopsy results were normal. The patient was treated with cimetidine, relieving her symptoms. In February 1983, CT was performed because of a rapidly growing pelvoabdominal mass.

A, the pelvic CT scan demonstrates a large pelvic mass. The patient then underwent exploratory laparotomy; a malignant right ovarian tumor containing signet ring cells suspicious for gastrointestinal tract origin was found.

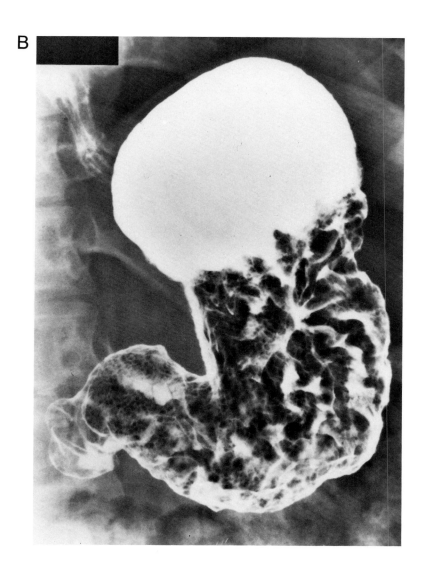

B, in March 1983, UGI series reveals prominent folds in the gastric body; they radiate to a linear collection of barium along the posterior wall.

At endoscopy, the prominent folds were seen radiating to a cleft-like ulcer next to a small depressed area covered with exudate. Biopsy results were initially normal. Repeat endoscopy with snare biospy of a prominent fold revealed signet ring adenocarcinoma.

In 1896, Krukenberg described an unusual ovarian tumor that subsequently proved to represent metastasis from the gastrointestinal tract. The term "Krukenberg's tumor" has come to be used for any metastatic lesion in ovary, particularly those from gastric or colon primaries. Not uncommonly, the ovarian mass accounts for the initial presentation. It is important to keep in mind that ovarian neoplasms may represent metastasis. A careful history of gastrointestinal symptomatology should be sought. When a CT scan is performed, careful attention should be paid to the stomach and colon.

A

B

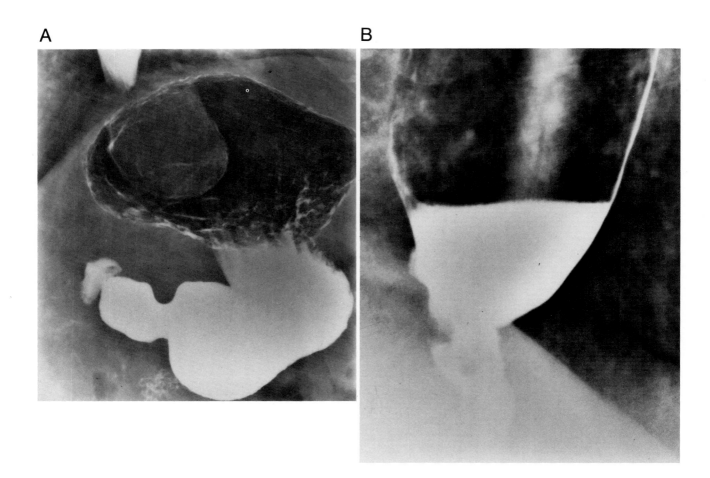

FIG 1–11.
Adenocarcinoma of the stomach. This 60-year-old man had a ten-week history of recurrent hiccups, chronic belching, and a 7.7-kg (17-lb) weight loss. Development of mild dysphagia to solid food prompted gastrointestinal workup.

A, a UGI series reveals a large smooth mass in the gastric fundus, most consistent with an intramural mass such as a leiomyoma.

B, however, malignant infiltration of the distal esophagus, resulting in proximal dilatation, suggests the true nature of the mass, namely, adenocarcinoma of the stomach with spread to the esophagus.

C and **D,** these CT scans are helpful because they show the contiguous involvement of fundus **(C)** and esophagogastric junction **(D).**

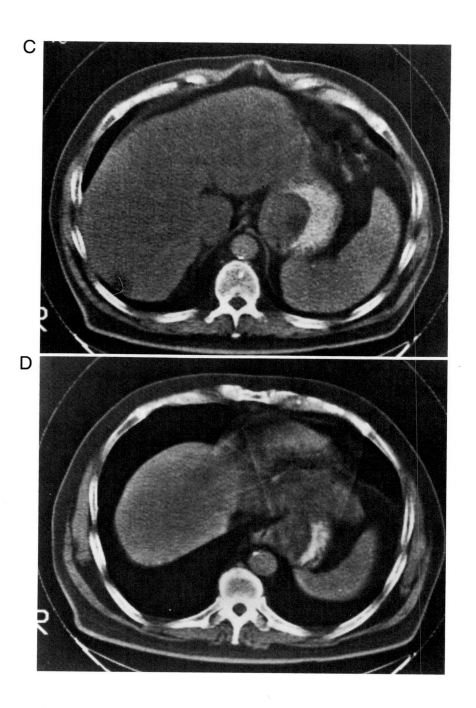

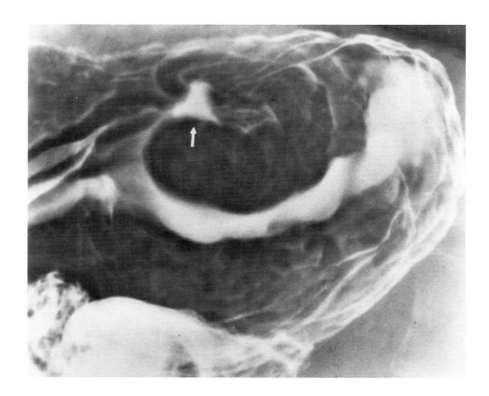

FIG 1–12.
Leiomyosarcoma of the stomach. This 68-year-old man presented initially with malaise. Workup revealed a gastric mass, which on endoscopic biopsy was called undifferentiated tumor.

The UGI series demonstrates a smooth submucosal mass with ulceration *(arrow)*.

Exploratory laparotomy revealed an intramural gastric mass with widespread hepatic and retroperitoneal metastases. The pathologic diagnosis was leiomyosarcoma.

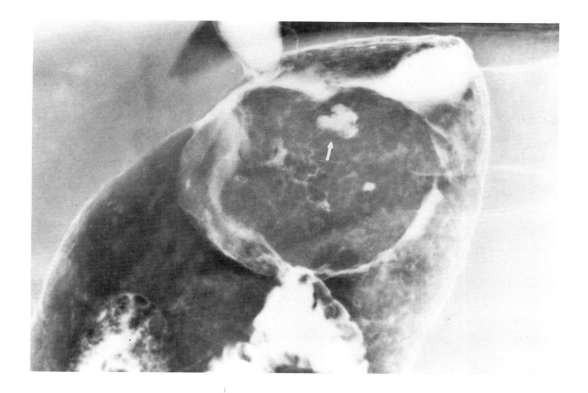

FIG 1–13.
Leiomyoma of the stomach. This 61-year-old man was evaluated because of UGI bleeding.

The UGI series reveals a submucosal mass with ulceration *(arrow)*. The endoscopic biopsy results were normal. Exploratory laparotomy revealed only the intramural mass; the abdomen was otherwise normal. Pathologically, the lesion was a leiomyoma.

This case and the case in Figure 1–12 illustrate the difficulty often encountered in distinguishing benign from malignant smooth muscle tumors, especially when the tumors are small.

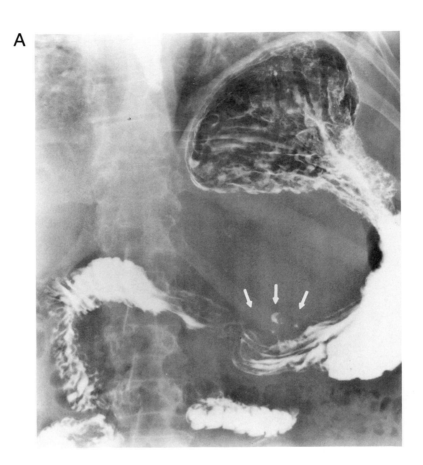

FIG 1–14.
Leiomyosarcoma of the stomach. This 67-year-old man complained of increasing abdominal girth and malaise.

A, a UGI series reveals extrinsic mass effect on the lesser curvature of the stomach, as well as stretching of the duodenum. There is a smaller intramural mass effect with central ulceration involving the antrum *(arrows).*

B, the CT scan shows a necrotic mass growing pre-dominantly exophytically from the posterior gastric antrum (*S,* stomach; *M,* mass).

C, a higher CT section shows a similarly low-attenuation metastasis in the left lobe of the liver, which accounts for some of the lesser-curvature mass effect on the UGI film.

Endoscopic biopsy confirmed leiomyosarcoma.

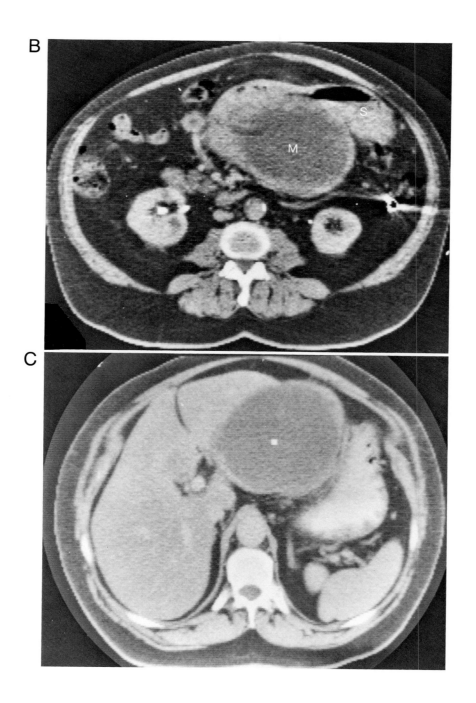

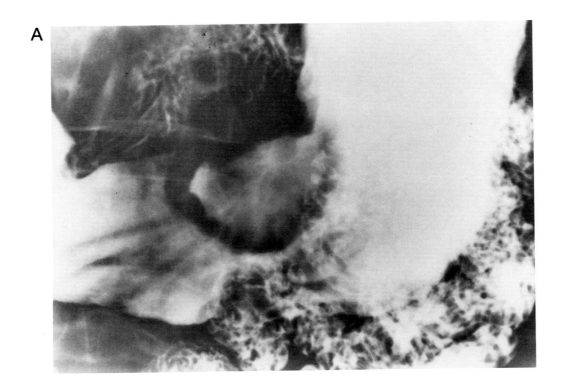

FIG 1–15.
Gastric lymphoma with recurrence. This 51-year-old woman was referred for treatment of an adenocarcinoma of the lung. On review of systems, she noted epigastric pain for three to four years and a 13.6-kg (30-lb) weight loss over two years.

A, a UGI series performed to evaluate these symptoms reveals an ulcerating tumor along the lesser curvature of the gastric body. The tumor has all the features of a Carman's (meniscus) sign (compare to Fig 1–6,**D**), which is most of-ten seen with gastric adenocarcinomas. Despite this and despite the neatness of being able to postulate only one disease affecting the stomach and secondarily the lung, endoscopic biopsy clearly established a diagnosis of large cell lymphoma of the stomach.

After the patient's lung cancer was excised, she was given chemotherapy for the lymphoma, but without response. The stomach mass was excised, and at operation there was no other evidence of disease. The patient was never able to tolerate oral feedings after surgery.

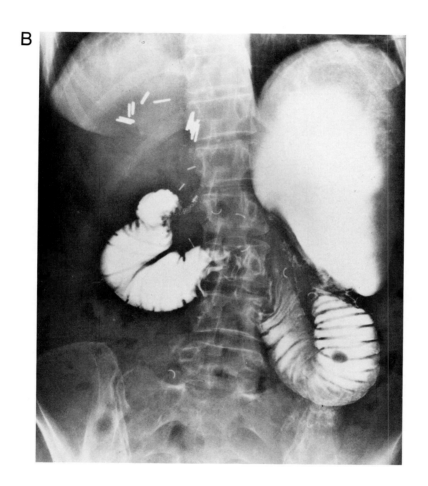

B, a UGI series performed three weeks after surgery for the stomach mass reveals almost complete obstruction of the efferent limb of the gastrojejunostomy. Reexploration revealed massive tumor recurrence with involvement of the efferent limb. This illustrates that large cell lymphoma can progress quite rapidly at times.

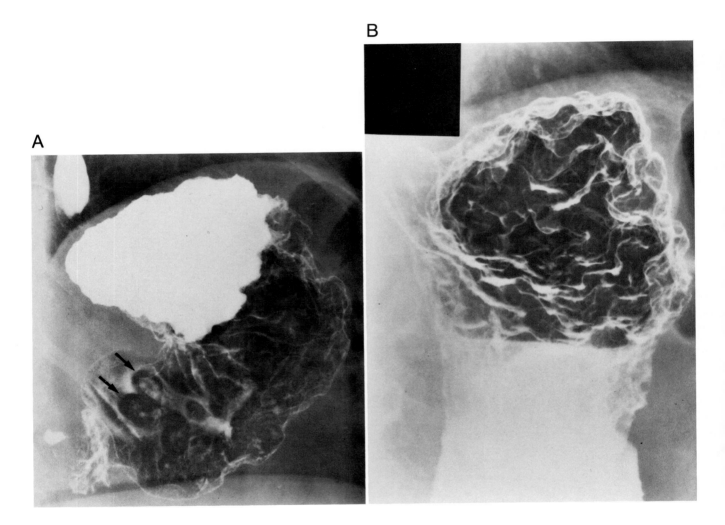

FIG 1–16.
Gastric lymphoma with response to treatment. This 66-year-old woman had a six-year history of diffuse large cell lymphoma. She initially presented with adenopathy and gastric involvement and achieved a complete remission with radiation therapy and chemotherapy. Two years later, disease recurred, but only in the nodes. Treatment again yielded complete remission. Three years later, stomach involvement was found.

A and **B,** the UGI series done at that time shows diffuse nodular thickening of the folds in the fundus and body, with some ulcerations *(arrows)*.

C

D

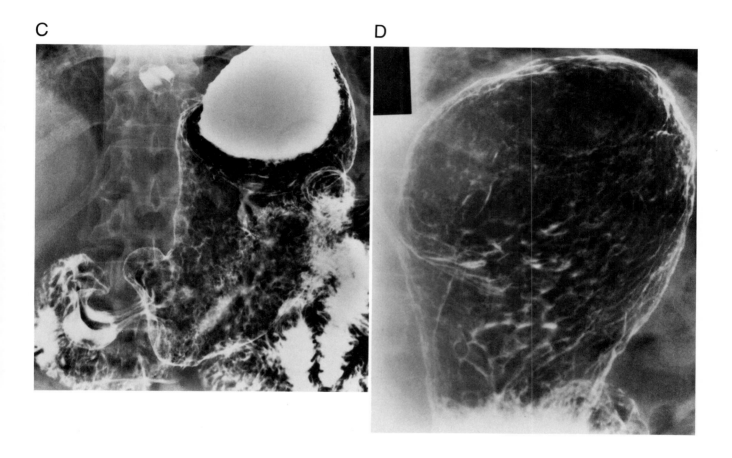

C and **D,** after three months of chemotherapy, a repeat UGI series shows at least partial regression of the fold thickening and ulceration.

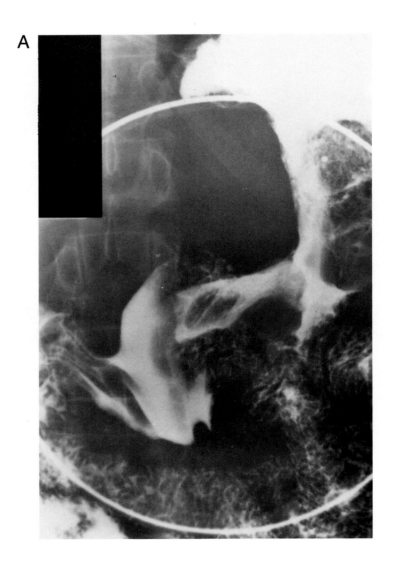

FIG 1–17.
Gastric lymphoma with response to treatment. This 46-year-old man presented with a one-month history of epigastric pain, vomiting, and weight loss.

A, a UGI series reveals large, infiltrated folds and luminal narrowing involving all but the fundus and distal antrum of the stomach. Biopsies revealed lymphoma, and the patient was treated with chemotherapy.

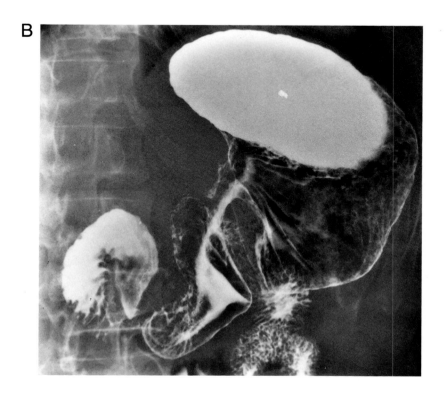

B, a repeat UGI series four months later demonstrates regression of the tumor bulk, with a stricture remaining in the proximal antrum. Biopsy results were normal at this time, and the appearance has remained stable to date, 16 months later.

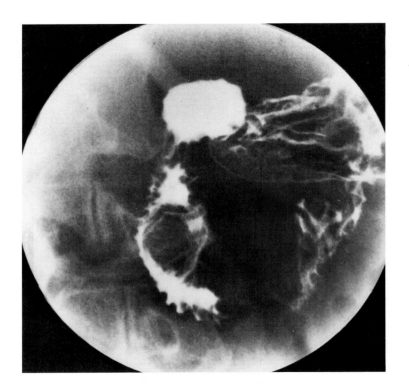

FIG 1–18.
Carcinoma of the ampulla of Vater. This 65-year-old woman presented with insidious onset of obstructive jaundice. A UGI series demonstrates a large, smooth filling defect in the descending duodenum at the expected location of the major papilla. Endoscopy confirmed the presence of a mass at the papilla. Biopsy results were positive for adenocarcinoma.

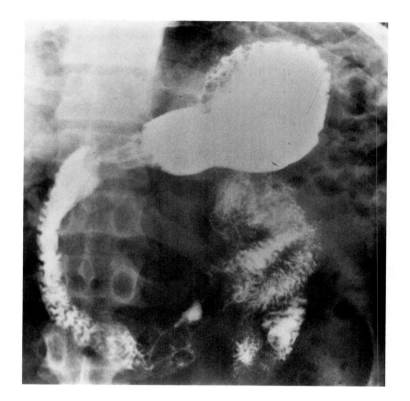

FIG 1–19.
Carcinoma of the duodenum. This 58-year-old man presented initially with epigastric pain and guaiac-positive stools. He was treated with an antiulcer regimen. He again sought medical attention ten months later, at which time he had pulmonary and hepatic metastases.

Review of UGI series from the time of his initial presentation reveals an ulcerating tumor mass circumferentially involving the fourth portion of the duodenum. Endoscopy then confirmed the extensive tumor in the duodenum, which histologically was adenocarcinoma.

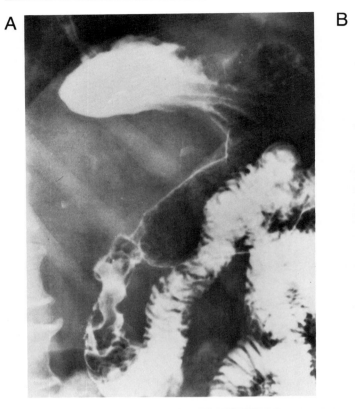

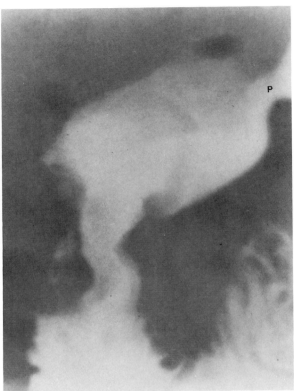

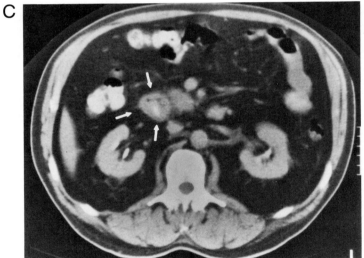

FIG 1–20.
Carcinoma of the duodenum. This 63-year-old man presented with a three-month history of weight loss and "weakness." Twenty years before, he had been treated for Hodgkin's disease with irradiation and chemotherapy, and there had been no evidence of disease since. He was now found to be anemic.

A and **B,** A UGI series reveals an annular, constricting, ulcerated lesion of the descending duodenum (*P,* pylorus).

C, A CT scan confirms the intrinsic circumferential nature of the tumor mass *(arrows)* lateral to the pancreas.

Endoscopic biopsy results were positive for adenocarcinoma. Whipple's operation was performed, and a primary carcinoma of the duodenum confirmed.

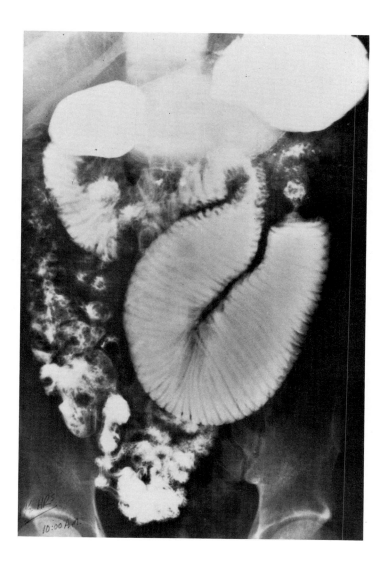

FIG 1–21.

Adenocarcinoma of the jejunum. This 37-year-old man experienced intermittent nausea and vomiting for one month, at which time the symptoms persisted and he sought medical attention.

A small bowel examination film demonstrates high-grade obstruction in the proximal jejunum secondary to an annular, constricting mass. An annular neoplasm 3 cm long was excised and liver metastases documented at surgery. Histologically, the tumor was an adenocarcinoma infiltrating through the bowel wall into the mesentery.

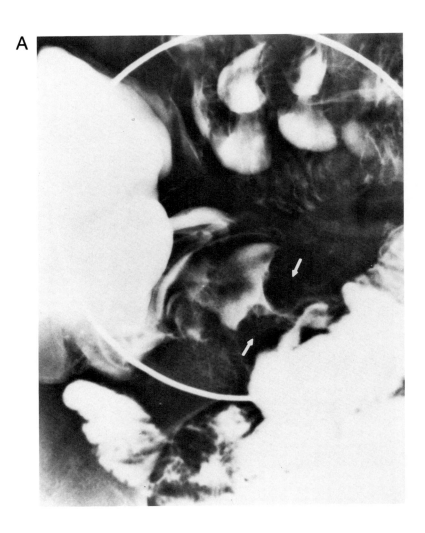

FIG 1–22.

Carcinoid tumor of the ileum with recurrence. This 62-year-old woman had a three-year history of carcinoid syndrome. When she first presented with diarrhea and flushing, she was found to have a primary ileal tumor and liver metastases.

A, a spot film from the small bowel series at her initial presentation shows an annular constricting lesion in the ileum *(arrows).*

The right colon and ileum were resected and treatment with 5-fluorouracil begun. A small bowel examination and CT scan at that time were normal, apart from the postoperative anatomy and the liver metastases. The patient underwent hepatic artery embolization, to which there was response.

B through **D,** although the lesions in the liver continued to respond and her syndrome was well controlled, the patient developed recurrent carcinoid tumor in the mesentery of the distal small bowel, illustrated on the small bowel examination film **(B),** the CT scan **(C),** and the angiogram **(D).** The distal small bowel loops are fixed in position and tethered toward a central point, seen in the right lower quadrant on both the CT scan and the barium study. The angiogram made by superior mesenteric artery injection demonstrates serpiginous encased vessels on the mesenteric side of the distal ileum *(arrows).*

B

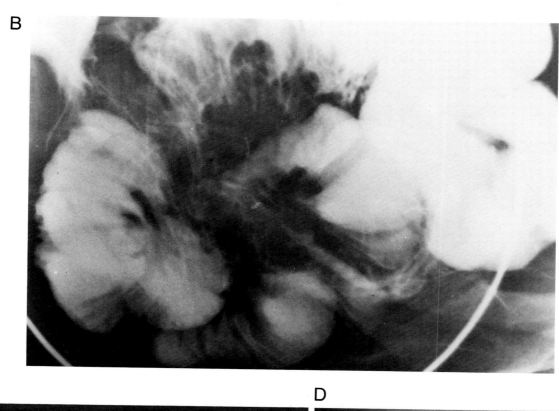

C

D

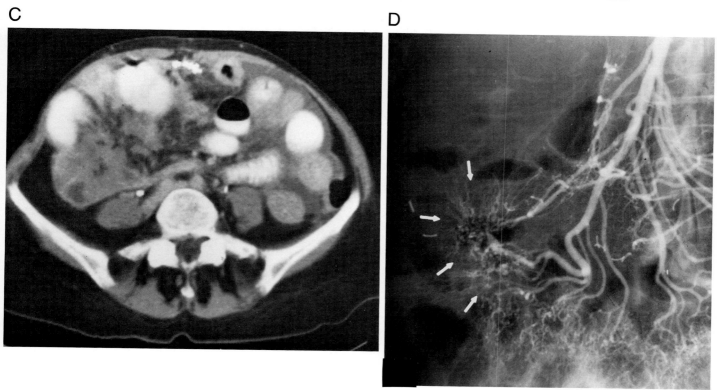

A

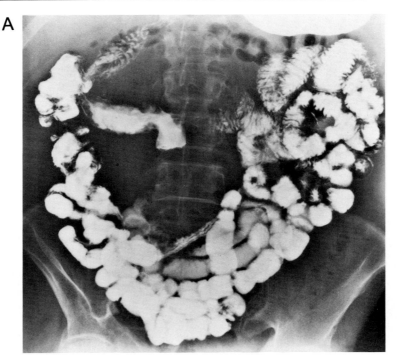

B

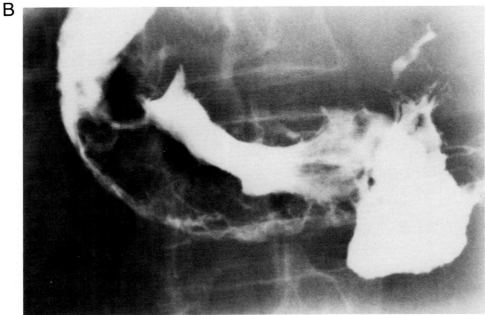

FIG 1–23.
Leiomyosarcoma of the duodenum. This 66-year-old man sought medical attention for a cough and fatigue. He was found to have an abdominal mass and anemia (hemoglobin, 5 g/100 ml).

A and **B,** the UGI films reveal a large mass involving the second and third portions of the duodenum, with extensive ulceration, particularly evident on spot film **(B)** of the duodenum.

C, the CT scan shows ascites and confirms the presence of a large soft tissue mass with necrosis.

D and **E,** angiograms demonstrate a large hypervascular mass with dual supply from the gastroduodenal **(D)** and superior mesenteric **(E)** arteries.

Endoscopic biopsy established the diagnosis of leiomyosarcoma.

C

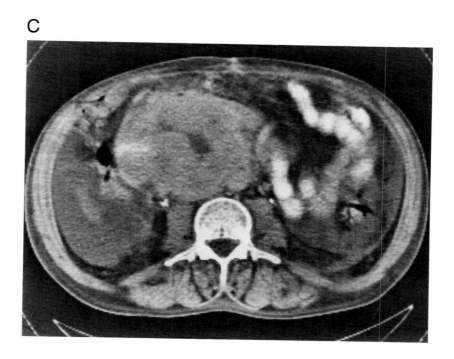

D

E

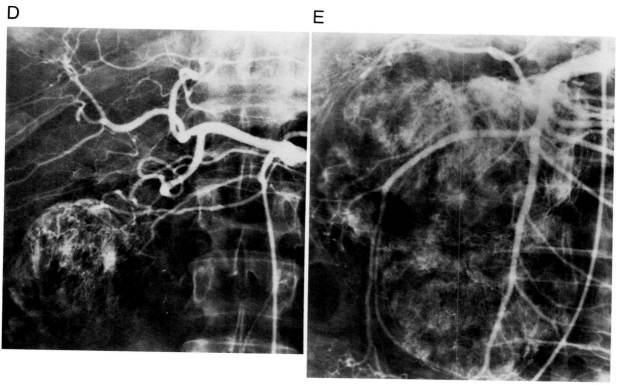

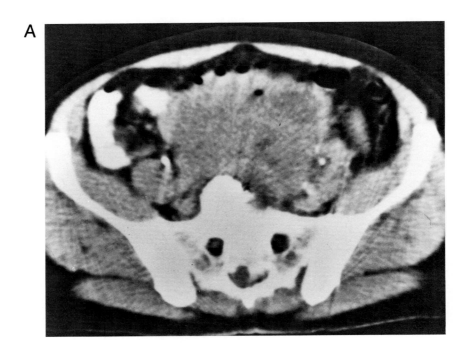

FIG 1–24.
Leiomyosarcoma of the jejunum. This 71-year-old man originally presented with a feeling of lower abdominal heaviness. On physical examination, he was found to have a large abdominopelvic mass. Percutaneous biopsy of the mass established the diagnosis of leiomyosarcoma. The origin was unclear. Barium study results were reportedly normal, apart from displacement and compression of the bladder, small bowel, and colon.

A, a CT scan at the time demonstrates a tiny amount of gas in the large mass. The tumor was considered inoperable, and chemotherapy was given.

There was a response to treatment. However, gastrointestinal bleeding became a significant problem.

B, a film from the small bowel series performed at this time demonstrates a focal segment of tethered small bowel in the pelvis that communicates freely into necrotic tumor.

C, a repeat CT scan shows barium and air in the tumor mass as well. It is likely that the mass grew exophytically from a primary origin in the wall of the small bowel.

B

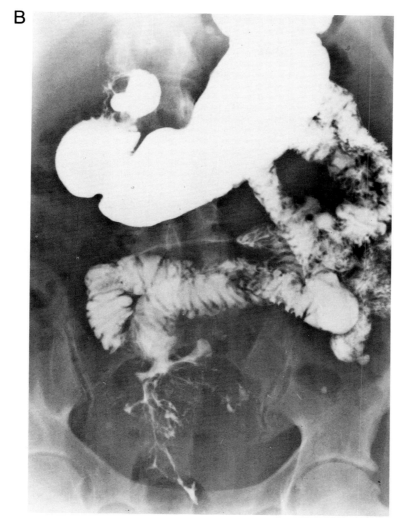

C

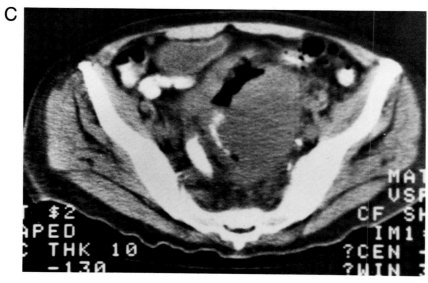

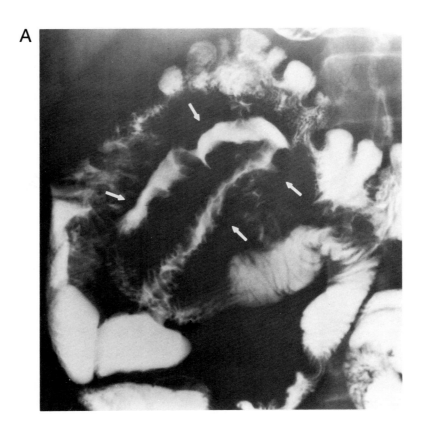

FIG 1–25.
Typical appearances of lymphoma of the small bowel.

 A, fixation of a loop of ileum with narrowing and efface-ment of the normal mucosal pattern *(arrows).*

 B, mesenteric tumor mass with excavation and com-munication with the small bowel.

 C, multiple nodules of varying size in the duodenal bulb. *(Continued.)*

B

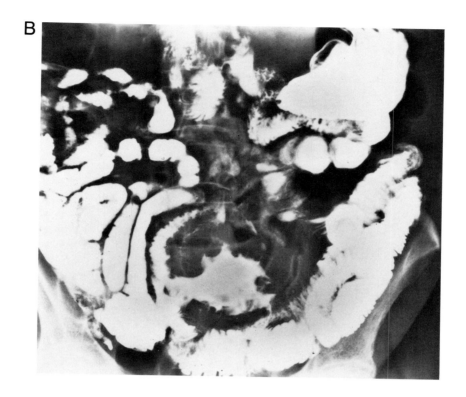

C

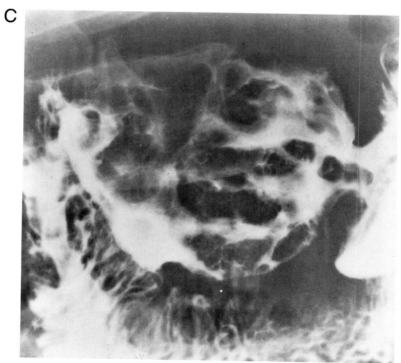

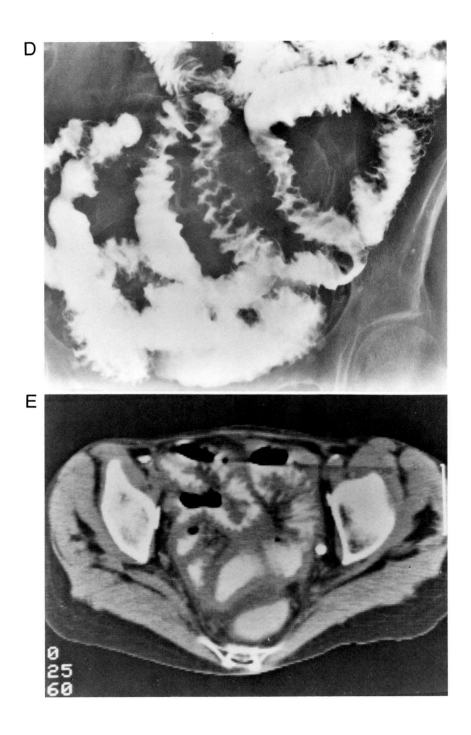

FIG 1–25 (cont.).
D and **E,** infiltration of the small bowel folds and wall seen
on small bowel series film and CT scan.

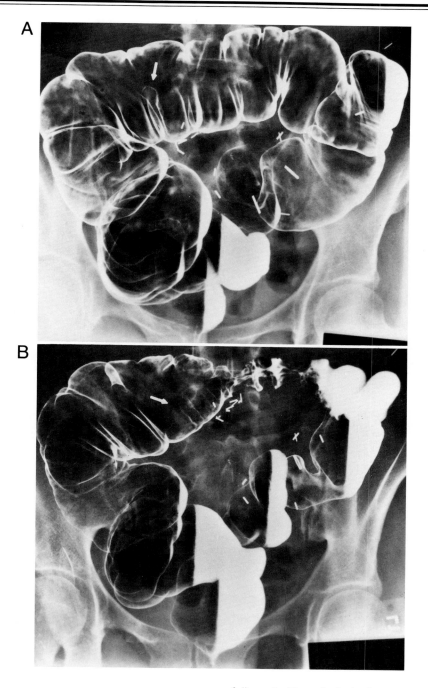

FIG 1–26.

Early metachronous carcinoma of the colon. This 43-year-old woman had had a perforated stage B2 carcinoma of the sigmoid colon excised at the age of 38. The following year, a rectal metastasis was excised, followed by the development of a left flank metastasis requiring excision of the splenic flexure and a portion of the stomach and small bowel. The patient remained well for four years and was followed with periodic barium enema examinations.

A, a small mass *(arrow)* arising from an interhaustral fold can be seen on the barium enema film.

B, in retrospect, the same fold, identified just proximal to the surgical clips, is already abnormal in this barium enema film from one year earlier. The fold is slightly widened and lobulated. The mass proved to be a Dukes B1 carcinoma, arising in an adenomatous polyp.

A

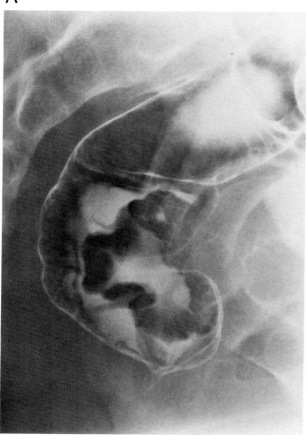

B

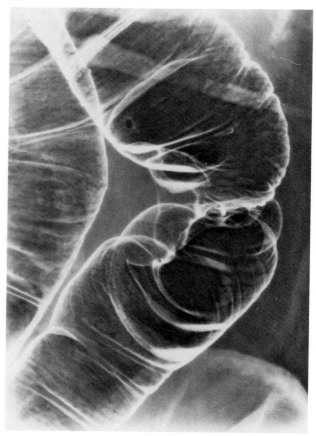

FIG 1–27.
Typical appearances of adenocarcinoma of the colorectum.

A, lobular tumor mass with large central ulceration in the rectum.

B, saddle-shaped mass in the descending colon.
C, fungating mass in the cecum.
D, apple core, or napkin ring, carcinoma of the transverse colon.

C

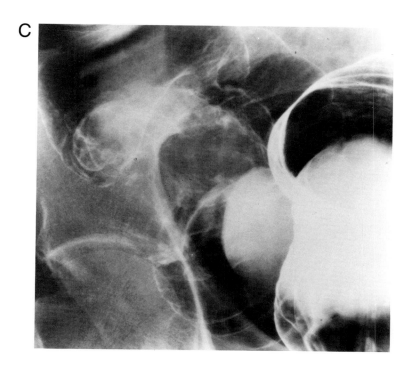

D

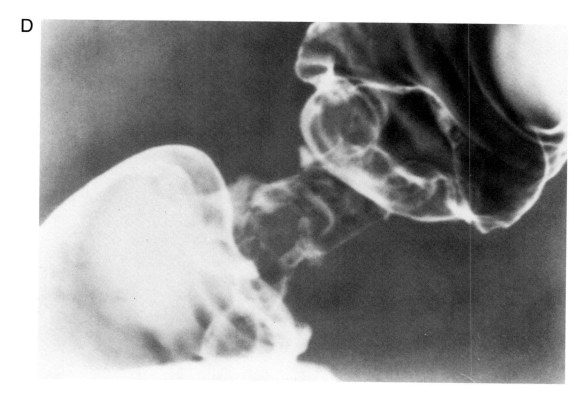

A

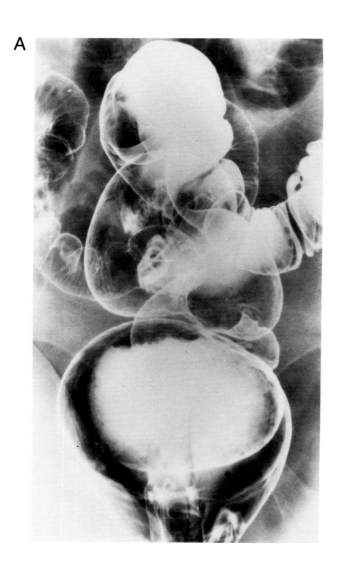

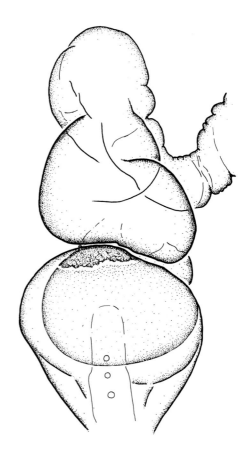

FIG 1–28.
Subtle appearances of carcinoma of the colorectum on double-contrast enema illustrated with corresponding drawings.

A, small mass deforming the barium pool in the rectum.
B, extra white line not readily explained as a luminal surface or fold. *(Continued.)*

B

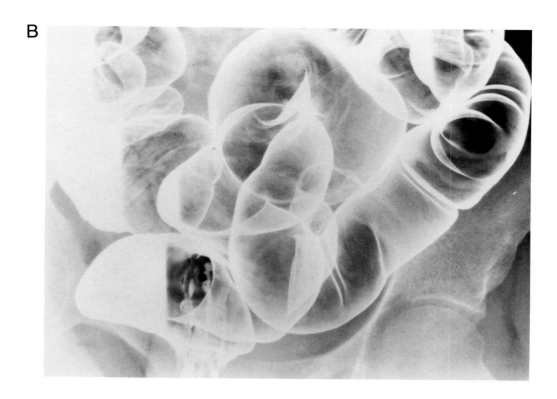

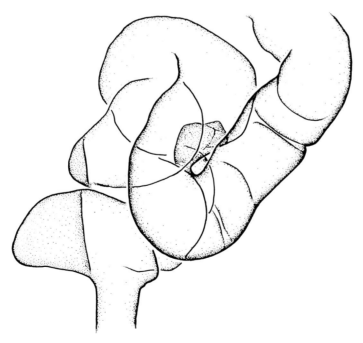

C

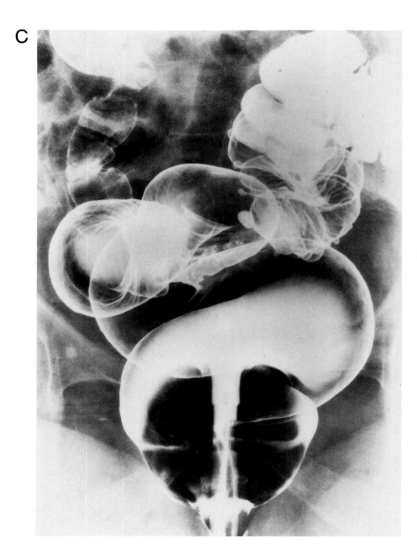

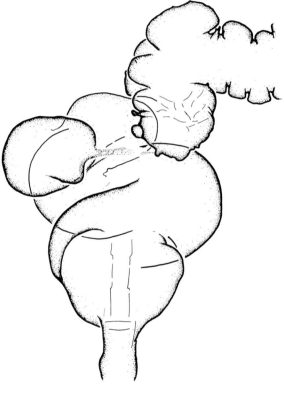

FIG 1–28 (cont.).

C, discontinuity of the lumen, representing a long annular lesion not coated by barium.

D, gray soft tissue mass within the expected black of the air-filled lumen.

D

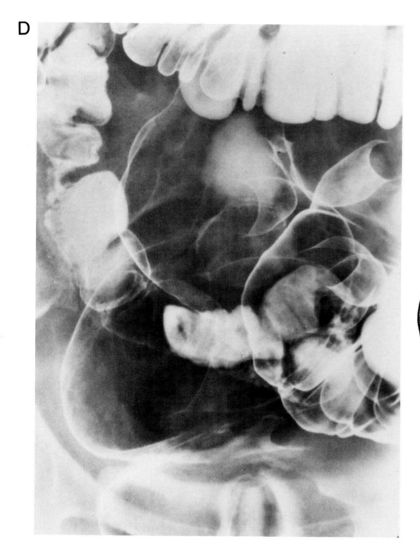

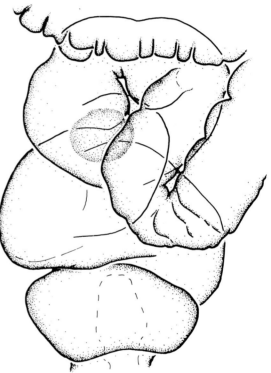

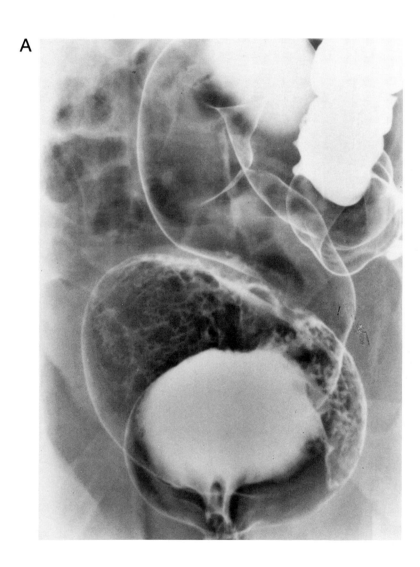

FIG 1–29.
Villous adenoma of the rectum. This 78-year-old woman presented with rectal bleeding.

Barium enema films (**A** and **B**) reveal a large, flat, reticular or villous tumor carpeting the anterior rectum.

B

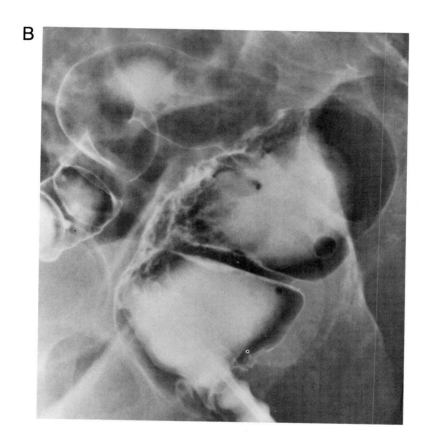

Biopsies disclosed a predominantly villous adenoma with focal areas of marked dysplasia. Although there might well have been invasive carcinoma in areas not sampled by biopsy, the patient was such a poor surgical risk that it was decided not to perform abdominoperineal resection.

It is of interest that in a recent series of 14 patients with carpet lesions such as this, only 1 patient harbored invasive carcinoma at surgery.[54]

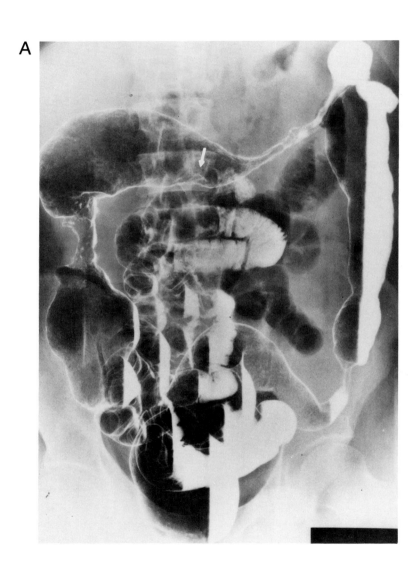

A

FIG 1–30.
Synchronous colon cancers in chronically active panulcerative colitis. This 45-year-old man had a 25-year history of ulcerative colitis but only sporadic medical follow-up, including no medical attention for the past several years.

He developed new rectal bleeding and was then evaluated with a barium enema examination (**A** and **B**), his first in 25 years. There are changes of chronically active ulcerative colitis throughout the colon, loss of haustral markings, and a coarse granularity to the en face mucosal appearance. In addition, there is an annular carcinoma in the as-

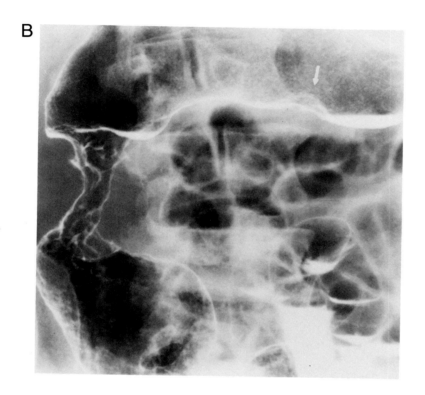

cending colon and a 2-cm, broad-based polyp in the proximal transverse colon *(arrow).*

The total colectomy specimen revealed a poorly differentiated adenocarcinoma of the ascending colon with transmural extension into the pericolic fat and 2/53 abnormal nodes; a moderately differentiated adenocarcinoma of the transverse colon with invasion into the muscularis propria; and chronic ulcerative colitis with multiple foci of epithelial dysplasia.

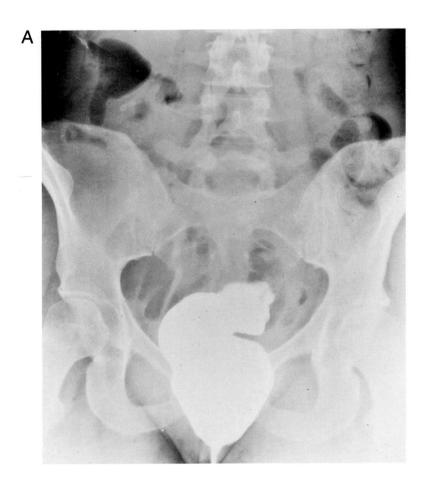

FIG 1–31.
Obstructing rectosigmoid cancer in a patient with unsuspected familial polyposis. This 23-year-old woman presented with bloody diarrhea. **A,** barium enema film reveals complete obstruction of the retrograde flow of barium at the rectosigmoid junction.

B

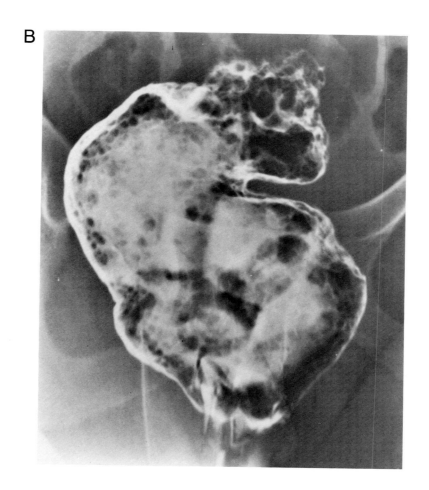

B, a lobular mass can be seen impressing the obstructed proximal margin. In addition, the double-contrast view of the rectum reveals multiple nodular filling defects compatible with extensive polyposis.

Although the patient had no family history of colorectal cancer or a polyposis syndrome, familial polyposis with an obstructing cancer at the rectosigmoid junction was subsequently confirmed.

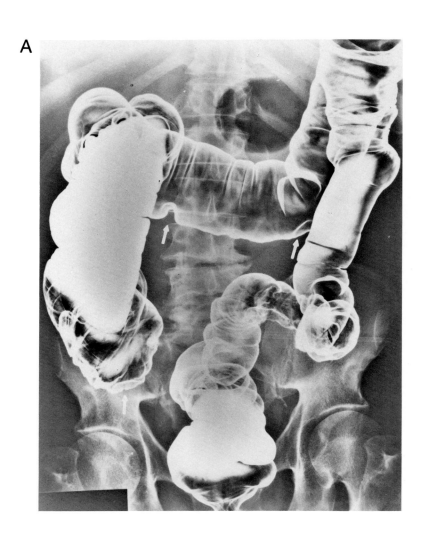

FIG 1–32.
Carcinoma of the colon with peritoneal metastases. This 64-year-old man presented with rectal bleeding and weight loss.

A and **B,** barium enema films demonstrate annular constriction of the sigmoid colon, compatible with a primary carcinoma of the colon.

C, in addition, an enema film reveals a mass in the pouch of Douglas, extrinsically impressing the anterior rectum, as well as multiple extramucosal masses involving the cecum and the transverse and descending colon (*arrows* in **A**). This is compatible with diffuse peritoneal spread, which is what was found at exploratory laparotomy performed for palliative removal of the primary tumor.

B

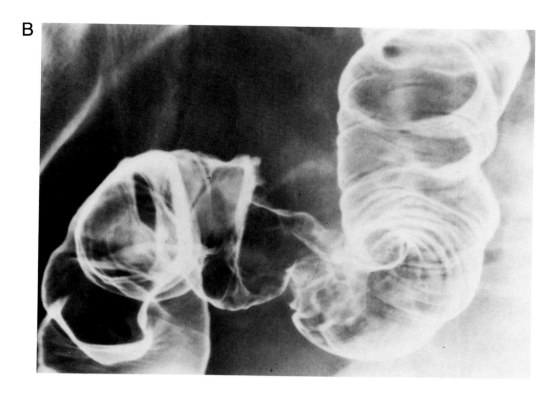

C

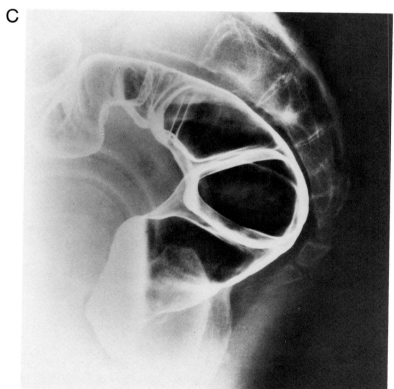

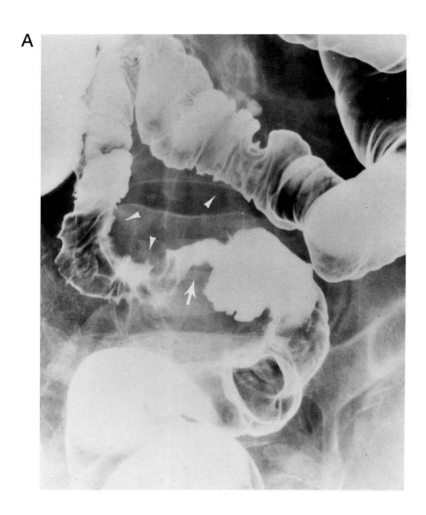

FIG 1–33.
Perforated adenocarcinoma of the sigmoid colon. This 55-year-old woman presented with fever, an elevated white blood cell count, and left lower quadrant pain. She was presumed to have peridiverticulitis.

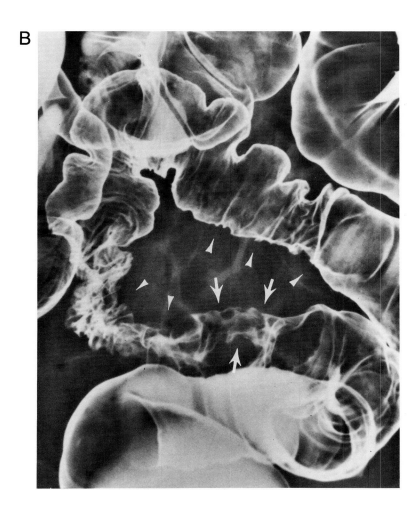

A and **B,** barium enema films demonstrate an annular, constricting tumor in the sigmoid colon *(arrows),* with associated pericolonic mass and spasm in the proximal sigmoid *(arrowheads),* compatible with a localized inflammatory process. A perforated carcinoma with pericolonic abscess was found at surgery.

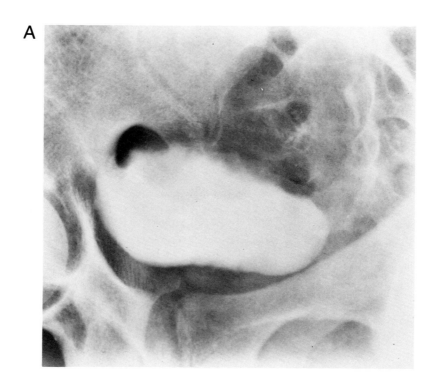

FIG 1–34.
Perforated carcinoma of the sigmoid colon. This 44-year-old man presented with complaints of urinary frequency and dysuria.

A, an intravenous urogram reveals persistent irregularity of the dome of the bladder. Cystoscopy confirmed the impression of bullous edema of the bladder wall.

B

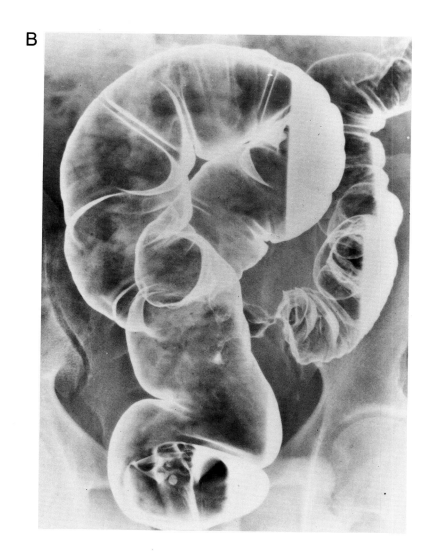

B, a barium enema film reveals carcinoma of the sigmoid colon with a sinus tract pointing toward the bladder.

At exploratory laparotomy, an inflammatory mass adherent to the dome of the bladder was found in association with the perforated cancer of the sigmoid colon.

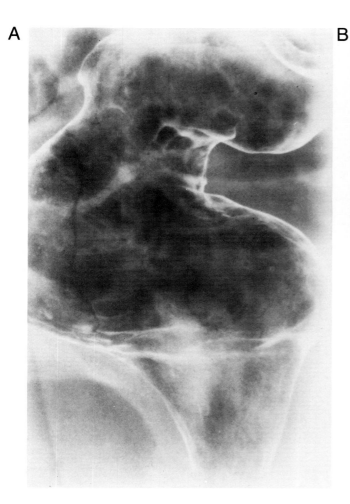

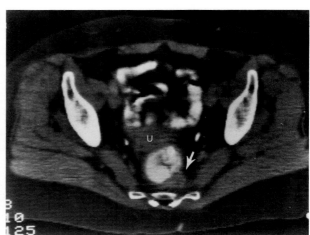

FIG 1–35.
Anastomotic recurrence after low anterior resection for rectal carcinoma. This 59-year-old woman had a low anterior resection for a Dukes C2 carcinoma of the rectosigmoid colon. Twenty-five of thirty nodes assessed for disease were abnormal.

A, the patient was followed with yearly barium enema examinations and CT scans. Three years after surgery, a film from a double-contrast enema examination reveals submucosal nodules on the left side of the anastomosis. Endoscopy was recommended.

B, this CT scan was reported as normal, but, in retrospect, a mass can be seen involving the left posterolateral wall of the rectum *(arrow)*, which is distended with contrast (*U,* uterus). Proctoscopy was not performed.

C, one year later, the barium enema film is grossly abnormal, showing an ulcerated mass that involves the left side of the rectum, centered at the anastomosis.

D, the CT scan at this time demonstrates a large mass involving the rectum as well as left internal iliac nodal metastases *(arrow)* (*U,* uterus).

At surgery, the tumor was found to be unresectable.

C

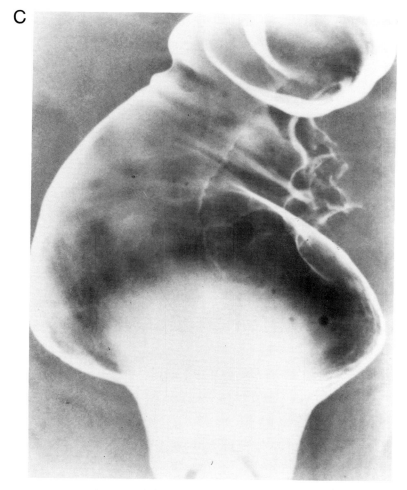

D

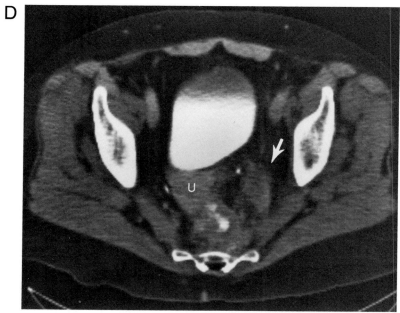

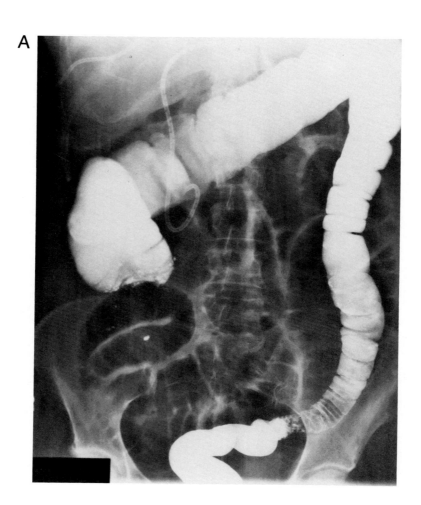

FIG 1–36.
Recurrent colon cancer at the ileocolonic anastomosis. This 68-year-old woman had had a Dukes C2 cancer of the cecum treated by right hemicolectomy. Eighteen months later, she presented with symptoms of partial obstruction of the small bowel.

A, a barium enema film demonstrates complete obstruction to retrograde flow at the presumed ileocolic anastomosis. There are multiple loops of dilated, gas-filled small bowel.

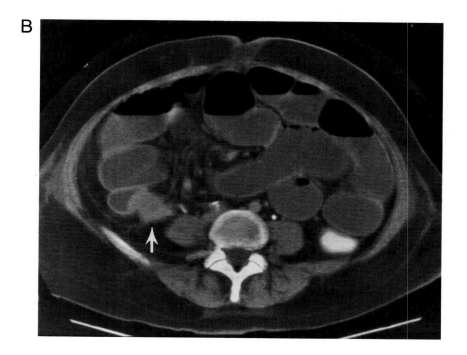

B, a CT scan demonstrates dilated loops of small bowel and a soft tissue mass *(arrow)* representing the recurrent obstructing tumor.

Exploratory laparotomy confirmed the presence of tumor at the anastomosis and complete obstruction of the small bowel.

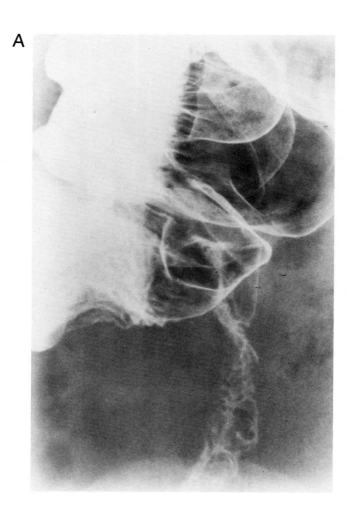

FIG 1–37.
Adenocarcinoma of the appendix with pseudomyxoma peritonei.

This 62-year-old man had a routine herniorrhaphy at the age of 55. Bits of omentum were removed, which were shown by histologic analysis to contain mucinous adenocarcinoma. The patient had experienced no symptoms of tumor involvement. A barium enema examination at that time was normal; the appendix was only partially filled with contrast. A CT scan was reported to be normal. The patient was not treated for adenocarcinoma and remained well. At the age of 60, he had a repeat barium enema examination.

A, this barium enema spot film shows nonfilling of the appendix and a mass impression on the cecal tip and terminal ileum.

Exploratory laparotomy revealed the tumor mass, along with mucinous tumor deposits scattered over the peritoneal surfaces. The resected ascending colon revealed mucinous adenocarcinoma arising in the appendix.

B through **D,** repeat CT scans have demonstrated very slowly progressive low-attenuation deposits *(cursors)* about the liver **(B)** and in the omentum and mesentery *(arrows* in **C** and **D**). The patient has remained without symptoms and has as yet received no treatment, eight years after the original diagnosis of adenocarcinoma.

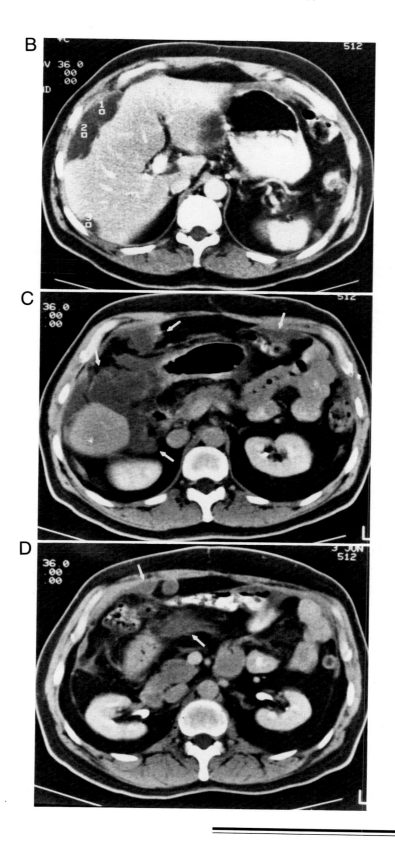

A

B

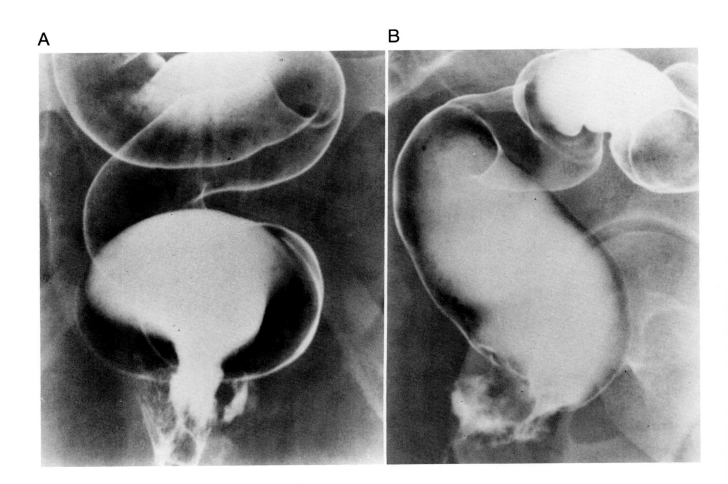

FIG 1–38.
Squamous cell carcinoma of the anal canal. This 57-year-old woman presented because of rectal pain on defecation. Physical examination disclosed an ulcerating mass in the anal canal. The mass proved to be a squamous cell carcinoma. Frontal and lateral views of barium enema (**A** and **B**) demonstrate deep posterolateral ulceration into the anal mass.

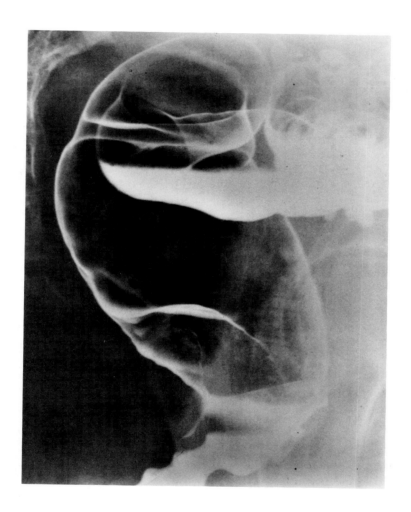

FIG 1–39.

Squamous cell carcinoma of the anal canal. This 65-year-old woman had a six-month history of rectal bleeding.

A film from the barium enema examination discloses a smooth mass in the inferior rectum, compatible with an intramural tumor. Some surface irregularity is seen.

Abdominoperineal resection was performed after proctoscopic biopsy and revealed squamous cell carcinoma. The specimen contained squamous cell carcinoma of the anorectal junction, transmurally invasive into the perirectal connective tissue and with a small central erosion of the mucosa.

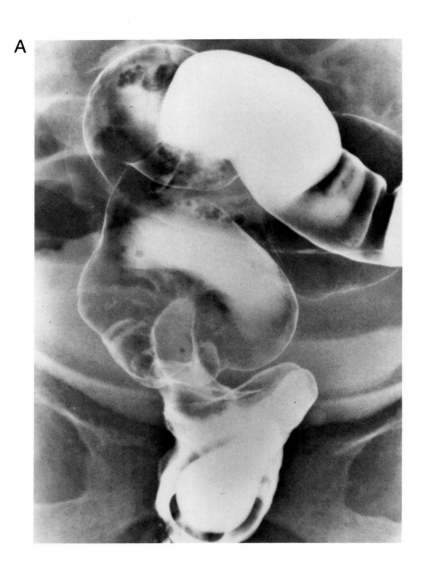

FIG 1–40.
Squamous cell carcinoma with basaloid features. This 59-year-old woman initially presented because of rectal bleeding. On physical examination, a mass was felt in the rectum; in addition, tumor was seen in the right posterior vagina.

A, a barium enema film obtained after IVP demonstrates smooth circumferential narrowing of the rectum.

B and **C,** these CT scans demonstrate mass involving the rectovaginal septum and extending toward the right pelvic sidewall (*R,* rectum; *V,* vagina).

Biopsies proved squamous cell carcinoma. The patient underwent radiation therapy and then posterior exenteration. The final pathologic specimen revealed moderately differentiated squamous cell carcinoma with basaloid appearance infiltrating the rectum, vagina, and rectovaginal septum, that is, "cloacogenic" carcinoma.

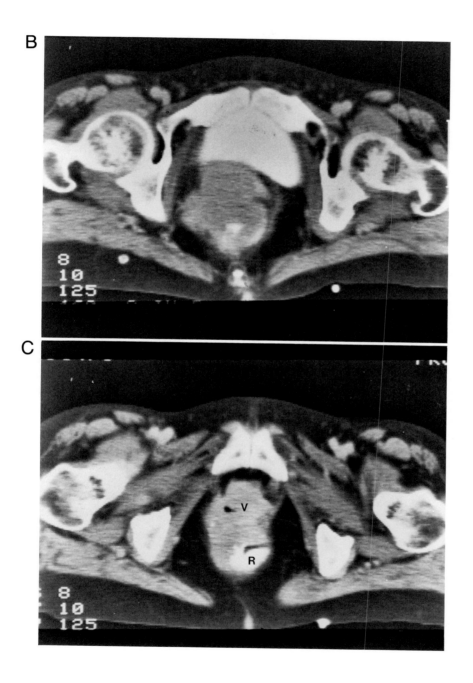

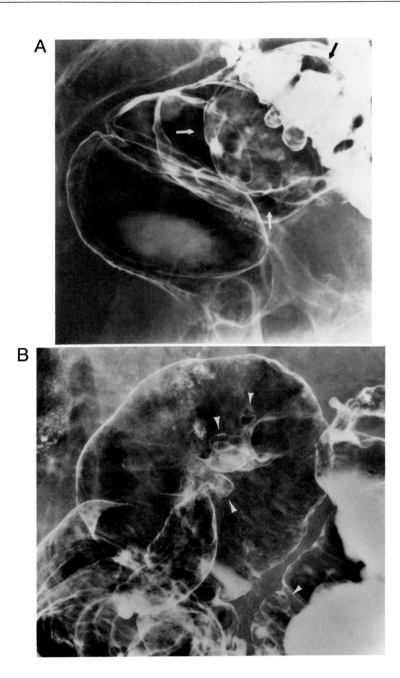

FIG 1–41.
Colorectal lymphoma. This 78-year-old woman had a five-year history of diffuse well-differentiated lymphoma, seen initially as a nasopharyngeal mass. She developed subcutaneous masses and, two years later, a sense of rectal urgency. The latter led to the discovery of multiple colon polyps, which also proved to be lymphoma. Chemotherapy was initially effective, but radiation therapy became necessary to control the growth of several subcutaneous masses and a lesion of the palate. Rectal symptoms recurred four years into her course of treatment.

A, a barium enema film at that time demonstrates a large, smooth mass filling the upper portion of the rectum *(arrows)*.

B, multiple polyps can be seen throughout the remainder of the colon as well *(arrowheads)*. The mass was treated with radiation therapy.

C

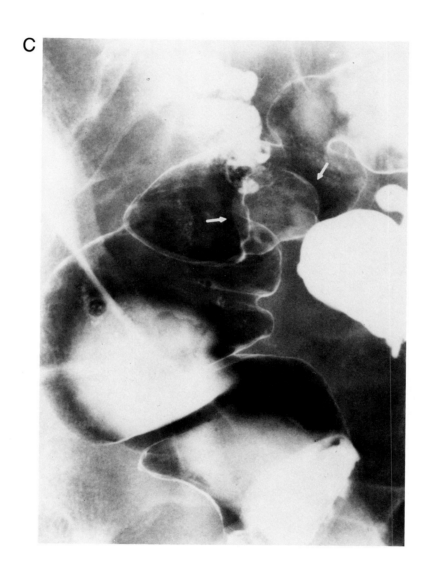

C, ten months later, the film from a repeat barium enema examination demonstrates considerable regression of the now clearly intramural mass *(arrows).*

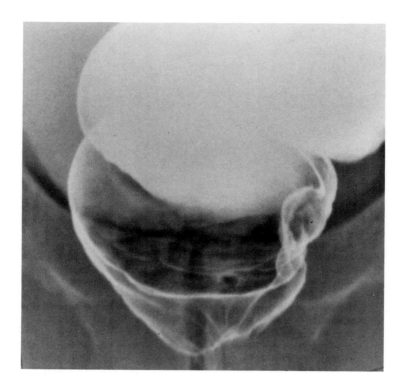

FIG 1–42.
Carcinoid tumor of the rectum. This 46-year-old man presented with a history of lower abdominal pain, which prompted evaluation of his colon and rectum.

A film from the barium enema examination demonstrates a submucosal mass 2 cm in diameter that involves the left lateral wall of the rectum. The mass was excised and found to be a carcinoid tumor. (From Dodd G.D., Zornoza J., in Margulis A.R., Burhenne J.H. (eds.): *Colon Malignancies in Alimentary Tract Radiology.* St. Louis, C.V. Mosby Co., 1983, p. 1206. Reproduced with permission.)

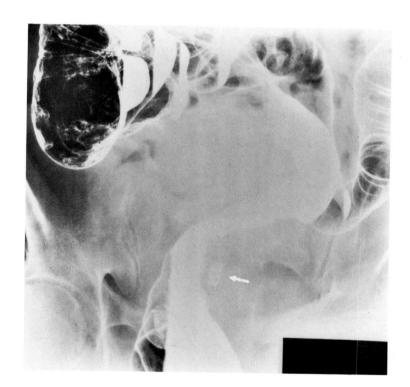

FIG 1–43.
Leiomyosarcoma of the rectosigmoid colon. This 52-year-old man presented with a six-month history of weight loss and with a palpable abdominal mass. A barium enema film reveals a large pelvic mass lifting the sigmoid, cecum, and small bowel out of the pelvis. Along the left lateral aspect of the rectosigmoid junction is an ulceration into the mass *(arrow)*. Percutaneous biopsy established the diagnosis of leiomyosarcoma. The tumor was excised, along with the involved rectosigmoid from which it arose.

A   B

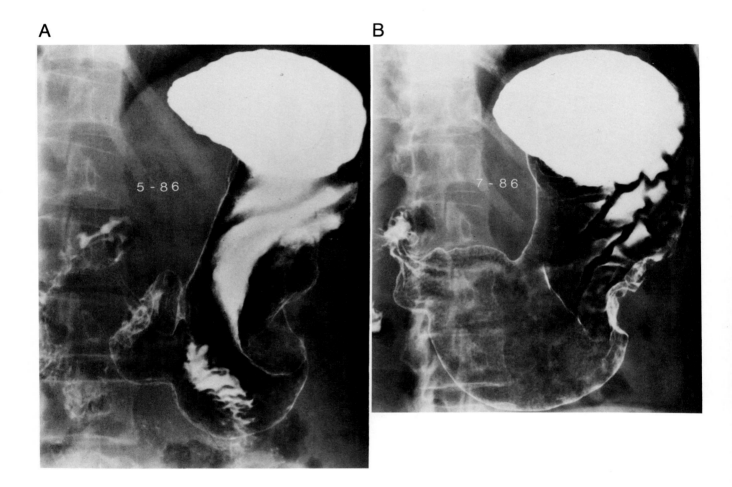

FIG 1–44.
Metastatic melanoma to the stomach. This 53-year-old woman presented with metastatic melanoma to several subcutaneous sites 22 years after resection of the primary skin lesion. She was noted to be anemic and reported a three-month history of vague epigastric discomfort.

A, a UGI film demonstrates a large intramural mass with a large central ulcer crater along the greater curvature of the stomach.

The remainder of the gastrointestinal tract was normal. Endoscopic biopsy proved metastatic melanoma.

B, as the patient responded to systemic chemotherapy two months later, the mass and the central ulceration became smaller.

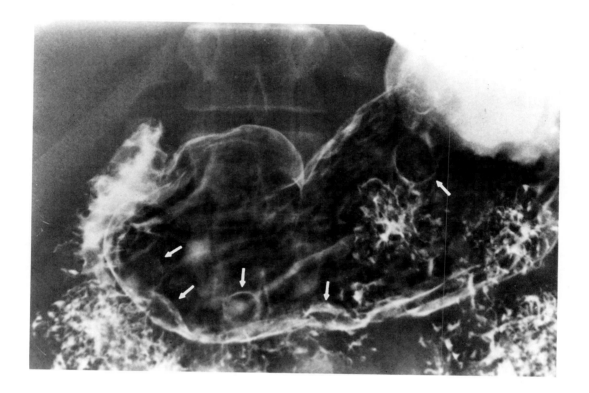

FIG 1–45.
Kaposi's sarcoma metastatic to the stomach. This 31-year-old homosexual man originally presented with malaise and scattered skin lesions, which proved to be Kaposi's sarcoma. Immunologic tests confirmed the diagnosis of acquired immunodeficiency syndrome. The patient had no gastrointestinal symptoms.

A UGI series was performed to look for occult metastases. The film shows multiple ulcerated submucosal nodules in the stomach *(arrows)*, entirely consistent with the diagnosis of metastatic Kaposi's sarcoma. Endoscopic biopsy provided histologic confirmation.

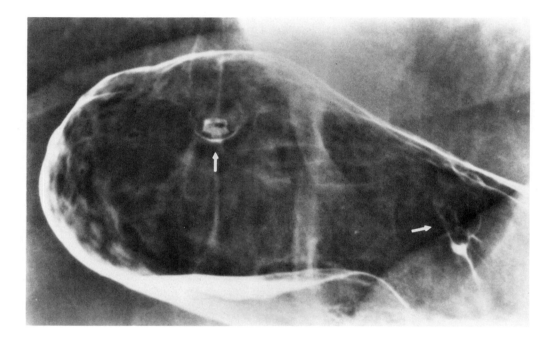

FIG 1–46.
Bronchogenic carcinoma metastatic to the stomach. This 62-year-old woman with adenocarcinoma of the lung metastatic to the mediastinum, right adrenal, and brain complained of nausea and vomiting.

A UGI film reveals two small, ulcerated nodules in the fundus of the stomach *(arrows).*

Endoscopic biopsy confirmed the radiologic impression of metastatic disease to the stomach. It is possible that these lesions were an incidental finding, unrelated to the patient's complaint of nausea and vomiting.

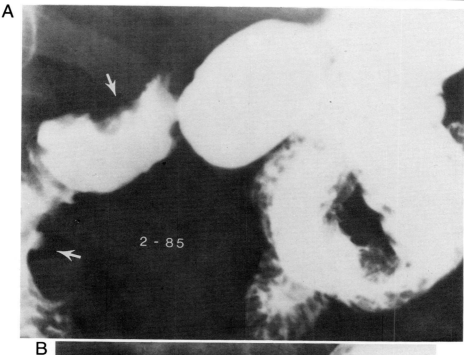

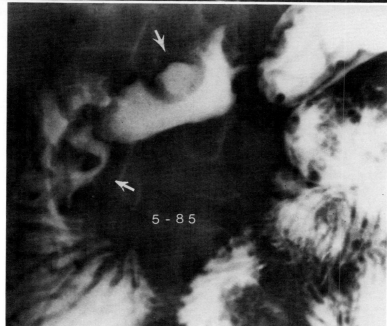

FIG 1–47.

Melanoma metastatic to the duodenum, with progression. This 41-year-old man had a melanoma of the right shoulder removed five years before he developed overt metastases. He was first found to have metastatic disease in his brain, and three months later he developed a complete obstruction of the small bowel due to tumor. The bowel lesion was excised two months prior to the UGI film in **A.**

A, this UGI film, performed when the patient was without symptoms, shows two submucosal ulcerated nodules involving the duodenum *(arrows).*

B, a follow-up UGI film three months later shows growth of the metastatic deposits, with larger areas of ulceration *(arrows).* The patient was still without symptoms but did have positive test results for occult blood in his stool.

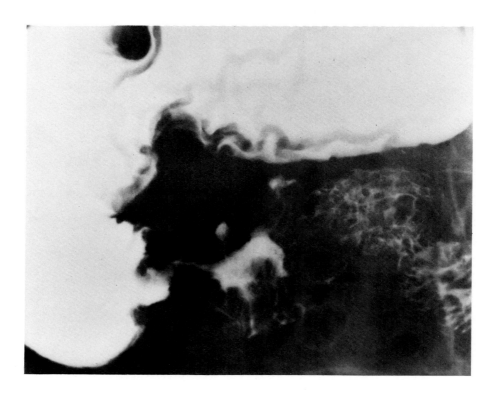

FIG 1–48.
Colon cancer metastatic to the root of the mesentery and duodenum. This 72-year-old woman had had a carcinoma of the cecum excised five years prior to the current evaluation. She had developed pulmonary metastases three years after her initial surgery; these metastatic lesions were very slowly progressive. The patient remained well for two years, until the rather acute onset of nausea and vomiting.

A UGI film reveals malignant obstruction of the third portion of the duodenum. At surgery, there was a large mass in the root of the mesentery, encircling the third portion of the duodenum. Biopsies confirmed metastatic colorectal carcinoma.

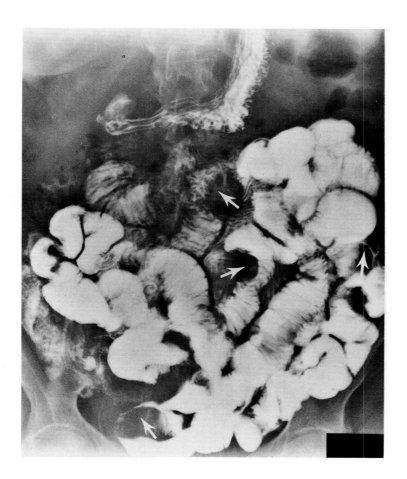

FIG 1–49.
Colon cancer metastatic to the small bowel. This 71-year-old woman with carcinoma of the transverse colon was noted to have peritoneal and mesenteric metastases at the time of primary tumor surgery.

Ten months later, a small bowel examination was performed because of nausea and vomiting. A film from this examination shows no evidence of obstruction, but multiple extramucosal mass impressions on the small bowel *(arrows)*, representing serosal metastases, can be appreciated.

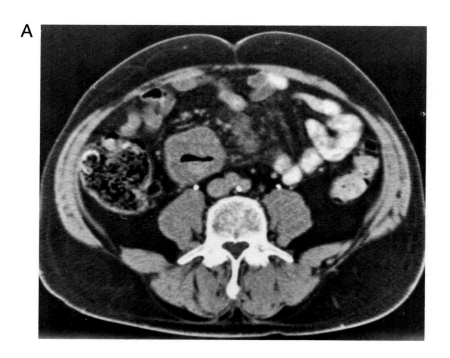

FIG 1–50.
Melanoma metastatic to the small bowel. This 66-year-old man had a two-year history of melanoma, which had first been seen in the neck. There was first a local recurrence and then pulmonary metastases, treated successfully with surgery and chemotherapy, respectively. Six months later, disease recurred again in the skin. The patient first reported no symptoms but on systems review admitted to mild epigastric discomfort.

A, a CT scan demonstrates diffuse thickening of the wall of an isolated loop of small bowel, as well as abnormal midline soft tissue in the adjacent mesentery.

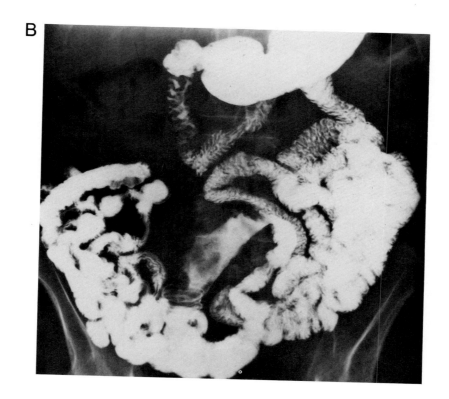

B, the small bowel examination confirms the presence of a solitary loop of encased and excavated small bowel corresponding to that seen on CT. No other lesions were seen.

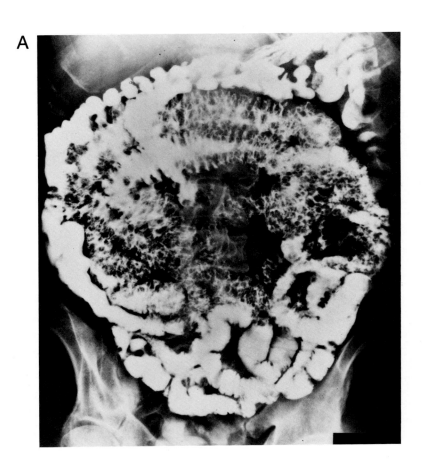

FIG 1–51.

Melanoma metastatic to the small bowel. This 56-year-old man was found to be anemic and hypoproteinemic during an admission for an acute inferior wall myocardial infarction. Upper gastrointestinal endoscopy disclosed multiple gastric and duodenal polyps, biopsy of which showed "undifferentiated neoplasm."

A and **B,** films from small bowel examination disclose multiple polypoid filling defects throughout the small bowel, with less involvement of the terminal ileum. The initial impression was lymphoma.

Repeat biopsy was read as "adenocarcinoma." The patient subsequently had a cardiac arrest and could not be resuscitated. Autopsy was performed. (**A** and **B** from ACR Multisystems Symposia Syllabus, 1986, pp. 49–50. Reproduced by permission.)

C, an autopsy segment of small bowel, studded with small polypoid masses, is seen (see also Color Plate 1).

Ultrastructural analysis of these "polyps" revealed multiple melanosomes, and the final pathologic diagnosis was metastatic melanoma. The patient's family subsequently related that he had had a "benign" growth removed from his back 18 months before.

B

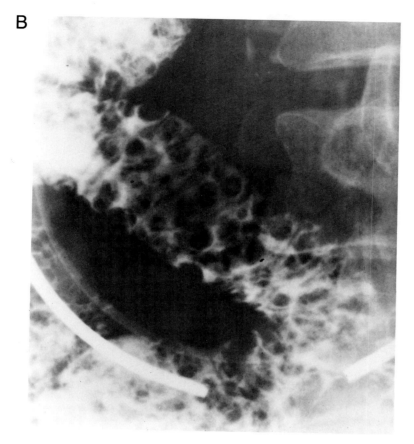

C

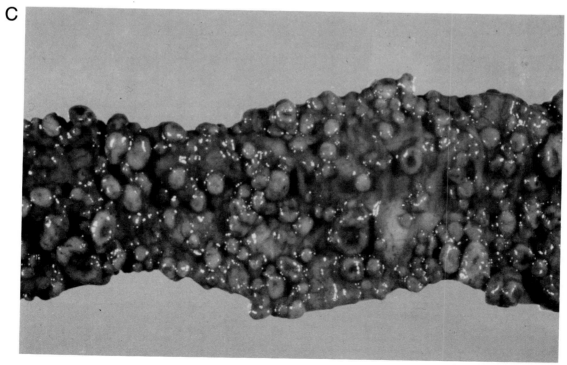

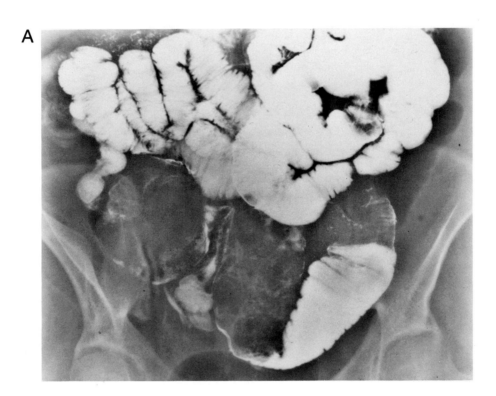

FIG 1–52.
Melanoma metastatic to the small bowel. This 45-year-old woman developed metastases to skin and lung eight months after wide excision of a malignant melanoma on her right forearm. In the course of her treatment, she developed a venous thrombosis of the left axillary vein, which was treated by anticoagulation. A week later, she developed bloody diarrhea. Colonoscopy revealed a 4- to 5-cm mass in the ascending colon, biopsies of which proved metastatic melanoma.

A, this film from a small bowel study reveals three very large intraluminal masses.

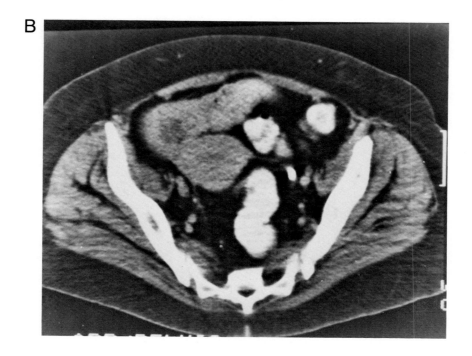

B, a CT scan demonstrates soft tissue expanding a loop of bowel.

The patient eventually required surgery to control the bleeding. All the masses were grossly intraluminal, with little growth into the bowel wall. Histologically, each metastasis was covered with normal mucosa, confirming submucosal origin.

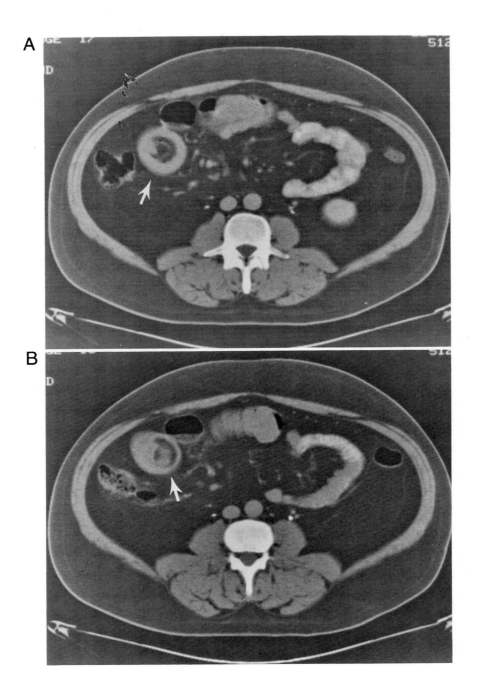

FIG 1–53.
Melanoma metastatic to the small bowel, with ileoileal intussusception. This 43-year-old man had a right leg melanoma metastatic to the right groin and to the lungs and brain. He had had some response to local and systemic therapy when he began to have diarrhea and gastrointestinal blood loss.

A and **B,** the CT scans demonstrate an enteroenteric intussusception in the right lower quadrant *(arrows).*

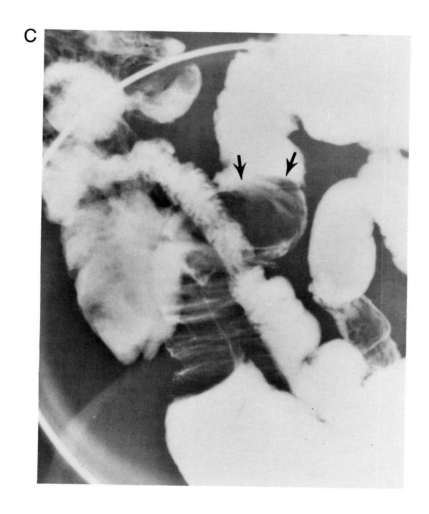

C, a spot film from a small bowel series confirms the intussusception in the distal ileum and demonstrates the lead point to be a 3-cm polypoid mass *(arrows).* Other findings compatible with hematogenous metastases to the bowel were seen as well.

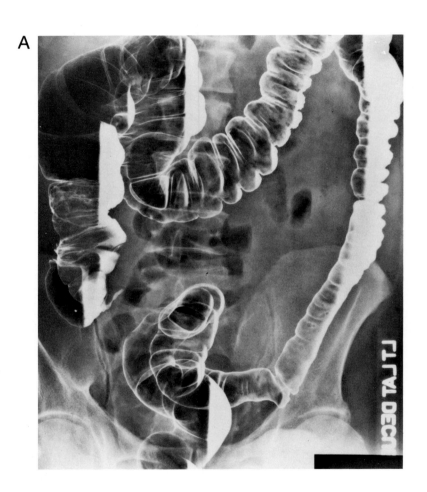

FIG 1–54.

Melanoma metastatic to the small bowel, with ileocolic intussusception. This 50-year-old man developed a subcutaneous metastasis on his back six years after having had extensive local surgery and neck dissection for a right facial melanoma. Workup at the time disclosed pulmonary and left adrenal metastases. The patient had vague abdominal pain, and a gastrointestinal evaluation was performed.

A, a barium enema film shows a large mass in the proximal ascending colon, compatible with ileocolic intussusception.

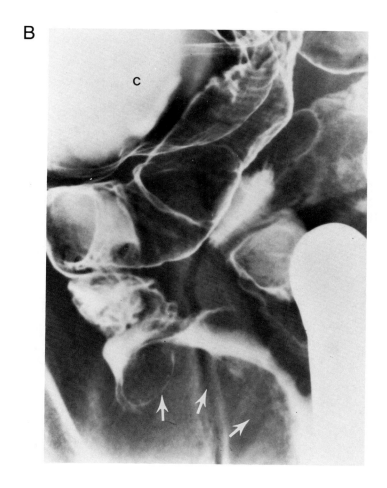

B, on a subsequent barium enema film, the intussusception has been reduced, and a large mass involving a segment of terminal ileum *(arrows)* approximately 25 cm proximal to the ileocecal valve is seen (**C,** cecum). This was undoubtedly the lead point for the original intussusception.

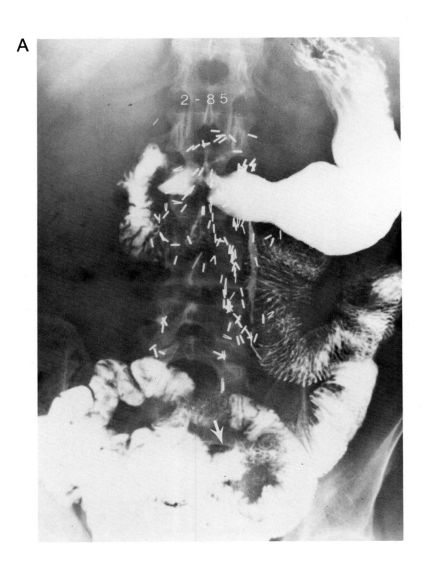

FIG 1–55.
Testicular tumor metastatic to the mesentery and small bowel.

    This 39-year-old man had had a left testicular tumor at the age of 27 treated with excision, radiation therapy, and lymph node dissection and a right testicular tumor at the age of 33 treated by excision alone. The pathology was embryonal cell tumor and teratoma on the left and embryonal cell tumor and seminoma on the right. At the age of 38, the patient had a cholecystectomy, at which time biopsy of a node revealed seminoma. Computed tomography confirmed paraaortic adenopathy, and chemotherapy was begun.

    A, because of abdominal pain, he had UGI and small bowel examination. An ulceration without significant mass effect is seen involving the proximal jejunum *(arrow).*

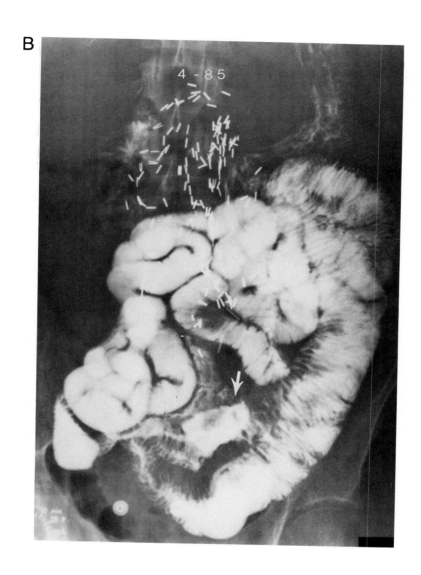

B, two months later, the ulceration is larger, and there is evidence of mass displacing other loops of bowel. *(Continued.)*

C

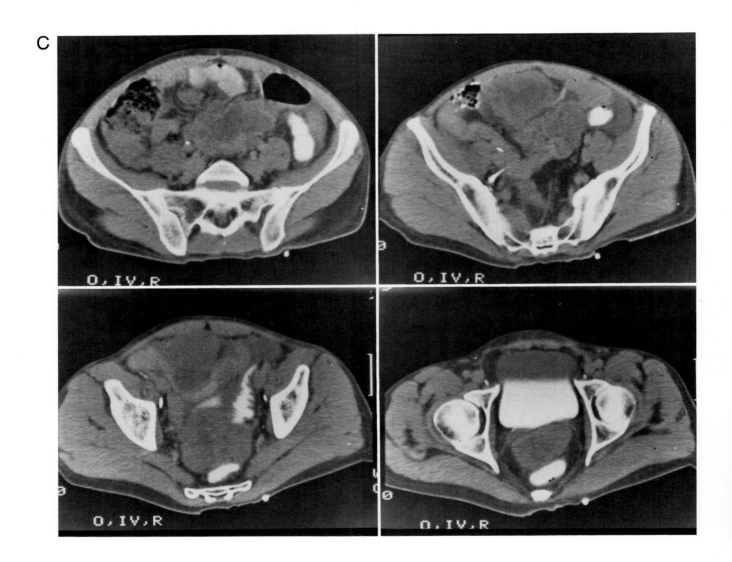

FIG 1–55 (cont.).
C, four images from a CT scan at this time reveal bulky tumor in the mesentery and in the pouch of Douglas.

The CT scan in this case demonstrates the extent of involvement to be much greater than would have been supposed from results of the small bowel series of the same date.

D

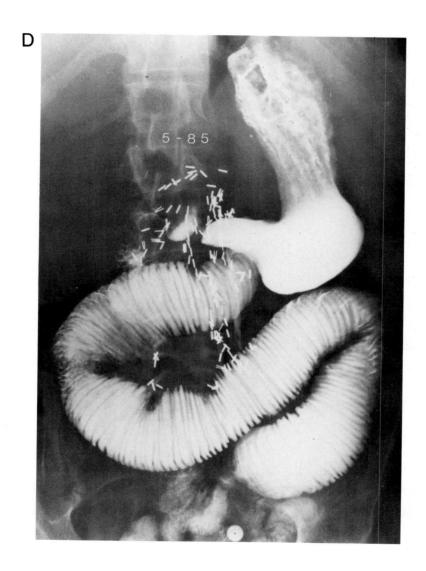

D, one month later, the patient developed a high-grade bowel obstruction at the site of prior ulceration.

Testicular tumors other than choriocarcinoma rarely metastasize hematogenously to the bowel but instead invade directly from contiguous areas of nodal involvement.[71]

A

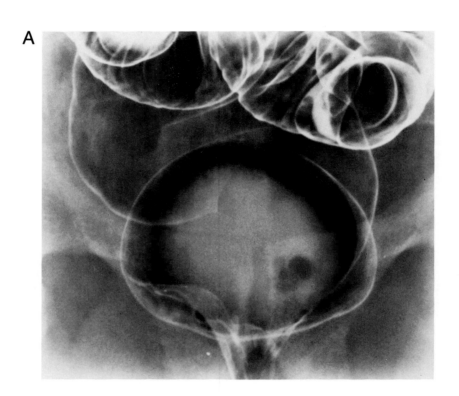

FIG 1–56.
Kaposi's sarcoma metastatic to the rectum. This 30-year-old homosexual man had a one-year history of swollen lymph nodes in his neck and groin and a recent development of skin lesions, which proved to be Kaposi's sarcoma. He had no gastrointestinal complaints.

A, a barium enema film reveals a submucosal mass along the right lateral wall of the rectum and a polypoid fill-ing defect anteriorly (patient is prone).

B, the CT scan confirms thickening of the right rectal wall. Proctoscopic biopsies of both lesions revealed Kapo-si's sarcoma.

C, this CT scan demonstrates bilateral enlarged pelvic nodes, often seen in patients with acquired immunodefi-ciency syndrome, not always representing metastases.

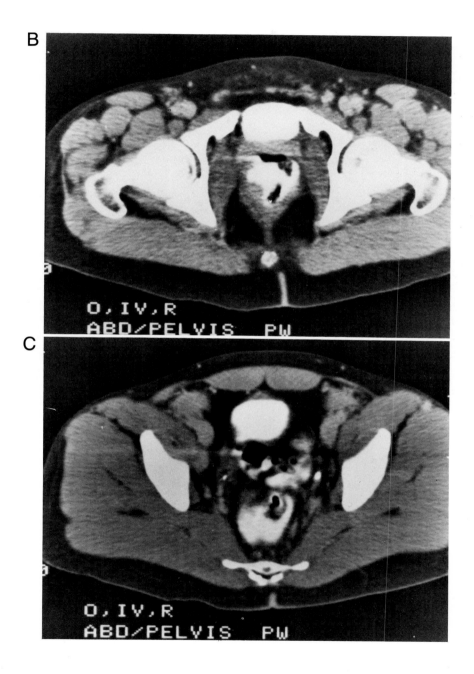

A

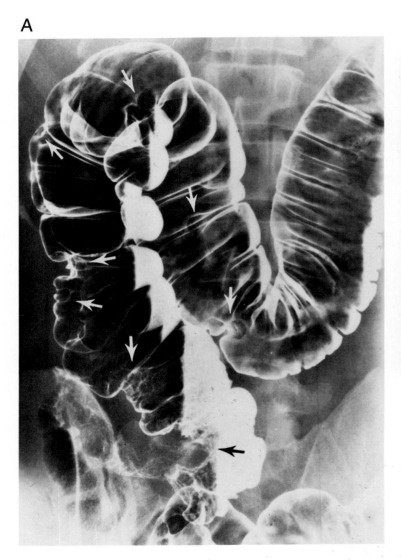

B

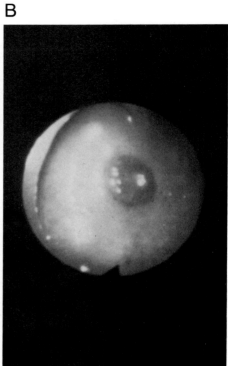

FIG 1–57.
Kaposi's sarcoma metastatic to the large bowel. This 31-year-old homosexual man with Kaposi's sarcoma related to acquired immunodeficiency syndrome had a barium enema examination as part of a routine evaluation.

A, the enema film reveals multiple irregular masses *(ar-* *rows)* scattered throughout the colon, compatible with Kaposi's sarcoma metastatic to the large bowel. His stomach was also involved (see Fig 1–45).

B, an endoscopic photograph shows one of the ulcerated submucosal metastases in the rectum (see also Color Plate 2).

A

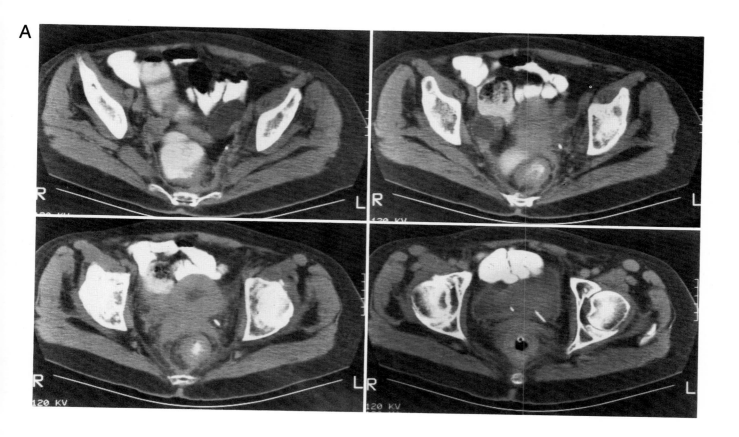

FIG 1–58.
Breast cancer metastatic to the rectum. This 63-year-old woman had a six-year history of metastatic carcinoma, presumed to represent a breast primary. She originally presented with a left axillary node that showed estrogen receptor–positive carcinoma; a breast lesion could not be found.

She had bone metastases at presentation and later developed liver metastases.

Five years later, she developed circumferential narrowing of the rectum, seen on both CT **(A)** barium enema **(B)** **(B,** see following page). *(Continued.)*

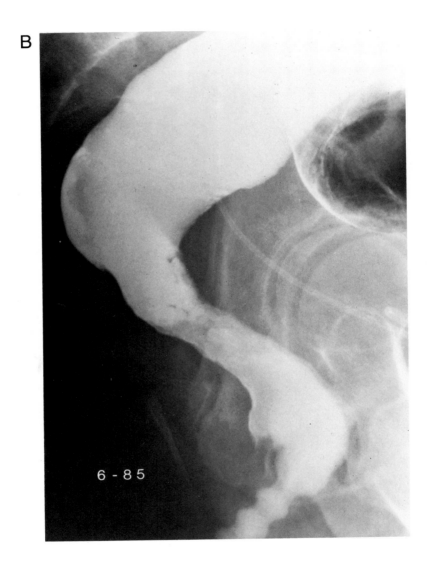

FIG 1–58 (cont.).
Proctoscopic biopsies revealed metastatic carcinoma. Ten months later, the relatively smooth rectal narrowing has markedly progressed **(C).**

C

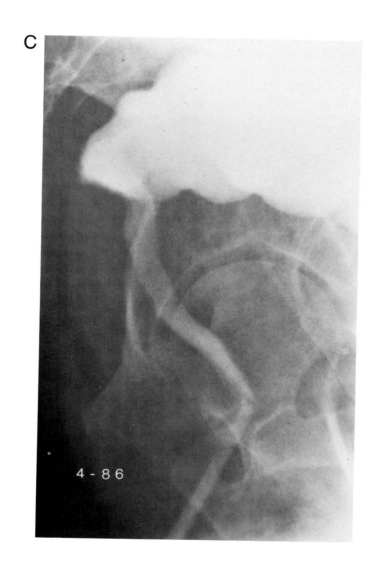

4 - 86

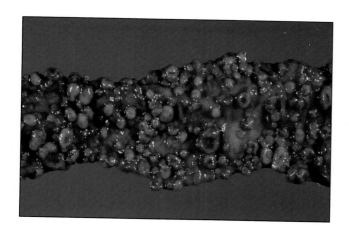

PLATE 1

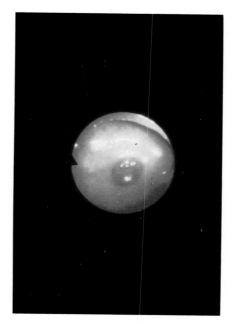

PLATE 2

2

Pancreatic Neoplasms

Ali Shirkhoda, M.D.

ANATOMICAL CONSIDERATIONS AND DIAGNOSTIC APPROACH

The development of increasingly sophisticated diagnostic technology over the past decade has significantly altered our understanding of the pancreas. Radiologic modalities, more specifically, computed tomography (CT) and ultrasonography, have emerged as a keystone in the diagnostic evaluation of this gland.[1–3]

The pancreas is a U-shaped, horizontal gland that is retroperitoneal but predominantly anterior to the midcoronal plane of the body. The entire gland is within the anterior pararenal space, along with such structures as the ascending and descending colon and duodenum and the major peripancreatic arteries and veins. The pancreas has an intimate relationship with the stomach and duodenum, and its body is separated from the gastric antrum by the omental bursa. It is bounded posteriorly by the anterior renal fascia and anteriorly by the posterior parietal peritoneum. It is outlined anteriorly-superiorly by the lesser sac and posteriorly-inferiorly by the reflection of the main peritoneal cavity forming the transverse mesocolon.

The size of the normal gland varies, mostly related to the patient's age. A large pancreas, which may be considered normal in a young adult patient, could represent pancreatitis or diffuse carcinoma in an older individual. Likewise, a small pancreas is considered normal in an elderly patient but may reflect atrophy in a younger one.[4] The pancreas typically tapers from its head to its tail, with the maximum respective widths of head, body, and tail being 3, 2.5, and 2 cm.[5] The normal main pancreatic duct is approximately 3 mm wide in the gland's head and up to 2 mm wide in the body and tail.[6]

Because there is no pancreatic capsule, ultrasound cannot define the margins of the gland as it does in the liver and kidney. Therefore, ultrasonic localization of the pancreas depends on identification of the major vascular landmarks[7] that lie in close proximity to the gland (aorta and vena cava, splenic and portal veins, and superior mesenteric, splenic, and hepatic arteries). Occasionally, a water-filled stomach and semierect position will help in identifying the gland.[8] In patients with suspected pancreatic disease who undergo sonographic evaluation, one should look for the size and configuration of the pancreas, presence of a focal mass or changes in the parenchymal texture, the caliber of the pancreatic duct, and the appearance of the biliary system and the hepatic parenchyma. Hessel et al. found ultrasound to have a sensitivity of 69% and a specificity of 82% for the detection of pancreatic abnormality.[3] The major causes of suboptimal evaluations are interference from intestinal gas, presence of ascites, and obesity.[4] Administration of metoclopramide HCl has been advocated to overcome the gas in the stomach and duodenum.[9]

Computed tomography is the initial diagnostic procedure of choice in patients with suspected pancreatic abnormality.[3] A study done at M. D. Anderson Hospital found the overall accuracy in detecting pancreatic carcinoma to be 96% for CT and 84% for ultrasound. However, after nondiagnostic studies were included, CT accuracy fell only 1%, to 95%, but ultrasound accuracy fell to 54%.[10] Although usually the pancreas is easily seen and well defined on CT, occasionally it may be quite difficult to identify the gland with this modality. Adequate orally administered contrast material, bolus intravenous contrast, and thin slices (usually 5-mm collimation without interval gaps) are keys in examining the gland. Inadequate visualization of the pancreas, a problem faced more often with older or cachectic patients, may be solved by recognizing the major pancreatic vascular landmarks, particularly the superior mesenteric artery and vein and the splenic and portal veins.[7] By use of a 5-mm collimation, the pancreatic duct may be seen in up to 70% of patients.

Endoscopic retrograde cholangiopancreatography (ERCP), which has an accuracy rate of nearly 95%,[11,12] can image the first recognizable changes of pancreatic adenocarcinoma. However, after the introduction of CT and ultrasound, the role of this diagnostic modality changed, and its primary indications are now (1) further investigation of a case in which there is strong suspicion of pancreatic disease but there is a normal, equivocal, or technically unsatisfactory computed tomogram or sonogram; (2) precise diagnosis of an isolated pancreatic mass demonstrated by CT or sonogram; and (3) guidance for percutaneously directed biopsy of pancreas or for cytologic examination of aspirated pancreatic juice.[13]

Classifications to be considered in the evaluation of the pancreas for neoplastic involvement are shown in Table 2–1.[14–16]

EXOCRINE MALIGNANT AND BENIGN NEOPLASMS

Cancer of the pancreas has increased 300% in incidence during the last 40 years, and the current 9.7 cases per 100,000 population account for 10% of all digestive organ cancers.[17] The mean five-year survival of patients with pancreatic carcinoma is 1% to 2% with a mean survival time of four months from the time of diagnosis.[16, 18–21] The tumor is fourth among cancers causing death in men and is fifth most common in women.[22, 23] At the time of diagnosis, in fact, approximately 90% of the patients

TABLE 2–1.

Classification of Neoplasms of the Pancreas*

Exocrine
  Malignant
    Ductal adenocarcinoma (including mucin-producing adenocarcinoma, adenosquamous carcinoma, and sarcomatoid carcinoma), acinar lesions, pancreaticoblastoma
  Benign
    Microcystic adenoma, mucinous cystic neoplasms, solid and papillary epithelial neoplasms
Endocrine
  Insulinoma, gastrinoma, glucagonoma, vipoma, somatostatinoma, carcinoid, tumors producing other hormones, multiple endocrine neoplasia
Rare
  Pancreatic lymphoma, pancreatic sarcoma, metastasis to pancreas, pancreatic hemangioma, pancreatic lymphangioma, lipomatous hypertrophy of the pancreas

*Adapted from Walker[14] and Cubilla and Fitzgerald.[15]

have incurable disease.[24] Surgery is the only hope of cure, but only 8% to 18% of patients with pancreatic carcinoma have lesions in which en bloc resection is potentially curative.[25–27] The "curative" surgery increases the mean survival time to approximately one year, but almost all patients will be dead two years postoperatively.[16, 26, 27]

Ductal adenocarcinoma, which accounts for approximately 75% to 90% of all pancreatic neoplasms, can be divided into three histologic subtypes.[21] The typical mucin-producing adenocarcinoma accounts for 85% of cases, whereas adenosquamous carcinoma and sarcomatoid cystadenocarcinoma each account for less than 5% of ductal adenocarcinomas.[15]

Pancreatic adenocarcinoma (Figs 2–1 to 2–13) occurs in the head of the gland in most patients, and the body is more often involved than the tail. In the Memorial Sloan-Kettering series, cancer originated in the pancreatic head in 61% of patients (Figs 2–2 to 2–9), in the body in 13% (Fig 2–10), and in the tail in 5% (Fig 2–13). The remaining 21% of patients had tumor at multiple sites within the gland (Figs 2–11 and 2–12).[28]

The cystic neoplasms are uncommon, slow-growing tumors that can effectively be treated by excision (Figs 2–14 to 2–17). The two types of cystic tumor are malignant mucinous cystic tumor (cystadenocarcinoma), which accounts for 1% to 2% of malignant lesions, and benign microcystic adenoma (glycogen-rich cystadenoma). Cystadenocarcinoma is commonly seen in middle-aged women, usually occurring in the body and tail of the pancreas (Fig 2–15). The tumor is typically encapsulated and large, measuring up to 10 cm, and sometimes has a calcified wall. Because of thin septa, it can simulate a pseudocyst. The microcystic adenomas, which account for 10% of benign cystic pancreatic lesions, are large and occur predominantly in women.[29] They are characterized by lobulation, a thick fibrous capsule, and an internal architecture that consists of numerous cysts of varying sizes.[28] They should also be differentiated from pancreatic pseudocyst (Figs 2–16 and 2–17) and necrotic adenocarcinoma.

Initial symptoms in carcinoma of the pancreas frequently are vague and do not suggest a specific etiology. Pain is the most common symptom, followed by weight loss, mild indigestion, steatorrhea secondary to pancreatitis, and, occasionally, diabetes mellitus.[30–34] Usually, carcinoma of the pancreatic head is symptomatic early on because of invasion of the duodenum or common bile duct. Direct spread of tumor, especially in the early stages, is common since there is no pancreatic capsule. Distant metastases occur, in order of decreasing frequency, in the liver, regional nodes, peritoneum, and lungs.[35]

Conventional radiology has little to offer in the diagnosis of pancreatic carcinoma and generally is limited to barium study of the upper gastrointestinal tract. On plain films, one occasionally might see ascites, a distended gallbladder, or, rarely, metastases to bone or lung.[13] On barium examination, the large tumors in the body and tail of the pancreas may cause extensive mass effect on the posterior gastric wall,[36] with occasional invasion of the stomach.[37] Invasion of the splenic vein is not uncommon and can produce collaterals and varices in and around the gastric wall. Carcinoma of the head of the pancreas may be detectable in about 25% of patients by using conventional barium study of the duodenum.[38] The changes include extrinsic pressure, encasement or mucosal invasion, and occasional barium reflux into the pancreatic or biliary duct.[7] Because of the intimate relationship of the pancreas and the colon by way of the transverse mesocolon and the phrenicocolic ligament, tumors in the body of the pancreas may spread directly to the transverse mesocolon and colon and be reflected in abnormal changes on barium enema examination. Occasionally ascites, which is often due to peritoneal carcinomatosis, causes displacement of the bowel.

Ultrasound evaluation of the pancreas has a relatively high rate of failure, varying according to the equipment, the expertise of the sonographer, and the patient's anatomy. However, its advantages of wide availability, variable scanning planes, and the ability to evaluate the biliary tract for evidence of obstruction make it uniquely useful for initial evaluation of patients with nonspecific abdominal symptoms or jaundice of unknown etiology. During pancreatic sonography, one should evaluate the size of the pancreas and search for the presence of a mass, dilated pancreatic or biliary ducts, ascites, splenic enlargement, and metastases to the liver and regional nodes.[1, 39] The pancreatic carcinomas are usually hypoechoic, and very infrequently they may generate a few echoes or be frankly echogenic.[40] The pancreatic duct can be identified in 60% to 84% of normal subjects and in 60% to 97% of patients with carcinoma.[41, 42] Normally, it should not exceed a 2-mm width in the body of the pancreas.[41] Occasionally, ductal dilatation is the only manifestation of carcinoma in the pancreatic head; the finding of such dilatation associated with a dilated common bile duct is referred to as the *double-barrel sign*.

Computed tomography is the primary diagnostic modality for evaluation of the pancreas. Many believe that all patients suspected of having pancreatic carcinoma, whether they are jaundiced or not, must be evaluated by CT. On CT scan, the carcinoma is seen as either enlargement of the gland, distortion of its contour, alteration of its density, or evidence of tumor invasion into such adjacent structures as the gastrointestinal tract, spleen, kidneys, adrenals, blood vessels, and common bile duct. In the early stages of tumor, the pancreatic mass may be poorly defined, and there may be only an apparent thickening of the celiac axis, the superior mesenteric artery, or both of these structures (Fig 2–1).[43] The density of the tumor is either equal to or less than that of the pancreas. However, by the use of intravenous contrast, there will be enhancement of the normal pancreas and better visualization of the tumor (Fig 2–13,B). Also, since splenic vein obstruction by direct tumor invasion is a frequent finding in carcinoma of the body and tail, CT with bolus intravenous contrast will illustrate enhancing collaterals involving the short gastric or left gastric veins. These pathways may result in extensive varices in the stomach.[44, 45]

Cancer of the pancreas usually does not calcify; however, carcinoma can occur in a previously calcified gland. Pancreatic calcifications per se are indicative of benign disease in more than 95% of cases. A pattern of tumoral calcification has been described in about 10% of cystic neoplasms of the pancreas. Because of the rich vascular and lymphatic supply of the gland and lack of a capsule, regional metastases may occur early within the peripancreatic nodes. These enlarged nodes may become inseparable from the primary pancreatic carcinoma.

In a study of 141 cases of pancreatic lesions, Luning et al. advocate that the diagnosis in suspected cases of pancreatic lesions should begin with CT and be followed by CT-guided fine-needle aspiration biopsy.[46]

Magnetic resonance imaging (MRI) has been used for the diagnosis of pancreatic carcinoma and for its differentiation from pancreatitis.[47] However, it has not yet replaced CT in the evaluation of the pancreas. In a recent study, normal and abnormal pancreases were compared using MRI. The T_1 and T_2 relaxation times and MR signal intensities showed no specific pattern to allow consistent differentiation between normal and diseased pancreatic tissue or to distinguish between tumor and inflammation.[48, 80] Details of this newer modality are discussed in Chapter 12.

ENDOCRINE NEOPLASMS OF THE PANCREAS

The islet cell tumors of the pancreas are either hormonally active or inactive and are either malignant or benign. Those that are hormonally active are often small at the time of clinical presentation and are frequently diagnosed by angiography. However, CT remains the initial radiologic approach in the evaluation because it is noninvasive and can detect approximately one third of both primary tumors and hepatic metastases. Also, because the islet cell tumors can occur as part of the multiple endocrine neoplasia (MEN) syndrome, the abdominal CT should include examination of the adrenals. Bilateral enlarged adrenal glands may be seen in those cases in which the islet cell tumor is producing adrenocorticotropic hormone.[13, 50]

The islet cell tumors of the pancreas are generally called *apudomas*.[51] The normal amine-precursor uptake and decarboxylation (APUD) cells found in the pancreatic islets include the beta (or B) cells, which produce insulin; alpha (or A) cells, which produce glucagon; G cells, which produce gastrin; D cells, which produce somatostatin; pp cells, which make pancreatic polypeptide; and D cells, which produce vasoactive intestinal polypeptide (VIP). The commonly seen islet cell tumors are insulinoma, glucagonoma, gastrinoma, and vipoma. Somatostatinoma is the rarest type of apudoma.

Insulinomas are islet cell tumors arising from the B cells of the pancreas and can be seen alone or as part of MEN syndrome.[52, 53] They are the common-

est type of islet cell tumors, occurring in all ages and with even distribution throughout different parts of the pancreas. Nearly 90% of these tumors are benign, but about 10% can be malignant.[54] However, 80% of those that are malignant are functional, hormone-producing tumors. Association of insulinoma with MEN syndrome is in the range of 5% to 10%. Diagnosis of these cases is generally based on the high level of serum insulin and on angiography, which has an accuracy of more than 90%.[55] On CT, the tumor is seen to have either the same density as the normal pancreas or it is denser; rarely, it may be of lesser density (Fig 2–22). It typically causes little or no distortion of the pancreas. In most cases, it shows a greater degree of contrast enhancement than does the remainder of the pancreas on dynamic CT images.[56] In those cases in which the tumor is inactive, the patients present with abdominal mass (Fig 2–18), which can be associated with biliary obstruction.

Glucagonoma arises from the A cells of the islets of Langerhans and secretes glucagon, which is a polypeptide maintaining hepatic glucose production. These tumors may exhibit features of benign adenoma or may have histologic characteristics of carcinoma. The malignant lesions appear to be more common in this type of apudoma.[57] Patients, who are predominantly women, present with skin lesions, anemia, weight loss, and symptoms of diabetes (Fig 2–19). These symptoms may be present for many years before the discovery of tumor. Because most of these tumors are malignant in character and because the liver is the primary target for metastatic disease, the liver should be thoroughly investigated during CT evaluation of the pancreas.[58] Treatment is usually surgical removal of the primary tumor.

Gastrinoma originates in one of the nonbeta islet cells (G cells) of the pancreas and was originally described by Zollinger and Ellison in 1955.[59] In patients with Zollinger-Ellison syndrome, there is overwhelming peptic ulcer disease in nearly 75% of cases, gastric hypersecretion, and pancreatic neoplasm. The gastrin can be produced by both the primary pancreatic neoplasms and their metastases. The gastrinoma can also arise from the G cells of the stomach or the duodenum and be presented as hyperplasia or as a neoplasm.[53] The gastrinomas are seen as solitary tumor in about 50% of cases but are multiple in 30% and are seen as microadenomatosis throughout the pancreas in about 20%.[60] Nearly 60% of the tumors are malignant. The microscopic appearances of malignant and benign gastrinomas may be similar, and the only certain way to establish malignancy is the demonstration of metastases.[61] Upper gastrointestinal study generally shows the ulcer in nearly 75% of patients, and angiography helps to demonstrate the hypervascular tumor in about 30% to 50%.[61] Depending on the size of the neoplasm, CT may help show the primary tumor[62] and any metastases to regional lymph nodes or to the liver. Treatment is gastrectomy; if this radical surgery is not done, there is nearly a 50% incidence of recurrent ulcer. Gastrinoma like insulinoma can be a part of MEN type I (Wermer's) syndrome. In fact, the islet cell tumor in this syndrome usually produces gastrin rather than insulin, and the release of gastrin is significantly stimulated by the hyperplastic parathyroid glands.[63] Hypergastrinemia in this syndrome is usually related to hyperplasia or multiple adenomas of the islet cell tissue. Multiple endocrine neoplasia type I syndrome is present in 20% to 30% of patients with Zollinger-Ellison syndrome. Extrapancreatic islet cell adenomas in the wall of the stomach or small bowel are common.[62] Also, the primary tumor has been seen to arise in lymph nodes outside the pancreas.

The vipomas are tumors that originate in one of the nonbeta islet cells (D_1 cells); patients present with profuse watery diarrhea, hypokalemia, and achlorhydria. This symptom complex is often referred to as *pancreatic cholera syndrome*.[64] Patients usually have symptoms for months or even years before the diagnosis is established. The tumor is in the body and tail of the pancreas in about 80% of patients (Fig 2–20); it is benign in about 43%, is malignant in about 37%, and presents as diffuse hyperplasia in about 20%.[53, 64, 65] Angiographically, a vascular lesion with large feeding vessels and dense capillary stain is present.[66] In larger tumors, the mass is easily diagnosable by CT. The high VIP levels in the plasma may also be assessed by radioimmunoassay.[67]

Multiple Endocrine Neoplasia Syndrome

Wermer's syndrome (MEN type I) is an inherited disorder associated with the autonomous release of excessive hormone from multiple neoplastic or hyperplastic sites. These sites include the famous three Ps: parathyroid, pancreas, and anterior pituitary gland (Figs 2–21 and 2–22). Abnormalities may be present in the adrenal cortex or in the thyroid gland.[68] Occasionally, patients have a carcinoid tumor in the gastrointestinal tract. Ballard et al. reviewed 85 cases of MEN type I syndrome and reported the prevalence of endocrine involvement to be parathyroid, 88%; pancreatic islet cells, 81%; an-

terior pituitary, 65%; adrenal cortex, 38%; and thyroid, 19%.[69] It has been reported that gastrinoma and insulinoma are the two most common islet cell tumors.[70] In some instances, the islet cell elaborates both gastrin and insulin, or it secretes a variety of polypeptides (VIP, glucagon, etc.).[71,81,82] The clinical manifestations of an islet cell abnormality frequently do not arise until five to ten years after the patient exhibits evidence of hyperparathyroidism.[70]

Islet cell tumors, particularly those that are malignant, may calcify,[83] in which case they are seen on the plain film. However, angiography and CT are most commonly used for their diagnosis. The tumors are usually hypervascular and occasionally associated with venous occlusion. They can extend into the splenic or portal vein and be associated with gastric varices.[84] In one report, abdominal CT was able to detect about 70% of the islet cell tumors subsequently documented at laparotomy.[85] On CT, the tumor is seen typically as a mass, sometimes as an irregularity of pancreatic contour or an area of low density, and rarely as a small cyst.[49] Magnetic resonance imaging may be able to demonstrate an islet cell tumor on the basis of tissue characterization.[86]

RARE PANCREATIC TUMORS

The pancreas can be infiltrated by lymphoma (Fig 2–23) or leukemia (Fig 2–24), the involvement manifested by a diffusely enlarged organ. Usually, however, the peripancreatic nodes are involved, and the findings may be indistinguishable from those in primary pancreatic carcinoma.[50] In approximately 35% of cases, the pancreas is discovered to be infiltrated by lymphoma at autopsy, mostly from adjacent nodes.[73] In Burkitt's lymphoma, the pancreas can be involved in up to 82% of cases; when there is diffuse infiltration, the disease can simulate pancreatitis.[74] On sonogram, the enlarged peripancreatic nodes are seen as focal hypoechoic pancreatic enlargement, and CT will show a locally or diffusely enlarged pancreas.[75] Neither of these features can be distinguished from primary pancreatic abnormality.[72]

Primary sarcoma of the pancreas (Figs 2–25 and 2–26) is extremely rare,[76] but metastatic sarcoma to the pancreas (Fig 2–27) is not unusual.[77, 78] These tumors cannot be distinguished from a primary neoplasm of the pancreas, and tissue should be obtained. However, their favorable response during treatment of the primary tumor will favor a diagnosis of metastasis.

Metastasis to the pancreas is not uncommon (Figs 2–28 and 2–29); in one series, 3% of 500 cancer autopsies demonstrated pancreatic metastases.[79] The primary tumor may be of the lung, breast, kidney, or gastrointestinal tract, or it may be melanoma.[77,78] The incidence of metastatic melanoma to the pancreas has been reported to be as high as 37.5%.[80] Metastases to the pancreas can be seen on CT as a single pancreatic mass or as multiple pancreatic masses.[77] In the latter, the entire pancreas is diffusely studded with discrete metastatic nodules (see Fig 4–30). When metastasis involves the head of the pancreas, the patient may present with jaundice. Presumably, the metastases are deposited in the pancreas by a hematogenous route. The intrapancreatic location of the lesions, as evidenced by biliary and pancreatic ductal obstruction, supports this assumption.[77] Because metastatic deposits in the pancreas are commonly of small size, and organ-related symptoms are infrequent, ultrasound can be very helpful in illustrating these lesions.[78] However, since there is no bulging of the contour of the pancreas in these cases, dynamic CT with bolus contrast injection may be very helpful in identifying the intrapancreatic lesion.[56] By catheterization of the proper feeding arteries, the pancreatic metastases can be treated by intraarterial chemotherapy.

REFERENCES

1. Lee J.K.T., Stanley R.J., Melson G.L., et al.: Pancreatic imaging by ultrasound and computed tomography: a general review. *Radiol. Clin. North Am.* 16:105–117, 1979.
2. Simeone J.E., Wittenberg J., Ferrucci J.R. Jr.: Modern concepts of imaging of the pancreas. *Invest. Radiol.* 15:6–18, 1980.
3. Hessel S.J., Siegelman S.S., McNeil B.J., et al.: A prospective evaluation of computed tomography and ultrasound of the pancreas. *Radiology* 143:129–133, 1982.
4. Donovan P.J.: Technique of examination and normal pancreatic anatomy, in Siegelman S.S. (ed.): *Computed Tomography of the Pancreas.* New York, Churchill Livingstone, 1983, pp. 1–32.
5. Kreel L., Haertel M., Katz D.: Computed tomography of the normal pancreas. *J. Comput. Assist. Tomogr.* 1:290–299, 1977.
6. Hadidi A.: Pancreatic duct diameter: sonographic measurement in normal subjects. *Journal of Clinical Ultrasound* 11:17–22, 1983.
7. Freeny P.C., Lawson T.L.: *Radiology of the Pancreas.* New York, Springer-Verlag New York, 1982, pp. 26–50.
8. Clark L.R., Jaffe M.H., Choyke P.L., et al.: Pancreatic imaging. *Radiol. Clin. North Am.* 23:489–501, 1985.
9. DuCret R.P., Jackson V.P., Rees C., et al.: Pancreatic sonography: enhancement by metoclopramide. *AJR* 146:341–343, 1986.
10. Kamin P.D., Bernardino M.E., Wallace S., et al.: Comparison of ultrasound and computed tomography in the detection of pancreatic malignancy. *Cancer* 46:2410–2412, 1980.
11. Ralls P.W., Halls J., Renner I., et al.: Endoscopic retrograde cholangiopancreatography of ductal abnormalities in differentiating benign from malignant disease. *Radiology* 134:347–352, 1980.
12. Reuben A., Cotton P.B.: Endoscopic retrograde cholangiopancreatography in carcinoma of the pancreas. *Surg. Gynecol. Obstet.* 148:179–184, 1979.
13. Lawson T.L., Berland L.L., Foley W.D.: Malignant neoplasms of the pancreas, liver, and biliary tract, in Bragg D.G., Rubin P., Youker J.K. (eds.): *Oncologic Imaging.* New York, Pergamon Press, 1985, pp. 282–342.
14. Walker P.D.: Pancreas, in Karcioglu Z.A., Someren A. (eds.): *Practical Surgical Pathology.* Lexington, Mass., Collamore Press, 1985, pp. 309–338.
15. Cubilla A.L., and Fitzgerald P.J.: Surgical pathology of tumors of the exocrine pancreas, in Moossa A.R. (ed.): *Tumors of the Pancreas.* Baltimore, Williams & Wilkins Co., 1980, pp. 159–193.
16. Cubilla A.L., Fitzgerald P.J.: Pancreas cancer: I. Duct adenocarcinoma: a clinical-pathologic study of 380 patients. *Pathol. Annu.* 13:241–289, 1978.
17. Malagelada J.R.: Pancreatic cancer: an overview of epidemiology, clinical presentation and diagnosis. *Mayo Clin. Proc.* 54:459–467, 1979.
18. Krain L.S.: The rising incidence of carcinoma of the pancreas: real or apparent? *J. Surg. Oncol.* 2:115–124, 1970.
19. Krain L.S.: The rising incidence of cancer of the pancreas: further epidemiologic studies. *J. Chronic Dis.* 23:685–690, 1971.
20. Charity Hospital Tumor Registry: *Charity Hospital Tumor Registry 1948-1975: Report.* New Orleans, Charity Hospital of Louisiana at New Orleans, 1979.
21. Cubilla A.L., Fitzgerald P.J.: Cancer of the pancreas (nonendocrine): a suggested morphologic classification. *Semin. Oncol.* 6:285–297, 1979.
22. Hermann R.E., Cooperman A.M.: Current concepts in cancer: cancer of the pancreas. *N. Engl. J. Med.* 301:482–485, 1979.
23. Berg J.W., Connelly R.R.: Updating the epidemiologic data on pancreatic cancer. *Semin. Oncol.* 6:275–284, 1979.
24. Moossa A.R.: Pancreatic cancer: approach to diagnosis, selection for surgery and choice of operation. *Cancer* 50:2689–2698, 1982.
25. Edis A.J., Kiernan P.D., Taylor W.F.: Attempted curative resection of ductal carcinoma of the pancreas: review of Mayo Clinic experience, 1951–1975. *Mayo Clin. Proc.* 55:531–536, 1980.

26. Jain K.M., Brief D.K., Nozick J.: Carcinoma of the pancreas: fifteen years' experience. *Am. Surg.* 45:15–20, 1979.

27. Sato T., Saitoh Y., Noto N., et al.: Factors influencing the late results of operating for carcinoma of the pancreas. *Am. J. Surg.* 136:582–586, 1978.

28. Fitzgerald P.J.: Pathology (nonendocrine), in Cohn I., Hastings P.R. (eds.): *Pancreatic Cancer.* UICC Technical Report Series. Geneva, International Union Against Cancer, 1981, pp. 13–30.

29. Parienty R.A., Ducellier R., Lubrano J.M., et al.: Cystadenomas of the pancreas: diagnosis by computed tomography. *J. Comput. Assist. Tomogr.* 4:364–367, 1980.

30. Macchia B., Bobruff J., Grissier V.W.: Positional relief of pain: important clue to clinical diagnosis of carcinoma of the pancreas. *JAMA* 182:6–8, 1962.

31. Gambill E.: Pancreatitis associated with pancreatic carcinoma: a study of 26 cases. *Mayo Clin. Proc.* 46:174–177, 1971.

32. Gambill E.: Pancreatic and ampullary carcinoma: diagnosis and prognosis in relationship to symptoms, physical findings and elapse of time in 252 patients. *South. Med. J.* 63:1119–1122, 1970.

33. Niccolini D.G., Graham J.H., Banks P.A.: Tumor-induced acute pancreatitis. *Gastroenterology* 71:142–145, 1976.

34. Van Waes L., Van Maele V., Demeulenaere L., et al.: Carcinoma of the pancreas presenting as relapsing pancreatitis. *Am. J. Gastroenterol.* 68:88–90, 1977.

35. Hoover H.: Carcinoma of the pancreas: clinical aspects, in Siegelman S.S. (ed.): *Computed Tomography of the Pancreas.* New York, Churchill Livingstone, 1983, pp. 61–82.

36. Eaton S.B. Jr., Ferrucci J.T. Jr.: *Radiology of the Pancreas and Duodenum.* Philadelphia, W.B. Saunders Co., 1973.

37. Chait H., Faegenbury D.H.: Illusory neoplasms of the stomach and duodenum as a manifestation of carcinoma of the pancreas. *Radiology* 74:771–777, 1960.

38. Kreel L.: The pancreas: newer radiological methods of investigation. *Postgrad. Med.* 43:14–23, 1967.

39. Cotton P.B., Lees W.R., Vallon A.G., et al.: Grayscale ultrasonography and endoscopic pancreatography in pancreatic diagnosis. *Radiology* 134:453–459, 1980.

40. Weinstein D.P., Wolfman N.T., Weinstein B.J.: Ultrasonic characteristics of pancreatic tumors. *Gastrointest. Radiol.* 4:245–251, 1979.

41. Shawker T.H., Garra B.S., Hill M.C., et al.: The spectrum of sonographic findings in pancreatic carcinoma. *J. Ultrasound Med.* 5:169–177, 1986.

42. Ohto M., Saotome N., Saisho H., et al.: Real-time sonography of the pancreatic duct: application to percutaneous pancreatic ductography. *AJR* 134:647–652, 1980.

43. Megibow A.J., Bosniak M.A., Ambos M.A., et al.: Thickening of the celiac axis and/or superior mesenteric artery: a sign of pancreatic carcinoma on computed tomography. *Radiology* 141:449–453, 1981.

44. Johnston F., Myers R.T.: Etiologic factors and consequences of splenic vein obstruction. *Ann. Surg.* 177:736–739, 1973.

45. Muhletaler C., Gerlock A.J. Jr., Goncharenko V., et al.: Gastric varices secondary to splenic vein occlusion: radiographic diagnosis and clinical significance. *Radiology* 132:593–598, 1979.

46. Luning M., Kursuwe R., Lorenz D., et al.: Improved diagnostic evaluation of mass occupying lesions of the pancreas by CT-directed fine needle biopsy [abstract]. *AJR* 146:428, 1986.

47. Anacker H., Rupp N., Reiser M.: Magnetic resonance (MR) in the diagnosis of pancreatic disease. *Eur. J. Radiol.* 4:265–269, 1984.

48. Tscholakoff D., Hricak H., Thoeni R., et al.: MR imaging in the diagnosis of pancreatic disease. *AJR* 148:703–709, 1987.

49. Stark D.D., Moss A.A., Goldberg H.I., et al.: Magnetic resonance and CT of the normal and diseased pancreas: a comparative study. *Radiology* 150:153–162, 1984.

50. Stephens D.H., Sheedy P.F.: CT evaluation of the pancreas, in Margulis A.R., Burhenne H.J. (eds.): *Alimentary Tract Radiology.* St. Louis, C.V. Mosby Co., 1979, vol. 3, pp. 251–274.

51. Pearse A.G.E.: The APUD cell concept and its implications in pathology. *Pathol. Annu.* 9:27–41, 1974.

52. Pearse A.G.E.: Common cytochemical and ultrastructural characteristics of cells producing polypeptide hormones (the APUD series) and their relevance to thyroid and ultimobranchial C cells and calcitonin. *Proc. R. Soc. Lond. (Biol.)* 170:71–80, 1968.

53. Welbourn R.B.: Current status of the apudomas. *Ann. Surg.* 185:1–12, 1977.

54. Howard J.M., Moss N.H., Rhoads J.E.: Hyperinsulinism and islet cell tumors of the pancreas. *Int. Abstr. Surg.* 90:417, 1950.

55. Fulton R.E., Sheedy P.F., McIlrath D.C., et al.: Preoperative angiographic localization of insulin-producing tumors of the pancreas. *AJR* 123:367–377, 1975.

56. Hosoki T.: Dynamic CT of pancreatic tumors. *AJR* 140:959–965, 1983.

57. Mallinson C.N., Bloom S.R., Warin A.P., et al.: A glucagonoma syndrome. *Lancet* 2:1–5, 1974.

58. McGavran M.H., Unger R.H., Recant L., et al.: A glucagon-secreting alpha-cell carcinoma of the pancreas. *N. Engl. J. Med.* 274:1408–1413, 1966.

59. Zollinger R.M., Ellison E.H.: Primary peptic ulcerations of the jejunum associated with islet cell tumors of the pancreas. *Ann. Surg.* 142:709–723, 1955.

60. Ellison E.H., Wilson S.D.: The Zollinger-Ellison syndrome: re-appraisal and evaluation of 260 registered cases. *Ann. Surg.* 160:512–530, 1964.

61. Isenberg J.I., Walsh J.H., Grossman M.I.: Zollinger-Ellison syndrome. *Gastroenterology* 65:140–165, 1973.

62. Doppman J.L.: Multiple endocrine syndromes—a

nightmare for the endocrinologic radiologist. *Semin. Roentgenol.* 20:7–16, 1985.

63. Jensen R.T., Gardner J.D., Raufman J.P., et al.: Zollinger-Ellison syndrome: current concepts and management. *Ann. Intern. Med.* 98:59–75, 1983.

64. Schein P.S., DeLellis R.A., Kahn C.R., et al.: Islet cell tumors: current concepts and management. *Ann. Intern. Med.* 79:239–257, 1973.

65. Verner J.V., Morrison A.B.: Endocrine pancreatic islet disease with diarrhea. Report of a case due to diffuse hyperplasia of nonbeta islet tissue with a review of 54 additional cases. *Arch. Intern. Med.* 133:492–499, 1974.

66. Gold R.P., Black T.J., Rotterdam H., et al.: Radiologic and pathologic characteristics of the WDHA syndrome. *AJR* 127:397–401, 1976.

67. Bloom S.R., Polak J.M., Pearse A.G.E.: Vasoactive intestinal peptide and watery-diarrhea syndrome. *Lancet* 2:14–16, 1973.

68. Wermer P.: Genetic aspects of adenomatosis of endocrine glands. *Am. J. Med.* 16:363–371, 1954.

69. Ballard H.S., Fame B., Hartsock R.J.: Familial multiple endocrine adenoma-peptic ulcer complex. *Medicine* (Baltimore) 43:481–516, 1964.

70. Dodds W.J., Wilson S.D., Thorsen M.K., et al.: MEN I syndrome and islet cell lesions of the pancreas. *Semin. Roentgenol.* 20:17–63, 1985.

71. Lamers C.B., Buis J.T., van Tongeren J.: Secretin-stimulated serum gastrin levels in hyperparathyroid patients from families with multiple endocrine adenomatosis type I. *Ann. Intern. Med.* 86:719–724, 1977.

72. Carroll B.A., Ta H.N.: The ultrasonic appearance of extranodal abdominal lymphoma. *Radiology* 136:419–425, 1980.

73. Burgener F.A., Hamlin D.J.: Histiocytic lymphoma of the abdomen: radiographic spectrum. *AJR* 137:337–342, 1981.

74. Francis I.R., Glazer G.M.: Case report. Burkitt's lymphoma of the pancreas presenting as acute pancreatitis. *J. Comput. Assist. Tomogr.* 6:395–397, 1982.

75. Glazer H.S., Lee J.K.T., Balfe D.M., et al.: Non-Hodgkin lymphoma: computed tomographic demonstration of unusual extranodal involvement. *Radiology* 149:211–217, 1983.

76. Berman J.L., Levene N.: Sarcoma of the pancreas. *Arch. Surg.* 73:894–896, 1956.

77. Rumancik W.M., Megibow A.J., Bosniak M.A., et al.: Metastatic disease to the pancreas: evaluation by computed tomography. *J. Comput. Assist. Tomogr.* 8:829–834, 1984.

78. Wernecke K., Petters P.E., Galanski M.: Pancreatic metastases: US evaluation. *Radiology* 160:399–402, 1986.

79. Willis R.A.: *The Spread of Tumors in the Human Body.* New York, Butterworth, 1975, p. 216.

80. Patel J.K., Didolkar M.S., Pickren J.W., et al.: Metastatic pattern of malignant melanoma: a study of 216 autopsy cases. *Am. J. Surg.* 135:807–810, 1978.

81. Thomas M.L., Lamb G.H., Barraclough M.A.: Angiographic demonstration of a pancreatic "vipoma" in the WDHA syndrome. *AJR* 127:1037–1039, 1976.

82. Oberg K., Walinder O., Bostrom H., et al.: Peptide hormone markers in screening for endocrine tumors in multiple endocrine adenomatosis type I. *Am. J. Med.* 73:619–630, 1982.

83. Imhof H., Frank P.: Pancreatic calcifications in malignant islet cell tumors. *Radiology* 122:333–337, 1977.

84. Bok E.L., Cho K.J., Williams D.M., et al.: Venous involvement in islet cell tumors of the pancreas. *AJR* 142:319–322, 1984.

85. Stark D.D., Moss A.A., Goldberg H.I., et al.: CT of pancreatic islet tumors. *Radiology* 148:485–488, 1984.

86. Pogany A.C., Kerlan R.K. Jr., Karam J.H., et al.: Cystic insulinoma. *AJR* 142:951–952, 1984.

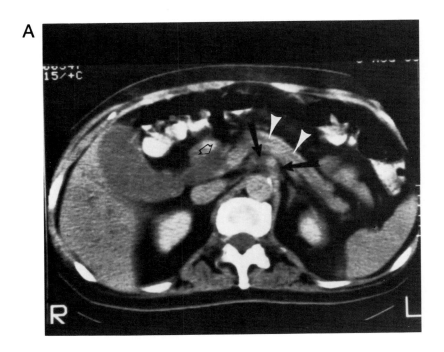

FIG 2–1.
Apparent thickening of celiac and superior mesenteric arteries in pancreatic carcinoma (two cases).

A, a 63-year-old man who presented with persistent nausea and some weight loss underwent a thorough workup that included abdominal CT. The CT scan showed equivocal enlargement of the head of the pancreas (not illustrated) associated with a dilated common bile duct *(open arrow)* and pancreatic duct *(arrowheads)*. On this image, one of the findings in pancreatic carcinoma is well illustrated: there is obliteration of the fat around the superior mesenteric artery behind the pancreas *(arrows)*, giving an appearance of thickening of the artery. Eventually, percutaneous needle aspiration biopsy was performed, and pancreatic adenocarcinoma was confirmed.

B and **C,** a CT scan of a patient with a history similar to that in **A** shows a hypodense mass in the body of the pancreas *(arrows* in **B**). Notice tumor infiltration around the superior mesenteric artery.

On the latter image **(C),** which shows the area 1 cm above the preceding view, there is apparent thickening of the celiac artery. *Arrowheads* point to the enhanced lumen of the vessel.

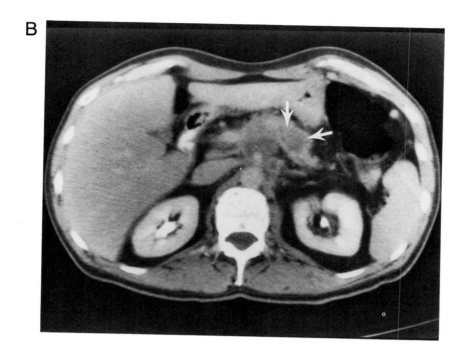

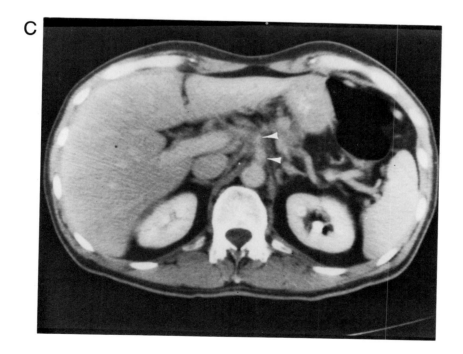

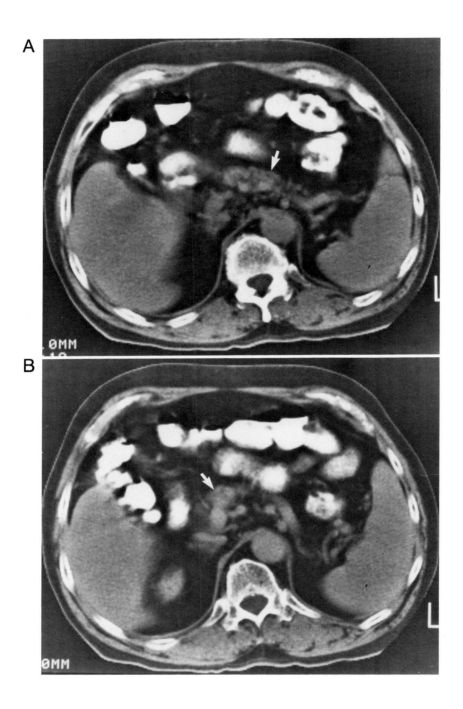

FIG 2–2.
Occult carcinoma of the pancreas (two cases).

A through **C,** this patient presented with abdominal pain and had an elevated bilirubin titer on laboratory examination.

The first CT scan **(A)** shows a normal pattern to the body and tail of the pancreas *(arrow).* Image **B** shows a subtle but real change in architecture in the head of the pancreas *(arrow)* just anterior to the portal vein. Because of the relative subtleties of this diagnosis, an ERCP series was performed.

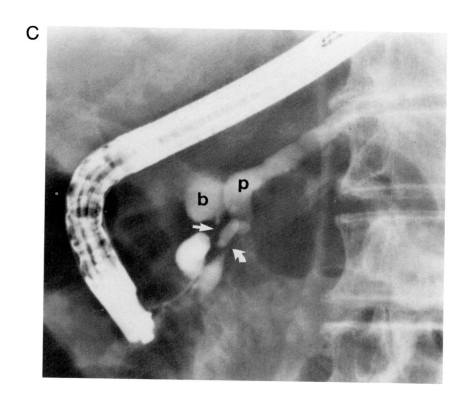

The ERCP series **(C)** reveals the portions of a pancreatogram and cholangiogram that show a dilated common bile duct *(b)* as well as a dilated pancreatic duct *(p)*. The narrowing of the common bile duct is shown by the *straight white arrow,* and the narrowing of the pancreatic duct is shown by the *curved white arrow.*

At surgery, adenocarcinoma was found and Whipple's operation performed. (**A** through **C** courtesy of M.A. Mauro, M.D., Department of Radiology, University of North Carolina, Chapel Hill, N.C.) *(Continued.)*

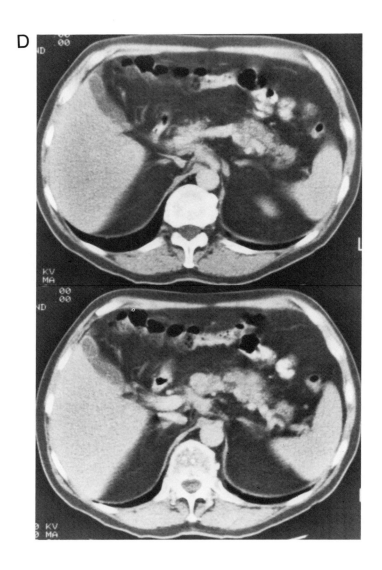

FIG 2–2 (cont.).
D through **F**, in another case, a 76-year-old man with bloating abdominal pain and weight loss had CT examination of the abdomen **(D)**, which was reported normal. An ERCP film **(E)** shows narrowing of the pancreatic duct in the head *(arrows)*, along with slight dilatation of the duct in the body. A CT scan was repeated **(F)** using 5-mm collimation without interval. A small enhancing mass is seen in the pancreatic head, of which a biopsy specimen was taken using CT guidance. The diagnosis was well-differentiated pancreatic adenocarcinoma. Retrospectively in **D,** the fat around the mesenteric and celiac vessels is obliterated, a finding that should alarm the radiologist. (**D** through **F** courtesy of Chandra S. Katragadda, M.D., Spohn Hospital, Corpus Christi, Tex.)

E

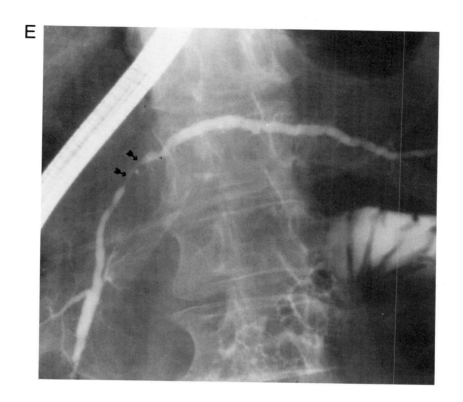

F

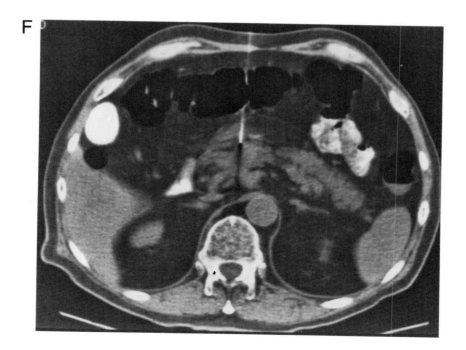

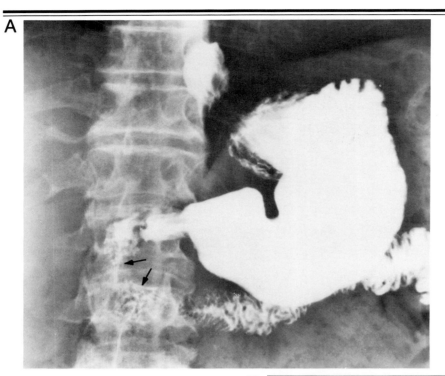

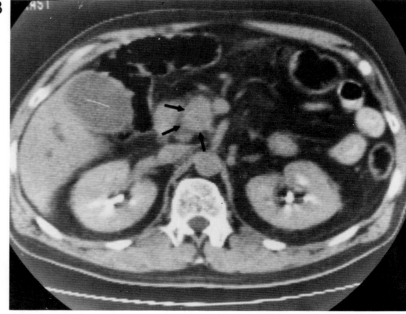

FIG 2–3.

Carcinoma of the pancreatic head. A 61-year-old man had an upper gastrointestinal barium study because of an 18-kg (40-lb) weight loss over three months and gradual onset of jaundice.

A, On this film, taken with the patient supine, there is, in addition to a small hiatal hernia, minimal widening of the duodenal loop with padding effect *(arrows)* on the medial wall of the lower descending and proximal transverse duodenum. In light of the clinical history, this finding warranted further investigation by CT.

B through **D,** a CT scan shows a 3-cm mass in the head of the pancreas *(black arrows* in **B)** associated with marked dilatation of the pancreatic duct *(arrowheads* in **C),** common bile duct *(white arrows* in **C),** and intrahepatic bile ducts **(D).** Part of the splenic vein is seen behind the pancreas *(open arrows* in **C).**

At surgery, a nonresectable pancreatic carcinoma was discovered along with malignancy in the locally excised nodes. The patient underwent a Roux-en-Y cholecystojejunostomy.

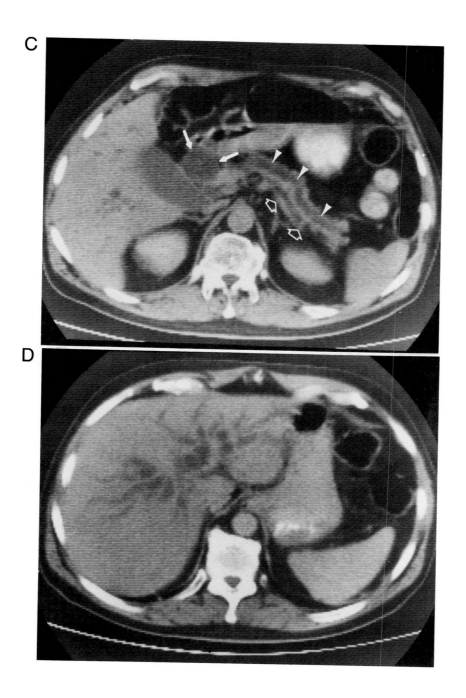

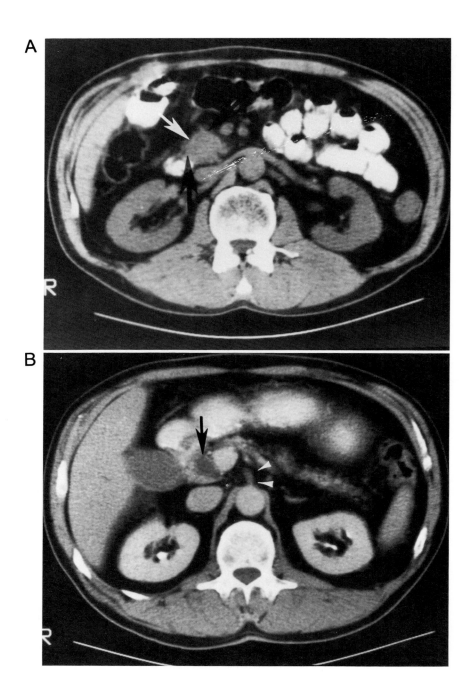

FIG 2–4.
Pancreatic carcinoma in the head with pancreatitis. A 64-year-old man presented with pruritus and jaundice and was found to have carcinoma of the head of the pancreas.

A, the initial CT scan of the abdomen reveals a mass measuring approximately 3 cm *(arrows)* in the head of the pancreas.

B, on the contrast-enhanced image 2 cm higher, the fat around the superior mesenteric artery appears to be free of abnormality *(arrowheads)*. The common bile duct is dilated *(arrow),* but there is no dilatation of the pancreatic duct.

Exploratory laparotomy confirmed carcinoma of the

C

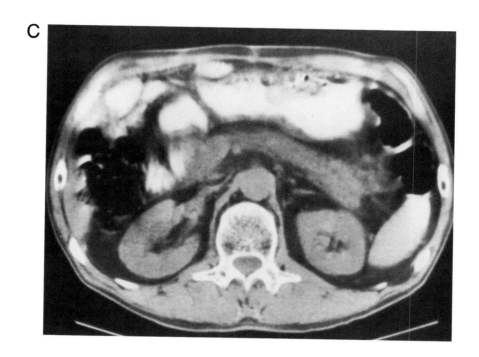

head of the pancreas. A biliary diversion was done, followed by cobalt therapy and chemotherapy. Eight months later, the patient presented with a decreasing energy level associated with vomiting.

C, a CT scan shows no significant change in the size of the mass in the pancreatic head; however, there is dif-

fuse enlargement of the pancreas with obliteration of the peripancreatic fat. The findings suggested diffuse pancreatitis. Because of severe vomiting, the patient had a second laparotomy, which showed the pancreatic mass had caused partial obstruction of the second portion of the duodenum. He underwent a gastrojejunostomy.

A

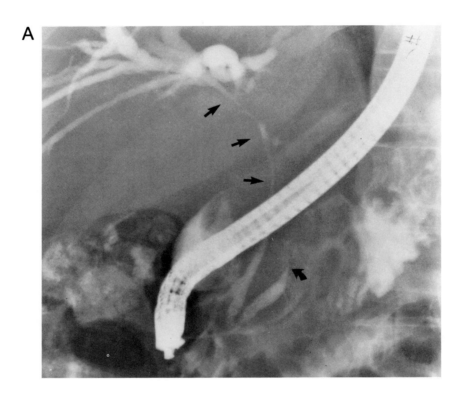

FIG 2–5.
Infiltrating carcinoma of the pancreatic head. This 60-year-old woman presented with painless jaundice. An ERCP series was done, followed by CT.

A, the ERCP film shows visualization of both the biliary and the pancreatic ductal systems. The cholangiogram re-veals narrowing of the proximal common hepatic and com-mon bile ducts *(straight arrows).* This is indicative of extrin-sic compression from tumor infiltration and nodes in the porta hepatis. The *curved arrow* points to an obstruction of the pancreatic duct, which indicates primary pancreatic car-cinoma.

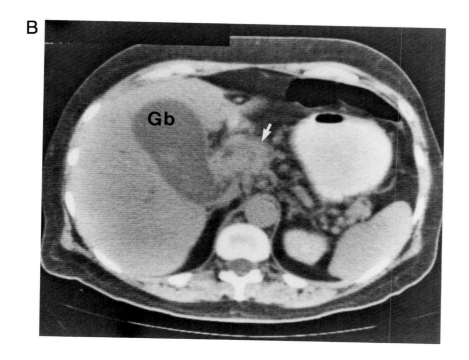

B, the CT scan shows dilatation of the gallbladder *(Gb)* as well as a mass *(arrow)* in the region of the neck of the pancreas.

At surgery, the patient was found to have a mass in the head and neck of the pancreas with diffuse infiltration and many nodes in the porta hepatis. There was also tumor infiltration around the duodenum and under the surface of the liver. Biliary diversion could not be performed. An endoprosthesis was placed two days after surgery. The patient then received radiation therapy for pain control. (Courtesy of M.A. Mauro, M.D., Department of Radiology, University of North Carolina, Chapel Hill, N.C.)

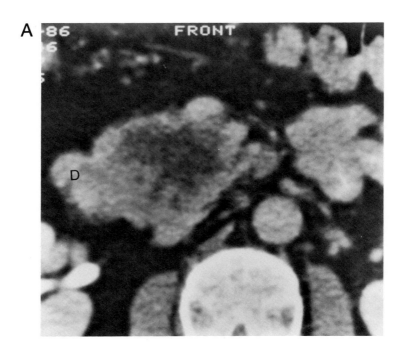

FIG 2–6.
Carcinoma of the pancreatic head with duodenal infiltration. This 64-year-old man presented with vague abdominal pain. Upper gastrointestinal barium study (not available) revealed an abnormal duodenum. Computed tomography was performed.

A, a large, partially necrotic tumor is seen in the head and uncinate process of the pancreas. It has infiltrated into the duodenum *(D)*. The tumor extends behind the superior mesenteric artery and vein.

B, 3 cm higher, the dilated pancreatic duct *(arrowheads)* is seen with the normal body of the pancreas. A portion of the head is outlined by *open arrows.* Duodenal infiltration is again seen.

C, transverse sonogram corresponding to the CT scan shown in **B** shows the tumor in the head *(arrows)* and its relationship with the duodenum *(D)*. The dilated pancreatic duct *(arrowheads)* is seen. *Open arrows* outline the anterior surface of the body of the pancreas.

Percutaneous aspiration biopsy specimens showed inflammatory cells in the first two passes and findings consistent with adenocarcinoma on the third pass.

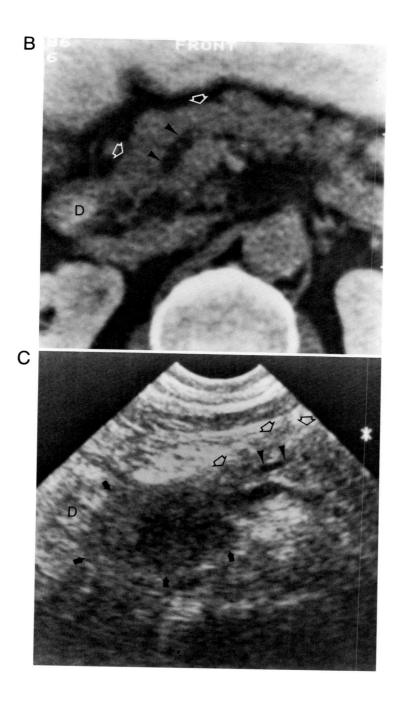

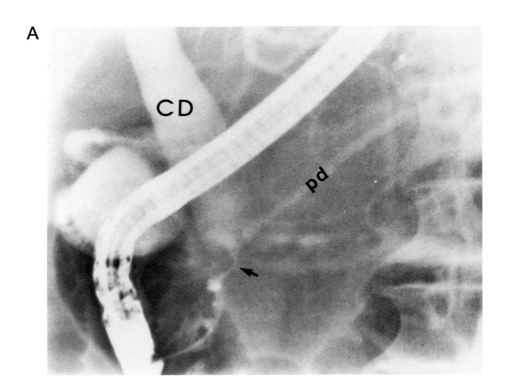

FIG 2–7.
Carcinoma of the pancreatic head. A 65-year-old man presented with pruritus, weight loss, and right upper quadrant pain. He was found to have an elevated alkaline phosphatase value. The CT scan showed a possible mass, and ERCP was performed.

A, the ERCP film reveals dilatation of the common bile duct *(CD).* The pancreatic duct *(pd)* is of normal size. The *arrow* points to the distal stricture of the common duct.

B

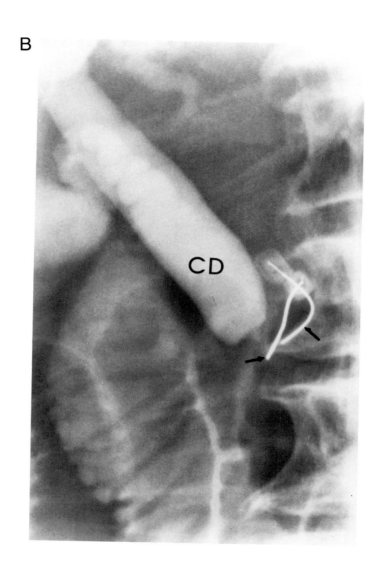

CD

B, after the endoscope was removed, two 22-gauge Chiba needles were used percutaneously *(arrows)* to biopsy the common bile duct **(CD)** at its distal narrowing. The retained contrast was used for guidance. The findings from this biopsy were positive for adenocarcinoma.

Operation again showed the adenocarcinoma of the pancreas. It was determined that the tumor was unresectable because of surrounding spread, and a choledochoduodenostomy was performed. (Courtesy of M.A. Mauro, M.D., Department of Radiology, University of North Carolina, Chapel Hill, N.C.)

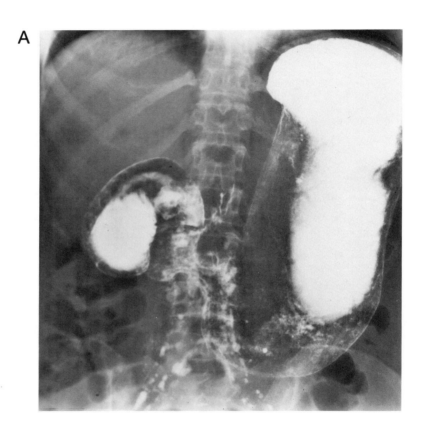

FIG 2–8.
Pancreatic carcinoma, simulating lymphoma. A 43-year-old woman with a history of ulcer disease and treated lymphoma developed a recent increase in nausea and crampy epigastric pain associated with occasional vomiting. The clinical evaluation, which included upper gastrointestinal endoscopy, was normal.

A, on the upper gastrointestinal series, there is a very distended stomach with almost no flow of barium beyond the descending duodenum.

B and **C,** an abdominal CT scan demonstrates retroperitoneal adenopathy *(arrows)* and fullness in the region of the head of the pancreas and porta hepatis. There is no dilatation of the intrahepatic biliary system.

B

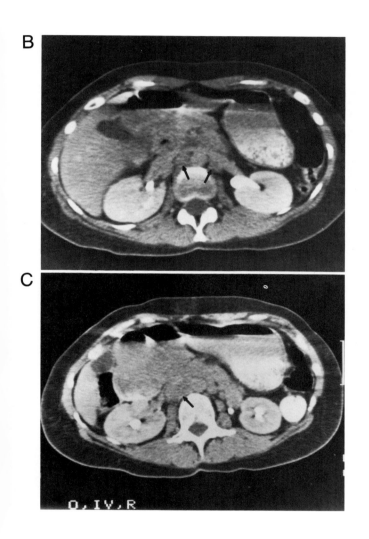

C

D

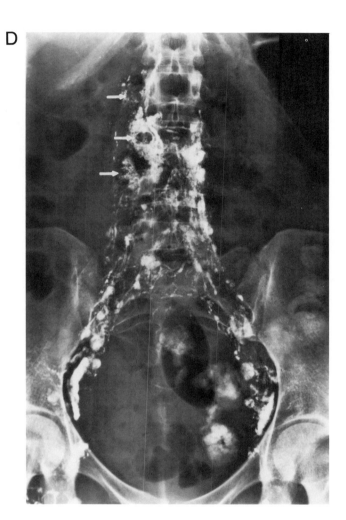

D, the lymphangiogram shows several nodes with abnormal architecture *(arrows).* The differential diagnosis was recurrent lymphoma vs. metastatic carcinoma.

At exploratory laparotomy, an approximately 8-cm mass in the head of the pancreas was discovered. The mass infiltrated the duodenum, and there were abnormal retroperitoneal lymph nodes. A diagnosis of pancreatic carcinoma with retroperitoneal adenopathy was established. In addition, there was evidence of metastases to the right ovary, proved by the surgical specimen from right oophorectomy.

A

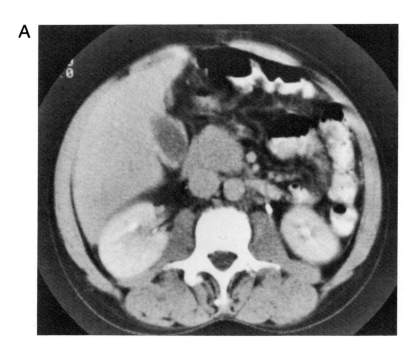

FIG 2–9.
Intrabiliary infiltrative carcinoma of the pancreas. A 50-year-old man with gradual onset of loss of appetite, weight loss, and jaundice underwent an upper gastrointestinal barium study, followed by abdominal CT examination and percutaneous transhepatic cholangiography (PTC). Results of the barium study of the upper gastrointestinal tract were unremarkable.

A, the CT scan shows enlargement of the head and uncinate process of the pancreas.

B, the contrast-enhanced liver images show marked dilatation of the intrahepatic biliary radicles with probable metastasis in the caudate lobe.

C, an attempt was made to perform PTC, and, with a great deal of difficulty, a small amount of bile could be as-pirated. No significant dilatation of the bile duct is seen. During the procedure, there was a fair amount of bleeding, and the study could not be continued. Intraluminal thrombus formation *(arrows)* was believed to be present.

The patient eventually underwent abdominal surgery, upon which a pancreatic mass was found. There was direct extension into the biliary duct system, and diffuse hepatic metastases were present. Bypass surgery was done with rebiopsy of the pancreatic mass and liver metastases.

It can retrospectively be seen that the situation in **B** is that of a dilated biliary system filled with tumor thrombus. Conforming to such an analysis, PTC was completed only with great difficulty, and no dilated ducts were demonstrated.

B

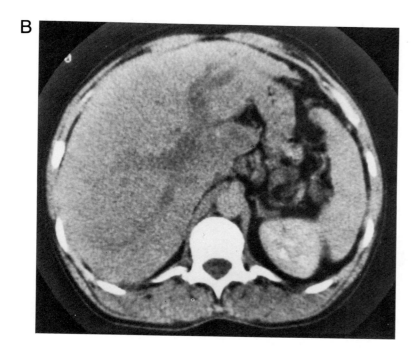

C

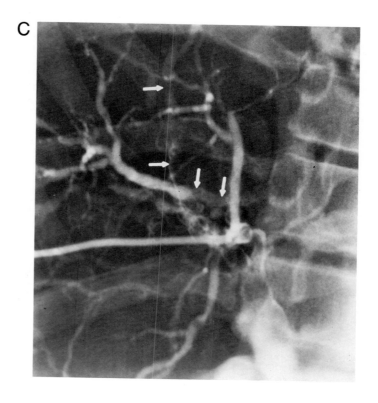

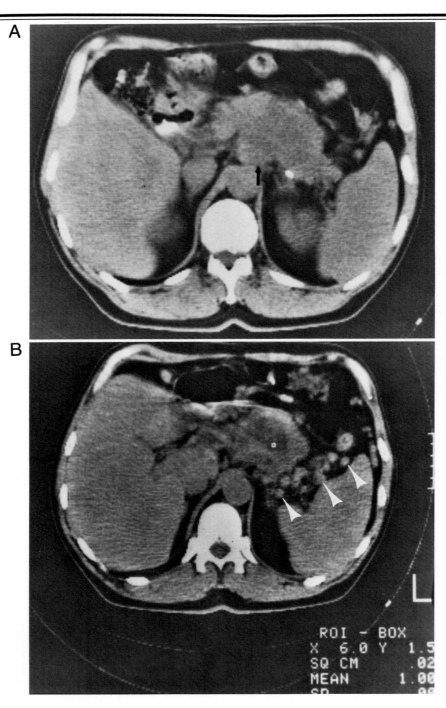

FIG 2–10.
Carcinoma of the pancreatic body. A 64-year-old man with a history of pancreatitis ten years before, presented with pain in the upper abdomen.

A, an abdominal CT scan reveals diffuse enlargement of the pancreas with areas of low attenuation. The plane of fat between the aorta and pancreas is totally obscured *(arrow).*

B, multiple collaterals are seen in the region of the splenic hilum and gastrosplenic ligament, suggesting splenic vein obstruction *(arrowheads).*

C, the ERCP film shows abrupt termination of the pancreatic duct in the region of the junction of the body and head of the pancreas *(arrow).* This corresponds well with the large mass in the body of the pancreas seen on CT. From these findings, the diagnosis of pancreatic carcinoma is most likely.

D, specimen from a percutaneous aspiration biopsy proved the diagnosis of pancreatic adenocarcinoma.

C

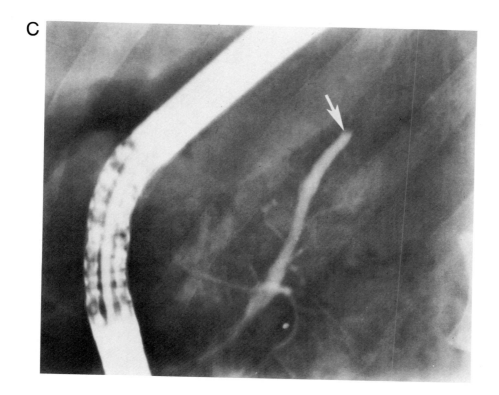

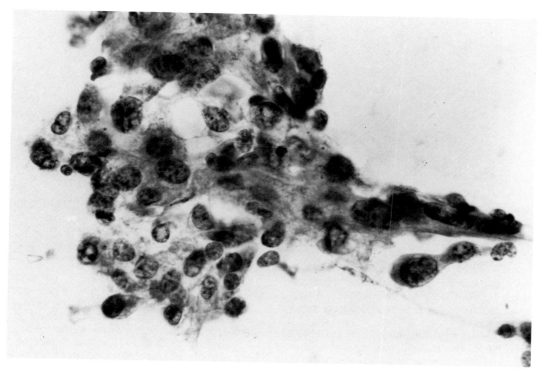

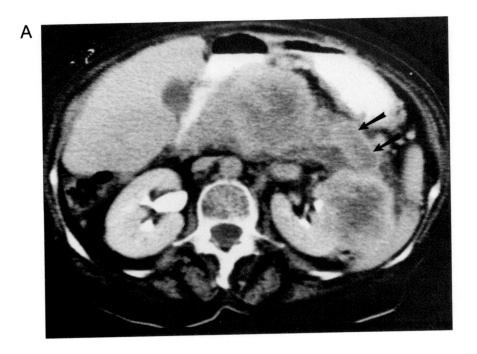

FIG 2–11.
Combined pancreatic carcinoma and renal cell carcinoma. A 59-year-old woman with low back pain and a 7.7-kg (17-lb) weight loss underwent intravenous pyelography (film not shown), which revealed a left renal mass.

A, a CT scan shows a necrotic tumor in the left kidney. In addition, there is a large mass occupying the body and head of the pancreas and dilatation of the pancreatic duct in the tail *(arrows)*. Few areas of low density in the liver were seen, compatible with hepatic metastases.

B, celiac arteriogram demonstrates encasement of the splenic artery *(arrows)* and splenic vein obstruction. The diagnosis of primary pancreatic carcinoma was strongly suggested.

C, image from selective left renal angiography demonstrates a hypervascular mass in the left kidney. The diagnosis of two primaries—renal cell carcinoma and pancreatic carcinoma—was strongly considered. Since the renal tumor was stage IV, interferon chemotherapy was considered appropriate. The diagnosis of pancreatic adenocarcinoma was established by percutaneous aspiration biopsy.

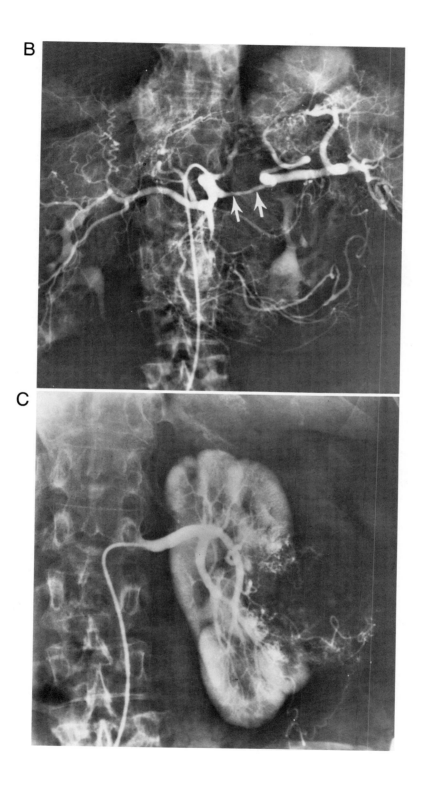

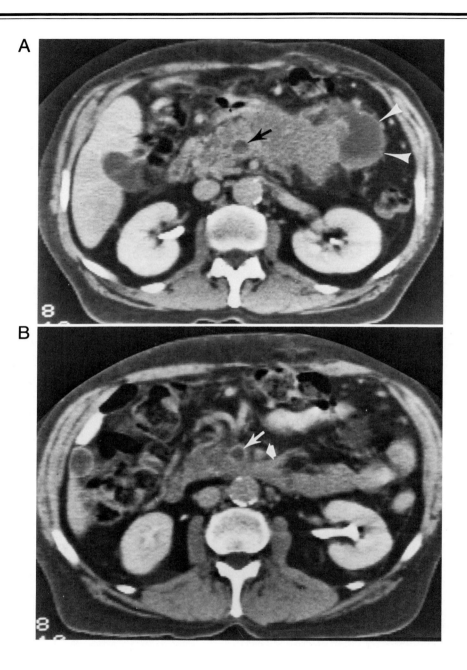

FIG 2–12.
Diffuse pancreatic carcinoma with thrombosis of superior mesenteric vein. A 65-year-old man was in excellent health until a month before presentation. During that month, he developed increasing abdominal pain and had a 2.3-kg (5-lb) weight loss.

A, the abdominal CT scan shows diffuse enlargement of the pancreas, with a cystic mass adjacent to the tail *(arrowheads)*. There is evidence of a filling defect throughout the superior mesenteric vein, consistent with thrombosis *(arrow)*.

B, this CT image was obtained 2.4 cm below that in **A** and shows the extent of thrombus in the superior mesenteric vein. The superior mesenteric artery is marked by a *fat arrow.*

The findings were thought to represent diffuse infiltrative carcinoma of the pancreas with a small pseudocyst. Percutaneous biopsy of the body of the pancreas established the diagnosis of adenocarcinoma. In this case, one should recognize the superior mesenteric vein thrombosis and not mistake it for an intrapancreatic low-density mass.

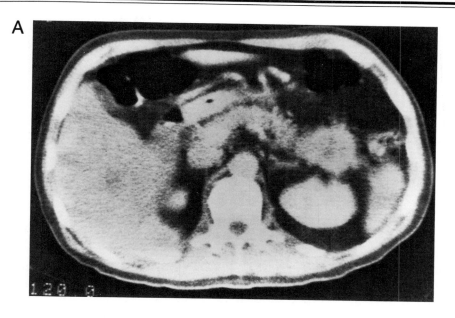

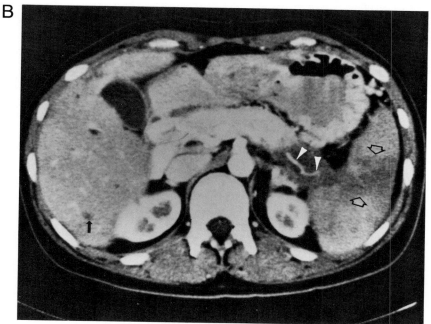

FIG 2–13.

Carcinoma of the tail of the pancreas (two cases).

A, a 67-year-old man with a history of peptic ulcer disease presented with a 9.9-kg (22-lb) weight loss over two months. Abdominal CT scan shows a well-defined mass in the tail of the pancreas, with normal body and head. There is evidence of liver metastasis. Percutaneous biopsy of the mass in the tail established the diagnosis of adenocarcinoma.

B, abdominal CT scan in another patient shows a well-

defined, low-density mass in the tail of the pancreas. The study, which was done with bolus contrast, shows significant enhancement of the normal pancreas, a single liver metastasis *(arrow),* and encasement of a branch of the splenic artery *(arrowheads).* The last has probably resulted in segmental hypoperfusion of the spleen *(open arrows).* Adenocarcinoma of the pancreas was proved. (**B** courtesy of Dr. Takayasu, National Cancer Center, Tokyo, Japan.)

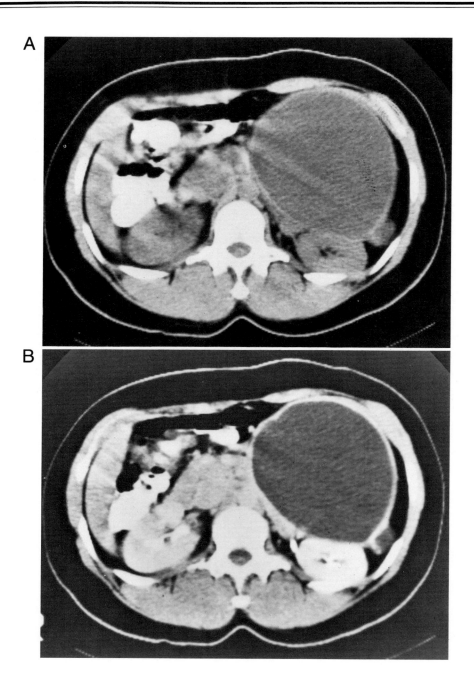

FIG 2–14.
Cystadenoma of the pancreas. A 45-year-old woman presented with gradually increasing abdominal girth and nausea. She had no history of alcohol abuse. An upper gastrointestinal barium study revealed a large retrogastric mass.

A, the unenhanced abdominal CT scan shows a very large cystic mass in the body and tail of the pancreas.

B, notice the significant degree of wall enhancement after intravenous contrast injection. There were no inflammatory changes in the anterior pararenal space or in the Gerota's fascia to suggest pseudocyst as a result of pancreatitis.

The diagnosis of pancreatic cystadenoma was established at surgery.

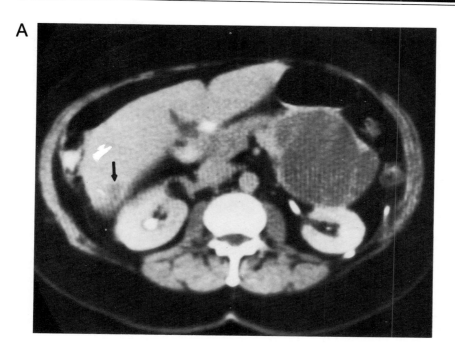

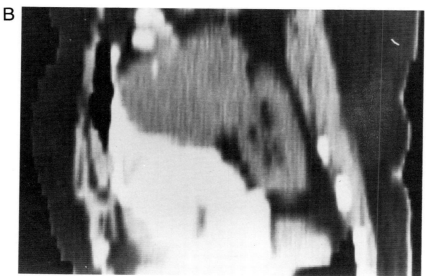

FIG 2–15.

Cystadenocarcinoma of the pancreas. A 70-year-old woman sought medical care because of a three-week history of severe indigestion associated with nausea and vomiting.

A, the enhanced abdominal CT scan reveals a large cystic mass in the body and tail of the pancreas, which has multiple septations. Several low-density lesions in the liver, one of which *(arrow)* is seen on this image, were considered to represent metastases. The pancreatic mass most likely represents a cystadenocarcinoma.

B, the sagittal reconstruction image from the unenhanced study was obtained through the tail of the pancreas and the left kidney. It shows the anteroposterior and craniocaudal dimensions of the mass and its relationship with the left kidney and peritoneum.

A CT-guided biopsy of the pancreatic mass was inconclusive; however, a subsequent biopsy of the hepatic lesion revealed adenocarcinoma. The patient was considered a candidate for chemotherapy.

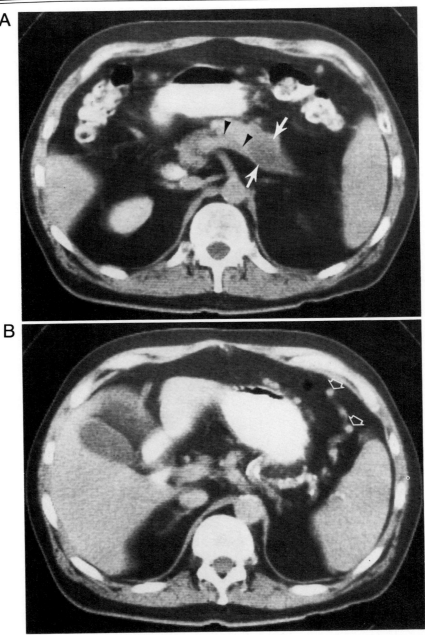

FIG 2–16.
Growing cystadenocarcinoma of the pancreas. A 63-year-old man presented with epigastric pain and weight loss.

A and **B,** the workup included abdominal CT, which reveals a cystic mass in the body and tail of the pancreas (*arrows* in **A**). The mass was called a pseudocyst. Results of other radiologic examinations were normal. Retrospective analysis of the images shows compression of the splenic vein *(arrowheads)* by the pancreatic mass and presence of some collaterals in the region of the gastrosplenic ligament *(open arrows).*

C, a repeat CT scan done five months later shows that the cystic mass has increased in size and has irregular bor-
ders and internal septations, suggesting the diagnosis of cystadenocarcinoma or possibly cystadenoma. Percutaneous biopsy proved the diagnosis of cystadenocarcinoma. (**C** courtesy of Mark Skolkin, M.D., St. Luke's Episcopal Hospital, Houston, Texas.)

D, two weeks later, an angiogram was done for preoperative evaluation. On this venous phase of the celiac arteriogram, occlusion of the splenic vein with presence of many collaterals *(open arrows)* is seen. The proximal splenic artery was encased. At surgery, pancreatic cystadenocarcinoma was discovered in the tail, with extension into the body of the pancreas and involvement of the splenic vessels.

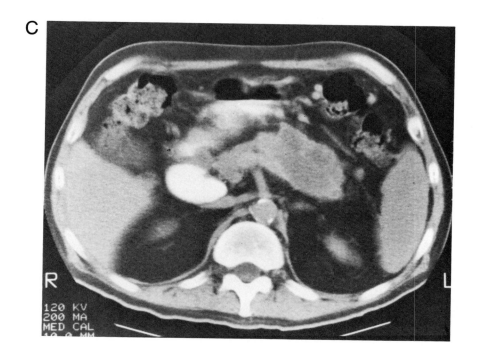

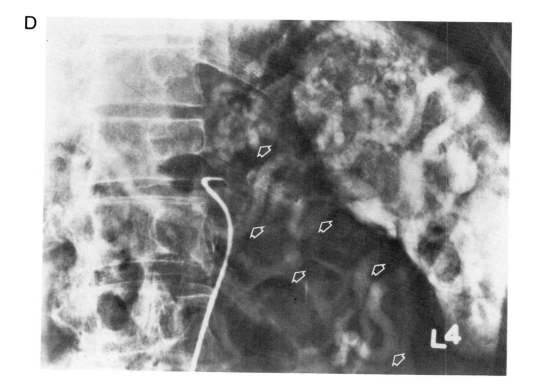

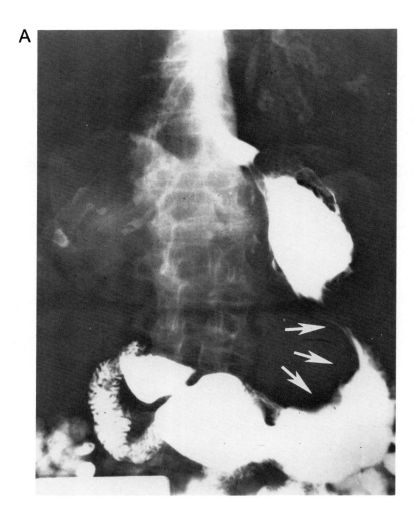

FIG 2–17.
Cystadenocarcinoma of the pancreas. An 83-year-old woman presented with gradual loss of appetite and a feeling of fullness in the epigastrium. She had no history of alcohol abuse.

A, the frontal view of an upper gastrointestinal barium study shows smooth mass effect on the lesser curvature of the stomach *(arrows).*

B

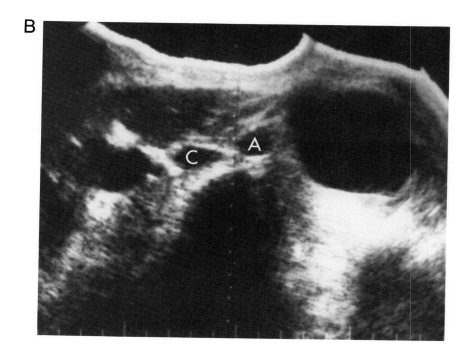

B, transverse sonogram shows the mass to be anechoic, with strong through-transmission. The aorta *(A)* and vena cava *(C)* are seen on this image. The body and tail of the pancreas could not be identified.

With the probable diagnosis of pancreatic pseudocyst, percutaneous aspiration biopsy was done with ultrasound guidance, and the specimen results were positive for carcinoma. There was no evidence of metastases. The patient wanted the tumor removed. The surgical specimen was diagnosed as pancreatic cystadenocarcinoma.

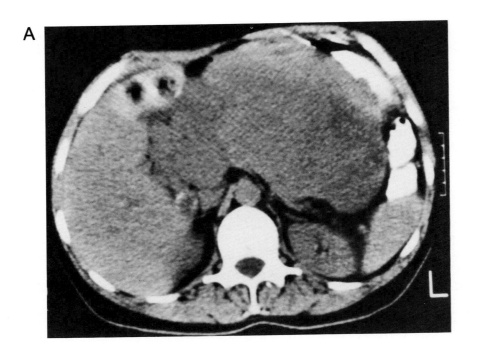

FIG 2–18.
Nonfunctioning islet cell tumor of the pancreas. A 46-year-old man sought medical attention because of a 9.1-kg (20-lb) weight loss and a palpable mass below the left rib cage. He had a history of occasional diarrhea with abdominal pain.

Radiologic evaluations comprised an upper gastrointestinal series, abdominal CT, and angiography. The only find-ing on barium study was a large mass displacing the adjacent stomach and bowel loops, with no wall infiltration.

A, the unenhanced abdominal CT scan confirms the location of the mass to be within the pancreas, with evidence of infiltration into the mesentery. The CT scan was also used for guided biopsy of the mass. Biopsy findings suggested the diagnosis of islet cell tumor.

B

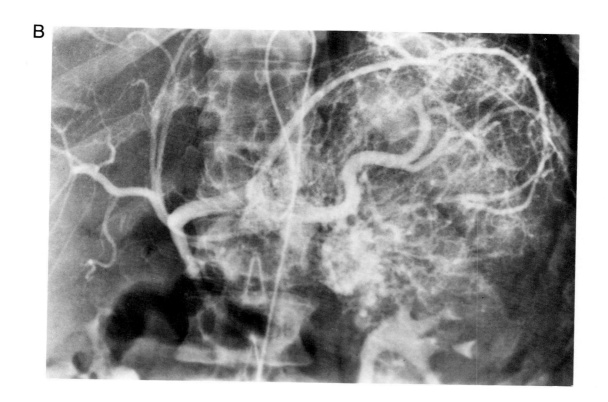

B, the celiac arteriogram shows a large, vascular tumor mass in the left upper quadrant, with arterial feeding from the left gastric and splenic arteries. Also, there were feeders from the pancreatic arcades and the superior mesenteric arterial branches. There was evidence of extension of the mass into the portal vein associated with portal vein thrombosis. *(Continued.)*

C

D

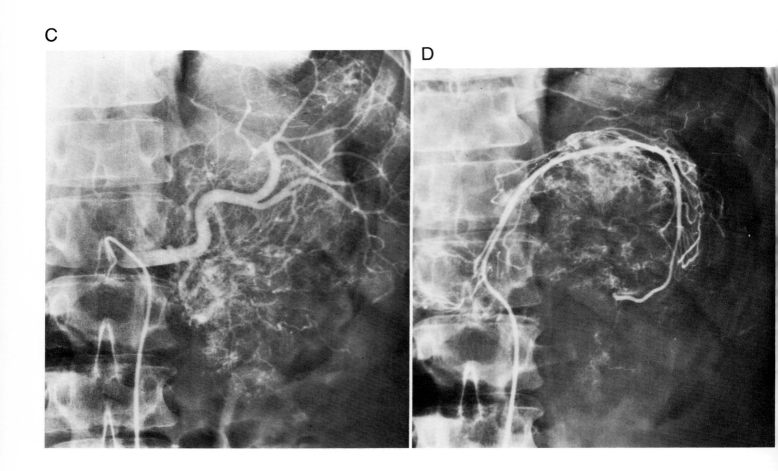

FIG 2–18 (cont.).
C and **D,** selective splenic **(C)** and left gastric artery **(D)** injections outline the tumor feeders in detail. These vessels were used to embolize the neoplasm.

E, a repeat CT scan was obtained after embolization and shows almost complete infarction of the spleen *(S).* Incidentally, note the central necrosis of the mass. Several embolizations and chemotherapy resulted in shrinkage of the tumor.

F, a T₂-weighted magnetic resonance image (TR/TE, 2,500/80) was obtained one year later and shows a significant decrease in the size of the tumor. The residual mass is seen *(arrows)* displaying high signal intensity. Incidentally, the gallbladder with two stones *(arrowheads)* is seen in the right upper quadrant.

E

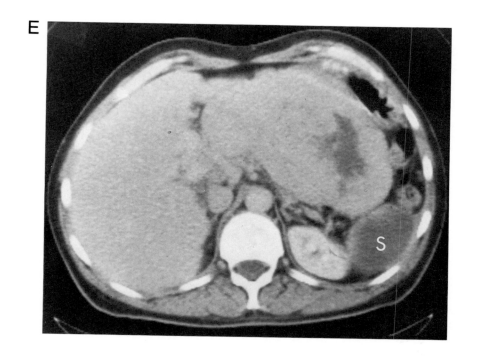

F

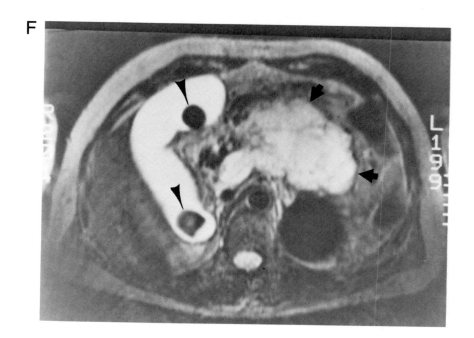

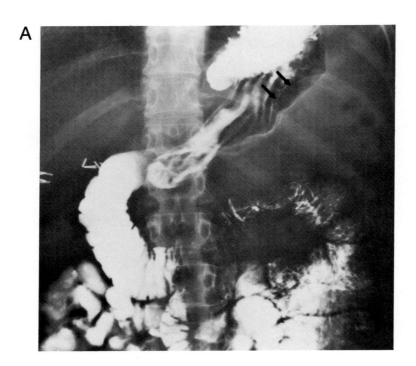

FIG 2–19.

Pancreatic glucagonoma. A 59-year-old woman presented in an outside hospital with black, tarry stools.

A, the upper gastrointestinal barium study shows a large retrogastric mass (*arrows* point to extrinsic mass effect on the stomach).

Exploration was done, and the pathologic diagnosis was undifferentiated small cell tumor of the pancreas. The patient was referred to M. D. Anderson Hospital, where the histologic material was reviewed, and a diagnosis of neuroendocrine tumor was favored. The patient's serum gluca-

gon level was elevated, and during hospitalization she developed a skin rash, described as typical for glucagonoma.

B, abdominal CT shows a large mass with areas of low density in the body and tail of the pancreas.

C, the CT scan at a higher level shows collateral vessels around the gastrosplenic and gastrohepatic ligaments. This development was due to the obstruction of the splenic vein. The patient received chemotherapy, and repeat CT of the abdomen showed a gradual decrease in the size of the mass. *(Continued.)*

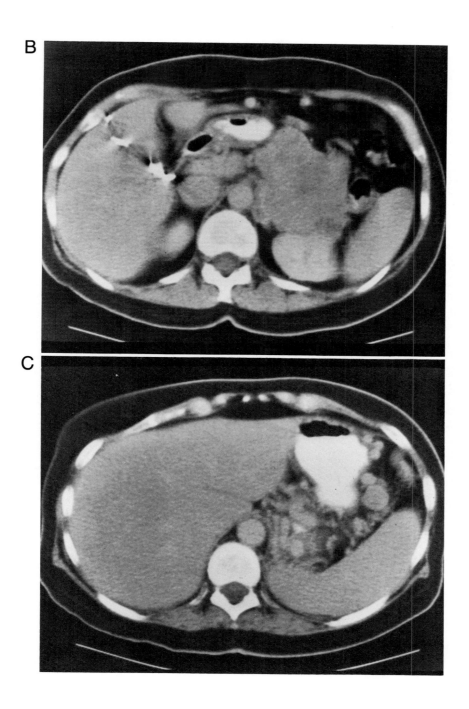

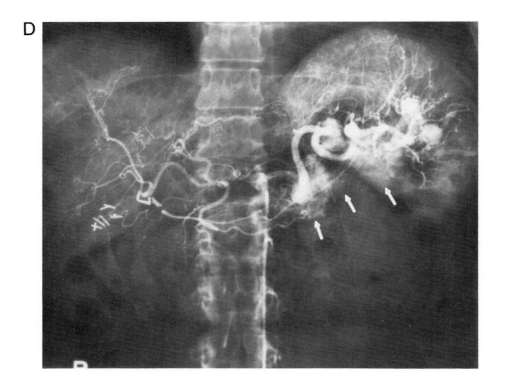

FIG 2–19 (cont.).
D and **E,** arteriography reveals a hypervascular tumor (*arrows* in **D**) in the body and the tail of the pancreas, with extension into the splenic hilum and obstruction of the splenic vein. The tumor has caused the development of numerous collaterals **(E).**

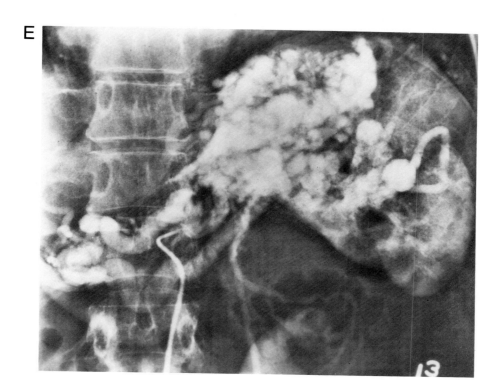

With the diagnosis of glucagonoma of the pancreas, the patient underwent further chemotherapy. The follow-up CT scan showed that the mass has responded to chemotherapy, with marked reduction in the size of the tumor. How-ever, because of the persistent symptoms, subtotal pancreatectomy was recommended. The spleen and the distal pancreas were removed, and the diagnosis of islet cell neoplasm was pathologically confirmed.

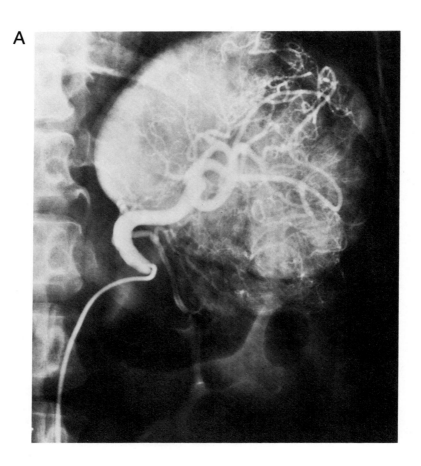

FIG 2–20.
Islet cell tumor of the pancreas (vipoma). A 50-year-old sea-man developed fever, chills, and diarrhea while overseas and was treated with the diagnosis of hepatitis. He came back to Texas, where he underwent an upper gastrointes-tinal barium study followed by abdominal ultrasound. The initial diagnosis was pancreatic carcinoma. His diarrhea and weight loss continued, and an open biopsy was performed. The diagnosis of islet cell tumor of the pancreas with liver metastases was established, for which appropriate chemo-therapy was given.

The patient did well for four years, until he began to experience nausea, vomiting, and diarrhea. The abdominal ultrasound revealed no significant change in the size of the pancreatic mass.

A, splenic arteriogram reveals a hypervascular mass in the tail of the pancreas. On hepatic arteriogram, multiple metastases were also documented throughout the liver; the metastases were repeatedly embolized.

Two years later, although his liver metastases were un-der control, the patient continued to have diarrhea. At this time, the serum VIP level was 987 pg/mL (normal, 0–170 pg/mL).

B, the abdominal CT scan shows a well-defined mass *(M)* in the body and tail of the pancreas and liver metas-tasis. The normal pancreatic head is seen *(p)*. Embolic par-ticles are noted in the liver.

C, with the diagnosis of vipoma, the patient underwent pancreatectomy and splenectomy. Even though there were liver metastases, they were considered to be inactive follow-ing repeated embolization. Notice the large mass *(M)* in the pancreatic body with the normal pancreatic head *(p)* (see also Color Plate 3).

Postoperatively, the patient did very well, with a re-markable recovery and an almost instant cessation of diar-rhea. Three months after surgery, his serum VIP level was 119 pg/mL. The patient is doing well eight years after the initial discovery of the tumor.

B

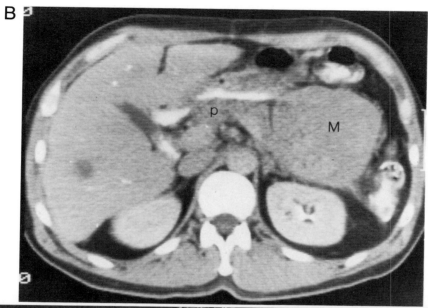

C

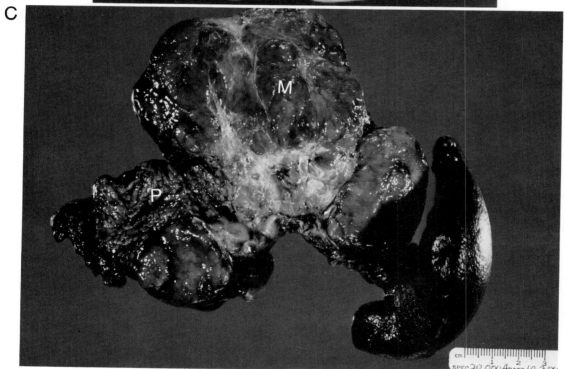

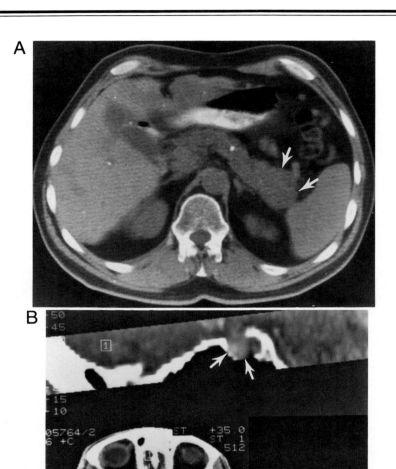

FIG 2–21.

Pancreatic islet cell tumor (MEN type I syndrome). A 48-year-old man with abdominal pain and a palpable liver was found to have significantly abnormal results on liver function tests. An abdominal CT showed extensive hepatic metastases, which were proved by biopsy to represent adenocarcinoma. The preoperative evaluation included barium enema, an upper gastrointestinal series, intravenous pyelography, and bone scans. The patient had a history of parathyroid adenomas excised six years earlier and multiple kidney stones removed three years earlier. A laparotomy was done in an outside hospital, and reportedly the surgeon felt a small mass in the pancreas.

At M. D. Anderson Hospital, hepatic arterial embolization was done for treatment of liver metastases. The serum glucagon level was 639 units (normal, < 150 units), and a diagnosis of glucagonoma was suggested.

A, abdominal CT shows enlargement of the tail of the pancreas *(arrows)*. The CT was done after liver embolization and therefore shows embolic particles in the hepatic parenchyma.

B, the patient also had bilateral gynecomastia and a serum prolactin level of 35 ng/ml (normal, < 20 ng/ml). Cranial CT shows a pituitary adenoma *(arrows)*.

C, his hypercalcemia recurred, and a transverse left parathyroid sonogram shows recurrent adenoma (*P,* recurrent adenoma; *T,* left lobe of thyroid; *C* and *J,* left carotid and jugular).

D, the abdominal film shows bilateral nephrocalcinosis and presence of catheter for chemotherapy within the hepatic artery.

Eventually, a pancreatic tumor was surgically removed. Pathology diagnosed malignant islet cell tumor with hepatic metastases.

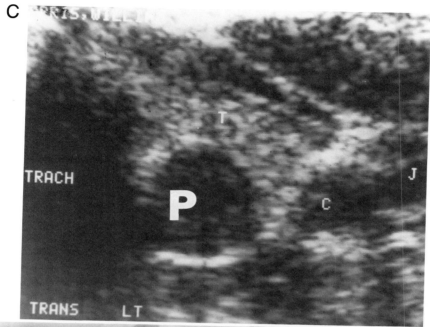

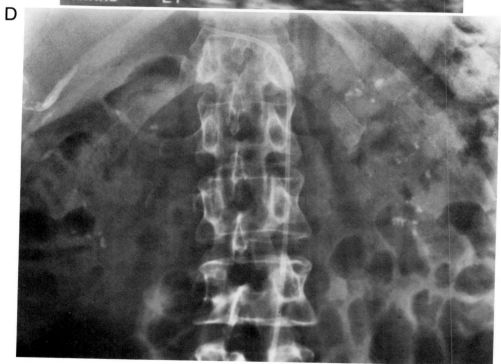

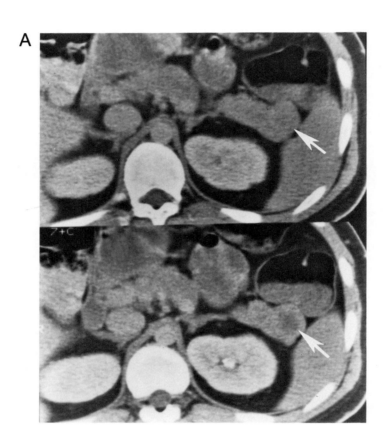

FIG 2–22.
Multiple pancreatic islet cell tumor in MEN type I syndrome. This 25-year-old man with a history of his father having had MEN type I syndrome (patient in Fig 2–21) underwent blood screening tests and was found to have hypercalcemia due to parathyroid adenoma, for which he underwent subtotal parathyroidectomy. He was also noted to have pituitary adenoma, and his serum gastrin and glucagon levels were elevated.

A, these CT scans, without and with contrast enhancement, show a well-defined, 2-cm nodule with central low density in the tail of the pancreas *(arrows)*. The body of the pancreas appears nonhomogeneous, but no nodule can be seen.

B and **C,** selective angiogram shows a 2-cm, round nodule *(open arrows* in **B**) in the region of the hilum of the spleen. The nodule that is best seen during the venous phase *(closed arrows* in **C**) corresponds to the abnormality of the pancreatic tail as seen on the CT scan.

The patient underwent conservative treatment and after two years had surgical exploration. *(Continued.)*

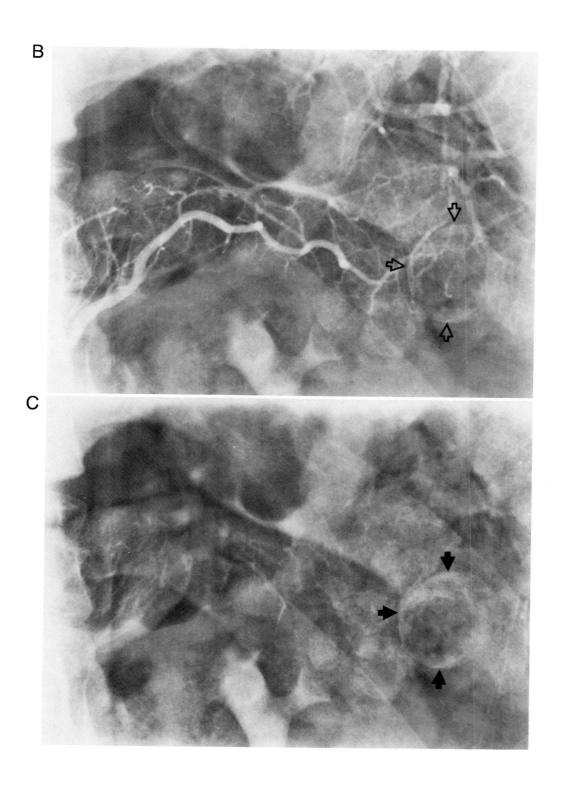

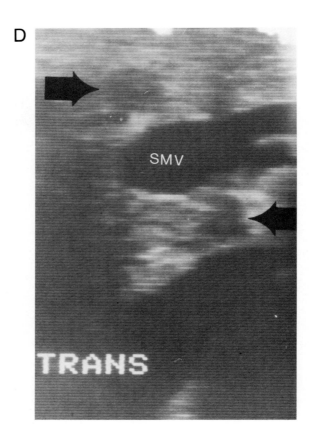

FIG 2–22 (cont.).
D, intraoperative sonogram showed multiple hypoechoic lesions throughout the entire pancreas. On this image of the head and uncinate process, two lesions *(arrows)* are seen anterior and posterior to the superior mesenteric vein *(SMV)*.

E

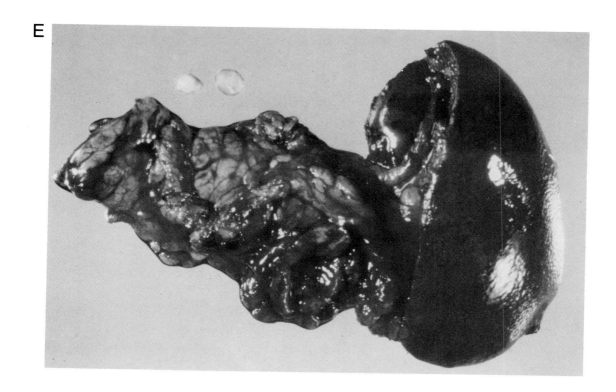

E, total pancreatectomy and splenectomy were done, and numerous islet cell tumors involving the entire pancreas were reported by the pathologist. One of the islet cells is dissected in this specimen (see also Color Plate 4).

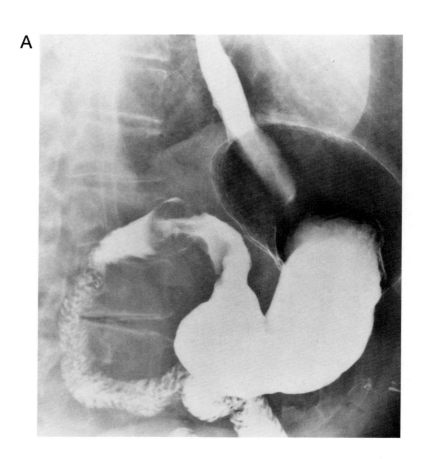

FIG 2–23.

Pancreatic lymphoma. An 89-year-old man presented with swelling above both eyes and a 4.5-kg (10-lb) weight loss. Biopsy of the right superior conjunctiva established the diagnosis of well-differentiated lymphocytic lymphoma, for which appropriate therapy was given. Five years later, he presented with a palpable abdominal mass.

A, on the upper gastrointestinal barium study, there is elevation of the gastric antrum and widening of the duodenal loop. Gastric tumor, retrogastric mass, and mass in the region of the pancreatic head were suggested. Endoscopy and biopsy suggested the diagnosis of gastric lymphoma.

B, the abdominal CT scan shows a large mass elevating the antrum of the stomach, with displacement of the duodenum and infiltration into the head of the pancreas. The body and tail of the pancreas are normal.

C, ten months after treatment, a repeat abdominal CT scan is within normal limits.

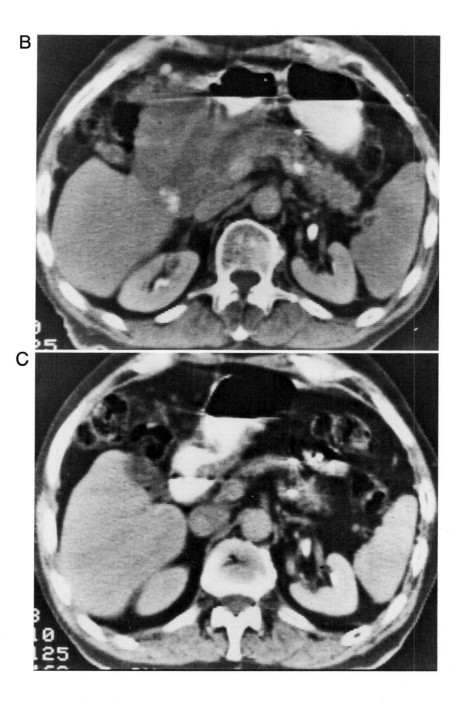

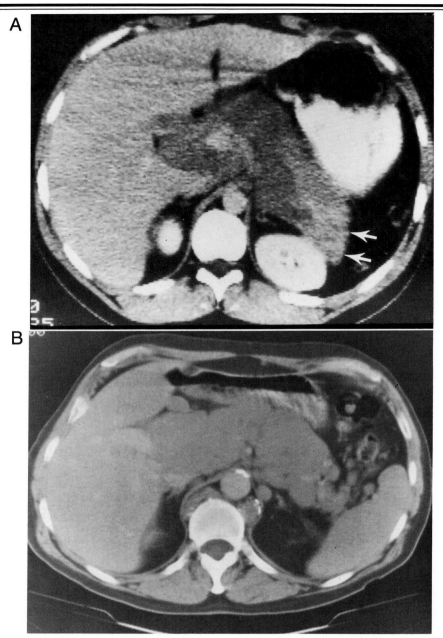

FIG 2–24.
Leukemic involvement of the pancreas and peripancreatic nodes (two cases).

A, a 32-year-old man presented with abdominal pain and weight loss. The chest radiograph showed mediastinal adenopathy extending down into the abdomen.

The abdominal CT scan reveals the adenopathy to be predominantly in the upper retroperitoneum and in the peripancreatic region. It appears that the pancreas is diffusely enlarged with areas of low density. However, only a portion of the normal pancreatic tail is seen on this image *(arrows).* The patient had a palpable node in the inguinal region; bi-opsy of the node established the diagnosis of hairy cell leukemia. The patient underwent chemotherapy.

B, this 57-year-old man with an eight-year history of chronic lymphocytic leukemia has been under treatment. At this time, he presented with cervical adenopathy and abdominal pain.

A CT scan of the upper abdomen shows massive peripancreatic adenopathy. There is also evidence of retrocrural adenopathy, which extended up into the mediastinum and neck.

Six months later and after chemotherapy, there was evidence of a decrease in the size of the nodes.

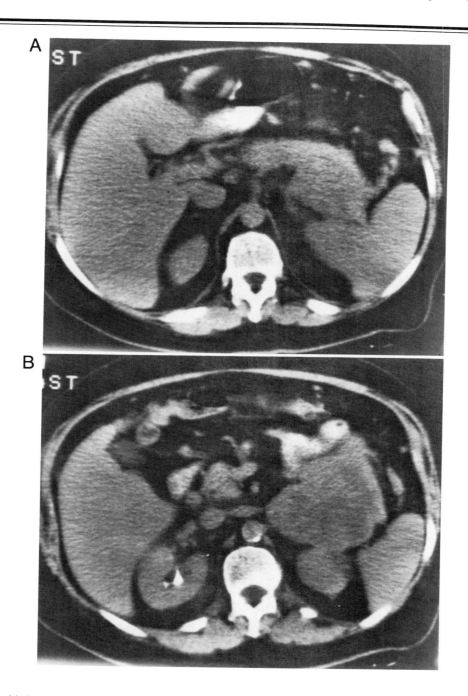

FIG 2–25.
Malignant fibrous histiocytoma of the pancreas. This 58-year-old man had a CT study in an outside institution because of new onset of weight loss. A percutaneous biopsy of an abdominal mass was reported as fibrosarcoma. He was referred to M. D. Anderson Hospital.

A, on this enhanced CT scan, a large mass is seen in the ventral aspect of the body and tail of the pancreas. On several images, no clear plane could be demonstrated between the pancreas and the mass.

B, this image, which was taken 16 mm below the image in **A,** shows an irregularly outlined mass with areas of low density.

A distal pancreatectomy, left colectomy, left nephrectomy, and splenectomy had to be done because of the extent of tumor. Pathologically, the tumor appeared to originate in the pancreas, encase the left adrenal, invade the left kidney, and extend to the pericolic fat. Histologic diagnosis was consistent with malignant fibrous histiocytoma.

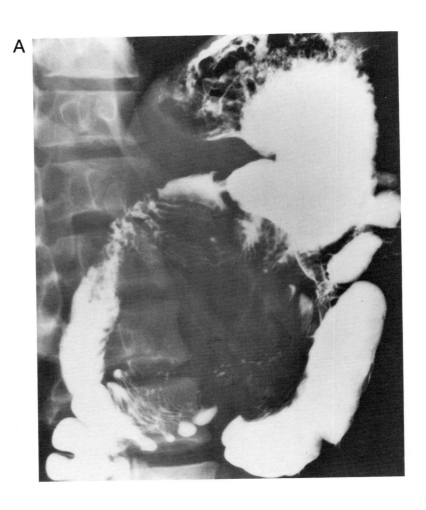

FIG 2–26.

Fibrosarcoma of the pancreas. A 23-year-old man had an upper gastrointestinal barium study in an outside hospital because of upper abdominal pain and a palpable mass.

A, on this steep oblique view of the upper gastrointestinal tract, which was done after barium enema and intravenous pyelography, widening of the duodenal loop and slight forward displacement of the stomach are seen.

B, the supine frontal view with compression pad reveals inferior displacement of the transverse colon and mass effect on the duodenum.

Because of continuous pain and with a probable diagnosis of pancreatic cyst, exploration was done and a 9 by 9 by 13 cm unresectable mass was found in the head of the pancreas. Biopsy proved the diagnosis of fibrosarcoma of the pancreas. The patient was referred to M. D. Anderson Hospital.

C, this CT scan shows a well-encapsulated, homogeneous mass *(M)* in the head of the pancreas, displacing the stomach and duodenum. The body and tail of the pancreas were normal (not shown) and there were no liver metastases.

B

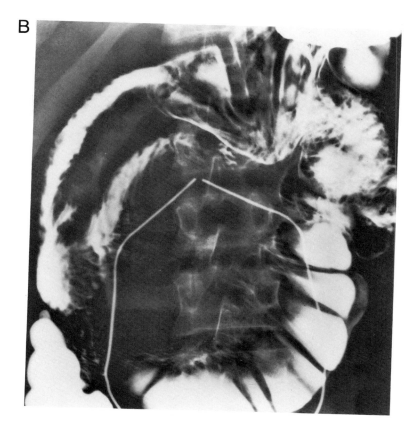

C

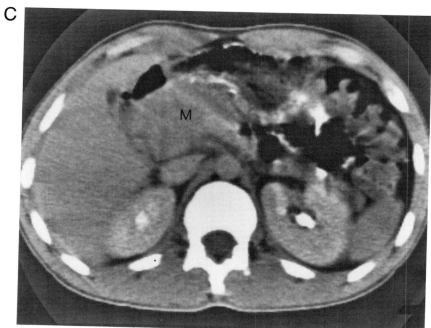

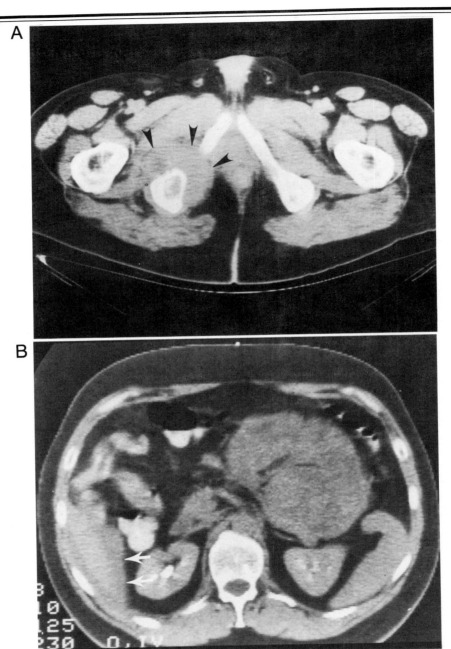

FIG 2–27.
Peripancreatic metastasis from soft tissue sarcoma. A 42-year-old man was diagnosed as having soft tissue Ewing's sarcoma in the right pelvis adjacent to the ischial tuberosity.

A, this CT scan of the pelvic tumor shows a soft tissue mass *(arrowheads)* with areas of necrosis and minimal adjacent cortical bone erosion. During chemotherapy, a large abdominal mass became palpable.

B, on this initial CT scan of the solid mass, it was thought that the mass originated in or invaded the pancreas. A small amount of ascites is also seen *(arrows)*. Percutaneous biopsy of the abdominal mass revealed metastatic sarcoma similar to the patient's primary pelvic neoplasm.

C, a repeat CT scan six months later demonstrates improvement of ascites and remarkable shrinkage of the mass with development of the cystic appearance. The density of the mass is 15 Hounsfield units, and on this image the mass appears to be separate from the pancreas. The patient underwent surgical exploration, and the tumor, along with the spleen and the tail of the pancreas, was excised. The pathologic diagnosis was peripancreatic metastatic small cell tumor consistent with Ewing's, without definite pancreatic involvement.

D, three months later, the follow-up CT scan shows local recurrence of metastasis with pancreatic infiltration, proved by biopsy.

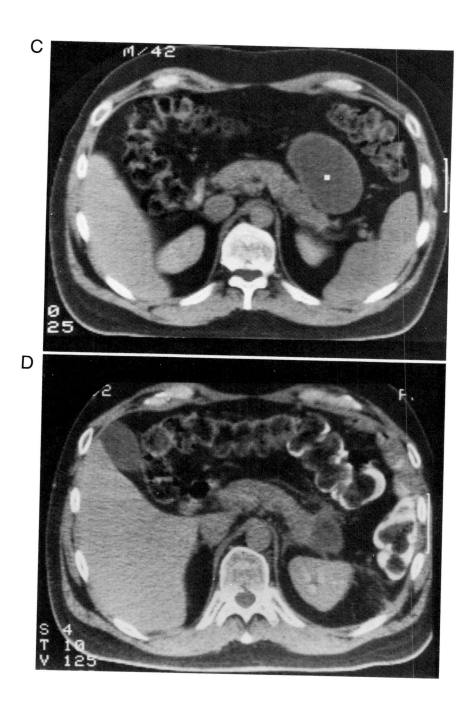

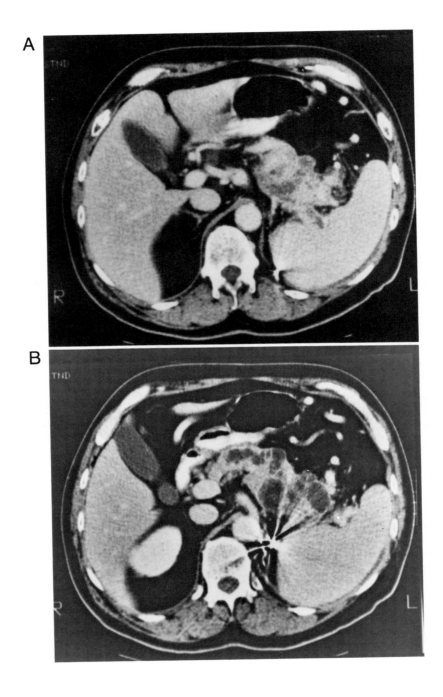

FIG 2–28.
Metastatic renal cell carcinoma to the pancreas. A 72-year-old man underwent radical left nephrectomy for renal cell carcinoma. He did well until five years later, when he had abdominal pain and was found to have guaiac-positive stool. Evaluation by barium enema was normal.

A and **B,** abdominal CT shows a large pancreas with multiple areas of low density. The tumor mass appears to

C

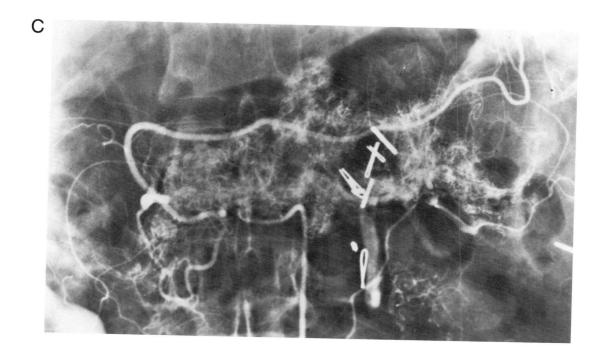

extend into the splenic hilum. The serum amylase level was normal, and there was no history of pancreatitis. A CT-guided biopsy of the pancreas revealed clear cell carcinoma compatible with pancreatic metastases from the patient's primary renal cell carcinoma.

C, angiography shows multiple hypervascular metastases in the pancreas. The catheter was positioned in the inferior pancreaticoduodenal artery for infusion of interferon.

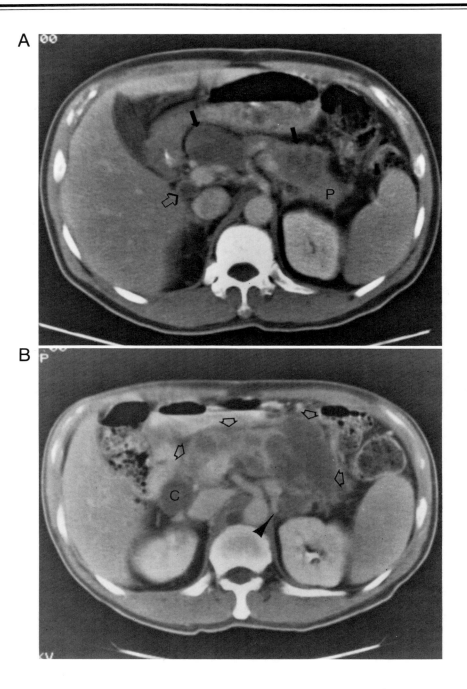

FIG 2–29.
Metastatic lung carcinoma to the pancreas. This is a 57-year-old man with squamous cell carcinoma of the lung who had pneumonectomy two months ago. Now he presents with increasing abdominal pain.

A, the CT scan shows multiple low-density masses *(arrows)* within and possibly around the pancreas *(P)*. The common bile duct *(open arrow)* is prominent.

B, three and one-half months later, repeat CT scan shows remarkable progression of the pancreatic disease *(open arrows)*. The common bile duct *(C)* is further dilated, and there is evidence of probable left adrenal metastasis *(arrowhead)*. Clinically, there was no evidence of pancreatitis.

Ultrasound-guided biopsy of pancreatic mass established the diagnosis of metastatic squamous cell carcinoma.

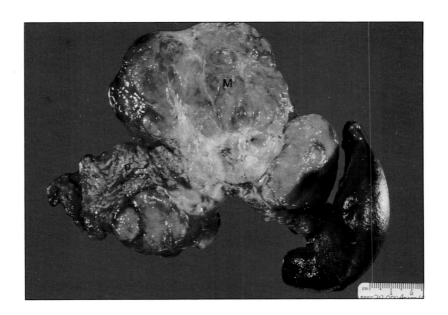

PLATE 3

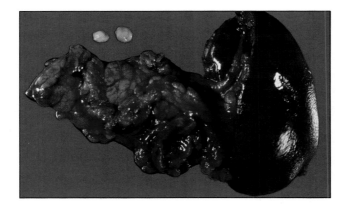

PLATE 4

3

Neoplasms of the Hepatobiliary System and Spleen

Pablo R. Ros, M.D.

James L. Buck, L.C.D.R., M.C., U.S.N.R.

Ali Shirkhoda, M.D.

HEPATOBILIARY SYSTEM

Radiology of the hepatobiliary system encompasses all imaging modalities, since the liver is one of the few organs in which nuclear medicine techniques and angiography still have diagnostic value and are significant in differentiating lesions. The roles of sonography and computed tomography (CT) in studying hepatic masses are well established. Magnetic resonance imaging (MRI) has found its principal upper abdominal use in the diagnosis of hepatic lesions.

It is in the study of primary liver neoplasms that an intelligent use of the different radiologic modalities may yield a specific diagnosis, relevant because different hepatic masses entail dramatically different prognoses. Malignant hepatic neoplasms accord, in general, a very short-term survival, and surgery may not even be attempted. On the other hand, benign neoplasms are frequently devoid of complications, and therefore resection may be unwarranted. Avoiding surgery in some benign neoplasms has recently become a particular issue because of the danger of contracting AIDS from the blood transfusions that are common during hepatic resections.

For all these reasons, we believe that it is necessary to be familiar with the underlying pathologic appearance of tumors of the liver and biliary system to better understand their radiologic presentation. We herein correlate these two facets, highlighting the key imaging features that may suggest a preoperative diagnosis. The various hepatobiliary neoplasms discussed here are outlined in Table 3–1.

Liver

The piece of clinical information that we consider most relevant in the differentiation of liver neoplasms is the age of the patient. Age originates the main division in hepatic tumors: pediatric and adult. Although there is some overlap, the tumors that occur in children are not seen in adults and vice versa. (Pediatric liver tumors are further discussed in Chapter 8.)

The next important datum is patient gender. As a general rule, malignant tumors are more frequently seen in men, benign ones in women. The presence of symptomatology is of value: benign tumors are in most cases asymptomatic and discovered incidentally, whereas malignant tumors almost al-

TABLE 3–1.

Classification of Hepatobiliary Neoplasms

Liver neoplasms
  Benign
    Hemangioma
    Focal nodular hyperplasia (FNH)
    Hepatocellular adenoma (HCA)
    Nodular regenerative hyperplasia (NRH)
    Infantile hemangioendothelioma (IHE)
    Mesenchymal hamartoma (MHL)
  Malignant
    Hepatocellular carcinoma (HCC)
    Fibrolamellar carcinoma
    Cholangiocarcinoma
    Angiosarcoma
    Undifferentiated (embryonal) sarcoma (UES)
    Hepatoblastoma
    Metastasis
    Lymphoma
  Focal fatty change
Gallbladder neoplasms
  Benign
    Adenomas
  Malignant
    Adenocarcinoma
    Metastasis
Bile duct neoplasms
  Benign
    Papilloma
    Cystadenoma
    Granular cell tumor
  Malignant
    Cholangiocarcinoma
    Ampullary carcinoma
    Metastasis
    Lymphoma

ways produce symptoms. The patient history may reveal such associations as hemochromatosis with hepatocellular carcinoma, thorium dioxide (Thorotrast) or vinyl chloride exposure with angiosarcoma, and contraceptive or anabolic steroid intake with adenoma.

Radiologically, there are many findings that are significant and that are to be taken into account in diagnosis. Among these findings are the solid vs. cystic nature of the mass, unifocal vs. multifocal presentation, calcification, homogeneity, intratumoral hemorrhage, pattern of enhancement, stellate areas of decreased density, shunting, compartmentalization, and portal invasion.

Plain films may play a significant role in detecting a right upper quadrant mass in a patient with abdominal pain, and thus in suggesting hepatic involvement and selecting sonography or CT as the next modality. Plain films of the abdomen are also helpful in demonstrating calcification (an important

finding in hepatic neoplasms), air in the biliary tree (which would indicate the presence of an enterobiliary fistula), and abnormalities in other areas of the abdomen, such as splenomegaly, ascites, and bone lesions.

The most valuable nuclear radiologic approaches in the workup of liver lesions are (1) studies utilizing technetium 99m–labeled red blood cells for the diagnosis of hemangioma, and (2) gallium scintigraphy, for the evaluation of HCC. Other uses of nuclear radiology in this area (e.g., monoclonal antibody imaging and single photon–emission computed tomography [SPECT]) are discussed in Chapter 13.

Sonography is able to demonstrate the internal nature of liver masses and detect the presence of septa, calcification, and areas of cystic transformation. Because of its ability to evaluate the hepatic texture, it may detect small lesions invisible by CT and other modalities. Sonography's ability to image vessels noninvasively can also be used in the study of liver neoplasms.

Computed tomography is probably the approach of choice for the evaluation of hepatic neoplasms because of its excellent depiction of abdominal anatomy (its imaging of other organs allowing disease staging), ability with enhancement to evaluate the vascularity of possible lesions, and superb demonstration of calcification.

Angiography is used in these lesions not only for interventional (embolization, ablation) and presurgical (vascular anatomy) purposes but also for diagnosis. Hypovascularity or hypervascularity, presence of normal vessels, arteriovenous shunting, delayed filling, venous pooling, and portal or hepatic vein invasion are important angiographic signs in defining the diagnosis.

Because of its high sensitivity, MRI is used in the evaluation of metastatic disease, and its ability to detect highly vascularized lesions with slow flow makes it helpful in the workup of possible hemangiomas.

Benign Tumors

Hemangioma.—Hemangioma is the most common benign tumor of the liver.[1] Its incidence in large autopsy series ranges from 0.5% to 10%, with a uniform geographic distribution and predominant occurrence in women (male/female ratio of 1:5). Although it affects all ages, it is rarely seen in young children.

Hemangiomas vary from several millimeters to several centimeters in diameter. They are usually solitary; multiple lesions are seen in about 10% of cases. Microscopically, hemangiomas are composed of vascular channels lined by endothelium. Typically, there are no symptoms; rupture and hemoperitoneum are very rare. A hemangioma can have a central area of fibrosis, and occasionally the tumor is entirely fibrotic.

Hemangioma may appear by plain films as an upper abdominal mass, more commonly on the right side. Calcification due to calcium deposition in an area of fibrosis or due to phleboliths may be seen.

Scintigraphy utilizing ^{99m}Tc–sulfur colloid or iminodiacetic acid (IDA) derivatives reveals a defect. Blood pool studies using ^{99m}Tc-labeled erythrocytes demonstrate the delayed filling of the initial defect[2] (Fig 3–1); this noninvasive approach has high specificity.[3] For identification of small hepatic hemangiomas, SPECT is a very sensitive modality; using red blood cells labeled in vitro with ^{99m}Tc, it can detect lesions as small as 1.0 cm.[4]

The usual sonographic features are those of a hyperechoic, sharply marginated mass with homogeneous internal pattern and some increased through-transmission.[1, 5] However, the sonographic appearance can vary from hyperechoic to mixed depending on the size, degree of fibrosis, presence of internal hemorrhage, and degree of cystic internal change (Fig 3–2). High-level echoes with acoustic shadowing can be seen if there are areas of calcification.

Unenhanced CT demonstrates a hypodense, well-marginated mass, usually near the surface of the liver, with central areas of markedly decreased attenuation corresponding to fibrosis or cystic change.[1] Calcification with irregular borders may be present. Dynamic CT offers another fairly specific method of diagnosis (Fig 3–2). Typically, there is contrast enhancement from the periphery to the center, lesions becoming isodense compared with the rest of the liver in delayed phase.[6] The presence of one or several enhancing nodules in the periphery during the early phase of contrast enhancement is common (Figs 3–2 and 3–3).

Prior to MRI, angiography was considered the most specific diagnostic method for hemangioma. The hepatic artery in these cases is normal in caliber due to lack of high-velocity arteriovenous shunting, and there are no tumoral vessels or early venous return. The presence of early pooling of contrast medium with a persistent very prolonged stain is characteristic of this entity and is responsible for the so-called cotton-wool appearance of hemangioma[7] (Figs 3–2 and 3–3).

Magnetic resonance imaging demonstrates cavernous hemangiomas with high degrees of sensitivity and specificity.[8] Cavernous hemangioma has a very high signal intensity on T_2-weighted images, whereas it is usually isointense with the liver on T_1-weighted images. These appearances probably reflect the large amount of slowly flowing blood within the intricate vascular channels of the tumor (see Fig 3–3).[9–11]

Focal Nodular Hyperplasia (FNH).—There is uncertainty about the nature of FNH: regenerative, hamartomatous, and neoplastic changes have been postulated. This condition, although rare, is twice as common as HCA. It is more common in women than in men, but this ratio is not as striking as in HCA. All ages are affected, although occurrence is predominantly in the third to fifth decades of life. Focal nodular hyperplasia is probably related to the use of contraceptive steroids.[12]

Grossly, FNH is a solitary and a firm *nodular mass*, frequently measuring less than 3 cm in diameter. It usually has a central stellate scar, and there are no areas of hemorrhage or necrosis. There is sharp demarcation by compressed liver but no true capsule. Microscopically, FNH is formed by normal hepatocytes abnormally arranged.

In 75% of cases, FNH is discovered incidentally. α-Fetoprotein and liver function values are within normal limits.

On plain films, there is evidence of a mass in the liver without calcification. This tumor may be pedunculated and project as an extrahepatic mass.

In approximately 50% of cases of FNH, there is normal accumulation of sulfur colloid (Fig 3–4).[13] In about 10% of cases, there is hyperconcentration of this radionuclide, indicating increased vascularity and possible higher concentration of Kupffer's cells. The tumor produces a defect in the scintiscan in about 40% of cases.

Sonographically, FNH appears as a well-demarcated hyperechogenic lesion (Fig 3–5). Homogeneous hypoechogenicity is rarely seen (Fig 3–4). The lack of anechoic areas reflects the solid nature of FNH and lack of central hemorrhage.

By CT, there is frequently a hypodense or isodense mass, with a hyperdense appearance following contrast injection. A central hypodense, irregular zone can be seen to correspond with the central fibrotic scar (Figs 3–4 and 3–5).[14] Occasionally the lesion will appear cystic on the CT study (Fig 3–6).

Magnetic resonance imaging can be helpful in diagnosing FNH and in distinguishing it from metastasis or other primary hepatic tumors such as hemangioma.[15] Focal nodular hyperplasia is usually either isointense or hypointense on T_1 images, and the central scar displays high signal intensity on T_2 images.

Angiographically, 80% to 90% of FNH cases are hypervascular. The fine radiations from the center to the periphery (centrifugal vascular supply) constitute the classic spoked-wheel pattern seen in as many as 70% of cases (Fig 3–5,D).[16] A very intense and homogeneous stain in the capillary phase without avascular zones is a reliable differential finding to distinguish FNH from HCA, since avascular zones are frequently seen in HCA.

Hepatocellular Adenoma (HCA).—Hepatocellular adenoma was extremely rare prior to 1960, after which its incidence increased, probably because of the widespread use of contraceptive steroids. It usually affects women of childbearing age, making it the most frequent tumor of the liver in women using contraceptive steroids.[12] It is practically not seen in men.

Hepatocellular adenomas are usually solitary, encapsulated, and large (average size, 8–10 cm). They are often subcapsular in location or pedunculated, facilitating local resection. They often present with foci of hemorrhage or necrosis. Microscopically, HCA is composed of sheets and cords of hepatocytes, mimicking normal liver; however, there are no portal or central veins or bile ducts. The vascular supply is received through the capsule.

Hepatocellular adenoma may be discovered incidentally as an asymptomatic hepatic mass, or it may produce right upper quadrant pain. Rupture with subsequent hemoperitoneum is not uncommon, and the possibility of this complication is the main reason for resection when the neoplasm is discovered serendipitously.

The plain film findings in HCA depend on the size of the tumor; presentation is often a nonspecific mass of soft tissue density without calcification. If the tumor is pedunculated, it may present as a right lower quadrant mass.

Sulfur-colloid scintigraphy commonly demonstrates a defect in the liver parenchyma (Fig 3–7). Although it is widely held that HCA does not accumulate ^{99m}Tc–sulfur colloid, uptake can be present.[17] Therefore, accumulation of activity by a hepatic tumor cannot be used as a definitive imaging criterion to exclude HCA in favor of FNH.

Sonographically, HCA may present as a well-defined, echogenic intrahepatic mass (Figs 3–7 and 3–8) with a central, single, large anechoic space or multiple, small, irregular anechoic areas.[18] The echogenicity of HCA is due to the presence of fat and glycogen within the tumor's hepatocytes. The areas of anechogenicity correspond to areas of hemorrhage, recent or old. Occasionally, in large adenomas, a central star-shaped area of decreased echogenicity, due to fibrosis, is detected (Fig 3–7).

On CT, HCA usually appears as a well-defined mass within the liver, commonly near its surface. The density varies from homogeneously hypodense (because of the fat and glycogen) to homogeneously isodense with the uninvolved liver parenchyma.[19] Unenhanced CT may demonstrate areas of increased density within a hypodense lesion, corresponding to recent intratumoral hemorrhage (Fig 3–9). This is a characteristic finding in HCA. Occasionally, HCA appears as a hepatic lesion with attenuation near water density because of massive necrosis. Computed tomography is able to identify hemoperitoneum secondary to rupture in HCA.

On MRI, HCA has an increased signal intensity on T_1- and T_2-weighted images because of its high glycogen and fat content.[20]

Hepatocellular adenoma is a hypervascular tumor, with large vessels on its periphery and centripetal flow (Fig 3–8). There is no arteriovenous shunting or vascular (portal or hepatic vein) invasion. In the capillary phase, there is an intense stain, and the tumors may contain small or large central avascular areas. The avascular areas are a helpful sign since they indicate the presence of the areas of hemorrhage common in HCA (Fig 3–9).

Nodular Regenerative Hyperplasia (NRH).—Nodular regenerative hyperplasia, also known as nodular transformation, is histologically characterized by diffuse involvement of the liver by hyperplastic nodules composed of cells resembling normal hepatocytes.[21] It occurs in men and women equally and is reported in all ages and races. Associated diseases are myeloproliferative syndromes and lymphoproliferative syndromes, among others. Various drugs have also been implicated, including steroids (particularly oral contraceptives) and antineoplastics.[22] The etiologic roles of these diseases and drugs and the exact incidence of NRH in these diseases are uncertain.

Grossly, the nodules range in size from a few millimeters to large masses. Structures such as bile ducts, portal veins, and hepatic artery branches may be trapped within the nodules. No significant fibrosis is found in or around the nodules, an important feature distinguishing NRH both from cirrhosis and hepatic FNH. Large nodules, viewed out of context of the diffuse nodularity, can histologically mimic HCA. Patients with NRH may have no symptoms or may present with idiopathic portal hypertension with varices, splenomegaly, or ascites.

The radiologic features of NRH reflect its composition by cells resembling normal hepatocytes and by the Kupffer's cells that may be present within or between the nodules. The nodules may take up ^{99m}Tc–sulfur colloid and have variable echogenicity on sonography. They are often hypodense on CT, without significant enhancement (Fig 3–10). Central hemorrhage within a large nodule may occur. Angiographically, the nodules are vascular and may fill in from the periphery, with hypovascular areas due to hemorrhage. These findings are nonspecific and may resemble some features of FNH, HCA, or metastases.[23]

Infantile Hemangioendothelioma (IHE).—Grossly, IHE may be round and smooth or multilobular and irregular. Although it has no true capsule, it tends to be well demarcated from surrounding liver since these tumors grow by compression rather than invasion. The tumor is reddish brown and is relatively soft and spongy. Central areas of large lesions tend to show evidence of infarction, hemorrhage, fibrosis, and foci of dystrophic calcification. Histologically, IHE consists of vascular spaces of variable size lined by fairly immature, plump endothelial cells, sometimes in multiple layers.

The most common clinical presentation is hepatomegaly with or without a palpable mass in an infant. High-output congestive heart failure occurs but is uncommon.[24] However, the presence of congestive heart failure with a liver mass strongly supports the diagnosis of IHE.[25]

Plain film may show a soft tissue mass with speckled calcification. Sonography is useful in localizing the mass to the liver and may show a hypoechoic, complex, or hyperechoic lesion. If there are large cystic components, the rare mesenchymal hamartoma is likely. Computed tomography using bolus intravenous contrast material with dynamic and delayed scans may show focal areas of low attenuation demonstrating early edge enhancement with variable delayed central enhancement. This pattern is similar to that of cavernous hemangioma in adults.[26] Radionuclide studies may be a useful adjunct to sonography and CT in demonstrating the hepatic origin of a lesion.

Angiography confirms the vascular nature of the mass but may be particularly useful in delineating the extent of the lesion when liver involvement is diffuse. There is often prolonged pooling of contrast material in vascular lakes or large areas of the tumor. Early arteriovenous shunting and enlarged tortuous feeding vessels are present in the cases with high-output congestive heart failure.

Mesenchymal Hamartoma (MHL).—Mesenchymal hamartoma of the liver is an uncommon cystic mass seen most often in infants.[27] It is thought to be a developmental anomaly rather than a true neoplasm and consists of an admixture of bile ducts and mesenchymal tissue. Before the term mesenchymal hamartoma was introduced, many synonyms were used: lymphangioma, bile cell fibroadenoma, hamartoma, cavernous lymphangiomatoid tumor, pseudocystic mesenchymal tumor, and cystic hamartoma.[28] The disease is usually manifested between the ages of four months and two years, with a few cases reported in newborns and in older patients. There is a slight male predominance.

Macroscopically, MHL is a solitary, round mass that is usually large and commonly located in the right lobe of the liver. On occasion, it is attached to the liver by a pedicle. The margin between the liver and the lesion is distinct, but typically a true capsule is not present. On the cut surface, there are multiple cysts in an edematous stroma. The cysts vary in size, from millimeters to 15 cm, and in number and distribution, being discrete or connected. Microscopically, MHL is characterized by an admixture of bile ducts in a prominent mesenchymal tissue. The cysts noted grossly are dilated bile ducts or fluid accumulations in the mesenchymal component.[29]

Clinically, there is usually a progressive painless abdominal enlargement, a palpable mass, or both, noted by the parents or on routine physical examination. Plain films of MHL demonstrate a large abdominal soft tissue mass usually involving the right upper quadrant; the mass may extend toward the pelvis and frequently crosses the midline. Calcification is usually not present.

Sulfur-colloid liver-spleen scintigraphy reveals a large defect and in general is a good adjunct to other imaging modalities to demonstrate the hepatic origin of the lesion.[30]

Ultrasound and CT findings reflect the spectrum of cystic changes observed pathologically, corresponding to the progressive accumulation of fluid in the bile ducts and degeneration of the mesenchyma.[31] On these two modalities, the appearance ranges from multiple small cysts in a solid mass, resembling Swiss cheese, to a multilocular cystic mass with intervening solid septa (Fig 3–11).[32]

Angiographically, MHL is a poorly vascularized tumor because of its cystic nature. The angiographic appearance ranges from a totally avascular mass producing displacement of major vessels in cases of cystic predominance to a hypovascular mass with fine tumor vessels (corresponding to the vascularization of the thick septa) surrounding avascular zones (corresponding to cysts).

Malignant Tumors

Hepatocellular Carcinoma (HCC).—Hepatocellular carcinoma, although rare in the United States, is one of the most frequent primary visceral malignancies in the world, with more than 1 million new cases per year. It has a bimodal geographic and age distribution; it is less common in the industrialized world, and relatively frequent in other areas (notably in sub-Saharan Africa and Asia).[33] In low-incidence areas, male predominance of HCC is 2.5 to 1, and the most common presentation is at 70 to 80 years of age, with rare occurrence at less than 40 years of age (c.f. in the fibrolamellar type below). In high-incidence areas, presentation is at 30 to 40 years of age, and men are affected eight times more commonly than women.

Grossly, there are three major forms: massive, nodular, and diffuse (cirrhotomimetic). If there is massive necrosis, HCC can appear cystic. Although vascular invasion (portal vein, hepatic veins, and inferior vena cava) is common,[34] invasion into the biliary system is rare. "Encapsulated" HCC may have a better prognosis than other types because of increased resectability.[35] Histologically, most HCCs are well differentiated.

In low-incidence areas, typically, onset of symptoms is insidious, whereas HCC usually has a very aggressive course and presents with rupture and massive hemoperitoneum in high-incidence areas. Jaundice is infrequent. Because of the production of hormones and pseudohormones by HCC, there are frequently paraneoplastic manifestations. Liver function tests are usually abnormal but the results indistinguishable from those in cirrhosis. α-Fetoprotein levels are consistently elevated.

By plain roentgenography, the findings are those of a nonspecific right upper quadrant mass of variable size. Calcification is almost never present in HCC, except in the fibrolamellar type. In patients with HCC and hemochromatosis, there are degenerative changes in joints (Fig 3–12).

Scintigraphy with ^{99m}Tc–sulfur colloid demonstrates a defect in a diffusely diseased liver (Fig 3–13),[36–38] which in a majority of cases will accumulate gallium.

Sonographically, the appearance of HCC is variable; however, this tumor frequently appears as a hypoechoic mass (Fig 3–12).[39] In about 25% of cases the tumor will be echogenic (Figs 3–14 and 3–15). The hyperechoic HCCs correlate with either fatty metamorphosis or marked sinusoidal dilatation.[40] Occasionally the tumor has a cystic sonographic appearance with irregularity in the wall (Fig 3–16). Ultrasonography is able to detect very small HCCs (2–3 cm), and it is advocated as the screening method, in combination with α-fetoprotein measurements, for HCC in high-risk patients.[41] By sonography, it is possible to noninvasively evaluate the presence of tumoral thrombi (Fig 3–17) in portal and hepatic veins as well as in the inferior vena cava.[42]

Computed tomography demonstrates a hepatic mass, generally of decreased attenuation, with rapid enhancement in dynamic scans.[43] Commonly, HCCs appear with large central areas of markedly decreased density, corresponding to necrosis (Fig 3–15).[44] They can be multicentric (Fig 3–18) or may appear cystic by both sonography and CT, making the differentiation from a cystic mass (e.g., cystadenoma, echinococcal cyst, biliary cyst) difficult (Figs 3–16 and 3–19). In patients with hemochromatosis, there is a very dense liver with an irregular contour, atrophy of the right lobe, prominence of the caudate lobe, and ascites—all signs of cirrhosis secondary to the iron deposition. The foci of HCC are seen as localized areas of hypodensity in the hyperdense liver. Computed tomography is helpful in the identification of encapsulated HCC (Fig 3–19). In these cases, a thin rim of low density is seen in the precontrast studies surrounding the HCC; this rim enhances after the administration of contrast material.

Hepatocellular carcinomas are very hypervascular tumors, with abnormal vessels (Figs 3–13 to 3–15), arteriovenous shunting, and vascular invasion.[45] Extension of HCC into the portal vein, hepatic veins, and inferior vena cava is commonly detected.[46] The sign of threads and streaks secondary to growth of HCC inside the portal vein is characteristic. Portal invasion can lead to cavernous transformation of the portal vein and thus to portal hypertension and esophageal varices (Fig 3–17).

On MRI,[47] HCC has a variable appearance. The signal intensity of the lesion may be low, high, or mixed. If there is steatosis in the HCC, there is high intensity; however, if fibrosis predominates, there is low intensity. The ring sign or peripheral halo characteristic of encapsulated HCC is detected more frequently by MRI than by CT.[48]

Fibrolamellar Carcinoma.—Fibrolamellar carcinoma (Fig 3–20) is considered by many authors to be a distinct entity and no longer a subtype of HCC. It is seen in adolescents and young adults, and there is no sex predominance. The most important differential point with typical HCC is fibrolamellar carcinoma's better prognosis.[49] Grossly, these tumors are firm and histologically show a characteristic lamellar fibrosis with no underlying cirrhosis. α-Fetoprotein levels are usually normal. The sonographic and CT findings reflect the tumor's homogeneous nature as seen on cut section and also its prominent fibrosis. By plain film calcification is frequently noted, and by sulfur-colloid scintigraphy there is a defect. Angiographically, a hypervascular mass with compartmentalization is the most common presentation.

Intrahepatic Cholangiocarcinoma.—Cholangiocarcinoma is considerably less common than HCC. It occurs more frequently in some Asian countries because of its association with the parasitic worm *Clonorchis sinensis.* In patients more than 60 years of age, it is more common in men than in women.[50]

There are several forms of cholangiocarcinoma according to the site of origin: (1) peripheral (10%), arising in the small intrahepatic ducts; (2) hilar, or Klatskin's tumor (25%); and (3) bile duct (65%). The intrahepatic forms (peripheral and hilar) are discussed here, and the bile duct form is discussed later. Cholangiocarcinoma is a firm, "woody" tumor with poor vascularity and, hence, infrequent areas of hemorrhage (Fig 3–21). Histologically, it is a well-differentiated adenocarcinoma that produces mucus but no bile.[51]

Cholangiocarcinoma is heralded by jaundice if it arises in the major ducts, such as the hepatic or the common bile duct. When it is peripherally located, its late discovery leads to a poor prognosis. α-Fetoprotein levels are usually within normal limits.

On plain films, intrahepatic cholangiocarcinoma presents as an upper abdominal mass. Calcification is frequent secondary to the tumor's secretion of mucus. There is focal defect by sulfur colloid and by IDA derivatives and there is no accumulation of gallium. The appearance of cholangiocarcinoma by sonography is that of a homogeneously hyperechoic mass, reflecting its uniform, firm nature.[52, 53] High-level echoes with shadowing, which represent calcified foci, are seen.[54]

Computed tomography shows a homogeneous, low-density mass, and areas of calcification are readily identified.[55–57] The angiographic appearance of the tumor is variable, with predominantly hypovascular or avascular patterns. Tumoral invasion of the portal or hepatic veins is uncommon.[58] Cholangiocarcinoma can be associated with thorium dioxide deposition (Fig 3–22).

Hepatic Sarcoma.—Angiosarcoma (Fig 3–23), is a rare tumor but is of special interest because of its association with previous exposure to thorium dioxide in approximately 50% of cases.[59] It is most commonly seen in adults in the sixth and seventh decades of life, and there is a male/female ratio of 4:1. Angiosarcoma is frequently a multicentric tumor with several well-circumscribed, purplish foci. Histologically, there are large sinusoidal spaces lined with sarcomatous cells. The prognosis is poor because there is rapid metastatic spread.

Plain films clearly demonstrate areas of increased density localized in the liver, spleen, and lymph nodes representing trapped thorium dioxide in the reticuloendothelial system.[60] However, in the angiosarcomas not secondary to thorium dioxide, the plain film appearance may be that of a nonspecific soft tissue mass in the liver.

Liver-spleen scintigraphy may reveal multiple defects in both the liver and spleen, corresponding to foci of angiosarcoma.[61] Computed tomography and ultrasound easily identify the dense and echogenic thorium dioxide and hypodense and echogenic parenchymal masses.[62, 63] Angiograms demonstrate hypervascular lesions with puddling of contrast.

Other sarcomas of the liver include leiomyosarcoma, fibrosarcoma, malignant fibrous histiocytoma, unclassified sarcoma, and embryonal rhabdomyosarcoma of bile ducts.[64] We have observed one case of primary osteosarcoma of the liver (Fig 3–23).

Undifferentiated (Embryonal) Sarcoma (UES).—Undifferentiated (embryonal) sarcoma is an uncommon malignant hepatic tumor of mesenchymal origin (Fig 3–24). The term has become generally accepted because the tumor is markedly undifferentiated and appears very primitive (i.e., embryonal). However, several synonyms have been used, including mesenchymal sarcoma, embryonal sarcoma, fibromyxosarcoma, mesenchoma, or simply primary sarcoma of the liver.[65] Although rare, UES is the fourth most common primary pediatric hepatic tumor (after hepatoblastoma, IHE, and HCC), occurring mostly in children six to ten years of age. However, there are cases reported in other age groups, particularly teenagers. The rarity of UES in patients less than five years old helps to distinguish this tumor from MHL, which, as previously mentioned, usually presents between the ages of four months and two years.

The usual presenting symptoms of UES are pain and abdominal mass. Patients may also have fever, jaundice, weight loss, and gastrointestinal complaints. α-Fetoprotein levels are usually not elevated.

Macroscopically, UES is a large, solitary, spherical mass with a variegated, predominantly yellowish to tan, glistening appearance with cystic areas on cut surface. Predominantly cystic tumors are more common than solid ones. The histologic pattern of UES is that of a rapidly growing, undifferentiated tumor with frequent mitoses. This rapid growth is probably responsible for the areas of necrosis and subsequent cystic degeneration. The abundant myxoid matrix of the tumor may be the cause of the hypodense appearance on CT scans.

Plain abdominal radiographs demonstrate a large noncalcified mass in the right upper quadrant, less commonly in the left upper quadrant, with displacement of the gastrointestinal tract. Liver scintiscans demonstrate a well-defined, photopenic intrahepatic mass. By sonography, the appearance ranges from a multiseptated cystic mass, with cysts of variable size (from a few millimeters to several centimeters), to a nonhomogeneous, predominantly echogenic mass. The hypoechogenicity nicely correlates with the degree of cystic change seen grossly. In solid UES, foci of calcification with high-level echoes and acoustic shadowing can be identified.[66]

By CT, UES appears as a hypodense mass compared with the normal liver, sometimes with density in the range of water.[66, 67] Septations are seen, frequently varying in number and thickness (Fig 3–24). Areas with muscle density are noted within the cystic tumors, corresponding to solid portions. A thin rim of dense tissue can be seen surrounding the cystic tumors, with increased absorption values after contrast injection, correlating with the tumoral pseudocapsule seen grossly. The tumors with values in the range of water by CT have cystic spaces filled with myxoid material, and the denser ones contain hemorrhagic and necrotic debris.

Angiographic studies demonstrate a large mass in the liver, with abnormal vessels. The mass can be hypovascular (decreased vascularity compared with normal liver), hypervascular (increased vascularity compared with normal liver), or avascular. Macroaneurysms can be seen, as well as arteriovenous shunting, pooling of contrast, and arterial encasement. The hypervascular pattern corresponds to predominantly solid tumors, and the most cystic UES demonstrates an avascular pattern.

Hepatoblastoma.—Hepatoblastoma is the most common primary liver neoplasm of childhood. It usually occurs in the first three years of life and may be present at birth. Although rarely, hepatoblastoma can appear in adolescents and adults. Hepatoblastoma is more frequent in males (2:1).[68]

Grossly, hepatoblastoma is usually a solitary mass (80% of cases), of large size, well circumscribed, and with a nodular or lobulated surface. Microscopically, epithelial (65%), mixed epithelial and mesenchymal (30%), and anaplastic (5%) types can be distinguished.

Clinically, patients with hepatoblastoma present with abdominal swelling, rarely accompanied by anorexia or weight loss. Signs of precocious puberty are occasionally encountered. Serum α-fetoprotein levels are elevated in most patients, and the levels closely parallel the course of the disease. Hepatoblastoma is usually a rapidly progressive malignancy, and lung metastases are common.

By plain radiographs, hepatoblastoma appears as a mass; frequently there is calcification, particularly in the mixed type (Fig 3–25). The calcifications are usually coarser than the ones seen in IHE.[69] By sonography, hepatoblastoma appears as an echogenic intrahepatic mass with foci of high-level echoes and shadowing corresponding to calcifications. Small hypoechoic areas are present, corresponding to hemorrhagic or necrotic spaces.[70, 71] Computed tomography demonstrates a solid, hypodense mass in the liver with minimal enhancement. Areas of nonhomogeneity are present more frequently in the mixed type. Computed tomography can detect more clearly than can sonography septations and lobulations. Hepatoblastoma appears hypointense on T_1-weighted MRI scans and hyperintense on T_2-weighted MRI scans. Magnetic resonance imaging nicely demonstrates the internal septations.

Angiographically, hepatoblastoma is usually a hypervascular mass, occasionally with a spoked-wheel pattern. Arteriovenous shunting is not commonly present, and invasion of vessels is rarely seen.[72]

Metastasis.—Hepatic metastases are common, accounting for 90% of all hepatic malignancies. The common primary sites are lung, colon, breast, and pancreas.[73]

The majority of these lesions are hypovascular. Hypervascular metastases are seen in pancreatic islet cell tumors, carcinoid (Fig 3–26), pheochromocytoma, renal cell carcinoma, and melanoma. Imaging studies of the liver are routinely performed in patients with known or suspected primary malignancies for the purpose of staging. For optimal screening, the imaging modality with the highest sensitivity should be utilized. However, specificity is important, because as many as 10% of adults have either a benign hepatic hemangioma or a simple liver cyst. Cost and efficiency are additional factors in choosing the best imaging modality. Liver metastasis detection rates of 93% for CT, 86% for scintigraphy, and 82% for ultrasound have been reported in patients with breast and colon carcinoma.[74]

Computed tomography remains accepted as the standard modality for detection and staging of metastatic disease in the liver. The CT appearance is widely variable, with lesions being solitary (Fig 3–27,A–C), multiple (Fig 3–27,D), or diffuse (Fig 3–28); small or large; regular or irregular in contour; and hypodense, isodense, or hyperdense. Lesions are homogeneous on CT. Contrast enhancement patterns also vary widely depending on the technique used to apply contrast medium (Figs 3–28 and 3–29). These characteristics can also vary between different lesions of the same histology.

Metastatic lesions with calcification are usually from mucinous adenocarcinoma of the colon (Fig 3–30). Other primaries include papillary serous ovarian cystadenocarcinoma, medullary carcinoma of the thyroid, renal cell carcinoma, and gastric malignancies. Treated metastases from any source may also calcify (Fig 3–31).

On unenhanced scans, most liver metastases are hypodense; 20% remain isodense.[75] Contrast-enhanced CT scanning increases the detection rate (see Fig 3–28). Rapid-infusion dynamic CT has a sensitivity of 91% to 98%, or more.[75–79] However, a few lesions will become isodense on enhanced scans and will be detected only on a precontrast study (Fig 3–29). Many of these lesions are hypervascular; therefore, obtaining both unenhanced and enhanced CT scans will increase the sensitivity of CT, particularly in patients with primary tumors that are hypervascular.[80]

In cases in which liver metastases have been detected by more conventional studies and a single hepatic lobe or segment found to be free of disease, partial hepatectomy may be contemplated for surgical cure. Under these circumstances, more sensitive staging can be done by means of delayed CT scanning or CT-angiography (Fig 3–32). Delayed (4–6 hr after contrast) CT was reported to detect more metastases than dynamic sequential CT in 7 of 15 patients, although no patients free of disease on dynamic CT were found to have lesions on delayed CT.[81] Computed tomography plus angiography can be done either during selective hepatic artery contrast injection or arterial portography by superior mesenteric artery injection (Fig 3–33). The latter should theoretically be more sensitive since normal liver is opacified by delivery of contrast via the portal system; thus, the metastases will be seen as hypodense lesions. In the former, on the other hand, direct opacification of metastatic foci by arterial contrast will show hyperdense lesions. In fact, since both primary and secondary hepatic neoplasms receive their blood supply almost exclusively from the hepatic artery, they are visualized as low-density areas on CT during portography. In 13 of 17 reported patients, CT–arterial portography detected more hepatic lesions than scintigraphy, ultrasound, conventional CT, or angiography.[82] Alternatively, intrahepatic arterial delivery of contrast medium is more sensitive than intravenous drip or bolus techniques for CT detection of hypervascular lesions.[76]

It is not possible to differentiate reliably among various hepatic metastases on the basis of the contrast enhancement pattern. Tumors of different histologies can demonstrate the same enhancement pattern, tumors of identical histology and size can demonstrate different enhancement patterns, and the enhancement pattern of a tumor changes with growth and size.[76, 83]

Organ-specific contrast agents such as ethiodized oil emulsions (EOEs) have been utilized to increase visualization of hepatic metastatic disease, showing significantly greater sensitivity than scintigraphy or CT utilizing iodinated water-soluble contrast.[85] However, the incidence of adverse reactions is higher with EOEs than with water-soluble contrast, and technical factors have limited their practical use.

In recent years, high-resolution real-time ultrasound has challenged CT as the most sensitive imaging modality in detecting small or diffuse hepatic masses (Fig 3–34).[86] However, the quality of the ultrasound examination depends on both the operator's expertise and the patient's body habitus or presence of overlying bowel gas. Attempts have been made to correlate sonographic appearance with histology in hepatic metastases. Cellular homogeneous masses usually produce a relatively sonolucent appearance, whereas nonhomogeneous arrays of fibrosis, calcification, or hypervascularity produce an echogenic appearance (Fig 3–35). Hemorrhagic lesions and metastases from gastrointestinal primaries tend to be echogenic, and necrotic masses tend to have a hypoechoic center. However, it should be noted that this correlation is far from perfect. Both hypervascular and hypovascular lesions can be either hyperechoic or hypoechoic.[87] Other studies have shown no correlation between histology and sonographic appearance of hepatic lesions.[88]

In cases of smooth, round, low-density hepatic lesions detected on CT, ultrasound is valuable in confirming the diagnosis of hepatic cysts as opposed to solid metastases.

Magnetic resonance imaging has been used in detection and characterization of liver tumors. The findings are based on both the elongation of T_1 and T_2 relaxation times of these lesions as well as on the strength of magnetic field (Fig 3–33,C–D).[48, 84]

Both CT and ultrasound have surpassed radionuclide liver scanning in sensitivity for detection of focal hepatic lesions.[74, 77] The development of SPECT has raised the sensitivity to between 85% and 87% vs. between 76% and 83% for planar scintigraphy,[79] but this sensitivity remains lower than that of CT. Radionuclide studies do have a particularly useful role in distinguishing focal fatty infiltration of the liver from metastases, as discussed later.

Lymphoma.—Primary lymphoma of the liver is very rare. Secondary liver involvement is more common, seen in both Hodgkin's and non-Hodgkin's lymphomas (Fig 3–36). One study of 323 lymphoma patients showed a sensitivity of 57% for CT and 71% for radionuclide scans in detecting hepatic involvement.[89] However, CT is the preferable examination, because it also provides information on abdominal lymph nodes. The CT findings are nonspecific, with the most common appearance being an infiltrative pattern with diffuse nonhomogeneity and normal or mildly increased liver size. Focal mass lesions are less common, but response to therapy is easily followed by CT in this form (Fig 3–36,D). The most common sonographic appearance is a fairly well defined hypoechoic mass without through-transmission. However, echogenic masses simulating metastases can be seen.

Focal Fatty Change

Focal fatty change of the liver is a well-recognized but poorly understood hepatocellular abnormality, most often associated with alcoholism, hepatitis, and obesity. It is also common in patients undergoing chemotherapy, in hyperalimentation, and in diabetes. It can take a diffuse or focal form

and may pose a diagnostic dilemma in liver imaging studies of cancer patients (Fig 3–37). The term focal fatty change or focal fatty liver is preferred to fatty infiltration since the latter has a pathologic implication of invasion or aggressiveness not seen in fatty liver. Computed tomography usually distinguishes focal fatty change from focal liver processes such as metastasis by the former's sharply marginated, geographic pattern and lack of mass effect on hepatic and portal veins. The change is usually nonspherical, with a density close to that of water; liver metastases, on the other hand, are usually round or oval, and unless cystic or necrotic, they have CT attenuation values closer to those of normal liver parenchyma than to those of water.[90]

Sonographically, focal fatty change appears as an area of increased echogenicity. Angulated, geometric margins between normal and fatty tissue and interdigitating margins with slender fingers of normal or fatty tissue (see Fig 3–37,C) are signs that may be useful for diagnosing the masslike areas in this abnormality and for distinguishing them sonographically from other hepatic masses.[91]

Also diagnostically useful is the fact that focal fatty change may resolve in days or weeks to a normal liver appearance on CT following better nutrition and complete abstinence from chemotherapy or alcohol. If CT and ultrasound are not diagnostic, and the lesions are more than 3 cm in diameter, normal findings on ^{99m}Tc-sulfur-colloid liver scan exclude space-occupying mass lesions such as metastases and confirm the diagnosis of focal fatty change.[90] Occasionally, percutaneous needle biopsy is needed to resolve diagnostic confusion.

Gallbladder

Benign Neoplasms

Benign neoplasms of the gallbladder are quite rare, and only adenoma is worth mentioning. Adenoma is usually an incidental finding of little clinical consequence. It may be associated with gallstones (<50% of cases) but is unlikely to cause symptoms by itself. Pathologically, gallbladder adenomas can be divided into tubular, papillary (i.e., villous), and mixed forms, analogous to colonic adenoma categories. However, unlike their colonic counterparts, gallbladder adenomas are believed to be an uncommon cause of invasive carcinoma.[92, 93] Unfortunately, however, these benign neoplasms are indistinguishable radiologically from small papillary adenocarcinomas. Multiple adenomas, which are seen in approximately one third of cases, may mimic cholesterol polyposis.

Malignant Neoplasms

Primary carcinoma of the gallbladder almost always arises from the epithelium and is usually some form of adenocarcinoma (although other histologic varieties are encountered). Almost all cases are associated with and, in fact, caused by cholelithiasis. For this reason, women are more likely to develop gallbladder carcinoma than men. Although gallbladder carcinoma is the most common neoplasm of the extrahepatic biliary tract, it is still a relatively uncommon malignancy.

In the past, gallbladder carcinoma was usually diagnosed intraoperatively, in patients undergoing cholecystectomy for presumed cholecystitis. At that time, the radiographic findings of gallbladder carcinoma were usually limited to a nonvisualizing oral cholecystogram. Now, however, with the aid of sonography and CT, a preoperative diagnosis of this malignancy is frequently made. Gallbladder carcinoma has a variety of appearances.[94, 95] It can appear as a persistent polypoid mass within the gallbladder lumen. Although several other conditions (including tumefacient sludge, hematoma, cholesterosis, and adenoma) can have this appearance, any persistent soft tissue mass within the gallbladder, particularly one that is associated with cholelithiasis (Fig 3–38, A–C), should be considered to be a carcinoma until proved otherwise. Another appearance of gallbladder carcinoma is that of either focal (Fig 3–38, D) or diffuse (Fig 3–38, E–F) thickening of the gallbladder wall. However, benign conditions such as adenomyomatosis and chronic cholecystitis,[96] particularly the uncommon xanthogranulomatous type,[97] can produce wall thickening that mimics carcinoma. Finally, the gallbladder (lumen and wall) may be entirely replaced by the carcinoma, producing the appearances of a solid subhepatic mass.[94, 95]

The important route of spread of gallbladder carcinoma is into the liver by direct extension, and this is present, at least microscopically, in the vast majority of cases. Regional nodal metastases to the cystic duct, common bile duct, and pancreaticoduodenal nodes are also quite common and contribute to the grim prognosis of this disease. Other modes of spread are intraluminal extension into adjacent extrahepatic bile ducts, direct extension into adjacent hollow viscera such as the duodenum or transverse colon, peritoneal implants, and distant hematogenous metastases.

Metastatic disease to the gallbladder is found fairly often in autopsy series, but, since this involvement is frequently asymptomatic, the clinical detection of gallbladder metastases is uncommon.[98] However, study may be done in an occasional patient because a gallbladder metastasis has caused acute cholecystitis (Fig 3–39).[99] Also, an abnormal gallbladder may be incidentally visualized during an examination of the abdomen performed for other reasons. In these instances, a diagnosis of metastatic disease can be made during life. The sonographic appearance of secondary malignancies is identical to that of primary carcinoma (see later discussion) with the exception that cholelithiasis is usually absent. The malignancy that is most likely to hematogenously metastasize to the gallbladder is melanoma (Fig 3–39),[100] although many other cancers have been reported in this context. Pancreatic, hepatobiliary, and other gastrointestinal carcinomas will more frequently involve the gallbladder by direct extension.[98]

Bile Ducts

Benign Neoplasms

Papillary adenoma *(papilloma)* is the most common of the generally uncommon benign biliary tumors. It usually occurs as a solitary polypoid lesion, but it may occur in a multifocal form termed *papillomatosis*. Histologically, these lesions are identical to the papillary adenomas of the gallbladder, but, whereas the gallbladder adenomas are uncommonly detected clinically, the biliary duct adenomas are more frequently discovered because they produce obstructive jaundice. Malignant degeneration of the solitary adenomas is unlikely, but because papillary adenoma cannot be distinguished from papillary carcinoma radiographically, resection is required nevertheless. Papillomatosis (Fig 3–40) is considered by some pathologists to be a premalignant condition, but even without malignant degeneration it can be fatal because of its propensity to recur and the difficulty of completely excising the tumors.

Cystadenoma of the biliary tract usually occurs in women and is analogous pathologically to the more common tumors of the same name involving the ovary and pancreas. It appears as a multiloculated cystic mass with variable amounts of solid tissue stroma.[101] Sonography and, to a lesser extent, CT will demonstrate the cystic nature of these tumors, but a cholangiogram will best demonstrate their origin in the bile duct wall. Malignant degeneration into a cystadenocarcinoma occurs infrequently, but unfortunately this change cannot be excluded on the basis of radiographic appearance (our unpublished data).

Granular cell tumor (formerly called *granular cell myoblastoma*) is a benign neoplasm of indeterminate cellular origin that occurs in many different soft tissue locations. In the biliary tract, the tumors are small, but the infiltration of the tumor within the bile duct wall produces a luminal narrowing and (often profound) biliary obstruction (Fig 3–41). Radiographically and even intraoperatively, granular cell tumor's appearance mimics that of the infiltrative form of cholangiocarcinoma, but its unique presentation in young, particularly black, women can lead to the correct diagnosis. Simple resection has been curative in all cases.[102]

Malignant Neoplasms

Lymphoma (Fig 3–42) and metastatic disease (Fig 3–43) involve the extrahepatic biliary ducts indirectly because of involvement of portal, common bile, or pancreaticoduodenal lymph nodes. Such involvement leads to extrinsic compression or actual invasion of the duct and is being recognized more frequently in recent years as a cause of jaundice in cancer patients.[103] However, the most important cause of secondary involvement of the extrahepatic duct remains local invasion by pancreatic carcinoma. This may cause stenosis or intraluminal filling defects within the common bile duct. Intrahepatic ducts may be similarly affected by HCC and metastatic disease of the liver.

As previously mentioned, cholangiocarcinoma is a term commonly used for adenocarcinoma of biliary ductal origin. Again, cholangiocarcinomas arising from the area of the hepatic duct bifurcation (Figs 3–44 and 3–45) are also called Klatskin's tumors. The carcinomas usually arise de novo, but they may be associated with other conditions that lead to chronic biliary inflammation, such as primary sclerosing cholangitis (Fig 3–46), Oriental cholangiohepatitis, choledocholithiasis, choledochal cyst (Fig 3–47), Caroli's disease, and biliary atresia. Also, as mentioned earlier, cholangiocarcinoma is one of several hepatic malignancies found in association with thorium dioxide exposure (Fig 3–22).[92] Cholangiocarcinomas are typically well-differentiated tumors histologically, but the frequent presence of local vascular and neural invasion and regional lymph node and hepatic metastases at the time of diagnosis leads to a very poor prognosis.[92]

Unlike adenocarcinoma of the gallbladder, these cancers are found more commonly in men than in women. Either the intrahepatic (10%–30% of cases) or extrahepatic ducts (70%–90% of cases) may be involved. Patients usually present with progressive obstructive jaundice and less commonly with symptoms of ascending cholangitis.[92]

The radiographic diagnosis of extrahepatic cholangiocarcinoma can be difficult. Most tumors are of an infiltrating type that produces an often severe ductal stenosis but a relatively small mass (Fig 3–48). Therefore, although CT and ultrasound will usually identify the level of biliary obstruction, a tumor mass will often not be seen.[57, 104] A recent report indicates that MRI may be more useful than CT or ultrasound in identifying cholangiocarcinoma.[105] Cholangiography, then, is often required to establish the diagnosis. The less common papillary variety of extrahepatic cholangiocarcinomas are more likely than other cholangiocarcinomas to be visible (as an intraluminal mass) on ultrasound or CT (Fig 3–48). Cholangiographically, a papillary cholangiocarcinoma will appear as a small polyp (indistinguishable from a papillary adenoma or sometimes even a calculus), a large intraluminal mass, or an indeterminate obstructing lesion.[106]

Ampullary carcinoma (Fig 3–49) is often considered a form of cholangiocarcinoma (although an adenocarcinoma in the ampullary region may actually originate in the duodenum or pancreas, in addition to the distal common bile duct or the ampulla proper). Because of the small size of the tumors at the time of presentation, cross-sectional imaging may fail to demonstrate a mass, and, again, cholangiography will be required for diagnosis. Cholangiography may reveal either a stricture or (occasionally) a filling defect in the most distal portion of the common bile duct. The presence of a polypoid mass in the duodenum and the coexistence of pancreatic duct dilatation help to establish the diagnosis.

SPLEEN

The spleen is a roughly oval organ that comprises the largest single collection of lymphocytes and reticuloendothelial cells in the body. However, it is supplied by arterial blood through the splenic artery and is therefore in the vascular rather than the lymphatic system.

Scintigraphy has been advocated as an excellent screening modality for splenic pathology.[107] In this study, ^{99m}Tc–sulfur colloid is used, and under normal circumstances homogeneous and equal uptake throughout the spleen is seen. Occasionally, because of an enlarged left lobe of the liver, variation in the shape of the spleen, accessory spleen, or large masses in adjacent organs simulating pathology, a misdiagnosis is made.[108] However, the recent development of SPECT has made the detection of smaller lesions more accurate (see Chapter 13).[109]

Sonography, however, is the most rewarding

noninvasive modality in the evaluation of the spleen. The normal spleen is usually as echogenic as the liver and homogeneous in nature.[110] Splenic lesions such as metastases and lymphoma are typically hypoechoic, but echogenic metastases are not uncommon, and focal echogenic lymphomatous deposits within the spleen have also been reported.[111]

On CT of the abdomen the spleen is seen, in virtually every patient, as a smoothly bordered, oblong or ovoid organ in the left upper quadrant. The density of the spleen is about 8 to 10 Hounsfield units less than that of the liver, which is the most dense visceral organ in the abdomen.[112] The spleen is optimally imaged by beginning with an unenhanced CT scan, followed by bolus intravenous contrast. However, it should be noted that dynamic CT of the spleen will occasionally show marked nonhomogeneity of the splenic parenchyma, probably because of variable rates of blood flow to the splenic red pulp.[113] Imaging in a later phase will demonstrate homogeneous density in the spleen, in most cases within 2 min of bolus injection (see Chapter 14).[114]

Ethiodized oil emulsion 13 (EOE-13) has been advocated as an intravenous contrast agent for evaluation of the spleen and liver. At 0.5 g of iodine/kg of body weight, it increases splenic enhancement by 52.3 Hounsfield units on average.[85] This contrast agent is extremely sensitive to tumor detection; however, it is neither currently available nor approved by the Food and Drug Administration.

In almost all patients, the splenic neoplasm is seen as an area of low-attenuation mass. The CT differential diagnosis of large, solitary or multiple splenic masses with low attenuation includes abscess, metastatic carcinoma, hematoma, angiosarcoma, Hodgkin's disease, hemangioma, lymphangioma, infarct, and splenic cyst.[115, 116] When the large mass is associated with retroperitoneal adenopathy, diagnosis of lymphoma is most likely.[117]

With its multiplanar capability, MRI is able to image the spleen in several projections. It is probably the most accurate way to evaluate the craniocaudal dimensions of the spleen. Unlike CT, it is noninvasive and does not require intravenous contrast, but like CT it is able to simultaneously evaluate the retroperitoneum for possible nodal disease in cases of lymphoma or leukemia and may be able to differentiate benign from malignant processes.[114]

The most common primary benign tumor of the spleen is hemangioma (Fig 3–50). These tumors are sometimes only a few millimeters in diameter, more often measuring 1 to 2 cm, but occasionally so large

as to cause splenomegaly.[116] Next in frequency are the lymphangiomas (Fig 3–51), which also may be very large and may present as multicentric lesions. Other benign tumors, such as fibroma, chondroma, and osteoma, are extremely rare. Occasionally, very well circumscribed but not encapsulated nodules made up of splenic tissue are seen within the splenic parenchyma; they have been called hamartomas, splenomas, splenic adenomas, and intrasplenic accessory spleen.[118]

The spleen is rarely the site of a primary malignant tumor, and most of the leukemias (Fig 3–52) and lymphomas, being multicentric in origin, are excluded from classification as primary splenic neoplasms. Rarely, lymphomas of different cell type, particularly non-Hodgkin's lymphoma, seem to originate in the spleen, and they have been called primary lymphomas of the spleen.[119, 120] Even in these unusual cases, there is often lymph node or bone marrow involvement by the disease. Bostick found only five primary splenic tumors among 17,707 autopsies and 68,820 surgeries, comprising two non-Hodgkin's lymphomas, two angiomas, and one epidermoid cyst.[121] Ninety percent of the primary malignant neoplasms of the spleen reported by Das Gupta et al. were non-Hodgkin's lymphomas.[122] In a review of 49 pathologic specimens, Ahmann et al. described four different patterns of splenic involvement by lymphoma (Fig 3–53): homogeneous enlargement with no masses, miliary masses measuring 1 to 5 mm, multiple masses measuring 2 to 10 cm, and a large solitary mass.[123] The masses, both multiple and single, were seen only in Hodgkin's disease and large cell lymphoma. Occasionally the masses are seen only on EOE-13 study (Fig 3–54).

Metastases to the spleen (Fig 3–55) are not uncommon, due to the high incidence of splenic involvement in melanoma.[124] However, metastases from other tumors are rare, occurring mainly in cancers of the lung, breast, stomach, and ovary and in chondrosarcoma and choriocarcinoma.[115] Usually, these lesions are of low density on CT and hypoechoic or occasionally echogenic on ultrasound.[110] Rarely conditions such as multiple myeloma will infiltrate the spleen and present as focal splenic lesions (Fig 3–56).

In hematologic conditions such as myelofibrosis and myeloid metaplasia, there is overgrowth of hematopoietic and connective tissue elements both within the bone marrow and at reticuloendothelial sites. The spleen may become very large (Fig 3–57), and at times the patient will present only with splenomegaly.

Acknowledgments

We thank the many radiologists and pathologists who sent their material to the Armed Forces Institute of Pathology since it is the basis for this study. We also thank John F. Rasmussen, M.D., of the Department of Radiology, University of Florida, for his valuable contribution in this chapter.

The opinions and assertions contained herein are the private views of the authors and are not to be constructed as official or as reflecting the views of the Departments of the Navy and Defense.

REFERENCES

1. Itai Y., Ohtomo K., Araki T., et al.: Computed tomography and sonography of cavernous hemangioma of the liver. *AJR* 141:315–320, 1983.
2. Moinuddin M., Allison J.R., Montgomery J.H., et al.: Scintigraphic diagnosis of hepatic hemangioma: its role in the management of hepatic mass lesions. *AJR* 145:223–228, 1985.
3. Rabinowitz S.A., McKusick K.A., Strauss H.W.: 99mTc red blood cell scintigraphy in evaluating focal liver lesions. *AJR* 143:63–68, 1984.
4. Brodsky R.I., Friedman A.C., Maurer A.H., et al.: Hepatic cavernous hemangioma: diagnosis with 99mTc-labeled red cells and single-photon emission CT. *AJR* 148:125–129, 1987.
5. Bree R.L., Schwab R.E., Neiman H.L.: Solitary echogenic spot in the liver: is it diagnostic of a hemangioma? *AJR* 140:41–45, 1983.
6. Mikulis D.J., Costello P., Clouse M.E.: Hepatic hemangioma: atypical appearance. *AJR* 145:77–78, 1985.
7. Takayasu K., Moriyama N., Shima Y., et al.: Atypical radiographic findings in hepatic cavernous hemangioma: correlation with histologic features. *AJR* 146:1149–1153, 1986.
8. Glazer G.M., Aisen A.M., Francis I.R., et al.: Hepatic cavernous hemangioma: magnetic resonance imaging. Work in progress. *Radiology* 155:417–420, 1985.
9. Itai Y., Ohtomo K., Furui S., et al.: Noninvasive diagnosis of small cavernous hemangioma of the liver: advantage of MRI. *AJR* 145:1195–1199, 1985.
10. Stark D.D., Felder R.C., Wittenberg J., et al.: Magnetic resonance imaging of cavernous hemangioma of the liver: tissue-specific characterization. *AJR* 145:213–222, 1985.
11. Ros P.R., Lubbers P.R., Olmsted W.W., et al.: Hemangioma of the liver. Magnetic resonance–gross morphologic correlation. *AJR* 149:1167–1170, 1987.
12. Knowles D.M. II, Casarella W.J., Johnson P.M., et al.: The clinical, radiologic, and pathologic characterization of benign hepatic neoplasms. Alleged association with oral contraceptives. *Medicine* (Baltimore) 57:223–237, 1978.
13. Biersack H.J., Thelen M., Torres J.F., et al.: Focal nodular hyperplasia of the liver as established by 99mTc sulfur colloid and HIDA scintigraphy. *Radiology* 137:187–190, 1980.
14. Welch T.J., Sheedy P.F. II, Johnson C.M., et al.: Focal nodular hyperplasia and hepatic adenoma: comparison of angiography, CT, US and scintigraphy. *Radiology* 156:593–595, 1985.
15. Mattison G.R., Glazer G.M., Quint L.E., et al.: MR imaging of hepatic focal nodular hyperplasia: characterization and distinction from primary malignant hepatic tumors. *AJR* 148:711–715, 1987.
16. Rogers J.V., Mack L.A., Freeny P.C., et al.: Hepatic focal nodular hyperplasia: angiography, CT, sonography and scintigraphy. *AJR* 137:983–990, 1981.
17. Lubbers P.R., Ros P.R., Goodman Z.D., et al.: Accumulation of technetium 99m sulfur colloid by hepatocellular adenoma: scintigraphic-pathologic correlation. *AJR* 148:1105–1108, 1987.
18. Sandler M.A., Petrocelli R.D., Marks D.S., et al.: Ultrasonic features and radionuclide correlation in liver cell adenoma and focal nodular hyperplasia. *Radiology* 135:393–397, 1980.
19. Mathieu D., Bruneton J.N., Drouillard J., et al.: Hepatic adenomas and focal nodular hyperplasia: dynamic CT study. *Radiology* 160:53–58, 1986.
20. Davis P.L., Moss A.A., Goldberg H.I., et al.: Nuclear magnetic resonance imaging of the liver and pancreas. *RadioGraphics* 4:159–169, 1984.
21. Sherlock S., Feldman C.A., Moran B., et al.: Partial nodular transformation of the liver with portal hypertension. *Am. J. Med.* 40:195–203, 1966.
22. Stromeyer F.W., Ishak K.G.: Nodular transformation (nodular "regenerative" hyperplasia) of the liver. A clinicopathologic study of 30 cases. *Hum. Pathol.* 12:60–71, 1981.
23. Dachman A.H., Ros P.R., Goodman Z.D., et al.: Nodular regenerative hyperplasia of the liver: radiographic description. *AJR* 148:717–722, 1987.
24. Ishak K.G., Rabin L.: Benign tumors of the liver. *Med. Clin. North Am.* 59:995–1013, 1975.
25. Dachman A.H., Lichtenstein J.E., Friedman A.C.: Infantile hemangioendothelioma of the liver: a radiologic-pathologic-clinical correlation. *AJR* 140:1091–1096, 1983.
26. Lucaya J., Enriquez G., Amat L., et al.: Computed tomography of infantile hepatic hemangioendothelioma. *AJR* 144:821–826, 1985.
27. Lanuza A., Perez-Candela V., Ceres L., et al.: Hepatic hamartoma in a newborn. *Pediatr. Radiol.* 9:111–112, 1980.
28. Wendth A.J. Jr., Shamoun J., Pantoja E., et al.: Cystic hamartoma of the liver in a pediatric patient. Angiographic findings. *Radiology* 121:440, 1976.
29. Ros P.R., Goodman Z.D., Ishak M.G., et al.: Mesen-

chymal hamartoma of the liver: radiologic-pathologic correlation. *Radiology* 158:619–624, 1986.

30. Siebert J.J., Soper R.T.: Preoperative diagnosis of benign hepatic hamartoma by correlation of radioisotopic and angiographic studies. *Pediatr. Radiol.* 4:149–152, 1976.

31. Rosenbaum D.M., Mindell H.J.: Ultrasonographic findings in mesenchymal hamartoma of the liver. *Radiology* 138:425–427, 1981.

32. Donovan T.A., Wolverson M.K., DeMello D., et al.: Multicystic hepatic mesenchymal hamartoma of childhood: CT and US characteristics. *Pediatr. Radiol.* 11:163–165, 1981.

33. Takashima T., Matsui I., Suzuki M., et al.: Diagnosis and screening of small hepatocellular carcinomas. *Radiology* 145:635–638, 1982.

34. Subramanyam B.R., Balthazar E.J., Hilton S., et al.: Hepatocellular carcinoma with venous invasion. *Radiology* 150:793–796, 1984.

35. Ebara M., Ohto M., Watanabe Y., et al.: Diagnosis of small hepatocellular carcinoma: correlation of MR imaging and tumor histologic studies. *Radiology* 159:371–377, 1986.

36. Desai A.G., Shaffer B., Park C.H.: Accumulation of bone-scanning agents in hepatoma. *Radiology* 149:292, 1983.

37. Lee V.W., O'Brien M.J., Devereux D.F., et al.: Hepatocellular carcinoma: uptake of ^{99m}Tc-IDA in primary tumor and metastasis. *AJR* 143:57–61, 1984.

38. Kudo M., Hirasa M., Takakuwa H.: Small hepatocellular carcinomas in chronic liver disease: detection with SPECT. *Radiology* 159:697–703, 1986.

39. Cottone M., Marceno M.P., Maringhini A., et al.: Ultrasound in the diagnosis of hepatocellular carcinoma associated with cirrhosis. *Radiology* 147:517–519, 1983.

40. Tanaka S., Kitamura T., Imaoka S., et al.: Hepatocellular carcinoma: sonographic and histologic correlation. *AJR* 140:701–707, 1983.

41. Sheu J.C., Chen D.S., Sung J.L., et al.: Hepatocellular carcinoma: US evolution in the early stage. *Radiology* 155:463–467, 1985.

42. Kauzlaric D., Petrovic M., Barmeir E.: Sonography of cavernous transformation of the portal vein. *AJR* 142:383–384, 1984.

43. Mathieu D., Grenier P., Larde D., et al.: Portal vein involvement in hepatocellular carcinoma. Dynamic CT features. *Radiology* 152:127–132, 1984.

44. LeBerge J.M., Lain F.C., Federle M.P., et al.: Hepatocellular carcinoma: assessment of resectability by computed tomography and ultrasound. *Radiology* 152:485–490, 1984.

45. Sumida M., Ohto M., Ebara M., et al.: Accuracy of angiography in the diagnosis of small hepatocellular carcinoma. *AJR* 147:531–536, 1986.

46. Takayasu K., Shima Y., Muramatsu Y., et al.: Angiography of small hepatocellular carcinomas: analy-

sis of 105 resected tumors. *AJR* 147:525–529, 1986.

47. Ohtomo K., Itai Y., Furui S., et al.: MR imaging of portal vein thrombus in hepatocellular carcinoma. *J. Comput. Assist. Tomogr.* 9:328–329, 1985.

48. Ohtomo K., Itai Y., Yoshikawa K., et al.: Hepatic tumors: dynamic MR imaging. *Radiology* 163:27–31, 1987.

49. Friedman A.C., Lichtenstein J.E., Goodman Z., et al.: Fibrolamellar hepatocellular carcinoma. *Radiology* 157:583–587, 1985.

50. Herba M.J., Casola G., Bret P.M., et al.: Cholangiocarcinoma as a late complication of choledochoenteric anastomoses. *AJR* 147:513–515, 1986.

51. Ros P.R., Buck J.L., Goodman Z.D., et al.: Intrahepatic cholangiocarcinoma: radiologic–pathologic correlation. *Radiology* (in press).

52. Machan L., Muller N.L., Cooperberg P.L.: Sonographic diagnosis of Klatskin tumors. *AJR* 147:509–512, 1986.

53. Meyer D.G., Weinstein B.J.: Klatskin tumors of the bile ducts: sonographic appearance. *Radiology* 148:803–804, 1983.

54. Subramanyam B.R., Raghavendra B.N., Balthazar E.J., et al.: Ultrasonic features of cholangiocarcinoma. *J. Ultrasound Med.* 3:405–408, 1984.

55. Itai Y., Araki T., Fururi S., et al.: Computed tomography of primary intrahepatic biliary malignancy. *Radiology* 147:485–490, 1983.

56. Carr D.H., Hadjis N.S., Banks L.M., et al.: Computed tomography of hilar cholangiocarcinoma: a new sign. *AJR* 145:53–56, 1985.

57. Thorsen M.K., Quiroz F., Lawson T.L., et al.: Primary biliary carcinoma: CT evaluation. *Radiology* 152:479–483, 1984.

58. Takayasu K., Muramatsu Y., Shima Y., et al.: Hepatic lobar atrophy following obstruction of the ipsilateral portal vein from hilar cholangiocarcinoma. *Radiology* 160:389–393, 1986.

59. Miller T.A., Ros P.R., Buck J.L., et al.: Angiosarcoma of the liver: radiologic-pathologic correlation. (Submitted for publication).

60. Levy D.W., Rindsberg S., Friedman A.C., et al.: Thorotrast-induced hepatosplenic neoplasia: CT identification. *AJR* 146:997–1004, 1986.

61. Whelan J.G. Jr., Creech J.L., Tamburro C.L.: Angiographic and radionuclide characteristics of hepatic angiosarcoma in vinyl chloride workers. *Radiology* 118:549–557, 1976.

62. Mahony B., Jeffrey R.B., Federle M.P.: Spontaneous rupture of hepatic and splenic angiosarcoma demonstrated by CT. *AJR* 138:965–966, 1982.

63. Silverman P.M., Ram P.C., Korobkin M.: CT appearance of abdominal Thorotrast deposition and Thorotrast-induced angiosarcoma of the liver. *J. Comput. Assist. Tomogr.* 4:655–658, 1983.

64. Goodman Z.D., Ishak K.G.: Non-parenchymal and metastatic malignant tumors of the liver, in Berk J.E.

(ed.): *Bockus Gastroenterology*, vol. 5: *Liver*. Philadelphia, W.B. Saunders Co., 1985, pp. 3377–3387.

65. Stocker J.T., Ishak K.G.: Undifferentiated (embryonal) sarcoma of the liver. Report of 31 cases. *Cancer* 42:336–348, 1978.

66. Ros P.R., Olmsted W.W., Dachman A.H., et al.: Undifferentiated (embryonal) sarcoma of the liver: radiologic-pathologic correlation. *Radiology* 160: 141–145, 1986.

67. Vermess M., Collier N.A., Mutum S.S., et al.: Misleading appearance of a rare malignant liver tumour on computed tomography. *Br. J. Radiol.* 57:262–265, 1984.

68. Giacomantonio M., Ein S.H., Mancer K., et al.: Thirty years of experience with pediatric primary malignant liver tumors. *J. Pediatr. Surg.* 19:523–526, 1984.

69. Dachman A.H., Parker R.L., Ros P.R., et al.: Hepatoblastoma: a radiologic-pathologic clinical correlation. *Radiology* 164:15–19, 1987.

70. Kaude J.V., Felman A.H., Hawkins I.F. Jr.: Ultrasonography in primary hepatic tumors in early childhood. *Pediatr. Radiol.* 9:77–83, 1980.

71. Miller J.H.: The ultrasonographic appearance of cystic hepatoblastoma. *Radiology* 138:141–143, 1981.

72. Smith W.L., Franken E.A., Mitros F.A.: Liver tumors in children. *Semin. Roentgenol.* 18:136–148, 1983.

73. Gilbert H.A., Kogan A.R.: Metastases: incidence, detection, and evaluation, in Weiss L. (ed.): *Fundamental Aspects of Metastasis*. New York, Elsevier North-Holland, 1976.

74. Alderson P.O., Adams D.F., McNeil B.J., et al.: Computed tomography, ultrasound and scintigraphy of the liver in patients with colon or breast carcinoma: a prospective comparison. *Radiology* 149: 225–230, 1983.

75. Alpern M.B., Lawson T.L., Foley W.D., et al.: Focal hepatic masses and fatty infiltration detected by enhanced dynamic CT. *Radiology* 158:45–49, 1986.

76. Moss A.A., Dean P.B., Axel L., et al.: Dynamic CT of hepatic masses with intravenous and intra-arterial contrast material. *AJR* 138:847–852, 1982.

77. Knopf D.R., Torres W.E., Fajman W.J., et al.: Liver lesions: comparative accuracy of scintigraphy and computed tomography. *AJR* 138:623–627, 1982.

78. Foley W.D., Berland L.L., Lawson T.L., et al.: Contrast enhancement technique for dynamic hepatic computed tomographic scanning. *Radiology* 147: 797–803, 1983.

79. Brendel A.J., Leccia F., Drouillard J., et al.: Single photon emission computed tomography (SPECT), planar scintigraphy, and transmission computed tomography: a comparison of accuracy in diagnosing focal hepatic disease. *Radiology* 153:527–532, 1984.

80. Bressler E.L., Alpern M.B., Glazer G.M., et al.: Hypervascular hepatic metastases: CT evaluation. *Radiology* 162:49–51, 1987.

81. Bernardino M.E., Erwin B.C., Steinberg H.V., et al.: Delayed hepatic CT scanning: increased confidence and improved detection of hepatic metastases. *Radiology* 159:71–74, 1986.

82. Matsui O., Kadoya M., Suzuki M., et al.: Work in progress: dynamic sequential computed tomography during arterial portography in the detection of hepatic neoplasms. *Radiology* 146:721–727, 1983.

83. Burgener F.A., Hamlin D.J.: Contrast enhancement of focal hepatic lesions in CT: effect of size and histology. *AJR* 140:297–301, 1983.

84. Ohtomo K., Itai Y., Furui S., et al.: Hepatic tumors: differentiation by transverse relaxation time (T2) of magnetic resonance imaging. *Radiology* 155:421–423, 1985.

85. Miller D.L., Vermess M., Doppman J.L., et al.: CT of the liver and spleen with EOE-13: review of 225 examinations. *AJR* 143:235–253, 1984.

86. Sheu J.C., Sung J.L., Chen D.S., et al.: Ultrasonography of small hepatic tumors using high-resolution linear-array real-time instruments. *Radiology* 150: 797–802, 1984.

87. Green B., Bree R.L., Goldstein H.M., et al.: Gray scale ultrasound evaluation of hepatic neoplasms: patterns and correlations. *Radiology* 124:203–208, 1977.

88. Scheible W., Gosink B.B., Leopold G.R.: Gray scale echographic patterns of hepatic metastatic disease. *AJR* 129:983–987, 1977.

89. Zornoza J., Ginaldi S.: Computed tomography in hepatic lymphoma. *Radiology* 138:405–410, 1981.

90. Halvorsen R.A., Korobkin M., Ram P.C., et al.: CT appearance of focal fatty infiltration of the liver. *AJR* 139:277–281, 1982.

91. Quinn S.F., Gosink B.B.: Characteristic sonographic signs of hepatic fatty infiltration. *AJR* 145:753–755, 1985.

92. Albores-Saavedra J., Henson D.E.: Tumors of the gallbladder and extrahepatic bile ducts, in *Atlas of Tumor Pathology*. Washington, D.C., Armed Forces Institute of Pathology, ser. 2, fasc. 22, 1986.

93. Christensen A.H., Ishak K.G.: Benign tumors and pseudo-tumors of the gallbladder. Report of 180 cases. *Arch. Pathol.* 90:423–432, 1970.

94. Yeh H.C.: Ultrasonography and computed tomography of carcinoma of the gallbladder. *Radiology* 133:167–173, 1979.

95. Weiner S.N., Koenigsberg M., Morehouse H., et al.: Sonography and computed tomography in the diagnosis of carcinoma of the gallbladder. *AJR* 142: 735–739, 1984.

96. Smathers R.L., Lee J.K.T., Heiken J.P.: Differentiation of complicated cholecystitis from gallbladder carcinoma by computed tomography. *AJR* 143: 255–259, 1984.

97. Duber C., Storkel S., Wagner P.K., et al.: Xanthogranulomatous cholecystitis mimicking carcinoma of

the gallbladder: CT findings. *J. Comput. Assist. Tomogr.* 8:1195–1197, 1984.

98. Phillips G., Pochaczevsky R., Goodman J., et al.: Ultrasound patterns of metastatic tumors in the gallbladder. *Journal of Clinical Ultrasound* 10:379–383, 1982.

99. Bundy A.L., Ritchie W.G.M.: Ultrasonic diagnosis of metastatic melanoma of the gallbladder presenting as acute cholecystitis. Case report. *Journal of Clinical Ultrasound* 10:285–287, 1982.

100. Shimkin P.M., Soloway M.S., Jaffe E.: Metastatic melanoma of the gallbladder. *AJR* 116:393–395, 1972.

101. Ishak K.G., Willis G.W., Cummins S.D., et al.: Biliary cystadenoma and cystadenocarcinoma: report of 14 cases and review of literature. *Cancer* 38:322–338, 1977.

102. Orenstein J.J., Brenner L.H., Nay H.R.: Granular cell myoblastoma of the extrahepatic biliary system. *Am. J. Surg.* 147:827–831, 1984.

103. Zeman R.K., Burnell M.I.: *Gallbladder and Bile Duct Imaging: A Clinical-Radiologic Approach.* New York, Churchill Livingstone, 1987.

104. Levine E., Maklad N.F., Wright C.H., et al.: Computed tomographic and ultrasonic appearances of primary carcinoma of the common bile duct. *Gastrointest. Radiol.* 4:147–151, 1979.

105. Dooms G.C., Kerlan R.K. Jr., Hricak H., et al.: Cholangiocarcinoma: imaging by MR. *Radiology* 159:89–94, 1986.

106. Nichols D.A., MacCarty R.L., Gaffey T.A.: Cholangiographic evaluation of bile duct carcinoma. *AJR* 141:1291–1294, 1983.

107. Drum D.E.: Current status of radiocolloid hepatic scintiphotography for space-occupying disease. *Semin. Nucl. Med.* 12:64–74, 1982.

108. Djang W.T., Young S.W., Castellino R.A., et al.: Computed tomography of the liver: evaluating focal defects on radionuclide liver-spleen scans. *AJR* 142:937–940, 1984.

109. Keyes J.W. Jr.: Perspectives on tomography. *J. Nucl. Med.* 23:633–640, 1982.

110. Mittelstaedt C.A.: Ultrasound of the spleen. *Seminars Ultrasound* 2:233–240, 1981.

111. Mittelstaedt C.A., Partain C.L.: Ultrasonic-pathologic classification of splenic abnormalities: gray-scale patterns. *Radiology* 134:697–705, 1980.

112. Piekarski J., Goldberg H.I., Royal S.A., et al.: Difference between liver and spleen CT numbers in the normal adult: its usefulness in predicting the presence of diffuse liver disease. *Radiology* 137:727–729, 1980.

113. Glazer G.M., Axel L., Goldberg H.I., et al.: Dynamic CT of the normal spleen. *AJR* 137:343–346, 1981.

114. Morehouse H.T., Thornhill B.A.: Splenic disease: a modern approach. *Postgraduate Radiology* 7:112–132, 1987.

115. Piekarski J., Federle M.P., Moss A.A., et al.: CT of the spleen. *Radiology* 135:683–689, 1980.

116. Ros P.R., Moser R.P. Jr., Dachman A.H., et al.: Hemangioma of the spleen: radiologic-pathologic correlation in ten cases. *Radiology* 167:73–77, 1987.

117. Meyer J.E., Harris N.L., Elman A., et al.: Large-cell lymphoma of the spleen: CT appearance. *Radiology* 148:199–201, 1983.

118. Rappaport H.: Tumors of the hematopoietic system, in *Atlas of Tumor Pathology.* Ser. 3, fasc. 8. Washington, D.C., Armed Forces Institute of Pathology, 1966, pp. 49 and 64.

119. Anderson W.A.D., Kissane J.M. (eds.): *Pathology.* St. Louis, C.V. Mosby Co., 1977, vol. 2, pp. 1489–1504.

120. Lessig H.J., Croll M.N., Brady L.W.: Primary splenic tumor diagnosed by preoperative sulfur colloid scan. *Applied Radiology* 6:207–208, 1977.

121. Bostick W.L.: Primary splenic neoplasms. *Am. J. Pathol.* 21:1143–1165, 1945.

122. Das Gupta T., Coombes B., Brasfield R.D.: Primary malignant neoplasms of the spleen. *Surg. Gynecol. Obstet.* 120:947–960, 1965.

123. Ahmann D.L., Kiely J.M., Harrison E.G. Jr., et al.: Malignant lymphoma of the spleen. A review of 49 cases in which the diagnosis was made at splenectomy. *Cancer* 19:461–469, 1966.

124. Shawker T.H.: Tumor invasion and dissemination, in Brascho D.J., Shawker T.H. (eds.): *Abdominal Ultrasound in the Cancer Patient.* New York, John Wiley & Sons, 1980, pp. 49–92.

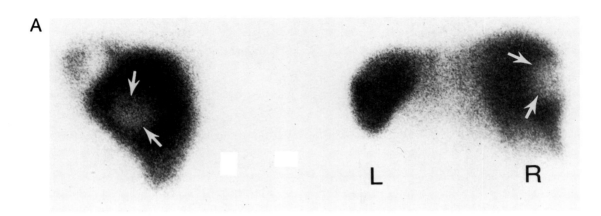

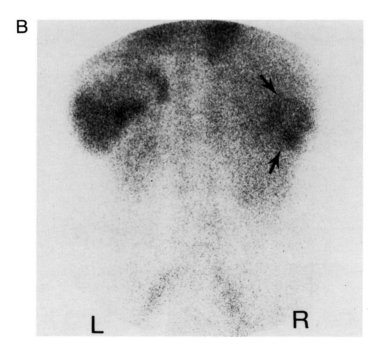

FIG 3–1.

Liver hemangioma (two cases).

A and **B,** this middle-aged woman had a previous history of breast carcinoma and mild right upper quadrant pain. A sulfur-colloid scintiscan **(A)** reveals a large single defect *(arrows)* in the right lobe of the liver (posterior and right lateral views). Posterior view scintiscan made with labeled red blood cells **(B)** shows uptake in delayed phases in the same area *(arrows),* suggesting that the liver lesion is a hemangioma.

C and **D,** this 48-year-old woman presented with mild abdominal pain and nausea. A scintiscan using ^{99m}Tc-red blood cells **(C)** demonstrates a defect in early phases *(arrows).* In late phases **(D),** there is filling of the previously seen defect *(arrows).* Small areas of nonhomogeneity are frequently seen and probably correspond to areas of fibrosis *(open arrow).*

C

D

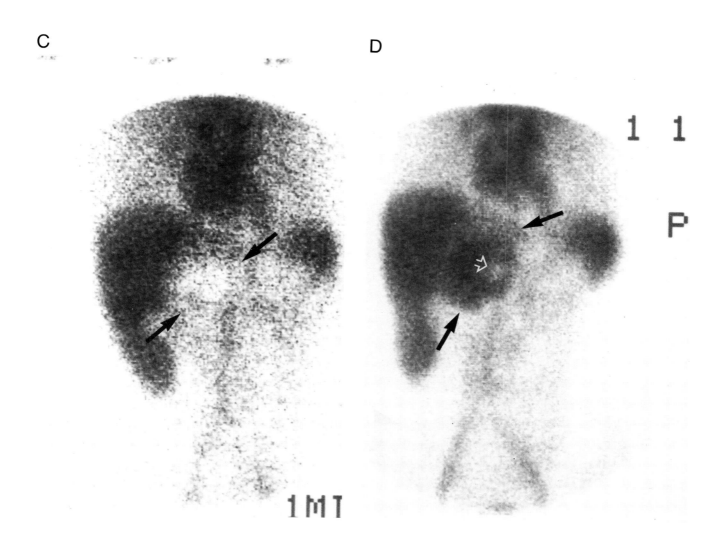

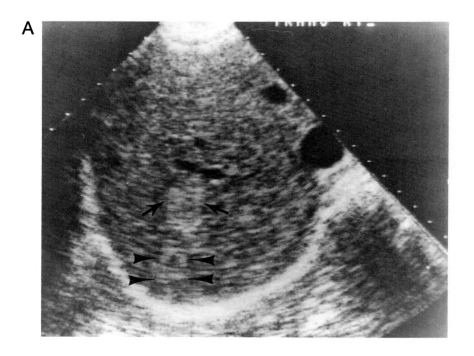

FIG 3–2.
Liver hemangioma (multiple cases).

A and **B,** a 47-year-old man with lung carcinoma. A right upper quadrant sonogram **(A)** demonstrates a mass *(arrows)* with a sharp contour, intense and homogeneous echogenicity, and faint acoustic enhancement *(arrowheads).* These characteristics are typical of hemangioma.

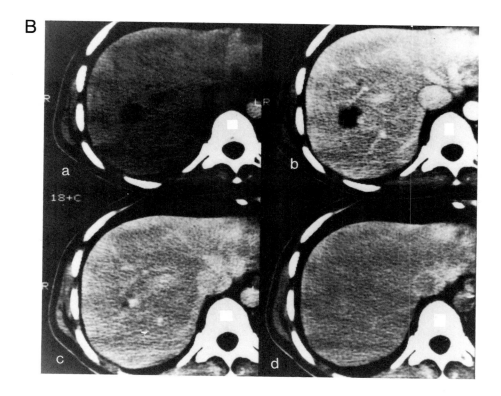

Sequential CT images **(B)** show gradual filling of the low-density lesion: *a,* unenhanced CT; *b,* early phase of intravenous contrast injection; *c,* 5 min after intravenous contrast injection; *d,* 5 min after *c.* Note total disappearance of lesion in *d. (Continued.)*

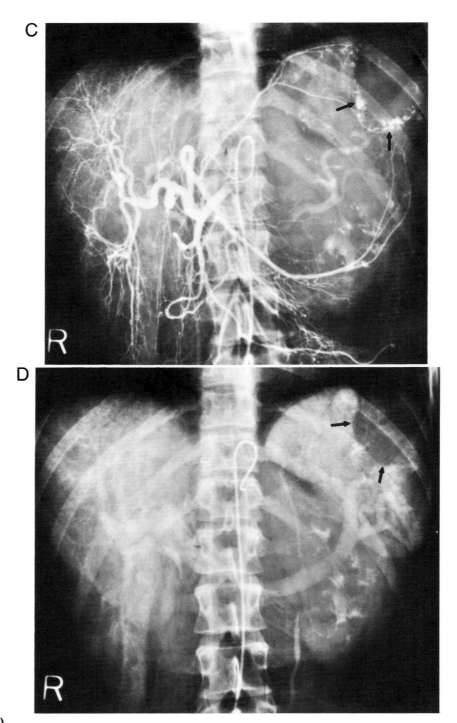

FIG 3–2 (cont.).

C and **D,** angiograms from another patient, one with diagnosed hemangioma of the left lobe of the liver. The typical appearance of hemangioma in the arterial phase is seen in **C:** *(1)* a normal hepatic artery, indicating lack of high-velocity shunting; *(2)* lack of tumoral vessels; and *(3)* early pooling of contrast medium *(arrows).*

In the late phase, shown in **D,** there is a persistent, prolonged stain. The avascular area *(arrows)* corresponds to fibrosis, necrosis, or internal hemorrhage.

E through **G,** a 58-year-old man one year after right colectomy for cecal adenocarcinoma.

Routine enhanced CT **(E)** demonstrates a low-density lesion *(arrows)* in the medial segment of the left lobe of the liver.

An oblique sonogram **(F)** shows the lesion *(arrows)* to be hypoechoic. *(Continued.)*

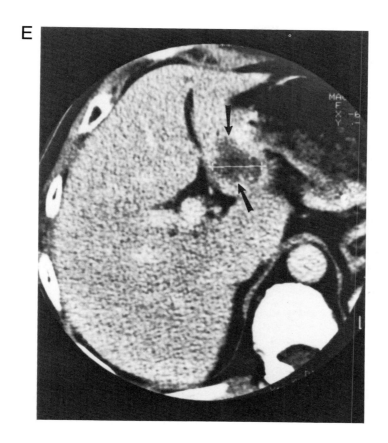

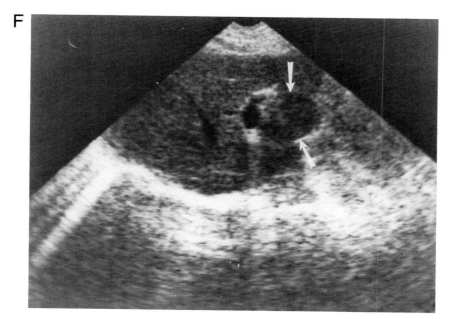

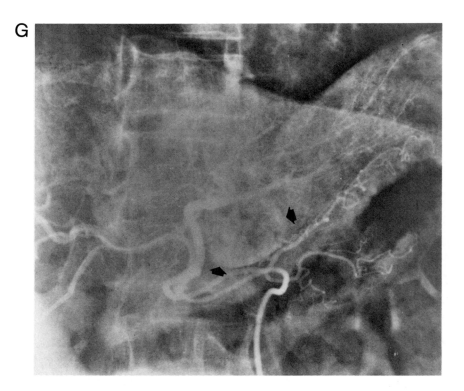

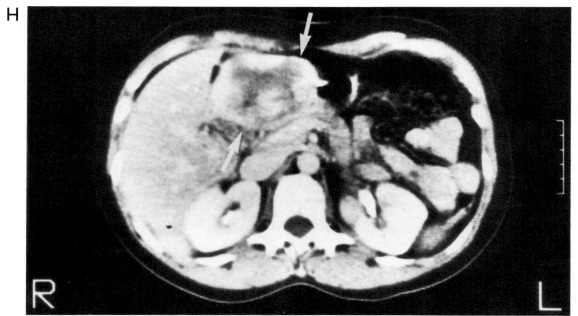

FIG 3–2 (cont.).

Angiography **(G)** shows early stain of the left lobe mass *(arrows)*. Notice the intense peripheral blush.

Open biopsy revealed hemangioma. This case illustrates the variable appearance of hemangioma by sonography and angiography.

H through **J,** a 48-year-old man who complained of mild abdominal pain underwent examination by enhanced CT.

Early CT scan after bolus contrast injection **(H)** reveals

a mass *(arrows)* with the characteristic pattern of enhancement from periphery to center. Note the nodular enhancement in the periphery.

There is homogeneous enhancement of the hemangioma in late phase **(I)** after contrast injection.

Radiograph of specimen injected with barium **(J)** demonstrates the peripheral distribution of vascularity in the resected hemangioma, correlating with the CT pattern of enhancement.

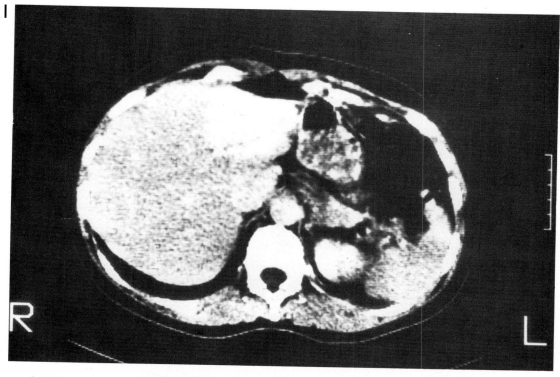

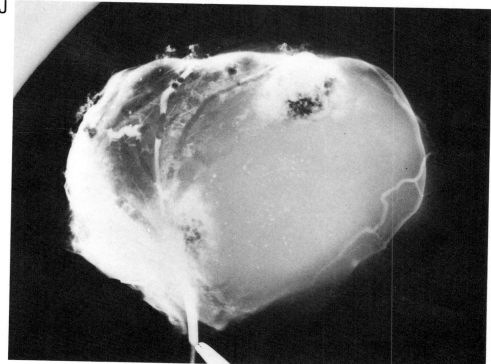

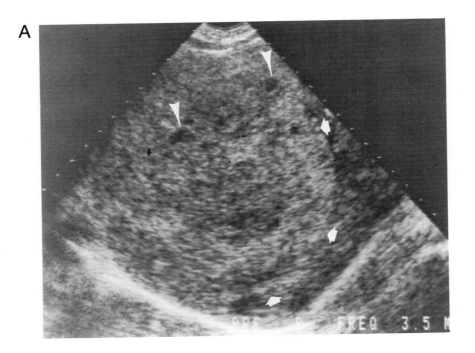

FIG 3–3.
Large cavernous hemangioma of the liver (multiple cases).

A through **E,** this 34-year-old woman had lower abdominal pain that required evaluation with ultrasound.

An incidental large hepatic mass was discovered on sonography **(A).** This mass *(arrows)* is hyperechoic with small cystic areas *(arrowheads).*

Unenhanced CT scan of the liver **(B)** demonstrates a hypodense mass in the right lobe with small areas of lower density likely corresponding to the cystic areas seen on sonography.

After contrast enhancement **(C),** there are several peripheral, ill-defined nodular enhancements *(arrows),* as commonly seen in hemangioma. *(Continued.)*

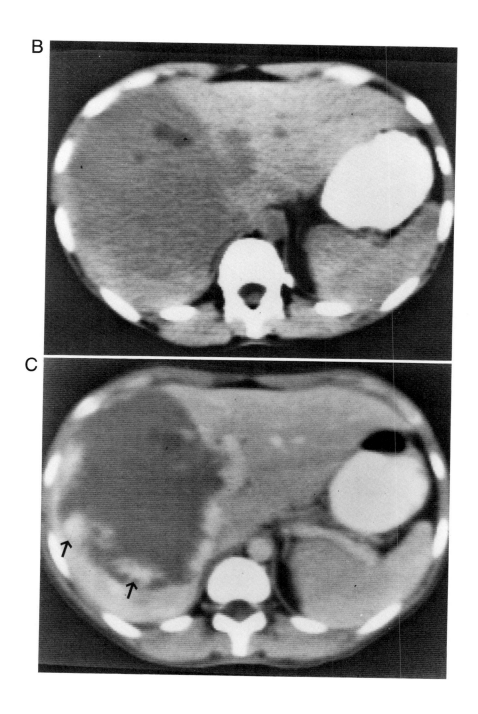

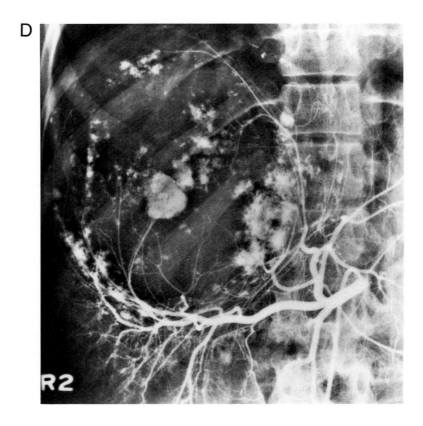

FIG 3–3 (cont.).
Angiographically **(D** and **E),** the characteristic cotton-wool appearance and delayed pooling are identified. The large avascular, hypodense, and echogenic areas likely correspond to the large areas of fibrosis commonly seen in hemangioma. *(Continued.)*

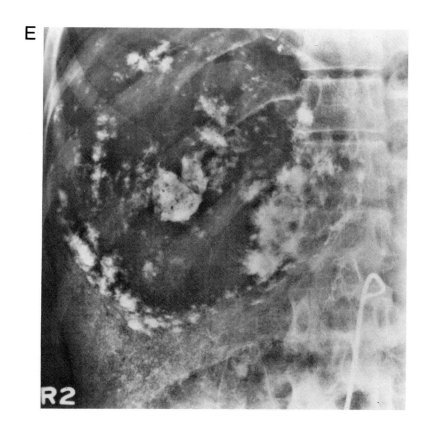

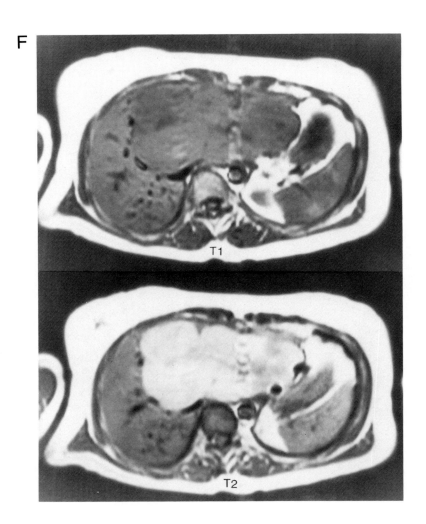

FIG 3–3 (cont.).
F and **G,** this woman with upper abdominal pain and reportedly abnormal CT results underwent MRI evaluation **(F)** in a 1.5-tesla magnet. In the T_1-weighted image (TR/TE, 800/25), there appears to be a large, well-marginated lesion with intermediate signal intensity within the left lobe of the liver. It is almost isointense with the liver. In the T_2-weighted image (TR/TE, 2,000/80), the lesion displays high signal intensity. This finding suggests the high vascularity of hemangiomas and helps to differentiate hemangioma from hypovascular liver lesions such as the majority of metastases.

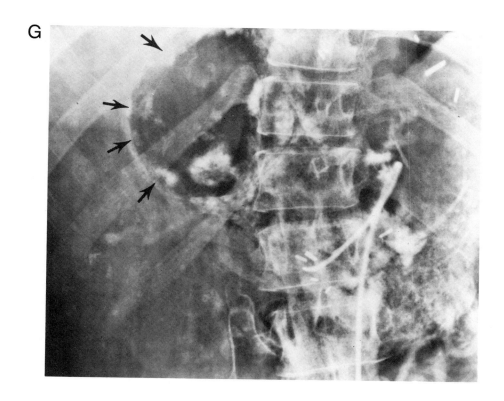

The capillary phase of a liver angiogram **(G)** shows enhancing nodules in the wall *(arrows)* with the cotton-wool appearance of the lesion. The findings are typical for hemangioma. *(Continued.)*

H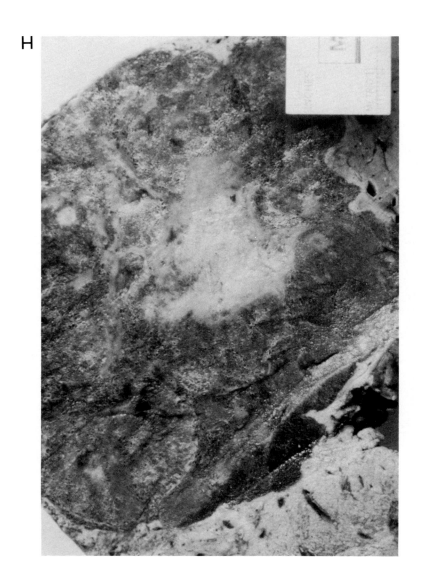

FIG 3–3 (cont.).
H and **I,** pathologic findings. Gross photography **(H)** of a large hemangioma *(cut section).* Note the large central area of fibrosis with smaller nodules of fibrosis distributed throughout the tumor (see also Color Plate 5). Hemangioma in the liver has a very sharp margin despite the lack of a capsule.

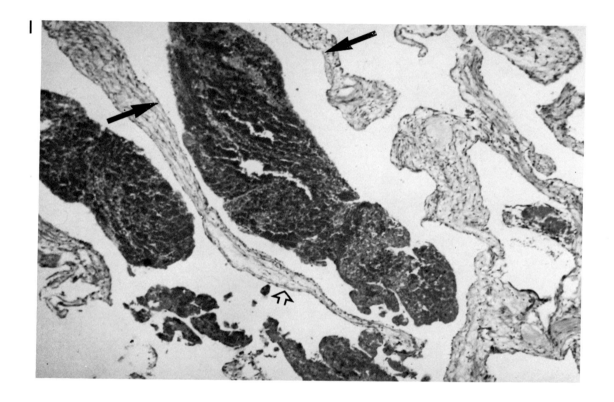

In the photomicrograph **(I)** of the typical appearance of hemangioma, observe the vascular channels *(arrows)* filled with red blood cells and lined by a single layer of endothelial cells *(open arrow)* (hematoxylin and eosin, ×60).

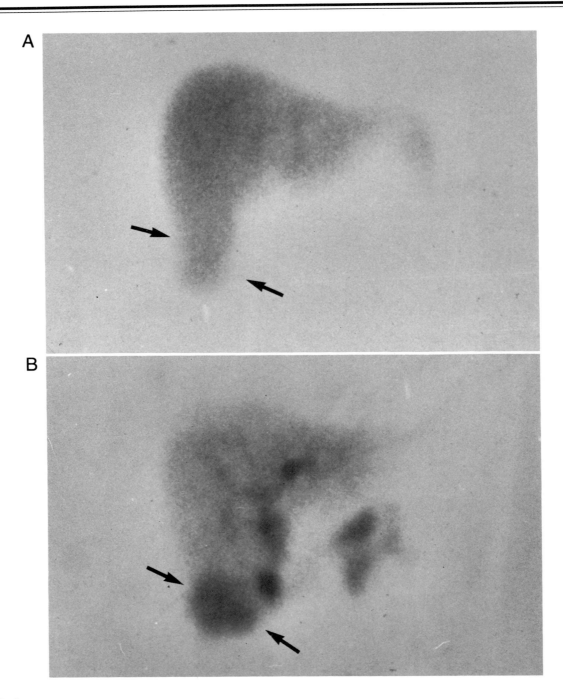

FIG 3–4.
Focal nodular hyperplasia (multiple cases).

    A and **B,** this 35-year-old woman presented with mild, diffuse abdominal pain. Liver-spleen scintigraphy **(A)** shows normal uptake of sulfur colloid in the liver, including in the elongated right lobe *(arrows)*. There is evidence of hyper-concentration of the IDA derivative **(B)** in the same region *(arrows),* likely due to increased hepatocytes in relation to surrounding normal liver. This area was proved to represent FNH.

    C and **D,** this 27-year-old woman presented with right upper quadrant pain, and liver abnormality was reported during gallbladder sonography. This anterior view sulfur-colloid liver scintiscan **(C)** is normal. Enhanced CT **(D)** shows a large, relatively isodense lesion in the right lobe of the liver *(open arrows)* displaying central hypodensity. Biopsy proved FNH. *(Continued.)*

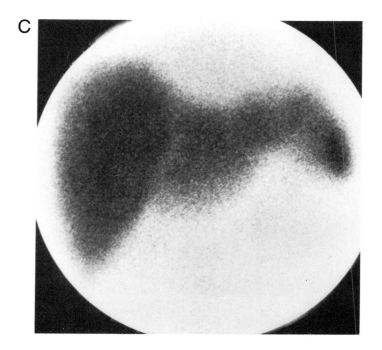

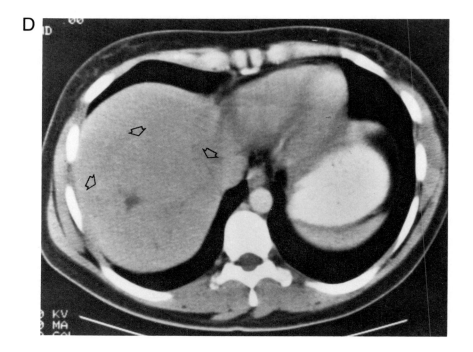

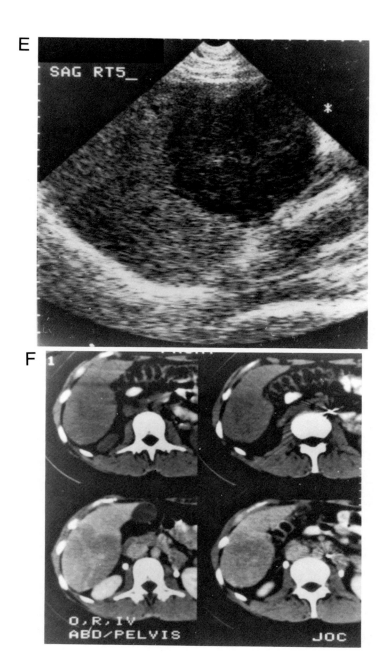

FIG 3–4 (cont.).
E through **H**, this 26-year-old woman treated six years previously for Hodgkin's lymphoma was found on physical examination to have a large liver.

A sonogram **(E)** shows a large, hypoechoic lesion within the right lobe of the liver. With the diagnosis of lymphoma, abdominal CT was done. The unenhanced *(top row)* and contrast-enhanced *(bottom row)* images **(F)** of the right lobe of the liver show a hypodense mass displaying minimal enhancement. Because of the enhancement, lymphoma became less likely and an angiogram was obtained.

Selective right hepatic arteriography **(G)** shows a very vascular mass with intense staining during the venous phase.

The catheter was placed in the superior mesenteric artery, and a CT-portogram was obtained during hand injection of contrast medium. The CT-portogram images **(H)** show well the opacification of the normal hepatic parenchyma and clearly delineate the borders of the mass.

Biopsy established the diagnosis of FNH. The tumor was excised.

G

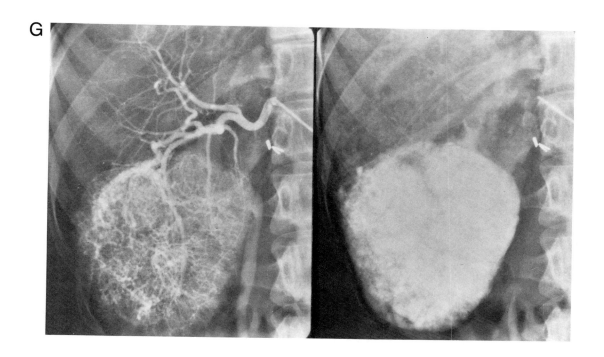

H

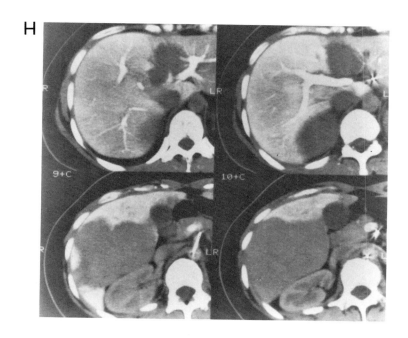

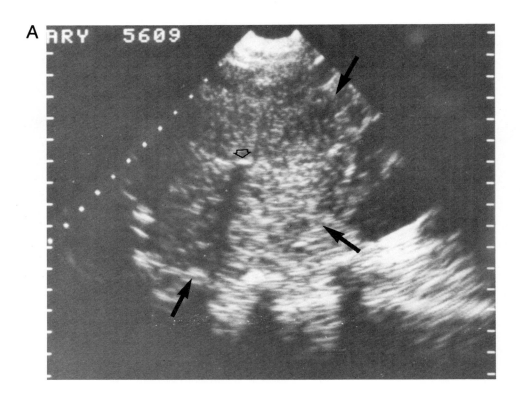

FIG 3–5.
Focal nodular hyperplasia. This 31-year-old woman presented with vague abdominal pain.

A, a sonogram of the liver demonstrates a large, echogenic lesion *(arrows)* with central acoustic shadowing
(open arrow). This corresponds to a large FNH with a central scar and with punctate calcifications.

B, a CT scan without contrast enhancement reveals a
large, hypodense lesion, homogeneous in nature except for
a spiculated area of further decreased density in its center
(open arrow). Note the displacement of a hepatic vein pos-
teromedially *(arrowhead)*.

C, after contrast enhancement, there is hyperdensity in
the FNH, reflecting its hypervascular nature. Note the avascular central fibrotic area and the lack of invasion of the
displaced hepatic vein. *(Continued.)*

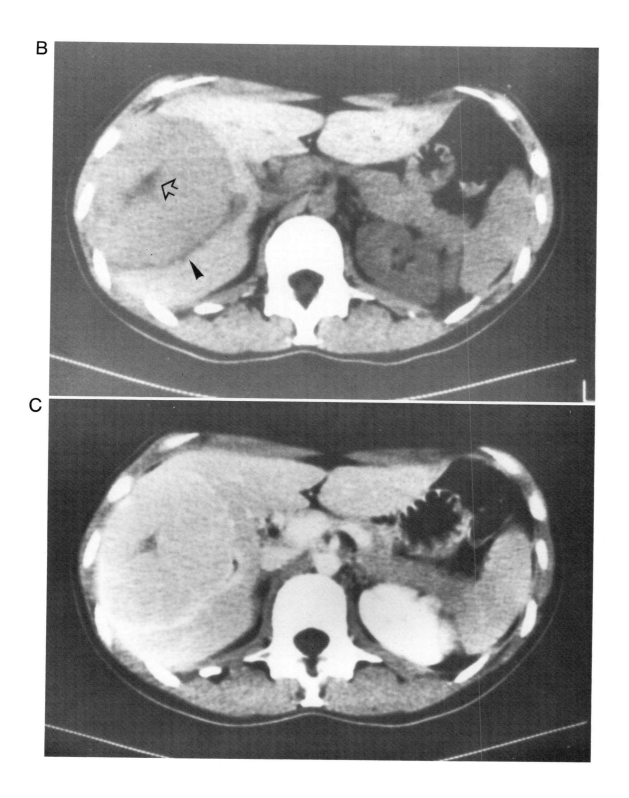

D

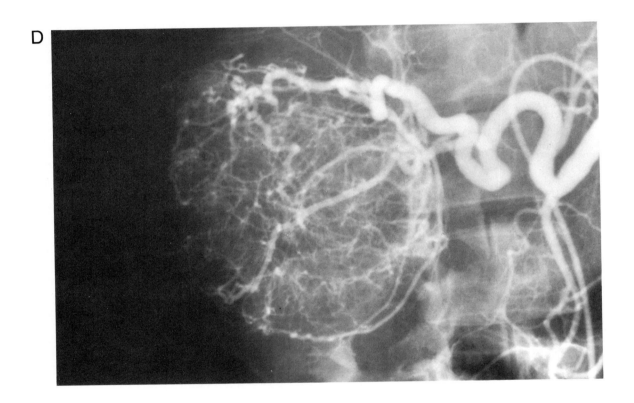

FIG 3–5 (cont.).
D, on angiography observe the hypervascular nature of FNH with fine radiating vessels in a spoked-wheel configuration.

E, the gross specimen demonstrates on cut section a central fibrotic scar, homogeneous appearance, and displaced hepatic vein inferiorly, correlating with CT and sonographic findings (see also Color Plate 6).

F, observe in this photomicrograph the lobular nature of FNH with multiple fibrous septa *(small arrows)* radiating from a central stellate scar *(large arrows).* Note the vascular structures in the central scar. This microscopic finding helps to explain the vasculature observed in the angiogram.

E

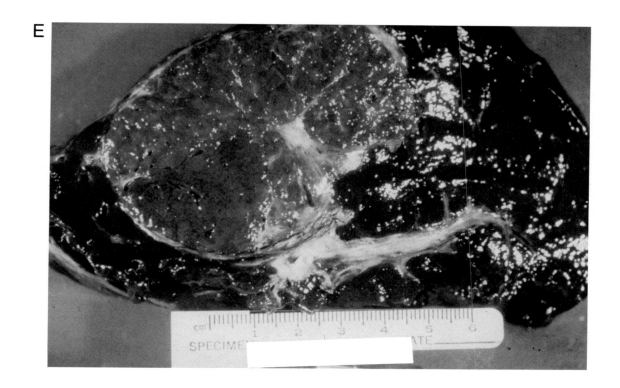

F

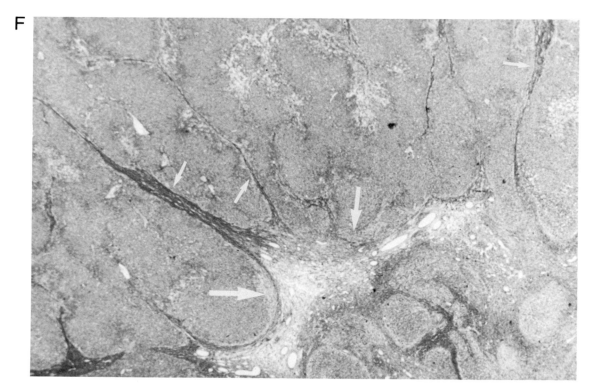

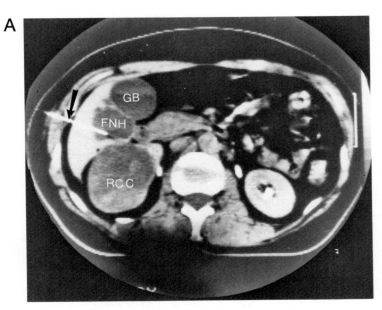

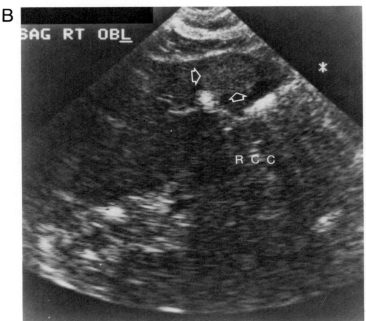

FIG 3–6.
Focal nodular hyperplasia and hypernephroma.

A, patient with right renal cell carcinoma *(RCC)* was found to have an incidental hypodense lesion *(FNH)* in the right lobe of the liver on enhanced CT (*CB*, gallbladder).

B, a parasagittal sonogram reveals a homogeneously hyperechoic lesion *(arrows)* within the right lobe of the liver (*RCC,* renal cell carcinoma).

C and **D,** angiography performed as part of the renal cell carcinoma workup demonstrates a hypervascular lesion *(arrows)* at the tip of the right lobe of the liver, with a homogeneous stain **(D)** in the capillary phase.

Focal nodular hyperplasia was proved both by percutaneous aspiration biopsy (needle indicated by *arrow* in **A**) and at the time of nephrectomy.

C

D

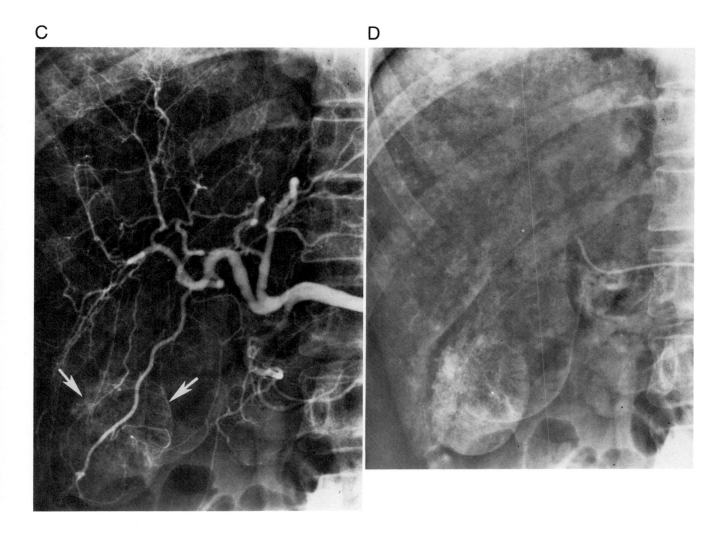

A

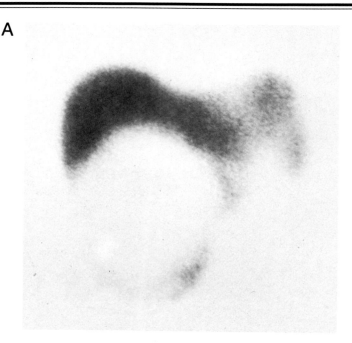

B

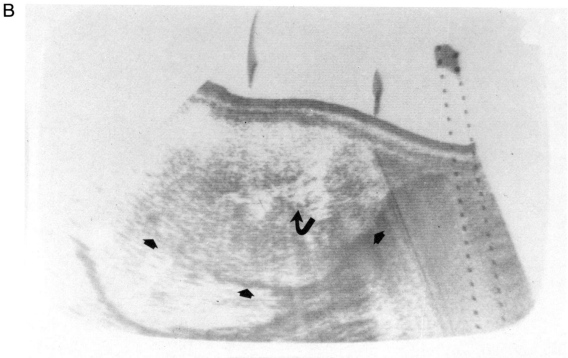

FIG 3–7.
Hepatocellular adenoma (two cases).

This 17-year-old girl had both pain and a large, palpable mass in the right lower quadrant.

A, anterior view from sulfur-colloid liver-spleen scintigraphy reveals a large defect within the right lobe of the liver. (**A** from *AJR* 148:15, 1987. Reproduced with permission.)

B, a sonogram demonstrates the well-defined echogenic mass *(arrows)* in the right hepatic lobe. The echogenicity is related to the fat and glycogen in the hepatocytes of this proved adenoma. The star-shaped area of decreased echogenicity *(curved arrow)* corresponds in this large adenoma to a central fibrotic area.

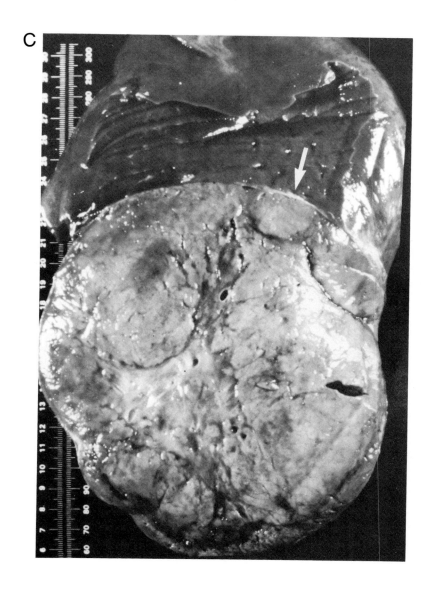

C, on the cut section of this large pedunculated adenoma, a thin capsule can be seen *(arrow)* in the superior portion of the tumor. *(Continued.)*

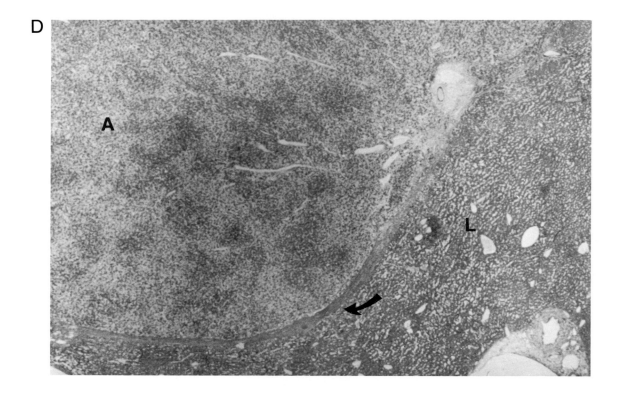

FIG 3–7 (cont.).
D, microscopically, the fibrous capsule *(curved arrow)* is easily detected. The cells in the adenoma *(A)* are pale compared with the normal hepatocytes *(L)* seen outside the capsule due to the high content of fat and glycogen in adenomas.

E

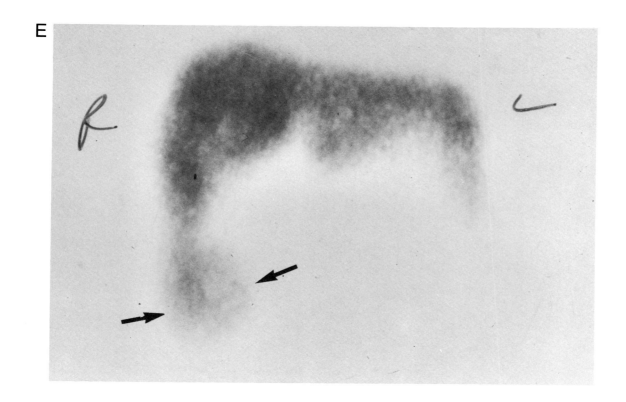

E, infrequently, HCA shows uptake of sulfur colloid, as in this second patient with pedunculated adenoma *(arrows).*

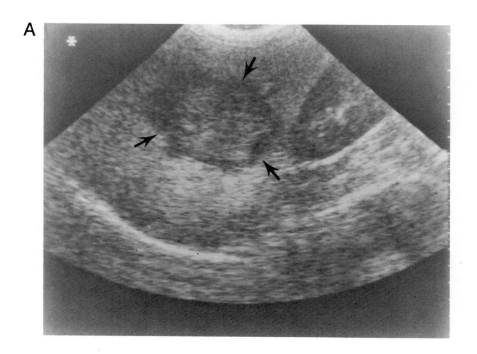

FIG 3–8.
Hepatocellular adenoma (two cases).
A and **B,** this 39-year-old woman with right upper quad-rant fullness underwent abdominal sonography. The longi-tudinal scan **(A)** shows an echogenic mass with hypoechoic halo *(arrows)* in the right lobe of the liver.

B

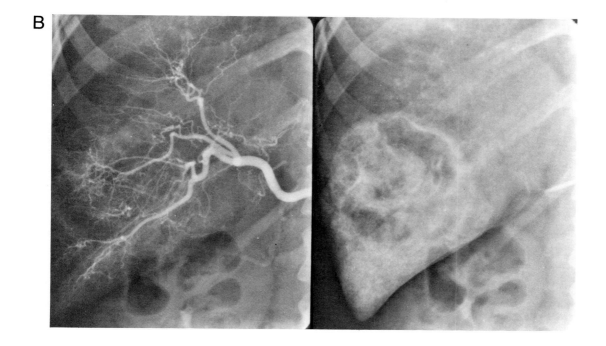

The angiogram **(B)** shows the mass to be vascular and to have a peripheral rim and central stain. Biopsy proved HCA. *(Continued.)*

C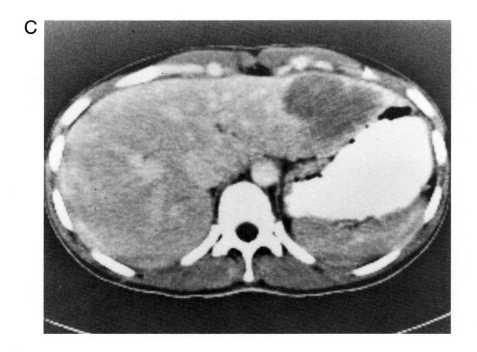

FIG 3–8 (cont.).
C through **E,** this 23-year-old woman had primary perineal sarcoma treated by resection. An abdominal CT scan **(C)** shows a hypodense lesion in the lateral segment of the left lobe of the liver. The mass displays abnormal vascularity on angiography **(D** and **E).** Since the patient had taken contraceptive pills for only six months, metastasis was considered more likely than adenoma. However, left hepatic segmentectomy proved the mass to represent adenoma.

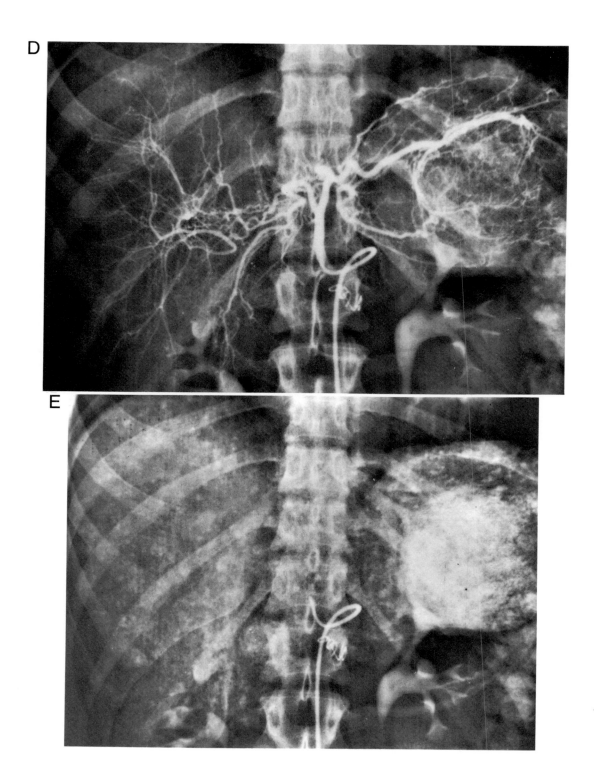

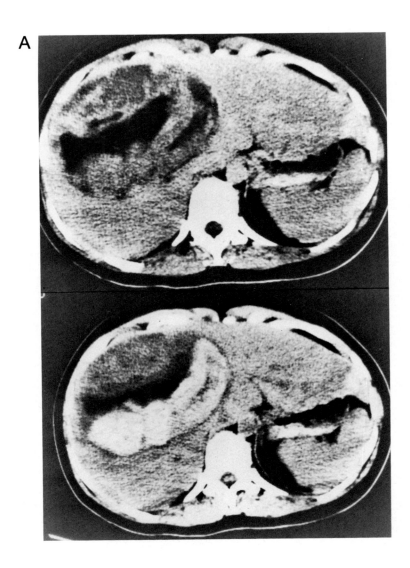

FIG 3–9.
Hepatocellular adenoma with hemorrhage. This 41-year-old patient presented with sudden-onset right upper quadrant pain.

A, unenhanced *(bottom)* and enhanced *(top)* CT scans reveal a large, well-defined, complex mass. Note the large area of increased density seen on unenhanced CT. This finding corresponds to internal bleeding.

B and **C,** angiography shows stretching of intrahepatic branches *(arrows)* and a relatively hypovascular mass, reflecting the cystic and hemorrhagic nature of the mass. Biopsy proved HCA.

B

C

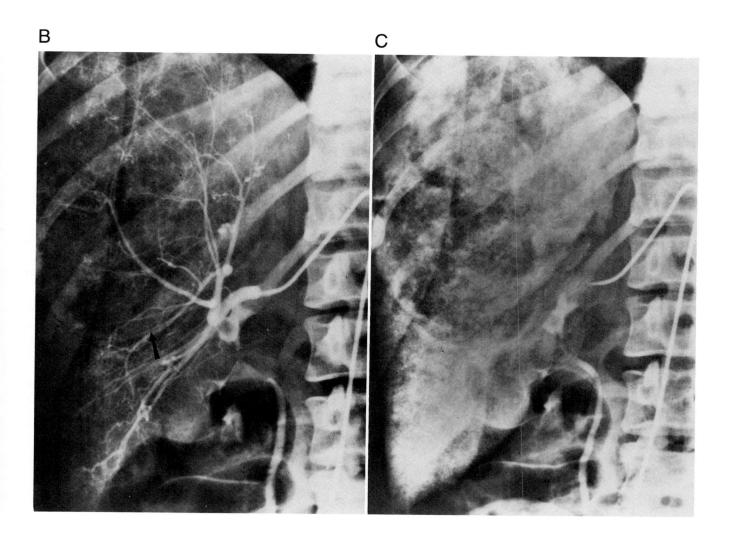

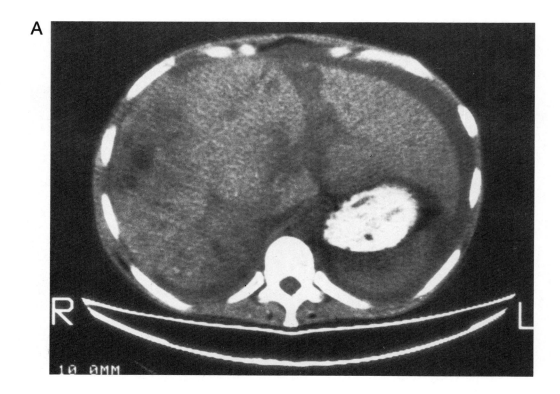

FIG 3–10.
Nodular regenerative hyperplasia.
    A, in this young man with ascites and portal hypertension, unenhanced CT of the liver demonstrates multiple low-density nodules within the hepatic parenchyma. (**A** from Dachman A.H., Ros P.R., Goodman Z.D., et al.: Nodular regenerative hyperplasia of the liver: radiographic description. *AJR* 148:717–722, 1987. Reproduced with permission.)

B

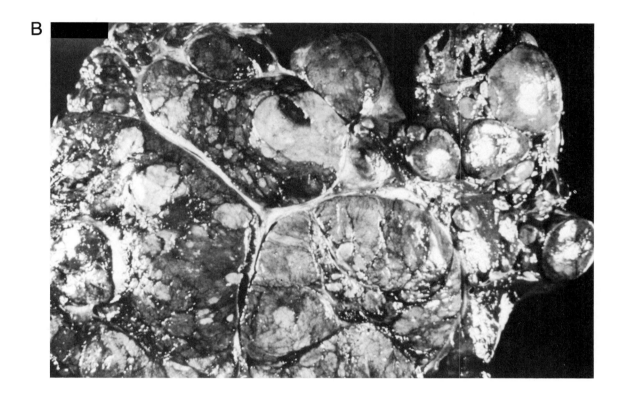

B, in a specimen (cut section) from another patient, observe the multiple nodules of variable size replacing a large area of the liver. (**B** courtesy of E.L. Barnes, M.D., Department of Radiology, Presbyterian University Hospital, Pittsburgh.)

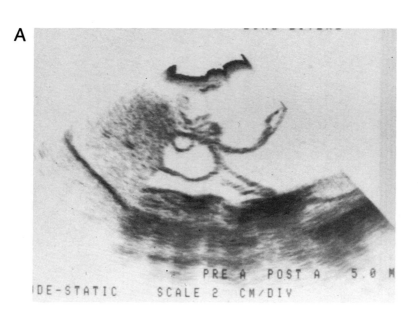

A

PRE A   POST A   5.0 M

DE-STATIC   SCALE 2   CM/DIV

FIG 3–11.
Mesenchymal hamartoma of the liver (MHL). This 15-month-old child presented with abdominal distension.

A, parasagittal sonogram in the right upper quadrant shows a multicystic mass with locules of variable size. This appearance may mimic loculated ascites.

B, computed tomography demonstrates a very large mass of water density compressing the kidneys and bowel posteriorly. There are multiple fine septations of higher density *(arrows)* in this MHL.

C, photomicrograph of this rare benign cystic hamartomatous tumor of the liver reveals abundant areas of degeneration with fluid accumulation. The areas are separated by thin strands of connective tissue. There are abnormal bile ducts *(arrow)* surrounded by primitive mesenchyma (hematoxylin and eosin, ×60).

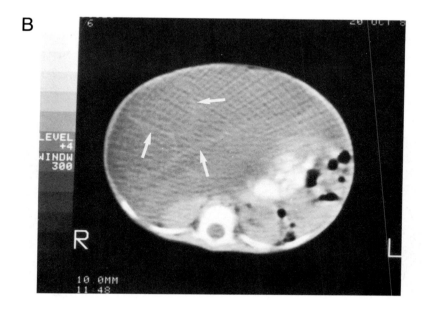

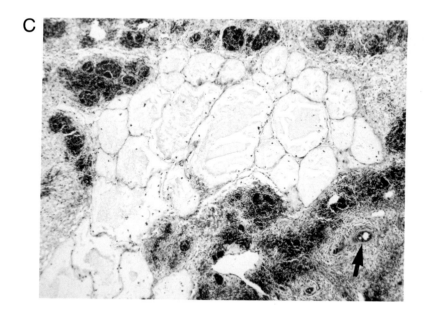

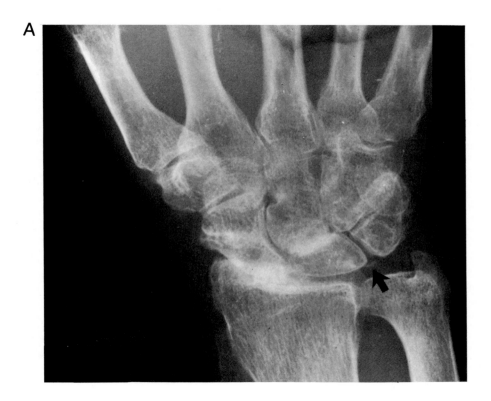

FIG 3–12.
Hepatocellular carcinoma and hemochromatosis.
   A, wrist radiograph in a 65-year-old man with hemochromatosis and right upper quadrant pain. Observe degenerative changes in the carpal bones and articular calcification *(arrow).*

B

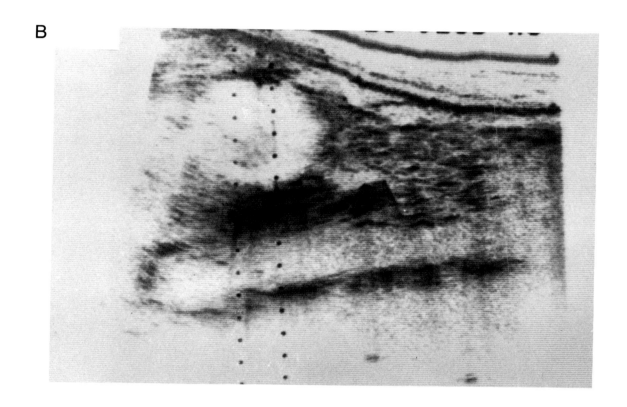

B, parasagittal midline sonogram demonstrates a hypoechoic, well-delineated, noncalcified mass in the left lobe of the liver. The hypoechoic appearance of the mass is usual in HCC. The presence of a hepatic mass in a patient with hemochromatosis should suggest this diagnosis.

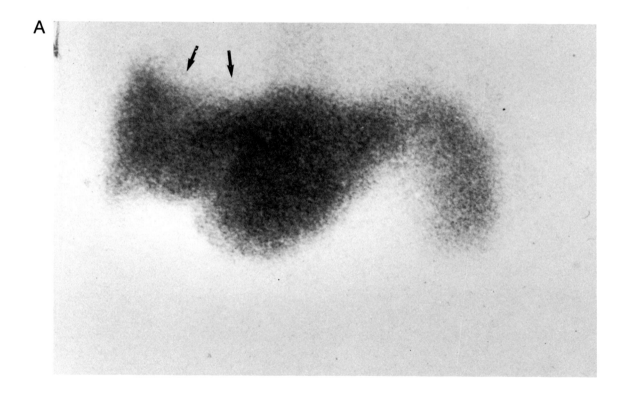

FIG 3–13.
Hepatocellular carcinoma and cirrhosis (two cases).

A and **B,** this 87-year-old man had hepatic cirrhosis, ascites, and esophageal varices. He underwent sulfur-colloid scintigraphy **(A).** There is an irregular area of filling defect *(arrows)* in the upper margin of the shrunken right lobe of the liver, suspicious for a mass. The enlarged spleen and hyperplastic left lobe are indicative of cirrhosis.

B

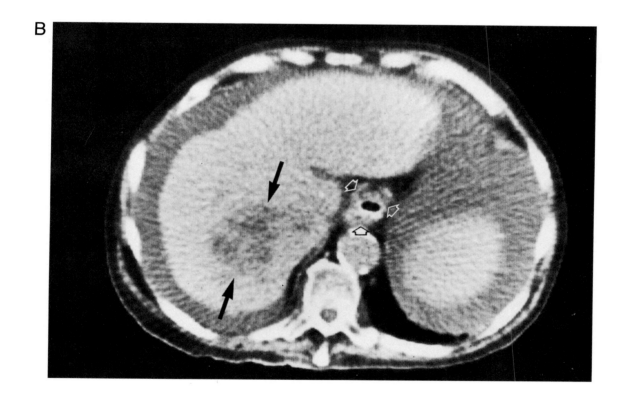

A CT scan **(B)** reveals an area of decreased density with ill-defined borders *(arrows),* confirming the scintigraphic findings. The CT scan also detects esophageal varices *(open arrows)* and ascites.

When sulfur-colloid scintigraphy detects any liver-contour abnormality in a patient with long-standing cirrhosis, HCC should be suspected, and CT or sonography is indicated to evaluate the abnormality. *(Continued.)*

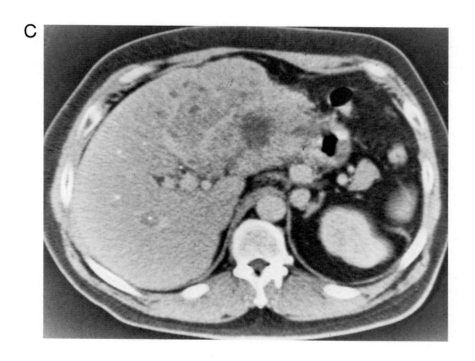

FIG 3–13 (cont.).
C and **D,** this 60-year-old man presented in his native country with epigastric pain. Cholelithiasis was discovered on so-

nography and surgical exploration performed. Biopsy of liver during cholecystectomy proved cirrhosis and HCC. The patient was referred to M.D. Anderson Hospital. A contrast-

D

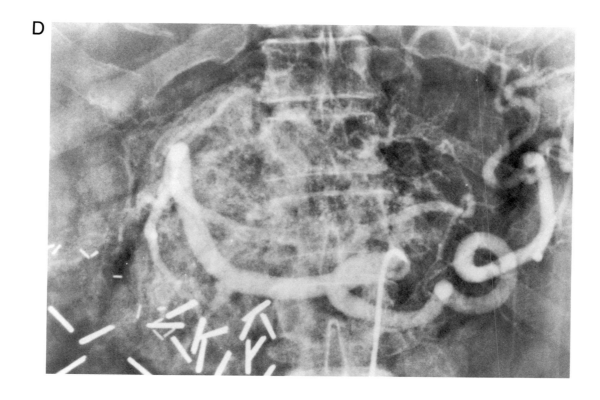

enhanced CT scan **(C)** shows an atrophic left lobe of the liver with a mass containing numerous areas of low density. A small lesion is also seen in the right lobe. An angiogram **(D)** shows a vascular lesion with areas of neovascularity.

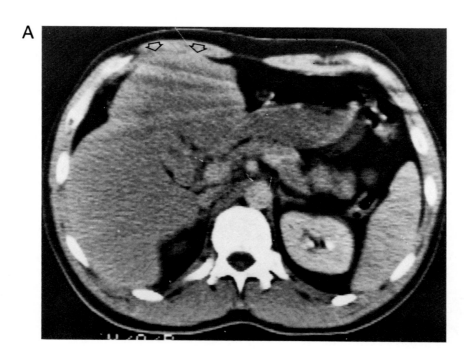

FIG 3–14.
Hepatocellular carcinoma and cirrhosis. This patient with known cirrhosis presented with weight loss.

A, the enhanced CT scan shows a somewhat irregularly prominent left lobe, isodense with the rest of the liver. Because of elevated serum α-fetoprotein values and the bulge on CT *(open arrows),* an abdominal sonogram was obtained.

B, longitudinal sonogram reveals a well-marginated hyperechoic mass *(arrows)* corresponding to the contour abnormality seen on CT.

C, arterial phase on a selective hepatic arteriogram confirms the presence of a hypervascular mass *(arrows),* with abnormal vessels. Biopsy proved HCC, and the patient had operation.

This case demonstrates that HCC can be isodense with the rest of the liver in CT scans. In these cases, if there are no gross contour abnormalities, sonograms and angiograms may better depict the neoplasm.

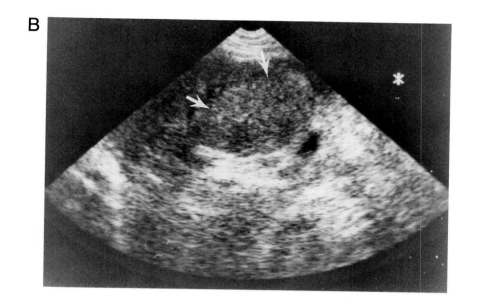

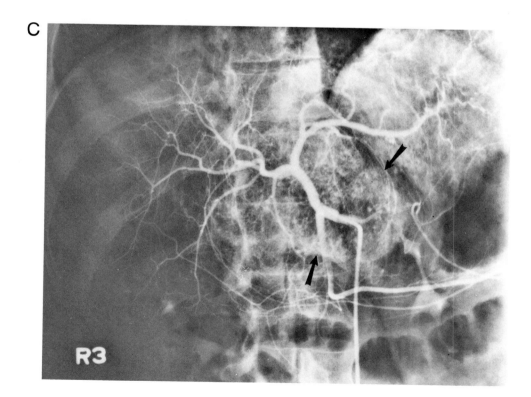

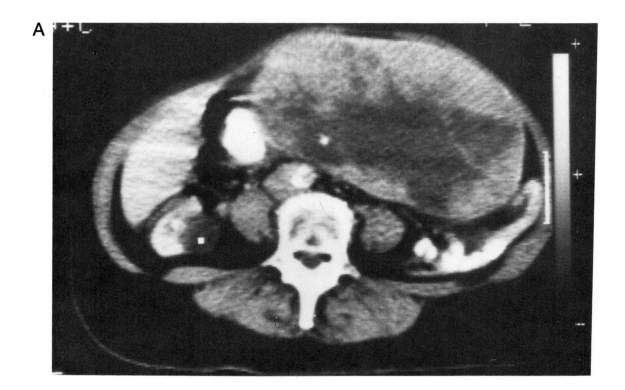

FIG 3–15.
Pedunculated hepatocellular carcinoma (two cases).

A, in this patient with a palpable midabdominal mass, a CT scan demonstrates a large pedunculated mass arising from the left lobe of the liver. Note the large central areas of markedly decreased density, corresponding to necrosis. The large areas of necrosis that are common in HCC will produce complex masses on CT scans and sonograms.

B through E, a 56-year-old woman presented with a palpable right lower quadrant mass.

Enhanced CT (B) demonstrates a dense bulging mass with a hypodense, irregular center (arrow) and a thin hyperdense rim corresponding to the capsule. It could not be determined whether or not the mass was from the liver.

Sagittal sonogram (C) demonstrates a hyperechoic mass, pedunculated from the inferior border of the right lobe of the liver and projecting below the level of right kidney (K). Note the thin hypoechoic halo (open arrows) in the periphery of the mass, corresponding to the capsule. The central hypoechoic area (arrow) corresponds to fibrosis or necrosis. (Continued.)

B

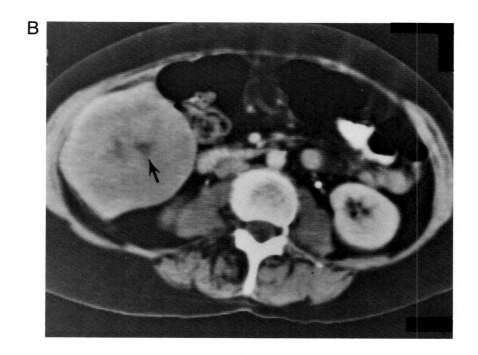

C

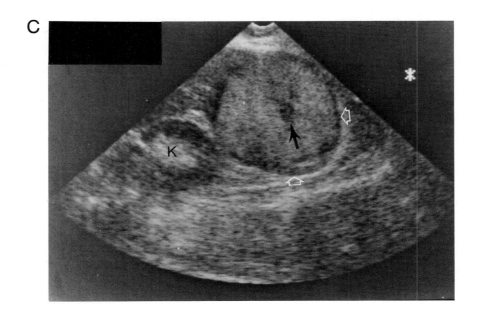

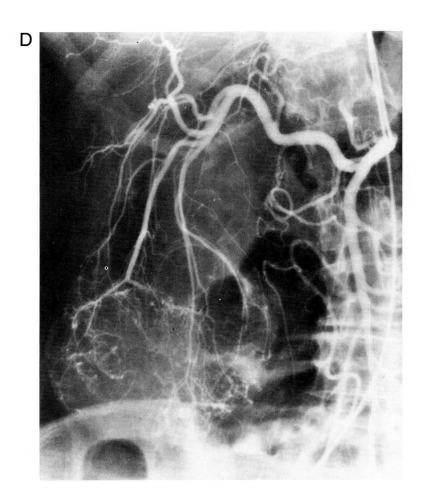

FIG 3–15 (cont.).
Arterial phase in a selective superior mesenteric artery an-giogram **(D)** reveals a hypervascular mass fed through a replaced right hepatic artery.

E

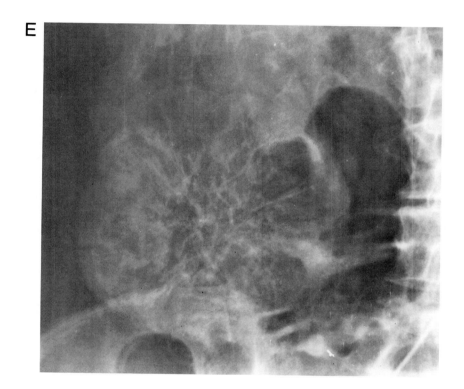

Capillary phase in the arteriogram **(E)** shows a thin avascular zone surrounding tissue, corresponding to the capsule noted on the sonogram and CT scan. The capillary pattern and the appearance of a spoked-wheel pattern suggested the diagnosis of FNH. However, surgery proved well-differentiated HCC.

These cases demonstrate the multifaceted appearance of HCC.

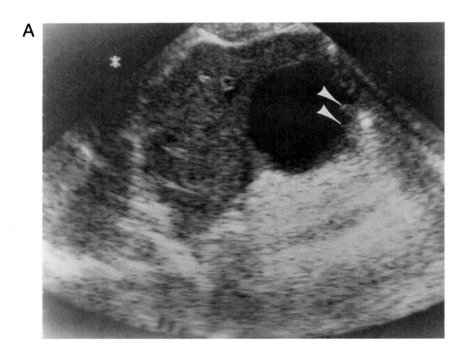

FIG 3–16.
Cystic or necrotic hepatocellular carcinoma (two cases).

A and B, this 33-year-old man with hypochromic anemia presented with abdominal pain.

A sonogram **(A)** demonstrates a cystic mass in the left lobe of the liver. On this midline sagittal view, note the acoustic enhancement; however, the inner wall is irregular with excrescences *(arrowheads),* suggesting that the lesion is not a simple cyst but probably cystic degeneration in a solid tumor.

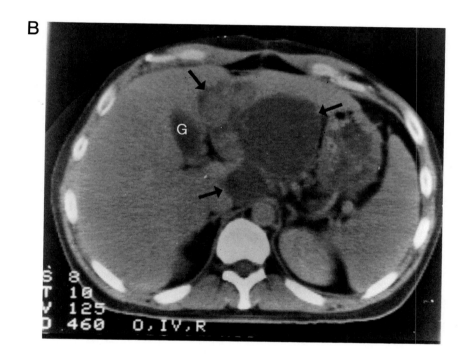

A CT scan **(B)** demonstrates a multifocal neoplasm *(arrows)* that has a large area of fluid density, correlating with the sonographic findings. Biopsy proved an HCC with marked necrosis (*G*, gallbladder). *(Continued.)*

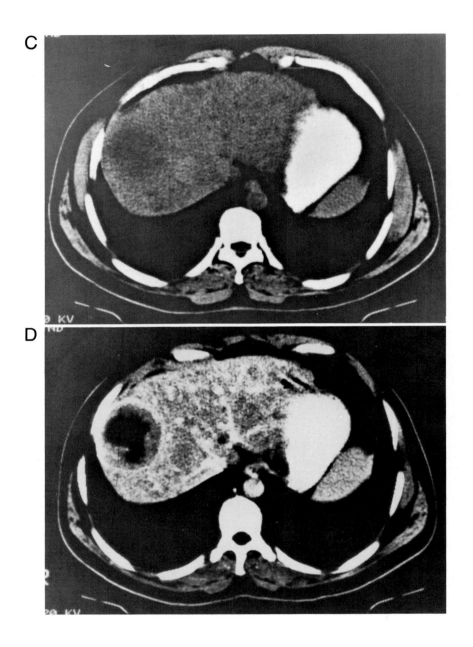

FIG 3–16 (cont.).
C and **D,** a 47-year-old man with generalized pruritus and upper abdominal pain underwent CT study of the abdomen.

Unenhanced **(C)** and enhanced **(D)** CT scans reveal a large low-density mass with enhancing thick wall within the right lobe of the liver.

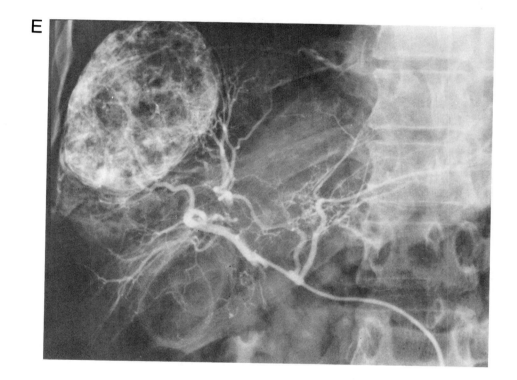

E, selective arteriogram shows a hypervascular lesion with numerous abnormal vessels. Percutaneous biopsy was consistent with moderately differentiated HCC.

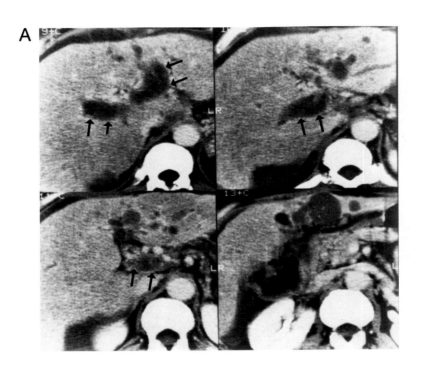

FIG 3–17.
Multicentric HCC with cavernous transformation of the portal vein. This 50-year-old man presented with weight loss and abdominal pain.

A, contrast-enhanced CT image of the liver shows multiple areas of low density within the hepatic parenchyma, along with intrahepatic ductal dilatation. There is lack of enhancement of the portal vein and its intrahepatic branches *(arrows),* suggesting thrombosis.

B, a sonogram demonstrates multiple hypoechoic lesions in the liver and numerous echoes within the portal vein *(arrows).* The common bile duct *(cursors)* is normal.

C, the capillary phase of a hepatic angiogram shows a vascular mass in the left lobe with multiple abnormal vessels. *(Continued.)*

B

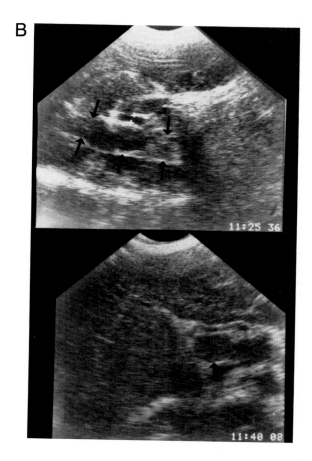

C

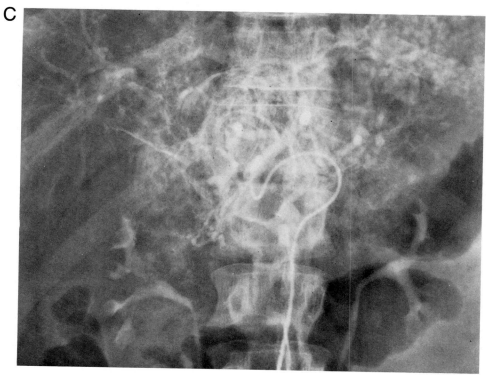

D

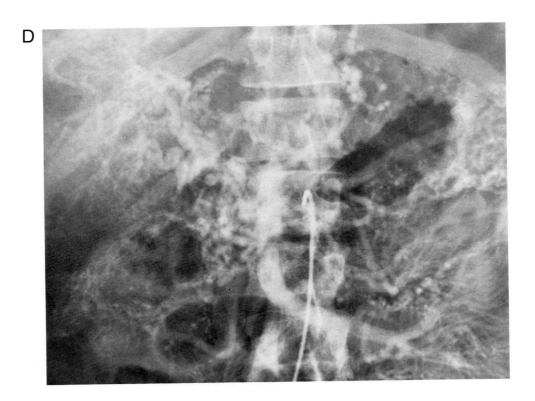

FIG 3–17 (cont.).
D, the venous phase of a superior mesenteric arteriogram reveals lack of filling of the portal vein and presence of numerous collaterals, all due to thrombosis and cavernous transformation of portal vein.

Percutaneous biopsy of the liver proved the diagnosis of HCC, for which the patient received chemotherapy.

E

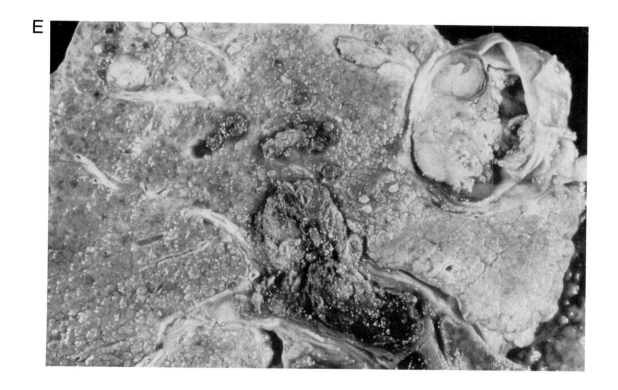

E, cut section of liver from a different patient with HCC shows tumoral invasion of the portal vein, portal branches, and hepatic veins (see also Color Plate 7).

A

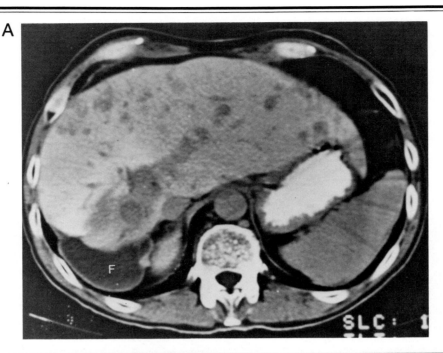

B

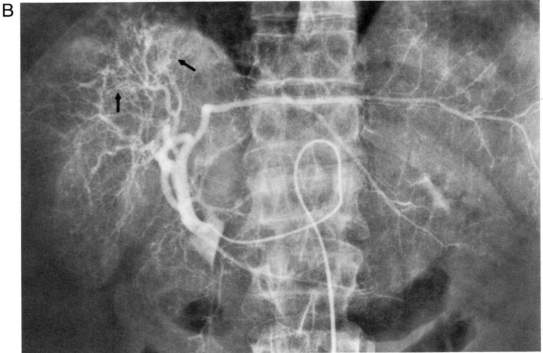

FIG 3–18.
Multicentric hepatocellular carcinoma. This 60-year-old man with hemochromatosis presented with abdominal fullness and a palpable liver.

A, a CT scan shows hypotrophic right lobe and hypertrophic left lobe of the liver. There are multiple irregular areas of decreased density throughout the liver. A subcapsular fluid collection *(F)* is seen posteriorly.

B, angiography by selective hepatic injection demonstrates multiple areas of abnormal vessels *(arrows).* It also showed arteriovenous shunting.

Multiple biopsies revealed multicentric HCC.

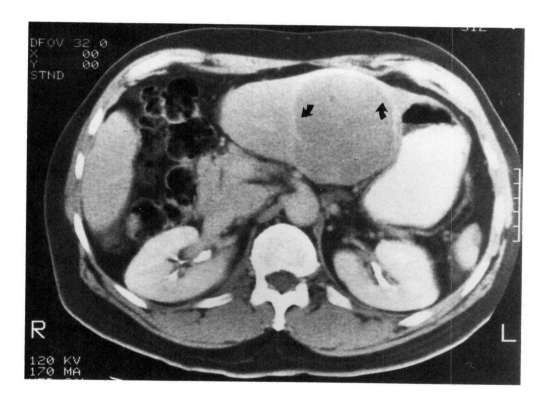

FIG 3–19.
Encapsulated HCC. In this 62-year-old man with chronic hepatitis and cirrhosis, enhanced CT demonstrates a mass within the left lobe of the liver. The mass has a capsule, seen as a fine band of increased density *(curved arrows)* surrounding the relatively hypodense mass.

Biopsy proved HCC. In HCC, distinguishing a capsule by imaging may be clinically important because encapsulated HCCs are easier to resect and entail a better prognosis.

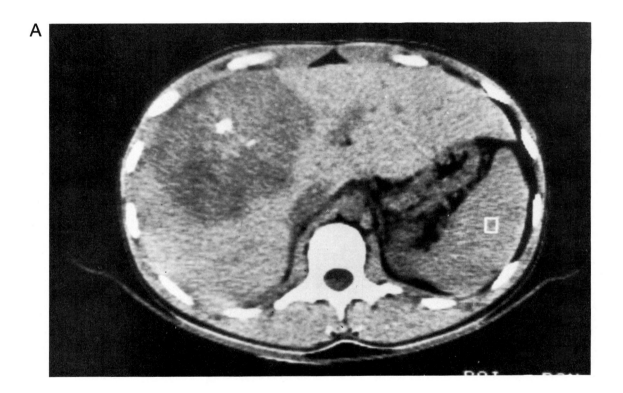

FIG 3–20.
Fibrolamellar carcinoma in a 20-year-old man with sharp pain in the right upper quadrant.

   A, unenhanced CT demonstrates a well-defined, hypodense mass in the liver. The mass has central spiculated calcification.

   B, contrast-enhanced CT, after bolus injection, shows marked enhancement corresponding to the hypervascular nature of this mass. Biopsy proved fibrolamellar carcinoma.

(**A** and **B** from Friedman A.C., Lichtenstein J.E., Goodman Z., et al.: Fibrolamellar hepatocellular carcinoma. *Radiology* 157:583–587, 1985. Reproduced with permission.)

   C, in the left photomicrograph, there is a typical HCC. Observe the cords of hepatocytes. In the right, there is a fibrolamellar carcinoma, with its characteristic lamellar fibrosis *(arrows)*. The cellular portion of the tumor is similar in appearance to an HCC; this is why some authors consider fibrolamellar carcinoma a subtype of HCC. *(Continued.)*

B

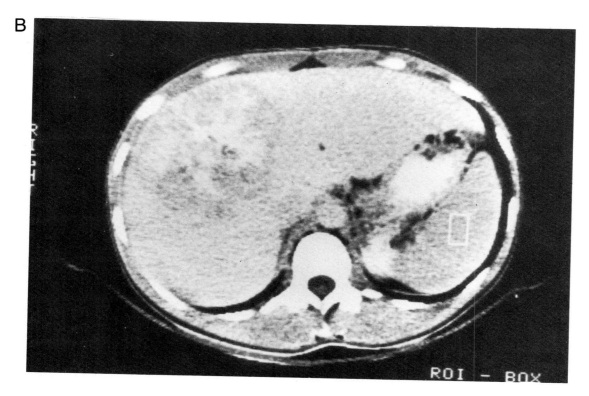

C

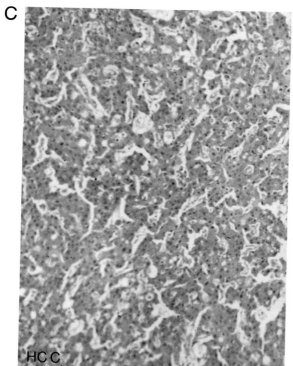

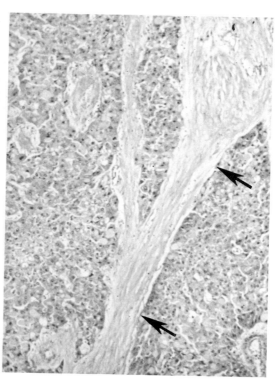

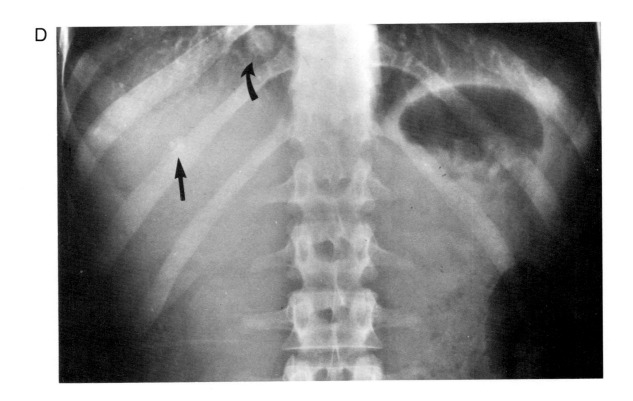

FIG 3–20 (cont.).
D, a plain radiograph demonstrates the calcification *(arrow)* that is common in fibrolamellar carcinoma and very unusual in HCC. Observe the pulmonary metastasis *(curved arrow).*

E, sulfur-colloid scintigraphy reveals a defect in the right lobe of the liver. This is an important differential finding with FNH, since FNH frequently shows normal uptake of the radionuclide.

F, there is marked hypervascularity and dense tumoral stain in this late-arterial-phase hepatic arteriogram. Serpiginous avascular areas can be observed within the tumor. This sign has been termed *compartmentalization,* which corresponds to bands of fibrosis. Note a satellite nodule of fibrolamellar carcinoma *(curved arrows).*

E

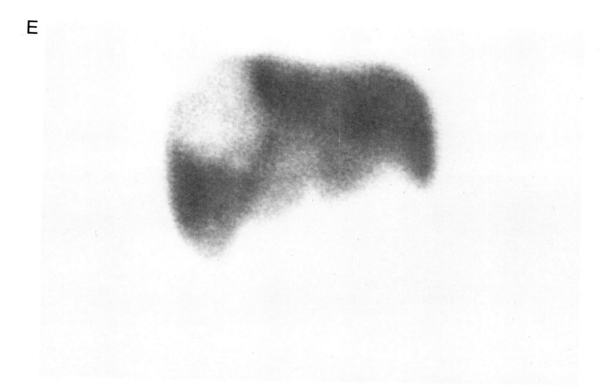

F

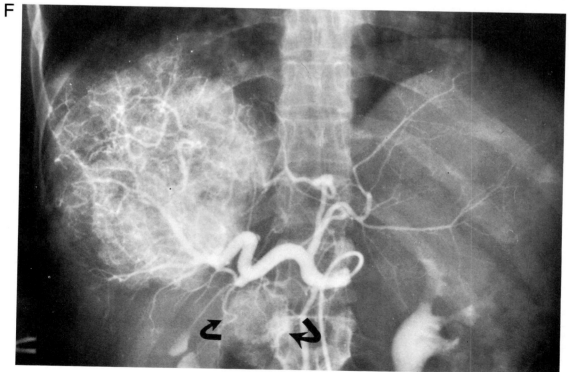

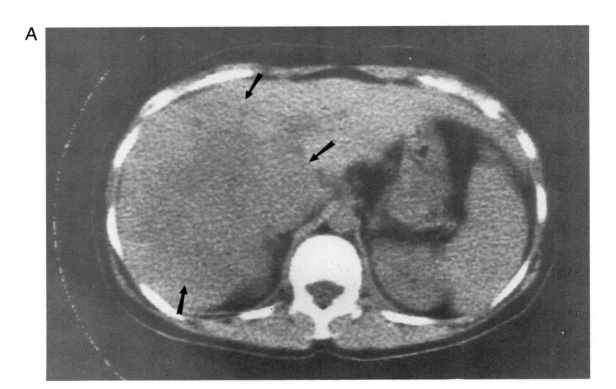

FIG 3–21.

Intrahepatic cholangiocarcinoma (multiple cases).

A, unenhanced CT of the abdomen in a middle-aged man with abnormal liver function tests demonstrates a large, ill-defined, homogeneous area of low density *(arrows)* in the right lobe of the liver. There is no dilatation of the intrahepatic biliary tree.

B and **C,** this 52-year-old man experienced left upper quadrant and epigastric discomfort for six months. The arterial phase **(B)** on common hepatic artery injection demonstrates in the left lobe of the liver a large lobulated area with intense stain *(arrows)* and with large avascular zones.

An oblique view of superselective left hepatic artery injection **(C,** capillary phase) reveals more clearly the extent of this intrahepatic mass with a large avascular zone. *(Continued.)*

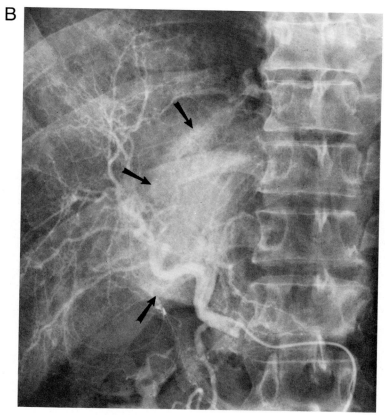

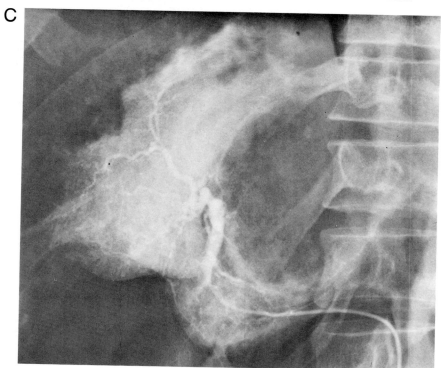

D

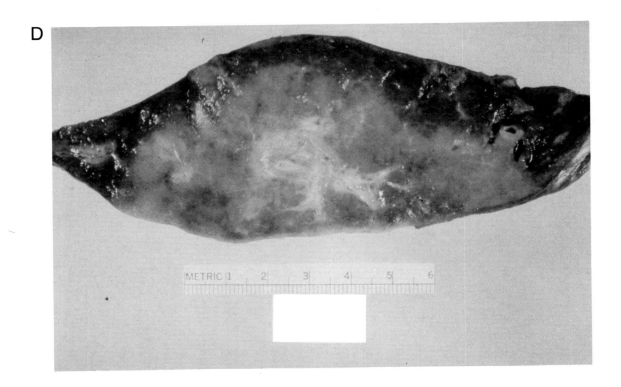

FIG 3–21 (cont.).
D through **F,** the typical gross appearance **(D)** of cholangiocarcinoma is seen in this cut section (different patient). There is a solid mass with prominent fibrous zones. Note the lack of intratumoral hemorrhage and the presence of satellite nodules (see also Color Plate 8).

A photomicrograph **(E)** demonstrates the fibrosis common in cholangiocarcinoma (hematoxylin and eosin, ×50).

Another photomicrograph **(F)** shows large areas of calcification *(arrows)* and mucoid material *(curved arrows),* both common in cholangiocarcinoma (hematoxylin and eosin, ×60).

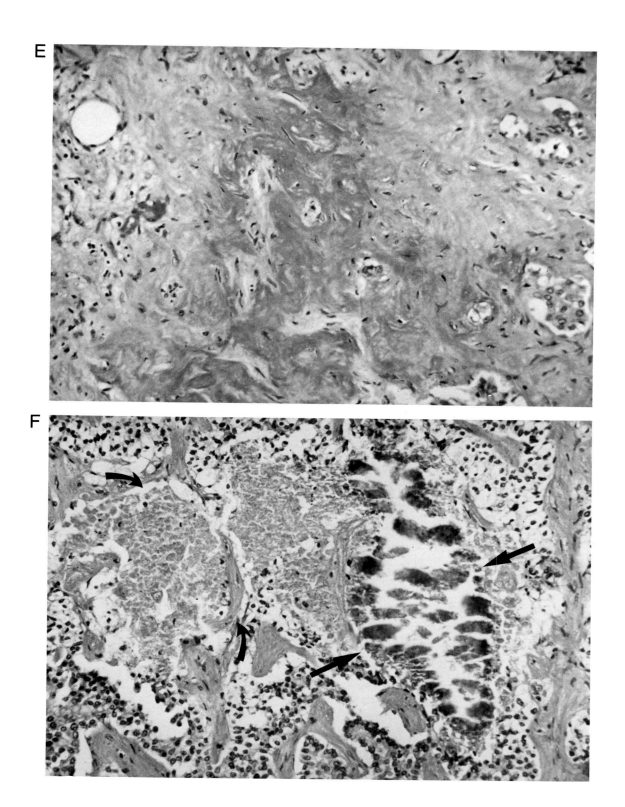

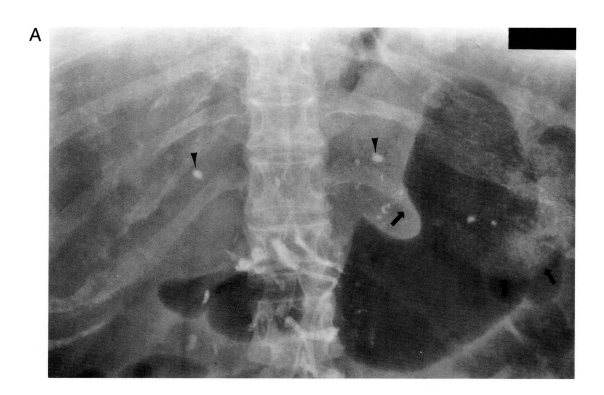

FIG 3–22.
Cholangiocarcinoma following use of thorium dioxide. This 57-year-old woman with mild epigastric pain underwent CT.

A, upper abdominal film before angiography shows diffuse punctate calcifications within the spleen *(arrows).* There are also denser calcifications between the liver and spleen *(arrowheads).* The patient had a history of thorium dioxide injection 36 years previously.

B, in the unenhanced portion of the CT study, there are serpiginous areas of increased density, seen primarily in the periphery of the liver. A large, irregular zone of decreased density is seen occupying most of the left lobe. Note the markedly increased density in the spleen *(S)* and in perihepatic lymph nodes *(arrowheads).* There is segmental dilatation of the intrahepatic biliary tree. The findings of dense spleen, linear hepatic densities, and nodal calcification are characteristic of thorium dioxide deposition.

C, after intravenous injection of contrast medium, the dilatation of the intrahepatic biliary tree is better seen.

Biopsy of the left hepatic mass proved cholangiocarcinoma.

Although thorium dioxide deposition is more often encountered in angiosarcoma, it is also associated with cholangiocarcinoma and HCC.

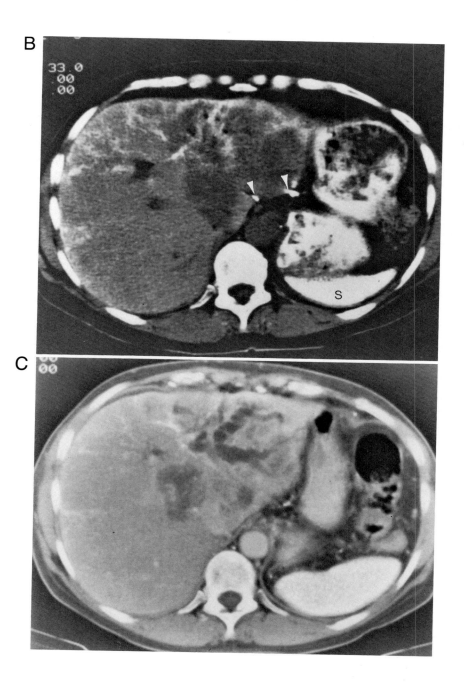

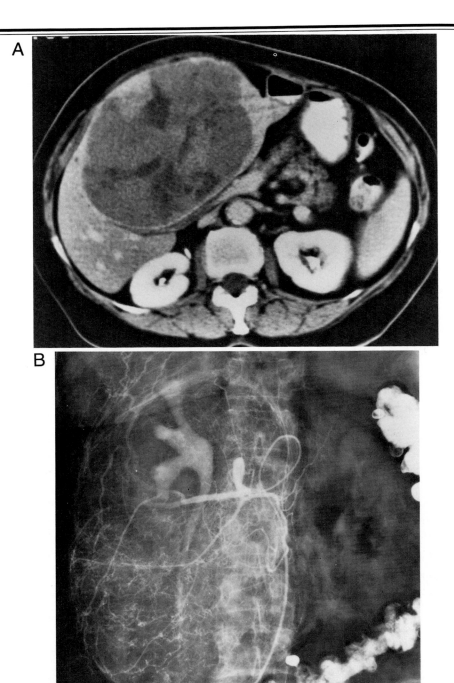

FIG 3–23.
Hepatic sarcoma (three cases).

A through **C,** this 72-year-old woman presented with progressive enlargement of the liver and a palpable right abdominal mass. Contrast-enhanced CT scan **(A)** shows a very large, well-defined mass predominantly in the left lobe of the liver. The tumor displays areas of low density.

Angiography **(B)** demonstrates the left lobe hepatic mass to extend over a length of approximately six vertebral bodies. It displays areas of neovascularity, particularly in the lower portion.

The patient had surgery, and on removal of the left lobe **(C),** the diagnosis of unclassified sarcoma was established (see also Color Plate 9).

D, this 81-year-old woman presented with weight loss. She had received thorium dioxide some 40 years ago. Unenhanced CT shows a very dense spleen with an area of low density in the liver containing numerous calcifications. Percutaneous biopsy established the diagnosis of angiosarcoma, and the patient was treated conservatively. *(Continued.)*

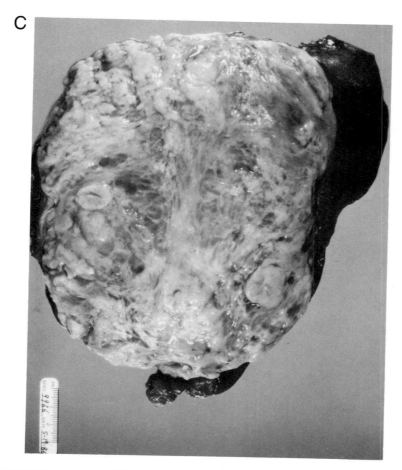

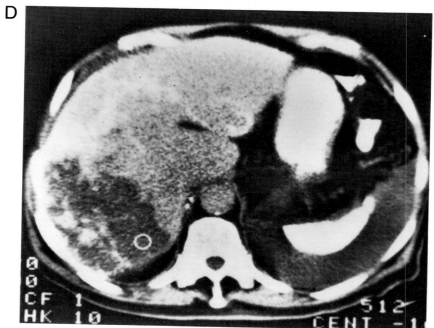

E

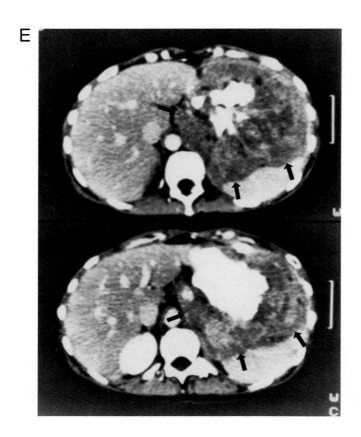

FIG 3–23 (cont.).
E through **G,** this 43-year-old woman with persistent abdominal pain was three months ago found to have a calcified area in the upper abdomen, the area having since grown. A CT scan **(E)** shows a very large soft tissue mass *(arrows)* with central dense calcification. The mass has displaced the spleen and aorta and could not be separated from the liver. Hepatic angiography **(F)** was done by celiac *(top)* and left hepatic *(bottom)* injection of contrast medium. This shows a very large, partially calcified mass that receives most of its blood supply from the left hepatic artery and some from the left gastric artery. The origin of the mass was thought to be in the liver, with gastric invasion. The patient received intraarterial chemotherapy and then underwent left hepatectomy with removal of the entire tumor **(G)** (see also Color Plate 10). The pathologic diagnosis was hepatic osteosarcoma.

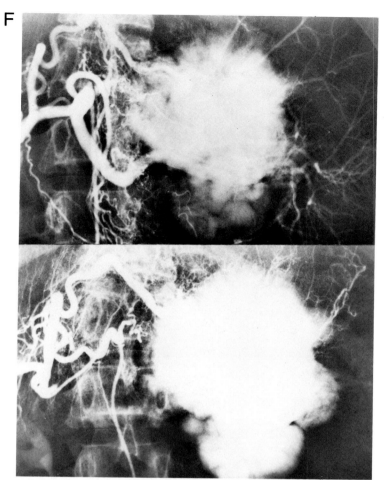

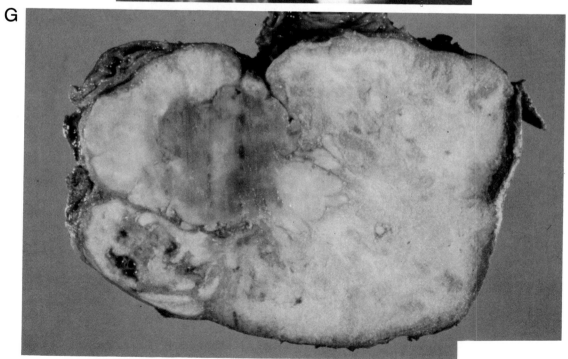

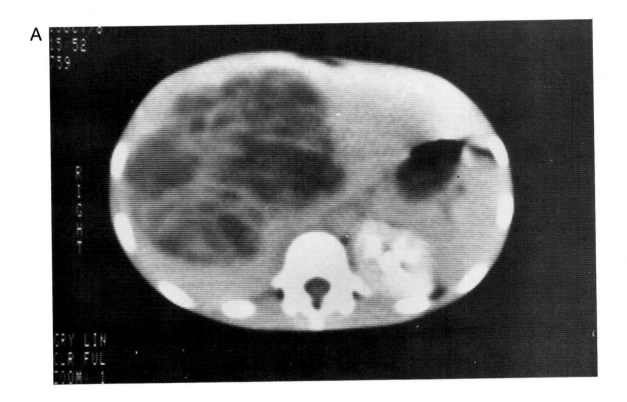

FIG 3–24.
Undifferentiated embryonal sarcoma (UES) (three cases).

A, a three-year-old boy presented with abdominal pain and a right upper quadrant mass. Enhanced CT shows a well-delineated, large, hypodense mass in the liver with dense septations of variable thickness. This is the most common appearance of UES.

B

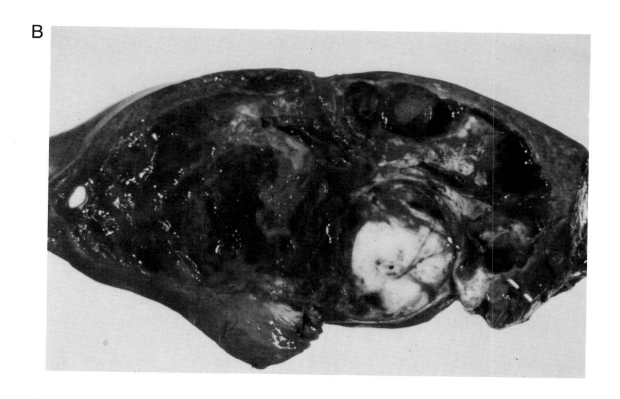

B and **C,** pathologic findings in another patient. Gross specimen (cut surface) **(B)** in another patient reveals a predominantly cystic UES containing necrotic debris, areas of fibrosis, and hemorrhagic fluid (see also Color Plate 11). *(Continued.)*

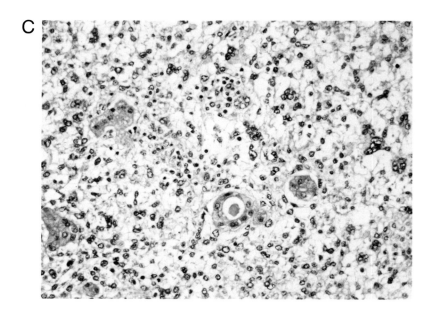

FIG 3–24 (cont.).
Photomicrograph of a UES **(C)** demonstrates very undifferentiated pleomorphic tumor cells in a loose myxoid matrix
(hematoxylin and eosin, ×20).

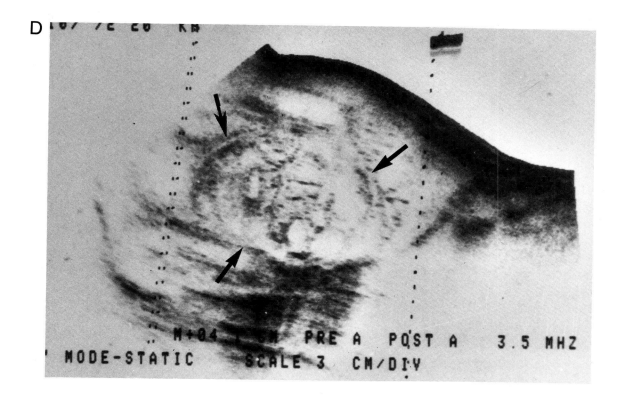

D, parasagittal sonogram in another child with UES shows a large, multiloculated cystic mass *(arrows)* within the liver. Occasionally, the UES will also be seen as a predominantly solid, echogenic mass.

(**A** and **B** from Ros P.R., Olmsted W.W., Dachman A.H., et al.: Undifferentiated (embryonal) sarcoma of the liver: radiologic-pathologic correlation. *Radiology* 160:141–145, 1986. Reproduced with permission.)

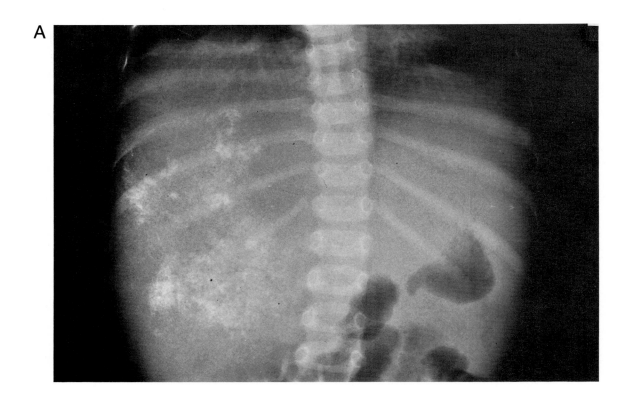

FIG 3–25.

Hepatoblastoma (multiple cases).

A, this 18-month-old boy presented with increased abdominal girth and weight loss. Plain radiography demonstrates extensive calcification in the right upper quadrant, proved to be within a mixed hepatoblastoma. A dense, coarse type of calcification is common in hepatoblastoma.

B, in a different patient with hepatoblastoma, CT reveals a large, solid, hypodense mass *(arrows)* with minimal enhancement and multiple calcifications of various sizes *(curved arrows).*

C, in the cut section of the gross specimen of a similar hepatoblastoma, note the tumor's large size, well-demarcated contour, and nodular surface.

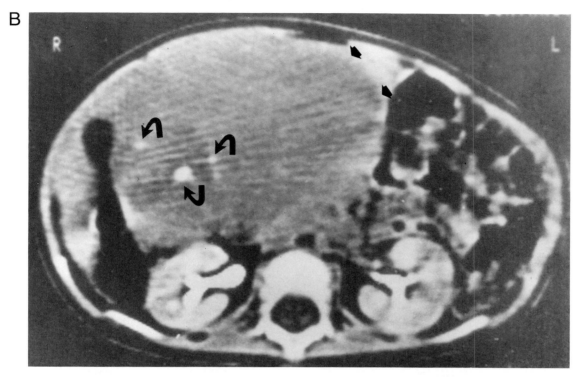

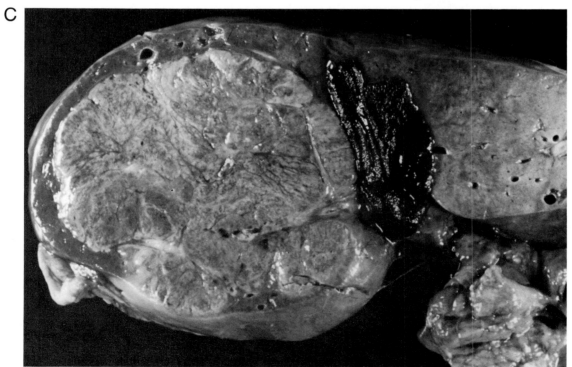

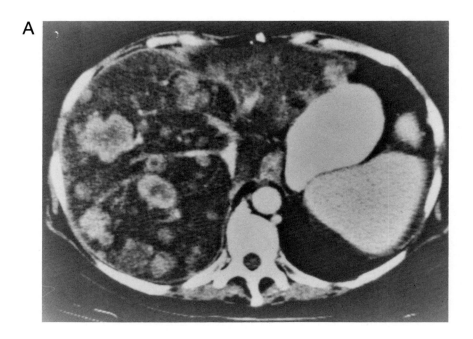

FIG 3–26.
Hypervascular diffuse liver metastasis. This patient had known carcinoid tumor and presented with hepatomegaly.

A, enhanced CT shows numerous enhancing, hypervascular metastases in the liver. There is diffuse fatty infiltration of the liver. The spleen is normal.

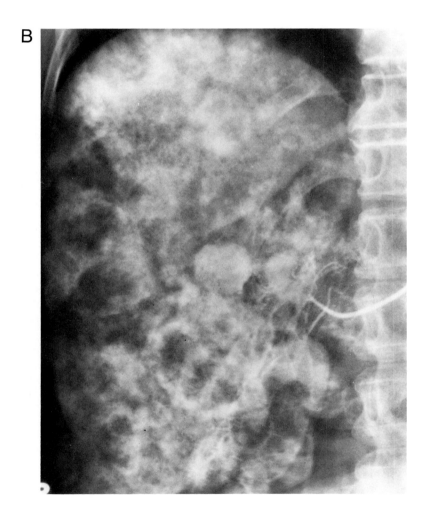

B, selective right hepatic arteriogram (venous phase) demonstrates dense capillary staining of numerous hepatic metastases.

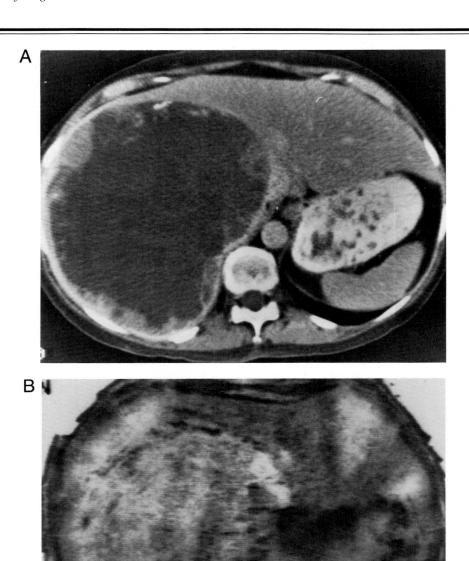

FIG 3–27.
Low-density large metastases (three cases).

A and **B,** this patient with granulosa cell tumor of the ovary presented with hepatomegaly. Enhanced CT **(A)** shows a large, well-encapsulated liver mass with nodules in the wall. This was thought to be a cystic metastasis; however, the sonogram **(B)** shows significant echoes within the mass.

C, a 33-year-old woman with a history of malignant melanoma of the head was discovered to have a solitary liver metastasis. Notice the multiloculated nature of the lesion and cystic areas. Melanoma usually results in numerous hepatic metastases.

D, this patient had leiomyosarcoma of the stomach. Computed tomography shows a large, low-density metastatic lesion in the right hepatic lobe, as well as several small nonhomogeneous masses in the remainder of the liver. Central low density is often associated with central necrosis and is very common in metastatic leiomyosarcoma.

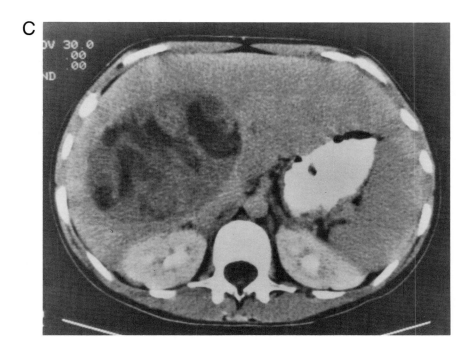

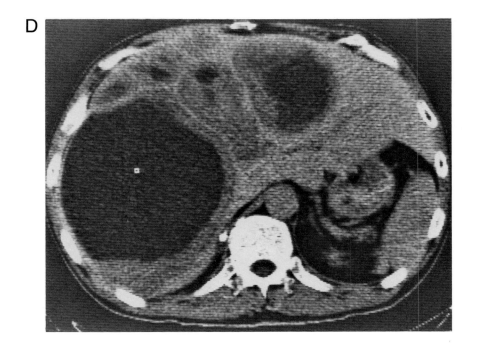

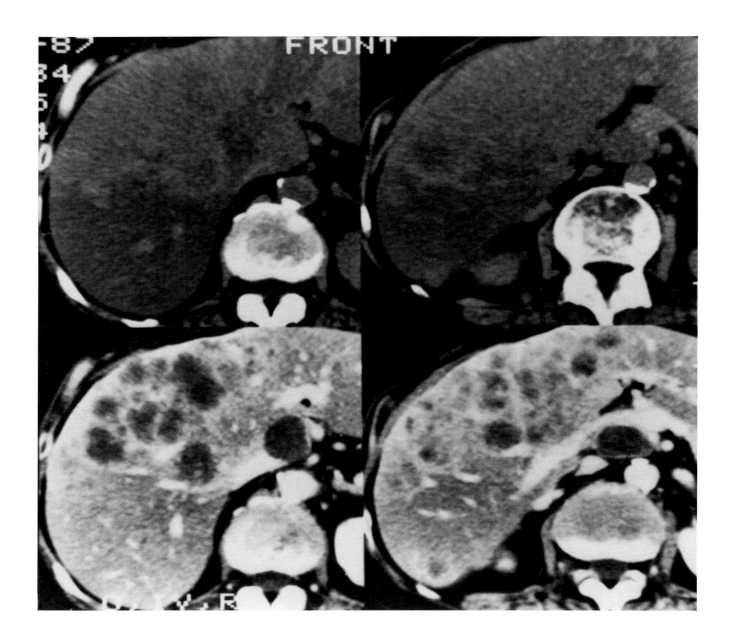

FIG 3–28.
Liver metastasis in a 55-year-old woman with a history of colon carcinoma excised two years earlier. She now presented with elevation of carcinoembryonic antigen levels.

A CT scan without contrast *(top row)* shows nonspherical hypodense regions in the posterior aspect of the right lobe of the liver with a somewhat segmental distribution, suggesting focal fatty change. Metastatic disease cannot be excluded.

Bolus contrast-enhanced CT *(bottom row)* clearly demonstrates multiple spherical, hypodense lesions in the midportion of the liver, typical of metastasis. These cannot be detected on the unenhanced CT scan.

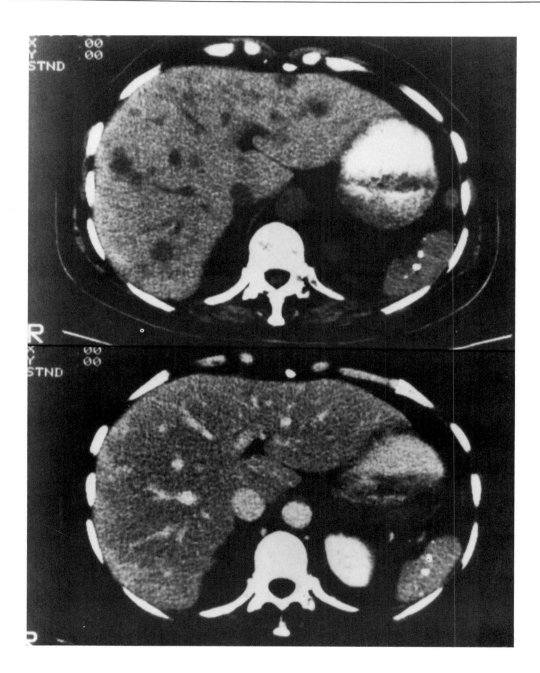

FIG 3–29.
Metastases masked on enhanced CT. This 62-year-old woman had breast carcinoma.

A CT scan without contrast *(top)* clearly shows numerous round, hypodense hepatic lesions, which are masked on contrast-enhanced CT (bolus technique, *bottom*), because they enhance to the same degree as liver parenchyma.

This case is not typical: breast metastases are usually hypovascular. This case is an example of the importance of using enhanced CT for the evaluation of metastasis. Plain and enhanced CT scans should be performed routinely to increase sensitivity in detection of metastatic foci.

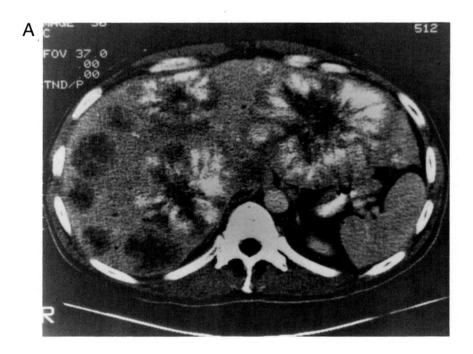

FIG 3–30.
Calcified liver metastases (two cases).

A, this patient had colonic adenocarcinoma. An unenhanced CT scan shows multiple low-density liver masses, several of them with peripheral calcification, representing metastatic foci.

B and C, this 46-year-old woman had a history of colon carcinoma excised two years ago. Because of mildly elevated carcinoembryonic antigen titers, a liver sonogram was made (B) and shows a single echogenic area *(arrow)* adjacent to the diaphragm at the dome. Since this was the only abnormal finding, CT was done (C) for guided biopsy. Calcified metastatic adenocarcinoma was proved.

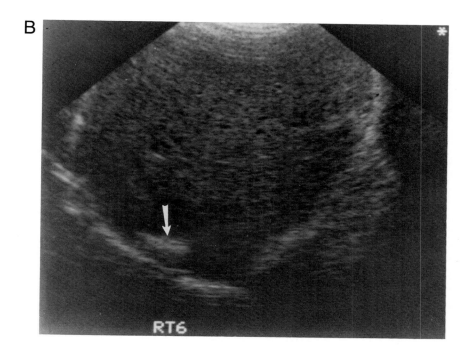

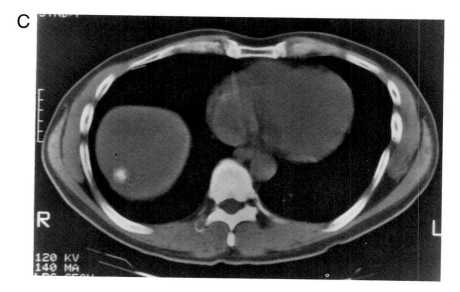

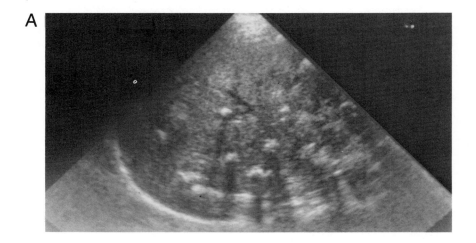

FIG 3–31.
Calcification of liver metastases following treatment. This patient had breast carcinoma treated with chemotherapy.

A, routine follow-up sonogram shows numerous bright, echogenic foci with acoustic shadowing within the liver.

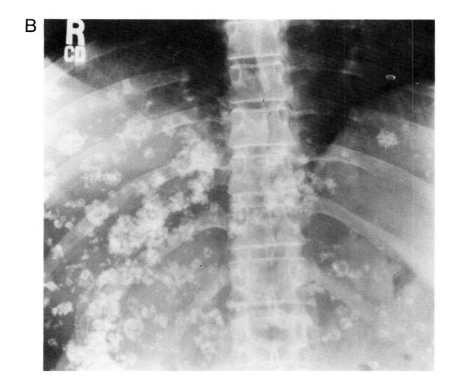

B, a plain film further confirms calcifications and their diffuse nature. The patient's liver enzyme values were normal, and one-year follow-up showed no change.

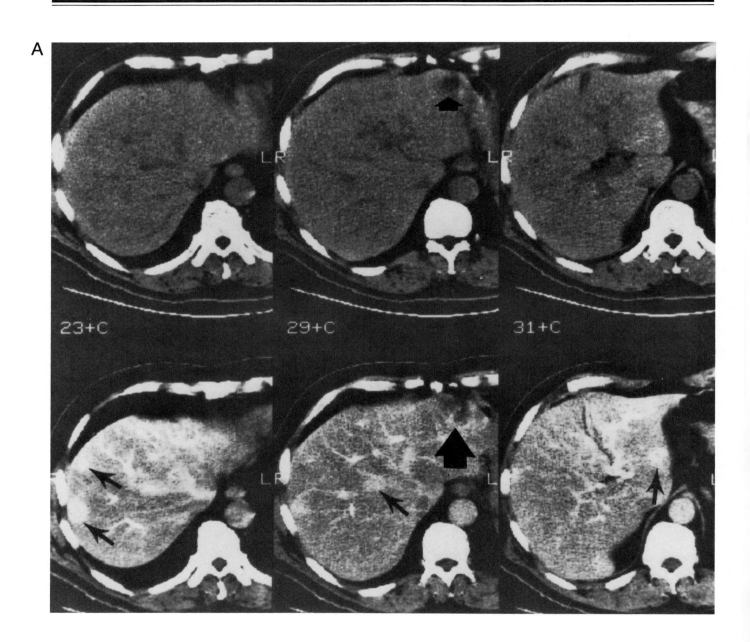

FIG 3–32.
Liver metastases (two cases of CT-angiography).

A, this 66-year-old man has colonic adenocarcinoma.

Unenhanced CT scan *(top row)* shows a single low-density lesion in the left lobe *(arrow).*

Enhanced CT scan *(bottom row)* was made during direct manual injection of contrast medium into the hepatic artery. This scan demonstrates multiple enhancing liver metastases *(arrows),* not detected on plain CT.

Nonenhancing left lobe lesion *(large arrow)* demonstrates that metastases of the same histologic type may have different enhancement patterns. This left lobe lesion is

also seen on the plain CT. Its lower density may represent necrosis.

B and **C,** in another patient, with breast carcinoma, enhanced CT **(B)** shows two lesions *(arrows)* in the left lobe of the liver. Repeat CT **(C)** during direct manual injection of contrast into the hepatic artery shows that almost the entire liver is involved by metastatic deposits (some of which are marked by *arrowheads*). Notice the diffuse fatty changes of the liver. (**B** and **C** from Lewis E., Bernardino M.E., Barnes P.A., et al.: The fatty liver: pitfalls in the CT and angiographic evaluation of metastatic disease. Reproduced by permission.)

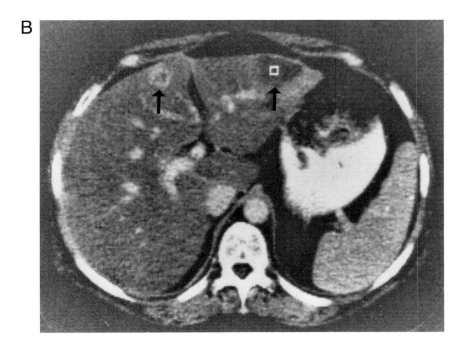

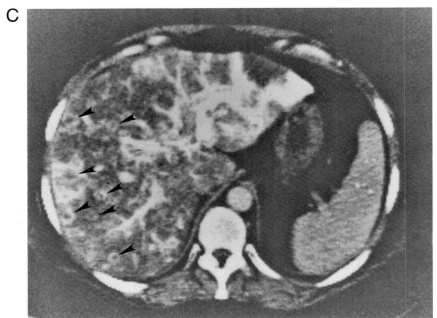

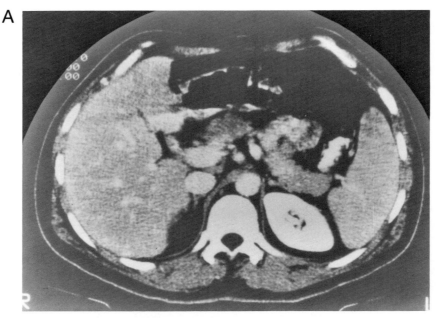

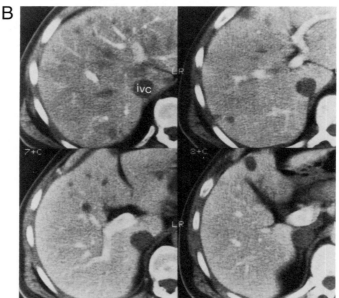

FIG 3–33.
Liver metastases (two cases).

A and **B,** a 41-year-old patient with colon carcinoma. A liver CT scan **(A)** made by bolus intravenous contrast technique appears normal.

Liver CT obtained during the portal venous phase of a selective manual superior mesenteric artery contrast injection **(B)** shows multiple small, hypodense metastases, previously undetected. Notice lack of opacification of the inferior vena cava *(IVC).*

Although time-consuming and expensive, CT-portography provides valuable clinical information when partial hepatectomy is being contemplated.

C and **D,** a 51-year-old man with known colon carcinoma evaluated due to rising serum carcinoembryonic antigen. T_1-weighted **(C)** magnetic resonance image of liver (TR/TE, 400/25) shows probable areas of low signal intensity within the liver. Notice the artifact from the pulsating aorta. T_2-weighted **(D)** image (TR/TE, 2,500/80) shows multiple metastases seen as areas of high signal intensity. This study was done in a 1.5-tesla magnet.

C
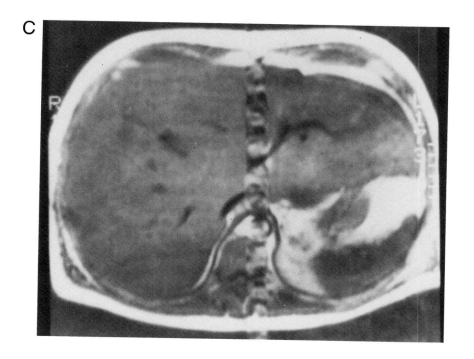

D
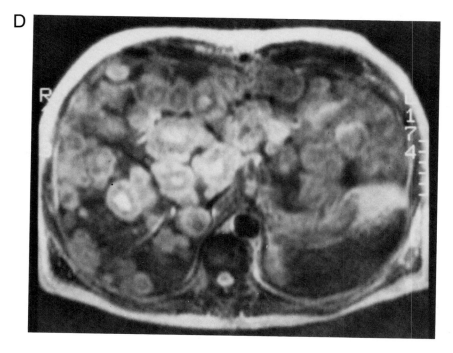

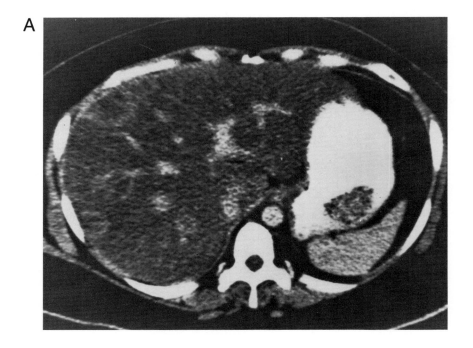

FIG 3–34.
Liver metastases (two cases).

 A and **B,** this patient had breast carcinoma and was receiving chemotherapy. A contrast-enhanced CT scan **(A)** shows nonhomogeneity and diffusely decreased density of the liver, the latter due to fatty change. Note several nodular, increased-density areas in the periphery of the liver with minimal enhancement.

B

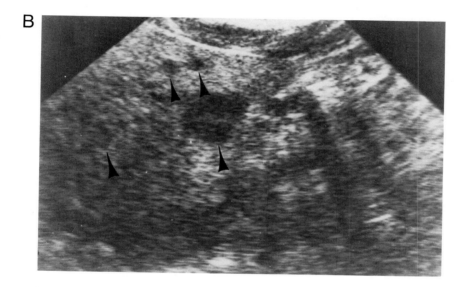

Transverse sonogram **(B)** shows nonhomogeneity and generalized increased echogenicity of the entire liver. In addition, there are several hypoechoic lesions *(arrowheads)* of variable size. These lesions were not demonstrated on CT study.

The findings by CT and ultrasound were proved to be due to diffuse metastatic disease from breast. *(Continued.)*

C

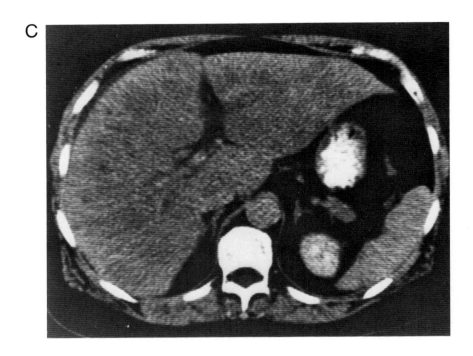

D

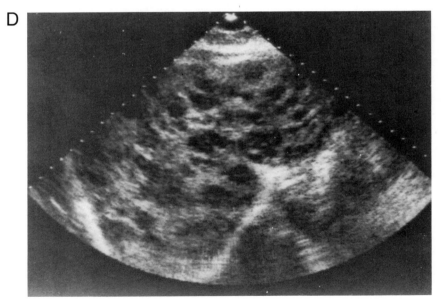

FIG 3–34 (cont.).
C and **D,** after intravenous pyelography, another patient with breast carcinoma had CT **(C),** which shows diffuse nonho-mogeneity of the liver without clear focal masses. The sono-gram **(D)** reveals numerous hypoechoic lesions represent-ing diffuse hepatic metastasis.

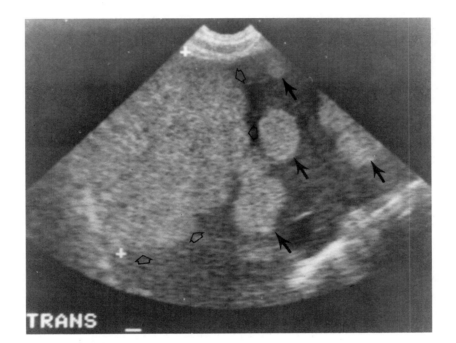

FIG 3–35.
Echogenic metastases. This 65-year-old man underwent re-section two years previously for malignant carcinoid of the lung.

An ultrasound scan shows one large *(open arrows)* and several small *(arrows)* echogenic, smoothly bordered masses in the liver, which were carcinoid metastases.

The hypervascular morphology of these lesions proba-bly accounts for their echogenic appearance.

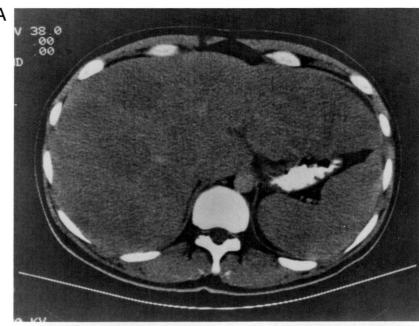

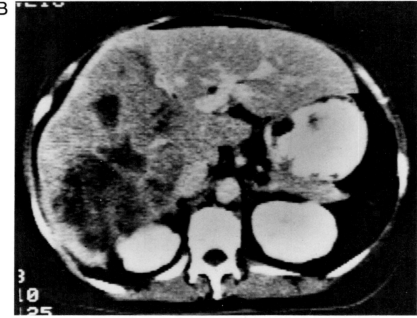

FIG 3–36.
Hepatic lymphoma (three cases).

A, this 26-year-old man had secondary liver involvement from non-Hodgkin's lymphoma. Enhanced CT (drip infusion) shows mild hepatomegaly with nonhomogeneous areas of slightly decreased density throughout the entire liver; these areas blend imperceptibly with normal liver. This represents the diffuse infiltrative form of hepatic lymphoma.

B and **C,** this patient with non-Hodgkin's lymphoma presented with hepatomegaly. An enhanced CT scan **(B)** shows a large mass in the right lobe with different degrees of hypodensity, lobulations, and a relatively well defined margin. The left lobe is normal. This represents the focal nodular or masslike type of lymphoma. A transverse sonogram **(C)** shows the mass in the right hepatic lobe *(arrows)* to be relatively homogeneous and hypoechoic. This appearance is due to the homogeneously cellular makeup of lymphomatous masses.

D, this 52-year-old man had lymphoma involving both the liver and the spleen. Computed tomography shows low-density hepatic and splenic lesions *(top),* decreased significantly in size and number following chemotherapy *(bottom).*

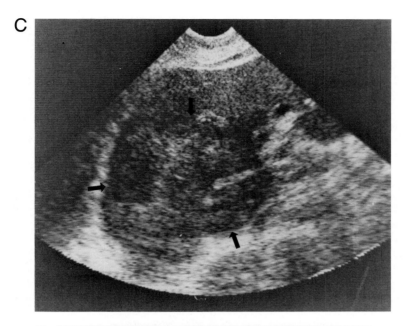

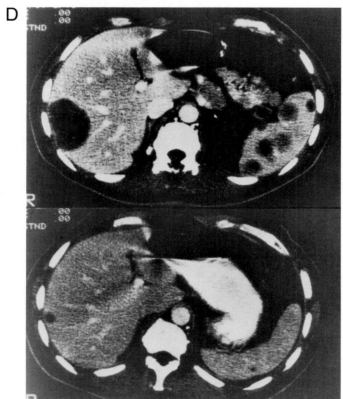

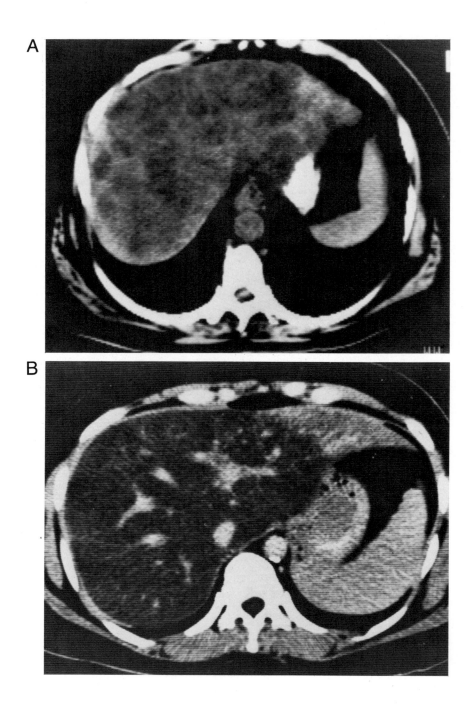

FIG 3–37.
Fatty liver (three cases).

A, this patient had a history of alcohol abuse. Computed tomography shows multiple ill-defined, hypodense hepatic lesions. Biopsy showed fatty change with no evidence of malignancy.

B, in a different patient, note the diffuse fatty change of the liver except for a portion of the lateral segment of the left lobe. Also, there is no mass effect on intrahepatic vascular structures. These findings are typical of diffuse fatty change.

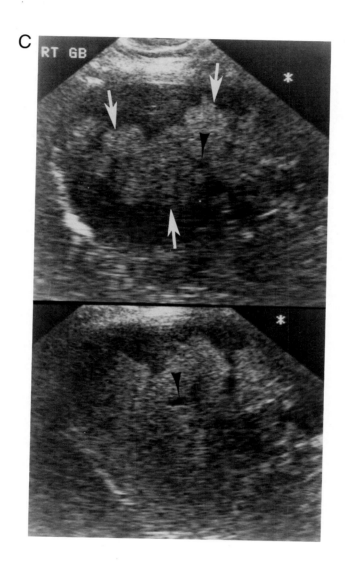

C, this patient with colon carcinoma and receiving chemotherapy had right upper quadrant pain, and sonography was done for gallbladder evaluation. There is an island area of increased echogenicity with geometric margins in the liver *(arrows)*. This configuration is typical of hepatic fatty change. Notice presence of vascular channels *(arrowheads)* within the echogenic area.

A

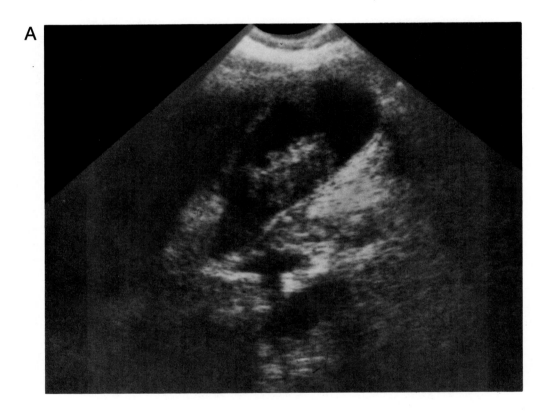

FIG 3–38.
Primary gallbladder carcinoma (four cases).

A, this 64-year-old woman presented with two-month history of right upper quadrant pain. Sonography reveals a solid mass projecting into the lumen and attached to the wall of the gallbladder.

At cholecystectomy, the mass in the wall of the gall-bladder was proved to be an adenocarcinoma.

B and **C,** this 62-year-old woman presented with mild epigastric pain and nausea. Sonography (results not shown) showed gallstones and abnormal liver. Unenhanced liver CT **(B)** shows calcification in the region of the gallbladder and numerous low-density hepatic lesions, which are better seen on contrast-enhanced CT **(C).** At surgery, the gallblad-der was seen to be replaced by cancerous tumor mass, and there were multiple nodules within the right lobe of the liver. The diagnosis was poorly differentiated adenocarcinoma of the gallbladder with liver metastasis. *(Continued.)*

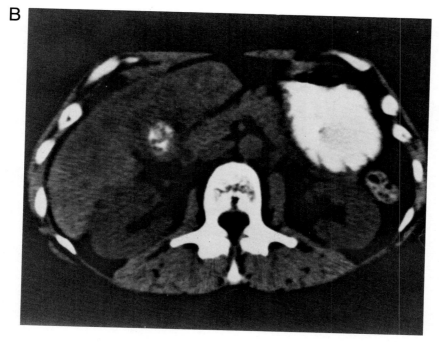

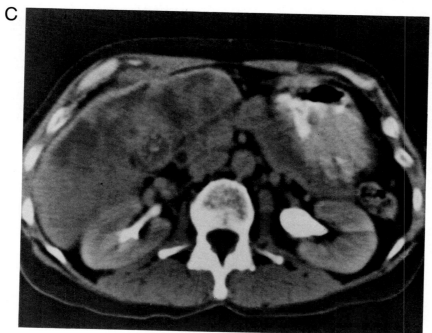

D

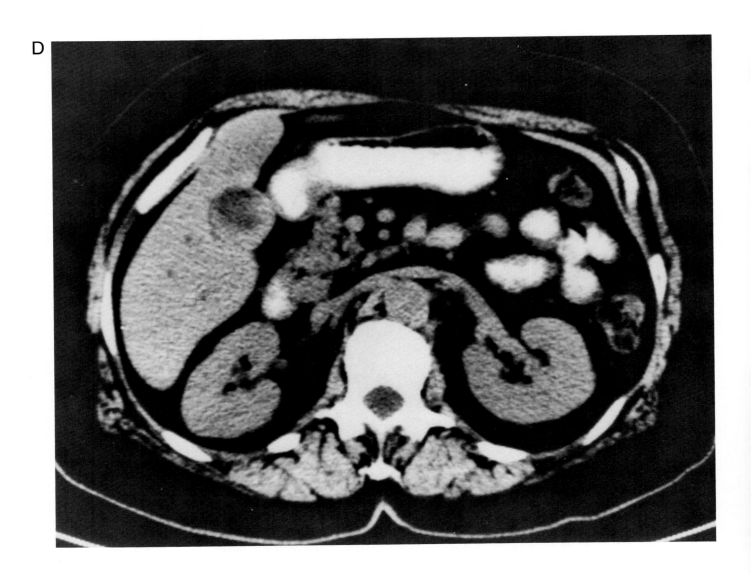

FIG 3–38 (cont.).
D, another patient, a 64-year-old woman who presented with chronic right upper quadrant pain and weight loss, was found to have localized thickening of the gallbladder wall on CT. At surgery, cholangiocarcinoma was found to involve the full thickness of the gallbladder wall.

E and **F,** this 75-year-old woman was admitted for evaluation of a one-month history of epigastric fullness, anorexia, and weight loss.

An abdominal sonogram **(E)** reveals an echogenic mass *(open arrows)* in the right upper quadrant. The mass has an anechoic center.

A CT scan **(F)** reveals a subhepatic mass with an area of central lucency.

Initially, the mass was believed to most likely be a necrotic lymphoma or leiomyosarcoma, but on laparotomy the tumor was found to be a poorly differentiated adenocarcinoma of the gallbladder that had infiltrated throughout the gallbladder wall and extended to the stomach and liver.

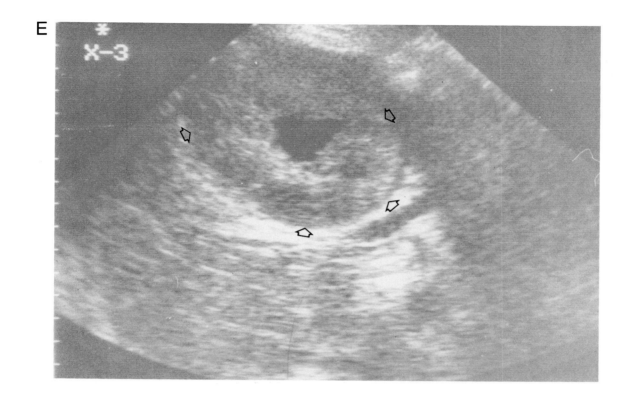

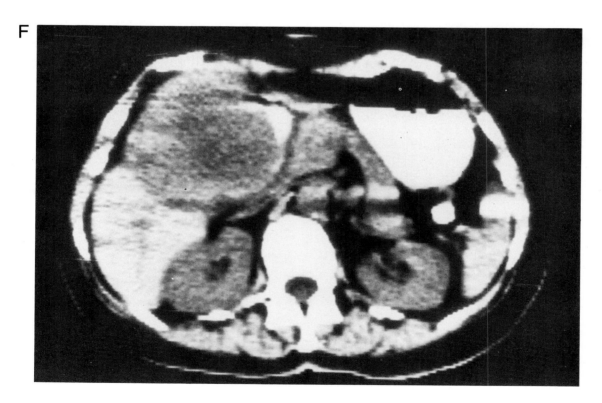

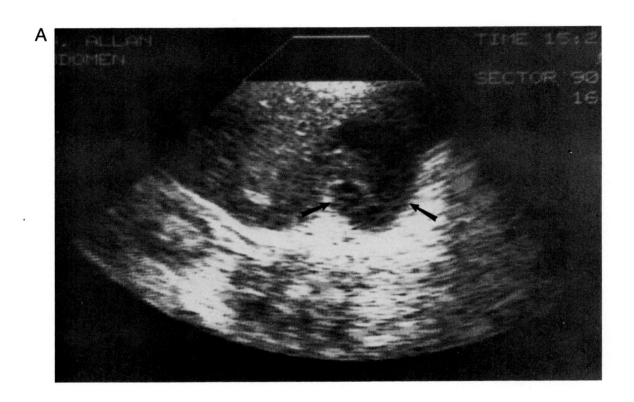

FIG 3–39.
Gallbladder metastasis (two cases).

A, this 64-year-old man presented at the emergency room with fever and severe right upper quadrant pain three years after a malignant melanoma was excised from his back. A clinical diagnosis of acute cholecystitis was made.

Sonogram revealed cholelithiasis (results not shown)

as well as a fixed, nonshadowing, echogenic lesion *(arrows)* within the lumen of the neck of the gallbladder.

At surgery, a necrotic mucosal nodule consistent with metastatic melanoma was found within the neck of the gallbladder. There was also evidence of acute and chronic cholecystitis.

B

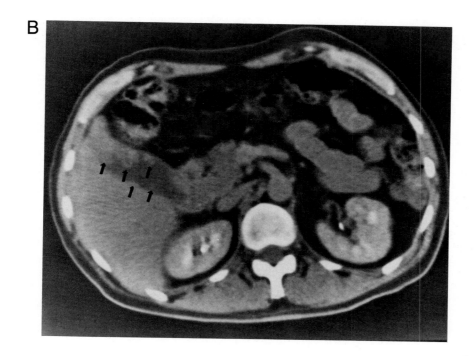

B, this 47-year-old man with known melanoma of the right shoulder has had several normal abdominal CT examinations during an 18-month follow-up. However, recently he had local recurrent tumor, and the CT showed liver metastases and numerous nodular densities *(arrows)* within the gallbladder wall, a finding that was not present four months ago and probably represents metastases. (**B** from Shirkhoda A., Albin J.: Malignant melanoma: correlating abdominal and pelvic CT with clinical staging. *Radiology* 165:75–78, 1987. Reproduced with permission.)

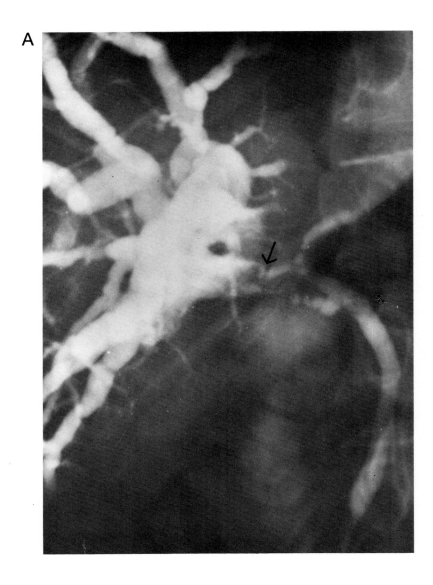

FIG 3–40.
Biliary papillomatosis. This 65-year-old man presented with pruritus and painless jaundice. Sonography (results not shown) revealed biliary ductal dilatation.

A, a percutaneous transhepatic cholangiogram reveals what appears to be stenosis *(arrow)* in the region of the biliary duct bifurcation.

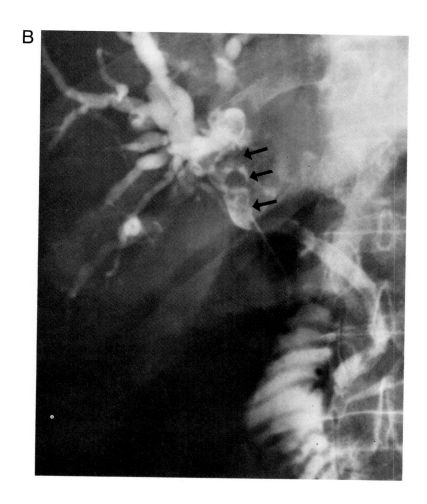

B, an intraoperative cholangiogram made shortly there-after reveals the obstructing lesion to actually be multiple intraluminal masses *(arrows).* The pathologic diagnosis was biliary papillomatosis.

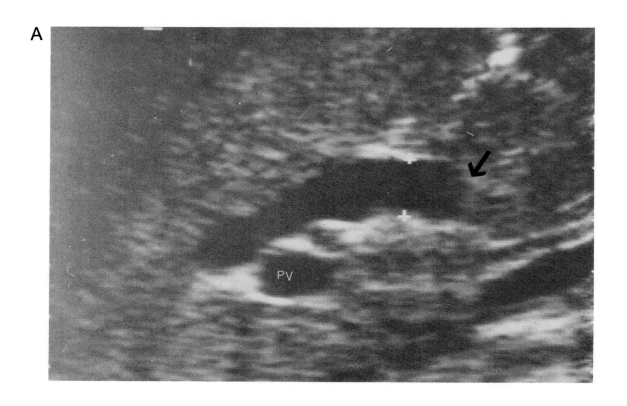

FIG 3–41.
Granular cell tumor of the distal common bile duct. This 41-year-old woman complained of recent-onset pruritus and jaundice.

A, an oblique sonogram shows a dilated common bile duct *(cursors,* 10 mm) with an abrupt termination *(arrow)* and no evidence of a calculus *(Pv,* portal vein).

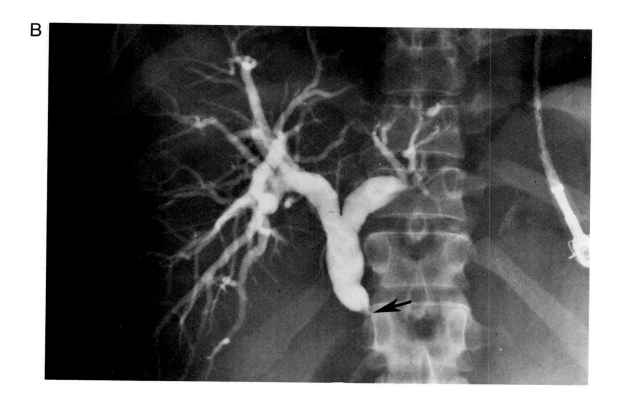

B, on a percutaneous transhepatic cholangiogram, the distal portion of the opacified duct *(arrow)* is seen to taper to a point.

At surgery, a granular cell tumor of the distal common bile duct was discovered and Whipple's operation performed.

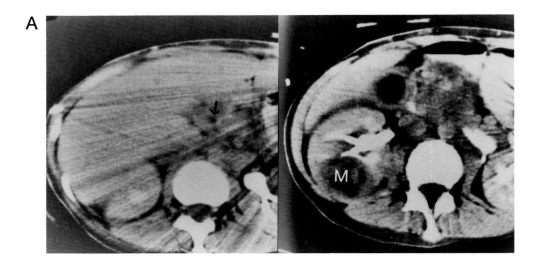

FIG 3–42.
Lymphomatous invasion of common bile duct. This 21-year-old woman with known Hodgkin's lymphoma presented with gradual-onset rising bilirubin titers.

A, two abdominal CT images show periaortic and porta hepatis adenopathy with minimal dilatation *(arrow)* of proximal common bile duct. The distal portion of the common bile duct is not seen. Notice many artifacts due to surgical clips from previous splenectomy. Also there is evidence of right renal mass *(M)* due to lymphomatous infiltration.

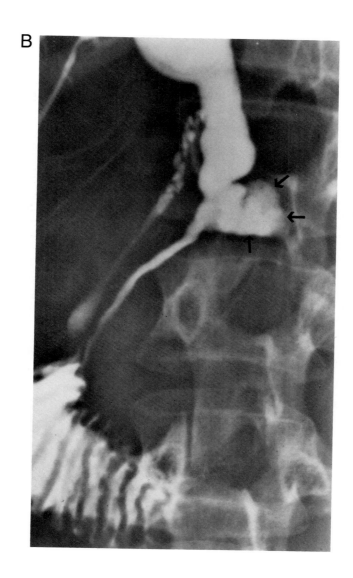

B, percutaneous transhepatic cholangiogram (PTC) shows a large false aneurysm *(arrows)*, probably due to ulceration of the wall of common duct and extension of contrast medium into adjacent nodes.

An earlier PTC revealed marked stenosis of the distal duct, which now, after chemotherapy, shows opening and flow of contrast into the duodenum.

A

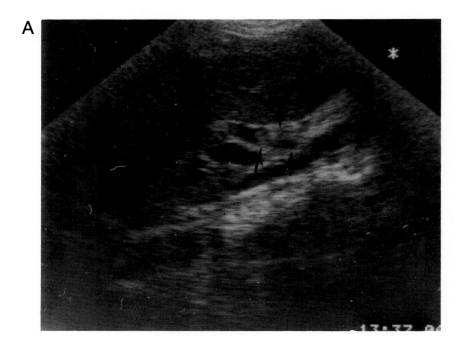

FIG 3–43.
Metastasis to the common bile duct. This 50-year-old woman with a history of colon carcinoma and partial hepatectomy for liver metastasis presented with gradual-onset jaundice.

A, a sonogram shows dilatation of the common bile duct and the presence of echogenic material *(arrows)* within the lumen of the common duct.

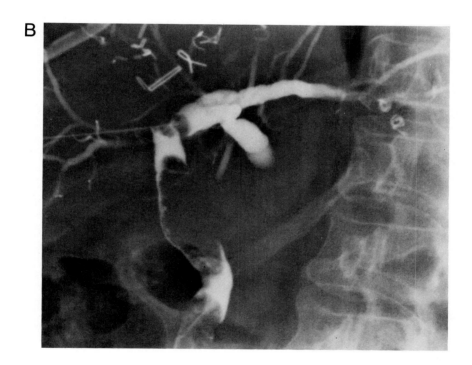

B, a PTC reveals an elongated filling defect within the lumen of a dilated common bile duct and involving its medial wall. Brush biopsy was done at the time of PTC and proved adenocarcinoma histologically similar to the colonic primary.

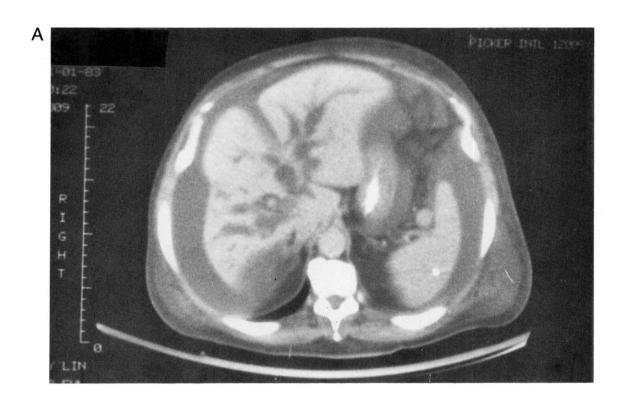

FIG 3–44.
Common hepatic duct cholangiocarcinoma (adenocarcinoma) (two cases).

A through **C,** this 72-year-old man presented with right upper quadrant pain, weight loss, ascites, and jaundice.

B

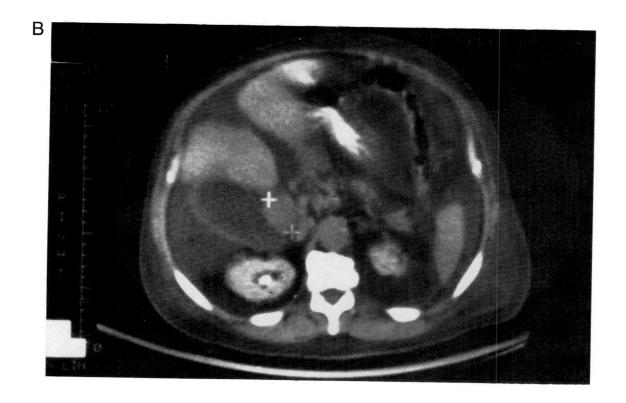

A CT scan **(A)** reveals ascites, dilated intrahepatic bile ducts, and a 4-cm soft tissue mass (*cursors* in **B**) distending the extrahepatic bile duct adjacent to the gallbladder. *(Continued.)*

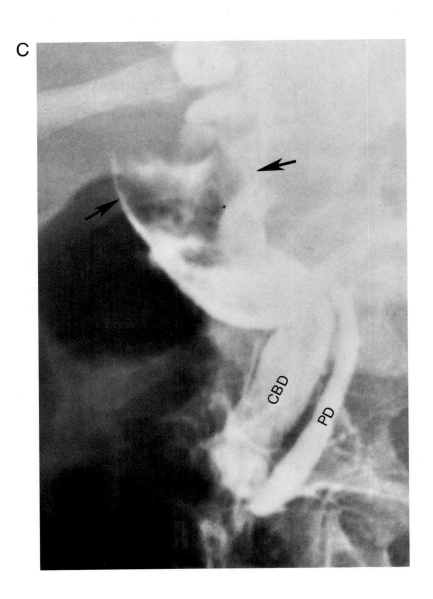

FIG 3–44 (cont.).
Endoscopic retrograde cholangiopancreatography (ERCP) **(C)** confirms the presence of a large intraluminal mass *(arrows),* which proved to be a poorly differentiated adenocarcinoma of the proximal common bile duct *(CBD)* and common hepatic duct *(PD,* pancreatic duct).

D and **E,** this 65-year-old man with a four-month history of upper abdominal pain underwent CT **(D),** which showed dilated intrahepatic bile ducts and fullness in the head of the pancreas and porta hepatis. On ERCP (not shown), the pancreas was normal, but a mass was visualized within the lumen of the common hepatic duct. At removal of the gallbladder, an intraoperative cholangiogram **(E)** was made. A lobulated filling defect *(arrows)* is seen in the common hepatic duct and extending into the right and left ducts. Biopsy of this mass established the diagnosis of well-differentiated papillary adenocarcinoma.

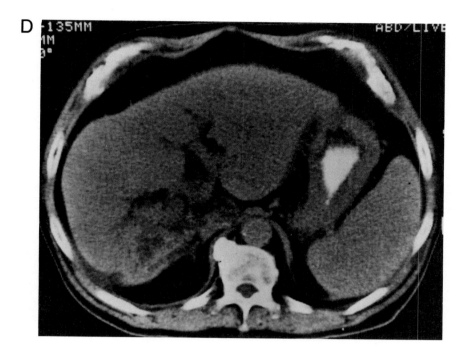

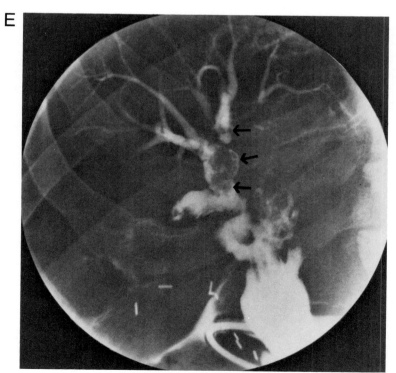

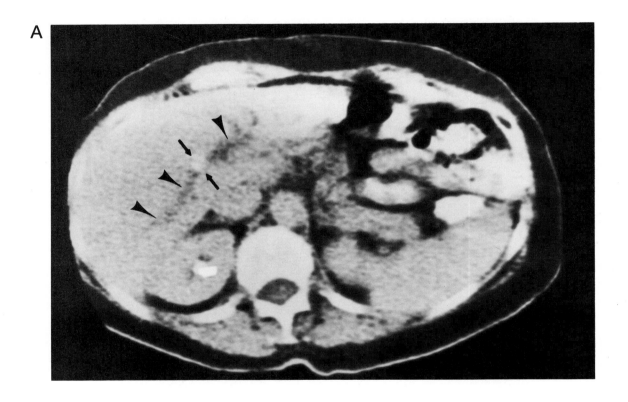

FIG 3–45.
Hilar cholangiocarcinoma (Klatskin's tumor). This 75-year-old woman presented with signs and symptoms of obstructive jaundice. A sonogram (not shown) revealed choleli-thiasis and no evidence of extrahepatic ductal dilatation.

A, a CT scan reveals multiple intrahepatic ductal dilatations *(arrowheads)* and a small area of calcification *(arrows)*. However, there was no evidence of a mass.

B

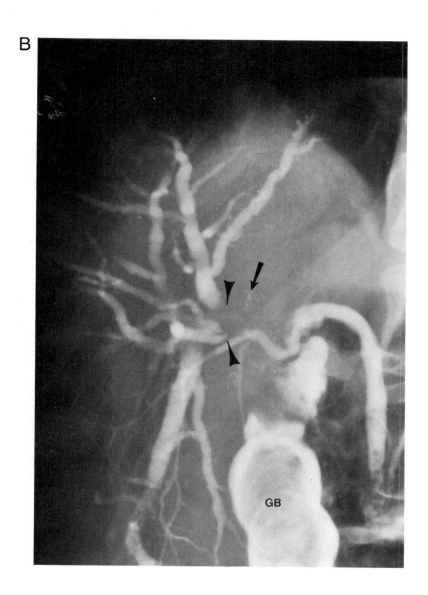

GB

B, an endoscopic retrograde cholangiogram reveals dilatation of the right intrahepatic ducts, proximal to stenosis in the central right hepatic duct. The left intrahepatic ducts were not visualized, thought to be due to a tumor in this area, one possibly containing a small calcification *(arrow)* and resulting in attenuation of the proximal ducts *(arrowheads)*. Large stones are seen in the gallbladder *(GB),* but the remainder of the extrahepatic tract was normal. Notice small filling defects in the distal common bile duct, which were thought to be air bubbles.

At surgery, an infiltrating adenocarcinoma at the junction of the hepatic ducts (Klatskin's tumor) was discovered. The calcification was most likely related to the tumor.

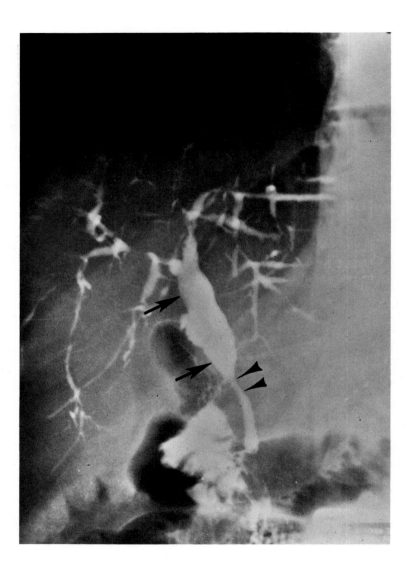

FIG 3–46.
Common bile duct adenocarcinoma in sclerosing cholangitis. This 41-year-old woman had a 23-year history of ulcerative colitis and a 7-year history of primary sclerosing cholangitis.

Because of worsening pruritus, a follow-up endoscopic retrograde cholangiogram was made. It reveals multiple areas of intrahepatic ductal stenosis, similar in appearance to prior studies and consistent with sclerosing cholangitis. However, the common bile duct is dilated *(arrows)* proximal to a new area of stenosis *(arrowheads)*.

After an attempted dilation of this stricture failed, a laparotomy was performed. Common bile duct biopsy revealed adenocarcinoma.

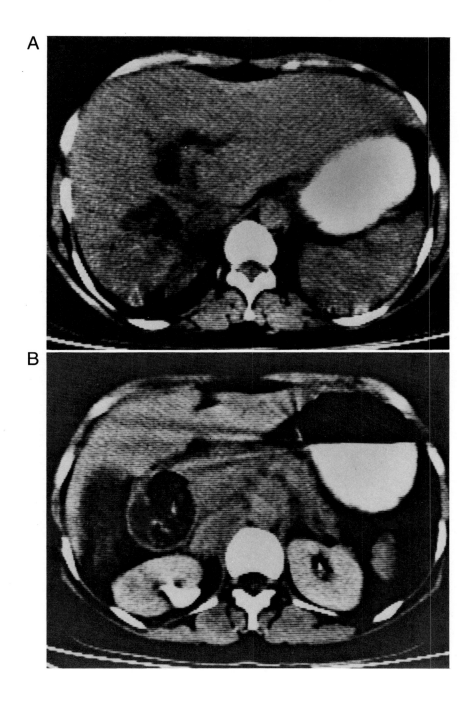

FIG 3–47.
Cholangiocarcinoma in a choledochal cyst (two cases).

   A through **D,** this 27-year-old woman was evaluated because of progressive onset of jaundice. When four years old, she had choledochoduodenostomy for obstructive jaun- dice, and choledochal cyst was discovered at the time of surgery. The enhanced CT scan of the liver **(A)** shows intra- hepatic biliary dilatation. There is evidence of a cystic mass below the porta hepatis **(B)** containing material of higher density. *(Continued.)*

C

D

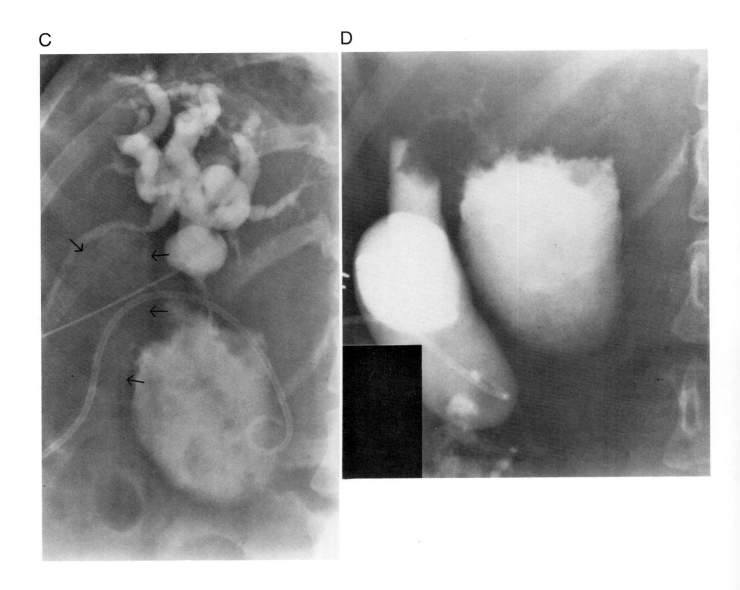

FIG 3–47 (cont.).
A percutaneous transhepatic cholangiogram **(C** and **D)** confirms the dilated biliary system and shows a stricture above the choledochal cyst. However, the contrast fills the cystic structure, which has an irregular wall. The gallbladder *(arrows)* is opacified with contrast in early phase. Cholangiocarcinoma at a choledochal cyst was proved at surgery.

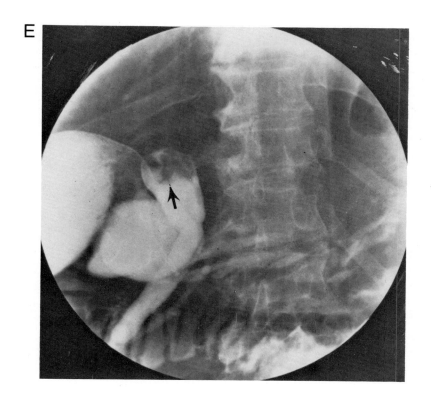

E, another patient, with elevated serum bilirubin titer, had endoscopic retrograde cholangiography, which shows filling of the gallbladder. But there is also filling defect within the lumen of the dilated hepatic duct *(arrow)*. Biopsy proved cholangiocarcinoma within an aneurysmally dilated common hepatic duct.

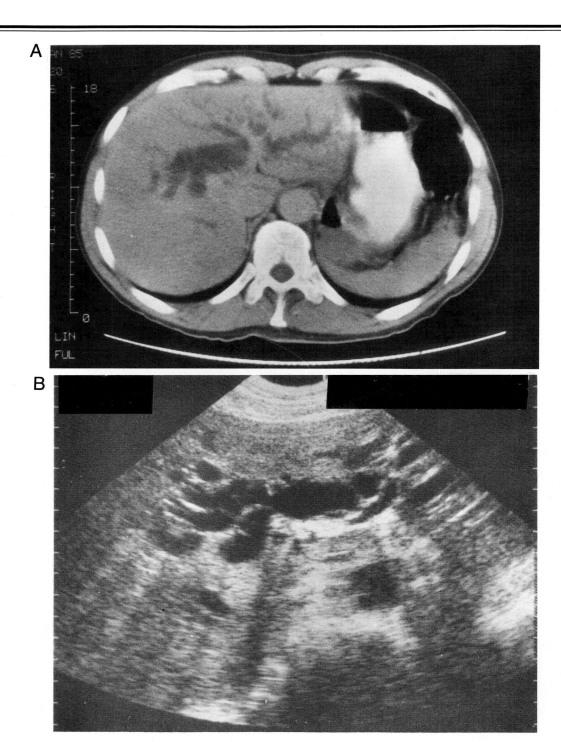

FIG 3–48.
Papillary adenocarcinoma of the common bile duct. This 61-year-old man presented with painless jaundice.

A, a CT scan reveals marked intrahepatic biliary ductal dilatation, but no obstructing lesion was identified.

B and **C,** a sonogram confirms the intrahepatic ductal dilatation **(B)** and also reveals a markedly enlarged common bile duct *(CBD)* with an apparent intraluminal soft tissue mass *(arrowheads* in **C**) at its point of obstruction.

D, a transhepatic cholangiogram confirms complete obstruction *(arrow).*

At surgery, a papillary adenocarcinoma involving both the proximal common bile duct and the cystic duct was found.

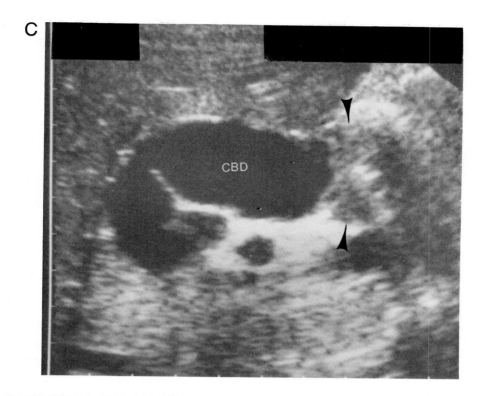

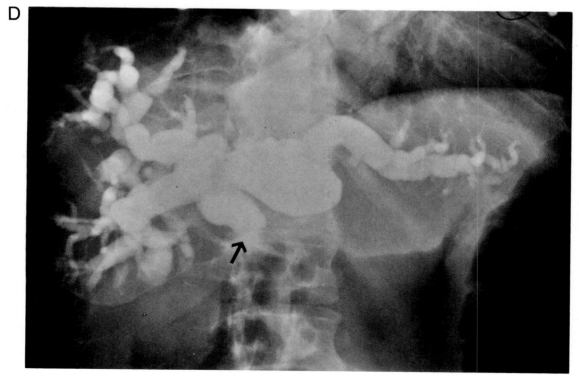

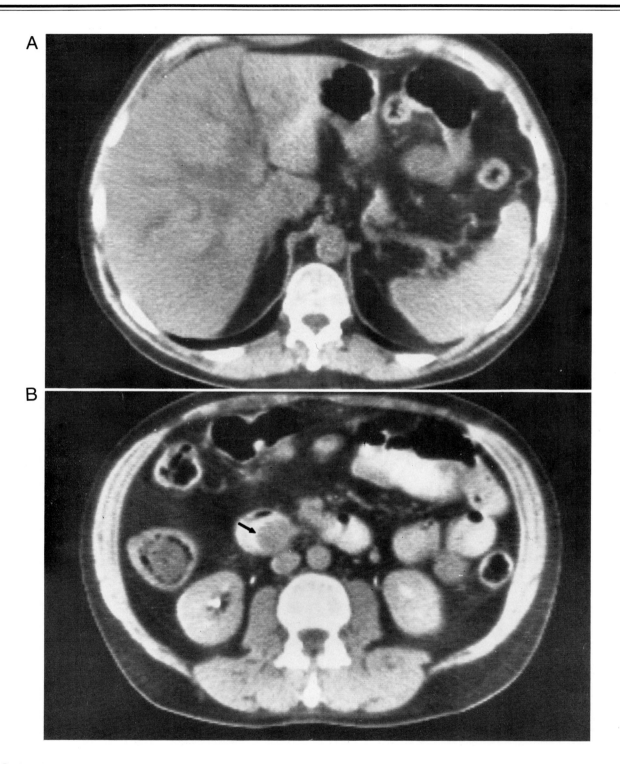

FIG 3–49.
Ampullary adenocarcinoma. This 53-year-old man had weight loss and progressive jaundice. An ultrasound examination (not shown) revealed intrahepatic and extrahepatic biliary ductal dilatation.

A and **B,** an abdominal CT study demonstrates intrahepatic biliary dilatation **(A)** and a mass (*arrow* in **B**) in the medial duodenal wall, adjacent to the ampulla of Vater.

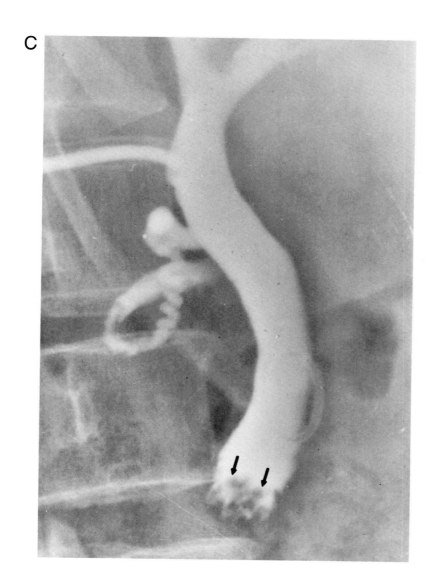

C, a percutaneous cholangiogram was then made. On this oblique view, an irregular filling defect *(arrows)* in the distal common bile duct is seen.

At surgery, a well-differentiated adenocarcinoma of the ampulla of Vater was completely excised.

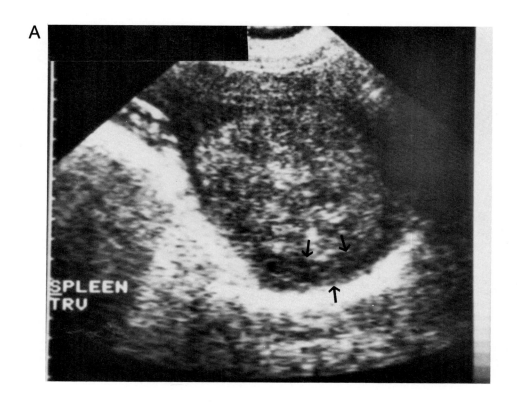

FIG 3–50.
Splenic hemangioma (two cases). These two patients presented with left upper quadrant fullness and underwent abdominal sonography.

A, there is a single large, solid mass occupying most of the spleen. There is a surrounding rim of hypoechogenic splenic tissue *(arrows).*

B, cut section of the resected spleen from this patient shows a large hemangioma *(arrows)* with surrounding normal spleen.

C, the sonogram from the second patient shows a complex mass within the spleen. Multiple predominantly anechoic, cystic areas *(arrowheads)* are noted, surrounded by echodense solid hemangiomas *(arrows).* (From Ros P.R., Moser R.P. Jr., Dachman A.H., et al.: Hemangioma of the spleen: radiologic-pathologic correlation in ten cases. *Radiology* 162:73–77, 1987. Reproduced with permission.)

B

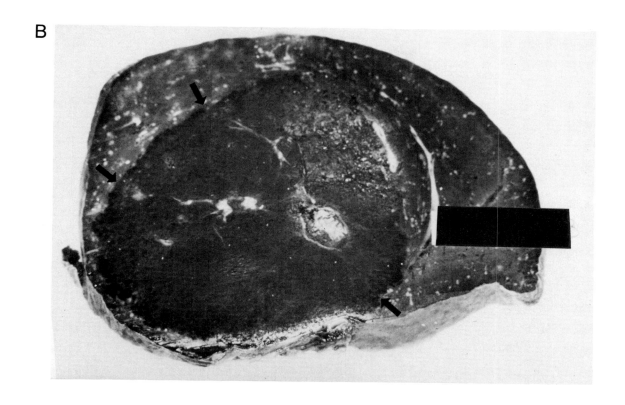

C

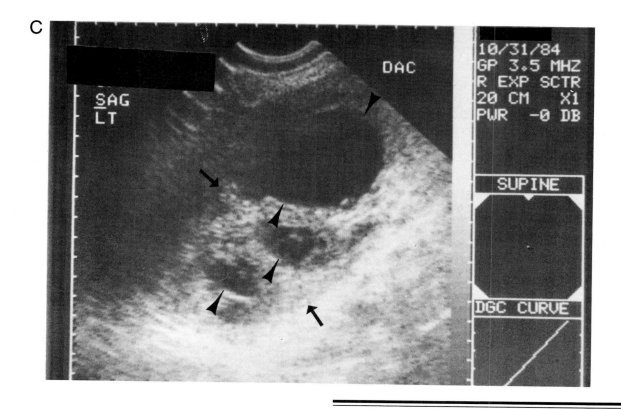

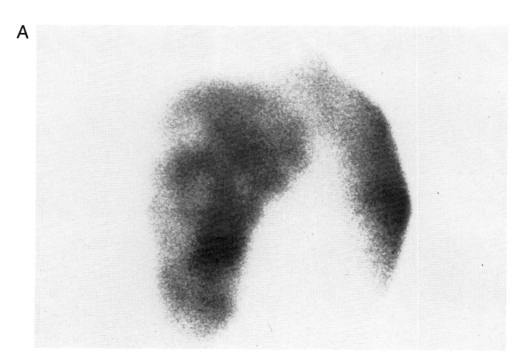

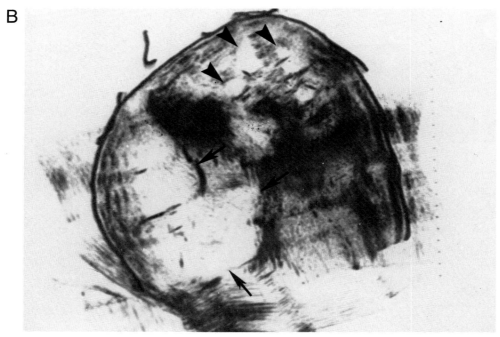

FIG 3–51.
Splenic lymphangiomatosis. This 20-year-old woman with a history of mediastinal cystic hygroma excised two years ago presented with splenomegaly.

A, posterior view of ^{99m}Tc-sulfur-colloid scan shows multiple filling defects within an enlarged spleen.

B, transverse right lateral decubitus sonogram shows cystic areas *(arrowheads)* within the spleen. In addition, a large multilocular cystic structure *(arrows)* is seen in the anterior and middle abdomen.

C

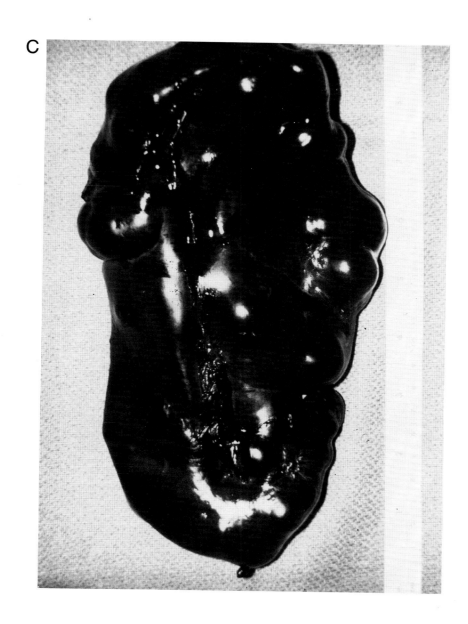

C, abdominal exploration showed large cysts in the omentum. The resected spleen contains multiple cysts and the pathologic diagnosis was lymphangiomatosis (see also Color Plate 12). (From Shirkhoda A., McCartney W.H., Staab E.V., et al.: Imaging of the spleen: a proposed algorithm. *AJR* 135:195–198, 1980. Reproduced with permission.)

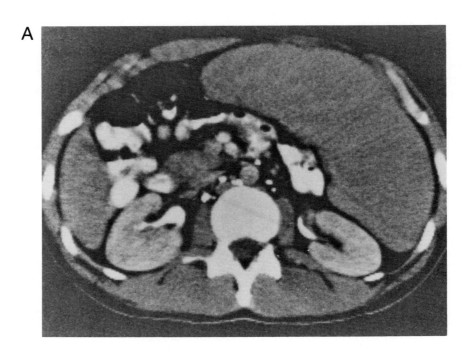

FIG 3–52.
Spleen in chronic myelogenous leukemia (two cases).

A, this 44-year-old patient with chronic myelogenous leukemia was found to have a very large spleen, extending from the diaphragm to the upper left iliac fossa. Notice that the density of the spleen is homogeneous, and there is no focal defect.

B and **C,** this 27-year-old woman had a ten-year history of chronic myelogenous leukemia. She re-presented with continuous fever and was found to be in blastic crisis, with severe neutropenia and thrombocytopenia. An abdominal CT scan **(B)** shows a very large spleen displaying diffuse decreased density except for the most medial part. A sonogram **(C)** reveals nonhomogeneous echo pattern throughout the large spleen. The patient died of pneumonia, and autopsy revealed leukemic infiltration of an extensively infarcted spleen. The low-density areas on CT and hypoechoic regions on sonography corresponded to the infarction.

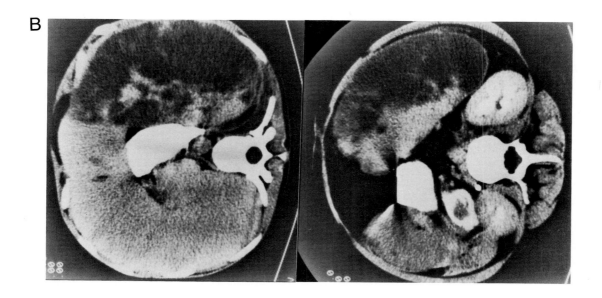

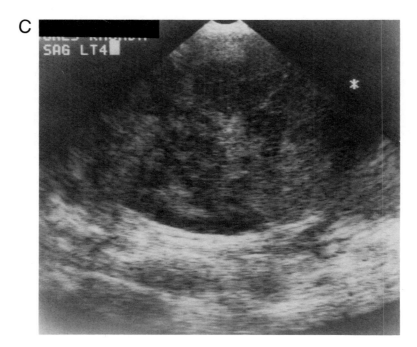

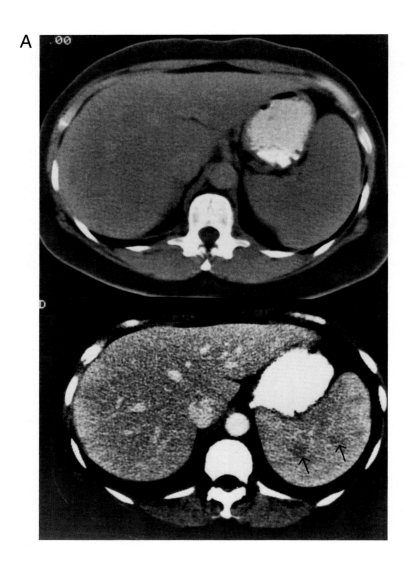

FIG 3–53.
Splenic lymphoma (multiple cases).

A and **B,** this patient with treated lymphoma underwent CT **(A)** of the abdomen and chest during follow-up. The top image is from the lower-thoracic CT, for which the patient was given drip infusion of contrast. The spleen appears normal. The bottom image is from bolus abdominal CT and shows multiple low-density lesions *(arrows)* in the spleen.

This finding was further proved by splenic sonography **(B),** whereby multiple hypoechoic lesions *(arrows)* consistent with lymphomatous infiltrate are seen.

C through **F,** this 34-year-old man with right upper quadrant pain was found during cholecystosonography to have a single hypoechoic liver lesion. A similar hypoechoic area *(arrowheads* in **C**) is also seen in the spleen *(S). (Continued.)*

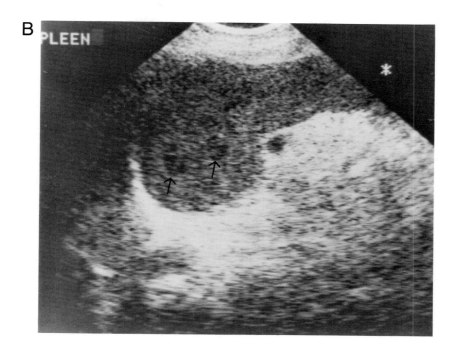

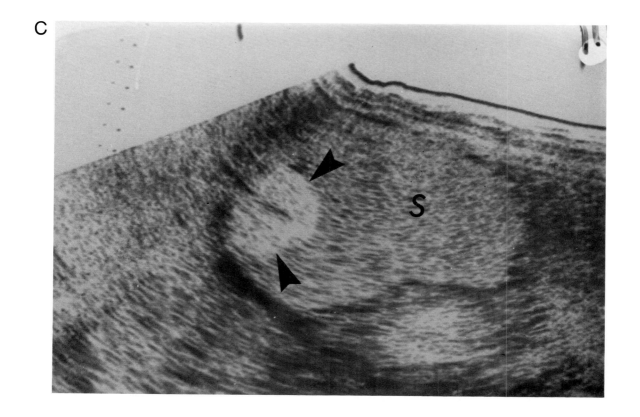

D

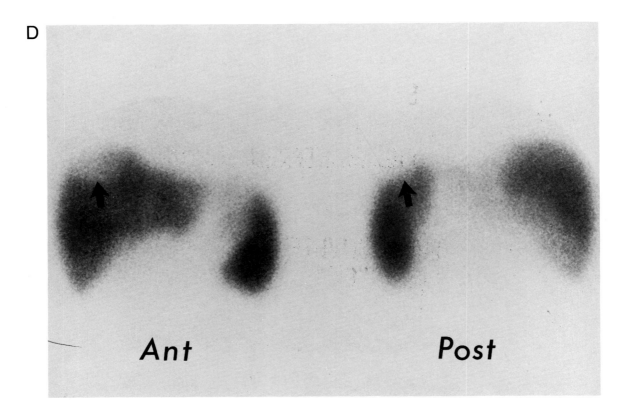

Ant   Post

FIG 3–53 (cont.).
A ⁹⁹ᵐTc-sulfur-colloid liver-spleen scan **(D)** proved these to be the only two lesions (*arrows* in **D**), and both were "hot" on anterior view gallium study (*arrows* in **E**). The total-body gallium scan was otherwise normal. Biopsy proved lym-phoma, and the patient had splenectomy **(F)** (see also Color Plate 13) and chemotherapy. (**C–F** from Shirkhoda A., McCartney W.H., Staab E.V., et al.: Imaging of the spleen: a proposed algorithm. *AJR* 135:195–198, 1980. Reproduced with permission.) *(Continued.)*

E

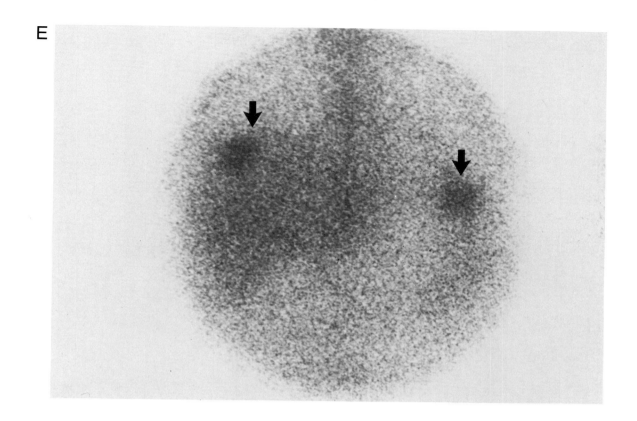

F

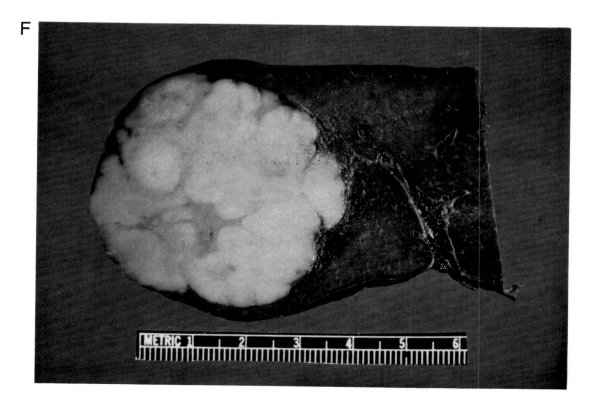

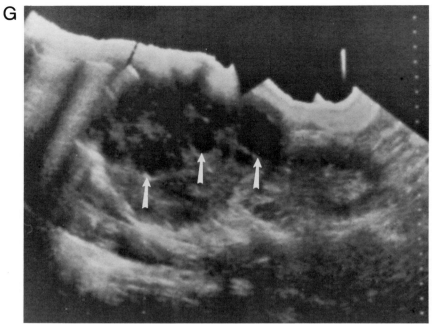

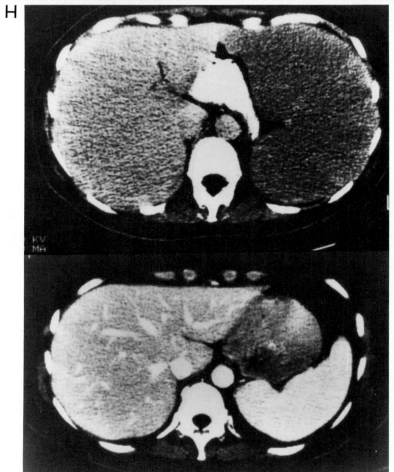

FIG 3–53 (cont.).
G, this sonogram in a 47-year-old patient with lymphoma shows multiple cystic lesions in the spleen *(arrows)*. The lesions were proved to represent lymphomatous infiltrate.

H, splenic lymphoma is seen in this patient as diffuse infiltration of the spleen resulting in splenomegaly and loss of normal density and enhancement *(top).* Four months later *(bottom),* after a period of treatment, the spleen is normal.

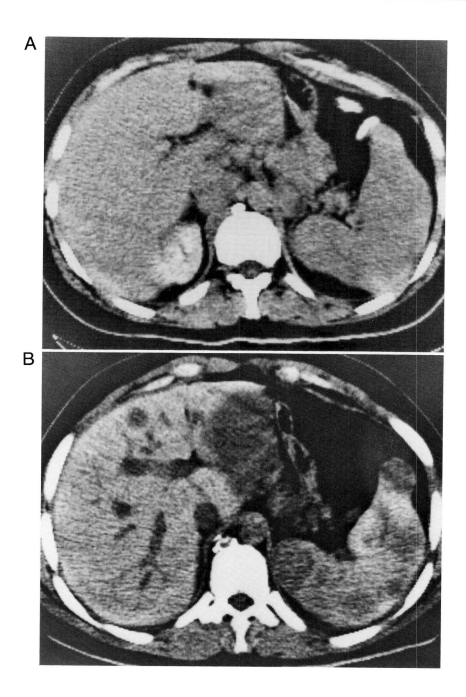

FIG 3–54.

Hepatosplenic lymphoma. This patient with a known diagnosis of non-Hodgkin's lymphoma was found to have abnormal liver enzyme values.

A, an enhanced CT scan (drip infusion) of the abdomen suggests a few enlarged nodes in the porta hepatis.

B, on the next day, the study was repeated following infusion of EOE-13. The CT scan shows multiple low-density lesions within the spleen, a single large one in the left lobe of the liver, and a few additional ones within the liver. Notice lack of enhancement of intrahepatic vascular channels with EOE-13.

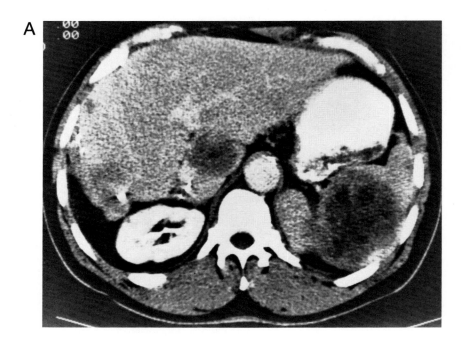

FIG 3–55.

Splenic metastases (multiple cases).

A, a 56-year-old man had colon carcinoma excised two years ago as well as right hepatectomy for metastasis. Metastases were later found in the spleen, liver, and adrenals.

B, this 37-year-old woman with ocular melanoma was found by follow-up CT examination to have metastasis to the liver and spleen. Notice the bull's-eye appearance of splenic metastasis on this contrast enhanced CT.

C, this 60-year-old woman with treated abdominal carcinomatosis due to primary ovarian carcinoma was found on follow-up CT two years later to have a single splenic lesion. Biopsy proved the lesion to be metastasis from the ovarian primary. *(Continued.)*

B

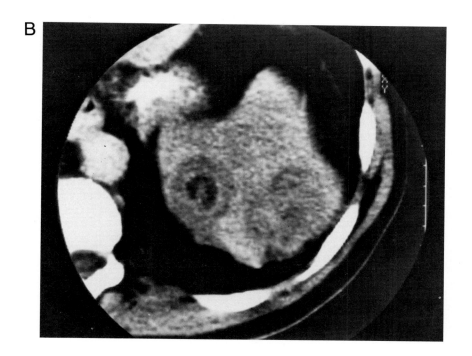

C

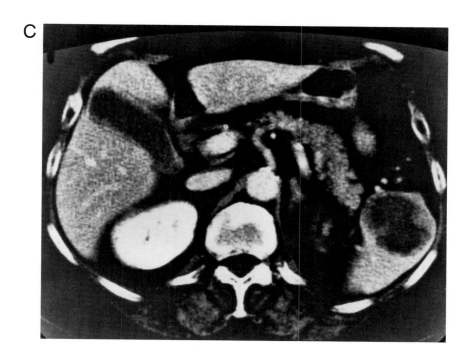

D

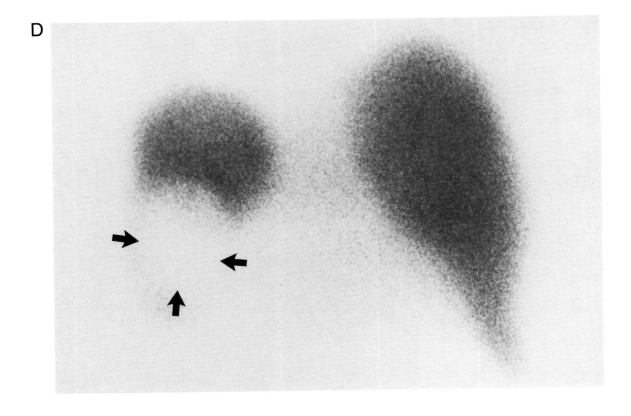

FIG 3–55 (cont.).
D and **E,** this woman with surgically treated ovarian carcinoma presented with splenomegaly and left upper quadrant pain. Posterior view liver-spleen scintiscan **(D)** shows a large defect in the lower part of the spleen *(arrows).*

E

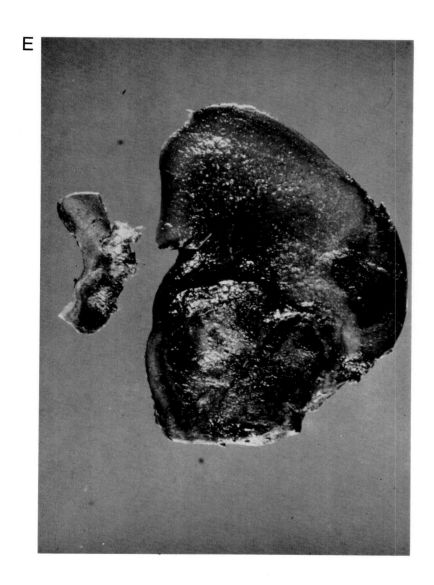

This defect was solid on ultrasound, and splenectomy **(E)** (see also Color Plate 14) proved it to represent metastatic ovarian carcinoma. (From Shirkhoda A., McCartney W.H., Staab E.V., et al.: Imaging of the spleen: a proposed algorithm. *AJR* 135:195–198, 1980. Reproduced with permission.) *(Continued.)*

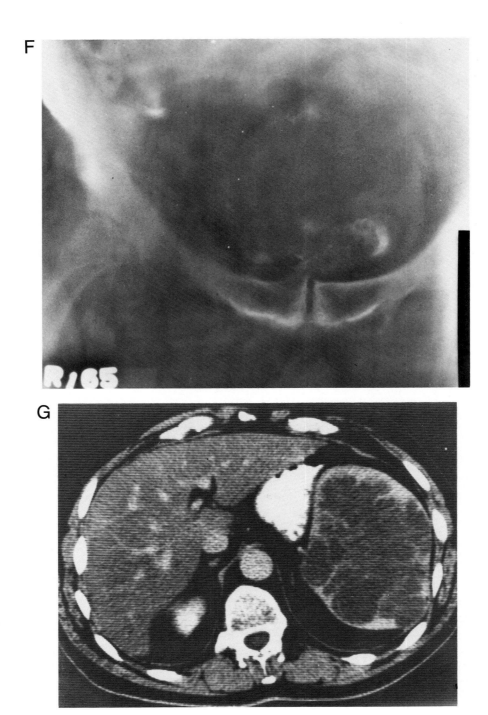

FIG 3–55 (cont.).
F and **G,** this 60-year-old man with a ten-year history of pubic chondrosarcoma **(F)** was discovered to have splenic metastasis six years after the diagnosis of bone tumor. A follow-up CT scan four years later **(G)** shows almost total replacement of the spleen by metastasis. There was also evidence of metastasis in the lungs.

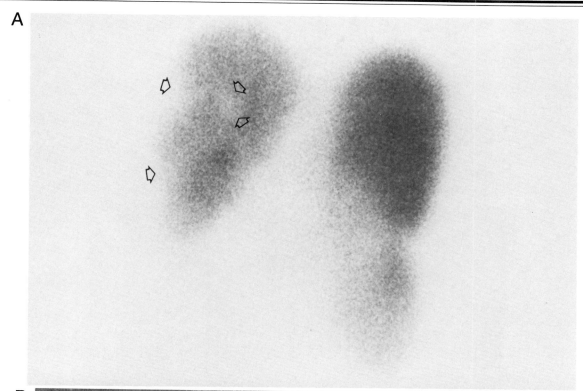

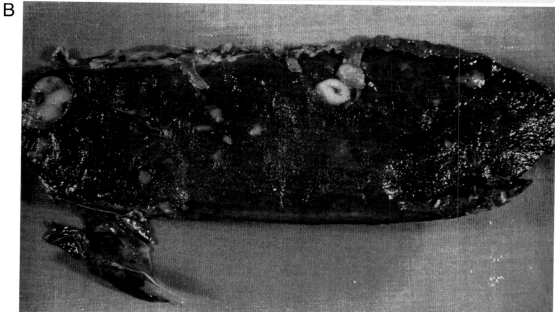

FIG 3–56.
Splenic myeloma. This 40-year-old woman with multiple myeloma was evaluated for hepatosplenomegaly.

A, posterior view ^{99m}Tc-sulfur-colloid scan shows one or possibly a few focal defects *(open arrows)* within the spleen. These defects were hypoechoic on sonogram.

B, after splenectomy, numerous areas of focal infiltration by plasma cells are seen (see also Color Plate 15). (From Shirkhoda A., McCartney W.H., Staab E.V., et al.: Imaging of the spleen: a proposed algorithm. *AJR* 135:195–198, 1980. Reproduced with permission.)

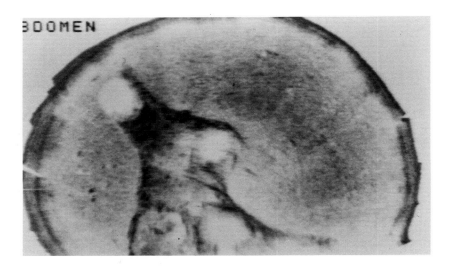

FIG 3–57.
Splenomegaly in myelofibrosis. This 52-year-old man is known to have had myelofibrosis for ten years, during which time he has been on chemotherapy. Recently his large spleen became larger, and he had shortness of breath.

Transverse abdominal sonogram just above the umbilicus shows a very large spleen with homogeneous echo pattern.

Splenectomy revealed a 7,000-g spleen measuring 34 × 17 × 10 cm with evidence of extramedullary hematopoiesis.

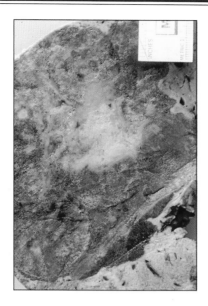

PLATE 5

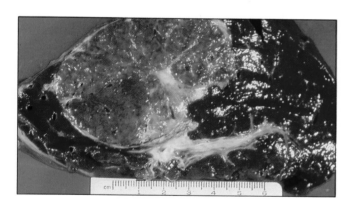

PLATE 6

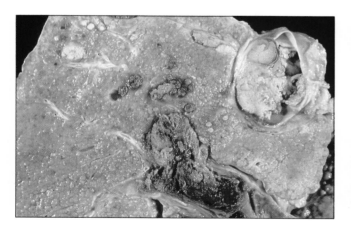

PLATE 7

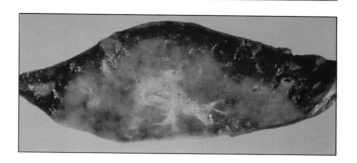

PLATE 8

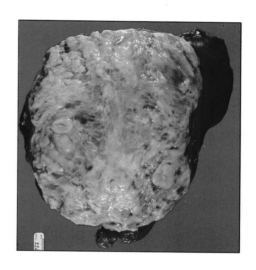

PLATE 9

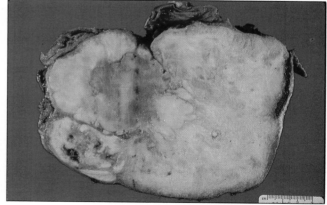

PLATE 10

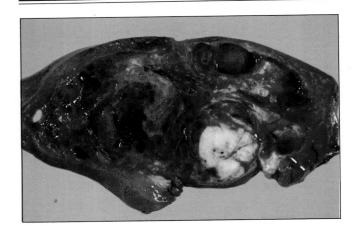

PLATE 11

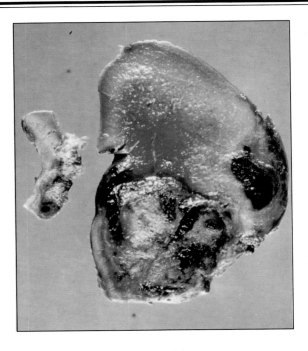

PLATE 14

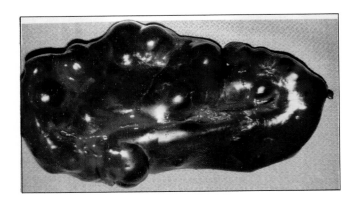

PLATE 12

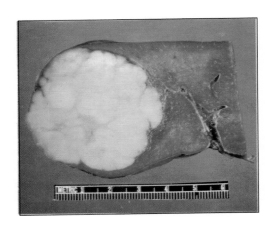

PLATE 13

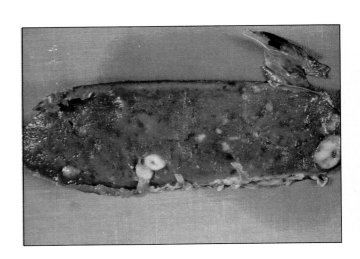

PLATE 15

4

Renal Masses

Chusilp Charnsangavej, M.D.

During the past ten years, new imaging modalities have modified the diagnostic approach to renal masses. Angiography was once used extensively in this context but has largely been replaced by ultrasonography and computed tomography (CT). An accurate assessment can be made with these less invasive techniques in the case of most renal masses. In certain lesions, however, diagnosis is difficult, and there is controversy about the proper diagnostic and therapeutic approaches.[1, 2] The diagnostic radiologist should not only be familiar with the clinical information about the patient but also understand the philosophy of the therapeutic approach of the referring physician. And because of the continuing changes in imaging modalities, the diagnostic approach should also be based on the quality and limitations of the various types of equipment and the radiologist's skill in their use.

Intravenous urography with nephrotomography has been and remains the primary screening approach for many urologic problems, particularly when a renal mass is suspected. Urography provides an overall view of the urinary tract and basic information about whether there is a mass and whether it is solid or cystic. This information will determine subsequent diagnostic approaches.

Ultrasonography is the study of choice for evaluation of a mass found on urography, since it is inexpensive, noninvasive, and accurate.[3] When the diagnosis of simple cyst is made by ultrasonography based on the strict sonographic criteria, no further

studies are needed. If a complicated cyst or complex mass is diagnosed, cyst puncture with cystography, CT, or both should be performed.[4] Since ultrasonography is operator dependent, its efficacy and reliability depend on the experience and effort of the individual examining the patient.

Computed tomography produces a unique cross-sectional image of the kidney and retroperitoneal spaces.[5, 6] Its ability to determine the density of a renal mass, whether the mass contains fat, blood or other fluid, or calcification, permits specific diagnosis. When a malignant tumor of the kidney is suspected, CT provides the best staging information; it outlines tumor involvement of the perirenal space, metastasis to lymph nodes, venous extension of tumor, or distant metastasis to the liver.[7-16]

Although CT is not operator dependent, the image quality can vary according to the generation of CT equipment used and the techniques of examination. The images obtained from state-of-the-art CT scanners are far superior to those made by early-generation equipment. Scanning without contrast enhancement followed by scanning with intravenous bolus contrast enhancement provides more information than scanning with contrast enhancement by intravenous drip infusion.[12, 17]

In general, when CT is performed to evaluate a known renal mass, examination without contrast enhancement and with bolus contrast enhancement should be done. When a vascular lesion is suspected, dynamic CT examination may be useful.

However, routine CT scanning without and with contrast enhancement may be impractical in a busy clinical practice, particularly when CT is used as a screening examination.

Magnetic resonance imaging (MRI) has been used in the diagnosis and staging of renal cell carcinoma, and the results have been compared with those in CT.[14] Among these tumors there are various MRI appearances, each with a different signal intensity; the most common is a mass with an intermediate intensity between that of renal cortex and that of medulla on T_1-weighted pulse sequence and increased intensity on T_2-weighted images. In general, although MRI shows venous invasion without the use of intravenous contrast medium and differentiates lymphadenopathy from small vascular lesions, neither CT nor MRI can differentiate stage I from stage II disease. The overall staging results with MRI are similar to those reported for CT scanning, and MRI may be used when there is contraindication for using iodinated contrast or when CT results are equivocal.

As previously mentioned, angiography's role in the differentiation of renal masses has diminished significantly in recent years. Yet angiography is still indicated in this context when ultrasonography and CT are inconclusive or lesions are of vascular origin. This modality may also be necessary for treatment planning, particularly when there are large, bulky tumors or local resection of the tumors is contemplated, and it is used in embolization of renal tumors. Angiography should be performed and interpreted in context, that is, in conjunction with other imaging findings. The location of the mass or masses should be well known for proper positioning of the patient for angiography. Selective angiography, angiography utilizing magnification techniques, or pharmacoangiography may be necessary for evaluation of a hypovascular mass or an intraparenchymal lesion.

Cyst puncture and cystography used to be routine in the evaluation of cystic masses until ultrasonography and CT were found to be highly accurate in the diagnosis of simple cysts. Cyst puncture is now reserved for complex or complicated cysts; aspirates are sent for chemical, culture and sensitivity, and cytologic analysis. Cystography, which involves injection of contrast material and air into the cyst, is occasionally used to evaluate the outline of the entire cyst to ensure that there is no mass in the cyst wall.

Percutaneous aspiration biopsy is not routinely performed in the evaluation of a renal mass. A solitary solid renal mass is usually managed directly by surgery. Biopsy is performed only when there are widespread metastases and tissue diagnosis is required before further management can be instituted. Percutaneous aspiration biopsy may also be warranted when there are infiltrative masses of the kidney, since the differential diagnosis of these masses includes metastases, infiltrative transitional cell carcinoma, lymphoma, and sarcomatous lesions.[18] Chemotherapy is perhaps preferable to surgery for many of these infiltrative masses.

DIAGNOSTIC APPROACH TO THE RENAL MASS

The renal cyst is one of the most common masses in the kidney and must be carefully distinguished from other solid masses. The ultrasonographic or CT diagnosis of a simple cyst should be based on adherence to strict interpretative criteria. By ultrasonography, a simple renal cyst (1) is an anechoic mass (with absence of internal echoes); (2) allows good through-transmission, with enhancement of sound beyond the far wall of the cyst; (3) allows clear demarcation of its far wall; and (4) is spherical or slightly ovoid.[3] By CT, a benign cyst is defined as a mass that shows (1) a homogeneous attenuation value near water density, (2) no enhancement when intravenous contrast material is used, (3) no measurable thickness of the wall, and (4) smooth and sharp interface with the renal parenchyma.[4] If these criteria are strictly observed, benign cysts can be accurately distinguished from other solid renal masses in 98% to 100% of the cases.

Complicated cystic lesions, defined as having a thick wall, are more difficult for the diagnostician. They may show internal echoes,[19–25] high-density cystic content on CT,[26–28] calcification in the wall,[29–32] or multiple septations.[33, 34] A complicated renal cyst may result from, among other things, hemorrhage in a simple cyst, an infected simple cyst, high protein content in cystic fluid, a multiseptated benign cyst, a multilocular cyst, tumor arising in a cyst, or necrotic, hemorrhagic tumor. Thus, whether or not further examinations are performed as well as which procedure or procedures are used (cyst puncture, angiography, or surgical exploration) depends on the clinical circumstances and the experience of the radiologist and referring physician.

Localized hydronephrosis may simulate a cystic lesion. Contrast enhancement of the parenchyma surrounding the hydronephrotic sac and layering of contrast material in the dilated collecting system are the clues to the diagnosis of localized hydronephrosis.

The tissue density and echogenicity of a mass are helpful in the differential diagnosis, particularly when the mass contains fat. Fat density on CT scan and a hyperechoic nature on sonogram most likely indicate angiomyolipoma,[35–37] although rare lesions such as lipoma, liposarcoma, and Wilms' tumor also may demonstrate fat density.[38–40] On the other hand, a high density of blood in the mass due to a hemorrhagic cyst or tumor can create diagnostic problems, as can tumoral calcification in papillary adenocarcinoma simulating calcification in tuberculous granuloma.

In the radiologic evaluation of a solid renal mass, certain appearances should be observed so that the origin of the mass—whether in the renal parenchyma, renal capsule, perirenal space, renal pelvis, or renal sinus—can be determined. A mass that originates in the renal parenchyma usually disrupts the normal outline or reniform shape of the kidney, and parenchymal beaks are often seen between the mass and normal parenchyma. In some cases, a small parenchymal mass that does not disrupt the cortical outline is difficult to differentiate from a mass arising from the renal pelvis, but intravenous urography or retrograde pyelography should permit a determination.

When a mass that has extraparenchymal origins involves the kidney, it usually has a broad-based attachment to the kidney. The kidney may be displaced, compressed, or effaced by the tumor but still maintain the reniform shape. Angiography can offer the clues to diagnosis since most of the blood supply to the mass arises from the extraparenchymal branches of the renal artery or from other branches of the abdominal aorta, and the renal parenchyma is usually intact.

A mass that originates in the renal pelvis or renal sinus, such as transitional cell carcinoma, lymphoma, metastatic tumor, or sarcoma, may obstruct the collecting system of the kidney or invade the renal parenchyma. The kidney may be enlarged because of the infiltrative process or displaced by the mass, but in most cases it maintains the reniform shape.

Although a large variety of renal tumors have been described, many of these tumors are rare and are often diagnosed in pathologic specimens as incidental findings. Discussion of these tumors is beyond the scope of this book. Only examples and discussion of common tumors or the ones that have been well described in the radiologic and urologic literature will be presented. Tumors of the kidney can be classified as shown in Table 4–1 according to histologic principles.

Tumors of Tubular Epithelium

Oncocytoma

Renal oncocytoma (also called renal oncocytic adenoma, adenoma with oncocytic features, and proximal tubular adenoma) is a rare, benign tumor composed of finely granular, eosinophilic cells without significant cellular or nuclear pleomorphism.[41–45]

TABLE 4–1.

Histologic Classification of Renal Tumors

Tissue Origin	Benign	Malignant
Tubular epithelium	Adenoma, oncocytoma	Renal cell carcinoma
Immature renal parenchyma	Multilocular cystic nephroma, congenital mesoblastic nephroma	Nephroblastoma (Wilms' tumor)
Mesenchymal origin	Fibroma, lipoma, leiomyoma, hemangioma, angiomyolipoma, juxtaglomerular tumor, medullary fibroma, neurilemoma, hemangiopericytoma	Fibrosarcoma, liposarcoma, leiomyosarcoma, angiosarcoma, neurosarcoma
Urothelium from the renal pelvis and calices		Transitional cell carcinoma, squamous cell carcinoma, adenocarcinoma
Metastatic tumors		
Unknown origin	Dermoid	Osteogenic sarcoma, primary lymphoma

The tumor is well defined, is fairly homogeneous, and often has central stellate scars (Fig 4–1). There is neither hemorrhage nor necrosis in these tumors. Vascular invasion and lymph node involvement are not features of renal oncocytoma, and the tumor does not recur after surgery.

On ultrasonography, there is a uniformly echogenic mass, and a small, central hypoechoic zone corresponds to any stellate scars. The usual CT finding is a well-circumscribed, hypodense mass with a central area that appears stellate (Figs 4–1 and 4–2).[46–48] On renal arteriography, a spoked-wheel arterial pattern and dense parenchymal stains, although not pathognomonic, are highly suggestive of renal oncocytoma (Fig 4–1).[47–50]

Renal Cell Carcinoma

Renal cell carcinoma (Figs 4–3 to 4–16) accounts for 85% of all kidney tumors. It is about two times more frequent in men than in women, and its peak incidence is in the seventh decade of life. The tumor is usually a solid, parenchymal mass, frequently with areas of hemorrhage and necrosis (Figs 4–3 to 4–8). Occasionally, it is a predominantly cystic necrotic tumor (Fig 4–10).

Clear cells, granular cells (acidophilic cells), or, infrequently, basophilic cells are the predominant components in renal cell carcinoma. The cells may be arranged in solid, cystic, tubular, or papillary patterns. In general, the clinical course in this disease does not significantly vary according to cell type or arrangement, except that the prognosis seems to be more favorable in papillary adenocarcinoma (Fig 4–11).[51] The most malignant form of renal cell carcinoma is the sarcomatoid variant, which is highly infiltrative and aggressive and carries a poor prognosis (Fig 4–9).[52–54] The pathologic staging adaptation commonly used in renal cell carcinoma is by Robson et al.[55] and Skinner et al.[56] In stage I, the tumor is confined to the renal capsule (Figs 4–3 and 4–4). Stage II neoplasms are those extending through the capsule into the perinephric fat (Fig 4–5). Regional lymph node metastasis (Fig 4–6) or tumor thrombus in the renal vein or inferior vena cava (Fig 4–7) defines stage III disease. In stage IV, there is direct tumor invasion of organs adjacent to the kidney, or there is distant metastasis (Fig 4–8).

Renal cell carcinoma is best evaluated by CT, which can readily demonstrate tumor extension into the perinephric fat, regional lymph node metastasis, and venous extension of disease.[8–12] According to the literature, the accuracy of CT in preoperative staging of renal cell carcinoma is 90% to 95%.[10–15]

However, recently Johnson et al., after reviewing 100 cases of renal adenocarcinoma, reported that perinephric invasion is the most difficult CT area for staging, accounting for more than one half of the CT errors in their study.[57] If one eliminates this error, the accuracy of CT in staging renal cell carcinoma rises to 98%. On CT, the tumors are usually less dense than normal renal parenchyma, both before and after contrast enhancement. Irregular hypodense areas that are due to necrosis or hemorrhage are often demonstrated in the mass (Figs 4–3 and 4–5). Acute hemorrhage from the tumor into the subcapsular or perirenal space infrequently occurs (Fig 4–16) and is sometimes seen on CT as a hyperdense mass similar to that seen in hemorrhage from other causes.[58]

Irregular tumoral calcification can be radiologically demonstrated in 20% to 30% of the tumors.[30–32] Most frequently, it is dystrophic, with irregular calcification inside the tumor (Fig 4–5).[31, 32, 59] On rare occasion, there is solid, dense calcification (Fig 4–15) simulating tuberculous granuloma, or peripheral linear calcification (Figs 4–13 and 4–14) simulating calcified benign cysts. Each of these two types of calcification can be seen in papillary adenocarcinoma.

Cystic tumors (Fig 4–10), tumors with a large necrotic area, and small tumor foci in the wall of cystic masses (Figs 4–11 and 4–12) are all rare. They may be difficult to diagnose[19–25] because on CT they may simulate benign or complicated cysts (Fig 4–13).

Hypervascular tumors with irregular tumor vascularity are demonstrated in 80% of renal cell carcinomas. Arteriovenous shunting and tumor extension into the renal vein are frequent. Approximately 15% of renal cell carcinomas are hypovascular, and about 5% are completely avascular (Fig 4–11).

Tumors of Immature Renal Parenchyma

Multilocular Cystic Nephroma

Multilocular cystic nephroma (Fig 4–17) occurs infrequently and is characterized by a well-circumscribed, encapsulated mass that contains multiple, noncommunicating, fluid-filled loculi.[60, 61] The cystic loculi are lined by epithelium, and the wall of the mass may contain foci of immature metanephric tissue and fibrous septa. The tumors are found mostly in two groups, namely, boys between three months and two years of age and women between 30 and 60 years of age.[62]

In multilocular cystic nephroma, ultrasonography demonstrates a complex renal mass that either has discrete septations dividing the mass into multiple small, sonolucent loculi or shows numerous internal echoes without definite loculi.[62, 63] The characteristic CT appearance is a well-defined mass with multiple cysts and thick septations.[62–64] The mass is frequently large, compressing or protruding into the renal pelvis. Calcification in the septa is common in these lesions. Angiography demonstrates a hypovascular mass, sometimes with stain in the septa.

Adult Wilms' Tumor

Wilms' tumor in adults simulates renal cell carcinoma (Fig 4–18), but the prognosis is worse than in the counterpart in children.[65] It may be confused with renal metastases, such as those from small cell lung carcinoma.

Tumors of Mesenchymal Origin

Angiomyolipoma

Angiomyolipoma, or renal hamartoma, is an uncommon, benign renal tumor composed of mainly fat cells intermixed with smooth muscle cells and aggregates of thick-walled blood vessels. There may be hemorrhage in the tumor itself or in the subcapsular or perinephric space. Two patterns of occurrence have been described in angiomyolipoma. In the first, which accounts for 80% of the cases, the tumor is solitary, nonhereditary, and found mostly in young to middle-aged women.[66, 67] In the second, multiple tumors and bilateral renal involvement are seen in patients in their early teens who have tuberous sclerosis.[68, 69]

Since angiomyolipoma contains three main tissue elements, imaging findings vary according to the amounts of these tissues in the lesion. A purely fatty tumor (lipoma) or a tumor that contains a great deal of fat displays hyperechoic density on ultrasonography and fat density on CT (Figs 4–19 to 4–21).[35–38, 70–72] A tumor in which there is hemorrhage or a large myomatous component may be hypoechoic, and it can be hyperdense or hypodense on CT depending on the age of bleeding (Fig 4–19).[35–37, 73] The more angiomatous elements there are, the more vascular the pattern on angiography.[35] If an angiomyolipoma does not contain enough fat to show fat density on radiologic examination, radiologic diagnosis is not possible (Fig 4–22).

Renal Sarcoma

Renal sarcomas are seen in 0.1% of autopsies and account for 1.1% of all malignant renal neoplasms. Leiomyosarcoma, fibrosarcoma, and liposarcoma are the most common malignant renal neoplasms of pure mesenchymal origin.[52–54] Radiologically, the diagnosis may be suggested if the tumor appears to originate in the renal capsule (Fig 4–23) or renal sinus (Fig 4–24) on CT and is hypovascular or avascular on angiography.[74] In cases of liposarcoma, the attenuation value of the tumor will suggest the diagnosis.

Tumors of Urothelial Origin

Transitional Cell Carcinoma

Transitional cell carcinoma is uncommonly seen in the renal pelvis and calices. This tumor occurs much more frequently in the bladder and is often multiple, so that when it occurs in a kidney, lesions involving the bladder, ureter, or contralateral kidney might be seen. Transitional cell carcinoma is malignant, ranging from low-grade to infiltrative, high-grade malignancy, and there may be distant metastases. The tumor is three to four times more common in men than in women, and the greatest number of cases occur when patients are between 40 and 70 years of age.[75–77]

Low-grade transitional cell carcinoma of the upper urinary tract can frequently be diagnosed by intravenous urography or retrograde pyelography (Fig 4–25). On CT, a low-grade tumor appears as a filling defect in the renal pelvis and is usually hypodense in comparison with the renal parenchyma; it may be slightly enhanced on intravenous bolus administration of contrast material.[78, 79] The tumor must be distinguished on CT from kidney stones and blood clots, both of which usually display a higher density. More infiltrative transitional cell carcinoma in the kidney is best diagnosed by CT.[80–83] When the tumor arises from the renal pelvis or calices and infiltrates into the renal parenchyma, local hydronephrosis or low density in the renal parenchyma with maintenance of the reniform shape of the kidney can be seen (Figs 4–26 and 4–27).

Diagnosis of transitional cell carcinoma by angiography alone can be difficult because the tumor is frequently hypovascular and obscured by the normal renal parenchyma. The tumor vascularity can be angiographically demonstrated only in a large, bulky lesion (Fig 4–26,D). Encasement of the renal vessels is characteristic of tumor invasion of the parenchyma (Fig 4–27,D) but is not pathognomonic, since other infiltrative tumors, such as sarcomatoid renal cell carcinoma (Fig 4–9,B), lymphoma (Fig 4–31), and metastasis from nonrenal primaries (Fig 4–23,C–D), can have a similar angiographic appearance.

Metastases to the Kidney

Kidney tumors that represent spread from non-renal primaries are relatively common at autopsy but are infrequently correctly diagnosed while a patient is alive. Neoplasms commonly metastatic to the kidney are melanoma, lymphoma, and carcinomas of the lungs, breasts, stomach, cervix, colon, and pancreas.[84-87] Spread is hematogenous, by direct invasion, by a lymphatic route, or by a combination of these routes.

Radiologic findings in tumor spread to the kidney vary according to the mode of spread. Hematogenous spread usually yields multiple and bilateral lesions (Fig 4–28).[88-90] A solitary metastasis is rare and cannot be radiologically distinguished from primary neoplasms of the kidney. Direct invasion of the kidney is most frequently seen in retroperitoneal sarcoma (Fig 4–29), lymphoma,[91-93] and pancreatic carcinoma (Fig 4–30). Computed tomography is the most sensitive modality in detecting renal metastasis.[84]

Metastasis by the lymphatic route can be seen in lymphoma (Figs 4–31 and 4–32) and urogenital tumors that spread into the renal sinus (Fig 4–33). In this type of metastasis, there is the appearance of infiltrating lesions, with invasion into the renal parenchyma, but the reniform shape of the organ is maintained. In the differential diagnosis of renal metastases, one should consider entities such as multicentric or bilateral renal cell carcinoma (Fig 4–34).

REFERENCES

1. Bosniak M.A.: Current radiological approach to renal cysts. *Radiology* 158:1–10, 1986.
2. Murphy J.B., Marshall F.F.: Renal cyst versus tumor: a continuing dilemma. *J. Urol.* 123:566–569, 1980.
3. Pollack H.M., Banner M.P., Arger P.H., et al.: The accuracy of gray-scale renal ultrasonography in differentiating cystic neoplasms from benign cysts. *Radiology* 143:741–745, 1982.
4. McClennan B.L., Stanley R.J., Melson G.L.: Computed tomography of the renal cyst—is cyst aspiration necessary? *AJR* 133:671–675, 1979.
5. Dunnick N.R., Korobkin M.: Computed tomography of the kidney. *Radiol. Clin. North Am.* 22:297–313, 1984.
6. Wadsworth D.E., McClennan B.L., Stanley R.J.: CT of the renal mass. *Urol. Radiol.* 4:85–94, 1982.
7. Mauro M.A., Wadsworth D.E., Stanley R.J., et al.: Renal cell carcinoma: angiography in the CT era. *AJR* 139:1135–1138, 1982.
8. Karp W., Ekelund L., Olafsson G., et al.: Computed tomography, angiography and ultrasound in staging of renal carcinoma. *Acta Radiol. (Diagn.) (Stockh.)* 22:625–633, 1981.
9. Wong W.S., Cochran S.T., Boxer R.J.: Radiographic grading system for renal cell carcinoma with clinical and pathological correlation. *Radiology* 144:61–65, 1982.
10. Levine E., Maklad N.F., Rosenthal S.J., et al.: Comparison of computed tomography and ultrasound in abdominal staging of renal cancer. *Urology* 16:317–322, 1980.
11. Jaschke W., van Kaick G., Peter S., et al.: Accuracy of computed tomography in staging of kidney tumors. *Acta Radiol. (Diagn.) (Stockh.)* 23:593–598, 1982.
12. Lang E.K.: Angio-computed tomography and dynamic computed tomography in staging of renal cell carcinoma. *Radiology* 151:149–155, 1984.
13. Weyman P.J., McClennan B.J., Stanley R.J., et al.: Comparison of computed tomography and angiography in the evaluation of renal cell carcinoma. *Radiology* 137:417–424, 1980.
14. Fein A.B., Lee J.K.T., Balfe D.M., et al.: Diagnosis and staging of renal cell carcinoma: a comparison of MR imaging and CT. *AJR* 148:749–753, 1987.
15. Cronan J.J., Zeman R.K., Rosenfield A.T.: Comparison of computerized tomography, ultrasound and arteriography in staging renal cell carcinoma. *J. Urol.* 127:712–714, 1982.
16. Probst P., Hoogewoud H.M., Haertel M., et al.: Computerized tomography versus angiography in the staging of malignant renal neoplasm. *Br. J. Radiol.* 54:744–753, 1981.
17. Baert A.L., Wilms G., Usewils R., et al.: Dynamic CT of the urogenital tract. *Urol. Radiol.* 4:69–83, 1982.
18. Shirkhoda A., Carrasco C.H., Charnsangavej C.: Percutaneous biopsy of adrenal and renal mass. *Semin. Intervent. Radiol.* 2:271–277, 1985.
19. Parienty R.A., Pradel J., Parienty I.: Cystic renal cancers: CT characteristics. *Radiology* 157:741–744, 1985.
20. Lang E.K.: Coexistence of cyst and tumor in the same kidney. *Radiology* 101:7–16, 1971.
21. Novetsky G.J., Berlin L., Epstein A.J., et al.: CT diagnosis of renal cyst wall tumor. *J. Comput. Assist. Tomogr.* 7:539–540, 1983.
22. Foster W.L. Jr., Vollmer R., Halvorsen R.A. Jr., et al.: Ultrasonographic findings of small hypernephroma associated with renal cyst. *JCU* 11:463–466, 1983.
23. Khorsand D.: Carcinoma within solitary renal cysts. *J. Urol.* 93:440–444, 1965.
24. Norfray J.F., Chan P.D., Failma F., et al.: Carcinoma in a renal cyst: computed tomographic diagnosis. *J. Urol.* 125:102–104, 1981.
25. Feldberg M.A.M., van Waes P.F.G.M.: Multilocular cystic renal cell carcinoma. *AJR* 138:953–955, 1982.
26. Fishman M.C., Pollack H.M., Arger P.H., et al.: High protein content: another cause of CT hyperdense benign renal cysts. *J. Comput. Assist. Tomogr.* 7:1103–1106, 1983.

27. Sussman S., Cochran S.T., Pagani J.J., et al.: Hyperdense renal masses: a CT manifestation of hemorrhagic renal cysts. *Radiology* 150:207–211, 1984.

28. Coleman B.G., Arger P.H., Mintz M.C., et al.: Hyperdense renal masses: a computed tomographic dilemma. *AJR* 143:291–294, 1984.

29. Jonutis A.J., Davidson A.J., Redman H.C.: Curvilinear calcifications in four uncommon benign renal lesions. *Clin. Radiol.* 24:468–474, 1973.

30. Babaian R.J., Lucey D.T., Fried F.A.: Significance and evaluation of calcification associated with renal masses. *Urology* 12:108–111, 1978.

31. Daniel W.W., Hartman G.W., Witten D.M., et al.: Calcified renal masses: a review of ten years experience at the Mayo Clinic. *Radiology* 103:503–508, 1972.

32. Weyman P.J., McClennan B.L., Lee J.K.T., et al.: CT of calcified renal masses. *AJR* 138:1095–1099, 1982.

33. Rosenberg E.R., Korobkin M., Foster W., et al.: The significance of septations in a renal cyst. *AJR* 144: 593–595, 1985.

34. Balfe D.M., McClennan B.L., Stanley R.J., et al.: Evaluation of renal masses considered indeterminate on computed tomography. *Radiology* 142:421–428, 1982.

35. Bosniak M.A.: Angiomyolipoma (hamartoma) of the kidney: a preoperative diagnosis is possible in virtually every case. *Urol. Radiol.* 3:135–142, 1981.

36. Hartman D.S., Goldman S.M., Friedman A.C., et al.: Angiomyolipoma: ultrasonic-pathologic correlation. *Radiology* 139:451–458, 1981.

37. Lee T.G., Henderson S.C., Freeny P.C., et al.: Ultrasound findings of renal angiomyolipoma. *JCU* 6:150–155, 1978.

38. Scheible W., Ellenbogen P.H., Leopold G.R., et al.: Lipomatous tumors of the kidney and adrenal: apparent echographic specificity. *Radiology* 129:153–156, 1978.

39. Kreel L., Bydder G.M.: Evaluation of retroperitoneal liposarcoma with computed tomography. *CT* 5: 111–117, 1981.

40. Parvey L.S., Warner R.M., Callihan T.R., et al.: CT demonstration of fat tissue in malignant renal neoplasms: atypical Wilms' tumors. *J. Comput. Assist. Tomogr.* 5:851–854, 1981.

41. Klein M.J., Valensi Q.J.: Proximal tubular adenomas of the kidney with so-called oncocytic features. *Cancer* 38:906–914, 1976.

42. Yu G.S.N., Rendler S., Herskowitz A., et al.: Renal oncocytoma: report of five cases and review of literature. *Cancer* 45:1010–1018, 1980.

43. Morales A., Wasan S., Bryniak S.: Oncocytomas: clinical, radiological and histological features. *J. Urol.* 123:261–264, 1980.

44. Liebes M.M., Tomera K.M., Farrow G.M.: Renal oncocytoma. *J. Urol.* 125:481–486, 1981.

45. Maatman J.J., Novick A.C., Tancinco B.F., et al.: Renal oncocytoma: a diagnostic and therapeutic dilemma. *J. Urol.* 132:878–881, 1984.

46. Levine E., Huntrakoon M.: Computed tomography of renal oncocytoma. *AJR* 141:741–746, 1983.

47. Quinn M.J., Hartman D.S., Friedman A.C., et al.: Renal oncocytoma: new observations. *Radiology* 153:49–53, 1984.

48. Bonavita J.A., Pollack H.M., Banner M.P.: Renal oncocytoma: further observations and literature review. *Urol. Radiol.* 2:229–234, 1981.

49. Wiener S.N., Berstein R.G.: Oncocytoma: angiographic features of two cases. *Radiology* 125:633–635, 1977.

50. Ambos M.A., Bosniak M.A., Valensi Q.J., et al.: Angiographic patterns in renal oncocytomas. *Radiology* 129:615–622, 1978.

51. Bard R.H., Lord B., Fromowitz F.: Papillary adenocarcinoma of kidney. *Urology* 19:16–19, 1982.

52. Farrow G.M., Harrison E.G., Jr., Utz D.C., et al.: Sarcomas and sarcomatoid and mixed malignant tumors of the kidney in adults—part 1. *Cancer* 22: 545–550, 1968.

53. Farrow G.M., Harrison E.G. Jr., Utz D.C., et al.: Sarcomas and sarcomatoid and mixed malignant tumors of the kidney in adults—part 2. *Cancer* 22:551–555, 1968.

54. Farrow G.M., Harrison E.G. Jr., Utz D.C., et al.: Sarcomas and sarcomatoid and mixed malignant tumors of the kidney in adults—part 3. *Cancer* 22:556–563, 1968.

55. Robson C.J., Churchill B.M., Anderson W.: The result of radical nephrectomy for renal cell carcinoma. *J. Urol.* 101:297–301, 1969.

56. Skinner D.G., Colvin R.B., Vermillion C.D., et al.: Diagnosis and management of renal cell carcinoma: a clinical and pathological study of 309 cases. *Cancer* 28:1165–1177, 1979.

57. Johnson C.D., Dunnick N.R., Cohan R.H.: Renal adenocarcinoma: CT staging of 100 tumors. *AJR* 148: 59–63, 1987.

58. Hilton S., Bosniak M.A., Megibow A.J., et al.: Computed tomographic demonstration of a spontaneous subcapsular hematoma due to a small renal cell carcinoma. *Radiology* 141:743–744, 1981.

59. Sniderman K.W., Kreiger J.N., Seligson G.R., et al.: The radiologic and clinical aspects of calcified hypernephroma. *Radiology* 131:31–35, 1979.

60. Baldauf M.C., Shulz D.M.: Multilocular cyst of the kidney. Report of three cases with review of the literature. *Am. J. Clin. Pathol.* 65:93–102, 1976.

61. Gallo G.E., Penchansky L.: Cystic nephroma. *Cancer* 39:1322–1327, 1977.

62. Madewell J.E., Goldman S.M., Davis C.J. Jr., et al.: Multilocular cystic nephroma: a radiologic–pathologic correlation of 58 patients. *Radiology* 146:309–321, 1983.

63. Banner M.P., Pollack H.M., Chatten J., et al.: Multilocular renal cysts: radiologic-pathologic correlation. *AJR* 136:239–247, 1981.

64. Parienty R.A., Pradel J., Imbert M.C., et al.: Com-

puted tomography of multilocular cyst nephroma. *Radiology* 140:135–139, 1981.

65. Byrd R.L., Evans A.E., D'Angio G.J.: Adult Wilms' tumor and effect of therapy on survival. *J. Urol.* 127:648–651, 1982.

66. Hajdn S.I., Foote F.W. Jr.: Angiomyolipoma of the kidney: report of 27 cases and review of the literature. *J. Urol.* 102:396–401, 1969.

67. Price E.B. Jr., Mostofi F.K.: Symptomatic angiomyolipoma of the kidney. *Cancer* 18:761–774, 1965.

68. Bissada N.K., White H.J., Sun C.N., et al.: Tuberous sclerosis complex and renal angiomyolipoma. *Urology* 6:105–113, 1975.

69. Chonko A.M., Weiss S.M., Stein J.H., et al.: Renal involvement in tuberous sclerosis. *Am. J. Med.* 56:124–132, 1974.

70. Shawker T.H., Horvath K.L., Dunnick N.R., et al.: Renal angiomyolipoma: diagnosis by combined ultrasound and computerized tomography. *J. Urol.* 121:675–676, 1979.

71. Sherman J.L., Hartman D.S., Friedman A.C., et al.: Angiomyolipoma: computed tomographic-pathologic correlation of 17 cases. *AJR* 137:1221–1226, 1981.

72. Hansen G.E., Hoffman R.B., Sample W.F., et al.: Computed tomography diagnosis of renal angiomyolipoma. *Radiology* 128:789–791, 1978.

73. Beh W.P., Barnhouse D.H., Johnson S.H. III, et al.: A renal cause for massive retroperitoneal hemorrhage—renal angiomyolipoma. *J. Urol.* 116:372–374, 1976.

74. Shirkhoda A., Lewis E.: Renal sarcoma and sarcomatoid renal cell carcinoma: CT and angiographic features. *Radiology* 162:353–357, 1987.

75. Batata M.A., Whitmore W.F. Jr., Hilaris B.S., et al.: Primary carcinoma of ureter: a prognostic study. *Cancer* 35:1626–1632, 1975.

76. Murphy D.M., Zincke H., Furlow W.L.: Primary grade I transitional cell carcinoma of the renal pelvis and ureter. *J. Urol.* 123:629–631, 1980.

77. Murphy D.M., Zincke H., Furlow W.L.: Management of high grade transitional cell cancer of the upper urinary tract. *J. Urol.* 125:25–29, 1981.

78. Pollack H.M., Arger P.H., Banner M.P., et al.: Computed tomography of renal pelvic filling defects. *Radiology* 138:645–651, 1981.

79. Parienty R.A., Ducellier R., Pradel J., et al.: Diagnostic value of CT numbers of pelvocalyceal filling defects. *Radiology* 145:743–747, 1982.

80. Baron R.L., McClennan B.L., Lee J.K.T., et al.: Computed tomography of transitional cell carcinoma of the renal pelvis and ureter. *Radiology* 144:125–130, 1982.

81. Gatewood O.M.B., Goldman S.M., Marshall F.F., et al.: Computed tomography in the diagnosis of transitional cell carcinoma of the kidney. *J. Urol.* 127:876–887, 1982.

82. Hartman D.S., Pyatt R.S., Dailey E.: Transitional cell carcinoma of the kidney with invasion of the renal vein. *Urol. Radiol.* 5:83–87, 1983.

83. Subramanyam B.R., Raghavendra B.N., Madamba M.R.: Renal transitional cell carcinoma: sonographic and pathologic correlation. *JCU* 10:203–210, 1982.

84. Choyke P.L., White E.M., Zeman R.K., et al.: Renal metastases: clinicopathologic and radiologic correlation. *Radiology* 162:359–363, 1987.

85. Olsson C.A., Moyer J.D., Laferte R.O.: Pulmonary cancer metastatic to the kidney—a common renal neoplasm. *J. Urol.* 105:492, 1971.

86. Klinger M.E.: Secondary tumors of the genito-urinary tract. *J. Urol.* 65:144–153, 1951.

87. Newsam J.E., Tulluch W.S.: Metastatic tumours in the kidney. *Br. J.Urol.* 38:1–6, 1966.

88. Bhatt G.M., Bernardino M.E., Graham S.D. Jr.: CT diagnosis of renal metastases. *J. Comput. Assist. Tomogr.* 7:1032–1034, 1983.

89. Ambos M.A., Bosniak M.A., Madayag M.A., et al.: Infiltrating neoplasms of the kidney. *AJR* 129:859–864, 1977.

90. Mitnick J.S., Bosniak M.A., Rothberg M., et al.: Metastatic neoplasm to the kidney studied by computed tomography and sonography. *J. Comput. Assist. Tomogr.* 9:43–49, 1985.

91. Horii S.C., Bosniak M.A., Megibow A.J., et al.: Correlation of CT and ultrasound in the evaluation of renal lymphoma. *Urol. Radiol.* 5:69–76, 1983.

92. Hartman D.S., Davis C.J. Jr., Goldman S.M., et al.: Renal lymphoma: radiologic-pathologic correlation of 21 cases. *Radiology* 144:759–766, 1982.

93. Jafris S.Z.H., Bree R.L., Amendola M.A., et al.: CT of renal and perirenal non-Hodgkin lymphoma. *AJR* 138:1101–1105, 1982.

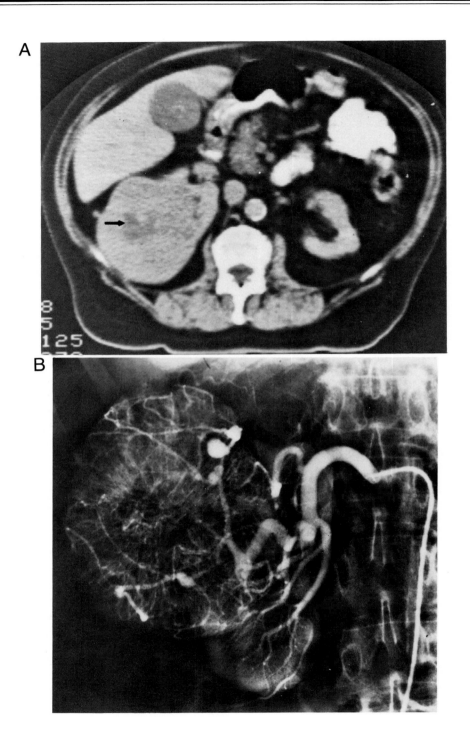

FIG 4–1.
Oncocytoma of the kidney. A 69-year-old woman with right upper quadrant pain was discovered to have a mass in the right flank. There was no history of hematuria.

A, the unenhanced CT scan demonstrates a large mass in the right kidney with low density *(arrow)* in the center.

B, a right renal arteriogram reveals a hypervascular mass with large vessels at the periphery focusing toward the center of the mass (i.e., a spoked-wheel pattern).

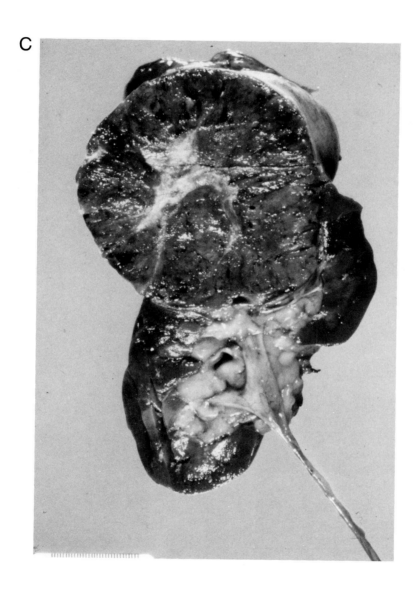

C, right nephrectomy was performed. There was a 12-cm mass in the right kidney without venous invasion or nodal metastasis. A central fibrotic scar, a typical appearance in oncocytoma, is seen. Histologic examination confirmed the diagnosis (see also Color Plate 16).

A

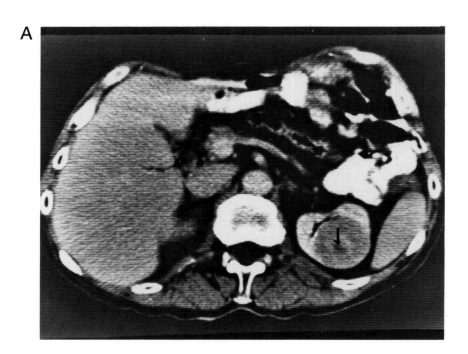

FIG 4–2.

Oncocytoma of the kidney. A 69-year-old man had prostatic carcinoma treated by radiation therapy to the pelvis two years earlier. Also, a melanoma of the left shoulder had been excised. During staging procedures, a mass in the left kidney was discovered.

A, the enhanced CT scan of the kidneys demonstrates a 4-cm, well-circumscribed mass that has low density at its center *(arrow).*

B, a left renal arteriogram reveals an intraparenchymal mass that displaces the vessels *(arrows).* A slight hypervascularity is seen but no definite spoked-wheel arrangement.

C, left nephrectomy was performed. A mass with central scarring was found, and the histologic diagnosis was oncocytoma (see also Color Plate 17).

When a tumor is small and confined within the renal parenchyma, it may be difficult to demonstrate tumor vascularity.

B

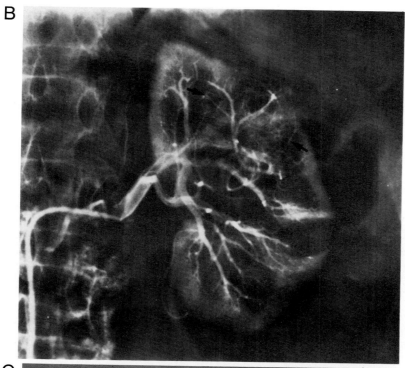

C

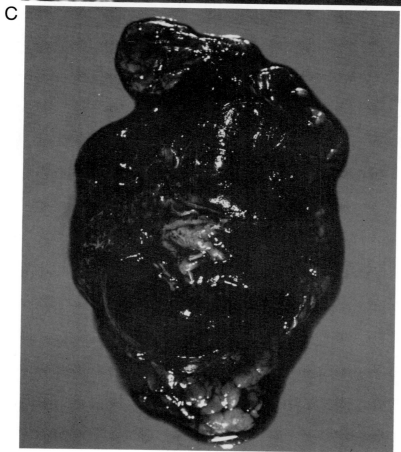

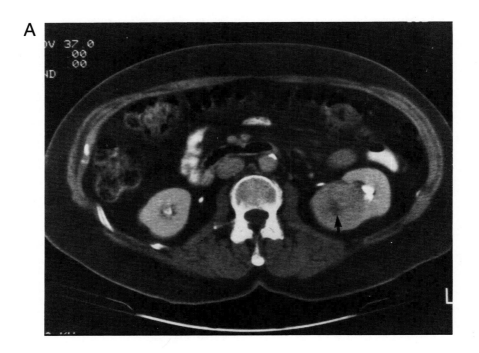

FIG 4–3.

Renal cell carcinoma. A mass in the left kidney was discovered in a 57-year-old woman during staging of carcinoma of the breast.

A, a CT scan of the kidneys made after administration of intravenous contrast material demonstrates a 4-cm mass in the lower pole of the left kidney. In the mass, there is a low-density center *(arrow)*.

B, a sonogram reveals a solid mass that has a hypoe-

choic area *(arrowhead)* at its center.

C, a left renal arteriogram shows a hypervascular, loculated mass extending toward the renal hilus. The tumor vascularity is unorganized, with no spoked-wheel pattern.

At surgery, a lobulated tumor with a necrotic area was found. The necrotic area corresponded to the low-density center noted on CT and ultrasound. The histologic diagnosis was renal cell carcinoma.

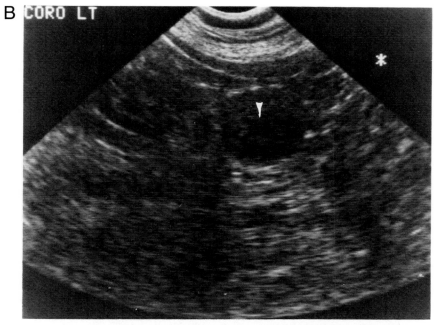

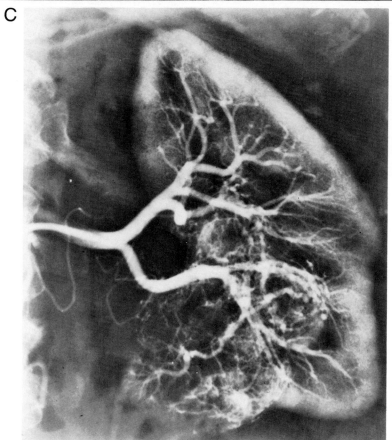

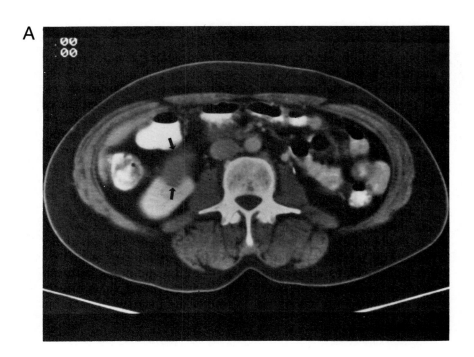

FIG 4–4.
Stage IB, hypovascular renal cell carcinoma. Stage IB squamous cell carcinoma of the cervix had been diagnosed in a 48-year-old woman in 1971, and treatment had been by irradiation. In 1978, a cyst in the upper pole of the right kidney had been diagnosed. On a routine follow-up CT scan, a mass was found in the lower pole of the right kidney.

A, renal CT was performed following administration of bolus contrast material. A 4-cm solid mass *(arrows)* is demonstrated.

B and **C,** there are two renal arteries supplying the right kidney. The mass is avascular and well circumscribed on both arterial and venous phases.

At surgery, this mass was found to be clear cell, renal cell carcinoma confined within the renal capsule.

B

C

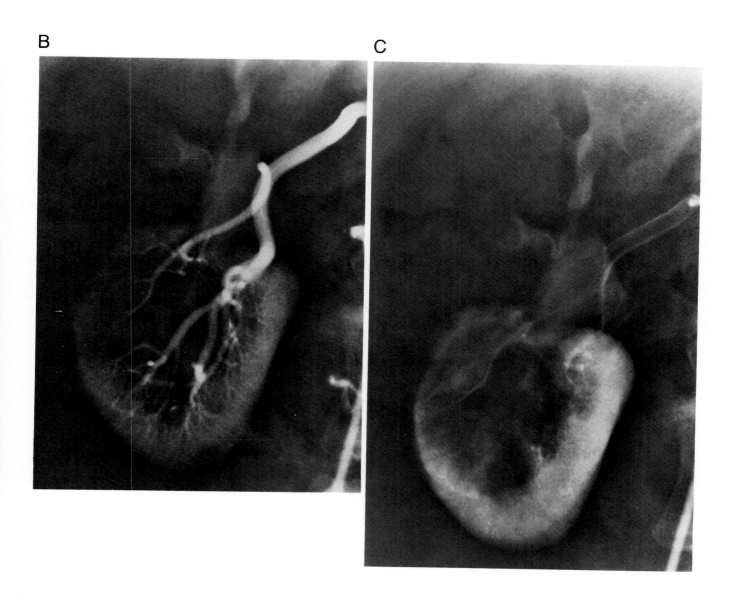

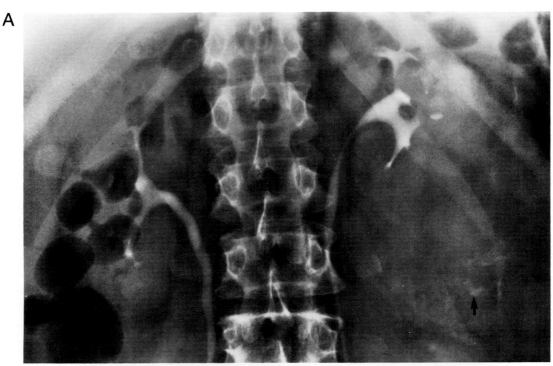

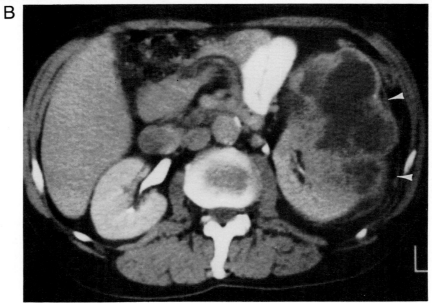

FIG 4–5.

Stage II renal cell carcinoma. A 59-year-old man presented with hematuria and a mass in the left flank.

A, an intravenous urogram demonstrates a large mass in the lower pole of the left kidney, with calcification *(arrow)* in the inferior portion of the mass.

B and **C,** the kidneys were assessed by CT. There is a large tumor with a large area of low density that is due to tumor necrosis. The tumor is poorly circumscribed and extends toward, but not beyond, the Gerota's fascia *(arrowheads).* Amorphous calcification *(arrow)* in the solid portion of the tumor is seen.

D, a sonogram of the left kidney shows many hypoechoic areas with thick irregular borders that indicate necrotic tumors. *(Continued.)*

C

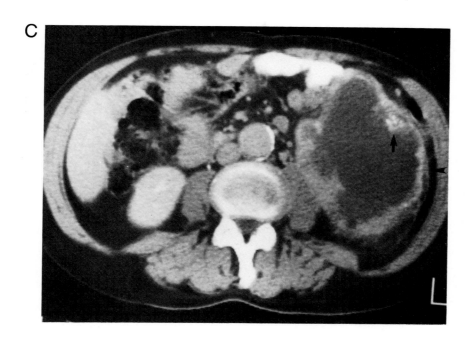

D

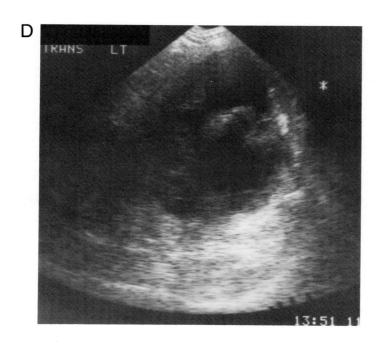

E

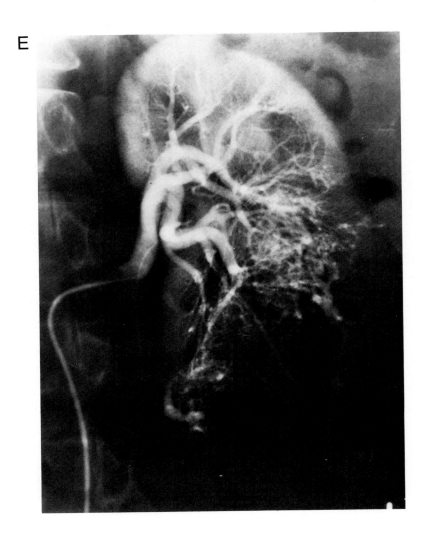

FIG 4–5 (cont.).
 E and **F**, left renal arteriograms in arterial and venous phases demonstrate a hypervascular mass with irregular tumor vascularity. A large area of avascularity corresponds to the necrotic portion of the tumor.

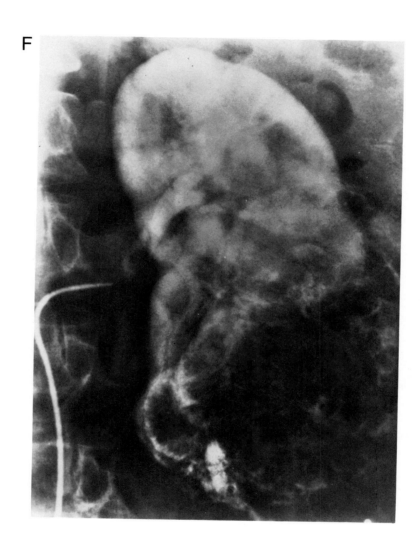

Tumor extension into the perirenal space is well demonstrated by CT, which was far superior to ultrasonography and angiography in this patient.

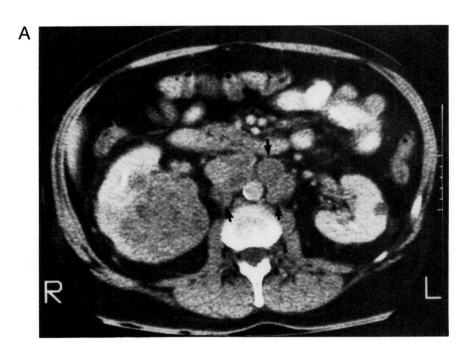

FIG 4–6.
Stage III renal cell carcinoma, with retroperitoneal nodal metastases. A 60-year-old man experienced right flank pain and hematuria.

A, a CT scan of the abdomen made after administration of intravenous contrast material demonstrates a poorly marginated, hypodense mass in the lower pole of the right kidney. There are a number of paraaortic and paracaval masses *(arrows)* compatible with nodal metastases. Note a small cyst in the left kidney.

B, a right renal arteriogram reveals a hypovascular mass in the lower pole. Staining and abnormal tumor vascularity are seen *(arrow).*

C, an inferior venacavogram shows lobulated extrinsic compression *(arrows)* of the vein by the enlarged lymph nodes. Biopsy proved the diagnosis of renal cell carcinoma. Nodal metastases are better demonstrated by CT than by angiography or venacavography.

B

C

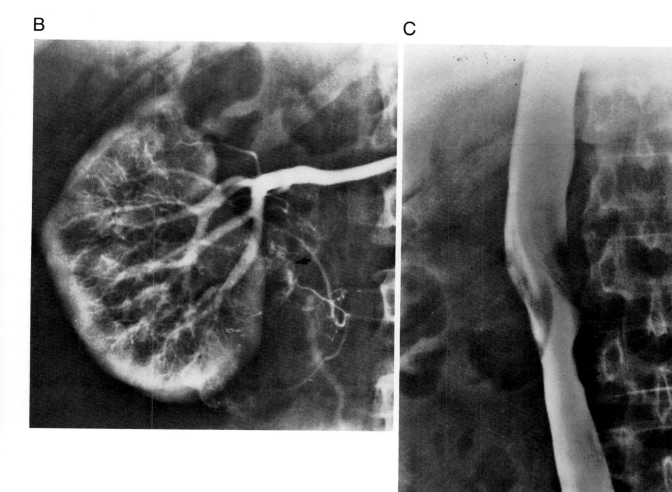

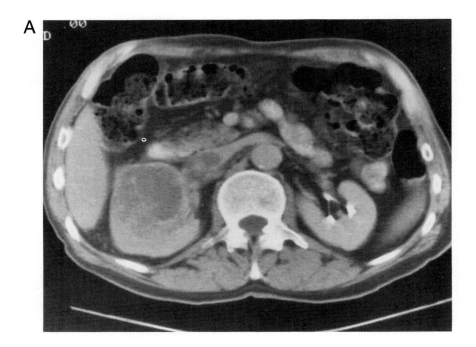

FIG 4–7.

Stage III renal cell carcinoma, with extension into the inferior vena cava. A 74-year-old man had a history of hematuria and right varicocele.

A, a CT scan of the abdomen made after administration of intravenous contrast material shows a hypodense mass in the right kidney. The low-density defect in the inferior vena cava is due to tumor thrombus extending into the vein.

B, a right renal arteriogram demonstrates a large, hy-pervascular mass in the midportion of the kidney.

C, an inferior venacavogram reveals a large tumor thrombus in the inferior vena cava.

When there is tumor thrombus from renal cell carcinoma, inferior venacavography should be performed to define the superior extent of the tumor. It may be necessary in some cases, in particular those in which the inferior vena cava is completely obstructed, to perform vena cavography from the jugular vein approach.

B

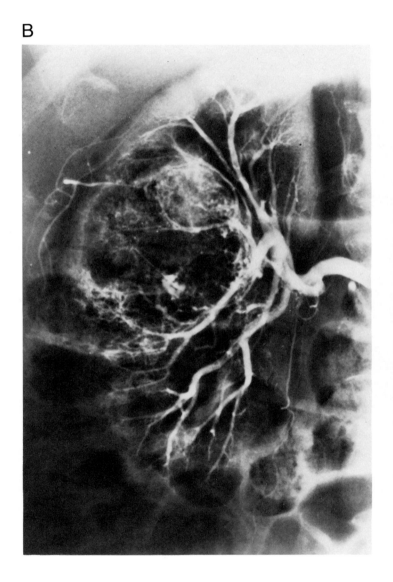

C

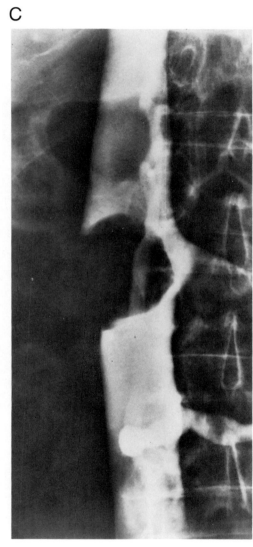

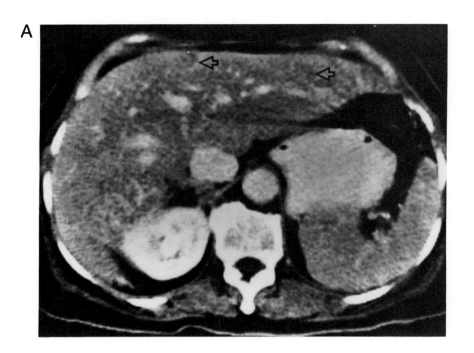

FIG 4–8.
Stage IV renal cell carcinoma, with hepatic metastasis. A 67-year-old woman presented with hematuria and a large mass in the right flank.

A and **B,** a CT scan of the abdomen made after bolus administration of contrast material **(A)** shows a few possible small nodules *(arrows)* in the liver. Delayed image **(B)** reveals the hepatic lesions and stasis of contrast in the right renal mass *(M).*

C, a sonogram of the liver demonstrates nonhomogeneous echo pattern with a few hypoechoic masses *(arrows)* in the right lobe. *(Continued.)*

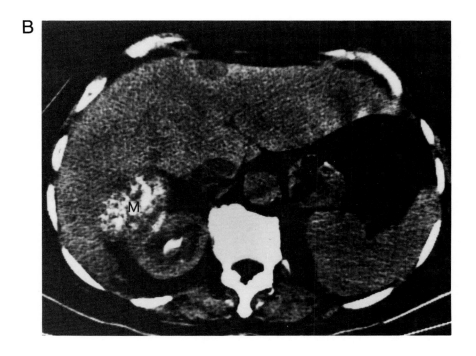

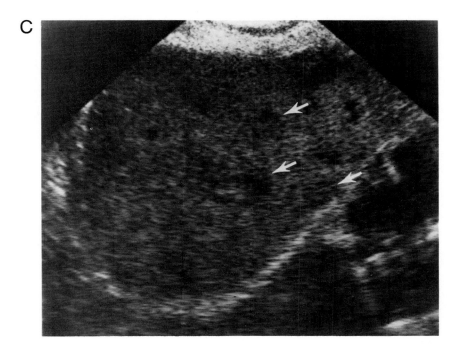

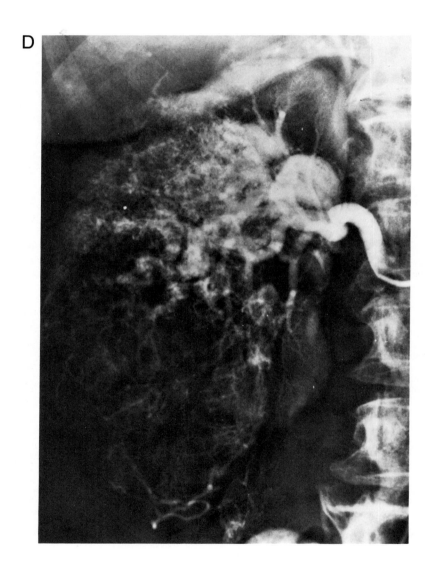

FIG 4–8 (cont.).
    D, a right renal arteriogram shows that a large hyper-vascular mass with arteriovenous shunting involves the right kidney, a typical appearance of renal cell carcinoma.

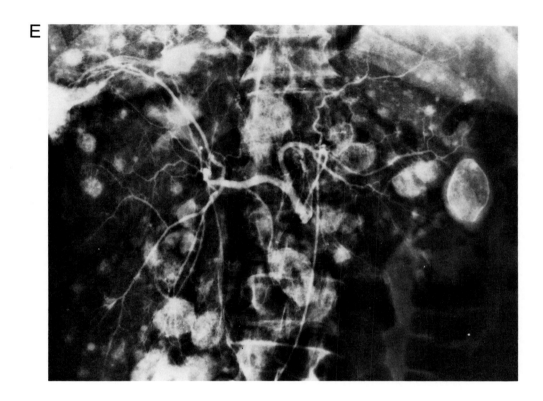

E

E, a proper hepatic arteriogram reveals multiple hypervascular metastases throughout the liver.

In hypervascular tumors, small metastases are best demonstrated by arteriography. At M. D. Anderson Hospital, selective hepatic arteriography is part of the presurgical workup in patients with renal cell carcinoma who have a large tumor.

A

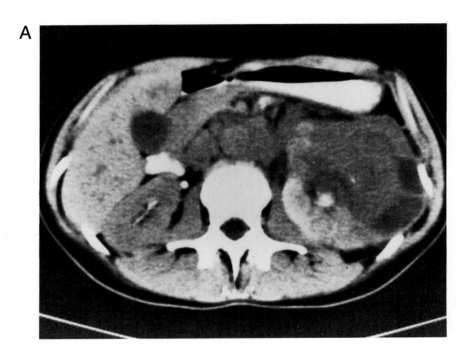

FIG 4–9.
Sarcomatoid renal cell carcinoma. A 30-year-old woman presented with a history of gross hematuria, weight loss, and fullness in the left upper quadrant.

A, a CT scan of the kidneys demonstrates a hypodense mass within the lower half of the left kidney. There is para-aortic adenopathy.

B, an arteriogram of the left kidney discloses a relatively vascular mass in the lower pole. The kidney is enlarged but maintains its reniform shape. The vessels are stretched and encased *(arrows),* giving an appearance of infiltrating neoplasm.

C, gross appearance of the left kidney at autopsy. The patient died less than one year after the diagnosis of sarcomatoid renal cell carcinoma was made by percutaneous needle biopsy. The kidney is enlarged but maintains its reniform shape. The infiltrative tumor *(arrows),* which was yellowish, occupies most of the kidney (see also Color Plate 18).

B

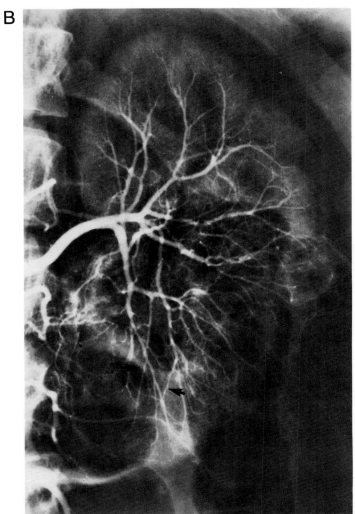

C

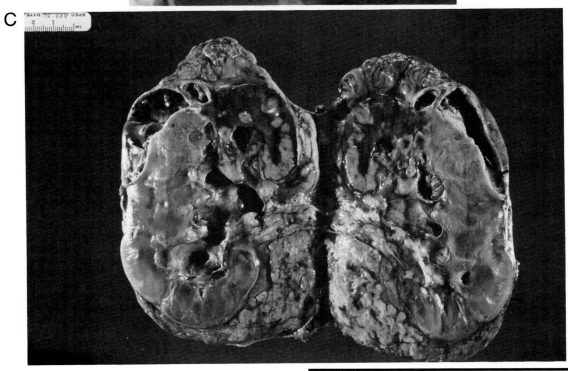

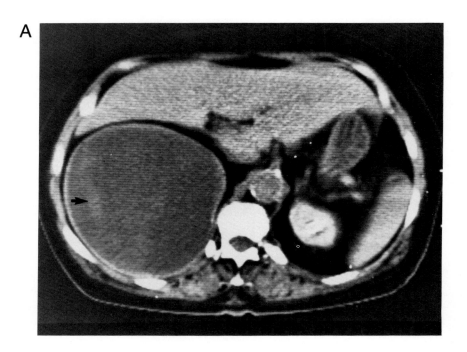

FIG 4–10.
Cystic, necrotic renal cell carcinoma. A 63-year-old woman presented because of hematuria and a feeling of fullness in the right side of the abdomen.

A, a CT scan demonstrates a large mass that is mainly hypodense and that arises from the upper pole of the right kidney. The mass has a thick wall and contains areas of ill-defined hyperdensity *(arrow).*

B

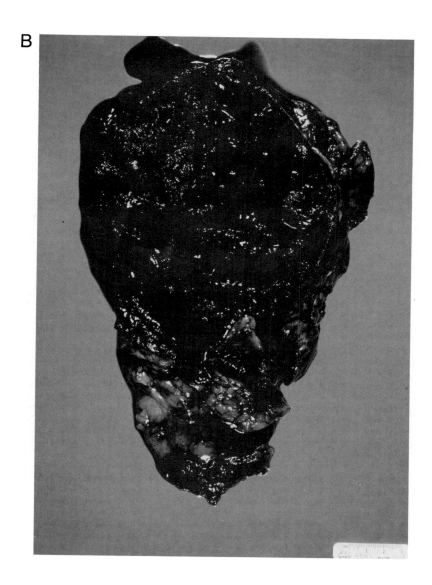

B, the pathologic specimen reveals a large, hemorrhagic, necrotic mass with irregular wall. Clear cell adenocarcinoma was identified in the wall of the mass (see also Color Plate 19).

Angiography performed on this patient demonstrated an avascular mass. This type of renal cell carcinoma may simulate a hemorrhagic cyst on CT or ultrasound. However, localized thickening in the wall of the mass should lead one to the diagnosis of tumor.

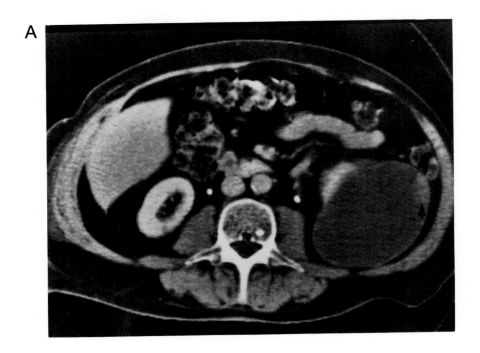

FIG 4–11.
Papillary renal cell carcinoma. A 62-year-old man had hematuria and a mass in the left flank.

   A, a CT scan of the abdomen shows a cystic mass arising from the left kidney. There is focal thickening *(arrow)* at various locations in the wall of the mass.

   B and **C,** left renal arteriograms demonstrate an avascular mass *(arrow).*

   Left nephrectomy was performed, and pathologic examination revealed a large necrotic tumor. Focal nodules in the wall of the cystic mass showed adenocarcinoma with papillary arrangement.

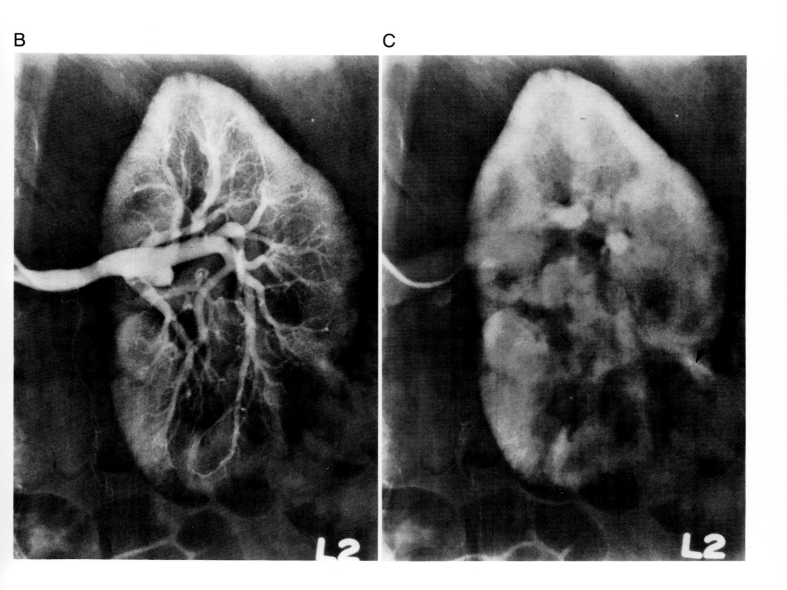

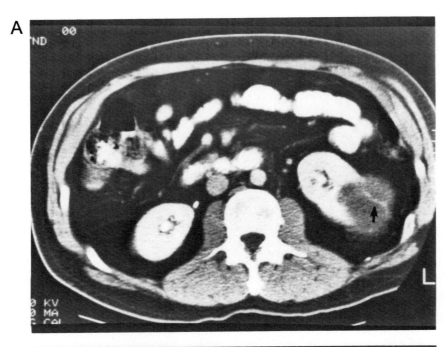

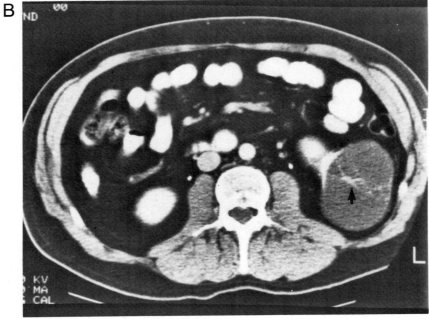

FIG 4–12.

Renal cell carcinoma in the wall of a cyst. In a 45-year-old man, a left kidney mass demonstrated by intravenous urography was diagnosed as a cyst on sonography. Follow-up urography three years later showed that the cyst had grown. There was no history of pain or hematuria.

A and **B,** computed tomography scans of the kidneys made after administration of contrast material show a cyst with multiple septation *(arrows)* at the lower pole of the left kidney. There is some enhancement at the superior portion of the cyst near the renal parenchyma.

C and **D,** left renal arteriograms demonstrate tumor vascularity *(arrows)* at the superior portion of the mass.

E, left radical nephrectomy was performed. The pathologic specimen reveals a renal cell carcinoma arising from the superior wall of the renal cyst. The fluid content of the cyst was yellowish and clear (see also Color Plate 20).

C

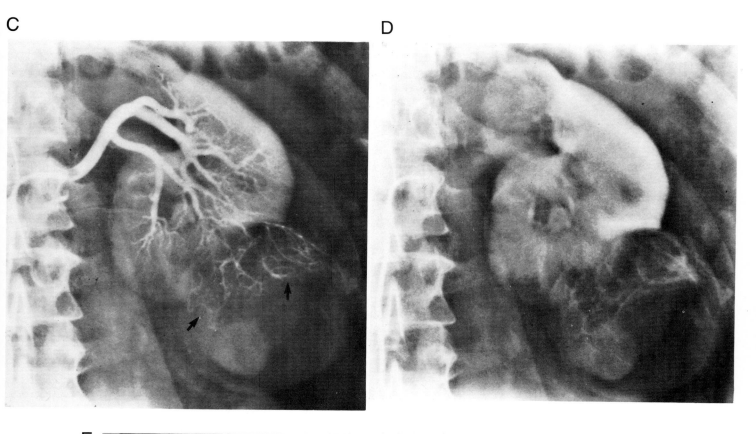

D

E

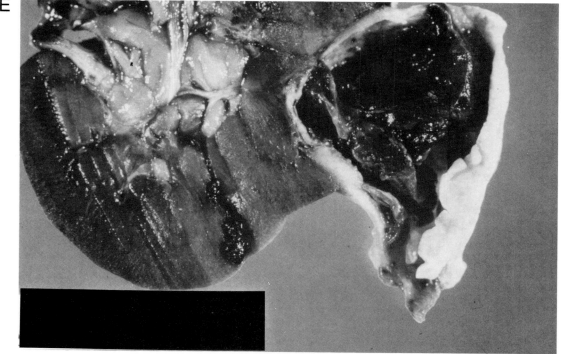

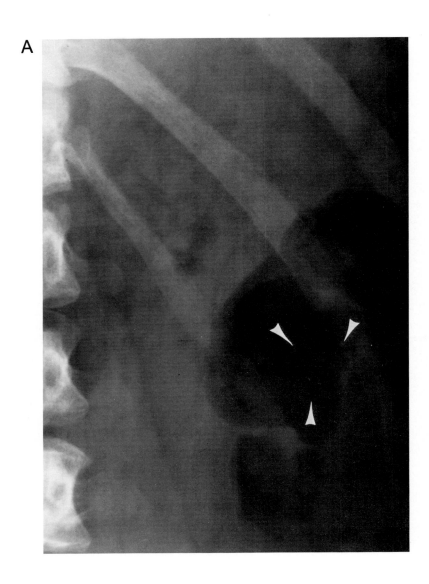

FIG 4–13.
Calcified cystic renal cell carcinoma. A 40-year-old woman with a history of breast carcinoma had a small, ringlike, linear calcification over the left kidney since six years previously. The calcification was thought to be a cyst.

A, a plain radiograph of the abdomen demonstrates a linear rim calcification *(arrowheads).* The size of this mass had not changed in six years.

B

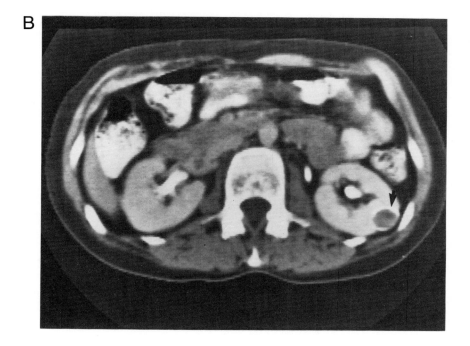

B, a CT scan of the abdomen reveals a small left renal mass with a thin rim of calcification *(arrow).* However, the content of the mass is solid, with a density of 62 Hounsfield units. *(Continued.)*

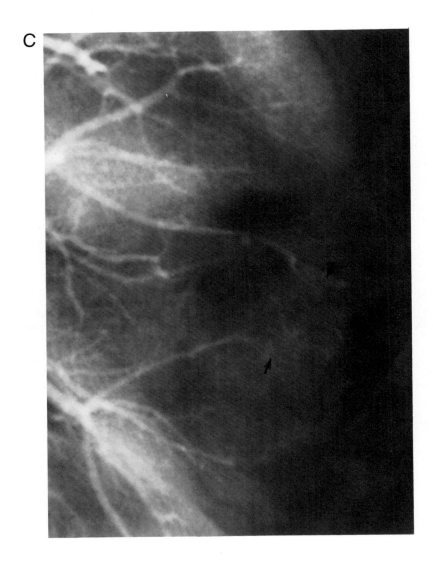

FIG 4–13 (cont.).
C, a magnification left renal arteriogram demonstrates   tumor vascularity in the mass *(arrows).*

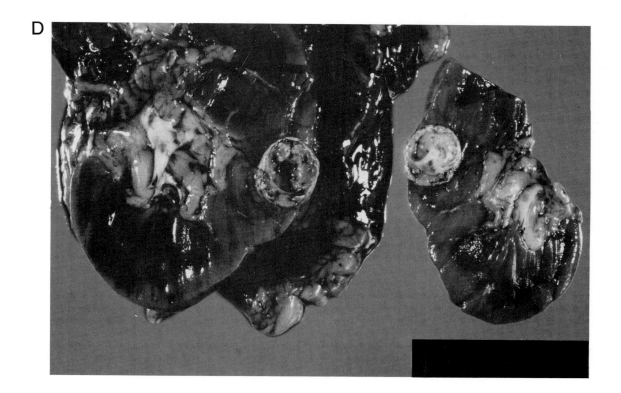

D, left nephrectomy was performed. Pathologic examination revealed a renal cell carcinoma in the calcified cyst (see also Color Plate 21).

A

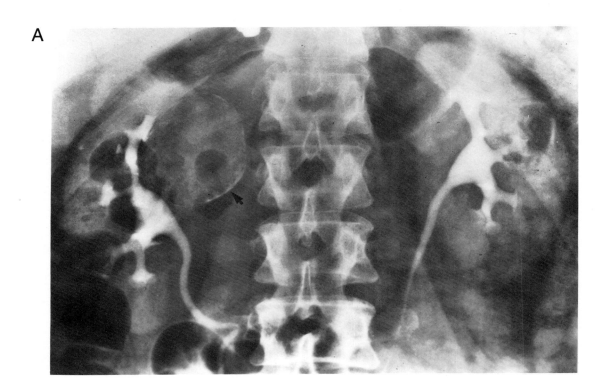

FIG 4–14.
Bilateral renal cell carcinoma. A 53-year-old veteran of the Korean War had a history of shrapnel injury to the chest and right upper back. When he sought medical attention for right flank pain, he was found to have a calcified mass in the right kidney.

A, an intravenous urogram reveals a mass with rim cal-

cification *(arrow)* in the upper pole of the right kidney.

B and **C,** abdominal CT scans demonstrate a solid mass with peripheral rim calcification *(arrows)* in the upper pole of the right kidney. In addition, there is a small solid mass in the upper pole of the left kidney *(arrowhead* in **C).** *(Continued.)*

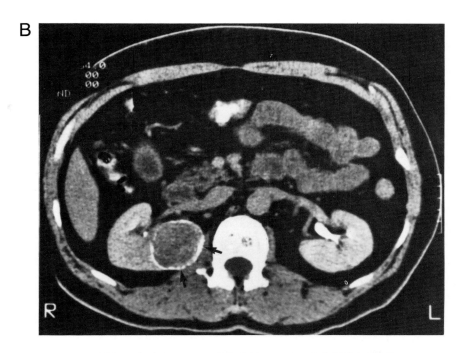

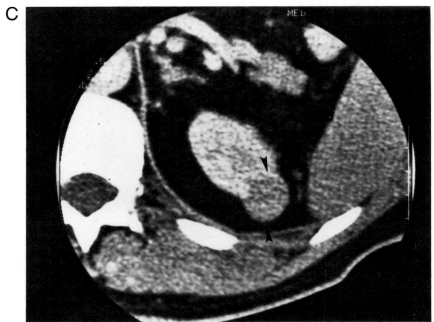

D

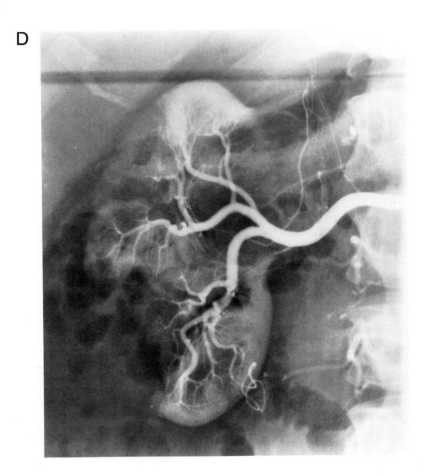

FIG 4–14 (cont.).
    D and **E,** right and left renal arteriograms show that two renal arteries supply each kidney. A selective arteriogram of the artery supplying the area of the tumors demonstrates the calcified mass in the right kidney to be avascular and the mass in the left kidney to be slightly hypervascular *(arrows).*

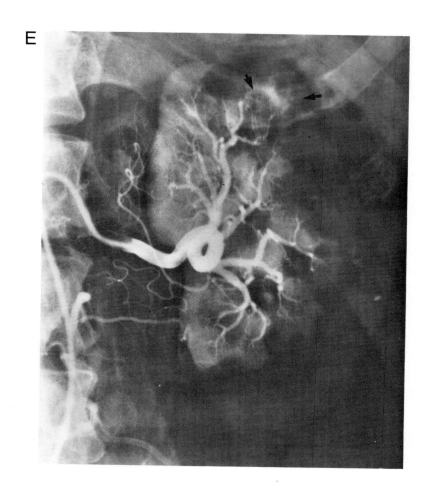

E

Both of the masses were excised and histologically shown to be hypernephroma. This case presents diagnostic difficulties because there are masses in both kidneys and a history of shrapnel injury. If either of the masses existed alone, one would consider hypernephroma the most likely diagnosis. However, when a history of shrapnel injury is significant, the mass in the right kidney would be taken to represent a calcified hematoma, and the surgical approach might be different.

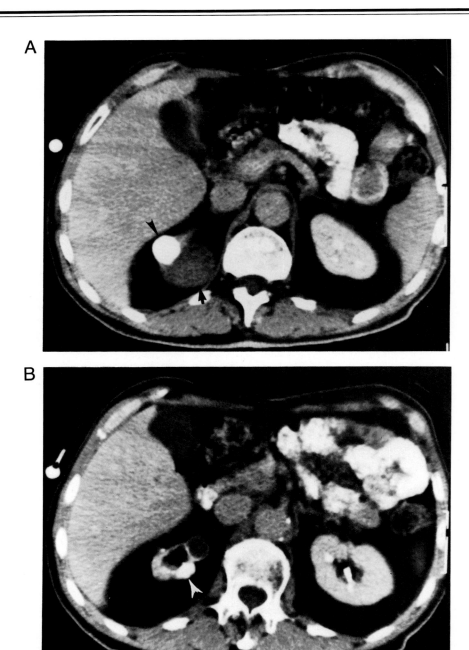

FIG 4–15.
Papillary adenocarcinoma (hypernephroma) of the kidney, with solid, dense calcification. A 72-year-old man had experienced hematuria for two months before this workup.

A and **B**, abdominal CT scans reveal a soft tissue mass *(arrow)* in the upper portion of the right kidney. There are areas of solid, dense calcification *(arrowheads)* in the mass. The parenchyma of the upper half of the right kidney is atrophic and contains an area of solid calcification. The pa-

renchyma of the lower half is normal.

C and **D,** an abdominal aortogram and a selective right renal arteriogram demonstrate small arteries supplying the upper half of the kidney and normal vascular supply in the lower half. There is no tumor vascularity.

Right nephrectomy was performed and revealed papillary adenocarcinoma of the upper portion of the kidney with multiple tumoral calcifications.

C

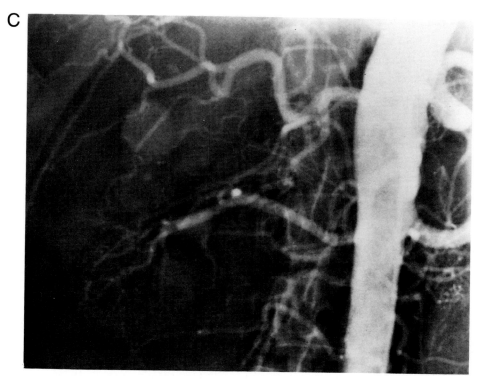

D

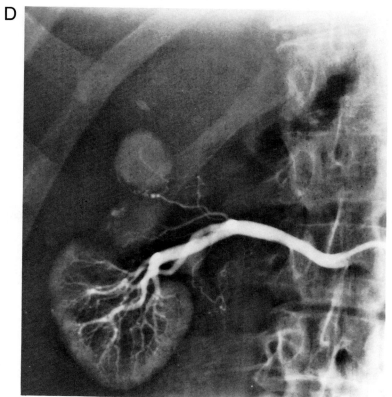

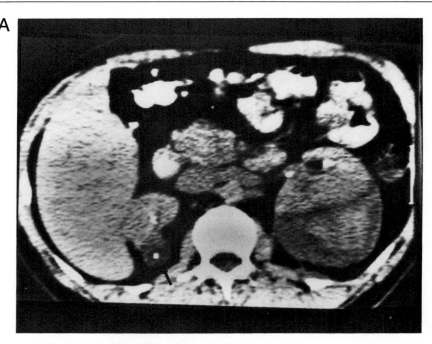

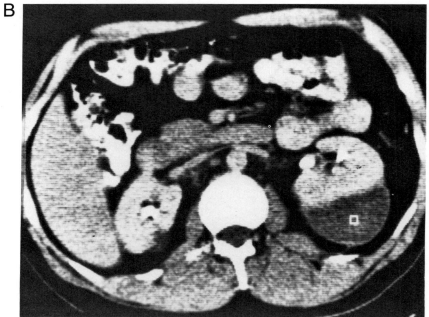

FIG 4–16.

Renal cell carcinoma with subcapsular hemorrhage. A 39-year-old man had a history of sudden-onset pain in the left flank. There was no hematuria.

A and **B,** renal CT scans reveal a subcapsular hematoma in the lower pole of the left kidney. There is no mass in the renal parenchyma associated with this subcapsular hematoma. However, a small, solid mass *(arrows)* is seen in the upper pole of the right kidney.

C and **D,** right and left renal arteriograms. The mass in the upper pole of the right kidney is hypervascular *(arrow).* There is an avascular mass displacing the left kidney upward, consistent with subcapsular hematoma.

Wedge resection of the mass at the upper pole of the right kidney and left nephrectomy were performed. The lesion from the right kidney was a renal cell carcinoma. In the left kidney, subcapsular hematoma was confirmed, and, although no tumor was grossly recognizable, histologic examination revealed a solid focus of renal cell carcinoma.

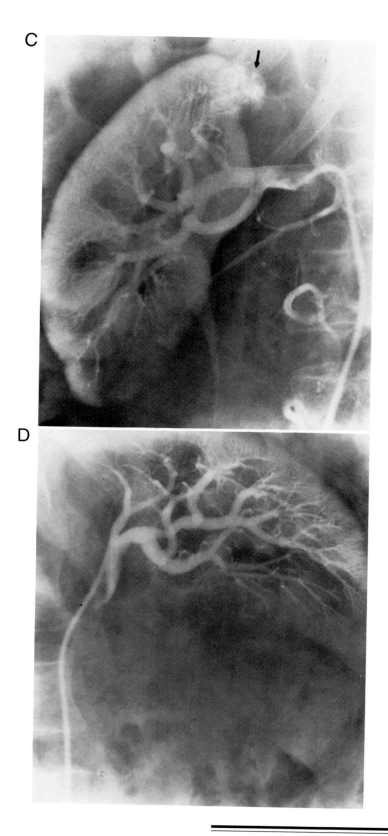

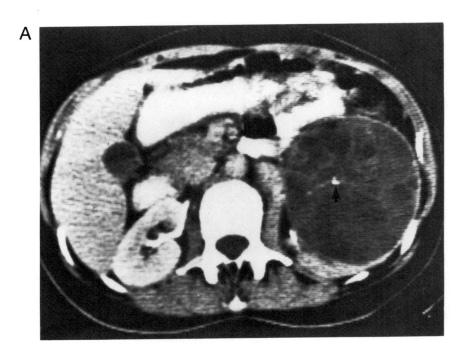

FIG 4–17.
Multilocular cystic nephroma. A 54-year-old woman presented with mild fever and left-sided abdominal pain. Diverticulitis was suspected, but during the workup a large mass in the left kidney was found on intravenous urography.

A, a CT scan of the abdomen demonstrates a large mass in the midportion of the left kidney. The mass is well encapsulated, and a clear margin separates it from the kidney parenchyma. Contained within the mass are multiple small cysts of water density. There is a focal area of calcification *(arrow)* in the septum in some of the small cysts.

B, left renal angiogram reveals a thick-walled avascular mass in the midportion of the left kidney.

C, left nephrectomy was performed. Pathologic examination shows a large, well-encapsulated mass containing multiple small cysts with thick fibrous septa, a typical appearance of multilocular cystic nephroma (see also Color Plate 22).

Even when CT and angiography demonstrate the typical appearance of multilocular cystic nephroma (which is a benign neoplasm), it may be difficult to exclude the possibility of multiloculated cystic hypernephroma. Multilocular cystic nephroma in most cases is treated by surgery.

B

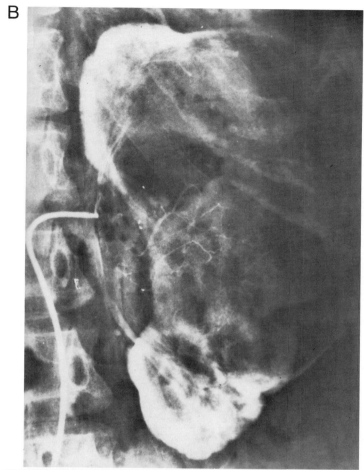

C

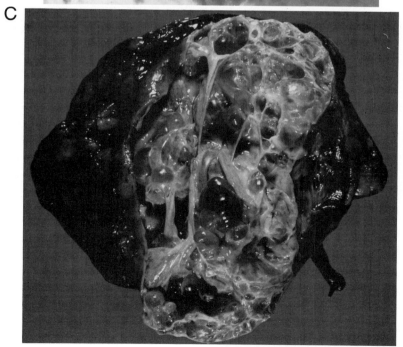

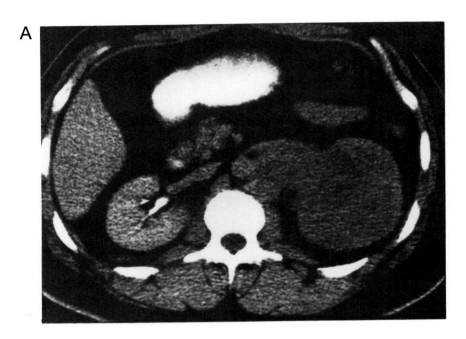

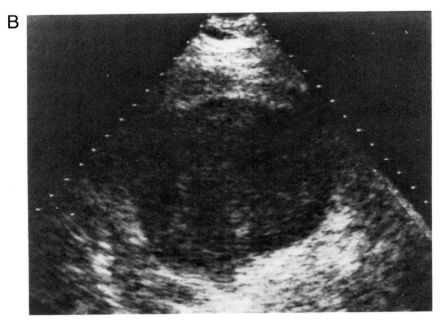

FIG 4–18.
Adult Wilms' tumor. A 28-year-old man had a history of pain in the left upper quadrant and fever for two months. There was recent onset of gross hematuria.

A, a CT scan of the abdomen demonstrates a mass in the left kidney and left paraaortic adenopathy.

B, a sonogram shows a solid, hypoechoic lesion.

C and **D,** left renal arteriograms demonstrate a hypo-vascular mass that occupies the middle portion of the kidney, sparing the superior and inferior poles *(arrows).* The renal artery is stretched and encased by the tumor. Residual barium from previous CT is seen in the colon.

The mass, because it was hypovascular, was considered to be an infiltrating neoplasm. Percutaneous biopsy yielded a histologic diagnosis of Wilms' tumor.

C

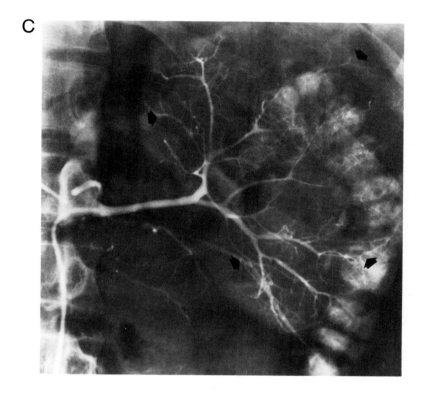

D

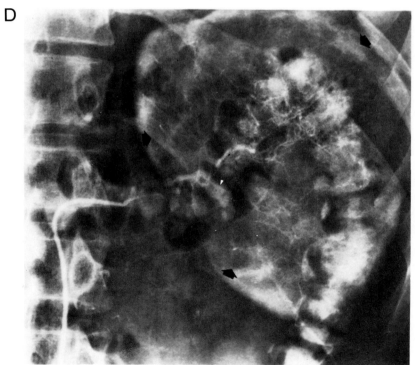

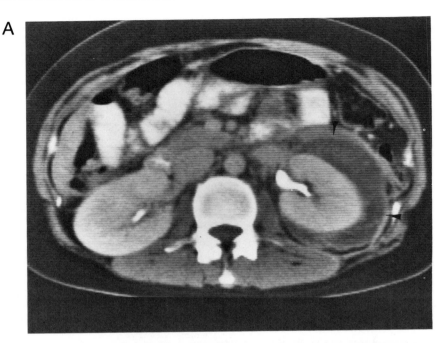

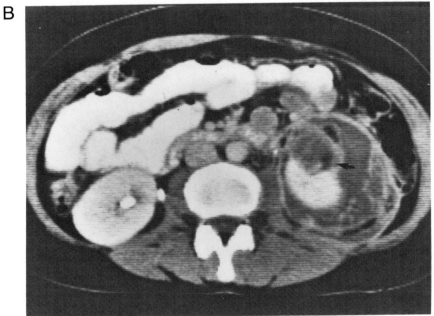

FIG 4–19.
Angiomyolipoma with perirenal hemorrhage. A 42-year-old woman presented with anemia and pain in the left flank.

A and **B,** renal CT scans demonstrate a hypodense collection *(arrowheads)* in the perirenal space of the left kidney. At the lower pole, there is a mass arising from the renal parenchyma; a small area of low density *(arrow* in **B)** in the mass is consistent with fat.

C, a sonogram of the left kidney reveals a hyperechoic mass *(arrow)* at the lower pole and hypoechoic collection *(arrowheads)* around the organ.

D, a left renal arteriogram demonstrates a mass in the lower pole that has abnormal vascularity and aneurysms *(arrow).* These findings are consistent with angiomyolipoma and perirenal hemorrhage.

The radiologic findings were confirmed on left nephrectomy.

C

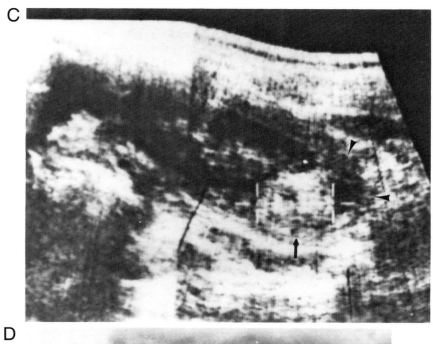

D

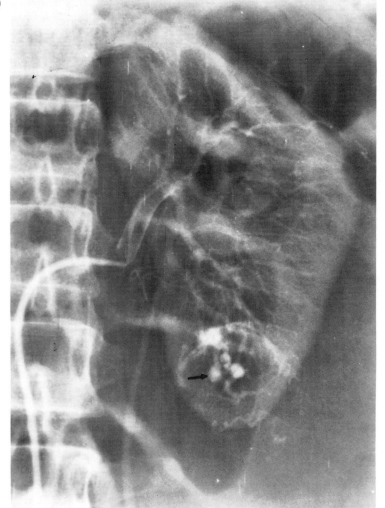

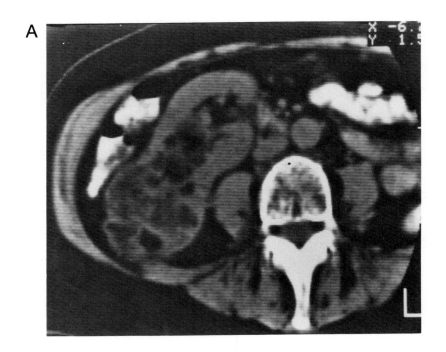

FIG 4–20.
Angiomyolipoma. A 61-year-old woman had a history of melanoma and Kaposi's sarcoma. On physical examination, a mass in the right upper quadrant was found.

A, a CT scan of the right kidney reveals a large mass arising from the posterior portion of the organ and extending into the perirenal space. In the mass there are hypodense areas consistent with fat density.

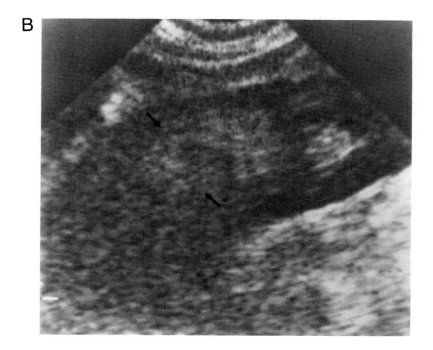

B, a sonogram of the right kidney shows the mass to be echogenic with hyperechoic areas *(arrows).*

Angiomyolipoma was cytologically confirmed on percutaneous aspiration biopsy.

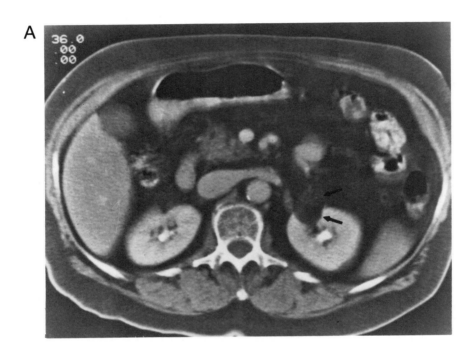

FIG 4–21.
Renal lipoma (two cases).

A, a 66-year-old woman had stage IB adenocarcinoma of the endometrium. Treatment was by total hysterectomy and bilateral salpingo-oophorectomy. A mass was discovered on routine follow-up CT.

The mass, which measured at fat density, originated in the renal parenchyma and protruded into the perirenal fat *(arrows).*

B and **C,** a middle-aged woman was found to have a left renal mass on routine intravenous urography. Coronal sonogram of the left kidney **(B)** shows a well-defined mass *(arrows)* within the renal parenchyma. A CT scan shows the mass **(C)** to be well defined with attenuation value of −70 Hounsfield units. There was no enhancement. With the presumptive diagnosis of a lipoma, it was elected to follow the patient by sonography.

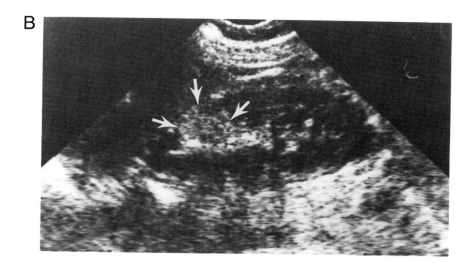

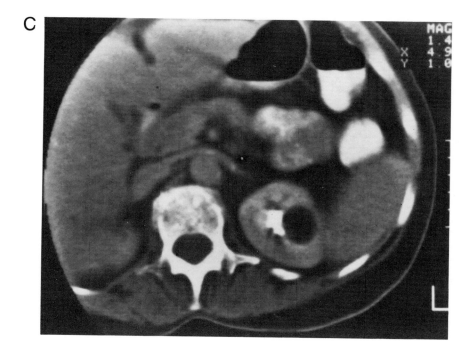

A

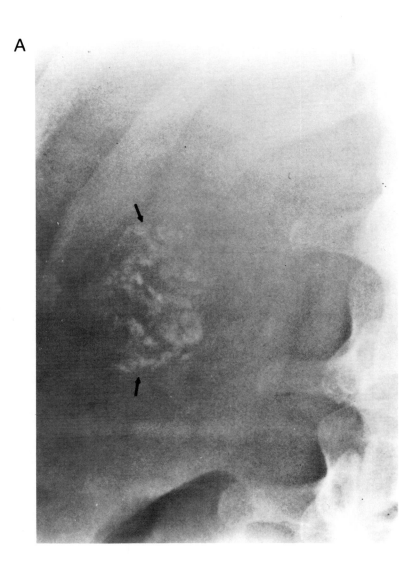

FIG 4–22.
Angiomyolipoma (hamartoma) of the kidney with calcification. A 32-year-old woman presented with hematuria. Intravenous urography demonstrated a calcified mass in the right kidney.

A, a plain film of the abdomen demonstrates a mass with multiple calcifications *(arrows).*

B, an intravenous urogram shows slight displacement of the middle group of calices.

C, right renal arteriogram reveals a hypovascular mass and displacement of intraparenchymal branches of the renal artery *(arrows).* Minimal abnormal vascularity is seen.

Right nephrectomy was performed. The histologic diagnosis was angiomyolipoma with calcification and prominent smooth muscle and fibrous tissue components.

B

C

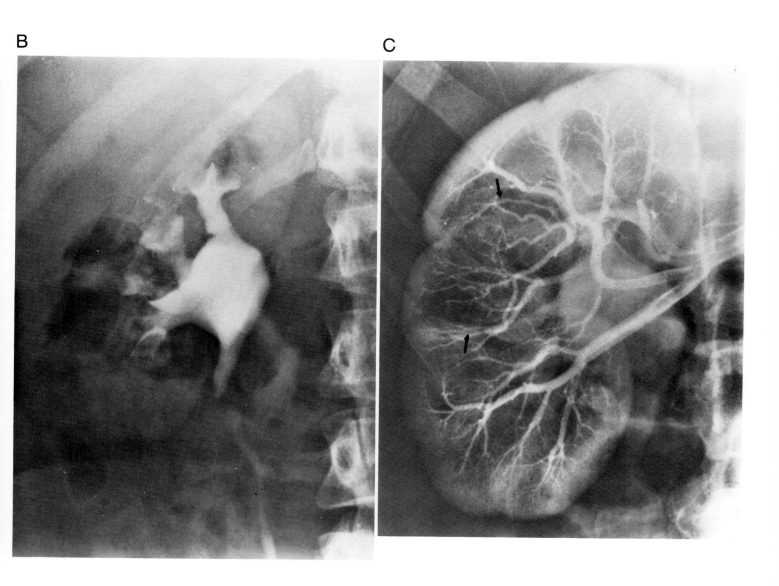

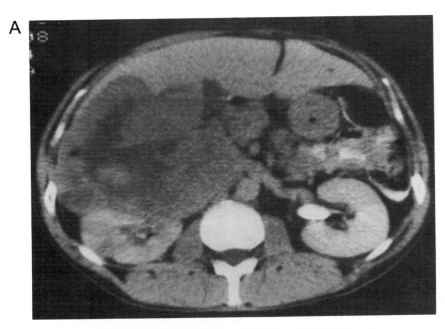

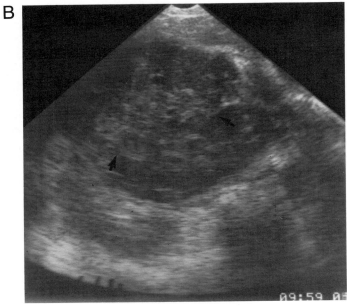

FIG 4–23.
Fibrosarcoma of the renal capsule. A 46-year-old man had experienced pain in the right flank and increasing abdominal girth for a month. A mass in the right side of the abdomen was found on physical examination.

A, an abdominal CT scan demonstrates a large mass arising from or attaching to the anterior surface of the right kidney. The renal parenchyma is mostly intact, although certain areas are locally invaded by the tumor.

B, a sonogram of the right kidney reveals a large, mostly hyperechoic mass anterior to the kidney. There is local invasion of the parenchyma *(arrows)*.

C
D

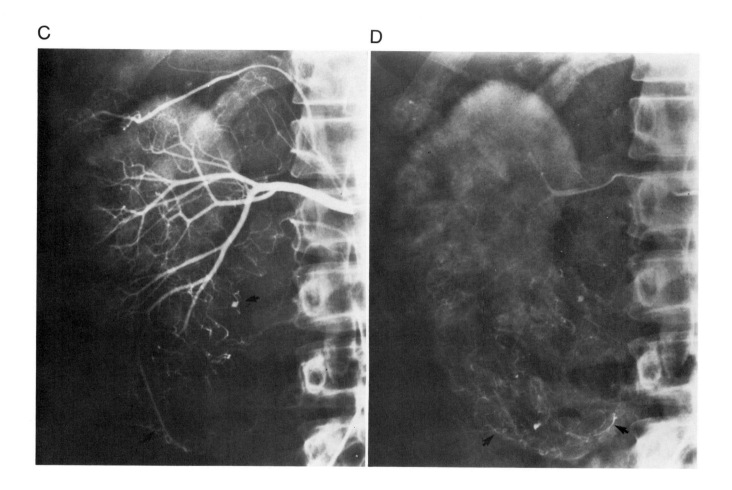

C and D, right renal arteriography demonstrates a large, moderately vascular mass, mostly extrinsic to the renal parenchyma. The blood supply to most of the mass was from the capsular arteries *(arrows)*. (C from Shirkhoda A., Lewis E.: Renal sarcoma and sarcomatoid renal cell carcinoma: CT and angiographic features. *Radiology* 162:353–357, 1987. Reproduced with permission.)

Since the epicenter of the mass was outside of the kidney and there was no parenchymal beak to suggest the parenchymal origin, this tumor should be considered mesenchymal (from the renal capsule or the perirenal space) in origin. Right nephrectomy was performed and the tumor seen to arise from the anterior surface of the kidney. The histologic diagnosis was fibrosarcoma.

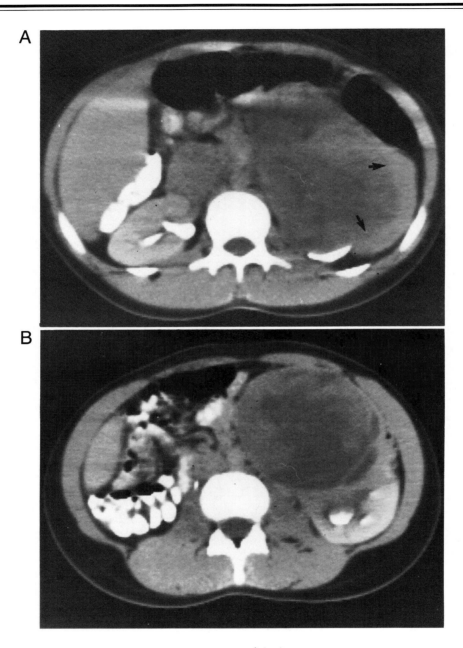

FIG 4–24.

Clear cell sarcoma of the kidney. A 20-year-old woman had experienced left abdominal fullness for two months before presentation and during that period had lost 9 kg. Intravenous urography revealed a mass in the left kidney.

A and **B,** abdominal CT scans demonstrate a large mass arising from the midportion and medial aspect of the left kidney. The renal parenchyma *(arrows)* is generally intact but laterally displaced.

C and **D,** left renal arteriograms reveal a large, moderately vascular tumor. The epicenter of the mass is in the renal sinus, and there is invasion of the renal parenchyma from the hilus *(arrows)*. The cortical outline of the kidney is intact.

E, left nephrectomy was performed. Most of the tumor is outside the kidney *(arrowheads)*. The tumor *(arrows)* appears to arise from the renal sinus with invasion of the kidney from its hilus. The histologic diagnosis was clear cell sarcoma (see also Color Plate 23).

Clear cell sarcoma is of mesenchymal origin, and in this patient, the tumor likely originated in the mesenchymal tissue of the renal sinus. Previously, clear cell sarcoma was considered a subgroup of Wilms' tumor. (**A–C** from Shirkhoda A., Lewis E.: Renal sarcoma and sarcomatoid renal cell carcinoma: CT and angiographic features. *Radiology* 162:353–357, 1987. Reproduced with permission.)

D

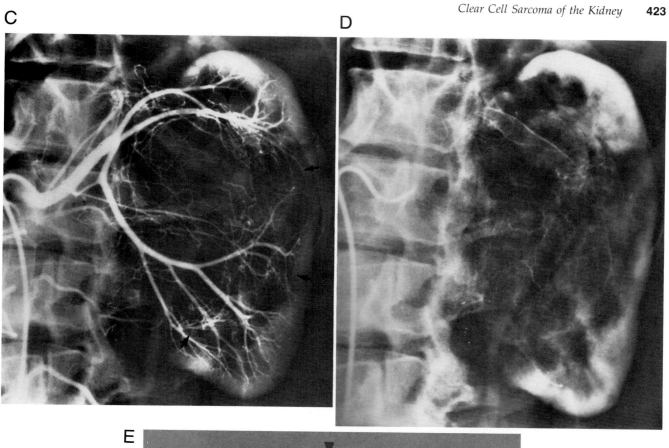

E

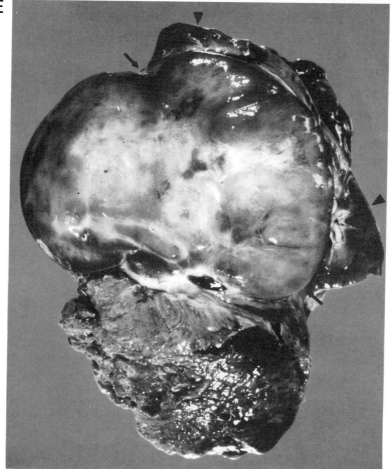

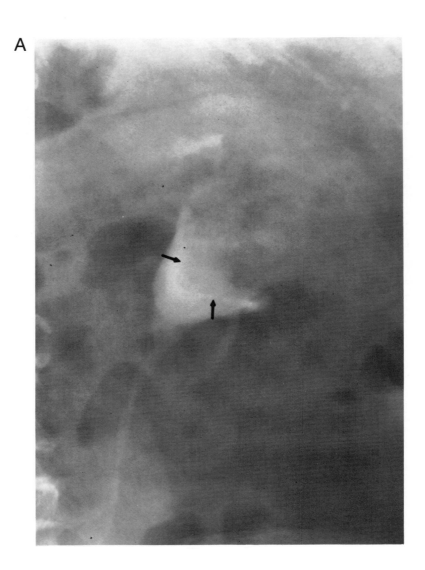

FIG 4–25.
Transitional cell carcinoma of the renal pelvis and ureter (multiple cases).

A and **B,** a 79-year-old man presented because of hematuria. An intravenous urogram **(A)** demonstrates a large filling defect in the left renal pelvis *(arrows).* A CT scan **(B)** reveals a soft tissue mass *(arrow)* in the pelvis of the left kidney. The density of the mass was measured at 38 Hounsfield units.

Left nephrectomy was performed. Transitional cell carcinoma of the renal pelvis with peripelvic fat infiltration (stage II) was found.

C and **D,** a 52-year-old man with low back pain and microscopic hematuria had a retrograde ureterogram **(C).** There are filling defects within the proximal right ureter, the largest one *(arrows)* being at the level of the iliac crest. A CT scan at the same level **(D)** shows the soft tissue density *(arrows)* within the dilated right ureteral lumen. This patient had a horseshoe kidney and extensive metastatic transitional cell carcinoma to the liver and lumbar vertebrae. He was treated by chemotherapy.

B

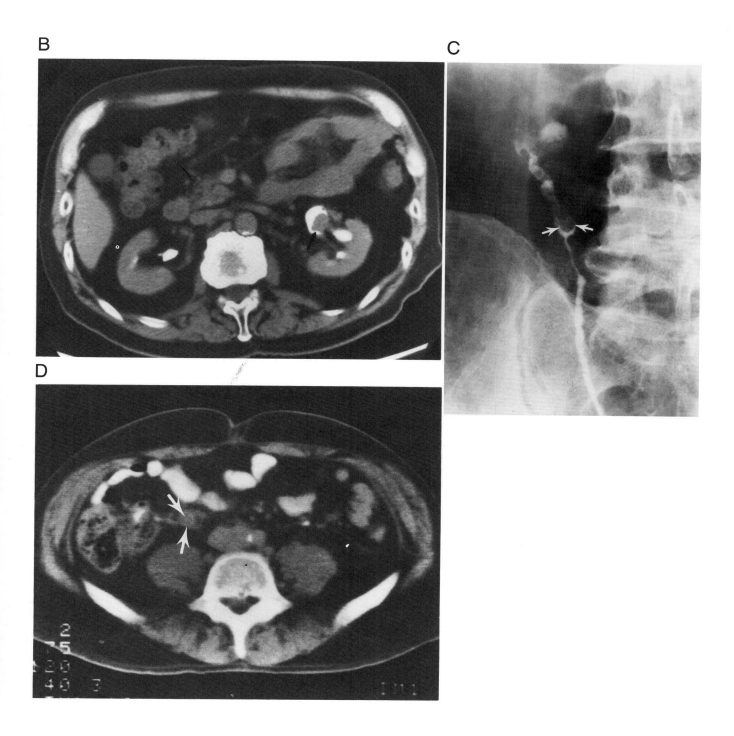

C

D

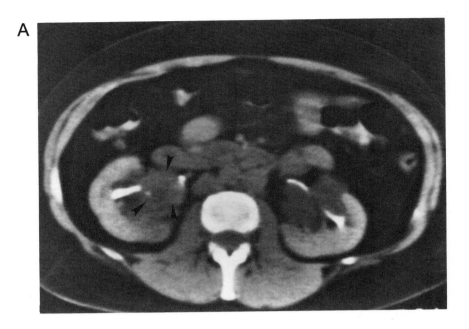

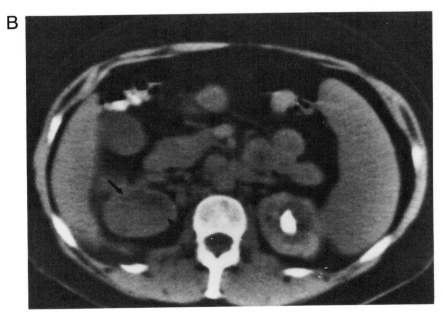

FIG 4–26.
Transitional cell carcinoma of the renal pelvis. A 63-year-old woman had a ten-year known history of parapelvic cyst. During the two years before her recent workup, she had experienced recurrent episodes of hematuria.

A and **B,** enhanced CT scans show a soft tissue mass in the right renal pelvis (*arrowhead* in **A**) in addition to parapelvic cysts. The soft tissue mass extends into and obstructs the calix of the upper pole (*arrows* in **B**) of the right kidney.

C, a retrograde pyelogram shows that the tumor in the renal pelvis extends into the upper-pole calix *(arrows).*

D, a right renal arteriogram demonstrates a hypovascular mass with tumor vascularity in the renal pelvis and in the upper portion of the kidney *(arrows),* corresponding to the CT findings. This appearance is consistent with transitional cell carcinoma involving the renal pelvis and extending into the upper-pole calix.

Right nephroureterectomy was performed, and the histologic diagnosis was transitional cell carcinoma.

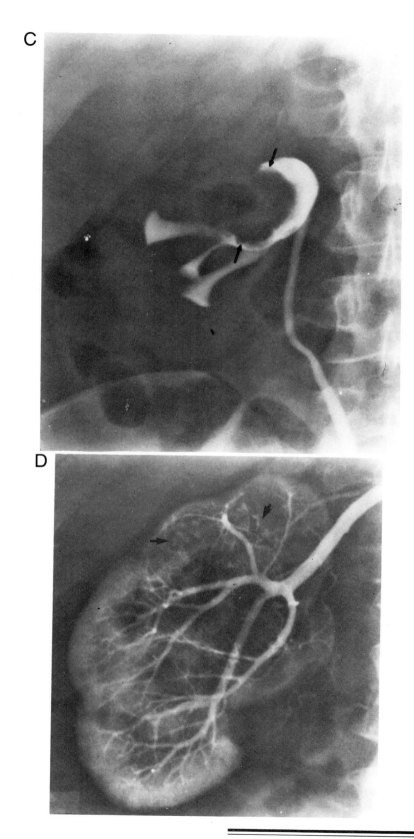

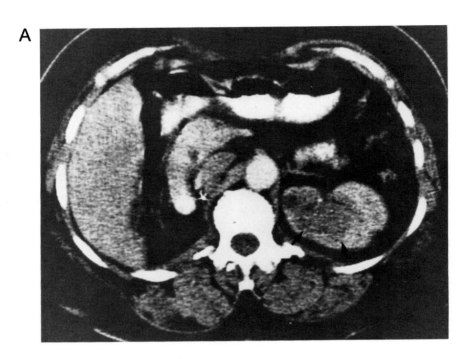

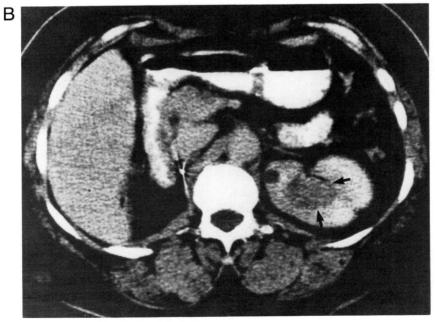

FIG 4–27.
Transitional cell carcinoma with invasion of renal parenchyma. A 62-year-old woman presented with a history of hematuria for the previous ten months. She had undergone a right nephrectomy 15 years earlier for a renal tumor. The final pathology of that kidney was not known.

A and **B,** renal CT scans reveal a mass arising from the renal pelvis and extending into the posterior portion of the parenchyma *(arrows).*

C

D

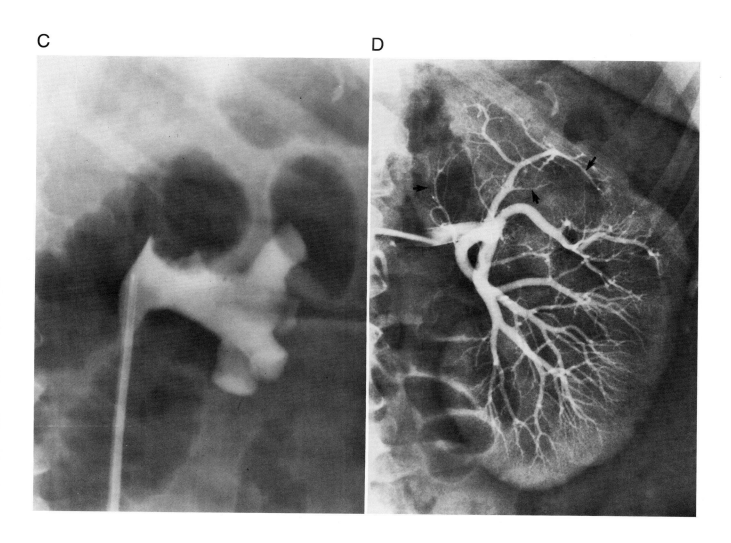

C, a left retrograde pyelogram demonstrates a large irregular filling defect in the renal pelvis; the defect obstructs the upper-pole calix.

D, a left renal arteriogram shows that in the upper pole, the parenchymal branches of the renal artery are displaced and encased *(arrows),* suggestive of parenchymal involvement.

Tissues obtained from retrograde examination and biopsy revealed a high-grade transitional cell carcinoma.

A

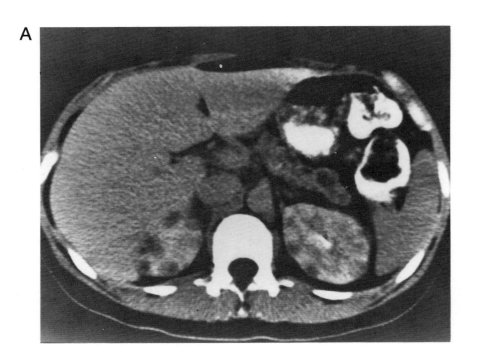

FIG 4–28.
Metastatic epithelioid sarcoma in the kidneys and pancreas. A 24-year-old woman had a five-year history of masses of the buttock, groin, scalp, and left breast. Biopsy of these masses showed epithelioid sarcoma. The patient was referred to M. D. Anderson Hospital for systemic chemotherapy.

A, CT scan of the abdomen reveals a number of small, low-density masses in both of the kidneys and in the pancreas.

B, five months later, a CT scan shows a number of circular calcifications *(arrowheads)* in both kidneys and in the pancreas. The masses in both kidneys grew progressively larger. The patient also developed obstructive jaundice, which required bypass surgery.

C, a plain film of the abdomen demonstrates calcifications in both kidneys.

Percutaneous biopsy of a skin lesion with similar circular calcification showed epithelioid sarcoma. Metastatic epithelioid sarcoma in the kidney and pancreas was confirmed at autopsy 15 months later.

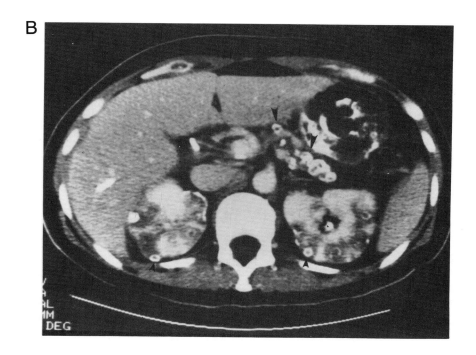

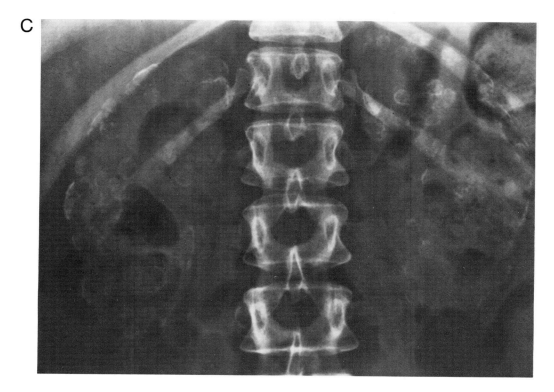

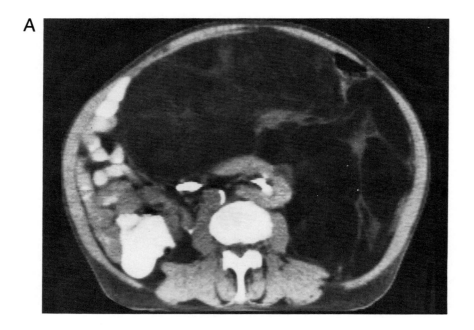

FIG 4–29.
Retroperitoneal liposarcoma. A 68-year-old man had a history of weight loss and increasing abdominal girth. A large soft tissue mass in the abdomen was discovered on palpation.

A, an abdominal CT scan demonstrates a large mass, mainly of fat density, that surrounds the left kidney and displaces the kidney across the midline of the body. Some solid component in the mass is seen in the lower part of the abdomen.

B

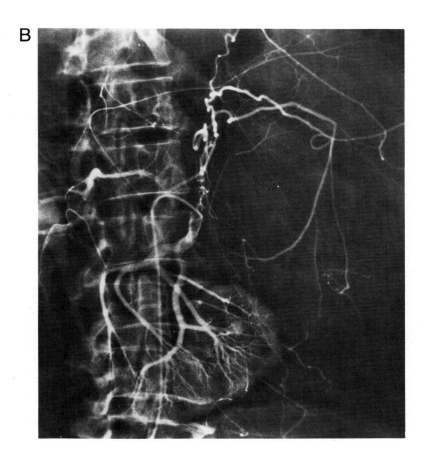

B, a left renal arteriogram reveals the mass surrounding the kidney, but there is no evidence of invasion of the renal parenchyma. Multiple capsular arteries supply the mass.

At surgery, retroperitoneal liposarcoma was found. The tumor was removed from the kidney without nephrectomy being required. Differentiation between a tumor arising from the renal capsule and tumor arising from the perirenal mesenchymal tissue can be extremely difficult despite the fact that these tumors receive their blood supplies from the capsular arteries. A diagnosis of capsular sarcoma is favored when the tumor is attached to the kidney by a broad base. A tumor that can be peeled away from the kidney, as in this case, is more likely to be of retroperitoneal origin.

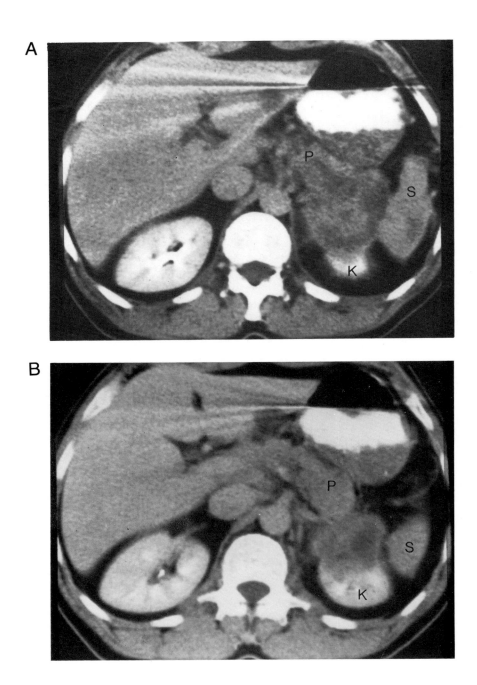

FIG 4-30.
Carcinoma of the pancreas with direct invasion of the kidney. A 58-year-old man had a history of pain in the left side of the back. On physical examination, a mass was found in the left upper quadrant of the abdomen.

A and **B,** abdominal CT scans show a mass that involves the tail of the pancreas *(P),* the spleen *(S),* and the superior pole of the left kidney *(K).*

C

D

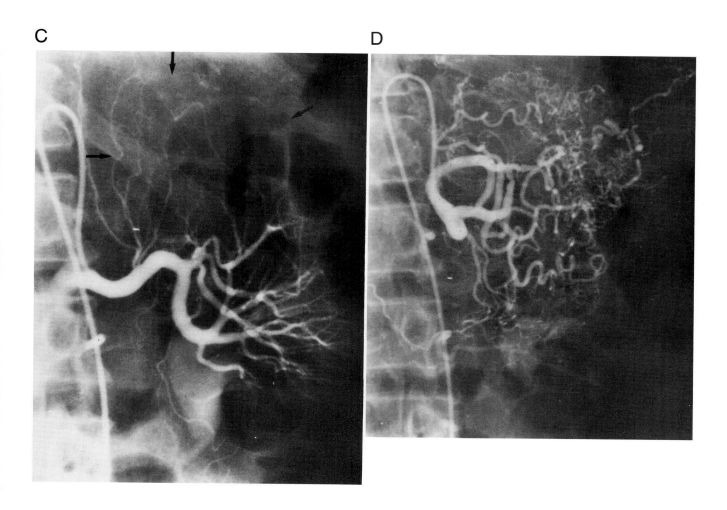

C, a left renal arteriogram reveals a hypovascular mass in the upper pole of the organ *(arrows).*

D, a splenic arteriogram demonstrates occlusion of the splenic artery with collaterals through the left gastric artery to supply the spleen.

It would have been difficult to localize the origin of this tumor mass on CT since the pancreas, spleen, and kidney were all involved. However, the aggressive nature of the tumor, with encasement and occlusion of the splenic artery, favored a diagnosis of carcinoma of the pancreas. Percutaneous biopsy confirmed this diagnosis.

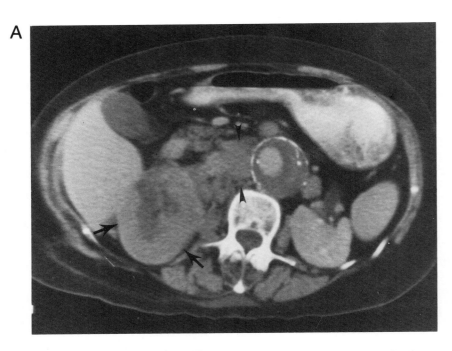

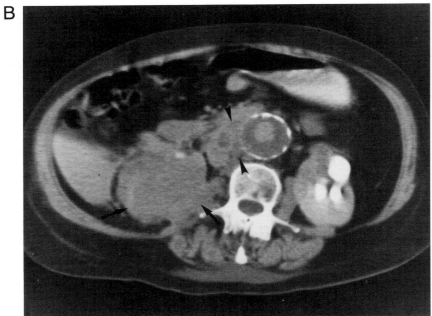

FIG 4–31.
Large cell lymphoma of the kidney. A 67-year-old woman presented with a history of dysuria and gross hematuria. She had experienced pain in the right flank associated with fever and night sweats during the previous few months.

A and **B,** abdominal CT scans show a large aneurysm in the abdominal aorta and a number of enlarged paracaval and aortocaval nodes *(arrowheads)*. A hypodense mass infiltrates throughout the kidney *(arrows),* but the reniform shape is maintained.

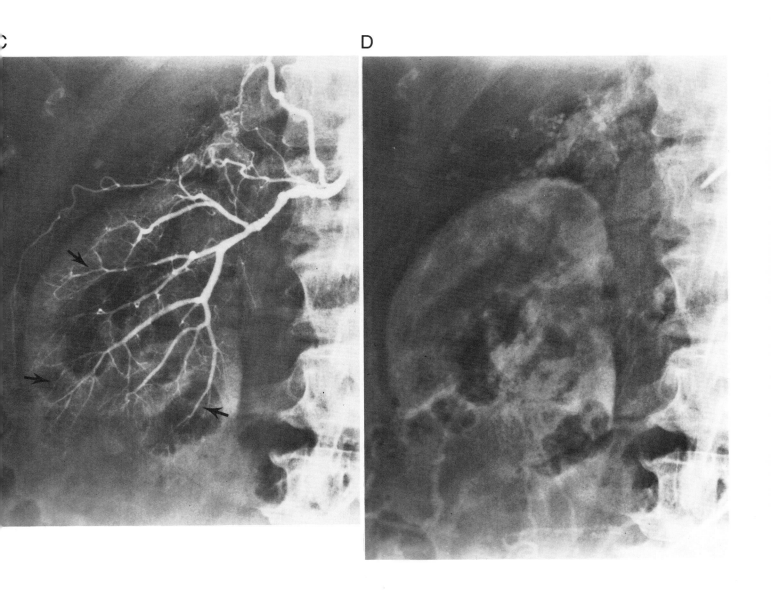

C and D, right renal arteriograms reveal stretching and encasement *(arrows)* of the intraparenchymal branches, compatible with infiltrative neoplasm.

Percutaneous aspiration biopsy of the renal mass was performed. The histologic and cytologic diagnoses were large cell lymphoma.

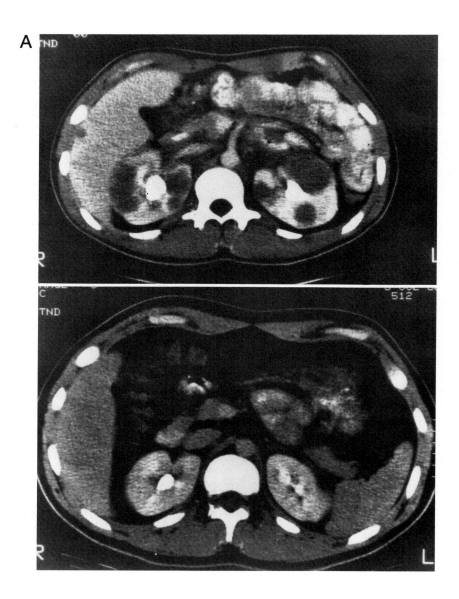

FIG 4–32.
Renal lymphoma (multiple cases).

A, a 17-year-old boy presented with episodes of fever and testicular enlargement. A testicular biopsy was consistent with lymphoblastic lymphoma. He was referred for further evaluation.

A contrast-enhanced CT scan of the abdomen shows retroperitoneal adenopathy with multiple low-density nodules within both kidneys *(top image)*. The attenuation values of the lesions were 72 to 78 Hounsfield units. With the diagnosis of renal lymphoma, the patient was treated and a repeat CT scan in 2 months *(bottom image)* was normal.

B

C

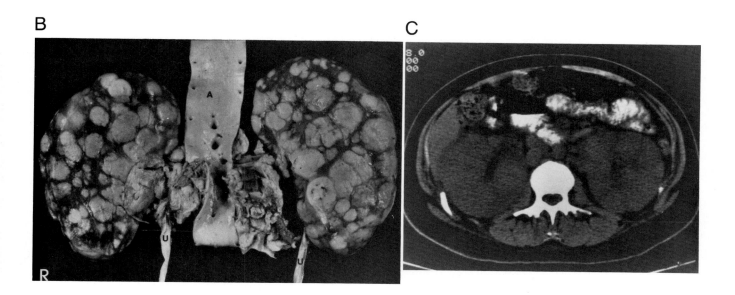

D

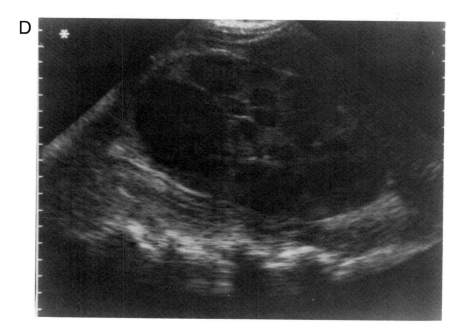

B, autopsy specimen in a 22-year-old man with the diagnosis of poorly differentiated lymphocytic lymphoma shows bilateral nodular renal involvement. (**B** from Shirkhoda A., Staab E., Mittelstaedt C.A.: Renal lymphoma imaged by ultrasound and gallium-67. *Radiology* 137:175–180, 1980. Reproduced with permission.)

C and **D,** a 22-year-old woman presented with a breast lump and vaginal bleeding. Endometrial biopsy was consistent with large cell lymphoma. The patient had abnormal renal function tests.

Unenhanced CT scan **(C)** shows bilateral nephromegaly, thought to be due to diffuse renal infiltration by lymphoma. There was also evidence of pelvic and retroperitoneal adenopathy. A sagittal sonogram of the right kidney **(D)** shows multiple hypoechoic masses throughout the kidney. There was total improvement of the renal masses after chemotherapy.

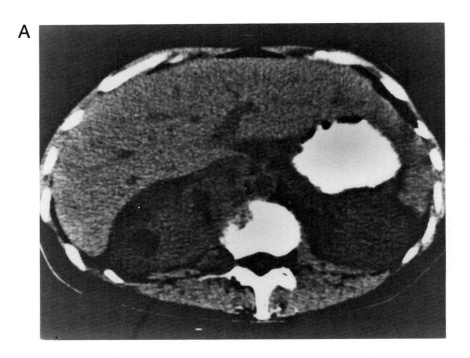

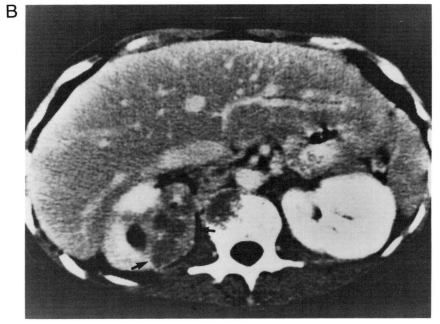

FIG 4–33.

Squamous cell carcinoma of the cervix metastatic to the kidney. A 42-year-old woman had undergone radiation therapy two years earlier for stage IB squamous cell carcinoma of the cervix. She presented because of recent-onset back pain.

A and **B,** abdominal CT scans were made without **(A)** and with **(B)** contrast enhancement. There is paracaval adenopathy with destruction of the vertebral body of L-1. The right kidney is involved by an infiltrative process *(arrows),* but the reniform shape is maintained.

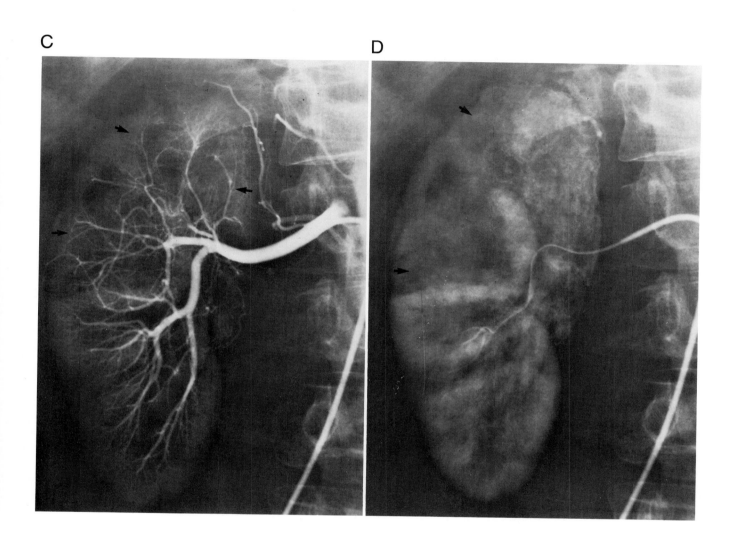

C and D, right renal arteriograms reveal an infiltrative neoplasm that involves the superior half of the organ *(arrows)*. There is minimal tumor vascularity. Differential diagnostic possibilities include lymphoma, invasive primary hypovascular renal tumor, metastasis.

Percutaneous aspiration biopsy of the right kidney yielded a squamous cell carcinoma compatible with metastasis from the cervix.

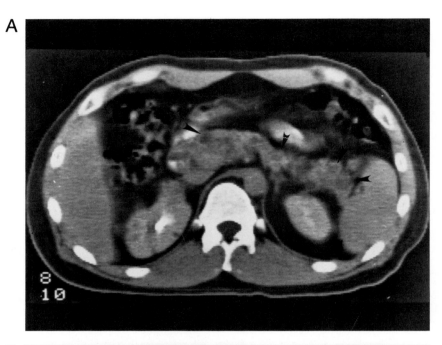

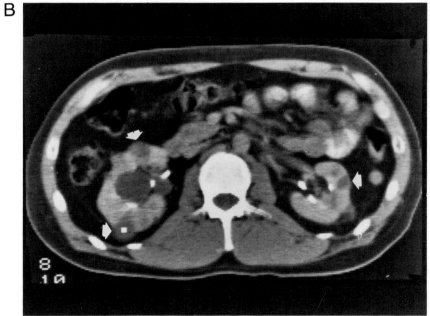

FIG 4–34.
Multiple renal tumors in von Hippel-Lindau disease. A 31-year-old man had had a left cerebellar hemangioblastoma excised ten years before this presentation. He now presented because of ataxia, and CT revealed a lesion in the right cerebellum.

A and **B,** abdominal CT scans demonstrate a number of cortical masses *(arrows),* many solid and some cystic, in both kidneys. In addition, there are a number of lesions *(arrowheads)* in the body and tail of the pancreas.

C

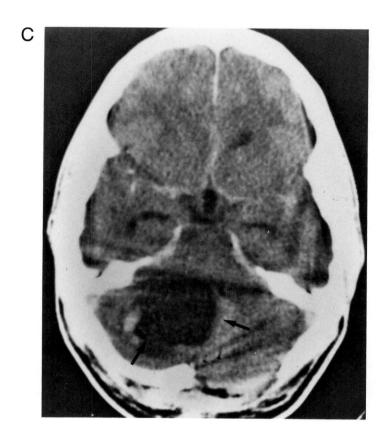

C, a contrast-enhanced CT scan of the brain demonstrates a low-density lesion *(arrows)* and several additional cystic lesions. *(Continued.)*

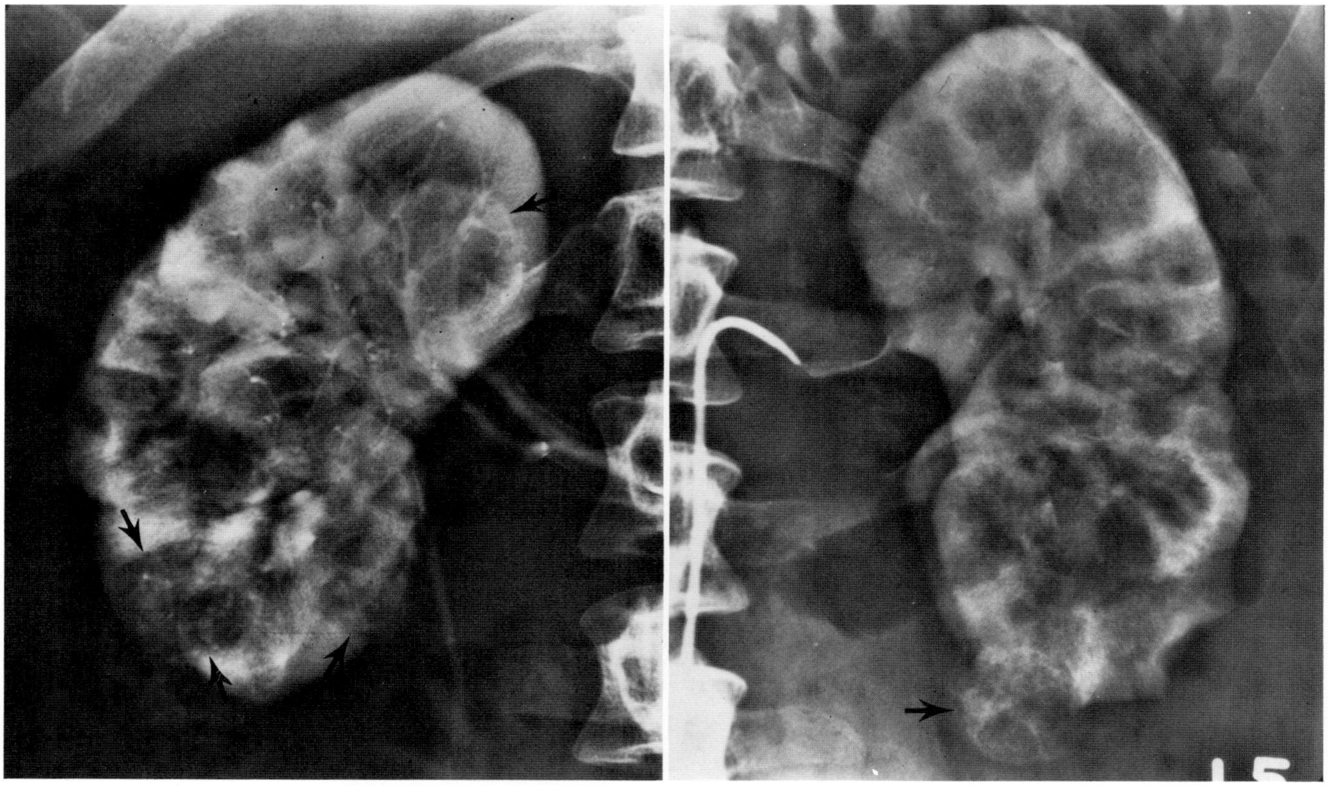

FIG 4–34 (cont.).

The clinical history and radiologic findings in this case are consistent with von Hippel-Lindau disease. This disease consists of cerebellar hemangioblastoma; there are angiomatous lesions of the retinas and cysts of the pancreas and kidneys (**D** and **E**), and frequently there is associated renal cell carcinoma. Renal cell carcinoma can be found in one half to two thirds of the patients.

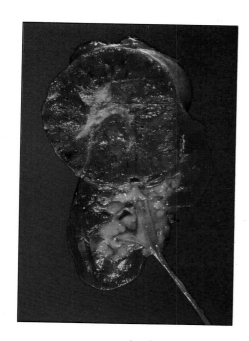

PLATE 16

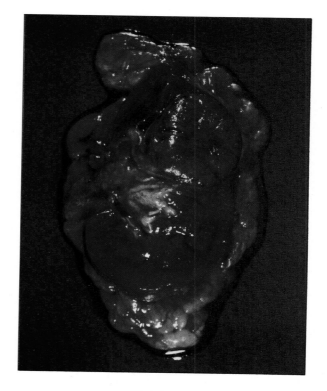

PLATE 17

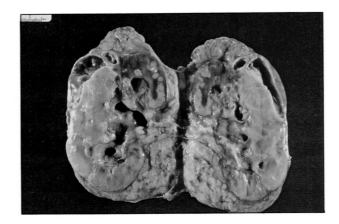

PLATE 18

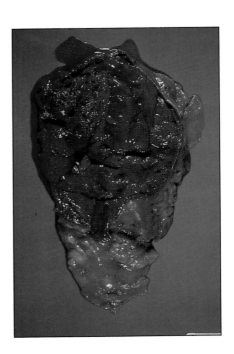

PLATE 19

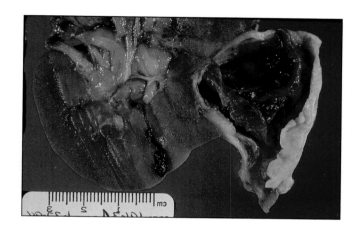

PLATE 20

PLATE 21

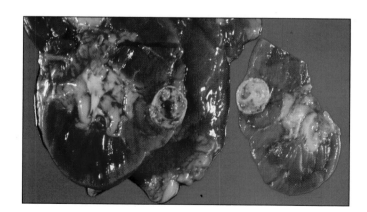

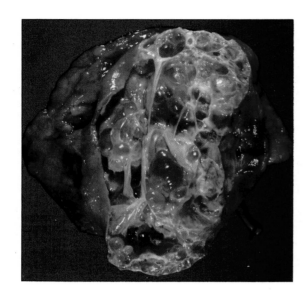

PLATE 22

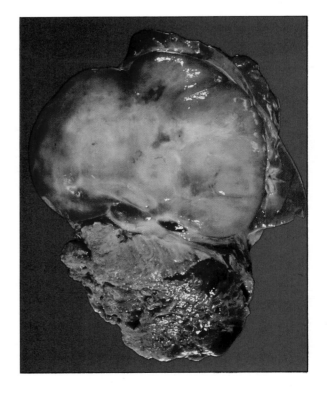

PLATE 23

5

Urinary Bladder and Male Genital Organs

Golden Pan, M.D.

Anita Thomas, M.D.

Ali Shirkhoda, M.D.

URINARY BLADDER

Neoplasms of the urinary bladder are the second most common group of urologic malignancies. The incidence of bladder cancer increases dramatically with age and reaches a peak in the sixth and seventh decades of life. Men are affected three to four times more commonly than women.[1]

Various chemical agents have been implicated as etiologic factors in industrialized countries. Cigarette smoking is a major cause of bladder cancer. Workers employed in the chemical, rubber, petroleum, leather, and photographic industries have been reported to have an increased risk as well. Other agents that have been implicated in the etiology of bladder cancer include caffeine, artificial sweeteners, phenacetin in large doses, and certain chemotherapeutic drugs.[2, 3]

Such conditions as chronic urinary tract infection, bladder calculi, bladder diverticula, extrophy of the bladder, and urachal remnants also have an associated risk of bladder cancer. The most common neoplasm in the first two conditions is squamous cell carcinoma, whereas transitional cell carcinomas are more common in diverticula, and the great majority of tumors found with bladder extrophy and urachal remnants are mucinous adenocarcinomas.[4–6] In many less industrialized countries, schistosomal infection of the bladder is the major cause of bladder cancer. These patients tend to be younger, and squamous cell carcinoma accounts for as many as 70% of the cases.[7]

Pathology and Staging

More than 90% of bladder tumors are of uroepithelial origins upon which type the staging system is based (Fig 5–1). These tumors most frequently are located at the trigone. The World Health Organization classification divides uroepithelial tumors into benign papillomas and carcinomas. In the first group are transitional cell papilloma, inverted papilloma, and squamous papilloma. Carcinomas are further divided by cell type into transitional cell, squamous cell, adenocarcinoma, undifferentiated, and mixed type (Figs 5–2 to 5–5). In industrialized countries, about 90% of the uroepithelial carcinomas originate as transitional cell carcinoma, and 70% have a papillary growth pattern. Squamous cell carcinomas account for 5% to 6% of bladder carcinomas, and adenocarcinomas 2% to 3%.[8, 9]

The nonepithelial benign tumors of the bladder

449

include leiomyomas, neurofibromas, hemangiomas, fibromas, myomas, lipomas, osteomas, chondromas, ganglioneuromas, pheochromocytomas, granular cell myoblastomas, and endometriosis. The classic presentation of bladder pheochromocytoma is symptoms of catecholamine release (headache, tachycardia, hypertension) on micturition (Fig 5–6). Bladder pheochromocytomas arise most commonly from the trigone area and most are benign, although metastases have developed in approximately 10% of the reported cases.[10]

Of the malignant nonepithelial tumors, leiomyosarcomas are the most common in adults (Fig 5–7). Rhabdomyosarcomas are the most common soft tissue tumor of children and, after the head and neck region, appear next most frequently in the genitourinary tract. Three histologic subtypes of rhabdomyosarcoma exist: embryonal, alveolar, and pleomorphic (undifferentiated). The sarcoma botryoides form of rhabdomyosarcoma is a morphological variant of the embryonal subtype and is common in young children; it appears as masses of vesicular clusters (Fig 5–8).[11] The list of other malignant tumors of the bladder includes other sarcomas (Figs 5–9 and 5–10), mesodermal mixed tumors, lymphoma (Fig 5–11), and metastasis (Figs 5–12 and 5–13).

The staging of bladder carcinomas involves clinical examination (cystourethroscopy and bimanual rectoabdominal palpation of the bladder and pelvis with the patient under anesthesia), radiologic studies to assess the extent of tumor spread, and pathologic examination of biopsy and surgical specimens.

In the United States, the staging system for uroepithelial carcinomas that is primarily used is that proposed by Jewett and Strong[12] and modified by Marshall (Fig 5–1).[13] In this system, stage 0 designates tumors involving only the mucosa and includes both papillary and flat in situ carcinomas. Stage A designates invasion into only the submucosa, and stage B is further invasion into the muscularis layer. Stage B is divided into B1 (Fig 5–14), superficial muscular invasion (less than halfway into the muscularis), and B2, deep muscular invasion (more than halfway). Stage C designates invasion into the perivesical fat or into but not beyond the capsules of adjacent organs (Fig 5–15). Stage D represents metastatic spread beyond the region of the bladder. In D1, the cancer, whether it is direct invasion or lymph node metastases, is confined to the pelvis below the level of the sacral promontory (Fig 5–16); in D2, there is spread beyond the pelvis. Outside of the United States, the tumor-node-metastasis (TNM) staging system of the Union Internationale Contre le Cancer (UICC) is more commonly used for bladder tumors. The TNM system provides for a more precise description of the extent of tumor; however, the two systems have nearly equivalent stages for the most clinically relevant levels.[14]

Tumors that have invaded the deeper layers of the bladder wall are more likely to have distant spread, and this likelihood increases with the depth of invasion. Regional lymph nodes are the major site of metastases, followed by skeleton, lung, and liver. The route of lymphatic drainage of the bladder is first to the perivesical lymph nodes, then to the middle and medial (obturator) groups of the external iliac nodes and the internal iliac, presacral, and common iliac lymph nodes. From there, drainage goes through the paraaortic lymph nodes.[15]

Radiologic Evaluation

The role of radiologic evaluation in bladder cancer has been directed primarily at assessing the extent of spread of these tumors that on other clinical grounds are likely to be invasive or to have metastases. The boundaries of tumor spread also can be better defined for planning radiation therapy. To a lesser extent, radiologic imaging is used for the detection of new or recurrent bladder tumors; in this capacity, most radiologic studies are at present limited by high cost or low sensitivity for small lesions.

In the initial workup of hematuria and lower urinary tract symptoms, the excretory urogram continues to play a major role. The cystogram is another conventional contrast study often used for evaluation of lower urinary tract disorders. These tests are capable of detecting the bladder tumors that may be responsible for the presenting symptoms, but they have a low sensitivity, particularly for small tumors. In addition, intravesical filling defects can be simulated by benign processes (Fig 5–17) such as cystitis cystica, blood clot, or nonradiopaque stones. In some large series, less than 40% of bladder tumors have been detectable as filling defects; other studies have suggested that the rate of detection of tumors greater than 5 mm exceeds 90%.[16, 17] Findings of hydronephrosis or nonfunctioning kidney secondary to obstruction from a bladder tumor are infrequent, estimated at less than 10% (Fig 5–14). Radiographically visible calcifications of bladder tumors are even more uncommon, seen in less than 1% (Fig 5–5).[17] Because of the low sensitivity, contrast radiography is not generally useful for the routine detection or follow-up of bladder tumors.[18]

Bipedal lymphangiography is capable of imaging

some of the regional lymph node groups that drain the bladder, and it can detect small metastases within normal-sized nodes. However, lymphangiography is unable to consistently demonstrate the perivesical, internal iliac, and presacral lymph nodes, which are also potential sites for lymphatic spread. Nonmetastatic causes of abnormal nodal architecture can cause false-positive studies, and observer variability between radiologic centers has also been a limiting factor. Published reports of the accuracy of lymphangiography in the staging of bladder cancer have varied from 72% to 91.6%, with sensitivity of 46% to 89% and specificity of 94% to 100%.[19, 20] In many centers, lymphangiography has been abandoned in favor of computed tomography (CT) for evaluating lymph node metastases. In fact, the two studies may be complementary in this role because of their different inherent strengths and weaknesses.[21]

Imaging of the primary bladder tumor by CT has been useful mainly for defining the tumor boundaries for radiation therapy and for staging the more advanced carcinomas. Computed tomography is also useful for follow-up after treatment with chemotherapy (Fig 5–18) or cystectomy (Fig 5–19). Rarely, as in urachal adenocarcinomas, a typical location or appearance on CT may suggest the histologic diagnosis (Fig 5–4).[22]

Computed tomography cannot differentiate between the layers of the bladder wall, and its accuracy in identifying tumor invasion of the perivesical fat is questionable. Microscopic invasion of the perivesical fat cannot be detected by CT, and cases with such invasion will therefore be understaged. Overstaging can result from an abnormal appearance of the perivesical fat due to previous radiation therapy or even cystoscopic procedures (Fig 5–20).[23]

Computed tomography of the pelvis and abdomen is capable of detecting enlarged pelvic and abdominal lymph node groups not seen with lymphangiography. The criteria for adenopathy vary from the strict definition of a node greater than 1.5 cm in diameter in the axial plane to "softer" findings of asymmetry of the soft tissues or the presence of a discrete nodule in the region of the major pelvic and abdominal lymph node chains. Assessment by CT of adenopathy in bladder cancer has the same inherent problems as in other diseases. False-positive results arise from benign causes of nodal enlargement, and CT cannot detect small foci of metastases within normal-sized nodes (Fig 5–21). Published reports of the overall accuracy of CT for the detection of lymph node metastases in bladder cancer have ranged from

79% to 92%, with sensitivity of 60% to 85% and specificity of 86% to 100%.[24–27]

Overall accuracy rates reported for CT staging of bladder tumors have ranged from 59% to 88%. However, the accuracy rates for individual stages vary considerably in these reports, and stage C, representing perivesical fat involvement, is probably the least accurate CT diagnosis, with accuracy rates of only 25% to 33%. Despite these problems, CT can significantly change the staging level in as many as 33% of selected patients, and therefore it does have some utility in advanced stages of bladder carcinoma.[24–28]

The sonographic evaluation of bladder carcinomas has many of the same limitations as CT. Three approaches have been used: transabdominal, transurethral, and transrectal. Transrectal sonography has a limited range and cannot image all of the bladder. It has been much more successful for evaluating the prostate.[29] Suprapubic transabdominal sonography provides good images of the distended bladder but is, in general, unable to reliably detect bladder lesions less than 5 mm in diameter.[30–32] The bladder wall appears on these scans as a single thickness of uniform echogenicity, and differentiation between the three layers of the wall is not possible. Deep tumor invasion of the bladder wall, however, can be assessed in these sonograms, and regional lymphadenopathy can also be identified. Accuracy rates as high as 85% have been reported for the sonographic detection of deep muscularis and perivesical fat invasion (Fig 5–12). Nevertheless, the results of transabdominal sonography are highly dependent on operator skill, and the combination of these limitations has thus far limited the role of this approach in the evaluation of bladder carcinomas.[30–32]

Transurethral intravesical sonography provides somewhat better resolution images of the bladder wall than is possible with the transabdominal approach. To some extent, superficial muscularis invasion (stage B1) can be distinguished from deep invasion (stage B2) and from extension into the perivesical fat (stage C) on these images (Fig 5–15). The study is normally performed at the time of cystoscopic evaluation of the bladder. To a certain degree, therefore, it must compete with the traditional and well-established urologic methods of tumor assessment by transurethral resection and pathologic examination. The full clinical utility of transurethral sonography for staging has yet to be demonstrated.[33–35]

Magnetic resonance imaging (MRI) of the pelvis yields a better resolution of the soft tissue structures than CT. Notably, with the use of both T_1- and T_2-weighted images with short TE (echo time), the boundaries are better defined (Fig 5–22). Stage C disease is therefore more likely to be accurately staged with MRI than with CT. Like CT, MRI is unable to resolve the layers of the bladder wall. Studies of MRI staging of bladder carcinomas have so far reported results similar to those for CT, except perhaps for improved results with stage C disease.[36] Like CT, MRI cannot differentiate benign from malignant adenopathy.[37]

PROSTATE

Prostate cancer is the second leading cause of cancer mortality among men in the United States. It is primarily a disease of older men, with a steep rise in the incidence after the age of 50. Autopsy studies indicate that approximately 10% to 30% of men over the age of 50 and virtually all men over the age of 90 have prostate cancer, most of which tumors were asymptomatic in life.

Many etiologic factors, such as the effects of heredity, hormones, sexual activity, diet, previous viral infections, and exposure to chemical agents, have been investigated, but so far no definite causes of prostate cancer have been found.[38, 39]

Pathology and Staging

The prostate is separated into median (periurethral), posterior, and two lateral lobes. With regard to function, three zones have been described: a central zone, a peripheral zone, and a preprostatic zone. The three zones are affected by different diseases. Benign prostatic hypertrophy occurs almost exclusively in the preprostatic region, whereas the peripheral zone is the area most susceptible to inflammatory processes and is also the site of origin of virtually all prostate carcinomas (Fig 5–23). The central zone, in contrast, is relatively free of disease.[40]

Almost all benign tumors of the prostate are prostatic hyperplasia, an entity that has several histologic subtypes. There is some doubt as to whether pure adenomas, leiomyomas, or fibromas of the prostate exist or are simply part of the spectrum of prostatic hyperplasia (Fig 5–24). Rare benign tumors of the prostate include papillary adenomas of the prostatic utricle, blue nevus, and carcinoid.

More than 95% of prostate cancers are adenocarcinomas arising from the glandular acini. Less common are carcinomas arising from within the prostatic ducts, which may be adenocarcinomas, transitional cell carcinomas, or a mixed type. Rare tumors include endometrioid and squamous cell carcinomas, carcinosarcomas, rhabdomyosarcomas (Fig 5–25), leiomyosarcomas, fibrosarcomas, malignant fibrous histiocytomas, and primary malignant melanomas.[41] Metastases to the prostate also occur.

Numerous grading systems have been created to correlate histologic patterns with clinical prognosis. There is a general correlation between histologic grade and tumor volume, which contributes to the prognostic value of histologic grading; poorly differentiated tumors are likely to be large in size and thus entail a poor prognosis.[42–44]

Prostate cancers spread by local invasion, through the lymphatics, and by hematogenous dissemination. Local invasion with obstruction of the bladder neck or distal ureters is common. Rarely, there is spread into the seminal vesicles or rectum; involvement of the urogenital diaphragm and external sphincter may occur late in the course of the disease.

Lymphatic invasion begins with the internal lymphatics of the prostate gland and proceeds through the drainage pathways into the internal iliac (including the medial chain or obturator group), external iliac, and presacral lymph nodes. From these primary nodal groups, tumor may travel into the common iliac, paraaortic, mediastinal, and supraclavicular nodes. The incidence of lymph node metastases increases with the greater size, greater local invasiveness, and worse histologic grade of the primary prostatic tumor.[15, 44]

Hematogenous metastases occur most commonly in the skeletal system. Approximately 85% of patients who die of prostate cancer will have had bone metastases. The lumbar spine is the site most frequently involved, followed in order by the pelvis, proximal femurs, thoracic spine, ribs, sternum, skull, and humeri. About 80% to 90% of these lesions are osteoblastic; most of the remainder are mixed, and less than 5% are the pure lytic type.[45]

The staging system for prostate cancer used in the United States is that developed by Whitmore[46] and modified by Jewett.[47] In this system, stage A represents small tumors localized to the prostate that are not clinically evident and that are discovered incidentally from prostatectomy for presumed benign hyperplasia. This stage is divided into A1 (focal disease) (Fig 5–26) and A2 (diffuse disease), with mortality rates of 2% and 20%, respectively.

Stage B disease represents those tumors evident on rectal examination but confined to the prostate gland. In stage B1, tumor is localized to one lobe; in stage B2, there is bilateral disease (Fig 5–27). Mortality in stage B1 prostate cancer is about 20%; in stage B2, it is about 70%.

Stage C cancers are those that have penetrated beyond the prostatic capsule. Stage C1 represents tumors with minimal extension beyond the capsule, and stage C2 designates tumors that are bulkier and that have caused bladder outlet obstruction or distal ureteral obstruction.

Stage D indicates distant metastases, with D0 representing cases of clinically localized prostate cancer and elevated serum acid phosphatase levels. In stage D1, metastases are confined to the pelvic region; in stage D2, there is evidence of more distant metastases, such as to bone or other organs (Figs 5–28 to 5–30). The vast majority of patients with stage D disease die within three years of the development of metastases. A clinical stage D3 is also sometimes used for cases in which relapse has occurred following therapy. These patients usually have highly malignant tumors, and most die within one year of relapse.[48, 49]

An equivalent sonographic staging system has also been proposed (Fig 5–23). Tumor size is more strictly defined in this system.

Radiologic Evaluation

Radiologic imaging has been used in prostate cancer for both detection of the primary neoplasm and evaluation of the extent of spread. Excretory urograms are often used as the initial study to assess for possible ureteral obstruction or bladder outlet obstruction. Radionuclide bone scanning is the most sensitive method for the detection of bone metastases. Some 10% to 50% of patients with bone metastases will have abnormal bone scans and normal bone radiographs. False-negative bone scans are uncommon, occurring in less than 2% of patients, and are often due to diffuse, symmetric metastases, which cause a "superscan." The incidence of occult bone metastases found on bone scans increases with the prescan clinical stage; up to 69% of patients with initial stage C2 disease have abnormal bone scans.[50–52]

Chest radiographs are an important part of screening for prostatic metastases but have a relatively low sensitivity. Autopsy series of patients who died of prostate cancer have shown that 23% to 74% have lung metastases, although in only 5% to 7% of these cases are such metastases detected on chest radiographs prior to death. The range of radiographic manifestations of prostate metastases in the chest includes reticular, reticulonodular, and nodular pulmonary disease, mediastinal adenopathy, and pleural effusions.[53, 54]

Bipedal lymphangiography has been used to detect lymphatic spread in prostate cancer. It is unable to consistently demonstrate the internal iliac and presacral nodes, however. This deficiency is of greater importance with prostate cancer since these nodal groups are more likely to be involved with lymphatic spread. Lymphangiography can miss up to one half of the histologically abnormal lymph nodes because of failure to opacify these nodal groups. This study is thus primarily useful in patients with advanced disease (stage C and above), in which multiple nodal chains are likely to be involved. When there is evidence of adenopathy, fine-needle aspiration biopsy can be useful; if the results are abnormal, a staging pelvic lymphadenectomy would be unnecessary.[55]

Computed tomography is better able than lymphangiography to detect lymphadenopathy in prostate cancer; it has accuracy rates of 73% to 88% in this disease. False-negative CT results arise from normal-sized nodes with small foci of metastases.[27, 56]

Computed tomography has not been as successful at imaging primary prostate cancers, since it does not have enough soft tissue resolution to differentiate localized neoplasms within the gland. It is capable to some extent of detecting tumor spread into the periprostatic fat, especially using thin (1.5-mm) sections. However, the CT appearance of periprostatic fat invasion may be mimicked by benign diseases such as prostatitis.[57]

Three approaches to sonographic imaging of the prostate gland have been used: transabdominal, perineal, and transrectal. Transabdominal and perineal sonography are capable of accurately assessing prostatic size, which may be useful in planning surgery or radiation therapy.[58] Transrectal sonography has revolutionized prostatic imaging and is capable of producing excellent images of this gland. It can detect approximately 90% of prostate cancers but has a false-positive rate of about 30%. The latter figure is, at present, a major limitation in applying this technique to mass screenings.[59] The prostatic capsule, seminal vesicles, symphysis pubis, surrounding musculature, and portions of the urinary bladder can all be imaged by this method. Resolution is in the range of 1 to 2 mm. The normal prostate appears on these scans as a homogeneous area of low to moderate acoustic reflectivity. In the region of the bladder neck (the preprostatic zone), the prostatic tissue forms a well-defined area that is hypoechoic relative to the rest of the gland. The prostatic capsule and pericapsular fat appear as densely echogenic structures. Areas of thick, dense echoes are usually from benign processes such as prostatic calcifications or deposits of corpora amylacea. Cysts appear as sharply marginated, purely hypoechoic areas. Benign hyperplasia typically appears as a diffuse homogeneous enlargement of the gland; however, it can have a nodular appearance with irregular echoes indistinguishable from carcinoma. Similarly, chronic prostatitis can mimic carcinoma on sonography. Focal prostate carcinomas are predominantly hypoechoic lesions (Figs 5–26 and 5–27). Larger carcinomas may be hyperechoic, probably because of infiltration of the normal prostate tissues and some associated desmoplastic reaction.[59,60] Generally, the overlap in sonographic appearance of benign with malignant disease is sufficient to warrant biopsy for all suspicious lesions.

Biopsy of palpable prostatic lesions can be done transrectally or through the perineum with either fine-needle aspiration or a cutting needle using finger guidance. Since many of the lesions detected by ultrasound cannot be palpated, transperineal and transrectal biopsy techniques with ultrasound guidance have been developed. Biopsies can be performed with the guidance of either longitudinal or axial transducers.[60]

With its improved soft tissue resolution, MRI is often capable of distinguishing neoplasms from normal prostatic tissue. On T_2-weighted studies, most prostate cancers appear as heterogeneous areas of high signal intensity when they are examined in a low- or intermediate-field magnet. But in a high-field 1- to 5-tesla unit, the carcinoma is seen as a hypointense focus.[61] However, there is a significant overlap for the MRI appearance of neoplasms and benign diseases, such as prostatic hyperplasia and chronic prostatitis. Early studies on MRI staging of prostate cancer indicate an overall accuracy of 83% to 89%, with a much-improved resolution of extracapsular extension compared with CT.[62, 63]

URETHRA

Neoplasms that involve the urethra are most likely to have spread secondarily from other sites such as the bladder or prostate. Primary carcinomas of the urethra are uncommon. In both sexes, chronic urethral infection or inflammation has an etiologic role. Most urethral carcinomas are of squamous cell type (Fig 5–31); the remainder are transitional cell carcinomas, adenocarcinomas, and undifferentiated carcinomas. Women have about a fivefold higher overall incidence of primary urethral carcinoma than men. There is an association in women between these cancers and urethral diverticula, and the majority of these carcinomas have been adenocarcinomas.[64]

Adenocarcinomas of the urethra are exceedingly rare in men, with less than 25 cases reported in the literature. They are thought to arise from the glands of Littre or Cowper in men and Skene's glands in women.[65] Among other malignant tumors of the urethra, 23 cases of primary malignant melanoma of the male urethra have been reported.[66]

The most common site of urethral carcinoma in men is the bulbar or bulbomembranous urethra. Transitional cell carcinomas occur mainly in this section of the urethra. Patients with cancer in this area often present with advanced-stage disease, with invasion into surrounding structures; these patients, thus, have a uniformly dismal prognosis (<16% survival). Lymphatic drainage is to the retropubic, retrofemoral, and external iliac lymph nodes. Carcinomas in the pendulous urethra may spread to involve the rest of the penis and then travel through the lymphatics into the inguinal nodes. Prognosis for these patients is much better, with about a 50% five-year survival.[67, 68]

Various benign polyps of the posterior urethra have been described. These tumors usually arise from or near the verumontanum. In young boys, the polyps are most often fibrovascular polyps, which are believed to be congenital. In adult males, adenomatous polyps predominate. These have been shown to be of prostatic epithelial origin, and patients often present with hematuria.[69, 70]

The diagnosis of a urethral neoplasm may sometimes be missed or delayed because of a presumption of benign stricture disease. Patients with urethral neoplasm most often present with symptoms of urinary obstruction or a palpable mass.[67, 68] Retrograde urethrography and voiding cystourethrography are useful in the screening evaluation of these patients, although the presence of a urethral filling defect is nonspecific. Corpus cavernosonography has been advocated for the detection of local spread into the penis.[71] Computed tomography, sonography, and MRI may be useful for defining the extent of tumor spread locally and through the lymphatics.

SEMINAL VESICLES

Primary tumors of the seminal vesicles are extremely rare. Approximately 60 cases of primary carcinoma of the seminal vesicles have been reported, but many of these have not stood up to strict pathologic review. Invasion of the seminal vesicles by an adenocarcinoma of the prostate or rectum occurs more commonly than do primary tumors. In a 1984 review, Benson et al. concluded that only 37 of the cases in the literature were acceptable as primary carcinomas of the seminal vesicles.[72] Most of these were papillary adenocarcinomas, since this histologic pattern resembles the mucosa of the seminal vesicles and is rarely encountered with prostate carcinomas.

Scattered case reports of other tumors of the seminal vesicles exist. Five cases of sarcoma have been reported, each of which was of a different histologic subtype.[73] Among benign tumors, eight cases of cystadenoma of the seminal vesicles exist in the literature.[74]

Patients generally present with symptoms of obstruction of the bladder outlet or the distal ureter and occasionally with lower abdominal or pelvic pain. A high, unilateral, palpable mass on rectal examination is the most common physical finding. The mean age in reported cases of carcinoma of the seminal vesicles is about 60 years.

The CT appearance of seminal vesicle carcinoma has been reported and is nonspecific, consisting of unilateral seminal vesicle enlargement. In the absence of obvious tumor involvement of the prostate, rectum, or bladder, a primary carcinoma of the seminal vesicle may be suggested by this appearance.[75]

PENIS

Carcinoma of the penis is a rare disease in the United States but is more prevalent elsewhere. It is primarily a disease of uncircumcised men and is associated with poor personal hygiene. The vast majority of cases are epidermoid carcinoma. Most patients present between the ages 50 and 80.[76]

Rare tumors of the penis include basal cell carcinoma,[77] melanoma,[78] and mesenchymal tumors, including fibrosarcoma, leiomyosarcoma, and hemangioendothelioma.[79] Kaposi's sarcoma may also be seen, especially in patients with acquired immunodeficiency syndrome (AIDS).

Metastatic lesions of the penis are usually from the genitourinary tract, especially bladder and prostate. Metastases from lung, pancreas, and testis have also been reported.[80]

Penile carcinoma is predominantly a dermatologic lesion. Often secondary infection is present, and inguinal nodes will be palpable on account of hyperplasia. For that reason, patients are usually evaluated for metastases after initial treatment of the skin lesion and appropriate antibiotic therapy.

The drainage of the penis is into the sentinel node at the base of the penis and then into inguinal nodes (Fig 5–32). From here, drainage is into the external iliac nodes. Tumors spread via the rich penile lymphatics and by direct invasion into the abdominal wall. Physical examination is useful for identifying inguinal adenopathy. Computed tomography and sonography are capable of identifying pelvic adenopathy, as well as other distant metastases. The role of MRI has yet to be evaluated, but as in other pelvic tumors, it should offer the advantage of excellent anatomical resolution.

TESTES

Testicular carcinoma is a disease of young men, with patients presenting at an average age of 32. Its incidence is 2.2 cases per 100,000 men.[81] Although it accounts for only 1% of cancers in men, it is a common cause of death from neoplasia in men aged 20 to 34 years. High cure rates are possible, especially with early detection. Unfortunately, testicular tumors are often missed on the initial physician's examination; they have been variously misdiagnosed as epididymitis, hydrocele, hernia, varicocele, spermatocele, or torsion.

There is an increased incidence of testicular carcinoma in cryptorchidism (Fig 5–33). Patients who have had one testicular tumor are at increased risk for the development of a contralateral tumor. In patients with testicular carcinoma and with bilateral cryptorchid testes, there is a 24% incidence of developing a contralateral tumor (Fig 5–34).[82] The etiologic factors are unknown.

About 95% of testicular tumors are of germ cell origin and are generally malignant. The non–germ cell tumors are of Sertoli or Leydig cell origin and are mostly benign. Seminomas account for approximately 40% of the germ cell tumors and occur mainly in middle age. The prognosis is generally good in testicular seminoma, with a cure rate of more than 95% for localized tumors (Fig 5–35). Twenty percent of the germ cell tumors are embryonal cell carcinomas, and these typically occur in a younger age group and entail a worse prognosis. Teratomas account for 5% to 10% of the germ cell tumors and can be well differentiated (mature form) and behave like a benign tumor (Fig 5–36) or can contain foci of malignant cells. Choriocarcinomas account for only about 1% to 3% of the germ cell tumors but have the most aggressive behavior and worst prognosis.

Overall, only about 60% of the germ cell tumors are of a single cell type, with the remainder occurring in mixtures of cell types (Fig 5–37). Teratocarcinomas (teratoma and embryonal carcinoma) are the most common variety of mixed tumor and have a malignant behavior.[76, 83]

In infancy and early childhood, the most common malignant testicular neoplasm is endodermal sinus tumor, or yolk sac tumor. It is also believed to be of germ cell origin. In adults, pure yolk sac tumors are rare, although yolk sac elements are often found in mixed testicular tumors. Endodermal sinus tumors may occur in ovaries and rarely in extragonadal sites such as the vagina, sacrococcygeal region, anterior mediastinum, retroperitoneum, pineal region, and liver (Fig 5–38).[84] The more common germ cell tumors also occur in similar extragonadal locations. These extragonadal tumors are thought to result from the failure of primordial germ cells to migrate from the urogenital ridge to the scrotum. They tend to carry a worse prognosis than similar tumors in the testes[85] and must be distinguished from metastases of occult or spontaneously regressed ("burned out") testicular primaries.

Metastatic disease can appear in the testes. Leukemia may show testicular relapse that often precedes hematologic relapse (Fig 5–39). In autopsy series, leukemic infiltration of the testes has been found in 27.7% to 92% of leukemia patients,[86] but in life this finding is usually not clinically obvious. Non-Hodgkin's lymphoma may be associated with primary or secondary involvement of the testes and is usually of the diffuse histiocytic or diffuse poorly differentiated lymphocytic type.[87] Rarely, other tumors, such as neuroblastoma,[88] prostate cancer, renal cell carcinoma, and primary gastrointestinal tumors, have been known to metastasize to the testes.[89]

Tumors of the paratesticular tissues are fairly rare. Most are benign and composed of connective tissue (Fig 5–40). Malignant paratesticular tumors are extremely rare and include rhabdomyosarcomas and fibrosarcomas.

The lymphatic drainage of the testes is into the nodes of the paraaortic chain near the renal hili, then to the supradiaphragmatic nodes in the mediastinum and supraclavicular fossa. Drainage goes first to the nodes at the level of L-1 to L-2 on the left and L-1 to L-3 on the right; extensive collateral lymphatics are present from T-11 to L-4, and the right testicular drainage may cross over directly to the left paraaortic nodes. Metastases to the inguinal or iliac nodes can occur if the tumor crosses the tunica albuginea or invades the epididymis.[83]

The malignant germ cell tumors have a variable tendency toward hematogenous metastasis. Seminomas rarely spread and are usually confined to the tunica albuginea, while choriocarcinomas have a tendency toward early hematogenous dissemination. Extranodal metastases occur most often in the lungs and liver and occur occasionally in the brain and skeleton. Less frequent sites of involvement include kidney, adrenal gland, inferior vena cava, muscle, spleen, stomach, seminal vesicle, prostate, and pericardium.[90]

High-resolution, small-part sonography has proved to be an excellent modality for examining the scrotal contents and is capable of providing detailed images of the testicular architecture. In particular, sonography is capable of distinguishing intratesticular from extratesticular masses, which is of diagnostic value since the majority of intratesticular masses are malignant, whereas the great majority of extratesticular masses are either inflammatory in nature or benign tumors.

Normal testes show a homogeneous echo pattern on sonography. Intratesticular tumors may appear as well-defined masses, as brightly echogenic foci, or as a diffuse abnormality in the echo texture of the testis. These sonographic findings can be mimicked, however, by such benign processes as abscess, infarction, and hemorrhage. Associated findings, such as epididymal changes, skin thickening, or hydrocele, usually indicate benign processes but are unreliable indicators since they can be mimicked by locally infiltrating neoplasms such as choriocarcinoma. Despite these limitations, sonography has a very low false-negative rate, and its overall accuracy in the detection of testicular neoplasms ranges from 80% to 90%.[83, 91]

It is not possible to predict tumor cell type by the sonographic appearance. Typically, however, seminomas tend to appear as hypoechoic, well-marginated masses (Fig 5–35), whereas the other testicular tumors tend to be more diffuse and often contain areas of hemorrhage, necrosis, or calcification. Leukemic or lymphomatous involvement of the testes (Fig 5–39) appears as focal or diffuse hypoechoic areas.[92]

A testicular primary should be searched for in young men presenting with retroperitoneal masses and in patients with apparent extragonadal germ cell neoplasms. Sonography is excellent for this purpose and may reveal a burned-out testicular tumor. These appear on sonography as hyperechoic foci (Fig 5–41).[93] Pathologically, the specimens in these cases reveal fibrous scars that may contain foci of immature bone, hyaline cartilage, or calcifications. It is postulated that these are tumors that have outgrown their blood supply and autoinfarcted.[83]

Computed tomography lacks enough soft tissue resolution to be of use in the evaluation of the scrotum but is the preferred method for evaluating the extent of metastatic disease. The results of several series from M. D. Anderson Hospital and other institutions suggest that CT is more accurate than lymphangiography in the detection of nodal metastases.[94, 95] In particular, CT can demonstrate metastases to renal hilar nodes or to the upper paraaortic regions that are not ordinarily opacified with bipedal lymphangiography. The mean attenuation values on CT of retroperitoneal masses have been used to predict the activity of metastatic neoplasms. A higher attenuation value is seen with actively malignant tissues than with benign masses.[96]

Metastatic lesions from testicular tumors are cystic or solid or have a mixed appearance on CT or sonography. On sonography, the margins may either appear sharp or ill defined, and bright echogenic foci may be seen.[97] Testicular tumors tend to produce bulky adenopathy (Fig 5–42), and tumor may completely replace nodal tissue. Following treatment, nodal metastases often show a dramatic decrease in size, but they may still contain some persistent abnormal soft tissue. In such cases, biopsy may be required to diagnose residual tumor activity.[98] Rarely, in patients with mixed germ cell tumors treated with chemotherapy, enlarging metastatic lesions appear that prove to contain only the benign elements of a mature teratoma, the so-called growing teratoma syndrome.[99]

Magnetic resonance imaging of the scrotal contents using surface coils is capable of producing high-resolution images that can distinguish the testes, epididymis, tunica albuginea, pampiniform plexus, and spermatic cord. Like sonography, MRI can define features of lesions within the scrotum, such as location (intratesticular or extratesticular)

and cystic or solid composition; simple fluid collections can also be distinguished from purulent or hemorrhagic material. So far, MRI of the scrotum has not appeared to have any additional specificity over what could be obtained less expensively with sonography. Advantages of MRI over sonography include a wider field of view, less dependence on operator skill, and greater ease of imaging in the patient with a painful scrotum.[100, 101]

REFERENCES

1. Silverberg E.: Cancer statistics, 1984. *CA* 34:7–23, 1984.
2. Lower G.M. Jr.: Concepts in causality: chemically induced human urinary bladder cancer. *Cancer* 49:1056–1066, 1982.
3. Fokkens W.: Phenacetin abuse related to bladder cancer. *Environ. Res.* 20:192–198, 1979.
4. Kaufman J.M., Fam B., Jacobs S.C., et al.: Bladder cancer and squamous metaplasia in spinal cord injury patients. *J. Urol.* 118:967–971, 1977.
5. Knappenberger S.T., Uson A.C., Meicow M.M.: Primary neoplasms occurring in vesical diverticula: a report of 18 cases. *J. Urol.* 83:153–159, 1960.
6. Jones W.A., Gibbons R.P., Correa R.J., et al.: Primary adenocarcinoma of the bladder. *Urology* 15:119–122, 1980.
7. El-Bolkainy M.N., Mokhtar N.M., Ghoneim M.A., et al.: The impact of schistosomiasis on the pathology of bladder carcinoma. *Cancer* 48:2643–2648, 1981.
8. Mostofi F.K., Sestermann I.A.: Pathology of epithelial tumors and carcinoma in situ of bladder, in Kuss R., Khoury S., Denis L.J., et al. (eds.): *Bladder Cancer: Part A. Pathology, Diagnosis, and Surgery.* New York, Alan R. Liss, 1984, pp. 75–80.
9. Koss L.G.: Tumors of the urinary bladder, in *Atlas of Tumor Pathology.* Washington, D.C., Armed Forces Institute of Pathology, ser. 2, fasc. 11, 1975.
10. Ochi K., Yoshioka A., Morita M., et al.: Pheochromocytoma of the bladder. *Urology* 17:228–230, 1981.
11. Baker M.E., Silverman P.M., Korobkin M.: Computed tomography of prostatic and bladder rhabdomyosarcomas. *J. Comput. Assist. Tomogr.* 9:780–783, 1985.
12. Jewett H.J., Strong G.H.: Infiltrating carcinoma of the bladder: relation of depth of penetration of the bladder wall to incidence of local extension and metastases. *J. Urol.* 55:366–372, 1946.
13. Marshall V.F.: The relation of the preoperative estimate to the pathologic demonstration of the extent of vesical neoplasms. *J. Urol.* 68:714–723, 1952.
14. Zingg E.J., Wallace D.M.A. (eds.): *Bladder Cancer.* New York, Springer-Verlag, 1985.
15. Jing B.D., Wallace S.: Lymphatic imaging of solid tumors, in Clouse M.E., Wallace S. (eds.): *Lymphatic*

Imaging: Lymphography, Computed Tomography, and Scintigraphy, ed. 2. Baltimore, Williams & Wilkins Co., 1985, pp. 378–383.

16. Hillman B.J., Silvert M., Cook G., et al.: Recognition of bladder tumors by excretory urography. *Radiology* 138:319–323, 1981.

17. Braband H.: The incidence of urographic findings in tumours of the urinary bladder. *Br. J. Radiol.* 34:625–629, 1961.

18. Walzer Y., Soloway M.S.: Should the follow-up of patients with bladder cancer include routine excretory urography? *J. Urol.* 130:672–673, 1983.

19. von Eschenbach A.C., Jing B.S., Wallace S.: Lymphangiography in genitourinary cancer. *Urol. Clin. North Am.* 12:715–723, 1985.

20. Strijk S.P., Debruyne F.M.J., Herman C.J.: Lymphography in the management of urologic tumors. Radiological-pathological correlation. *Radiology* 146:39–45, 1983.

21. Jing B.S., Wallace S., Zornoza J.: Metastases to retroperitoneal and pelvic lymph nodes. *Radiol. Clin. North Am.* 20:511–530, 1982.

22. Kwok-Liu J.P., Zikman J.M., Cockshott W.P.: Carcinoma of the urachus: the role of computed tomography. *Radiology* 137:731–734, 1980.

23. Lome L.G., Presman D.: Potential overstaging of bladder cancer by computerized tomography scanning. *J. Urol.* 132:758–761, 1984.

24. Koss J.C., Arger P.H., Coleman B.G., et al.: CT staging of bladder carcinoma. *AJR* 137:359–362, 1981.

25. Walsh J.W., Amendola M.A., Konerding K.F., et al.: Computed tomographic detection of pelvic and inguinal lymph-node metastases from primary and recurrent pelvic malignant disease. *Radiology* 137:157–166, 1980.

26. Morgan C.L., Calkins R.F., Cavalcanti E.J.: Computed tomography in the evaluation, staging, and therapy of carcinoma of the bladder and prostate. *Radiology* 140:751–761, 1981.

27. Arger P.H.: Computed tomography of the lower urinary tract. *Urol. Clin. North Am.* 12:677–686, 1985.

28. Sager E.M., Talle K., Fossa S., et al.: The role of CT in demonstrating perivesical tumor growth in the preoperative staging of carcinoma of the urinary bladder. *Radiology* 146:443–446, 1983.

29. Watanabe H., Mishina T., Ohe H.: Staging of bladder tumors by transrectal ultrasonotomography and U.I. Octoson. *Urol. Radiol.* 5:11–16, 1983.

30. Singer D., Itzchak Y., Fischelovitch Y.: Ultrasonographic assessment of bladder tumors: II. Clinical staging. *J Urol.* 126:31–33, 1981.

31. Kyle K.F.: Ultrasound in the staging of bladder tumours. A review after 6 years. *Br. J. Urol.* 54:65, 1982.

32. Brun B., Gammelgaard J., Christoffersen J.: Transabdominal ultrasonography in detection of bladder tumors. *J. Urol.* 132:19–20, 1984.

33. Abu-Yousef M.M., Narayana A.S., Brown R.C.,

et al.: Urinary bladder tumors studied by cystosonography: Part II. Staging. *Radiology* 153:227–231, 1984.

34. Schuller J., Walther V., Schmiedt E., et al.: Intravesical ultrasound tomography in staging bladder carcinoma. *J. Urol.* 128:264–266, 1982.

35. Rifkin M.D.: Ultrasonography of the lower genitourinary tract. *Urol. Clin. North Am.* 12:645–656, 1985.

36. Amendola M.A., Glazer G.M., Grossman H.B., et al.: Staging of bladder carcinoma: MRI-CT surgical correlation. *AJR* 146:1179–1183, 1986.

37. Heiken J.P., Lee J.K.T.: MR imaging of the pelvis. *Radiology* 166:11–16, 1988.

38. Hutchinson G.B.: Incidence and etiology of prostate cancer. *Urology* 17(suppl 3):4–10, 1981.

39. Bouffioux C.R.: Etiological and epidemiological considerations in prostatic cancer. *Scand. J. Urol. Nephrol.* [suppl] 55:9–16, 1980.

40. McNeal J.E.: Normal and pathological anatomy of prostate. *Urology* 17(suppl 3):11–16, 1981.

41. Mostofi F.K., Price E.B.: Tumors of the male genital system, in *Atlas of Tumor Pathology.* Washington, D.C., Armed Forces Institute of Pathology, 1973, ser. 2, fasc. 8, pp. 177–258.

42. Gleason D.F., Mellinger G.T.: The Veterans Administration Cooperative Urological Research Group: prediction of prognosis for prostatic adenocarcinoma by combined histological grading and clinical staging. *J. Urol.* 111:58–64, 1974.

43. Mostofi F.K.: Problems of grading carcinoma of prostate. *Semin. Oncol.* 3:161–169, 1976.

44. Catalona W.J.: *Prostate Cancer.* New York, Grune & Stratton, 1984, pp. 15–32.

45. Jacobs S.C.: Spread of prostatic cancer to bone. *Urology* 21:337–344, 1983.

46. Whitmore W.F. Jr.: The natural history of prostatic cancer. *Cancer* 32:1104–1112, 1973.

47. Jewett H.J.: The present status of radical prostatectomy for stages A and B prostatic cancer. *Urol. Clin. North Am.* 2:105–124, 1975.

48. Blackard C.E., Byar C.P., Jordan W.P.: Veterans Administration Cooperative Urological Research Group. Orchiectomy for advanced prostatic carcinoma: a reevaluation. *Urology* 1:553–560, 1973.

49. Slack N.H., Mittelman A., Brady M.F., et al.: The importance of the stable category for chemotherapy treated patients with advanced and relapsing prostate cancer. *Cancer* 46:2393–2402, 1980.

50. Schaffer D.L., Pendergrass H.P.: Comparison of enzyme, clinical radiographic and radionuclide methods of detecting bone metastases from carcinoma of the prostate. *Radiology* 121:431–434, 1976.

51. Lund F., Smith P.H., Suciu S.: Do bone scans predict prognosis in prostatic cancer? A report of the EORTC protocol 30762. *Br. J. Urol.* 56:58–63, 1984.

52. Pollen J.J., Gerber K., Ashburn W.L.: The value of nuclear bone imaging in advanced prostatic cancer. *J. Urol.* 125:222–223, 1981.

53. Apple J.S., Paulson D.F., Baber C., et al.: Advanced prostatic carcinoma: pulmonary manifestations. *Radiology* 154:601–604, 1985.

54. Lindell M.M., Doubleday L.C., von Eschenbach A.C., et al.: Mediastinal metastases from prostatic carcinoma. *J. Urol.* 128:331–334, 1982.

55. Johnson D.E., von Eschenbach A.C.: Role of lymphangiography and pelvic lymphadenectomy in staging prostate cancer. *Urology* 17(suppl 3):66–71, 1981.

56. Levine M.S., Arger P.H., Coleman B.G., et al.: Detecting lymphatic metastases from prostatic carcinoma: superiority of CT. *AJR* 137:207–211, 1981.

57. Emory T.H., Reinke D.B., Hill A.L., et al.: Use of CT to reduce understaging in prostatic cancer: comparison with conventional staging techniques. *AJR* 141:351–354, 1983.

58. Greenberg M., Neiman H.L., Brandt T.D., et al.: Ultrasound of the prostate. Analysis of the tissue texture and abnormalities. *Radiology* 141:757–762, 1981.

59. Lee F., Gray J.H., McLeary R.D., et al.: Prostatic evaluation by transrectal sonography: criteria for diagnosis of early carcinoma. *Radiology* 158:91–95, 1986.

60. Rifkin M.D.: Endorectal sonography of the prostate: clinical implications. *AJR* 148:1137–1142, 1987.

61. Carrol C.L., Sommer F.G., McNeal J.E., et al.: The abnormal prostate: MR imaging at 1–5 T with histopathologic correlation. *Radiology* 163:521–525, 1987.

62. Biondetti P.R., Lee J.K.T., Ling D., et al.: Clinical stage B prostate carcinoma: staging with MR imaging. *Radiology* 162:325–329, 1987.

63. Hricak H., Dooms G.G., Jeffrey R.B., et al.: Prostatic carcinoma: staging by clinical assessment, CT, and MR imaging. *Radiology* 162:331–336, 1987.

64. Tines S.C., Bigongiari L.R., Weigel J.W.: Carcinoma in diverticulum of the female urethra. *AJR* 138:582–585, 1982.

65. Ingram E.A., DePauw P.: Adenocarcinoma of the male urethra with associated nephrogenic metaplasia. *Cancer* 55:160–164, 1985.

66. Sanders T.J., Venable D.D., Sanusi I.D.: Primary malignant melanoma of the urethra in a black man: a case report. *J. Urol.* 135:1012–1014, 1986.

67. Hopkins S.C., Nag S.K., Soloway M.S.: Primary carcinoma of male urethra. *Urology* 23:128–133, 1984.

68. Anderson K.A., McAninch J.W.: Primary squamous cell carcinoma of anterior male urethra. *Urology* 23:134–140, 1984.

69. Eglen D.E., Pontius E.E.: Benign prostatic epithelial polyp of the urethra. *J. Urol.* 131:120–122, 1984.

70. Foster R.S., Garrett R.A.: Congenital posterior urethral polyps. *J. Urol.* 136:670–672, 1986.

71. Fujita J., Matsumoto K., Kakizoe T., et al.: Spongiosography for staging male urethral carcinoma. *Br. J. Urol.* 55:120, 1983.

72. Benson R.C. Jr., Clark W.R., Farrow G.M.: Carcinoma of the seminal vesicle. *J. Urol.* 132:483–485, 1984.

73. Chiou R.K., Limas C., Lang P.H.: Hemangiosarcoma of the seminal vesicle: case report and literature review. *J. Urol.* 134:371–373, 1985.

74. Lundhus E., Bundgaard N., Sorensen F.B.: Cystadenoma of the seminal vesicle. A case report. *Scand. J. Urol. Nephrol.* 18:341–342, 1984.

75. Sussman S.K., Dunnick N.R., Silverman P.M., et al.: Carcinoma of the seminal vesicle: CT appearance. *J. Comput. Assist. Tomogr.* 10:519–520, 1986.

76. Johnson D.E., Bracken R.B., Wallace S., et al.: Urologic cancer, in Clark R.L., Howe C.D. (eds.): *Cancer Patient Care at M. D. Anderson Hospital and Tumor Institute.* Chicago, Year Book Medical Publishers, 1976, pp. 361–414.

77. Bracken R.B., Diokno A.C.: Melanoma of the penis and urethra: two case reports and review of the literature. *J. Urol.* 111:198–200, 1974.

78. Fegen J.P., Beebe D., Persky L.: Basal cell carcinoma of the penis. *J. Urol.* 104:864–866, 1970.

79. Dehner L.P., Smith B.H.: Soft tissue tumors of the penis. A clinicopathologic study of 46 cases. *Cancer* 25:1431–1447, 1970.

80. Persky L., deKernion J.: Carcinoma of the penis. *CA* 36:258–273, 1986.

81. Clark B.G.: The relative frequency and age incidence of principal urologic disease. *J. Urol.* 98:701–705, 1967.

82. Frank I.N., Keys H.M., McCures C.S.: Urologic and male genital cancers, in *Clinical Oncology: A Multidisciplinary Approach.* New York, American Cancer Society, 1983, pp. 213–220.

83. Eftekhari F., Jing B.S., Wallace S.: Imaging in testicular tumors. *Revista Brasileira de Cancerologia* (in press.)

84. Talerman A.: Endodermal sinus (yolk sac) tumor elements in testicular germ-cell tumors in adults: comparison of prospective and retrospective studies. *Cancer* 46:1213–1217, 1980.

85. Burt M.E., Javadpour N.: Germ cell tumors in patients with apparently normal testes. *Cancer* 47:1911–1915, 1981.

86. Givler R.L.: Testicular involvement in leukemia and lymphoma. *Cancer* 23:1290–1295, 1969.

87. Tepperman B.S., Gospodarowicz M.K., Bush R.S., et al.: Non-Hodgkin lymphoma of the testis. *Radiology* 142:203–209, 1982.

88. Casola G., Scheible W., Leopold G.R.: Neuroblastoma metastatic to the testis: ultrasonic screening as an aid to clinical staging. *Radiology* 151:475–476, 1984.

89. Pienkos E.J., Jablokow J.R.: Secondary testicular tumors. *Cancer* 30:481–485, 1972.

90. Husband J.E., Bellamy E.A.: Unusual thoracoabdominal sites of metastases in testicular tumors. *AJR* 145:1165–1171, 1985.

91. Worthy L., Miller E.I., Chinn D.H.: Evaluation of extratesticular findings in scrotal neoplasms. *J. Ultrasound Med.* 5:261–263, 1986.

92. Lupetin A.R., King W. III, Rich P., et al.: Ultrasound diagnosis of testicular leukemia. *Radiology* 146:171–172, 1983.

93. Shawker T.H., Javadpour N., O'Leary T., et al.: Ultrasonographic detection of "burned-out" primary testicular germ cell tumors in clinically normal testes. *J. Ultrasound Med.* 2:477–479, 1983.

94. Thomas J.L., Bernardino M.E., Bracken R.B.: Staging of testicular carcinoma: comparison of CT and lymphangiography. *AJR* 137:991–996, 1981.

95. Lien H.H., Kolbenstvedt A., Talle K., et al.: Comparison of computed tomography, lymphography, and phlebography in 200 consecutive patients with regard to retroperitoneal metastases from testicular tumor. *Radiology* 146:129–132, 1983.

96. Husband J.E., Hawkes D.J., Peckham M.J.: CT estimates of mean attenuation values and volume in testicular tumors: a comparison with surgical and histologic findings. *Radiology* 144:553–558, 1982.

97. Grantham J.G., Charboneau J.W., James E.M., et al.: Testicular neoplasms: 29 tumors studied by high-resolution US. *Radiology* 157:775–780, 1985.

98. Libshitz H.I., Jing B.S., Wallace S., et al.: Sterilized metastases: a diagnostic and therapeutic dilemma. *AJR* 140:15–19, 1983.

99. Logothetis C.J., Samuels M.L., Trindade A., et al.: The growing teratoma syndrome. *Cancer* 50:1629–1635, 1982.

100. Baker L.L., Hajek P.C., Burkhard T.K., et al.: MR imaging of the scrotum: pathologic conditions. *Radiology* 163:93–98, 1987.

101. Rholl K.S., Lee J.K.T., Ling D., et al.: MR imaging of the scrotum with a high-resolution surface coil. *Radiology* 163:99–103, 1987.

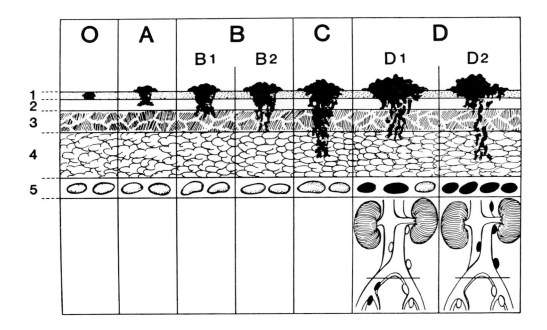

FIG 5–1.
Staging of uroepithelial carcinomas of the bladder, where *1* = mucosa, *2* = submucosa, *3* = muscularis, *4* = perivesical fat, and *5* = lymph nodes. (From Marshall V.F.: The relation of the preoperative estimate to the pathologic demonstration of the extent of vesical neoplasms. *J. Urol.* 68(4):714–723, 1952. © by Williams & Wilkins, 1988. Reproduced with permission.)

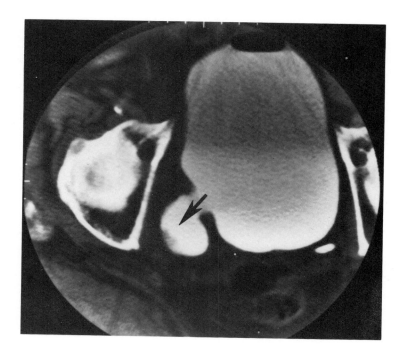

FIG 5–2.

Transitional cell carcinoma of the bladder in bladder diverticulum. This 72-year-old man with a history of heavy smoking and previous calculus in a bladder diverticulum presented with hematuria. He underwent cystoscopy, and a tumor was seen within a right-sided bladder diverticulum.

The CT scan, which was done following cystoscopy, shows a small mass *(arrow)* in the wall of the diverticulum. The tumor is confined to the wall, without any perivesical extension. Notice the residual air in the bladder from recent cystoscopy.

At surgery, it proved to be a stage B2 transitional cell carcinoma of the bladder. The pelvic nodes were normal.

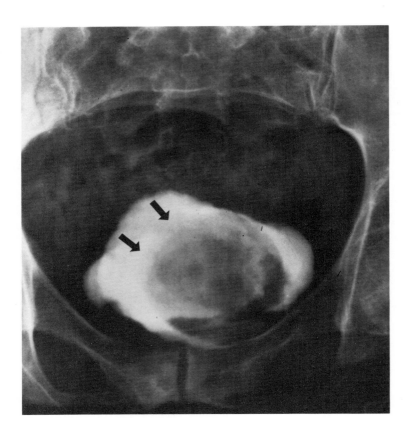

FIG 5–3.
Squamous cell carcinoma of the bladder. This 66-year-old woman with gross hematuria underwent intravenous pyelography and was discovered to have a large, fungating intravesical mass *(arrows).*

Biopsy of the tumor by transurethral approach showed a grade 2 squamous cell carcinoma, with invasion of the muscularis. There were also chronic inflammatory changes of the bladder wall. Cystectomy was performed.

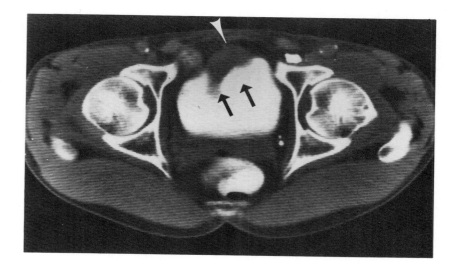

FIG 5–4.
Adenocarcinoma of a urachal remnant. This 56-year-old man presented with gross hematuria and was discovered on intravenous pyelography to have a filling defect in the bladder.

The CT scan shows a relatively well defined mass in the anterior wall of the bladder *(arrows)*. The mass is confined to the bladder wall with the exception of a small, streaky density extending to the abdominal wall *(arrow-head)*.

Based on the typical location of the tumor (midline and in the anterior superior wall of the bladder), urachal carcinoma was suspected and proved on biopsy. The pathologic report was consistent with a colloid mucinous adenocarcinoma of the urachal remnant. The patient underwent radiation therapy, followed by a partial cystectomy, and is in remission after four years.

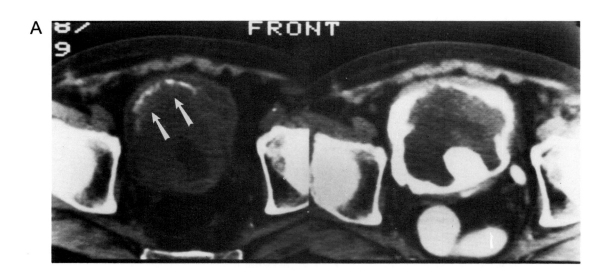

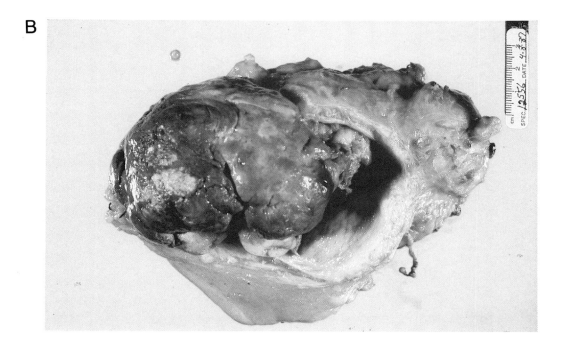

FIG 5–5.

Sarcomatoid carcinoma of the bladder. This 81-year-old man with gross hematuria was found on intravenous pyelography to have a large bladder mass.

A, the CT scan without intravenous contrast *(left)* shows a large mass with rim calcification *(arrows)* within the lumen of the bladder. There is no extension beyond the bladder wall. The enhanced CT scan *(right)* shows the lob-

ulated nature of the mass and minimal dilatation of the left distal ureter.

B, the patient had radical cystectomy, which revealed a large bulky intravesical tumor. Histologic diagnosis was consistent with high-grade sarcomatoid carcinoma of the bladder with areas of transitional cell carcinoma and squamous cell carcinoma differentiation (see also Color Plate 24).

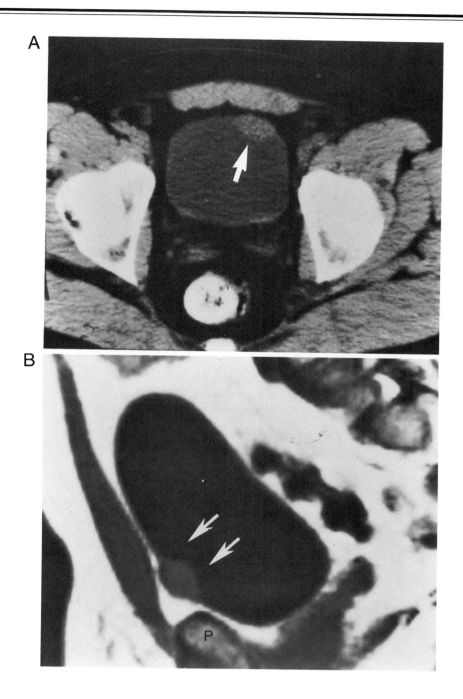

FIG 5–6.
Bladder pheochromocytoma. This 40-year-old man presented with episodes of headaches and hypertension. About one month earlier for the first time he experienced a severe pulsatile headache less than 1 min after voiding. The pain lasted for 5 hr. The same symptoms occurred in the subsequent mornings after voiding. The blood pressure following one episode was 214/122 mm Hg and in between episodes was 124/81 mm Hg.

A, pelvic CT scan shows a well-defined soft tissue mass *(arrow)* in the anterior wall of the bladder.

B, a midline sagittal T_1-weighted magnetic resonance image shows a mass with intermediate signal intensity *(arrows)* confined to the anterior and inferior wall of the bladder just above the pubis *(P)*. The perivesical fat is clear.

The bladder wall mass was surgically proved to be a pheochromocytoma.

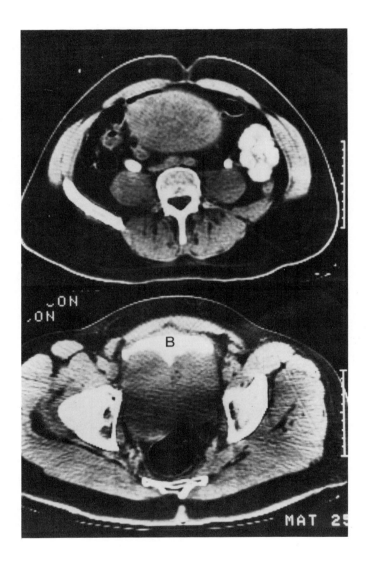

FIG 5–7.

Leiomyosarcoma of the bladder. This 59-year-old man with increased urinary frequency and dysuria was found to have a palpable lower abdominal mass.

The CT scan of the lower abdomen *(top image)* shows a large mass at the level of the aortic bifurcation. There is evidence of bilateral hydroureter. This mass is continuous with the one that is seen in the pelvis *(bottom image)* behind the bladder. The mass appears to be continuous with the bladder wall although predominantly extrinsic. The bladder *(B)* is displaced anteriorly.

At surgery, there was a large tumor arising from the posterior wall of the bladder. Radical cystectomy was performed and the tumor proved to be a myxoid leiomyosarcoma. The mucosa of the bladder was intact and there was no evidence of tumor invasion into adjacent organs or to the pelvic sidewalls.

A

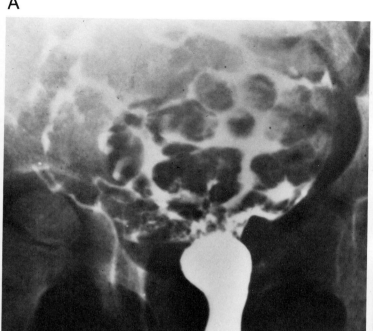

B

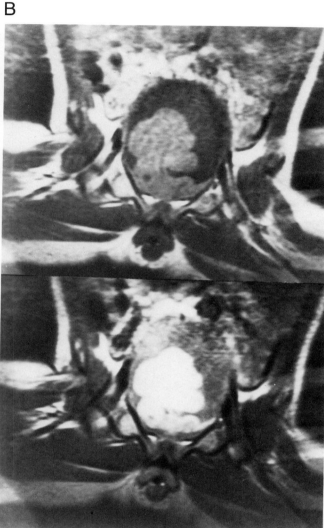

FIG 5–8.

Rhabdomyosarcoma of the bladder (two cases).

A, a 32-month-old child presented with hematuria, and a retrograde cystogram was made.

Multiple filling defects are seen within the lumen of the bladder. They are of varying sizes and appear to cluster together. Pathologic diagnosis was rhabdomyosarcoma of botryoides type. (**A** courtesy of Dominique Counet, M.D., Institut Gustave Roussy, Villejuif, France.)

B, an 18-month-old infant presented with voiding difficulty and a palpable suprapubic mass, which was believed to represent a distended bladder.

Coronal T$_1$-weighted *(top)* and T$_2$-weighted *(bottom)* pulse-sequence images obtained in a 1.5 T magnet show a large fungating intravesical mass displaying high signal intensity on T$_2$. It appears that the mass is originating from the base of the bladder. This was proved to represent sarcoma botryoides. (**B** courtesy of Abe Pera, D.O., Michigan State University, Department of Radiology, East Lansing, Mich.)

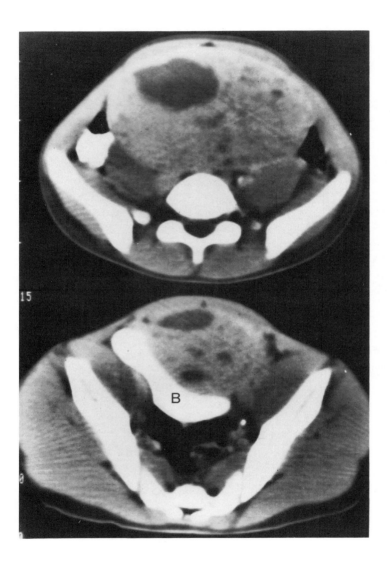

FIG 5–9.
Ewing's sarcoma of the bladder wall. A 13-year-old boy with lower abdominal pain and increasing urinary frequency was found to have a palpable lower abdominal mass.

The CT scan shows a large, partially necrotic mass extending from the dome of the bladder to the lower abdomen. The bladder *(B)* is displaced to the right. The mass is well defined and does not appear to extend to the adjacent organs.

At surgery, a large tumor was excised from the dome of the bladder, with most of the bladder preserved. The pathologic diagnosis was primary Ewing's sarcoma. The patient received several courses of adjuvant chemotherapy. (Courtesy of R.P. Chepey, M.D., Memorial Hospital, Corpus Christi, Tex.)

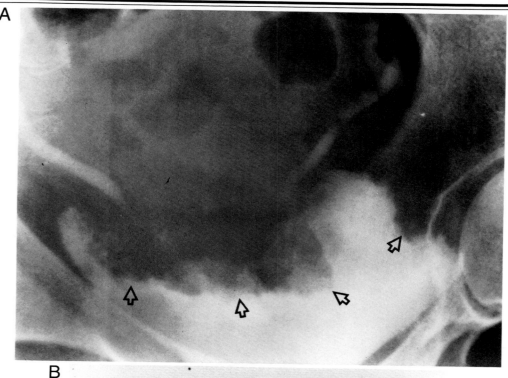

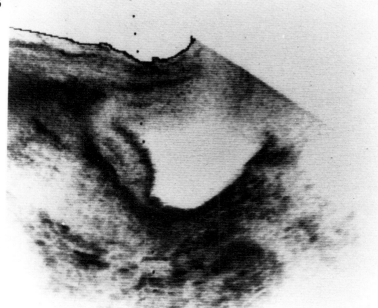

FIG 5–10.
Granulocytic sarcoma of the bladder (chloroma). A 29-year-old woman with a history of drug and alcohol abuse ending eight years earlier presented with dysuria and hematuria.

A, the oblique view of the bladder on the intravenous pyelogram shows a large filling defect at the dome of the bladder, mostly on the right side but with a smaller defect on the left *(arrows)*.

B, the sagittal midline sonogram demonstrates the hy-poechoic nature of the infiltrative mass, which is at the dome and extends into the anterior portion of the bladder wall. It is covered by an echogenic thick rim. The mass does not appear to go beyond the bladder wall. Cystoscopy and biopsy revealed an acute granulocytic leukemia (chloroma) of the bladder. There was no evidence of systemic leukemia. The patient was treated with chemotherapy and went into complete remission.

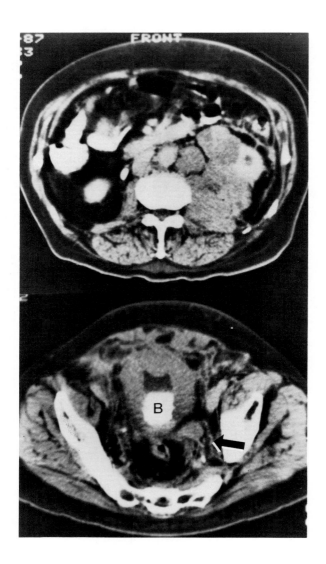

FIG 5–11.
Lymphoma of the bladder. This 75-year-old man presented with perineal pain and dysuria. The intravenous pyelogram (not shown) revealed a retroperitoneal mass and thickened bladder wall.

The abdominal CT scan *(top image)* shows a large retroperitoneal mass lateral to the aorta with probable infiltration into the left psoas muscle. The postcontrast pelvic CT scan *(bottom image)* shows the filled bladder *(B)* with circumferentially thickened walls and adjacent adenopathy *(arrow)*.

Cystoscopy of the bladder showed a diffuse infiltrative lesion of the bladder wall, which proved to be a large cell lymphoma (predominantly noncleaved cell type, considered to be a B-cell lymphoma). The patient was treated with chemotherapy.

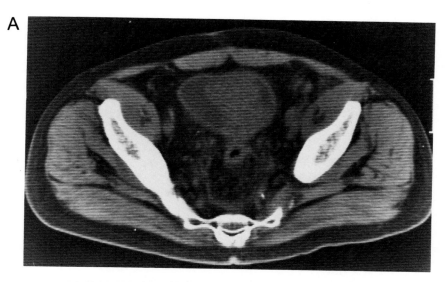

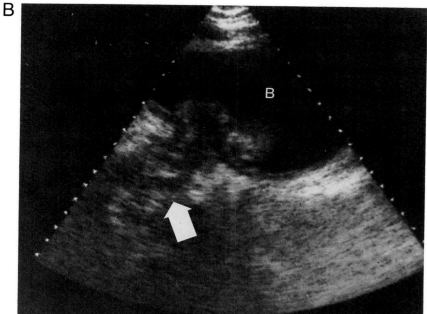

FIG 5–12.

Bladder invasion by colon carcinoma. This 58-year-old man with symptoms of dysuria was found on intravenous pyelography to have an intraluminal defect of the bladder.

A, unenhanced CT scan of the pelvis shows a large intravesical mass, which appears to arise from the posterior bladder wall. The mass is relatively well outlined and is homogeneous. The possibility of primary bladder neoplasm was considered.

B, a pelvic ultrasound was done for better evaluation of the bladder wall. This shows the tumor to merge into the posterior wall of the bladder *(B)*. There is a suggestion of contiguity of the tumor with the perivesical structures *(arrow)*.

The patient underwent an exploratory laparotomy and was found to have an adenocarcinoma of the sigmoid colon that extended directly into the base and trigone of the bladder. Cystectomy had already been rejected by the patient, and so he underwent palliative radiation therapy.

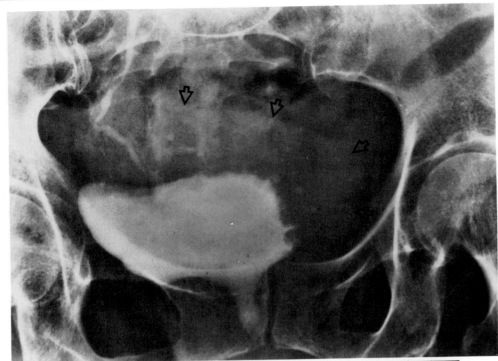

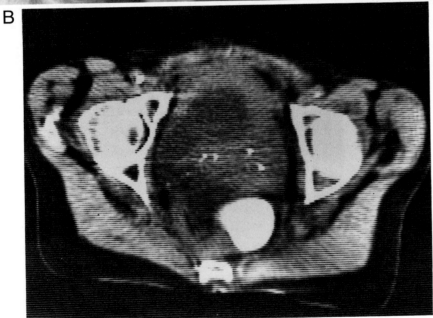

FIG 5–13.
Metastatic breast carcinoma to the bladder. This 47-year-old woman with a history of mastectomy for breast carcinoma presented with dysuria.

A, the pelvic view of the intravenous pyelogram shows marked thickening of the anterior and left lateral side of the bladder *(arrows),* with irregularity of the wall. Notice lateral deviation of the right ureter and lack of opacification of the left ureter. There was evidence of left hydronephrosis.

B, the CT scan of the pelvis shows almost-circumferential thickening of the bladder wall, predominantly in the left side.

Cystoscopy and biopsy revealed an adenocarcinoma histologically identical to the primary breast malignancy.

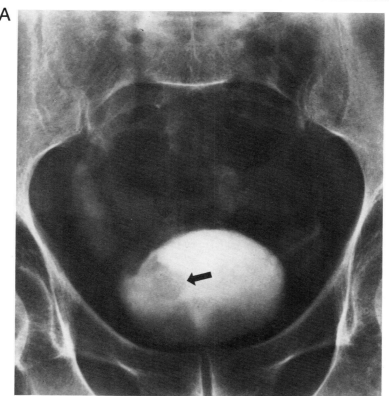

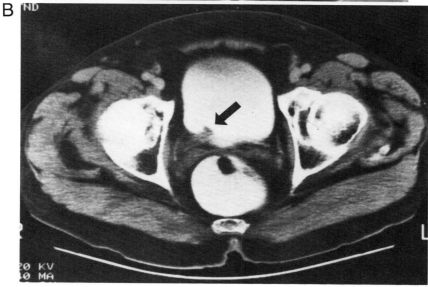

FIG 5–14.

Transitional cell carcinoma of the bladder, stage B1. This 68-year-old man with gross hematuria underwent intravenous pyelography.

A, the cone down view of the bladder from the pyelogram shows an intravesical filling defect *(arrow)* associated with distal right ureteral obstruction and right hydroureter.

B, the CT scan shows the tumor at the right ureteral orifice *(arrow),* with probable extension into the distal right ureter.

Radical cystectomy showed a transitional cell carcinoma with only superficial invasion of the muscularis, consistent with stage B1. Computed tomography is unable to differentiate the lower stages (from stage 0 to stage B2).

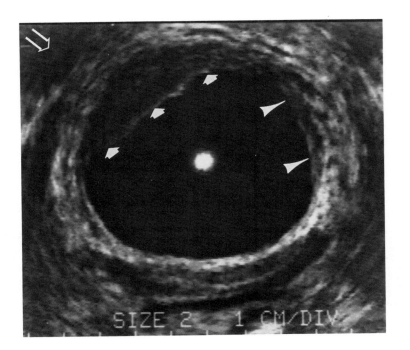

FIG 5–15.
Transitional cell carcinoma of the bladder, stage C. This 62-year-old woman with hematuria had intravenous pyelography, followed by cystoscopy, and was found to have a grade 3 transitional cell carcinoma of the bladder with full-thickness invasion into the perivesical space.

The intravesical sonogram shows a thick mass of low echogenicity at the right and anterior wall of the bladder *(arrows)*. The tumor appears to extend to the left side as a thin layer *(arrowheads)*. The mass in the right wall appears to extend through the full thickness of the bladder into the perivesical space *(open arrow)*.

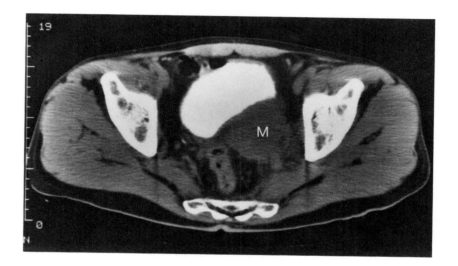

FIG 5–16.
Transitional cell carcinoma of the bladder, stage D1. This 55-year-old man with gross hematuria had cystoscopy and biopsy, which proved the diagnosis of transitional cell carcinoma of the bladder with invasion into the muscularis.

The CT scan shows thickening of the posterior and left bladder wall with an extrinsic mass *(M)* that directly extends into the left pelvic sidewall. This finding, which was best illustrated on CT scan, resulted in staging the tumor as D1. The patient was treated with chemotherapy.

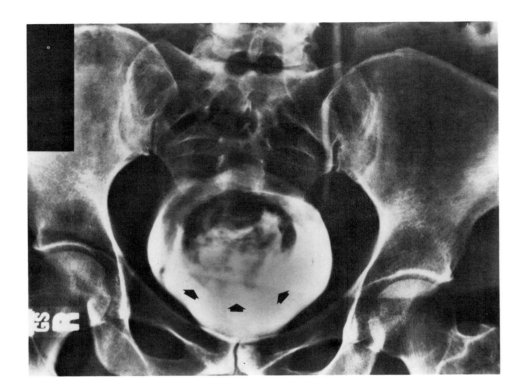

FIG 5–17.
Inflammatory pseudotumor of the bladder. This 44-year-old woman with gross hematuria underwent intravenous pyelography.

The pelvic film shows a large intravesical filling defect *(arrows)* with possible areas of ulceration. This was initially thought to represent a leiomyosarcoma.

The patient underwent partial cystectomy, and the pathologic diagnosis was inflammatory pseudotumor. There were changes of chronic and acute cystitis and marked fibroblastic proliferation. No further treatment was given.

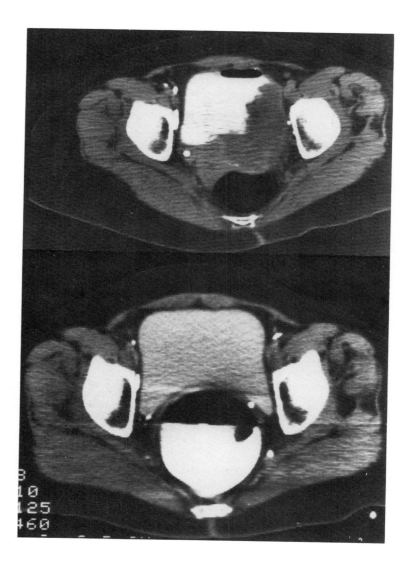

FIG 5–18.

Resolution of poorly differentiated transitional cell carcinoma of the bladder, stage D1. This 63-year-old man presented with hematuria and underwent cystoscopy and biopsy; he was found to have a poorly differentiated transitional cell carcinoma of the bladder with invasion into the muscularis. A lymphangiogram was done and showed metastasis to the pelvic lymph nodes, hence staging the tumor as D1.

The CT scan *(top)* shows infiltrative mass in the posterior and left side of the bladder wall. There is no evidence of direct extension of the tumor into the pelvic sidewall. The bulk of the tumor is extrinsic and impinges on the anterior wall of the rectum. Residual air in the lumen of the bladder is from the previous cystoscopy.

The patient received both intravenous and intraarterial chemotherapy, and a repeat CT scan *(bottom)* showed total disappearance of the bladder neoplasm. This was further confirmed by cystoscopy, and follow-up films of the lymphangiogram showed resolution of the lymph node metastases as well.

The patient remained free of disease for three years, when he developed a new transitional cell carcinoma of the bladder (moderately differentiated and minimally invasive into the muscularis). He underwent transurethral resection for this bladder tumor.

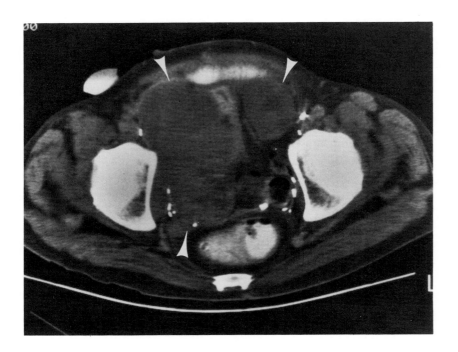

FIG 5–19.
Recurrent bladder carcinoma after radical cystectomy. This 70-year-old man, with a history of high-grade transitional cell carcinoma of the bladder invasive into the muscularis, had a radical cystectomy. Results of pelvic node dissection were negative for metastasis.

A CT scan five months following surgery shows extensive tumor recurrence in the pelvis, seen as large masses predominantly in the right side *(arrowheads).* The tumor displays areas of necrosis. There was simultaneous pulmonary metastasis, and the patient died one month later.

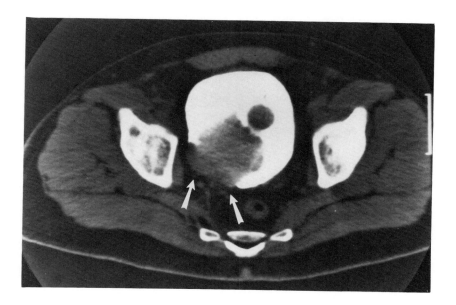

FIG 5–20.
Overstaging by CT of a papillary transitional cell carcinoma of the bladder. This 44-year-old man who presented with hesitancy and dribbling on micturition was found on intravenous pyelography to have an intravesical filling defect. He had a cystoscopy and biopsy of the mass.

The CT scan shows a large mass at the posterior and right lateral bladder wall. The mass appears to extend into the perivesical fat *(arrows),* suggesting stage C based on the CT findings.

However, resection of the bladder tumor showed only a grade 1 papillary transitional cell carcinoma without invasion into the submucosa (stage 0). The apparent perivesical mass resolved on a subsequent CT scan.

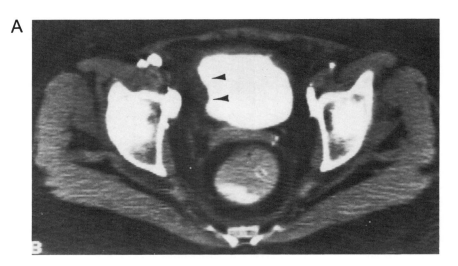

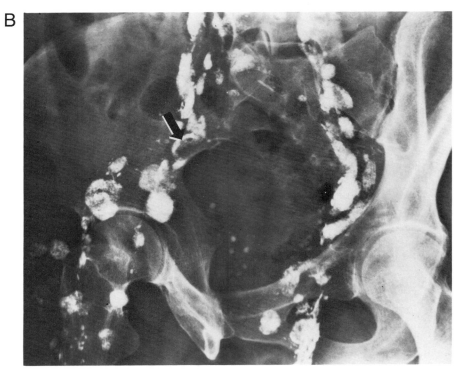

FIG 5–21.
Computed tomography vs. lymphangiography in staging bladder tumors. This 67-year-old woman underwent cystoscopy after an episode of hematuria. The diagnosis was a mixed cell tumor of the bladder (spindle cell, glandular, squamous, and small cell elements) invasive into the muscularis.

A, on the CT scan, thickening of the right bladder wall *(arrowheads)* is seen, with normal perivesical fat. Based on the CT image, the tumor was thought to be stage B. The opacified nodes do not appear to be abnormal.

B, however, the lymphangiogram showed a few abnormal nodes in the pelvis, including the one indicated by the *arrow* in the right external iliac region. Biopsy of this node proved metastasis. The tumor was therefore staged as D1, and the patient underwent radiation therapy and chemotherapy. However, she died one year later.

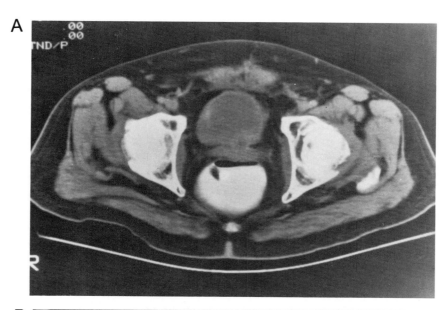

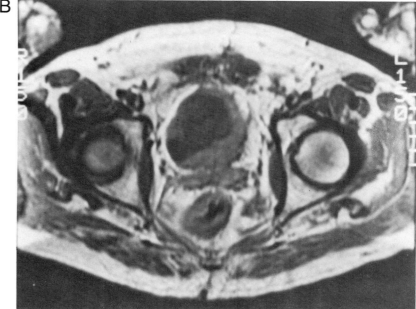

FIG 5–22.
Transitional cell carcinoma of the bladder. A 58-year-old man was diagnosed with stage B2 transitional cell carcinoma of the bladder 3 years ago. He had local resection followed by radiotherapy. He now presented with hematuria.

A, CT scan shows minimal irregularity of the posterior and left bladder wall, some of which could be postoperative.

B, axial proton-density MR image (TR/TE, 2,000/20) clearly shows tumor infiltration into the lateral and posterior bladder wall.

At cystoscopy, recurrent tumor was seen coming off the posterior lateral wall on the left and extending into the lumen of the bladder. Biopsy proved recurrent, invasive poorly differentiated carcinoma.

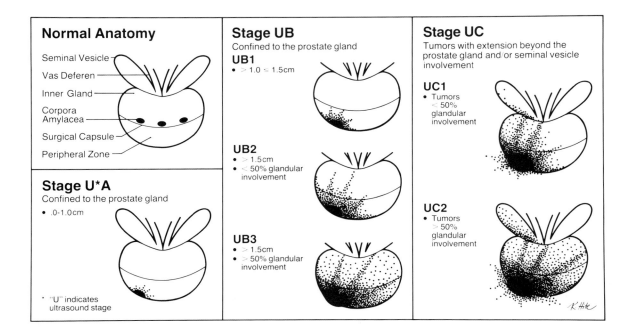

Normal Anatomy

Seminal Vesicle
Vas Deferen
Inner Gland
Corpora
Amylacea
Surgical Capsule
Peripheral Zone

Stage U*A
Confined to the prostate gland
• .0–1.0cm

* "U" indicates
  ultrasound stage

Stage UB
Confined to the prostate gland
UB1
• > 1.0 ≤ 1.5cm

UB2
• > 1.5cm
• < 50% glandular
  involvement

UB3
• > 1.5cm
• > 50% glandular
  involvement

Stage UC
Tumors with extension beyond the
prostate gland and/or seminal vesicle
involvement

UC1
• Tumors
  < 50%
  glandular
  involvement

UC2
• Tumors
  > 50%
  glandular
  involvement

FIG 5–23.
Ultrasound staging of prostate cancer. (Courtesy of Fred Lee   M.D., Department of Radiology, St. Joseph Mercy Hospital, Ann Arbor, Michigan.)

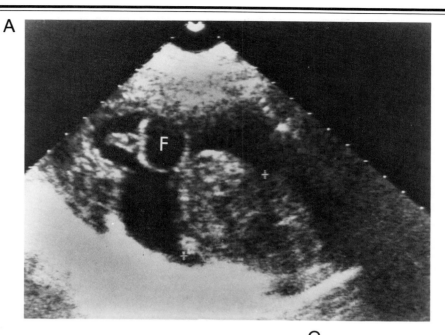

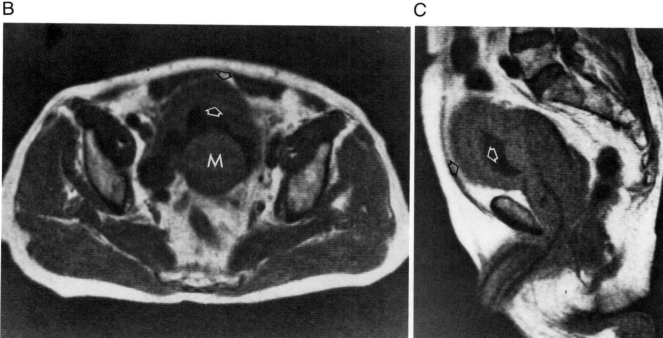

FIG 5–24.

Prostatic adenoma. This 75-year-old man was found to have a large prostate on physical examination.

A, midline sagittal sonogram demonstrates a large echogenic mass elevating the base of the bladder thought to represent hypertrophy of the median lobe of the prostate. There is a Foley catheter *(F)* within the lumen of the bladder.

B, and **C,** MRI study using T_1-weighted pulse sequence (TR/TE, 500/28) was done, showing a well-defined homogeneous mass *(M)* seen in both axial **(B)** and midline sagittal **(C)** views to elevate the base of the bladder. Notice significant hypertrophy of the bladder wall *(arrows)*. The signal intensity throughout the mass was homogeneous and thought to represent benign prostatic hypertrophy. This diagnosis was proved by transurethral resection of prostate. (Courtesy of Professor J.L. Lamarque, Hospital Lapeyronie, Montpellier, France.)

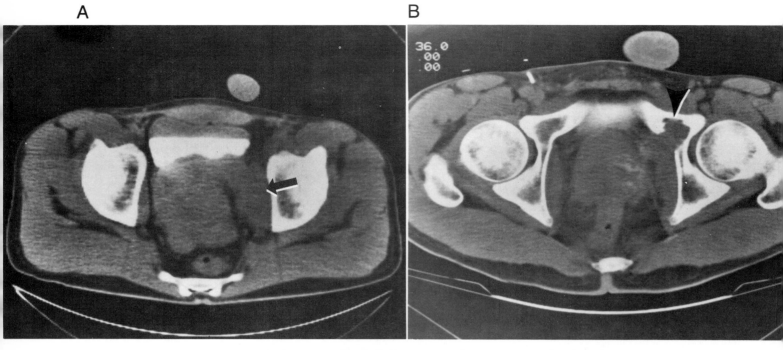

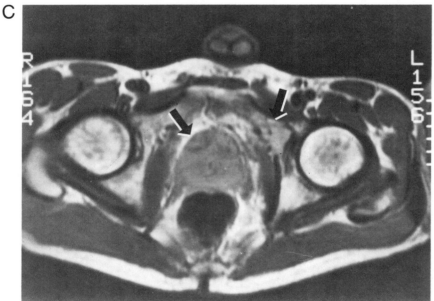

FIG 5–25.
Embryonal rhabdomyosarcoma of the prostate. A 22-year-old man with a history of left side and buttock pain and urinary incontinence underwent intravenous pyelography followed by CT scanning of the abdomen and pelvis.

A and **B**, the CT scans show a large prostatic mass with extension into the left pelvic sidewall *(arrow in* **A***)* and the left pubic ramus *(arrowhead in* **B***).*

C and **D**, the axial proton-density (TR/TE, 2,000/25) and sagittal T_2-weighted (TR/TE, 2,000/70) images show a large mass in the prostate with a mixed signal intensity *(ar-*

rows). The tumor extends beyond the prostatic capsule and elevates the bladder *(BL).*

E, subtraction angiogram of the anterior division branches of the left internal iliac artery demonstrates the tumor stain *(arrows).*

F, a CT-angiogram at the level of the prostatic tumor demonstrates an intense blush *(arrows).* The angiography catheter was left in place for chemotherapy. Biopsy of the tumor had shown an embryonal rhabdomyosarcoma of the prostate, and the patient was treated with systemic and intraarterial chemotherapy.

D

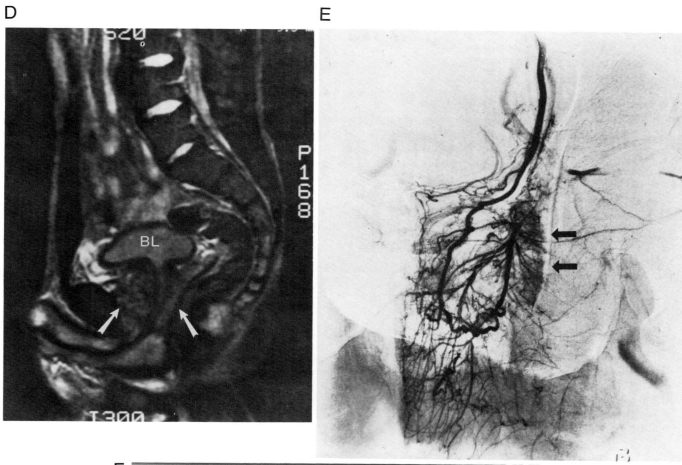

E

F

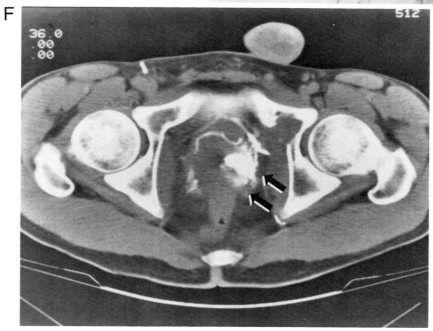

A

B

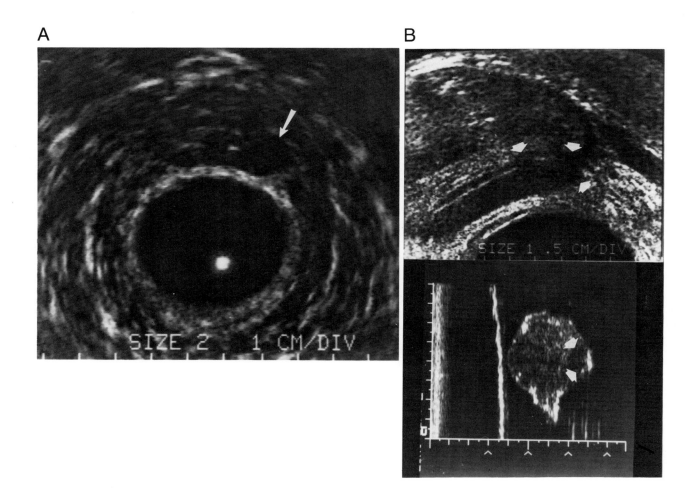

FIG 5–26.

Prostatic carcinoma, stage A1 (two cases).

A, this 56-year-old man was found on rectal examination to have a palpable prostatic nodule.

The transrectal sonogram reveals a small, hypoechoic lesion *(arrow)* confined to the left lobe of the prostate. Multiple ultrasound-guided needle biopsies of the lesion revealed a grade 1 adenocarcinoma.

B through D, this 74-year-old man was found on rectal examination to have a palpable prostatic nodule. **B,** the transrectal sonogram *(top image)* shows a small, hypoechoic lesion *(arrows)* within the left lobe. Upon biopsy with ultrasound guidance, diagnosis of moderately differentiated

adenocarcinoma was established. Radical prostatectomy was done and sonogram of the specimen *(bottom image)* reveals a similar hypoechoic lesion *(arrows)* within the posterior left lobe. **C,** surgical specimen shows a nodule of carcinoma measuring 1.8 cm in its greatest extent confirmed filling the posterior left lobe (see also Color Plate 25).

D, corresponding microscopic section confirmed the diagnosis of moderately differentiated adenocarcinoma (see also Color Plate 26). (Case **B–D** courtesy of Robert Bree, M.D., William Beaumont Hospital, Department of Diagnostic Radiology, Royal Oak, Michigan.)

C

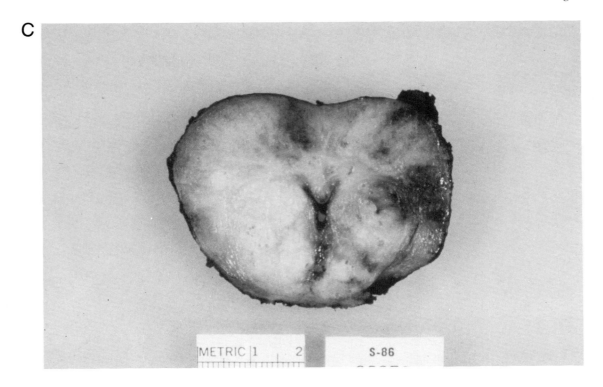

D

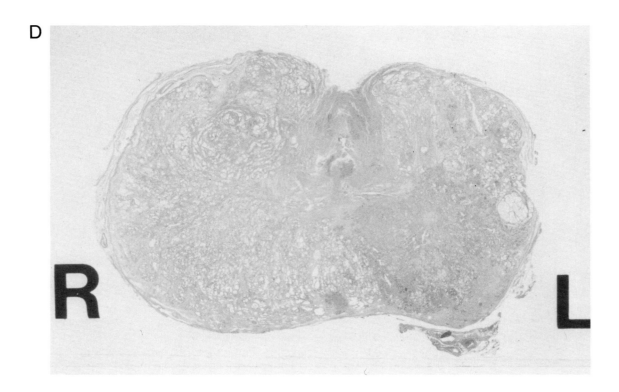

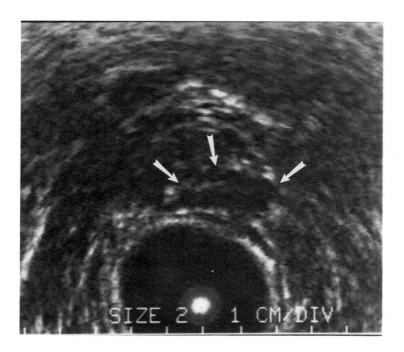

FIG 5–27.
Carcinoma of the prostate, stage B2. A 72-year-old man had a transurethral resection of the prostate seven years earlier and at that time was incidentally found to have a stage A1 adenocarcinoma of the prostate. This was left untreated until a palpable prostate mass was found on a follow-up examination.

A preoperative transrectal sonogram shows a hypoechoic mass *(arrows)* predominantly in the left lobe of the prostate but crossing the midline into the right side. Ultrasound-guided needle biopsy of this area showed grade 3 adenocarcinoma involving both prostatic lobes, indicating stage B2 disease. Results of a staging pelvic lymphadenectomy were normal.

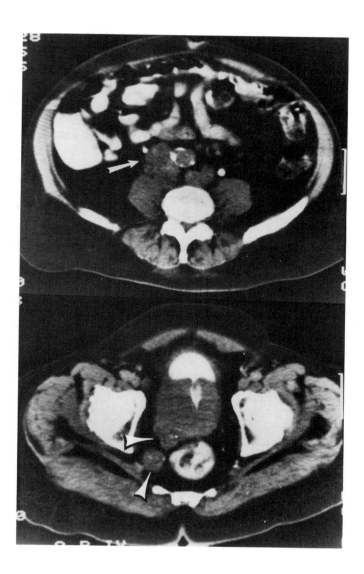

FIG 5–28.
Recurrent prostatic carcinoma, with local invasion and paraaortic adenopathy (stage D2). A 76-year-old man presented with acute urinary retention. He had 13 years previously undergone orchiectomy for prostate cancer.

The abdominal CT scan *(top image)* shows paraaortic adenopathy *(arrow)*. The pelvic CT scan *(bottom image)* shows a large prostatic mass extending into the bladder neck and the right seminal vesicle. There is a large node in the right internal iliac region *(arrowheads)*.

A transurethral prostate resection showed grade 4 adenocarcinoma in 90% of the prostate shavings. The patient also had osseous metastases and was treated with systemic chemotherapy and external irradiation.

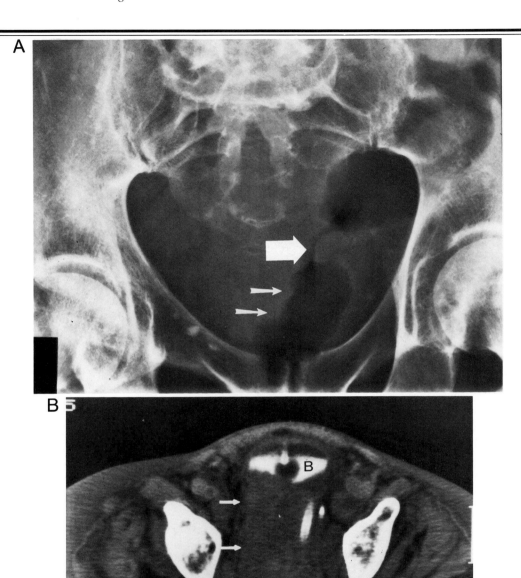

FIG 5–29.
Prostate carcinoma invading the rectum. A 68-year-old man presented with hematuria and partial obstruction of the colon.

A, the pelvic film shows narrowing of the rectosigmoid colon due to what appears to be an infiltrative process in the wall *(arrows).* The barium was passed with a great deal of difficulty at the point of maximum narrowing *(large arrow).*

B, the CT scan shows a very large tumor involving the prostate and the rectosigmoid colon. The bladder *(B),* which contains a Foley catheter, is displaced anteriorly and appears to be infiltrated by the neoplastic process.

Colonoscopy showed extrinsic compression of the sigmoid colon by a large mass, which biopsy proved to be grade 4 adenocarcinoma of the prostate. The patient had diffuse osseous metastasis and died shortly after diagnosis.

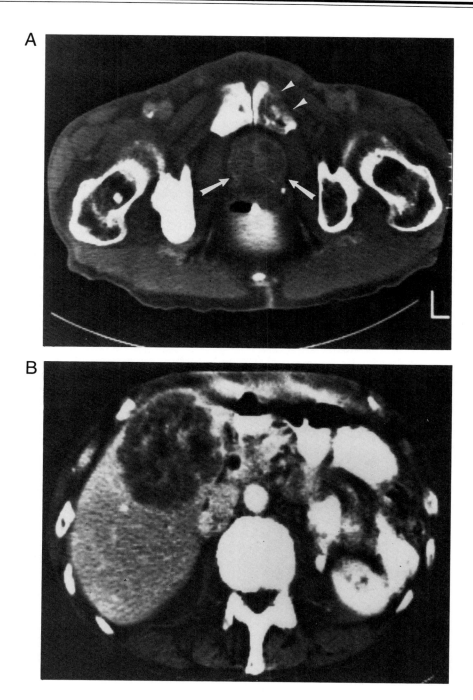

FIG 5–30.
Prostatic carcinoma with osseous and hepatic metastases, stage D2.

A, this patient with known invasive carcinoma of the prostate *(arrows)* developed mixed lytic and blastic osseous metastasis *(arrowheads)*, which failed to respond to chemo-therapy. The tumor extended to the rectum.

B, three months later, while the patient was receiving chemotherapy, abdominal CT scan showed a hepatic lesion proved to represent a metastatic carcinoma of the prostate. The patient died shortly thereafter.

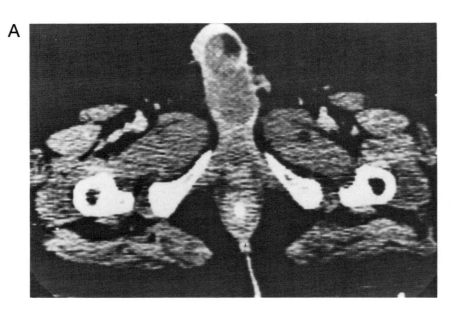

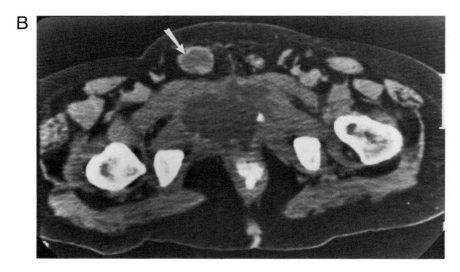

FIG 5–31.
Squamous cell carcinoma of the urethra. This 61-year-old man presented with urinary retention. On physical examination, a large mass was found at the penile-scrotal juncture. Biopsy of the mass proved poorly differentiated squamous cell carcinoma of the urethra.

A, a CT scan shows a low-density mass filling the body of, and causing expansion of, the penis. On the left surface, there is some irregularity, probably due to ulceration or biopsy.

B, the tumor mass extends to the proximal urethra and beyond the lumen, infiltrating into the adjacent muscle. A metastatic nodule *(arrow)* is present in the right spermatic cord.

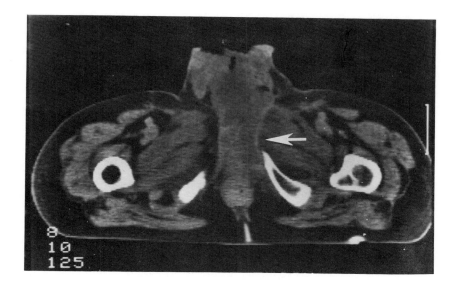

FIG 5–32.

Locally recurrent penile carcinoma. This 73-year-old man was treated with a penectomy for epidermoid carcinoma of the penis. He presented one and one-half years later with locally recurrent disease.

A CT scan through the pelvis shows tumor extending into the penile base *(arrow)*.

A

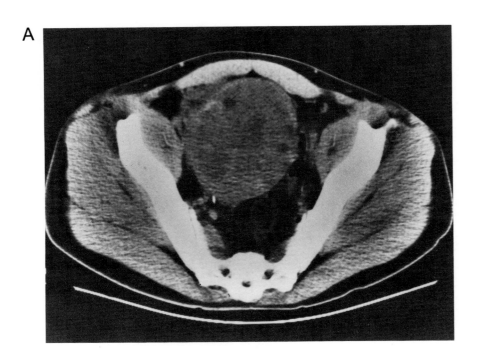

FIG 5–33.
Germ cell tumor in an undescended testis. A 29-year-old man presented with a three-month history of right lower quadrant and suprapubic pain. He was found to have an undescended right testis and a palpable pelvic mass.

A, a pelvic CT scan shows a large, well-defined soft tissue mass within the pelvis. It has areas of low density, probably representing necrosis.

B, coronal magnetic resonance images using T₁-weighted (TR/TE, 800/25) and T₂-weighted (TR/TE, 2,000/80) pulse sequences show the mass *(arrowheads)* with areas of high and intermediate signal intensities. Notice presence of one testes within the scrotum *(arrows).*

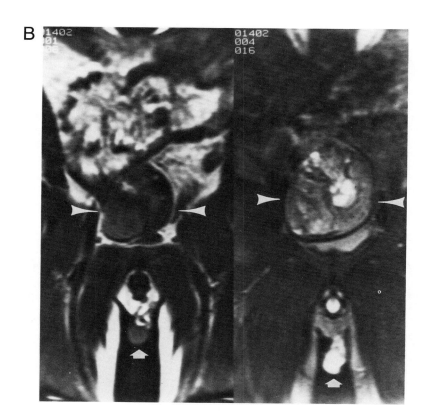

The serum human chorionic gonadotropin (HCG) and α-fetoprotein (AFP) levels were extremely elevated—1,734 million international units (IU)/mL (normal, 0–3 million IU/mL in males) and 958 ng/mL (normal, 0–3 ng/mL in males), respectively. Based on the undescended testis and the elevated hormone titers, the tumor was presumed to be a germ cell tumor, and the patient was treated with a chemotherapy protocol. In two months, the HCG level had dropped to 1,335 million IU/mL and the AFP to 351 ng/mL. Biopsy proved the diagnosis of mature teratoma.

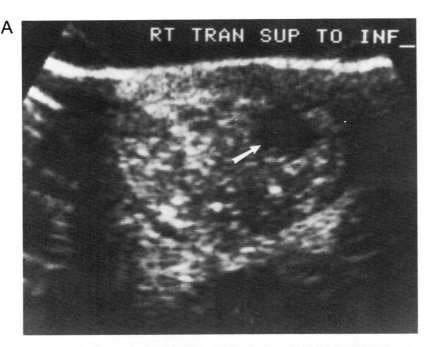

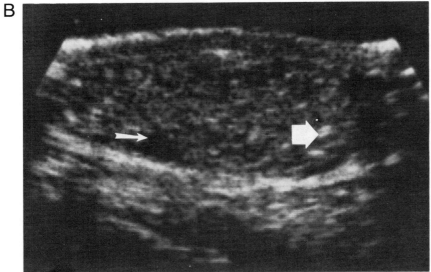

FIG 5–34.
Seminoma arising in contralateral testis following orchiectomy. This 24-year-old man was treated two years prior to admission for mixed germ cell carcinoma of the left testis. He presented this time with a right testicular nodule.

A, a sonogram shows a well-defined, hypoechoic area *(arrow)* within the right testis.

B, a sagittal view through the same testis also shows multiple echogenic areas *(wide arrow)* in addition to the hypoechoic area *(arrow).*

The pathologic specimen showed multiple foci of pure seminoma. Patients with one testicular tumor are at increased risk for contralateral tumor and should be followed with ultrasound.

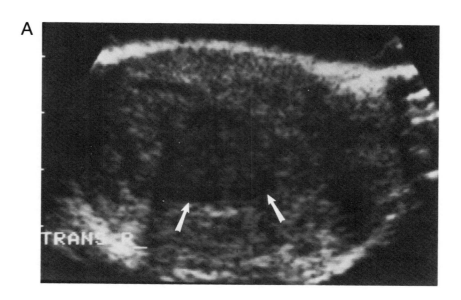

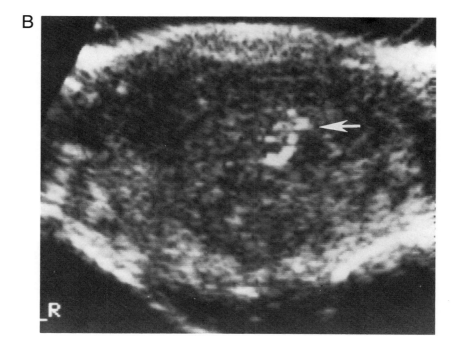

FIG 5–35.
Seminoma with hemorrhage. This 26-year-old man presented with a palpable right testicular mass.

A, a sonogram shows a well-defined, hypoechoic mass *(arrows)* with adjacent halo.

B, an image obtained more superiorly in the testis shows irregular areas and intense echogenicity without shadowing *(arrow).*

The pathologic specimen revealed pure seminoma with extensive tumor necrosis and a focal area of hemorrhage.

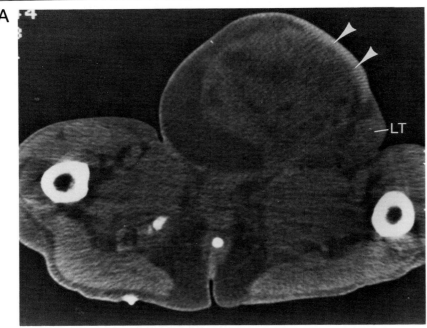

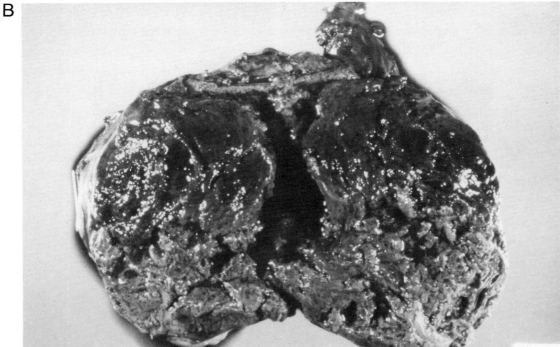

FIG 5–36.
Testicular teratoma. This 55-year-old man five years earlier was found to have a mass in the right testis. He had adamantly refused surgery and instead sought out various holistic cancer treatments around the world. The size of the mass had dramatically increased in the year before he finally came to surgery.

A, the preoperative CT scan shows a very large mass in the right scrotum *(arrowheads)* with areas of low attenuation. There is evidence of hydrocele. The left testis *(LT)* is squeezed to the side by the very large right scrotal sac. The testicular mass has areas of low density, which may represent necrotic areas. There was no evidence of calcification.

The patient underwent right radical orchiectomy and was found to have a mature teratoma.

B, the surgical specimen shows a very large mass with areas of cystic changes. The histologic diagnosis was mature teratoma of the right testis (see also Color Plate 27).

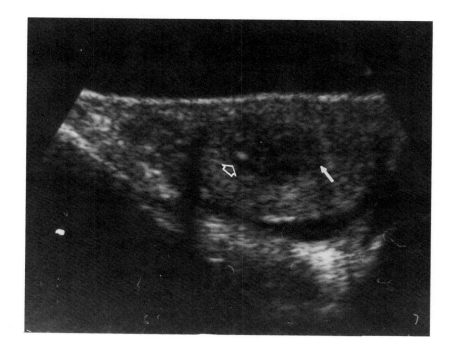

FIG 5–37.

Mixed germ cell tumor. This 21-year-old man presented with neck swelling. Physical examination revealed enlarged supraclavicular nodes, and a chest radiograph showed mediastinal adenopathy. An abnormal nodule was palpated in the left testis.

A transverse sonogram shows a well-defined lesion that is predominantly hypoechoic *(arrow)* but that contains a single echogenic focus *(open arrow)*.

Following orchiectomy, a mixed germ cell tumor (containing embryonal, yolk sac, and immature teratoma elements) was found in the inferior pole of the left testis. A hemorrhagic area was present within the tumor, corresponding to the echogenic focus seen on sonogram.

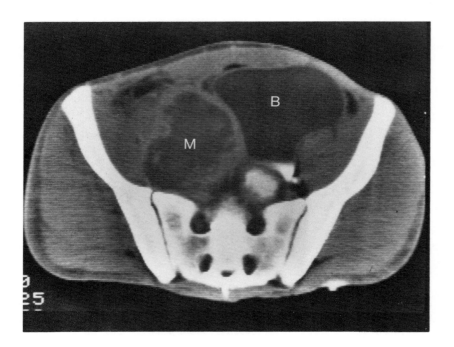

FIG 5–38.

Endodermal sinus tumor. This 52-year-old man with a history of intravenous drug abuse presented with deep venous thrombosis of the right lower extremity. A pelvic mass was palpable.

The pelvic CT scan shows a large mass *(M)* in the right, with areas of low density, presumably representing necrosis. The mass has displaced the urinary bladder *(B)* to the left. There was also evidence of retroperitoneal adenopathy.

At surgery, the necrotic mass was discovered to invade the right psoas muscle. It proved to be an endodermal sinus tumor, for which the patient received chemotherapy.

A

B

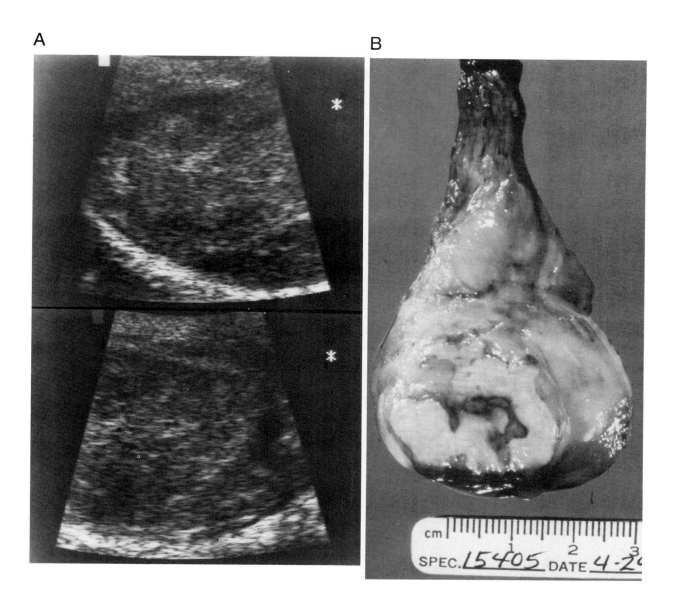

FIG 5–39.
Leukemic infiltration of the testis. This 14-year-old boy with a three-year history of acute lymphoblastic leukemia and three episodes of relapse and remission presented with an enlarged, painful right testis.

A, parasagittal sonograms through the upper and lower right testis demonstrate marked nonhomogeneity of echo pattern. This was considered to be due to leukemic infiltrate, which was proved at orchiectomy.

B, surgical specimen proved to represent diffuse infiltration of the testis and the spermatic cord by leukemic cells (see also Color Plate 28).

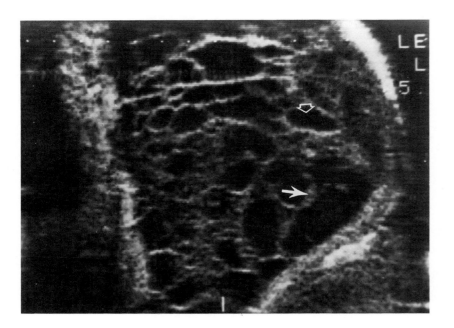

FIG 5–40.

Adenomatoid tumor. This 51-year-old man presented with scrotal swelling of many years' duration. Physical examination revealed a massive hydrocelelike mass that did not transilluminate. The swelling extended through the external ring into the area of the inguinal canal. Ultrasound examination was performed and showed a large mass filling the scrotum. A normal right testis was imaged; however, no definite left testis could be found.

A sonogram through the right hemiscrotum shows multiple cystic areas *(open arrow)* divided by thick septations *(closed arrow).*

Orchiectomy revealed an adenomatoid tumor of the epididymis with marked reactive fibrosis and organizing hemorrhage. This is an atypical appearance of an adenomatoid tumor, which is usually much smaller and often hyperechoic. The cystic appearance is due to the associated bleeding and hematoma formation.

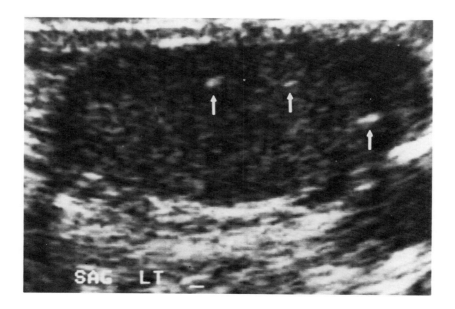

FIG 5–41.

Burned-out primary tumor. This 22-year-old man underwent exploratory laparotomy because of an abdominal mass. Laparotomy revealed a nonseminomatous germ cell tumor. The patient was referred to M. D. Anderson Hospital and received five courses of chemotherapy. Subsequently, an ultrasound examination of the testes was performed.

A sagittal scan shows multiple well-defined areas of calcification *(arrows).*

An orchiectomy was performed and several irregular areas of scarring were present in the cut specimen. Histology revealed a burned-out, or differentiated, occult primary tumor.

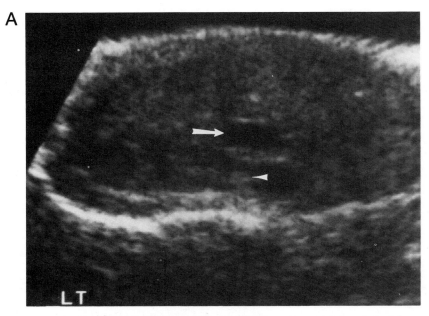

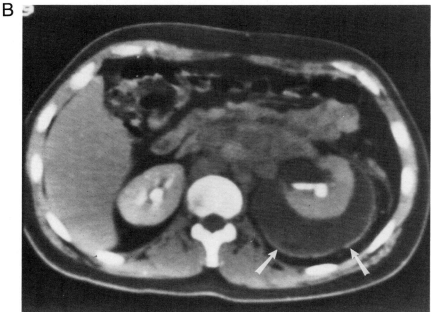

FIG 5–42.
Mature teratoma and retroperitoneal adenopathy. This 22-year-old man presented with a three-month history of an enlarged left testis. Physical examination revealed a large abdominal mass, as well as a left testicular nodule.

A, a testicular sonogram shows well-defined cystic spaces *(arrow)* and a small tumor nodule *(arrowhead)*.

B, an abdominal CT scan shows extensive paraaortic adenopathy encasing the great vessels and causing a left-sided hydronephrosis and subcapsular urinoma *(arrows)*.

A chest radiograph showed massive mediastinal adenopathy, as well as multiple parenchymal metastases. The patient underwent an orchiectomy, which revealed a focal mature teratoma of the testis with glandular epithelium, cartilage, and a focal necrotic area. The patient was treated with chemotherapy and responded well, with clearing of the chest metastases.

This case demonstrates a testicular primary that had matured by the time of orchiectomy and that was associated with widespread metastatic disease.

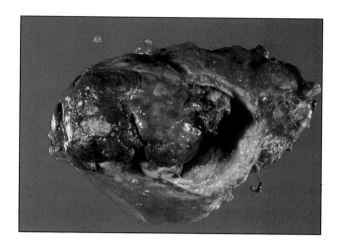

PLATE 24

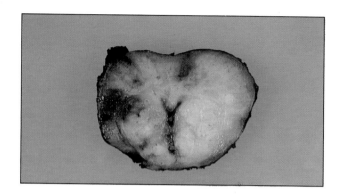

PLATE 25

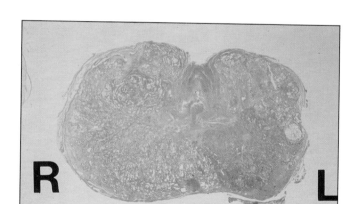

PLATE 26

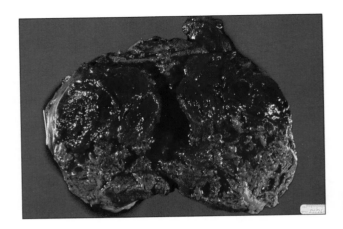

PLATE 27

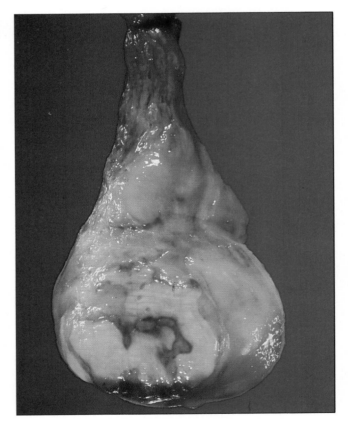

PLATE 28

6

Gynecologic Neoplasms

Errol Lewis, M.D.

Anita Thomas, M.D.

In the United States, gynecologic malignancies account for 28% of all cancers in the female (endometrium, 13%; ovary, 6%; cervix, 6%; other sites, 3%). Most cases are diagnosed clinically, since patients often present with advanced disease. The radiologist is thus chiefly concerned at diagnosis with establishing the extent of involvement by tumor. However, the radiologist's role in the diagnosis and management of patients with gynecologic malignancies has become a far more active one with the use of radiology in such procedures as transcatheter intraarterial infusion and occlusion, percutaneous aspiration and injection of cystic or necrotic neoplasms, and other procedures such as nephrostomy.

Non-cross-sectional noninvasive modalities, such as plain films, intravenous urography, barium enema, and upper gastrointestinal studies, can accurately detect gross mass in soft tissue but not lesser soft tissue involvement, and they can define metastases to bone but not to pelvic and retroperitoneal lymph nodes. Ultrasound and computed tomography (CT) have superseded these older modalities in both the diagnosis and staging of pelvic malignancies, because they not only are noninvasive but can determine the entire extent of intrapelvic disease and define the presence of extrapelvic spread. A third cross-sectional technique, magnetic resonance imaging (MRI), is increasing in importance in gynecologic oncology as its capabilities become better defined. It will be discussed in detail in Chapter 12.

The gynecologic neoplasms are summarized in Table 6–1.

NEOPLASMS OF THE OVARY

In the United States, carcinoma of the ovary is the fourth most common cause of cancer deaths in females. It has been estimated that 19,000 new cases will be diagnosed in 1988.[1] Most cases are advanced at presentation because of the silent nature of the disease. Five-year survival is only 30%.[2] The incidence peaks in the perimenopausal and postmenopausal years and is greatest in the highly industrialized nations.[3]

Eighty-eight percent of ovarian cancers originate in the coelomic epithelium, a thin layer of mesothelium covering the ovary.[4, 5] Serous cystadenomas and serous cystadenocarcinomas (Figs 6–1 and 6–2) account for about 40% of epithelial ovarian neoplasms; mucinous, endometrioid, and mesonephric tumors account for about 30%, 10%, and 5%, respectively; and undifferentiated adenocarcinomas account for the remaining 15%. Most of the serous tumors are malignant. The mucinous tumors, however, are usually benign but may become very large, sometimes rupturing into the peritoneal cavity and producing

TABLE 6–1.

Gynecologic Neoplasms

Ovary		
Primary epithelial tumors	Serous tumors	
	Mucinous tumors	
	Endometrioid tumors	
	Clear cell tumors	
Sex cord, stromal tumor	Granulosa-stromal cell tumor	
	Sertoli-Leydig cell tumors	
Germ cell tumors	Teratoma	
	Dysgerminoma	
	Choriocarcinoma	
	Endodermal sinus tumor	
Metastases		
Fallopian tube		
Benign	Epithelial tumors	
	Mesodermal tumors	
	Mesotheliomas	
	Teratoma	
Malignant	Adenocarcinoma	
	Sarcomas	
	Lymphomas	
Uterus		
Benign	Leiomyomas	
	Adenomyosis	
	Mesodermal tumors	
Malignant	Adenocarcinoma	
	Adenoacanthoma	
	Adenosquamous cell tumors	
	Primary squamous cell tumors	
	Clear cell carcinoma	
	Sarcoma	
		Leiomyosarcoma
		Endometrial stromal tumor
		Malignant mixed muellerian tumors
	Metastases	
Cervix		
Benign	Leiomyoma	
Malignant	Carcinoma	
		Squamous
		Verrucous
		Adenocarcinoma
Vagina		
Benign	Granular myoblastoma	
Malignant	Carcinoma	
	Melanoma	
	Sarcoma	
	Metastases	
Vulva		
Benign cystic	Bartholin's cyst	
	Keratinous cyst	
	Mesonephric cyst	
	Cyst of the canal of Nuck	
Benign solid	Connective tissue tumor	
	Epithelial tumor	
Malignant	Squamous cell tumor	
	Paget's disease	
	Melanoma	

pseudomyxoma peritonei. The endometrioid tumors are identical to and may be associated with endometrial carcinoma,[6] and the mesonephric, or clear cell, tumors resemble genitourinary tract epithelial neoplasms. Mixtures of histologic types are frequently seen, but the classification of a tumor is by the predominant cell type.[7]

Stromal cell ovarian neoplasms include the estrogenic granulosa-theca cell tumors (Fig 6–3) and the androgenic Sertoli-Leydig cell tumors. They are malignant in approximately 10% of cases. The estrogenic tumors may be associated with endometrial hyperplasia or with sexual precociousness or pseudoprecociousness, and the androgenic tumors may be associated with virilization.

The germ cell ovarian tumors are most frequently seen in young adults. These include benign teratoma, or dermoid cyst, which has well-differentiated components and is very common. Only 1% to 2% of these cysts become malignant, and 10% to 15% are bilateral. In dysgerminoma, the germ cells have not differentiated into embryonic or intraembryonic structures. These neoplasms are usually unilateral (90%) and carry a fairly good prognosis.[8] Choriocarcinoma and endodermal sinus tumors are typically very malignant; they arise from cells undergoing extraembryonal differentiation.

Ovarian carcinoma spreads within the pelvis and abdomen, following the dynamics of the distribution of ascites. The most common sites of metastasis are the pouch of Douglas, the right lower quadrant, the sigmoid colon, and the right paracolic gutter.[9] Metastases along the diaphragm are also common, and right-sided malignant pleural effusions are frequently seen (Fig 6–4). Liver metastases are seen in approximately 10% of cases.[10] The lymphatic drainage of the ovary is via the paraaortic nodes, from the aortic bifurcation to the renal pelvis, and to the middle chain of the external iliac nodes. However, if the ovarian capsule is invaded, the iliac or inguinal nodes may be involved; anastomoses exist between the ovarian lymph vessels and those of the uterus and fallopian tubes. In a lymphangiographic series by Athey et al., 70% of patients with nodal metastases from ovarian carcinoma had abnormal paraaortic nodes, 58% had abnormal iliac nodes, and 27% had abnormal inguinal nodes.[11]

Conventional radiographs are usually low yield in the diagnosis of ovarian neoplasms. However, the visualization of a calcified tooth is pathognomonic of teratoma; fat and calcium are also suggestive of this neoplasm (Fig 6–5). Serous cystadenomas display psammomatous calcification on plain radiography in 20% of cases (Fig 6–6). Ascites may also be seen in advanced carcinomatosis. Conventional radiographs can image pleural effusions and pulmonary metastases and occasionally define abnormal bowel loops or skeletal metastases.

Tethering of mucosal folds on a barium examination is indicative of tumor extension to bowel, and ovarian tumors account for the greatest number of cases in the female of direct invasion of bowel by a primary.[12] Excretory urography may reveal a pelvic mass that displaces or obstructs the ureters or that displaces the bladder.

Ultrasound is often the initial study in the workup of a pelvic mass. In early disease, it is useful in differentiating adnexal and uterine pathology. The sonographic appearance of ovarian neoplasms varies widely, and the ultrasonic characteristics cannot predict the histologic type.[13] In general, however, the more cystic a mass appears on ultrasound, the more likely it is a benign tumor, particularly a serous cystadenoma (Fig 6–7). Suggestive of a malignant mass are thick septations, solid nodules, multilocular masses larger than 5 cm, or a mass fixed to the uterus or sidewall (Fig 6–1).

The ultrasonic appearance of dermoids varies according to the composition of the various tissue components and can range from completely solid to cystic.[14] If hair or calcification is present within the tumor, intense echoes and distal shadowing are seen. Because of the intense echoes that result from hair and fat, it may be impossible to differentiate a dermoid mass from adjacent gas-filled bowel, so that even a clinically palpable mass may not be imaged.[15] Or, the highly echogenic interface may allow only partial imaging of the mass, yielding the well-known "tip of the iceberg" sign. In these tumors, there may be fluid-fluid interface that can be observed on ultrasound to shift in relation to a change of position of the patient (Fig 6–5).

Ultrasonography is a very good modality for identifying ascites (Fig 6–6), extrapelvic disease, hydronephrosis, liver metastases, and paraaortic adenopathy (Fig 6–8). But it yields high false-negative rates in omental and peritoneal disease.[16] The presence of ascites can aid in detecting peritoneal implants adherent to the diaphragm or on the surface of the liver.[17] Ultrasound can be used to assess the response of a neoplastic mass to chemotherapy and also in follow-up to determine the presence of recurrent disease (Fig 6–9).[18] At M. D. Anderson Hospital, it is also used to localize the peritoneal instillation of viral oncolysate (Ralph S. Freedman, M.D., 1986, personal communication, Department of Gynecology, The University of Texas M. D. Anderson Hospital and Tumor Institute at Houston).

Computed tomography is useful in defining the nature of a mass and can accurately determine the presence of fat, fluid interface, and dental calcification in dermoids (Fig 6–5)[19] or amorphous psammomatous calcification in serous adenocarcinoma. It can suggest invasion of adjacent structures and identify adenopathy, ascites, and peritoneal implants larger than 2.0 cm in diameter (Fig 6–4).[20] Omental involvement is often seen in advanced ovarian disease, with pancaking of involved bowel (Fig 6–10). For identification of spread of pelvic tumor to the adrenals (Fig 6–11) or liver or for evaluation of subcapsular hepatic metastases (see Fig 6–4), CT is the preferred modality.[21]

Computed tomography is effective in guiding fine-needle biopsy of lymph nodes.[22] The major limitation of CT is its inability to detect peritoneal implants less than 2 cm in diameter.[23] Computed tomography is not accurate enough to replace the second-look operation in the assessment of residual tumor, but it may be used as a guide in the search for recurrent disease.[24]

Magnetic resonance imaging has demonstrated great potential for the evaluation of adnexal masses.[25] Its ability to image anatomy in the coronal, sagittal, and axial projections is particularly useful in visualizing the relationship of an adnexal mass with the uterus and pelvic sidewall. The masses are usually best seen by using T_2-weighted pulse sequence when the tumor displays high signal intensity compared with the surrounding muscle and adipose tissue. T_1-weighted images will usually improve tissue characterization.[26] In ovarian cystic teratomas, more than 80% of which occur during the reproductive years, MRI is the procedure of choice because radiation hazards are thus avoided.[27]

Metastases to the ovaries are not uncommon. They most frequently derive from primaries in the gastrointestinal tract, breasts, lungs, reticuloendothelial system, or kidneys (Fig 6–12). *Krukenberg's tumor* is the term used to describe all ovarian metastases from carcinoma of the gastrointestinal tract (Fig 6–13).[28] These metastases tend to be homogeneous and bilateral.[29, 30] Because the survival rate of children with acute lymphocytic leukemia is increasing, leukemic relapse in the ovaries is being identified more frequently (Fig 6–14)[31]; disease is present in the ovaries in up to 50% of cases in autopsy series.[32] In lymphoma, the ovaries can be the main site of dis-

ease.[33, 34] The ovaries are most easily identified by ultrasound, and leukemic or lymphomatous involvement typically produces bilaterally enlarged, hypoechoic ovaries.

NEOPLASMS OF THE UTERUS

Leiomyomas are the most common benign tumors of the female genital tract; they are found in 20% to 40% of women more than 33 years of age. These tumors are the most common cause, excluding pregnancy, of an enlarged uterus. They are classified by their location and can be subserosal, intramural (Fig 6–15), or pedunculated. The pedunculated fibroids sometimes are seen as an adnexal mass (Fig 6–16). Complications of leiomyomas include tumor degeneration (especially during pregnancy [Fig 6–16]), infection, and bleeding. On conventional radiography, fibroids may appear as a pelvic mass that indents and displaces bladder and bowel. Irregular and coarse calcifications are sometimes identified (Fig 6–17). Ultrasound is often utilized in the workup of an enlarged uterus, and its diagnostic accuracy for fibroids is between 65% and 93%.[35–37] The ultrasonic appearance of fibroids depends on the type of stromal tissue and the presence of calcification (Fig 6–17). The mass cannot usually be separated from the uterus, and the outline of the uterus is often distorted. Cystic areas may be seen if hyalinization and liquefaction occur in the fibroids. Fibroids become more sonolucent during pregnancy (Fig 6–16). Care should be taken to not misdiagnose the echo-free fundus of a retroverted uterus as a fibroid.[38, 39]

Fibroids are indicated on CT by a lobulated, enlarged uterus that may contain areas of calcification.[40] The attenuation values are generally similar to that of normal uterus,[41] but areas of necrosis or degeneration may result in a low-attenuation mass. Adenomyomatosis may result in a false-positive diagnosis of fibroids.

Endometrial carcinoma is the most common malignancy of the female pelvis. In the United States each year, 38,000 new cases are diagnosed,[42] and the disease accounts for 3,000 deaths. There is an increased incidence in women with late menopause, obesity, diabetes, and a history of irregular menstrual periods. Unlike ovarian carcinoma, most uterine carcinomas are diagnosed at an early stage, and five-year survival is 75% to 78%.[43] Postmenopausal bleeding is the typical reason for presentation, and the tumor is usually diagnosed by a dilation and curettage.

Ninety percent of endometrial carcinomas are adenocarcinomas (Figs 6–18 and 6–19).[44] Less common varieties of tumors include adenoacanthomas, papillary carcinoma, clear cell carcinoma, and secretory and mucinous adenocarcinomas. Sarcomas make up 5% of all uterine cancers[45]; the different types are leiomyosarcoma, endometrial stromal sarcoma, and mixed mesodermal sarcoma. All of the sarcomas carry a poor prognosis.

Although advanced cases are uncommon, endometrial carcinoma may extend into the cervix (stage II) or pelvis (stage III) or metastasize to pelvic or retroperitoneal nodes, bladder, rectum, lung, bone, or brain (stage IV) (Figs 6–20 and 6–21). Pyometra or hematometra is seen when the tumor obstructs the cervix.

Earlier investigations showed that ultrasound cannot determine the degree of myometrial invasion, and therefore it may not help to distinguish stage I and II disease.[46] However, more recently, it has been shown that myometrial invasion by endometrial carcinoma can be accurately detected by high-resolution sonography.[47] By using a transvaginal transducer, one can minimize factors, such as obesity and uterine retroflexion, that can hamper the accuracy of conventional scanning. Findings indicative of fluid collection within the endometrial cavity of a postmenopausal woman suggest carcinoma (Fig 6–18).[48] However, such fluid collection may also be seen secondary to radiation fibrosis or postsurgical scarring.

Computed tomography typically shows endometrial tumors as areas of decreased attenuation (Fig 6–19). The administration of intravenous contrast material is important in delineating the mass,[49] although CT cannot accurately show the degree of myometrial invasion.[50] Computed tomography is helpful in assessing advanced disease and can differentiate stage II from stage III and IV tumors by showing parametrial extension and extrapelvic spread (Figs 6–20 and 6–21).[51] It is also useful in planning irradiation portals.

Magnetic resonance imaging can display an endometrial tumor with a very high degree of accuracy, but it may not be able to differentiate carcinoma from either blood clot or benign adenomatous hyperplasia. It should be noted that the incidence of lymph node metastases increases from approximately 3% with superficial invasion of myometrium to more than 40% with deep invasion and that MRI is highly accurate (92%) in the staging of endometrial carcinoma (Fig 6–19).[52]

GESTATIONAL TROPHOBLASTIC DISEASE

Gestational trophoblastic disease comprises hydatidiform mole (80%), in which the molar tissue is only in the endometrial cavity; chorioadenoma destruens (15%), in which the molar tissue invades the myometrium locally; and choriocarcinoma (5%), which metastasizes. A complete mole consists of diffuse hydropic villi and atypical trophoblastic tissue. Complete moles probably arise de novo,[53] and about 20% become invasive.[54] A partial mole consists of focal hydropic villi, trophoblastic proliferation, and a fetus of XXY karyotype.[55, 56] The incidence of malignant transformation in a partial mole is less than with a complete mole.[57] Most choriocarcinomas follow a molar pregnancy, but they may also be seen after a normal term pregnancy, an abortion, or a tubal pregnancy.

Ultrasound is the best diagnostic modality for the evaluation of a suspected molar pregnancy. The most common pattern is multiple sonolucent areas in a vesicular, or grapelike, pattern. Attention should be directed to determining if hydropic changes are focal or diffuse because of the different prognoses between complete and partial moles.[58] If a fetus is present, the mole is unlikely to be a complete one. Theca-lutein cysts are seen in the ovaries in 15% to 50% of patients screened by ultrasound.[59, 60] Invasive mole and choriocarcinoma both demonstrate abnormal echoes within the myometrium on ultrasound (Fig 6–22).

Ultrasound may also be used to follow treatment of trophoblastic disease. Following evacuation of the uterus, the sonolucent areas are no longer identified. The uterus gradually decreases in size, although it remains enlarged for several weeks to months. Measurement of human chorionic gonadotropin levels is more sensitive than ultrasound in detecting recurrent or residual disease.[61] Computed tomography is the best method for detecting liver or brain metastases of choriocarcinoma, which occur in 10% of cases.[62] Conventional chest films can identify lung metastases. Both lung and brain metastases have a tendency to bleed (Fig 6–23).

NEOPLASMS OF THE CERVIX

Cervical cancer is the second most common malignancy in women between 15 and 34 years of age.[63, 64] Most cases are asymptomatic; approximately one third of patients present with vaginal bleeding and leukorrhea. Between 1945 and 1975, the incidence of invasive cervical carcinoma dropped by half,[63] whereas the incidence of in situ lesions increased.[65] These changes are probably related to the introduction of the Papanicolaou smear in 1945. However, approximately 20% of women delay seeking medical attention for at least six months following the onset of symptoms.

Squamous cell carcinoma accounts for 95% of all invasive tumors of the cervix.[66] Most of the remaining invasive cervical cancers are adenocarcinomas that arise from the endocervical columnar cells. These particular tumors can become quite large, at which point they are seen as barrel-shaped tumors confined to the cervix.[67, 68] Clear cell carcinoma of the cervix is only rarely seen; it occurs in adults and is thought in some cases to be related to in utero exposure to diethylstilbestrol.[69] Other rare tumors of the cervix include adenocystic, verrucous, basal cell, and glassy cell carcinomas.

The conventional radiographic techniques only rarely detect metastases from cervical tumors, with an incidence of 1% on chest radiography, 3.4% on barium enema, and 7.3% on excretory urography.[70] Excretory urography demonstrates deviation of the ureters and hydronephrosis in 20% of cases. Changes that occur after irradiation, as well as related complications, can be detected on urography. These include an elevated, small, thick-walled bladder and bowel changes such as a narrow, rigid rectum, increased pelvic fat, and a widened presacral space.[71] Barium examinations as well as retrograde cystography may be helpful in detecting the rectovaginal and vesicovaginal fistulas that occur in 1.2% of patients and that occur more frequently when hysterectomy is combined with radiation therapy (Fig 6–24).[72] Bony changes such as radionecrosis and aseptic necrosis of the femoral head can be detected by routine radiography.[73]

The lymphatics of the uterine cervix form a rich plexus and drain to the lymph nodes of the external iliac and hypogastric chain as well as the presacral area. Lymphangiography is the only radiologic modality that visualizes the internal architecture of lymph nodes and vessels. A nodal defect not traversed by lymphatic channels is the most reliable criterion for the diagnosis of metastatic disease in a patient with a known primary neoplasm. Lymphangiography is also the only radiologic modality that can detect metastases in normal-sized nodes. This detection of abnormal nodes in the pelvis or retroperitoneum is obviously extremely important, as it would dictate a change of therapy, including extension of radiotherapy portals.

The yield of lymphangiography in the detection of metastases in patients with stage I carcinoma of the cervix is small.[74] In this group of patients, the metastases are usually in the pelvis and most likely would be included within the radiotherapy portal. In a study of 103 patients at M. D. Anderson Hospital, lymphangiography had a sensitivity of 77%, a specificity of 98%, and an overall accuracy of 87%. However, there was also a 12% rate of false-negative results,[75, 76] which highlights the opinion that only a diagnosis of a definitely positive node is of clinical significance, since microscopic neoplastic foci cannot be detected by lymphangiography and not all the involved pelvic and paraaortic lymph nodes are opacified.

Sonography offers little diagnostically in patients with cervical carcinoma, especially in early-stage cases. However, should physical examination be extremely difficult because of large exophytic fungating masses, there may be a role for ultrasound (Fig 6–25). Large masses of the cervix with extension to the parametrium and pelvic nodes (i.e., stage III or IV carcinomas) can be demonstrated by ultrasound (Figs 6–25 and 6–26). Involvement of the pelvic wall, bladder, or rectum may be difficult to define by ultrasonography. The kidneys should be routinely examined for hydronephrosis, which indicates stage III disease.[46, 77]

On CT examination, a primary neoplasm of the cervix is frequently seen as a mass of low density, best visualized at the level of the femoral heads (Fig 6–27). Extension into the parametrium is determined by soft tissue extension of tumor to the internal obturator muscle or to the piriform muscles. Bladder and rectal invasion are difficult to assess. Such invasion may be manifested by irregular thickening of adjacent walls with obliteration of the posterior perivesical and anterior rectal fat planes. Computed tomography's main role in cervical carcinoma is to determine the extent of disease by defining the size of the tumor, the size of the uterus, and the degree, if any, of endometrial invasion (Fig 6–28), parametrial and pelvic sidewall extension, and pelvic adenopathy (Fig 6–29). Extrapelvic metastases to the liver, skeleton, and paraaortic lymph nodes are readily detected, as is hydronephrosis.[78–82] In their 1981 series of 75 patients, Walsh and Goplerud found that CT was inaccurate in differentiating stage IB from stage IIB but was extremely accurate in the diagnosis and staging of advanced lesions (i.e., those beyond stage IIIB).[79] This study, as well as others, reports CT to be about 90% accurate with advanced lesions. However, a diagnostic difficulty with CT is its inability to differentiate tumor recurrence from radiation fibrosis, which are both imaged as soft tissue masses with irregular margins within the pelvis. The differentiation can be made only by a needle biopsy, preferably done under CT guidance.

The lymph nodes most frequently involved by metastases of cervical carcinoma are the obturator, hypogastric, external, and common iliac. Lymph nodes larger than 1.5 cm in diameter are considered to be abnormal by CT criteria. However, because of the high incidence of secondary infection in carcinoma of the cervix, they might reflect nodal hyperplasia rather than metastasis. Any diagnosis should therefore be confirmed by biopsy or lymphangiography (Fig 6–29). It is well known that metastasis in normal-sized nodes may escape detection by CT. However, there are reports discussing CT recognition of lymph node metastases.[81, 82] Whitley et al. reported a sensitivity of 80%, specificity of 83%, and accuracy of 83%,[81] whereas Walsh et al., in a series of 75 patients, found an accuracy of 74%.[82] Computed tomography also plays a role in mapping radiotherapy portals and in detecting pelvic sidewall and retroperitoneal disease. Postirradiation changes within the pelvis can also be determined by CT.

The role of MRI in cervical carcinoma has yet to be fully defined. However, a cervical mass may be demonstrated as an area of increased intensity.[83–85] This modality's future role may be in differentiating stage IIA and IIB lesions. Because of its ability to scan in both sagittal and coronal planes, MRI is able to define uterine, vaginal, and rectal extension (Fig 6–24). In addition, it is thought that MRI is far better able than CT to differentiate between uterine invasion and an obstructed uterus with hematometra or hydrometra (Fig 6–28). To date, MRI cannot distinguish benign from malignant involvement of nodes, but it is hoped that MRI will aid in the detection of abnormal nodes within the pelvis.

The interventional radiologist now plays an active role in the therapeutic management of patients with large, bulky, extensive tumors of the cervix through the intraarterial infusion of high-dose cisplatin, bleomycin, vincristine, and mitomycin C. In a trial of this combination at our institution, there was a reduction of 50% or more in the size of the pelvic mass in all seven patients enrolled. If apparently uncontrollable bleeding from tumors develops, it can be controlled with embolization using Ivalon particles, absorbable gelatin sterile (Gelfoam) cubes, or a stainless steel coil.[86–89]

Radiologic techniques are also utilized in pa-

tients with cervical tumors when ureteral obstruction requires nephrostomy. The fistula created can subsequently be converted into an internal ureteral stent.[90] Finally, needle aspiration biopsies under CT or fluoroscopic guidance have been extremely accurate in the pretreatment staging of carcinoma of the cervix. An overall accuracy of 68%, sensitivity of 58%, and specificity of 100% can be obtained without significant complications. A biopsy finding positive for disease obviates exploratory laparotomy or lymphadenectomy (see Fig 6–29). It should be emphasized that only positive biopsy results are of clinical significance, because the predictive value of a normal test result is only 42%.[91]

NEOPLASMS OF THE VAGINA, VULVA, AND FALLOPIAN TUBES

Cancer of the vagina is a disease of older women and accounts for 1% to 2% of all gynecologic cancers. About 95% of cases are squamous cell carcinomas (Figs 6–30 and 6–31). Clear cell carcinoma (following maternal use of diethylstilbestrol), melanoma, and sarcoma botryoides make up most of the remainder. The vagina is more commonly involved by metastases (Fig 6–32) than by primaries, and those metastases are usually from the cervix, endometrium, ovary, or bowel. Primary vaginal carcinoma spreads mainly by local invasion into adjacent organs: bladder, rectum, paracolpial tissue, and pelvic sidewall lymph nodes. The spread of upper vaginal lesions is similar to that of cervical lesions, with lymphatic drainage to the obturator and iliac nodes, whereas lesions of the distal third of the vagina metastasize to the regional nodes of the groin.[92–95]

Like cancer of the vagina, cancer of the vulva affects older women. It accounts for 4% of all cancers in females.[96] More than 90% of invasive vulvar carcinomas are squamous cell in type (Fig 6–33). Other less common malignancies include Bartholin's gland carcinoma (Fig 6–34), basal cell carcinomas, adenocarcinoma, sarcomas, Paget's disease, malignant melanoma, and verrucous carcinoma. The principal means of spread is lymphatic, usually to the inguinal and femoral nodes (Fig 6–33).[97–100]

Carcinoma of the fallopian tubes is the rarest gynecologic malignancy. Early diagnosis is usually difficult; invariably, diagnosis is made at the operating table in patients thought to have another neoplasm. Fallopian tube cancer is histologically similar to ovarian cancer, and most cases are pure adenocarcinomas. Also like ovarian carcinoma, it spreads to the omentum and retroperitoneal nodes, although its spread is rather unpredictable.[101–105]

Ultrasonography, CT, and lymphangiography are useful for determining nodal involvement from tumors of the vagina, vulva, and fallopian tubes, since spread is both local and by the lymphatic system. Ultrasonography and CT can define both intrapelvic and extrapelvic extension and aid when necessary in radiotherapy planning (Fig 6–33).

Magnetic resonance imaging, by providing a high-resolution sagittal image, can often be helpful in evaluating the extent of tumor and the tumor's relationship with the bladder, rectum, and adjacent soft tissue in vaginal neoplasm (Fig 6–31).

REFERENCES

1. American Cancer Society: *Cancer Facts and Figures 1988*. New York, American Cancer Society, 1988.
2. Cutler S.J., Myers M.H., Green S.B.: Trends in survival rates of patients with cancer. *N. Engl. J. Med.* 293:122–124, 1975.
3. Wynder E., Dodo H., Barber H.: Epidemiology of cancer of the ovary. *Cancer* 1:352–370, 1969.
4. Hertig A., Gore H.: *Tumors of the Female Sex Organs: Part 3. Tumors of the Ovary and Fallopian Tubes.* Washington, D.C., Armed Forces Institute of Pathology, 1959.
5. Rutledge F.N., Fletcher G.H., Smith J.P., et al.: Gynecologic cancer, In Clark R.L., Howe C.D. (eds.): *Cancer Patient Care.* Chicago, Year Book Medical Publishers, 1976, pp. 263–308.
6. Lang P.: Endometriosis-like formations. *Acta Obstet. Gynecol. Scand.* 34:111–119, 1955.
7. Seror S., Scully R., Sobin L.: *Histologic Typing of Ovarian Tumors.* Geneva, World Health Organization, 1973.
8. Linto E.B.: Dysgerminoma of the ovary. *J. Reprod. Med.* 26:255–260, 1981.
9. Meyers M.A.: Distribution of intraabdominal, malignant seeding: dependency on dynamics of flow of ascitic fluid. *AJR* 119:198–206, 1973.
10. Lewis E., Zornoza J., Jing B.S., et al.: Radiologic contributions to the diagnosis and management of gynecologic neoplasms. *Semin. Roentgenol.* 17:251–268, 1982.
11. Athey P.A., Wallace S., Jing B.S., et al.: Lymphangiography in ovarian carcinoma. *AJR* 132:915–918, 1979.
12. Meyers M.A.: Metastatic seeding along the small bowel mesentery. *AJR* 123:67–73, 1975.
13. Moyle J.W., Rochester D., Sider L., et al.: Sonography of ovarian tumors: predictability of tumor type. *AJR* 141:985–991, 1983.
14. Sandler M.A., Silver T.M., Karo J.J.: Gray-scale ultrasonic features of ovarian teratomas. *Radiology* 131:705–709, 1979.
15. Callen P.W.: *Ultrasonography in Obstetrics and Gynecology.* Philadelphia, W.B. Saunders Co., 1983, p. 220.
16. Reguard C.K., Mettler F.A., Wicks J.D.: Preoperative sonography of malignant ovarian neoplasms. *AJR* 137:79–82, 1981.
17. Paling M.R., Shawker T.H.: Abdominal ultrasound in advanced ovarian carcinoma. *Journal of Clinical Ultrasound* 9:435–441, 1981.
18. Paling M.R., Shawker T.H., Dwyer A.: Ultrasonic evaluation of therapeutic response in tumors: its value and implications. *Journal of Clinical Ultrasound* 9:281–288, 1981.
19. Friedman A.C., Pyatt R.S., Hartman D.S., et al.: CT of benign cystic teratomas. *AJR* 138:659–665, 1982.
20. Mamtora H., Isherwood I.: Computed tomography in ovarian carcinoma: patterns of disease and limitations. *Clin. Radiol.* 33:165–171, 1982.
21. Snow J.H. Jr., Goldstein H.M., Wallace S.: Comparison of scintigraphy, sonography, and computed tomography in the evaluation of hepatic neoplasms. *AJR* 132:915–918, 1979.
22. Dunnick N.R., Fisher R.I., Chu E.W., et al.: Percutaneous aspiration of retroperitoneal lymph nodes in ovarian cancer. *AJR* 134:109–113, 1980.
23. Johnson R.J., Blackledge G., Eddleston B., et al.: Abdomino-pelvic computed tomography in the management of ovarian carcinoma. *Radiology* 146:447–452, 1983.
24. Choyke P.L., Thickman D., Kressel H.Y.: Controversies in the radiologic diagnosis of pelvic malignancies. *Radiol. Clin. North Am.* 23:531–549, 1985.
25. Dooms G.C., Hricak H., Tscholakoff D.: Adnexal structures: MR imaging. *Radiology* 158:639–646, 1986.
26. Mitchell D.G., Mintz M.C., Spritzer C.E., et al.: Adnexal masses: MR imaging observations at 1.5 T, with US and CT correlation. *Radiology* 162:319–324, 1987.
27. Togashi K., Nishimura K., Itoh K., et al.: Ovarian cystic teratomas: MR imaging. *Radiology* 162:669–673, 1987.
28. Hale RW: Krukenberg tumor of the ovaries: a review of 81 records. *Obstet. Gynecol.* 23:221–225, 1968.
29. Gross B.H., Moss A.A., Mihara K., et al.: Computed tomography of gynecologic disease. *AJR* 141:765–773, 1983.
30. Cho K.C., Gold B.M.: Computed tomography of Krukenberg tumors. *AJR* 145:285–288, 1985.
31. Zarrouk S.O., Kim T.H., Hargreaves H.K., et al.: Leukemic involvement of the ovaries in childhood acute lymphocytic leukemia. *J. Pediatr.* 100:422–424, 1982.
32. Viadana E., Bross I.D.J., Pickren J.W.: An autopsy study of the metastatic patterns of human leukemias. *Oncology* 35:87, 1978.

33. Paladugu R.R., Bearman R.M., Rappaport H.: Malignant lymphoma with primary manifestation in the gonad: a clinicopathologic study of 38 patients. *Cancer* 45:561–571, 1980.

34. Gompel C., Silverberg S.G.: *Pathology in Gynecology and Obstetrics*, ed. 7. Philadelphia, W.B. Saunders Co., 1974.

35. Morley P., Barnett E.: The use of ultrasound in the diagnosis of pelvic masses. *Br. J. Radiol.* 43:602–616, 1970.

36. Cochrane W.J., Thomas M.A.: Ultrasound diagnosis of gynecologic pelvic masses. *Radiology* 110: 649–654, 1974.

37. Fleischer A.C., James A.S., Millis J.D., et al.: Differential diagnosis of pelvic masses by gray-scale sonography. *AJR* 131:469–476, 1978.

38. Walsh J.W., Taylor K.J.W., Wasson J.F., et al.: Gray-scale ultrasound in 204 proved gynecologic masses: accuracy and specific diagnostic criteria. *Radiology* 130:391–397, 1979.

39. Callen P.W., DeMartini W.J., Filly R.A.: The central uterine cavity echo: a useful anatomic sign in the ultrasonographic evaluation of the female pelvis. *Radiology* 131:187–190, 1979.

40. Tada S., Tsukioka M., Ishi C., et al.: Computed tomographic features of uterine myoma. *J. Comput. Assist. Tomogr.* 5:866–869, 1981.

41. Walsh J.W., Rosenfield A.T., Jaffe C.C.: Prospective comparison of ultrasound and CT in the evaluation of gynecologic pelvic masses. *AJR* 131:955–960, 1978.

42. Creasman W.T., Weed J.C.: *Cancer of the Endometrium.* Chicago, Year Book Medical Publishers, 1980.

43. Boronow R.C.: Endometrial cancer, not a benign disease. *Obstet. Gynecol.* 47:630–634, 1976.

44. Scully R.E.: Cancer of the uterine corpus—pathologic types. *Int. J. Radiat. Oncol. Biol. Phys.* 6:361–364, 1980.

45. Morrow C.P., Townsend D.E.: *Synopsis of Gynecologic Oncology.* Clinical Monographs in Obstetrics and Gynecology. New York, John Wiley & Sons, 1981.

46. Requard C.K., Wicks J.D., Mettler F.A.: Ultrasonography in the staging of endometrial adenocarcinoma. *Radiology* 140:781–785, 1981.

47. Fleischer A.C., Dudley B.S., Entman S.S., et al.: Myometrial invasion by endometrial carcinoma: sonographic assessment. *Radiology* 162:307–310, 1987.

48. Breckenridge J.W., Kurtz A.B., Ritchie W.G., et al.: Postmenopausal uterine fluid collection: indicator of carcinoma. *AJR* 139:529–534, 1982.

49. Hamlin D.J., Burgener F.A., Beecham J.B.: CT of intramural endometrial carcinoma: contrast enhancement is essential. *AJR* 137:551–554, 1981.

50. Hasumi K., Matsuzawa M., Chen H.F., et al.: Computed tomography in the evaluation and treatment of endometrial carcinoma. *Cancer* 50:904–908, 1982.

51. Walsh J.W., Goplerud D.R.: Computed tomography of primary, persistent, and recurrent endometrial malignancy. *AJR* 139:1149–1154, 1982.

52. Hricak H., Stern J.L., Fisher M.R., et al.: Endometrial carcinoma staging by MR imaging. *Radiology* 162:297–305, 1987.

53. Reynolds S.R.M.: Hydatidiform mole: a vascular congenital anomaly. *Obstet. Gynecol.* 47:224–250, 1976.

54. Lewis J.L. Jr.: Current status of treatment of gestational trophoblastic disease. *Cancer* 38:620–626, 1976.

55. Szulman A.E., Surti U.: The syndromes of hydatidiform mole: I. Cytogenetic and morphologic correlations. *Am. J. Obstet. Gynecol.* 131:665–671, 1978.

56. Szulman A.E., Surti U.: The syndromes of hydatidiform mole: II. Morphologic evaluation of the complete and partial mole. *Am. J. Obstet. Gynecol.* 132:20–27, 1978.

57. Vassilakos P., Riotton G., Kajii T.: Hydatidiform mole: two entities. A morphologic and cytogenic study with some clinical considerations. *Am. J. Obstet. Gynecol.* 127:167–170, 1977.

58. Reid M.H., McGahan J.P., Oi R.: Sonographic evaluation of hydatidiform mole and its look-alikes. *AJR* 140:307–311, 1983.

59. Cadkin A.V., Saggagha R.E.: Ultrasonic diagnosis of abnormal pregnancy. *Clin. Obstet. Gynecol.* 20:265–277, 1977.

60. Baird A.M., Beckly D.E., Ross F.G.M.: The ultrasound diagnosis of hydatidiform mole. *Clin. Radiol.* 28:637–645, 1977.

61. Requard C.K., Mettler F.A.: The use of ultrasound in the evaluation of trophoblastic disease and its response to therapy. *Radiology* 135:419–422, 1980.

62. Goldstein D.P., Berkowitz R.S.: The management of gestational trophoblastic neoplasms. *Current Problems in Obstetrics and Gynecology* 4:1–42, 1980.

63. Silverberg E.: *Cancer Statistics 1982.* New York, American Cancer Society, 1982.

64. Barran B.A., Richart R.M.: An epidemiologic study of cervical neoplastic disease: based on a self-selected sample of 7,000 women in Barbados, West Indies. *Cancer* 27:978–984, 1971.

65. DiSaia P.J., Creasman W.T.: *Clinical Gynecologic Oncology.* St. Louis, C.V. Mosby Co., 1981.

66. Gusberg S.B., Frick H.C.: *Corscaden's Gynecologic Cancer,* ed. 5. Baltimore, Williams & Wilkins Co., 1978.

67. Moier R.C., Norris H.J.: Existence of cervical intraepithelial neoplasia with primary adenocarcinoma of the endocervix. *Obstet. Gynecol.* 56:361–364, 1980.

68. Moyer E.G., Galindo J., Davis J.: Adenocarcinoma of the uterine cervix: incidence and role of radiation therapy. *Radiology* 121:725–729, 1976.

69. Herbst A.L., Cole P., Norusis M.J., et al.: Epidemiologic aspects and factors related to survival in 384 Registry cases of clear cell adenocarcinoma of the vagina and cervix. *Am. J. Obstet. Gynecol.* 135:876–886, 1979.

70. Griffin W.G., Parker R.G., Taylor W.J.: An evalua-

tion of procedures used in staging carcinoma of the cervix. *AJR* 127:825–827, 1976.

71. Green B., Libshitz H.I.: Bladder and ureter, in Libshitz H.I. (ed.): *Diagnostic Roentgenology of Radiotherapy Change.* Baltimore, Williams & Wilkins Co., 1979, pp. 123–136.

72. Strockbine M.F., Hancock J.E., Fletcher G.H.: Complications in 831 patients with squamous cell carcinoma of the intact uterine cervix treated with 3,000 rads or more whole pelvis irradiation. *AJR* 108:293–304, 1970.

73. Cunningham J.J., Fuks Z.Y., Castellino R.A.: Radiographic manifestations of carcinoma of the cervix and complications of its treatment. *Radiol. Clin. North Am.* 12:93–108, 1974.

74. Piver S., Wallace S., Castro J.: The accuracy of lymphangiography in carcinoma of the uterine cervix: the accuracy of lymphangiography in carcinoma of the uterine cervix. *AJR* 111:278, 1971.

75. Wallace S., Jing B.S.: Carcinoma, in Clouse M.E. (ed.): *Clinical Lymphangiography.* Baltimore, Williams & Wilkins Co., 1977, sect. 7, pp. 185–273.

76. Wallace S., Jing B.S., Zornoza J., et al.: Is lymphangiography worthwhile? *Int. J. Radiat. Oncol. Biol. Phys.* 5:1873–1876, 1979.

77. Sanders R.C., James A.E. Jr. (eds.): *Principles and Practice of Ultrasonography in Obstetrics and Gynecology,* ed. 2. New York, Appleton-Century-Crofts, 1980.

78. Kilcheski T.S., Arger P.H., Mulhern C.B., et al.: Role of computed tomography in the presurgical evaluation of carcinoma of the cervix. *J. Comput. Assist. Tomogr.* 5:378–383, 1981.

79. Walsh J.W., Goplerud D.R.: Prospective comparison between clinical and CT staging in primary cervical carcinoma. *AJR* 137:997–1003, 1981.

80. Ginaldi S., Wallace S., Jing B.S., et al.: Carcinoma of the cervix: lymphangiography and computed tomography. *AJR* 136:1087–1091, 1981.

81. Whitley N.O., Brenner D.E., Francis A., et al.: Computed tomographic evaluation of carcinoma of the cervix. *Radiology* 142:439–446, 1982.

82. Walsh J.W., Amendola M.A., Hall D.J., et al.: Recurrent carcinoma of the cervix: CT diagnosis. *AJR* 136:117–122, 1981.

83. Bryan P.J., Butler H.E., LiPuma J.P., et al.: NMR scanning of the pelvis: initial experience with a 0.3 T system. *AJR* 141:1111–1118, 1983.

84. Hricak H.J., Alpers C., Crooks L.E., et al.: Magnetic resonance imaging of the female pelvis: initial experience. *AJR* 141:1119–1128, 1983.

85. Johnson I.R., Symonds E.M., Worthington B.S., et al.: Imaging ovarian tumours by nuclear magnetic resonance. *Br. J. Obstet. Gynaecol.* 91:260–264, 1984.

86. Morrow C.P., DiSaia P.J., Mangan C.F., et al.: Continuous pelvic arterial infusion with bleomycin for squamous carcinoma of the cervix recurrent after irradiation therapy. *Cancer Treat. Rep.* 61:1403–1405, 1977.

87. Swenerton K.D., Evers J.A., White G.W., et al.: Intermittent pelvic infusion with vincristine, bleomycin, and mitomycin C for advanced recurrent carcinoma of the cervix. *Cancer Treat. Rep.* 63:1379–1381, 1979.

88. Ohta A.: Basic and clinical studies on the simultaneous combination treatment of cervical cancer with a carcinostatic agent and radiation. *Tokyo Ika Daigaku Zasshi (Journal of Tokyo Medical College)* 36:529, 1978.

89. Oku T., Iwasaki M., Tojo S.: Study on surgical chemotherapy for advanced carcinoma of the uterine cervix, particularly on the problem of clinical effect and drug concentration. *Acta Obstetrica et Gynaecologica Japonica* (English edition) 31:1833, 1979.

90. Pfister R.C., Yoder I.C., Newhouse J.H.: Percutaneous uroradiologic procedures. *Semin. Roentgenol.* 16:135–151, 1981.

91. Edeiken-Monroe B.S., Zornoza J.: Carcinoma of the cervix: percutaneous lymph node aspiration biopsy. *AJR* 138:655–657, 1982.

92. Perez C.A., Anneson A.N., Galakatos A., et al.: Malignant tumors of the vagina. *Cancer* 31:36–55, 1973.

93. Pride G.L., Buchles D.A.: Carcinoma of the vagina 10 or more years following pelvic irradiation therapy. *Am. J. Obstet. Gynecol.* 127:513–517, 1977.

94. Pride G.L., Schultz A.E., Chuprevich T.W., et al.: Primary invasive squamous carcinoma of the vagina. *Obstet. Gynecol.* 53:218–225, 1979.

95. Rutledge F.: Cancer of the vagina. *Am. J. Obstet. Gynecol.* 97:635–655, 1967.

96. DiSaia P.J., Creasman W.T., Rich W.M.: An alternative approach to early cancer of the vulva. *Am. J. Obstet. Gynecol.* 133:825–832, 1979.

97. Chamlian D.L., Taylor H.B.: Primary carcinoma of the Bartholin's gland. *Obstet. Gynecol.* 39:489–494, 1972.

98. Charpentier-Arnavon P., Prade M., Michel G.: Basal cell carcinoma of the vulva—report of nine cases. *Arch. Anat. Cytol. Pathol.* 28:139–154, 1980.

99. Creasman W.T., Gallager H.S., Rutledge F.: Paget's disease of the vulva. *Gynecol. Oncol.* 3:133–148, 1975.

100. Curry S.L., Wharton J.T., Rutledge F.: Positive lymph nodes in vulvar squamous carcinoma. *Gynecol. Oncol.* 9:63–67, 1980.

101. Sedlis A.: Carcinoma of the fallopian tube. *Surg. Clin. North Am.* 58:121–129, 1978.

102. Yoonessi M.: Carcinoma of the fallopian tube. *Obstet. Gynecol. Surv.* 34:257–270, 1979.

103. Finn W.F., Javert C.T.: Primary and metastatic cancer of the fallopian tube. *Cancer* 2:803–814, 1949.

104. Jones O.V.: Primary carcinoma of the uterine tube. *Obstet. Gynecol.* 26:122–129, 1965.

105. Dodson M.G., Ford J.H., Averette H.E.: Clinical aspects of fallopian tube carcinoma. *Obstet. Gynecol.* 36:935–938, 1970.

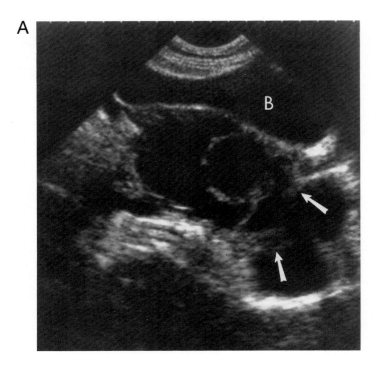

FIG 6–1.
Ovarian carcinoma (two cases).

    A and **B,** a 54-year-old woman presented with discomfort and swelling in the abdomen.

    A sagittal sonogram **(A)** through the bladder *(B)* demonstrates a large, multiseptated cystic mass in the pelvis. Solid tumor nodules *(arrows)* are visible.

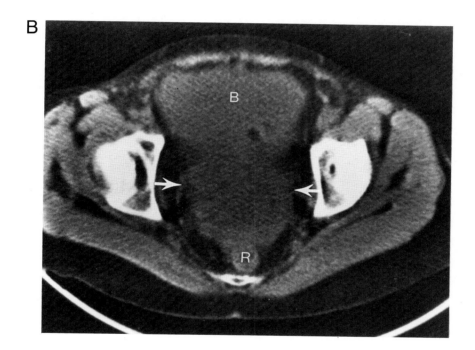

The corresponding unenhanced CT scan **(B)** shows a large pelvic mass *(arrows)* between the bladder *(B)* and rectum *(R)*.

At surgery, the patient was found to have a large pelvic tumor and a "frozen" pelvis. Biopsy proved the diagnosis to be papillary cystadenocarcinoma of the ovary. The ovarian tumor involved the bladder, rectum, and small bowel. *(Continued.)*

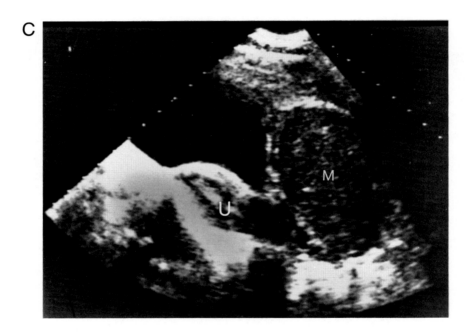

FIG 6–1 (cont.).
C through **E,** a sagittal sonogram **(C)** shows a large echogenic mass *(M)* predominantly in the left side of the pelvis. The uterus *(U)* appears normal.

Coronal MR image **(D)** using T$_1$-weighted pulse sequence (TR/TE, 500/28) shows the mass *(arrows)* to be within the left side of the pelvis extending into the midline and displacing the bladder *(B)* to the right. There appear to be multiple tumoral vessels within the mass.

Midline sagittal MR image **(E)** using moderately T$_2$-weighted pulse sequence (TR/TE, 1,000/50) shows the intermediate signal intensity within the mass *(white arrows)* with the presence of multiple vessels. The high signal intensity *(black arrow)* within the uterine cavity represents hemorrhage.

At surgery, an inoperable pelvic neoplasm, diagnosed as primitive mixed carcinoma of the left ovary, was found. **(C–E** courtesy of Professor J.L. Lamarque, Hospital Lapeyronie, Montpellier, France.)

D

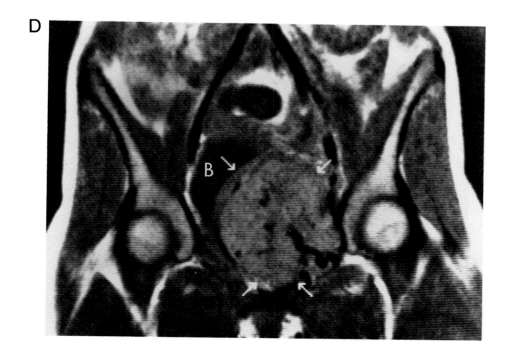

E

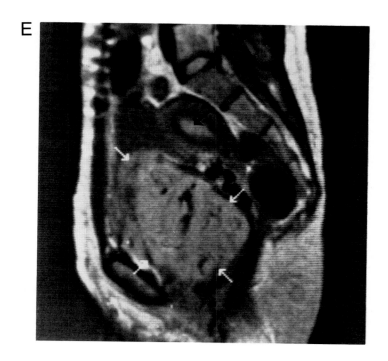

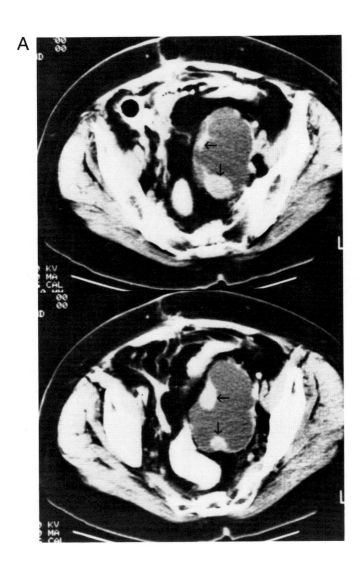

FIG 6–2.

Ovarian serous cystadenocarcinoma with peritoneal and subcutaneous metastasis. This 61-year-old woman underwent exploratory laparotomy with the diagnosis of small bowel obstruction. The serosa of the resected ileum was nodular, and pathologic diagnosis was metastatic serosal carcinoma. A mass was palpable in the pelvis. She was referred to M. D. Anderson Hospital.

A, pelvic CT images show a large, predominantly cystic mass with nodules in the wall *(arrows)* located in the left adnexa. The patient had surgery, and the diagnosis of serous cystadenocarcinoma was proved. This was followed by chemotherapy.

Two years later she presented with a palpable nodule in the anterior abdominal wall.

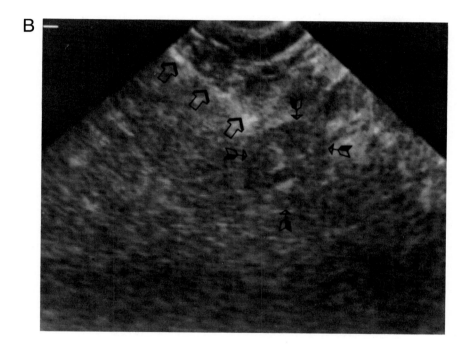

B, sonography proved the subcutaneous nature of this nodule *(four arrows),* and ultrasound-guided percutaneous needle aspiration *(three arrows)* proved the nodule to represent metastatic serous cystadenocarcinoma.

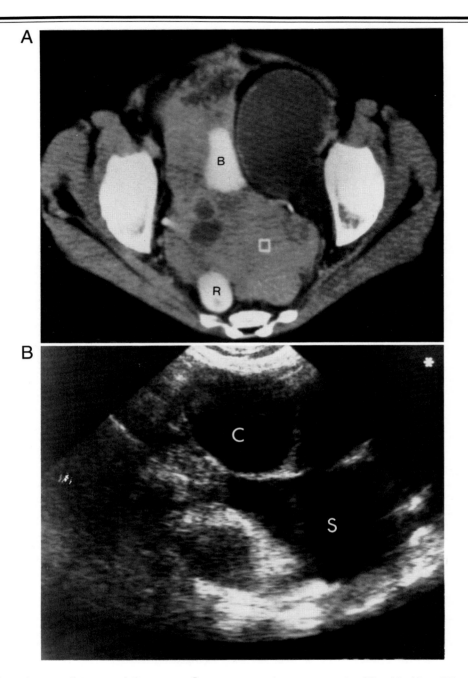

FIG 6–3.
Recurrent granulosa-theca cell tumor of the ovary. Seventeen years before this presentation, the patient underwent exploratory laparotomy for a right adnexal mass, which was diagnosed as granulosa-theca cell tumor. Seven years after the laparotomy, she had a total hysterectomy with removal of the left ovary, which was reported to contain a dermoid cyst with a cystic teratoma. She presented with weakness, indigestion, weight loss, and abdominal swelling and discomfort.

A, the CT scan shows a large mass with both solid and cystic components. The bladder *(B)* and rectum *(R)* are markedly displaced.

B, a sagittal sonogram obtained to the left of the midline demonstrates the cystic component *(C)* anteriorly and the solid component *(S)* posteriorly.

At surgery, a large tumor arising from the pelvis and involving the sigmoid colon was found. The tumor could not be entirely removed because it invaded both pelvic sidewalls. The pathologic diagnosis was recurrent granulosa-theca cell tumor.

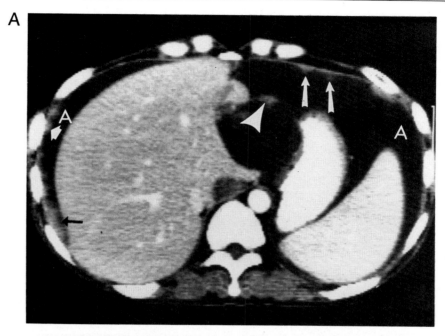

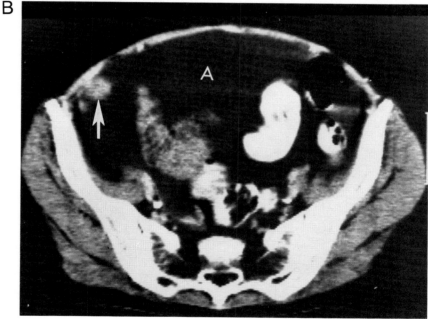

FIG 6–4.

Recurrent ovarian mesonephroid carcinoma metastatic to the peritoneal cavity. A 38-year-old woman presented with a history of abdominal discomfort and increasing abdominal girth, and she was found to have right pleural effusion. Exploratory laparotomy revealed a large ovarian mass and ascites. The pathology was that of mesonephroid carcinoma of the ovary with positive ascitic fluid results. A hysterectomy, bilateral salpingo-oophorectomy, and omentectomy were performed, followed by chemotherapy.

A, a CT examination eight months later showed recurrent ovarian carcinoma. There is a large amount of ascites *(A)* in the abdomen and pelvis, as well as multiple metastatic peritoneal implants *(arrows)*. Metastatic nodules were also present on the gastrohepatic ligament *(arrowhead)*.

B, peritoneal implants *(arrow)* are clearly seen because of surrounding ascites *(A)*.

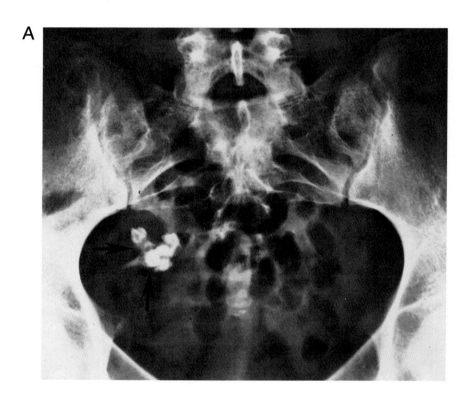

FIG 6–5.
Mature cystic teratoma of the right ovary. A 19-year-old woman was referred to our hospital after a right adnexal mass was found on routine pelvic examination.

A, a conventional radiograph of the pelvis shows several well-formed toothlike structures *(arrows)* in the right side of the pelvis.

B, a CT scan shows a right adnexal mass *(arrows)* containing fat *(F),* soft tissue *(S),* and calcified densities.

C, a sagittal sonogram demonstrates the right adnexal mass, which contains calcification *(arrows)* with distal shadowing *(open arrows).*

A 5 × 5 cm cystic ovarian mass was surgically removed. The pathologic diagnosis was mature cystic teratoma.

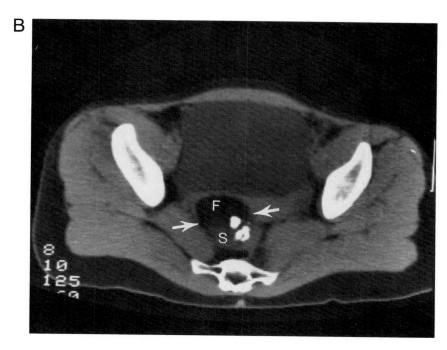

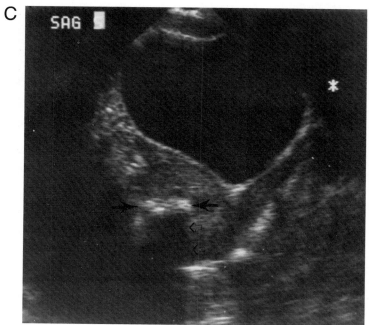

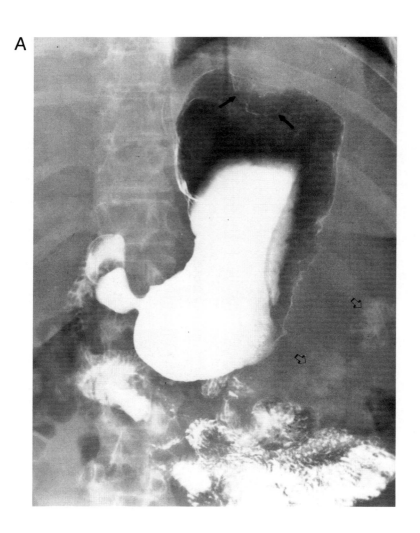

FIG 6–6.

Recurrent ovarian carcinoma with psammomatous calcification. A 32-year-old was treated with bilateral salpingo-oophorectomy and chemotherapy for papillary serous adenocarcinoma of the ovary. Five years later, she was referred to M. D. Anderson Hospital for management of progressive abdominal disease.

A, an upper gastrointestinal film shows an extramural lesion *(arrows)* compressing the gastric fundus, with amorphous calcification *(open arrows)* in a left upper quadrant mass.

B, a transverse right abdominal sonogram shows a large amount of ascites *(A)* throughout the abdomen. Multiple echogenic masses, typical of psammomatous calcification *(arrows),* were located on the surface of the liver.

C, a transverse sonogram of the pelvis demonstrates a cystic mass *(M),* proved to represent recurrent tumor, to the right of the bladder *(B).*

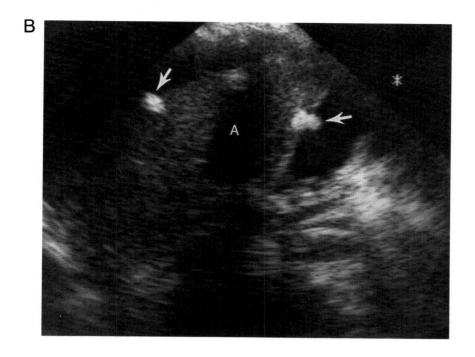

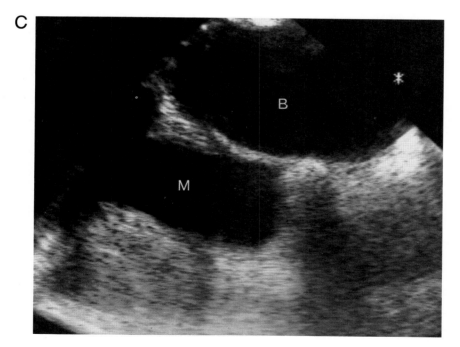

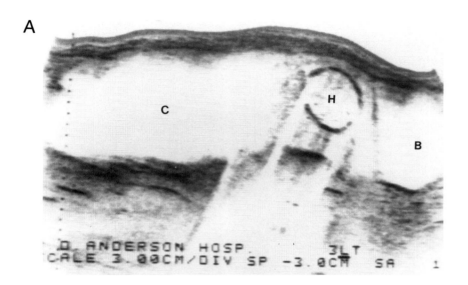

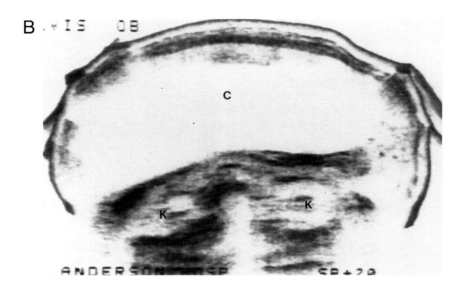

FIG 6–7.
Serous cystadenoma coexistent with a uterine pregnancy. A gravida 3, para 2 31-year-old woman presented to her physician with a history of fainting. Physical examination revealed a large pelvic mass, which increased in size over the next week. Ultrasound showed a left ovarian mass measuring 10 × 10 cm. One week later, the mass was reported to measure 15 × 25 cm. Ultrasound at that time showed a pregnancy of 20.5 weeks' gestational age.

A, a sonogram demonstrated a live fetus of 20.5 weeks' gestational age. The sagittal sonogram shows the head of the fetus *(H)* superior to the bladder *(B).* A large extrauterine cystic mass *(C)* is present superiorly.

B, the transverse scan demonstrates the large cystic mass *(C)* occupying most of the abdomen *(K,* kidneys).

At surgery, a 25 × 20 × 10 cm cystic mass compatible with a serous cystadenoma was found. There was no evidence of malignancy.

A

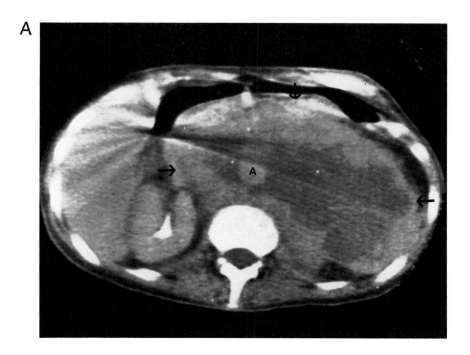

B

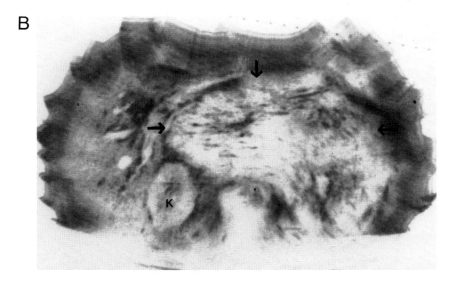

FIG 6–8.

Recurrent dysgerminoma. A 23-year-old woman presented with increasing abdominal girth and a history of removal of the left ovary two years previously for ovarian dysgerminoma.

A, the CT examination shows a huge mass of mixed attenuation *(arrows)* filling the entire retroperitoneum and encasing the major vessels (*A,* aorta).

B, the corresponding static sonogram demonstrates the large, solid mass *(arrows)* seen on CT. The mass is also displacing the right kidney *(K)*.

At surgery, it was confirmed that the mass was due to recurrent dysgerminoma. The mass filled the entire left upper quadrant and the lesser sac and surrounded the aorta and inferior vena cava. Treatment was by irradiation, and the patient is well six years later.

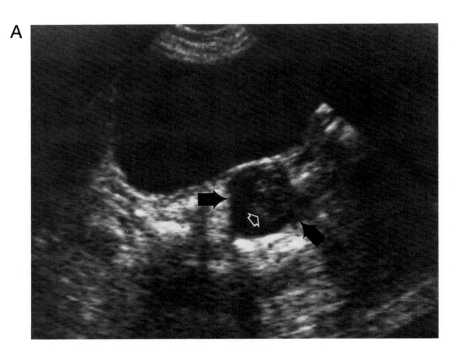

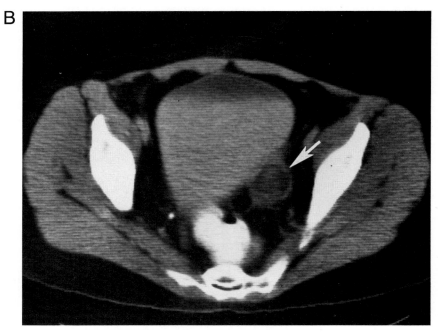

FIG 6–9.
Recurrent ovarian carcinoma. A 45-year-old woman underwent surgery, irradiation, and chemotherapy for papillary serous adenocarcinoma involving both ovaries. One year later, she presented with a palpable adnexal mass.

A, a transverse sonogram of the pelvis shows a complex, predominantly cystic mass *(arrows)* in the left adnexa. A solid mural nodule *(open arrow)* is visible.

B, the CT delineation of the mixed-density mass *(arrow)* is comparable to the sonographic appearance. A CT-guided biopsy confirmed the diagnosis of recurrent ovarian carcinoma.

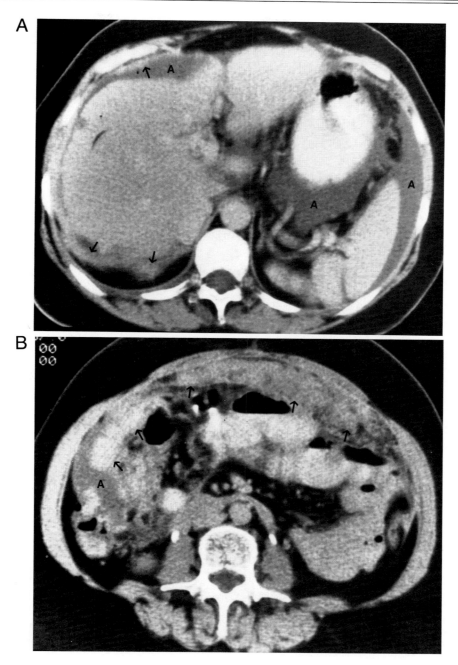

FIG 6–10.

Abdominal carcinomatosis from ovarian cancer. A 59-year-old woman underwent abdominal hysterectomy and bilateral salpingo-oophorectomy for stage III mixed adenocarcinoma of the ovary. The small amount of residual disease was treated with chemotherapy. The patient was without evidence of disease until four years later, when she presented because of increasing abdominal girth.

A, a CT examination showed advanced, recurrent ab-dominal carcinomatosis. Ascites *(A)* surrounds the liver and spleen and extends into the lesser sac. Peritoneal implants *(arrows)* are identified along the edge of the liver.

B, there is advanced peritoneal disease, with pancak-ing of the omentum *(arrows),* as well as ascites *(A).*

Exploratory laparotomy revealed extensive abdominal disease. There were multiple metastatic plaques on all se-rosal surfaces, and approximately 2 L of ascites was re-moved.

A

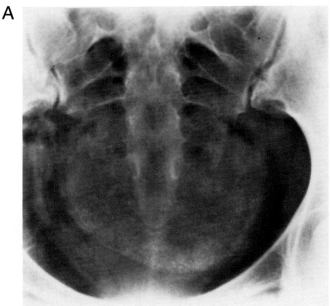

B

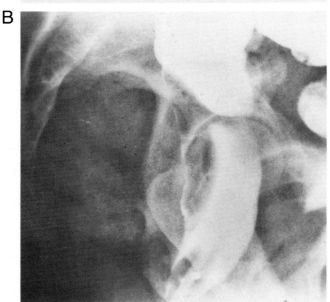

FIG 6–11.

Presacral teratoma with distant metastases. This 43-year-old woman was found on routine physical examination to have a large pelvic mass. Chest radiography showed pulmonary metastases.

A and **B,** on the plain radiograph **(A),** a large pelvic mass is seen. Areas of fine calcification are predominantly in the peripheral aspect of the mass. Lateral view from a barium enema examination **(B)** shows the presacral nature of the mass, which displaces the rectum anteriorly without invasion.

C, this CT study reveals the mass to be behind the bladder and anterior to the sacrum. It is well circumscribed with areas of increased density, but the appearance is not typical for teratomatous calcification. The posterior portion of this mass is denser and has a thicker wall. Intravenous pyelography showed extrinsic mass effect on the bladder without any evidence of wall invasion.

D, abdominal CT, done as a part of routine workup, discloses a left adrenal mass.

The patient underwent surgery, and the large cystic mass, measuring 10 × 11 × 7 cm, was excised from the presacral area. Also, a 5 × 7 cm mass was removed from the region of the left adrenal gland. The pathology report listed adenocarcinoma arising from the presacral teratoma with metastases to the left adrenal and lungs. The patient underwent chemotherapy.

C

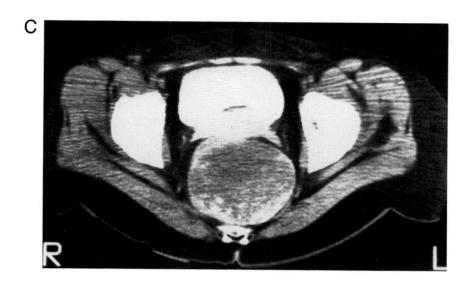

D

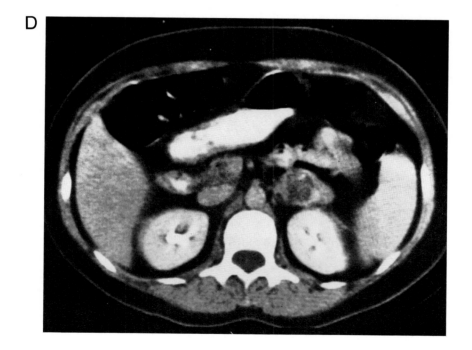

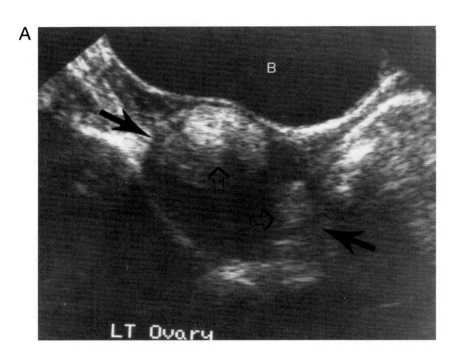

FIG 6–12.

Metastases of renal cell carcinoma to the left ovary. A 60-year-old woman with confirmed renal cell carcinoma and lung metastases had nephrectomy and interferon therapy. The initial CT examination showed a benign liver cyst. The patient subsequently developed a paraspinal metastasis, and a left adnexal mass was palpated on pelvic examination.

A, a sagittal sonogram through the bladder *(B)* demonstrates a complex mass *(arrows)* with solid nodules *(open arrows).*

B, the corresponding CT scan shows both the solid and cystic components of the left adnexal mass.

C, a percutaneous biopsy done under ultrasonic guidance proved renal cell carcinoma metastatic to the ovary (see also Color Plate 29). There are cells with vacuolated cytoplasm and eccentric nuclei, characteristic of renal cell carcinoma.

B

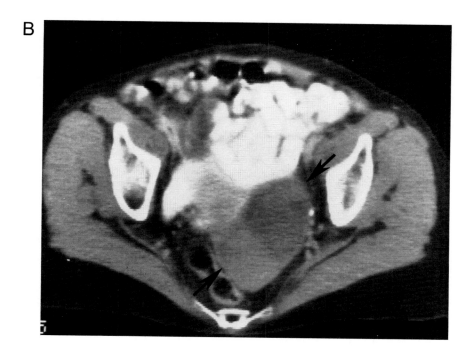

C

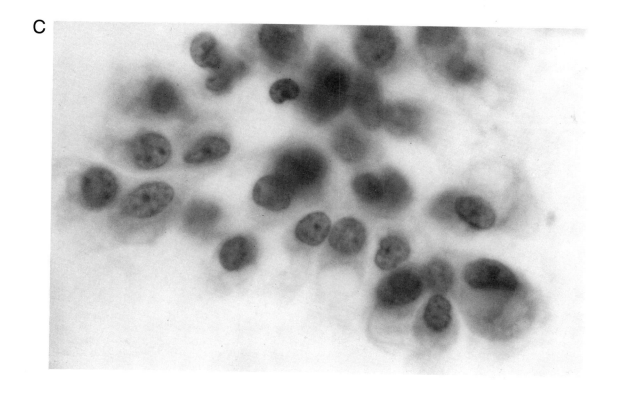

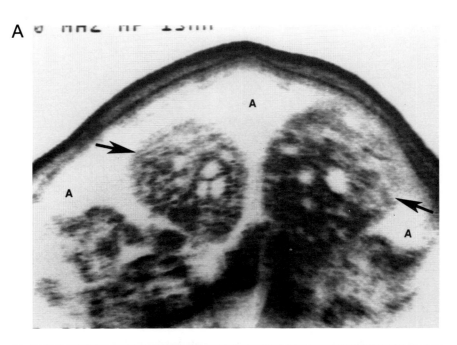

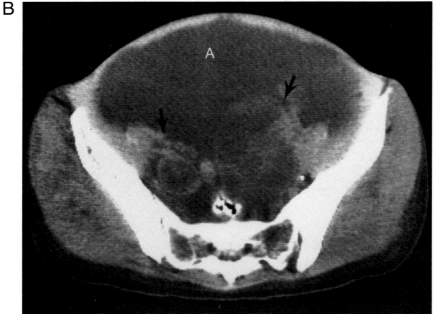

FIG 6–13.
Krukenberg's tumor of the ovary. Eight months after a 33-year-old woman had a total gastrectomy for gastric carcinoma, she presented with abdominal swelling and ascites.

A, the abdominal sonogram shows ascites *(A),* within which two large, complex masses *(arrows)* arise from the pelvis.

B, the corresponding CT scan shows the two masses *(arrows),* which were interpreted to surround the ovaries, and the large collection of ascites *(A).* Such bilateral ovarian masses are compatible with Krukenberg's tumor.

The patient died shortly thereafter, and autopsy confirmed the diagnosis of bilateral Krukenberg's tumors from gastric metastasis. The ovaries weighed 300 and 500 g.

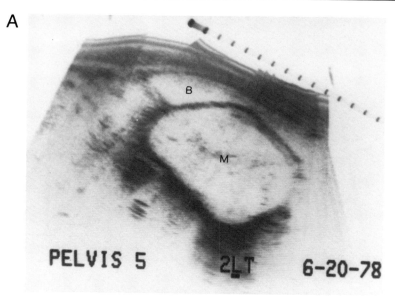

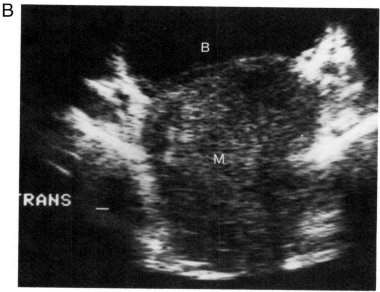

FIG 6–14.

Leukemic involvement of the ovaries (two cases).

A, this eight-year-old girl had a known diagnosis of acute lymphocytic leukemia. Treatment was by systemic and intrathecal chemotherapy. While in complete remission for three years, she developed abdominal fullness. Ultrasound exam showed bilaterally enlarged ovaries. This sagittal scan to the left of midline shows a large hypoechoic mass *(M)* posterior to the bladder *(B)*. Surgical exploration proved leukemic infiltration of the ovaries.

B, another child, a ten-year-old girl with a seven years' diagnosis of acute lymphocytic leukemia, was in complete remission when she presented with a left lower quadrant mass. The transverse sonogram shows a large mass *(M)* with medium-level echoes posterior to the bladder *(B)* and probable infiltration of the bladder wall. The uterus and ovaries could not be identified. The sonographic diagnosis was leukemic involvement of the ovary. At laparotomy, a 7 × 7 × 3 cm hemorrhagic mass was discovered adherent to the bladder and the uterus, eroding the anterior wall of the vagina and obstructing the left ureter. Cystostomy proved the involvement of the bladder wall. The uterus and right ovary were normal. The pathologic diagnosis was leukemic infiltrate of the left ovary with areas of hemorrhage and necrosis. (From Shirkhoda A., Eftekhari F., Frankel L.S., et al.: Diagnosis of leukemic relapse in the pelvic soft tissues of juvenile females. *Journal of Clinical Ultrasound* 14:191–195, 1986. Reprinted by permission.)

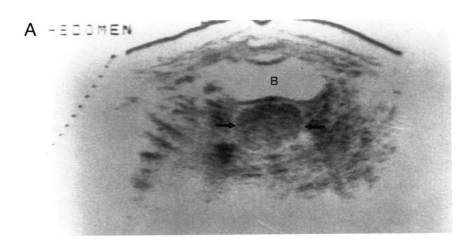

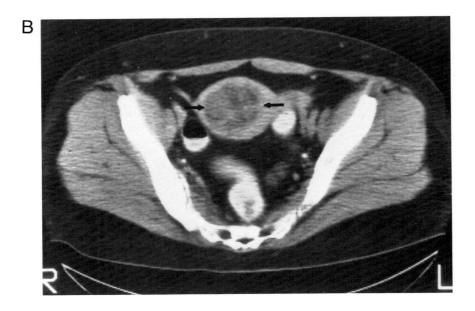

FIG 6–15.

Intramural myoma. This 51-year-old woman had a known diagnosis of Gardner's syndrome. Pelvic examination revealed an enlarged uterus.

A, the transverse sonogram through the bladder *(B)* shows an echogenic mass *(arrows)* within the uterus.

B, the corresponding CT examination demonstrates a mass *(arrows)* of inhomogenious low attenuation within the uterus. These findings corresponded with those of ultrasound. The diagnosis was a uterine fibroid.

A hysterectomy revealed a 7 × 6 × 5 cm intramural myoma.

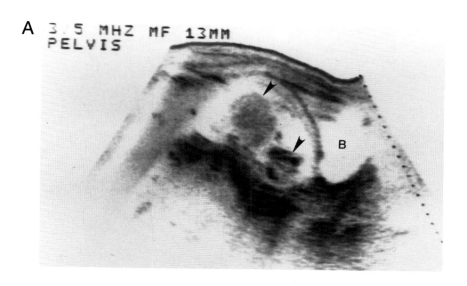

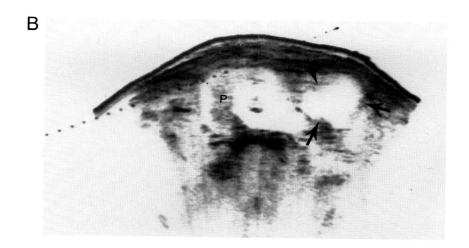

FIG 6–16.

Degenerated, pedunculated fibroid coexistent with pregnancy. A 32-year-old woman who was 13 weeks' pregnant (gravida 1) presented to our institution with a left adnexal mass.

A, the sagittal sonogram of the pelvis, taken through the bladder *(B)*, shows a live fetus *(arrowheads)*.

B, the transverse sonogram shows a left cystic adnexal mass *(arrows)*. Placenta *(P)* is seen in the lateral wall of the uterine cavity. An ovarian mass of uncertain etiology was diagnosed.

The patient was operated on, at which time a degenerated, pedunculated fibroid measuring 11 × 6 × 6 cm was found on the anterior surface of the uterus.

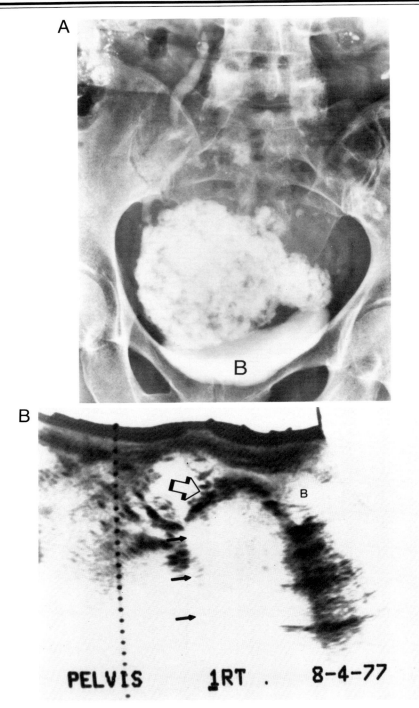

FIG 6–17.
Calcified uterine fibroids. On physical examination, a 77-year-old woman was found to have a firm, globular mass involving the uterus.
    A, on excretory urography, a large calcified mass is seen superior to the bladder *(B).*

B, a sagittal sonogram through the urinary bladder *(B)* shows a heavily calcified mass *(large arrow)* with distal shadowing *(small arrows),* findings consistent with a calcified fibroid.
Conservative management by follow-up alone was used.

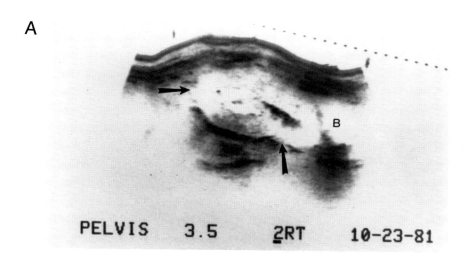

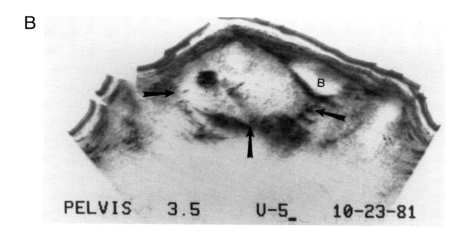

FIG 6–18.

Endometrial carcinoma with hematometra. An 80-year-old woman presented with a large pelvic mass. The physical examination distinguished a 20-cm mass in the pelvis and a 1-cm mass in the posterior vagina.

A, the midline sagittal sonogram reveals a 15 × 9 × 12 cm uterine mass *(arrow)* extending above the filled urinary bladder *(B).*

B, a transverse scan demonstrates the large mass *(arrows)* with marked irregularity of the central endometrial canal. Both cystic and echogenic areas are present because of hemorrhage and debris (*B,* bladder).

When a transvaginal biopsy of the mass was performed, 1 L of blood drained from the uterine cavity. The diagnosis was adenocarcinoma of the endometrium. The patient refused surgery and died of disease.

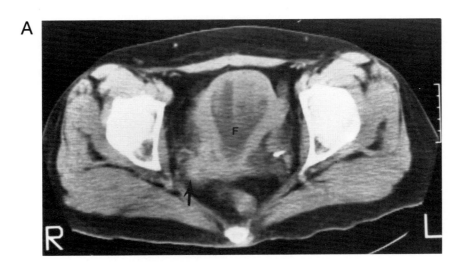

FIG 6–19.

Endometrial carcinoma (two cases).

A and **B,** this 43-year-old woman presented with a pelvic mass and a history of cervical carcinoma treated by radiotherapy five years previously.

A, the CT scan reveals an enlarged uterus with a thickened, irregular, nodular wall. The central low density *(F)* is due to blood, secretions, or both. Posteriorly on the right side *(arrow),* there is tumor extension into the fat. The patient underwent hysterectomy and subsequent chemotherapy.

B, the surgical specimen is shown here (see also Color Plate 30). The uterus measured 8 × 6.5 × 5 cm. The central endometrial cavity is filled by a 7 × 5 × 3 cm tumor *(arrows)* proved to be adenocarcinoma. It is attached to the uterine fundus, and there is invasion of the myometrium.

The patient is well, and there has been no clinical evidence of tumor recurrence in two years' follow-up.

C, another patient, a 74-year-old woman with endometrial carcinoma, underwent MRI evaluation as a part of staging tumor workup. The midline T$_2$-weighted sagittal image (TR/TE, 2,000/90) shows infiltration of the anterior wall of the uterus by the neoplasm *(arrows).* The tumor clearly invades the anterior myometrium, causing loss of the normal three different layers, as seen here in the posterior wall *(open arrows).* Also, the endometrial cavity *(EC)* is seen; it may contain some blood product. (**C** courtesy of Steven Harms, M.D., Department of Radiology, Baylor University Medical Center, Dallas, Tex.)

B

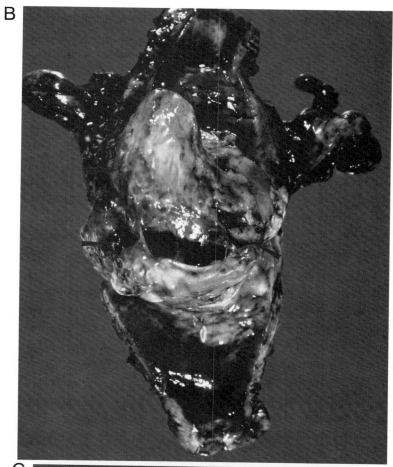

C

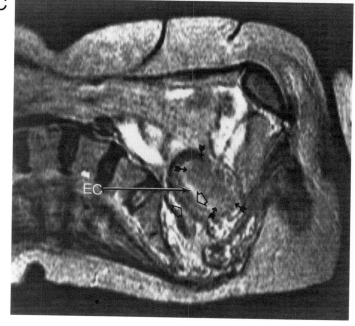

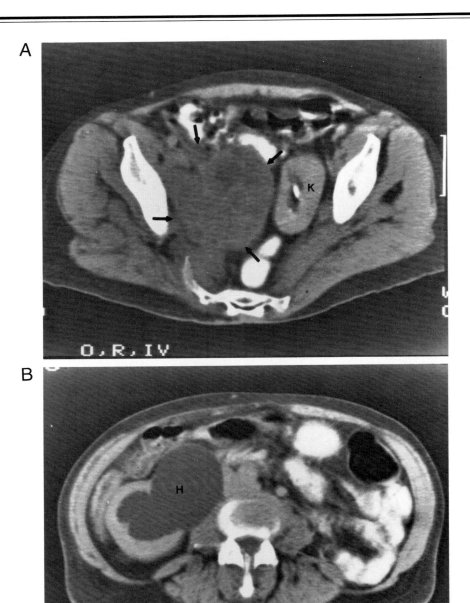

FIG 6–20.
Recurrent endometrial carcinoma, producing hydronephrosis. A gravida 3, para 3 68-year-old woman presented with a pelvic recurrence of endometrial adenocarcinoma. She had undergone hysterectomy and bilateral salpingo-oophorectomy five years earlier; the surgical specimen at that time showed only superficial myometrial invasion.

A, the CT examination shows a large mass *(arrows)* in the pelvis. The mass is inseparable from the adjacent pelvic wall and iliac adenopathy. The tumor also extends posteriorly to the region of the sacrum. Incidentally, note a left pelvic kidney *(K).*

B, higher in the abdomen, a CT image shows marked hydronephrosis *(H)* of the right kidney, secondary to the large pelvic tumor. Percutaneous biopsy proved the recurrent adenocarcinoma.

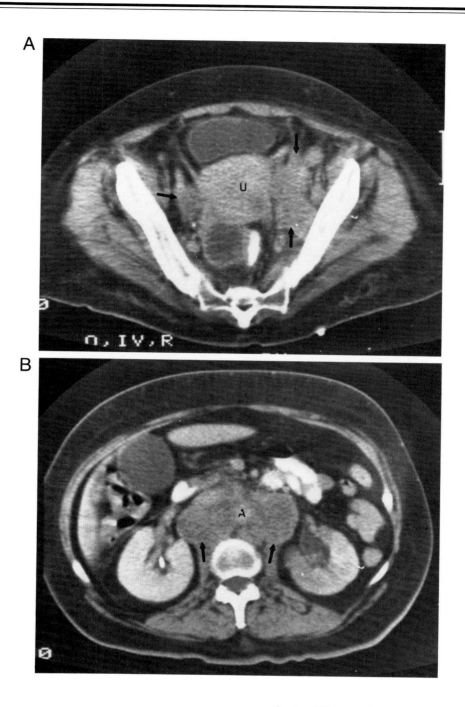

FIG 6–21.

Endometrial carcinoma with extensive pelvic and retroperitoneal adenopathy. A 62-year-old woman presented with a several-month history of abnormal vaginal bleeding, pelvic pain, and a 9.1-kg (20-lb) weight loss. She underwent a dilation and curettage, which showed a grade 3 adenocarcinoma of the endometrium.

A, the CT scan demonstrates a prominent uterus *(U)* infiltrated by tumor. There is bilateral iliac adenopathy *(arrows)*, more on the left than on the right.

B, the higher CT scan shows massive paraaortic adenopathy *(arrows)* engulfing the major vessels and causing left hydronephrosis *(A,* aorta).

Treatment was by chemotherapy.

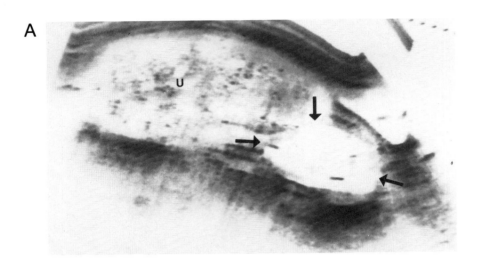

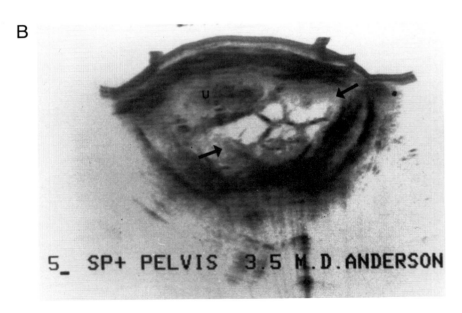

FIG 6–22.
Hydatidiform mole with theca-lutein cysts. A 19-year-old woman had a one-day history of vaginal bleeding and passage of a small amount of tissue from the vagina. She also had a history of amenorrhea for a few weeks.

A, the sagittal sonogram through the bladder and lower abdomen demonstrates an enlarged uterus *(U)* containing multiple echoes with sonolucent areas. A cystic mass *(arrows)* is present inferiorly.

B, the transverse scan in the mid-pelvis demonstrates a multiseptated cyst *(arrows)* inferior and lateral to the large uterus *(U).* The sonographic findings are compatible with hydatidiform mole associated with a theca-lutein cyst.

The uterus was evacuated, and the diagnosis was consistent with molar pregnancy. Subsequent to evacuation, the patient's human chorionic gonadotropin (HCG) titer was rising, and she was treated with methotrexate and actinomycin D.

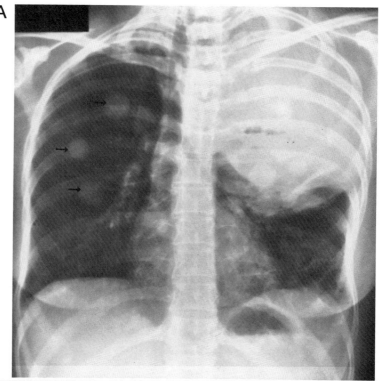

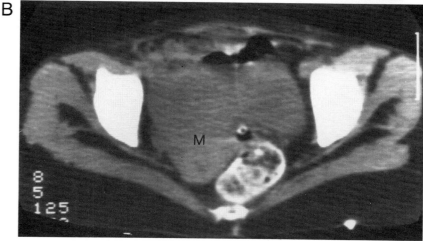

FIG 6–23.

Choriocarcinoma of the uterus, with pulmonary metastases. A 30-year-old gravida 3, para 1, abortion 1 woman was referred because of hemoptysis and lung mass. She also showed left-sided Horner's syndrome and had a palpable pelvic mass. A percutaneous biopsy of the left upper lobe mass revealed choriocarcinoma. The patient had undergone uterine evacuation five years previously for a molar pregnancy.

A, the chest roentgenogram reveals a large mass involving the left upper lung, with multiple small right paren-

chymal metastases *(arrows)*.

B, a CT scan reveals presence of a pelvic mass *(M)* behind the unopacified bladder, proved to represent choriocarcinoma.

Chemotherapy was begun, and subsequently the patient became extremely short of breath and hypoxic. The follow-up chest roentgenogram showed diffuse parenchymal infiltrate, consistent with intraparenchymal bleeding from the metastasis of choriocarcinoma. The patient's condition continued to deteriorate, and she soon died. The primary and hemorrhagic metastases were proved at autopsy.

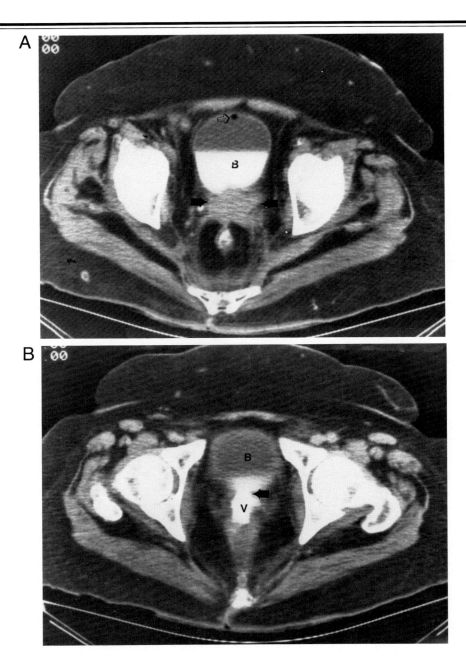

FIG 6–24.
Complicated squamous cell carcinoma of the cervix (two cases).

A, through **C,** a 49-year-old woman was referred with a diagnosis of stage IIIB squamous cell carcinoma of the cervix. She had received external-beam radiotherapy. Some time after the initiation of radiotherapy, the patient developed a rectovaginal fistula, then a rectovesicovaginal fistula. After the development of the latter, she underwent a transverse loop colostomy.

A, the CT scan demonstrates an irregularly shaped mass *(arrows)* in the region of the cervix. There is a small bubble of air *(open arrow)* in the bladder *(B)* because of the fistula.

B, on another CT scan, the fistula *(arrow)* between the bladder *(B)* and vagina *(V)* is seen to cause the contrast to leak into the vagina.

C, a lateral pelvic film made after rectal administration of contrast medium demonstrates a complex fistula between the bladder *(B)*, vagina *(V)*, and rectum *(R)* and a sinus tract *(arrows)* into the presacral space.

D, another patient with carcinoma of the cervix was evaluated by MRI. The T$_2$-weighted axial image (TR/TE, 2,000/80) shows direct extension of the tumor *(arrows)* into the anterior and right lateral wall of the rectum *(R)*. (**D** courtesy of Shirley McCarthy, M.D., Department of Radiology, Yale University, New Haven, Conn.)

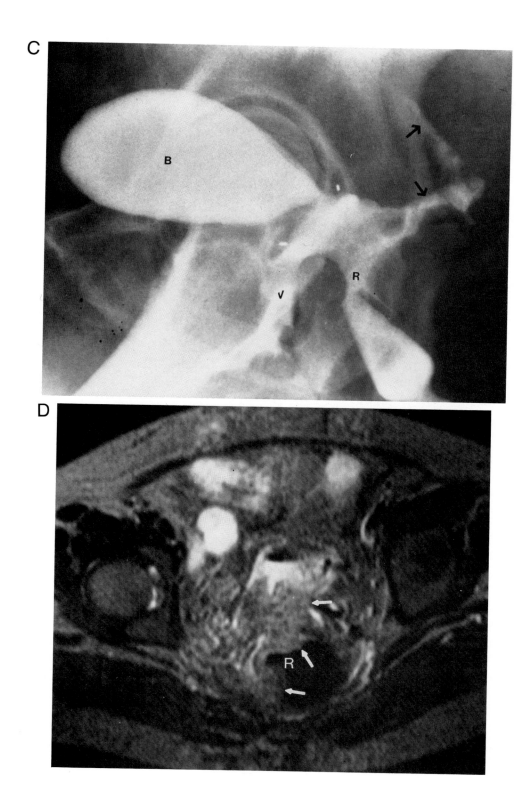

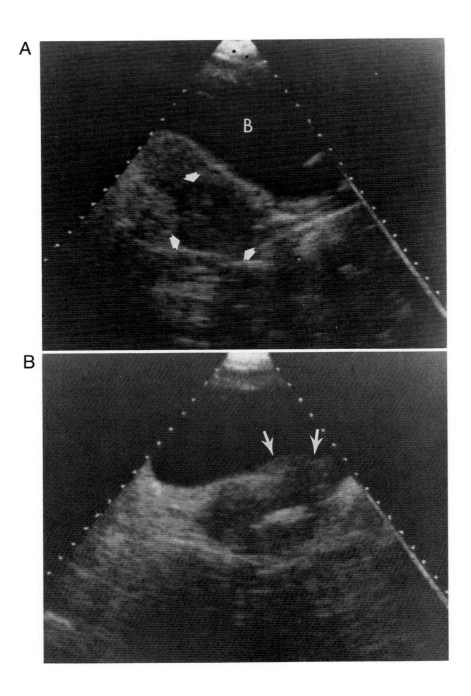

FIG 6–25.
Invasive adenosquamous carcinoma of the cervix. A 27-year-old gravida 0 woman presented with a watery vaginal discharge. Relief was not achieved by treatment with metronidazole and other vaginal preparations. Pelvic examination revealed a 3 × 3 cm mass involving the cervix. Biopsy of the mass revealed adenosquamous carcinoma.

A, the sagittal scan through the bladder *(B)* shows a hypoechoic mass *(arrows)* in the cervix.

B, the transverse scan reveals invasion *(arrows)* of the posterolateral wall of the bladder, proved by cystoscopy.

C

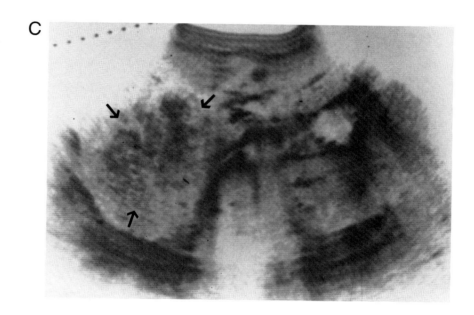

C, a transverse sonogram of the abdomen shows an echogenic hepatic mass, proved to be metastasis *(arrows).* There was also left hydronephrosis. The lesion proved to be stage IIIB carcinoma of the cervix.

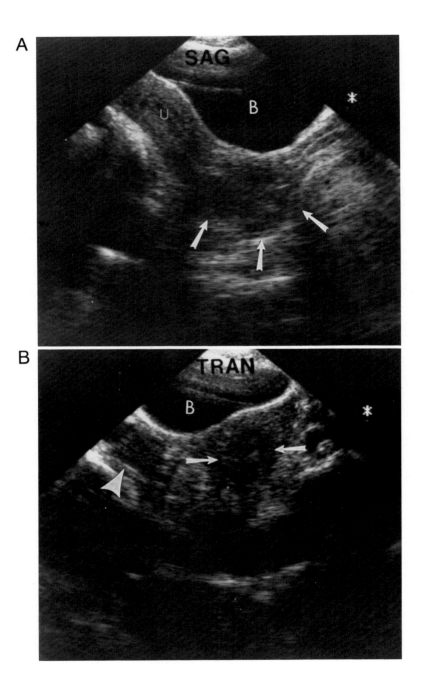

FIG 6–26.
Small cell carcinoma of the cervix. A 29-year-old gravida 2, abortion 2 woman presented with intermenstrual bleeding while on birth control pills. Physical examination showed a large mass in the cervix.

A, the sagittal midline sonogram through the bladder *(B)* reveals a hypoechoic mass *(arrows)* in the cervix. The normal uterus *(U)* is seen.

B, the transverse scan shows right iliac adenopathy *(arrowhead).* The upper portion of the cervical mass *(arrows)* is shown *(B, bladder).*

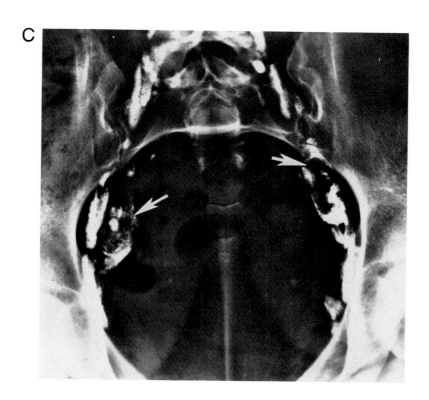

C

C, the lymphangiogram shows metastases in the iliac nodes *(arrows)* bilaterally.

Pelvic radiotherapy and systemic chemotherapy did not prevent subsequent hepatic and skeletal metastasis.

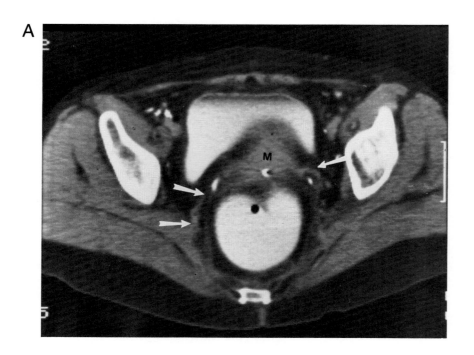

FIG 6–27.
Squamous cell carcinoma of the cervix (two cases).

A and **B,** a gravida 10, para 2 44-year-old woman presented with vaginal bleeding. Physical examination showed an ulcerative mass in the cervix with thickening of the left parametrium and nodularity of the right side. The lesion was clinically staged as IIB.

The CT scan **(A)** shows a small mass *(M)* in the cervix with periureteral extension, thickening of the adnexa *(arrow),* and thickened nodular right uterosacral ligament *(paired arrows).*

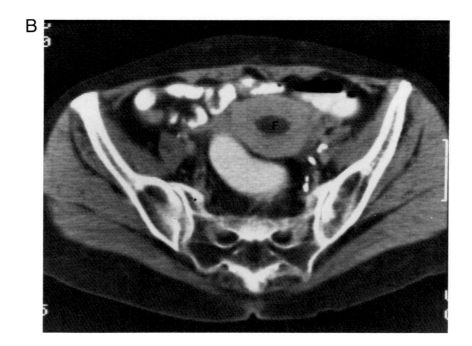

The scan of the uterus **(B)** shows retained secretions *(F)* within the endometrial cavity.

The clinical staging was confirmed by the CT scan. Bi-opsy proved diagnosis of squamous carcinoma of the cervix. (*Continued.*)

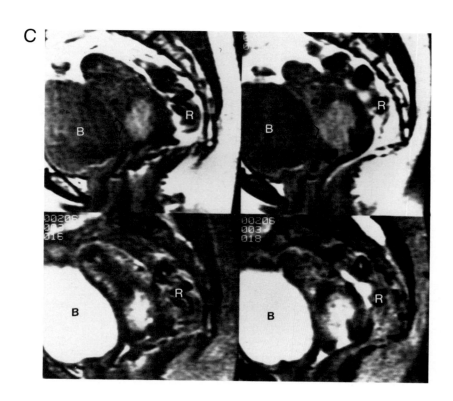

FIG 6–27 (cont.).

C through **E,** a 47-year-old woman was found to have an irregular cervical mass.

Multiple sagittal midline magnetic resonance images **(C)** using T₁-weighted (*top row,* TR/TE, 800/25) and T₂-weighted (*bottom row,* TR/TE, 2,000/80) images demonstrate an infiltrating mass *(open arrow)* in the region of the uterine cervix extending superiorly into the uterus body. The mass displays higher signal intensity on T₂. There is no evidence of obstruction of the endometrial cavity. The tumor does not appear to extend anteriorly into the bladder *(B)* or

posteriorly into the rectum *(R).*

Axial proton-density (*top row,* TR/TE, 2,000/40) and T₂-weighted (*bottom row,* TR/TE, 2,000/80) images **(D)** demonstrate the high-signal-intensity mass *(open arrows)* to be confined to the uterine cervix. A single enlarged node *(arrow)* is seen in the right iliac region.

Bipedal lymphangiography **(E)** demonstrates multiple abnormal nodes in the right external iliac region *(arrows)* corresponding to the abnormal findings on MRI.

Biopsy proved squamous cell carcinoma of the cervix.

D

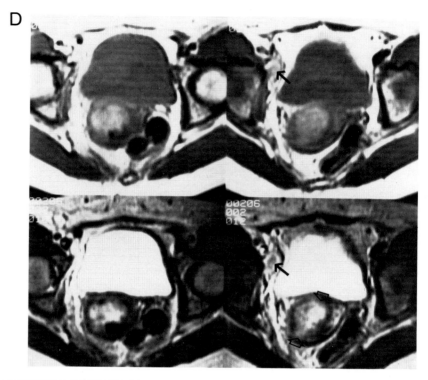

E

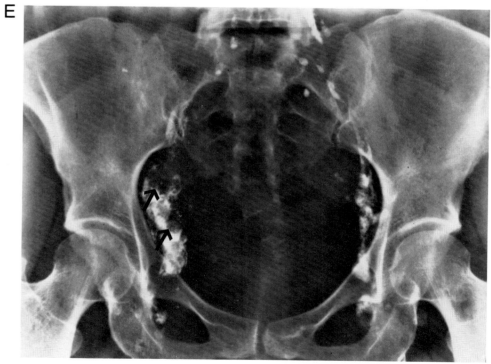

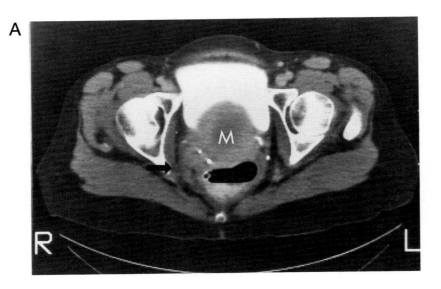

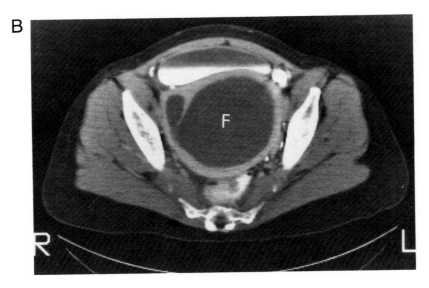

FIG 6–28.
Adenosquamous carcinoma of the cervix (two cases).

A through **C,** a 50-year-old woman was referred because of class III findings on a Papanicolaou smear and a history of light-brownish vaginal discharge. On physical examination, the uterus, which was not tender, was the size of an eight- to ten-week pregnancy. The uterus could not be probed.

The CT scan **(A)** shows a large cervical mass *(M)* with extension to the right pelvic sidewall *(arrow).*

The scan of the uterus **(B)** shows marked distention of the endometrial cavity with fluid *(F).*

The CT findings were confirmed by a transverse sonogram **(C)**, which shows fluid *(F)* in the endometrial cavity *(B, bladder).*

Biopsy showed poorly differentiated adenosquamous carcinoma of the cervix with metastases to the vagina. Obstruction of the cervical os by the tumor and cervical stenosis had caused the hydrometra.

D, MRI was done in another patient, who had cervical carcinoma invading the rectum. On this midline sagittal T_2-weighted image (TR/TE, 2,000/80), the primary tumor is seen as an ill-defined mass *(open arrows)* with intermediate signal intensity. It infiltrates into the anterior wall of the rectum *(arrowheads)* and because of obstruction of the cervical canal has resulted in dilatation of the uterus. The air-fluid *(AF)* level in the distended uterus proved to be due to infection. The normal bladder *(B)* is seen anteriorly. (**D** courtesy of Shirley McCarthy, M.D., Department of Radiology, Yale University, New Haven, Conn.)

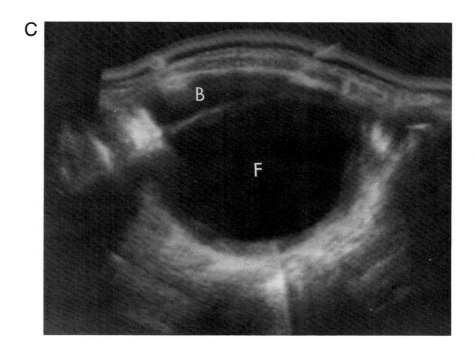

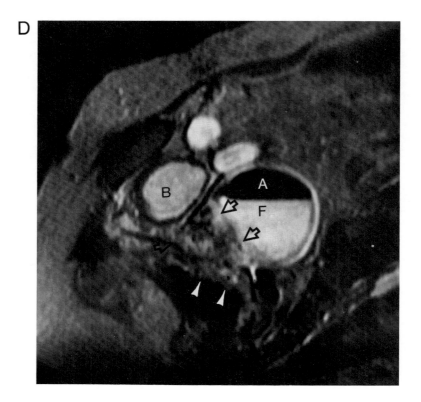

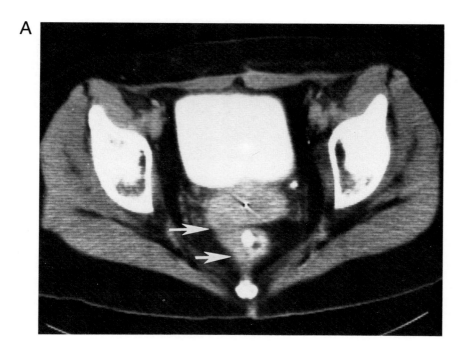

FIG 6–29.
Recurrent cervical cancer. A gravida 2, para 2 35-year-old woman presented with stage I adenocarcinoma of the cervix. After both external (4,000 cGy) and intracavitary radiotherapy, the patient was without symptoms for approximately two years, when she developed back pain of increasing severity.

A, a CT scan shows a soft tissue mass involving the cervix, with marked thickening *(arrows)* of the right uterosacral ligament.

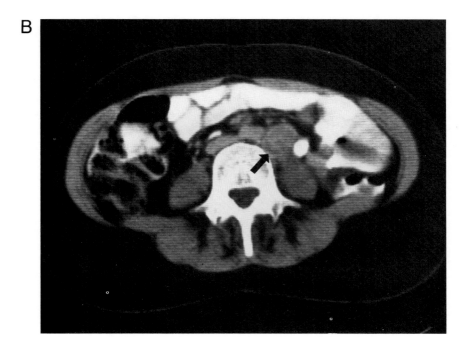

B, left paraaortic adenopathy *(arrow)* is also seen.

A percutaneous needle aspiration under CT guidance confirmed that the paraaortic node was involved by metastatic carcinoma of the cervix.

The patient responded well to six courses of 5-fluoro-uracil, doxorubicin, and cisplatin, but one year later she presented with metastases in the right breast, left supraclavicular nodes, and left thigh.

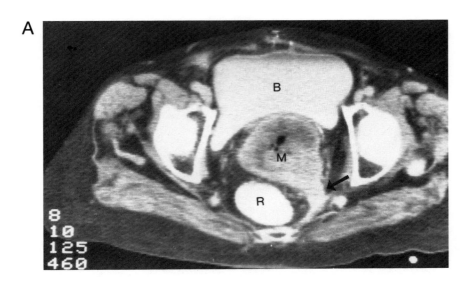

FIG 6–30.
Squamous cell carcinoma of the vagina. A 75-year-old woman presented with a history of vaginal discharge, pain on defecation, and constipation. She had history of total abdominal hysterectomy and bilateral salpingo-oophorectomy for a fibroid uterus. On examination, she was found to have a large tumor mass in the vaginal vault invading the rectovaginal septum and the left parametrial tissues.

A, the CT scan demonstrates a large mass of mixed attenuation *(M)* between the rectum *(R)* and bladder *(B)* with extension to the left pelvic sidewall *(arrow)*. A small collection of air due to the recent biopsy was present.

B, the more inferior scan shows the large mass *(M)* in the vagina displacing the rectum *(arrow)*.

A regimen of intraarterially infused mitomycin C, bleomycin, and cisplatin was begun. After several courses of chemotherapy, the tumor was markedly reduced in size.

C, a follow-up CT scan shows marked reduction in the size of the tumor with minimal residual soft tissue density *(arrows)* between the bladder *(B)* and rectum *(R)*. There was no definite residual tumor on biopsy.

B

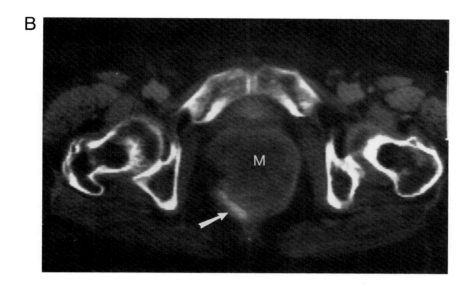

C

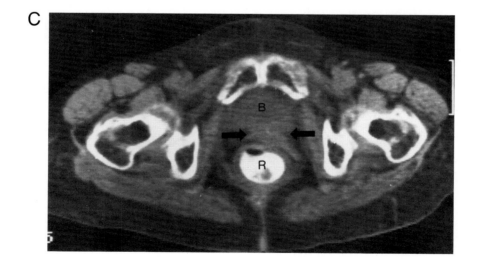

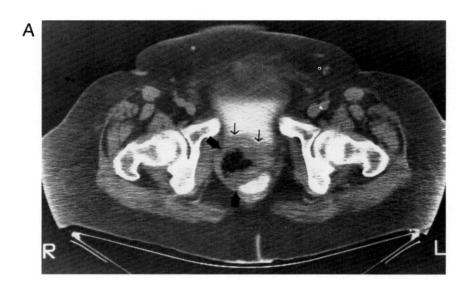

FIG 6–31.
Squamous carcinoma of the vagina (two cases).

A, this 70-year-old woman presented with vaginal spotting. She had a history of total abdominal hysterectomy and bilateral salpingo-oophorectomy 24 years prior to this presentation for atypical hyperplasia of the cervix. On examination, a necrotic tumor mass was present in the vaginal vault, with involvement of the right vaginal sidewall and floor of the vagina. Cystoscopic examination showed invasion of the bladder by tumor.

The CT scan demonstrates a large necrotic mass *(large arrows),* with collection of air, involving the vaginal wall. Because of anterior invasion, the tissue planes between the vagina and bladder are obliterated, and there is irregularity of the posterior wall *(small arrows)* of the bladder.

B and **C,** another patient, a 69-year-old woman with the biopsy-proved diagnosis of vaginal carcinoma, was referred for MRI study. On midline sagittal T_1-weighted image (TR/TE, 500/24) **(B),** there is a soft tissue mass with intermediate signal intensity *(arrows)* filling the space between the rectum *(R)* and the bladder *(BL).* This mass has replaced the normal collapsed vagina. The normal uterus *(U)* is seen in the midline. On T_2-weighted axial images (TR/TE, 2,000/60) **(C),** the vaginal tumor displays areas of high and low signal intensity *(arrows)* infiltrating into the perirectal fat *(R,* rectum). The top transverse image in **C** corresponds with the level of the *single long arrow* in **B** and shows the uterine cervix *(dotted arrow).* (**B** and **C** courtesy of Steven Harms, M.D., Department of Radiology, Baylor University Medical Center, Dallas, Tex.)

B

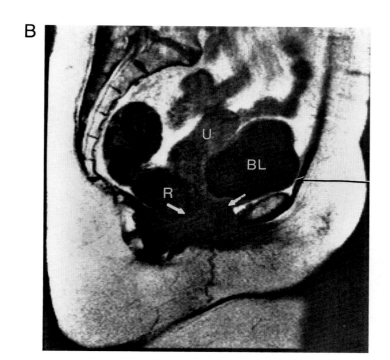

C

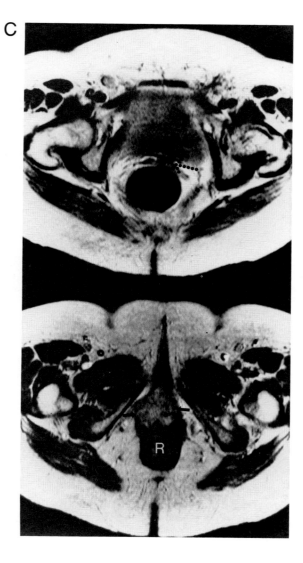

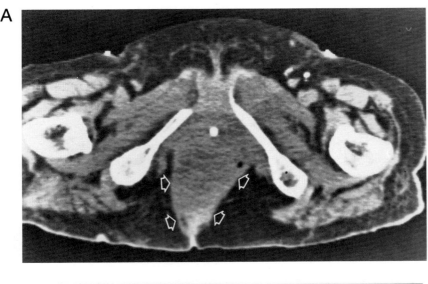

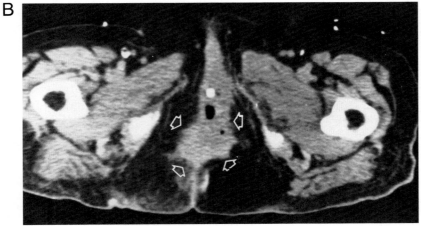

FIG 6–32.
Squamous cell carcinoma of the cervix, metastatic to the vagina and vulva. A 58-year-old gravida 16, para 15 woman presented with stage IIA squamous cell carcinoma of the cervix. After treatment with 4,000 cGy to the whole pelvis followed by intracavitary therapy, the patient did well for approximately one year, when she noted a mass involving the vulva and vagina. Physical examination revealed an exophytic, friable tumor that extended from the urethra to the left lateral border of the labia majora and inferiorly to the introitus on the left. Biopsy revealed recurrent grade 3 squamous cell carcinoma.

A and **B,** two years after the initial presentation, the CT scan shows a large soft tissue mass *(open arrows)* that in-volves the urethra, vagina, and introitus and that extends posteriorly around the rectum.

C and **D,** the computed angiotomogram preparatory to selective intraarterial chemotherapy demonstrates enhancement *(arrows)* due to the blood supply to the hypervascular components of the tumor. This procedure is to assure the proper delivery of chemotherapy via the arterial blood supply to the neoplasm.

Following excellent response to a regimen of intraarterial mitomycin C, bleomycin, and cisplatin, the patient underwent total pelvic exenteration and radical vulvectomy with reconstruction of the vagina with bilateral gracilis myocutaneous flaps. At present, the patient is alive and well.

C

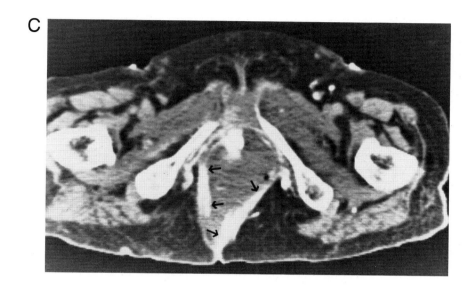

D

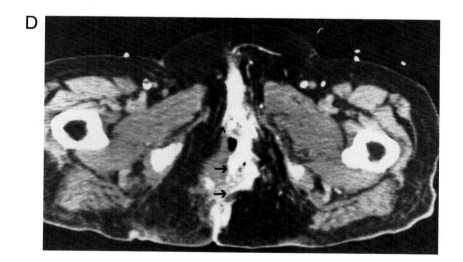

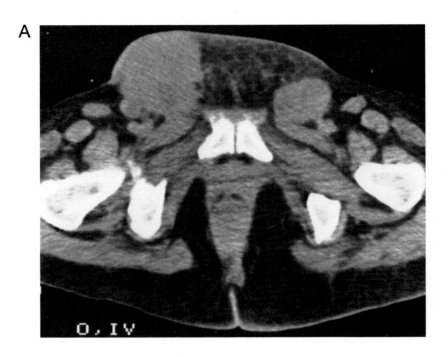

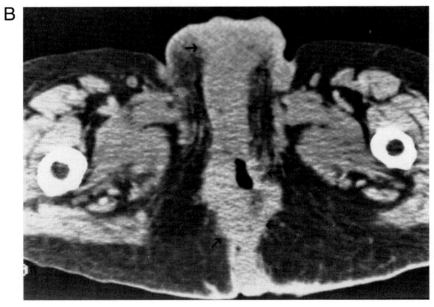

FIG 6–33.
Invasive vulvar carcinoma. A gravida 1, para 1 41-year-old woman presented with a vulvar mass and palpable inguinal nodes. There was drainage at both sites, and the initial diagnosis was lymphogranuloma venereum. Examination revealed an exophytic, necrotic, friable tumor involving the labia bilaterally, the perineal body, and the perianal area. Bimanual examination revealed involvement of the vagina and rectovaginal septum. The pathologic diagnosis was stage IV vulvar squamous cell carcinoma.

A through **C,** the CT images show extensive adenopathy in the inguinal areas *(large arrows)* and pelvis. By direct extension, the tumor involves the rectovaginal junction on both sides and infiltrates into the perineum and to the left buttock (*arrows* in **C**).

D, the lateral barium enema image reveals involvement of the wall of the rectum *(arrows)*. There is tumor for a distance of approximately 5 cm. (*Continued.*)

C

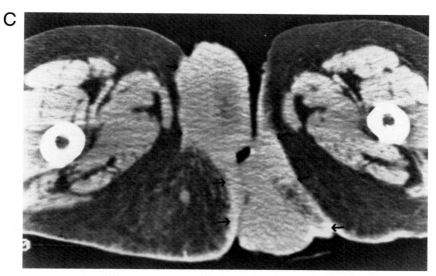

D

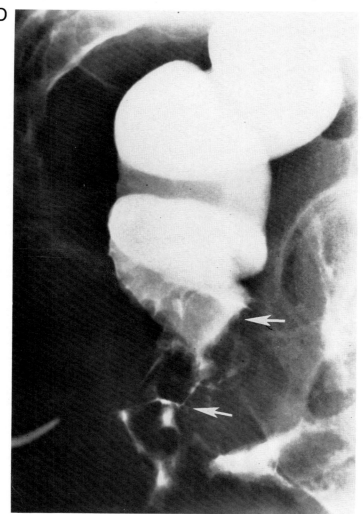

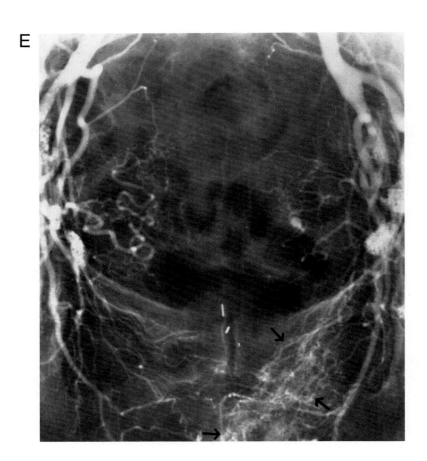

FIG 6–33 (cont.).

E, bilateral iliac arteriogram demonstrates areas of hypervascularity and neovascularity *(arrows)* in the region of the vulva and inguinal areas, particularly in the left. The main blood supply is from the internal pudendal arteries.

In view of the extensive perineal and nodal involvement, traditional radiotherapy or surgery would have been inadequate. Intraarterial chemotherapy with mitomycin C, bleomycin, and cisplatin was used in an attempt to reduce the size of the tumor.

F through **H,** follow-up CT scans show marked tumor response after several courses of chemotherapy The images were used for radiation therapy planning.

Chemotherapy was followed by radiotherapy, and there was dramatic response after both treatments.

F

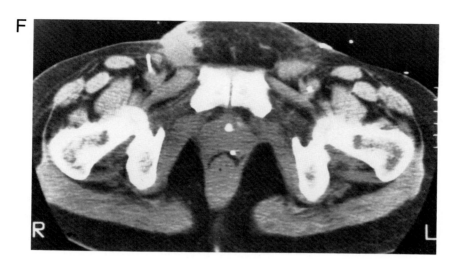

G

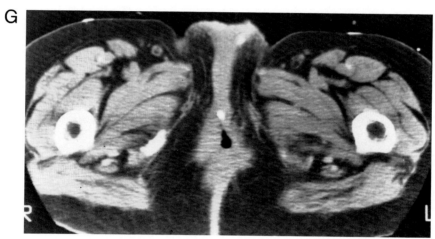

H

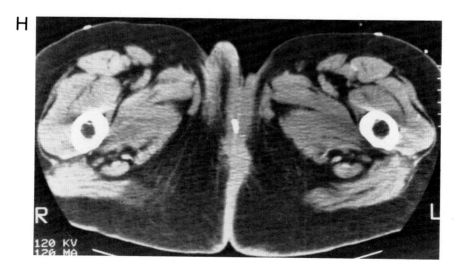

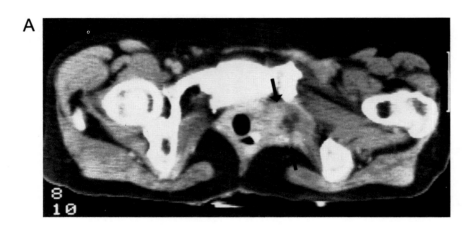

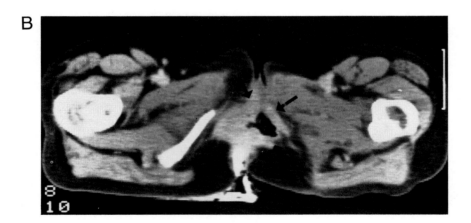

FIG 6–34.

Recurrent carcinoma of Bartholin's gland. Twenty years before presentation, this patient underwent a total abdominal hysterectomy for carcinoma in situ of the cervix. Sixteen years after that surgery, she was diagnosed as having squamous cell carcinoma of the left Bartholin's gland, which was treated with left hemivulvectomy and inguinal node dissection, followed by radiotherapy. The present workup was initiated because of a recurrent mass in the area of the left Bartholin's gland.

A and **B,** the CT scans show a soft tissue mass *(arrows)* with an area of decreased attenuation on the left side of the vaginal wall. The mass appears to also involve the internal obturator muscle, and there is a suggestion of bone involvement.

Muscle involvement and bone involvement were confirmed at surgical exploration. The mass measured 3 × 2 cm and was fixed to the pubic bone. It was deemed inoperable.

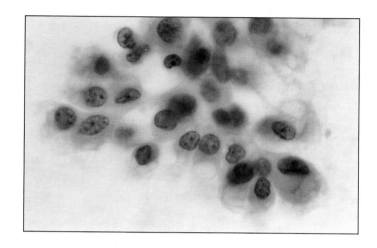

PLATE 29

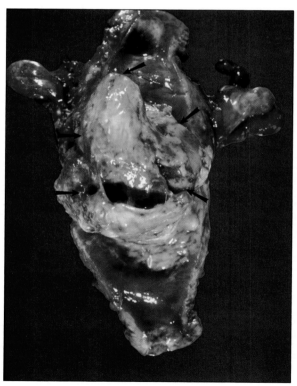

PLATE 30

7

Adrenal Gland Neoplasms

Ali Shirkhoda, M.D.

The diagnosis and differentiation of adrenal masses have always been difficult for clinicians because of the deep-seated location of the glands. The two adrenals are within the perirenal fat inside the Gerota's fasciae, superior, anterior, and medial to the kidneys. Their location and the infrequency of their tumor-related functional disturbance often delay recognition of involvement by primary or metastatic disease.

Adrenal lesions are not commonly encountered in the routine practice of radiology, but they are now being identified more frequently because of the availability of computed tomography (CT), ultrasound, and, more recently, magnetic resonance imaging (MRI).[1] The large number of imaging techniques used to demonstrate adrenal lesions, in fact, reflects the limitations of any given method. In patients in whom there is chemical or clinical evidence of adrenal dysfunction, morphological delineation of the gland is particularly valuable.

The conventional methods such as plain abdominal films, excretory urography, and, particularly, angiography do provide significant information for the diagnosis and management of adrenal masses. The plain abdominal film may show an adrenal mass with calcification in patients with cyst, teratoma, carcinoma, or neuroblastoma. However, calcification is unusual in pheochromocytoma, is rare in adenoma, and does not occur in hyperplasia.[2] Approximately 15% of adrenal tumors larger than 15 cm in diameter display areas of calcification. Urography combined with tomography may show adrenal masses larger than 2 cm in diameter and can be up to 70% accurate in diagnosing adrenal tumors.[3] This study is recommended only when such modalities as CT and ultrasound are not available.

Vascular studies are not usually used as the primary modality in diagnosing adrenal masses. Angiography is commonly employed preoperatively for documentation of adrenal masses, particularly of the vascular neoplasms such as pheochromocytoma and adrenal cortical carcinoma. However, according to several investigators, the angiographic appearance of adrenal tumors is not helpful in distinguishing the histology of the neoplasm, and the presence of tumor vessels does not necessarily imply that the adrenal mass has a malignant nature.[4-7] Venography is used to identify smaller tumors, since they usually act as an avascular, space-occupying lesion. By this technique, lesions as small as 5 mm can be recognized, and, in cases of functioning adenoma, blood samples can be collected for hormone analysis.[6, 8]

Such imaging techniques as adrenal scintigraphy, ultrasonography, and CT have been used more frequently, and CT in particular has replaced many other diagnostic methods. In one series, radionuclide studies with a high degree of specificity demonstrated whether the underlying adrenal mass was due to hyperplasia, carcinoma, or adenoma in nearly 95% of patients with Cushing's syndrome.[9] More recently, agents such as iodine 131–*meta*-iodobenzyl-guanidine (^{131}I-MIBG) have been used to make specific diagnosis of and also to localize and treat adrenergic tumors such as pheochromocytoma.[10-12]

However, radionuclide studies of adrenals are lengthy and deliver a large amount of radiation to the glands.[13]

Ultrasonography of the adrenals requires expertise but can determine whether the nature of an adrenal mass is cystic or solid. The accuracy of ultrasound in these studies is 70%, with a sensitivity of 79% and a specificity of 61%.[14] The role of ultrasound is generally that of a screening procedure.

Scanning by CT, which is now widely used as the initial diagnostic modality in the evaluation of the adrenals, can detect the normal glands in nearly 100% of patients.[15] It is advisable to scan the patient's adrenal region at a slice thickness of 4 to 7 mm without any interval between images. Abrams et al. reported a sensitivity of 84%, specificity of 98%, and overall accuracy of 90% for CT of the adrenals,[14] but those parameters are now probably even higher with the development of new-generation scanners. The very high accuracy of CT means that it is the first and often the only diagnostic modality used in patients suspected of having adrenal neoplasm.[16, 17] Except in cases of microscopic lesions (e.g., metastases that do not alter the configuration of the glands), a normal CT study rules out adrenal tumor at a high confidence level.

Magnetic resonance imaging is able to show the normal adrenal glands in 95% of subjects.[19] This modality is now widely advocated for diagnosis and differentiation of various adrenal masses.[1] It is able to display different signal intensities on different pulse sequences based on the nature of the adrenal mass. In particular, its sensitivity in differentiating adrenal metastases, adenoma, and pheochromocytoma has been emphasized.[1, 20]

This chapter discusses and illustrates neoplasms of the adrenal glands. Pediatric tumors (e.g., neuroblastoma) are discussed in Chapter 8. The value of MRI is further emphasized in Chapter 12.

BENIGN ADRENAL NEOPLASMS

Benign neoplasms in the adrenal glands are either functional or nonfunctional. Increasingly, the latter tumors are being discovered incidentally through the use of sophisticated radiologic examinations, in particular high-resolution CT.

Cortical Adenomas

Nonfunctional cortical adenomas are usually single and unilateral (Figs 7–1 and 7–2), although occasionally they are bilateral (Fig 7–3). They represent a localized overgrowth of cortical cells that is probably due to the alteration of the cortical structure associated with advancing age. They are the most common primary adrenal lesion; as seen grossly or examined microscopically at autopsy, they occur in 3% to 64% of the population.[21, 22] The nonfunctional adenomas are frequently reported to be present in patients with hypertension (Fig 7–4), cardiovascular disease, or renal cell carcinoma.[21, 23]

Functional cortical adenomas may produce one of a variety of endocrine disorders, including virilization, hyperaldosteronism (Fig 7–5), and Cushing's syndrome. Cortical adenomas account for 10% of Cushing's syndrome cases[15]; as a result of adrenocorticotropic hormone suppression, the contralateral gland is usually smaller than normal.

The cortical adenomas may calcify (Figs 7–1 and 7–2) and should be differentiated from such other calcified adrenal lesions as adrenal carcinoma (Figs 7–29 and 7–30), pheochromocytoma, and such conditions as hemorrhage, cyst, and granuloma. Those that are not calcified may prove enigmatic in a cancer patient and would require additional studies such as MRI (Fig 7–4) or biopsy. It has been shown that MRI is able to distinguish adrenal adenomas from metastasis, carcinoma, and pheochromocytoma. This is accomplished by evaluating the ratio of the signal intensity of the adrenal mass to that of the liver (see Figs 7–4 and 7–21)[20] or retroperitoneal fat.[19]

The subject of incidental discovery of adrenal nodule and its management will be discussed at the end of the chapter. However, unlike metastases, adenomas are usually less than 3 cm in diameter (Fig 7–3).[24] Large adenomas are extremely rare (Fig 7–4), although examples as large as 7.5 cm have been reported.[25]

Aldosteronoma is functioning adrenal adenoma associated with clinical symptoms of hyperaldosteronism. Between 65% and 75% of cases of primary hyperaldosteronism are associated with unilateral benign cortical adenoma.[26, 27] Other causes of aldosteronism are malignant tumors and hyperplasia of the zona glomerulosa. Typically, the adenoma is a unilateral, small tumor, often less than 1 cm (Figs 7–5 and 7–6) and rarely more than 2.5 cm in diameter. Multiple or bilateral adenomas are occasionally found. Adrenocortical carcinoma is an uncommon cause of primary aldosteronism; however, approximately 5% of patients in a large series were found to have malignant tumor.[28]

Hyperaldosteronism, or Conn's syndrome, is

characterized by hypertension, hypokalemia, increased aldosterone production, and absent or subnormal plasma renin activity. Size and density of aldosteronomas are the two major factors that might contribute to the difficulty in their diagnosis by CT. Their usually small size (<1 cm) necessitates fine collimation and overlapping CT cuts to achieve a high detection rate. These cortical adenomas have a high cholesterol content, which may yield low CT attenuation values,[29] as in a cyst.[8] Although venous sampling remains the most sensitive test, CT can detect aldosteronomas in 70% to 80% of patients.[8, 30] If CT results are normal or nondiagnostic, or if confirmation of adrenal CT results seems necessary, adrenal venous sampling (Fig 7–5) should be the next procedure.[19]

Myelolipoma, Cysts, and Hemorrhage

Other benign adrenal nodules such as myelolipoma and adrenal cysts have distinctive characteristics on CT.

Myelolipoma (Fig 7–7) of the adrenal gland is a rare, benign, biochemically nonfunctioning tumor made up of both fat and myeloid and erythroid elements. Although most of these tumors are small and reported in autopsy series, larger lesions may become symptomatic or present as a palpable mass. The CT and ultrasound appearances of a fatty adrenal mass with or without associated calcification should suggest the diagnosis.[31, 32] Rarely, it may become necessary to do fine-needle aspiration biopsy to establish the diagnosis (and eliminate the need for surgery).[33]

Adrenal cysts (Fig 7–8) are usually well-defined, homogeneous masses that can easily be aspirated for diagnostic confirmation.[34] They can be very large and be surrounded by fibrous tissue with calcification. Occasionally, it is difficult to differentiate an adrenal cyst from a renal cyst on axial CT scanning and parasagittal sonography becomes necessary.

Adrenal hemorrhage (Fig 7–9), which can be spontaneous or result from trauma, is more common in infants because of the large size of their adrenal glands.[35] Ultrasound usually shows a mass with internal echo, occasionally with separation of clot and serum. In fresh hemorrhage, CT will show the high density of blood.

Pheochromocytoma

Pheochromocytomas are functioning tumors that most commonly occur in the adrenal medulla. In adults, about 90% of pheochromocytomas are located within the adrenal gland (Figs 7–10 and 7–11); in children, about 30% are extraadrenal. Extraadrenal pheochromocytomas can be found anywhere from the base of the skull to the anus but are most frequently seen in the organs of Zuckerkandl, mediastinum, or urinary bladder.[36–39] Pheochromocytomas are bilateral in 5% to 10% of cases and multicentric in 10%.[40, 41] In children, the incidence of bilateral disease is 20%.

These tumors are malignant in 10% to 30% of cases in adults (Fig 7–12),[42] and the incidence of malignancy is higher in children.[36] They secrete abnormal amounts of catecholamines and are associated with a rare but dramatic syndrome of variable hypertension and episodic attacks of tachycardia, diaphoresis, and anxiety.[43, 44] Pheochromocytomas can be associated with neurofibromatosis; they can also be an integrated part of the multiple endocrine neoplasia (MEN) type IIA or IIB syndrome (Fig 7–13),[38, 45] in which bilateral tumors (Fig 7–14) are the rule rather than the exception, occurring in 75% of cases.[46] The MEN type IIA syndrome is characterized by medullary thyroid carcinoma, pheochromocytoma, and parathyroid hyperplasia or adenoma (Fig 7–13). Patients with MEN type IIB syndrome also have medullary thyroid carcinoma and pheochromocytoma, but associated multiple mucosal neuromas, ganglioneuromatosis of the gastrointestinal tract, a marfanoid body habitus (Fig 7–14), and absence of parathyroid hyperplasia[47, 48] are distinctive in these cases. With MEN type I syndrome, there are reported cases of pheochromocytoma,[49] neurofibromatosis, von Hippel-Lindau disease,[50] and carcinoids of the gastrointestinal tract and bronchus.[49, 51]

Intravenous pyelography (Fig 7–10) has been useful in suggesting the diagnosis of pheochromocytoma,[3] angiography (Fig 7–11) in confirming the diagnosis,[52] and scintigraphy (Figs 7–12 and 7–13) in detecting the site or sites of involvement.[10, 53] The tendency for patients to have a marked increase in blood pressure after injection of contrast material into a blood vessel feeding the tumor can be considered either a deleterious effect of the procedure or a valuable provocative test.[54]

The newly introduced scintigraphy that uses ^{131}I-MIBG to image pheochromocytomas is an excellent way to diagnose and properly localize the tumor regardless of its location or size (Figs 7–12 and 7–13). This agent is an adrenergic tissue-localizing radiopharmaceutical that has a sensitivity of 87% and specificity of 99%[18]; it can show tumors as small as

0.2 g[10] and can also be used to detect metastatic malignant pheochromocytoma.[55] As previously mentioned, it has been more recently introduced as a treatment agent into the protocols for such adrenergic tumors as neuroblastomas.[11] McEwan et al.[11] recommend ^{131}I-MIBG imaging even in cases of CT-proved adrenal masses because it serves to (1) provide information about the function of the mass, (2) screen multifocal or bilateral disease, and (3) exclude metastases.

Computed tomography (Figs 7–10 to 7–14) appears to be as accurate as angiography in detecting tumors but without the corollary complications of an iatrogenic hypertension.[53] When there is strong clinical and biochemical evidence of pheochromocytoma and normal or equivocal findings on CT, angiography may become essential to determine an extraadrenal source for tumor, particularly if the organs of Zuckerkandl, pelvis,[56, 57] and chest[58] have been searched by CT. Even under these circumstances, using ^{131}I-MIBG provides more specific information.[18] On CT scan, the pheochromocytoma is typically a well-encapsulated neoplasm of medium size, occasionally with areas of low density (Figs 7–11 and 7–13) and rarely with calcification (Fig 7–12). Ultrasound for detection of this neoplasm can be rewarding provided it is done by an experienced sonographer. On MRI, the pheochromocytoma displays high signal intensity on T_2-weighted spin-echo scans.[1, 20, 59, 60] This modality is the noninvasive way to approach adrenal glands for pheochromocytoma or to search extraadrenal sites, particularly when CT scanning is not desirable.[61]

METASTASES, LYMPHOMA, AND SARCOMA

The adrenal gland has been shown to be a prime site, in relation to its unit weight, for metastases from many malignant tumors.[62] It has been demonstrated that only a small amount of residual adrenal tissue is needed to maintain normal adrenal function[63]; thus, the vast majority of adrenal metastases are silent since they fail to destroy enough tissue to cause symptoms. Typically, they are discovered either incidentally during radiologic survey to assess the extent of tumor spread or at autopsy.

Adrenal metastases occur more frequently in the medullary portion of the gland than in the cortex by a factor of 10 to 1.[64] The most frequent origins are primary breast cancer, lung cancer, and melanoma (Figs 7–15 to 7–21), followed by malignant neoplasms in the stomach, kidneys, pancreas, and colon.[65] In the Abrams et al. series of 1,000 autopsies, adrenal metastases were found in 53% of cases of primary breast carcinoma and in 35% of cases of primary lung carcinoma.[65] There were microscopic or very small metastases, not identifiable by available imaging modalities, in a significant number of these cases. As the length of survival increases among cancer patients, the frequency of detectable adrenal metastases is expected to rise.

Silent adrenal masses that are discovered during the assessment of patients with malignant disease mandate a tissue diagnosis for optimal management (Fig 7–22). Discovery of adrenal metastases may radically alter the initial therapy of certain primary tumors. Since 2% to 3% of the general population has benign adrenal adenoma, many of the cases detectable by abdominal CT, confirmation by pathology of the nature of the adrenal nodule is of prime importance.[23, 24]

Adrenal lymphoma is rarely an isolated lesion. At autopsy the adrenals are seen to be involved in as many as 25% of lymphoma cases, usually by contiguous spread from adjacent organs or nodes. However, the adrenals may contain heterotopic lymphoid elements that may be involved intrinsically by lymphoma.[66, 67] In our experience, their involvement is usually bilateral (Figs 7–23 to 7–26). Adrenal sarcoma is extremely rare (Fig 7–27), and, in most cases, the adrenals are invaded by retroperitoneal sarcomatous tumors.

The diagnostic approach to adrenal metastasis is similar to that for other adrenal masses and should be by CT scanning or ultrasound. In general, discovery of a solid adrenal mass is a nonspecific finding, and although the smaller-sized masses favor a diagnosis of benign adenoma,[24] in an oncologic patient biopsy should be done to rule out malignancy.

Magnetic resonance imaging has been shown to be helpful in differentiating adrenal lesions. Metastases (Fig 7–21), adrenal cortical carcinoma, and pheochromocytoma display a high signal intensity in the mass on T_2-weighted spin-echo scans, whereas adenomas show a low signal intensity similar to that of the liver when the same pulse sequence is used.[20]

ADRENAL CORTICAL CARCINOMA

The incidence of adrenal cortical carcinoma (Figs 7–28 to 7–33) is 1 per 1,700,000 of the general population, or 0.02% of all cancers.[68, 69] The mean age at occurrence is 38 years in males and 28 years in fe-

males. This malignant tumor is often locally extensive or even metastatic at the time of initial diagnosis. Upper abdominal pain and weight loss are frequent complaints at presentation.[70]

About one third of adult patients with adrenal cortical carcinoma have recognizable endocrine syndromes secondary to excess tumor steroid production.[71] In children, the incidence of functional tumor is much higher; according to one report, it can reach 100%.[72] These tumors can be associated with Cushing's syndrome (Figs 7–28 and 7–30), adrenogenital syndrome, or hyperaldosteronism. Those associated with Cushing's syndrome rarely produce the pure syndrome; frequently, there is some virilization, resulting in mixed syndrome. Androgenic effects such as virilization in girls and pseudoprecocious puberty in boys are by far the commonest types of endocrine symptoms seen.[72] Cushing's syndrome, feminization, and hyperaldosteronism are much less common.[73–75] Differentiation of a benign adrenal lesion from a malignant one in a child is difficult with all imaging modalities. Calcification of the tumor (Figs 7–29 to 7–31) and invasion of the kidney (Fig 7–32) may help to diagnose the malignant nature of an adrenal mass.[70, 72, 74, 76] The tumor size is usually very large, with capsular and vascular invasion, and there is a high incidence of recurrence after resection.[77]

Because of the large size of the primary neoplasm, one third to one half of patients with adrenal cortical carcinoma may have a palpable abdominal mass (Fig 7–30), its appearance on CT usually being different from other masses.[70, 71, 78] In one series of 49 cases, reported by King and Lack,[70] the size of the tumor ranged from 5 to 28.5 cm and weight ranged from 33 to 3,100 g. In a more recent study of 26 cases, tumors ranged from 3 to 22 cm.[80] The functioning tumors are usually smaller because they are discovered earlier.[80, 81] However, in the differential diagnosis of a large, bulky mass seen on CT with areas of low density in a patient otherwise without symptoms, one should consider such other conditions as metastases and pheochromocytoma. Computed tomography may also show evidence of direct venous extension of tumor (Fig 7–29), perhaps with occlusion of the renal vein or inferior vena cava. The inferior vena cava is better seen with ultrasound (Fig 7–31), but its visualization on CT can be improved if scanning is performed during and not after the intravenous injection of contrast material.[72] On angiography, these tumors are hypervascular with areas of neovascularity (Figs 7–29, 7–30, and 7–32). Angiography is occasionally used for diagnostic purposes, but it is commonly used for embolization and infarction of the neoplasm.

In all age groups, CT should be the initial diagnostic modality for evaluation of patients suspected of having adrenal cortical carcinoma. This diagnostic modality is also able to define postsurgical local recurrences (Fig 7–33) or metastases.[77]

INCIDENTAL ADRENAL NODULE

The incidentally discovered adrenal nodule in any patient poses an enigma as to its etiology. However, because of the adrenals' susceptibility to metastatic involvement, the possibility of metastasis should be considered seriously when an adrenal nodule or mass is discovered in a cancer patient. These nodules are being detected more frequently because of the increasing use of CT and MRI, with increased numbers of both benign and malignant adrenal lesions seen on workup for metastatic disease.

Adrenal masses in an adult may be cortical adenomas (Figs 7–1 to 7–4), cortical carcinomas (Figs 7–28 to 7–32), pheochromocytomas (Figs 7–10 to 7–14), ganglioneuromas, cysts (Fig 7–8), myelolipomas (Fig 7–7), adenolipomas, or metastases (Figs 7–15 to 7–22) from other tumors.[82]

Unsuspected adrenal masses have been reported in 0.6% of CT studies of the upper abdomen.[83, 84] Among 73 reported patients with adrenal masses incidentally discovered on CT, 3 (4%) had a clinically unsuspected, biochemically active pheochromocytoma.[35, 76, 83, 84] The rest of the masses proved to be lesions for which surgery would not be needed, including 18 (25%) clinically and biochemically silent cortical adenomas, 15 (21%) metastases from known malignancies, 7 cysts, 3 myelolipomas, 1 focal cortical hyperplasia, 1 lymphoma, 1 nonfunctional pheochromocytoma, and 1 lesion shown by surgery to be a neoplasm of the pancreatic tail rather than an adrenal mass. The remaining 23 patients were followed for up to three years without any changes on subsequent CT scans or referable clinical findings.

When an adrenal nodule or mass is incidentally discovered, the first question should be whether the mass is functional or nonfunctional. If the mass produces hormones in sufficient quantity to cause symptoms, it should in most cases be removed whether it is a cortical adenoma, carcinoma, or pheochromocytoma.[85] This removal may be surgical or by means of arterial embolization, as in some cases of adrenal cortical carcinoma. However, nonfunctional masses may be benign or malignant and those that are not malignant may be left in place. Special attention should be paid to cortical carcinomas because, when steroid production is subject to greater scrutiny, the proportion of hormone-producing adrenal cortical carcinomas increases. In other words, when the urinary steroid excretions of patients with clinically nonfunctional carcinoma are examined, many of the patients are found to be producing adrenal steroids in excess.[86, 87] In most cases of patients with Cushing's syndrome caused by adrenal cortical carcinoma, women outnumber men approximately 6 to 4.[88, 89] Among patients with clinically nonfunctional carcinomas, however, there are twice as many men as women. Nonfunctional carcinomas account for about 17% of such neoplasms in children and for about 60% in adults.[87–89]

Pheochromocytoma can also be discovered incidentally; unlike other benign lesions, it can be both elusive and potentially lethal. A 50-year autopsy series from the Mayo Clinic[90] described 41 patients with clinically unsuspected pheochromocytoma. Only 54% had a reported history of hypertension. Thus, the absence of hypertension does not exclude the diagnosis of pheochromocytoma in a patient with incidentally discovered adrenal mass (Fig 7–11,C). In a search for pheochromocytoma, a combination of 24-hr urine analyses for vanillylmandelic acid, metanephrines, and catecholamines should be conducted. Each of these tests is more than 95% sensitive[91]; however, among these, the test for elevated catecholamines has the highest sensitivity.[92]

If the lesion is clinically and biochemically silent, the size is perhaps the most important determinant of its nature. Adenomas usually have a diameter of 3 cm or less.[24] Larger adenomas (Fig 7–4) are extremely rare but have been reported in autopsy series.[25] Discovery of an adrenal nodule in a cancer patient may alter the initial therapy for certain primary tumors. Therefore, pathologic confirmation of the nature of the nodule is of prime importance,[93] particularly in light of the high frequency of incidental benign adrenal nodules in the general population, the marked propensity of certain neoplasms to metastasize to the adrenal gland, and our inability to distinguish metastases from primary adrenal neoplasms based solely on radiologic appearance.[21, 22, 35, 62] More recently, adrenal nodules have been assigned to different categories based on their MRI signal intensities.[59] However, those who advocate MRI have found a 21% to 31% overlap between malignant and benign adrenal nodules.[19, 20]

The association of benign nonfunctional adrenal nodules with advancing age, diabetes, hypertension (Fig 7–4), and various malignancies is well established.[23, 94–96] The prevalence of benign nonfunctional nodules (including nodular hyperplasia and adenoma) was 8% in one large prospective autopsy study[23] and 65.5% in another.[21] This inconsistency is attributable to the inclusion in the latter series of both microscopic adrenal cortical nodules as well as grossly visible lesions that deform glandular structure. Based only on microscopic findings, on the other hand, Commons and Callaway found cortical adenomas more than 3 mm in diameter in 2.9% of 9,866 consecutive autopsies,[22] and Kokko et al. found cortical adenomas larger than 5 mm in 1.4% of 1,495 cases.[97] The minimal size of an adrenal mass that can be resolved by CT is between 5 and 10 mm, depending on the scanner and technique, thus accounting for the discrepancy in prevalence between the imaging and microscopic series.

In the clinical study of malignant neoplasia, the proper approach in a case of incidental adrenal mass in the absence of other evidence of systemic metastases is first to test for evidence of adrenal hyperfunction using standard biochemical tests. If the mass is nonfunctional, CT-guided fine-needle aspiration is performed, and the aspirated material is immediately evaluated cytologically to be certain that the specimen is representative.[93–97] Under these circumstances, the nonfunctional pheochromocytoma may pose a problem; even though hypertensive episodes precipitated by needle aspiration are rare, the radiologist should be prepared to offer immediate treatment.[98]

The conservative approach of simply obtaining follow-up CT scans of the adrenal in two to three months in a cancer patient, looking for a change in the size of the mass, may lead to unnecessary delay in definitive treatment of those lesions that prove to be malignant (see Figs 7–19 and 7–20). However, a conservative "wait and see" attitude and serial follow-up CT or MRI examination at six months to two years is appropriate when there are nonfunctional small adrenal nodules and no evidence of carcinoma.[79, 84]

Mitnick et al. for one year monitored a series of patients in whom small, nonfunctional adrenal lesions were found incidentally, and they recommended CT criteria for establishing benignancy of adrenal lesions.[99] According to that study, tumors with a smooth contour, a well-defined margin, no growth on serial CT scans over one year, and a diameter less than 5 cm need not be followed further for possible malignancy. However, when the asymptomatic adrenal lesion is larger than 5 cm, there is a high incidence of malignancy and surgery is indicated.[79]

The cytologic appearances of adrenal adenomas and other benign nodules are characteristic.[24, 93] Once the pathologist becomes familiar with the distinctive elements, the lesions are easily recognized (Fig 7–3).

REFERENCES

1. Reinig J.W., Doppman J.L., Dwyer A.J., et al.: Distinction between adrenal adenomas and metastases using MR imaging. *J. Comput. Assist. Tomogr.* 9:898–901, 1985.
2. Kahn P.C.: The radiologic identification of functioning adrenal tumors. *Radiol. Clin. North Am.* 5:221–230, 1967.
3. Pickering R.S., Hartman G.W., Weeks R.E., et al.: Excretory urographic localization of adrenal cortical tumors and pheochromocytomas. *Radiology* 114:345–349, 1975.
4. Alfidi R.J., Gill W.M. Jr., Klein J.H.: Arteriography of adrenal neoplasms. *AJR* 106:635–641, 1969.
5. Colapinto R.F., Steed B.L.: Arteriography of adrenal tumors. *Radiology* 100:343–350, 1971.
6. Mitty H.A., Nicolis G.L., Gabrilove J.L.: Adrenal venography: clinical-roentgenographic correlation in 80 patients. *AJR* 119:564–574, 1973.
7. Jensen S.R., Novelline R.A., Brewster D.C., et al.: Transient renal artery stenosis produced by a pheochromocytoma. *Radiology* 144:767–768, 1982.
8. Geisinger M.A., Zelch M.G., Bravo E.L., et al.: Primary hyperaldosteronism: comparison of CT, adrenal venography, and venous sampling. *AJR* 141:299–302, 1983.
9. Thrall J.H., Freitas J.E., Beierwaltes W.H.: Adrenal scintigraphy. *Semin. Nucl. Med.* 8:23–41, 1978.
10. Sisson J.C., Frager M.P., Valk T.W., et al.: Scintigraphic localization of pheochromocytoma. *N. Engl. J. Med.* 305:12–17, 1981.
11. McEwan A.J., Shapiro B., Sisson J.C., et al.: Radioiodobenzylguanidine for the scintigraphic localization and therapy of adrenergic tumors. *Semin. Nucl. Med.* 15:132–153, 1985.
12. Lynn M.D., Shapiro B., Sisson J.C., et al.: Pheochromocytoma and the normal adrenal medulla: improved visualization with ^{123}I MIBG scintigraphy. *Radiology* 155:789–792, 1985.
13. Seabold J.E., Cohen E.L., Beierwaltes W.H., et al.: Adrenal imaging with ^{131}I-19-iodocholesterol in the diagnostic evaluation of patients with aldosteronism. *J. Clin. Endocrinol. Metab.* 42:41–51, 1976.
14. Abrams H.L., Siegleman S.S., Adams D.F., et al.: Computed tomography versus ultrasound of the adrenal gland: a prospective study. *Radiology* 143:121–128, 1982.
15. Wilms G., Baert A., Marchal G., et al.: Computed tomography of the normal adrenal glands: correlative study with autopsy specimens. *J. Comput. Assist. Tomogr.* 3:467–469, 1979.
16. Nielsen M.E. Jr., Heaston D.K., Dunnick N.R., et al.: Preoperative CT evaluation of adrenal glands in nonsmall cell bronchogenic carcinoma. *AJR* 139:317–320, 1982.
17. Sandler M.A., Pearlberg J.L., Madrazo B.L., et al.: Computed tomographic evaluation of the adrenal gland in the preoperative assessment of bronchogenic carcinoma. *Radiology* 145:733–736, 1982.
18. Ackery D.M., Tippett P.A., Condon B.R., et al.: New approach to the localization of pheochromocytoma: imaging with iodine-131-*meta*-iodobenzylguanidine. *Br. Med. J. (Clin. Res.)* 288:1587–1591, 1984.
19. Chang A., Glazer H.S., Lee J.K.T., et al.: Adrenal gland: MR imaging. *Radiology* 163:123–128, 1987.
20. Reinig J.W., Doppman J.L., Dwyer A.H., et al.: Adrenal masses differentiated by MR. *Radiology* 158:81–84, 1986.
21. Dobbie J.W.: Adrenocortical nodular hyperplasia: the ageing adrenal. *J. Pathol.* 99:1–18, 1969.
22. Commons R.R., Callaway C.P.: Adenomas of the adrenal cortex. *Arch. Intern. Med.* 81:37–41, 1948.
23. Ambos M.A., Bosniak M.A., Lefleur R.S., et al.: Adrenal adenoma associated with renal cell carcinoma. *AJR* 136:81–84, 1981.
24. Katz R.L., Shirkhoda A.: Diagnostic approach to incidental adrenal nodules in the cancer patient: results of a clinical, radiologic, and fine-needle aspiration study. *Cancer* 55:1995–2000, 1985.
25. Guerrero L.A.: Diagnostic and therapeutic approach to incidental adrenal mass. *Urology* 26:435–440, 1985.
26. Biglieri E.G.: A perspective on aldosterone abnormalities (review). *Clin. Endocrinol. Metab.* 5:399–410, 1976.
27. Neville A.M., Mackay A.M.: The structure of the human adrenal cortex in health and disease. *Clin. Endocrinol. Metab.* 1:361–395, 1972.
28. Salassa R.M., Weeks R.E., Northcutt R.C., et al.: Primary aldosteronism and malignant adrenocortical neoplasia. *Trans. Am. Clin. Climatol. Assoc.* 80:163–172, 1972.
29. Schaner E.G., Dunnick N.R., Doppman J.L., et al.: Adrenal cortical tumors with low attenuation coefficients: a pitfall in CT diagnosis. *J. Comput. Assist. Tomogr.* 2:11–15, 1978.
30. Shirkhoda A.: Current diagnostic approach to adrenal abnormalities. *J. Comput. Tomogr.* 8:277–285, 1984.
31. Behan M., Martin E.E., Muecke E.C., et al.: Myelolipoma of the adrenal: two cases with ultrasound and CT findings. *AJR* 129:993–996, 1977.
32. Friedman A.C., Hartman D.S., Sherman J., et al.: Computed tomography of abdominal fatty masses. *Radiology* 139:415–429, 1981.

33. Gould J.D., Mitty H.A., Pertsemlidis D.: Adrenal myelolipoma: diagnosis by fine-needle aspiration. *AJR* 148:921–922, 1987.

34. Scheible W., Coel M., Siemers P.T., et al.: Percutaneous aspiration of adrenal cysts. *AJR* 128:1013–1016, 1977.

35. Mittelstaedt C.A., Volberg F.M., Merten D.F., et al.: The sonographic diagnosis of neonatal adrenal hemorrhage. *Radiology* 131:453–457, 1979.

36. Reynes C.J., Churchill R., Moncada R., et al.: Computed tomography of adrenal glands. *Radiol. Clin. North Am.* 17:91–104, 1979.

37. Philips B.: Intrathoracic pheochromocytoma. *Arch. Pathol. Lab. Med.* 30:916, 1940.

38. Thomas J.L., Bernardino M.E.: Pheochromocytoma in multiple endocrine adenomatosis. *JAMA* 245:1467–1469, 1981.

39. Bloom D.A., Fonkalsrud E.W.: Surgical management of pheochromocytoma in children. *J. Pediatr. Surg.* 9:179–184, 1974.

40. Fries J.G., Chamberin J.A.: Extra-adrenal pheochromocytoma: literature review and report of a cervical pheochromocytoma. *Surgery* 63:268–279, 1968.

41. Welch T.J., Sheedy P.F., Van Heerdan J.A., et al.: Pheochromocytoma: value of computed tomography. *Radiology* 148:501–503, 1983.

42. Remine W.H., Chong G.C., Van Heerden J.A., et al.: Current management of pheochromocytoma. *Ann. Surg.* 179:740–748, 1974.

43. Engelman K.: Pheochromocytoma. *Clin. Endocrinol. Metab.* 6:769–797, 1977.

44. Laursen K., Damgaard-Pedersen K.: CT for pheochromocytoma diagnosis. *AJR* 134:277–280, 1980.

45. Mayorga L.M., Zabludowski J.R., Camera M.I., et al.: Bilateral pheochromocytoma localized by computed tomography [letter]. *Arch. Intern. Med.* 141:693, 1981.

46. Frier D.T., Thompson N.W., Sisson J.C., et al.: Dilemmas in the early diagnosis and treatment of multiple endocrine adenomatosis, type II. *Surgery* 82:407–413, 1977.

47. Brunt L.M., Wells S.A.: The multiple endocrine neoplasia syndromes. *Invest. Radiol.* 20:916–927, 1985.

48. Dodd G.D.: The radiologic features of multiple endocrine neoplasia types IIA and IIB. *Semin. Roentgenol.* 20:64–90, 1985.

49. Tateishi R., Wada A., Ishiguro S., et al.: Coexistence of bilateral pheochromocytoma and pancreatic islet cell tumor: a report of a case and review of the literature. *Cancer* 42:2928–2934, 1978.

50. Probst A., Lotz M., Heitz P.: Von Hippel-Lindau's disease, syringomyelia and multiple endocrine tumors: a complex neuroendocrinopathy. *Virchows Arch.* [Pathol. Anat.] 378:265–272, 1978.

51. Ram M.D., Rao K.N., Brown L.: Hypercalcitoninemia, pheochromocytoma and C-cell hyperplasia: a new variant of Sipple's syndrome. *JAMA* 239:2155–2156, 1978.

52. Christenson R., Smith C.W., Burko H.: Arterio-graphic manifestations of pheochromocytoma. *AJR* 126:567–575, 1976.

53. Stewart G.H., Bravo E.L., Haaga J., et al.: Localization of pheochromocytoma by computed tomography. *N. Engl. J. Med.* 299:460–461, 1978.

54. Zelch J.V., Meaney T.F., Belhobek G.H.: Radiologic approach to the patient with suspected pheochromocytoma. *Radiology* 111:279–284, 1974.

55. Francis I.R., Glazer G.M., Shapiro B., et al.: Complementary roles of CT and ^{131}I-MIBG scintigraphy in diagnosing pheochromocytoma. *AJR* 141:719–725, 1983.

56. Raper A.J., Jessee E.F., Texter J.H., et al.: Pheochromocytoma of the urinary bladder: a broad clinical spectrum. *Am. J. Cardiol.* 40:820–824, 1977.

57. Aron D.C., Marks W.M., Alper P.R., et al.: Pheochromocytoma of the broad ligament. Localization by computerized tomography and ultrasonography. *Arch. Intern. Med.* 140:550–552, 1980.

58. Shirkhoda A., Wallace S.: Computed tomography of juxtacardiac pheochromocytoma. *J. Comput. Tomogr.* 8:207–209, 1984.

59. Glazer G.M., Woolsey E.J., Burrello J., et al.: Adrenal tissue characterization using MR imaging. *Radiology* 158:73–79, 1986.

60. Fisher M.R., Higgins C.B., Andereck W.: MR imaging of an intrapericardial pheochromocytoma. *J. Comput. Assist. Tomogr.* 9:1103–1105, 1985.

61. Greenberg M., Moawad A.H., Wieties B.M., et al.: Extraadrenal pheochromocytoma: detection during pregnancy using MR imaging. *Radiology* 161:475–476, 1986.

62. Glomset D.A.: The incidence of metastasis of malignant tumors to the adrenals. *Am. J. Cancer* 32:57–61, 1938.

63. Cedermark B.J., Sjoberg H.E.: The clinical significance of metastases to the adrenal glands. *Surg. Gynecol. Obstet.* 152:607–610, 1981.

64. Willis R.S.: Secondary tumours of the kidneys, in *The Spread of Tumours in the Human Body,* ed. 3. New York, Butterworth, 1927.

65. Abrams H.L., Spiro R., Goldstein N.: Metastases in carcinoma: analysis of 1000 autopsied cases. *Cancer* 3:74–85, 1950.

66. Glazer H.S., Lee J.K.T., Balfe D.M., et al.: Non-Hodgkin lymphoma: computed tomographic demonstration of unusual extranodal involvement. *Radiology* 149:211–217, 1983.

67. Paling M.R., Williamson B.R.J.: Adrenal involvement in non-Hodgkin lymphoma. *AJR* 141:303–305, 1983.

68. National Cancer Institute: *Third National Cancer Survey: Incidence Data.* National Cancer Institute Monograph 41; DHEW publication no. (NIH) 75-787. Bethesda, Md., U.S. Department of Health, Education, and Welfare, 1975.

69. Hutter A.M., Kayhoe D.E.: Adrenal cortical carcinoma: results of treatment with OPDDD in 138 patients. *Am. J. Med.* 41:581–592, 1966.

70. King D.R., Lack E.E.: Adrenal cortical carcinoma: a

clinical and pathologic study of 49 cases. *Cancer* 44:239–244, 1979.

71. Nader S., Hickey R.C., Sellin R.V., et al.: Adrenal cortical carcinoma: a study of 77 cases. *Cancer* 52:707–711, 1983.

72. Daneman A., Chan H.S.L., Martin J.: Adrenal carcinoma and adenoma in children: a review of 17 patients. *Pediatr. Radiol.* 13:11–18, 1983.

73. Hayles A.B., Hahn H.B. Jr., Sprague R.G., et al.: Adrenal carcinoma and adenoma in children: hormone-secreting tumors of the adrenal cortex in children. *Pediatrics* 37:19–25, 1966.

74. Stewart D.R., Morris Jones P.H., Jolleys A.: Carcinoma of the adrenal gland in children. *J. Pediatr. Surg.* 9:59–67, 1974.

75. Zaitoon M.M., Mackie G.G.: Adrenal cortical tumors in children. *Urology* 12:645–649, 1978.

76. Korobkin M., White E.A., Kressel H.Y., et al.: Computed tomography in the diagnosis of adrenal disease. *AJR* 132:231–238, 1979.

77. Shirkhoda A.: Computed tomography after adrenalectomy in adrenal cortical carcinoma. *Urol. Radiol.* 7:132–137, 1985.

78. Dunnick N.R., Heaston D., Halvorsen R., et al.: CT appearance of adrenal cortical carcinoma. *J. Comput. Assist. Tomogr.* 6:978–982, 1982.

79. Bernardino M.E.: Management of the asymptomatic patient with a unilateral adrenal mass. *Radiology* 166:121–123, 1988.

80. Hamper U.M., Fishman E.K., Hartman D.S., et al.: Primary adrenocortical carcinoma: sonographic evaluation with clinical and pathologic correlation in 26 patients. *AJR* 148:915–919, 1987.

81. Denis R.K., Ernest E.L.: Adrenal cortical carcinoma: a clinical and pathologic study of 49 cases. *Cancer* 44:239–244, 1979.

82. Karsner H.T: Tumors of the adrenal, in *Atlas of Tumor Pathology.* Washington, D.C., Armed Forces Institute of Pathology, 1950, sect. 8, fasc. 29.

83. Glazer H.S., Weyman P.J., Sagel S.S., et al.: Non-functioning adrenal mass: incidental discovery on computed tomography. *AJR* 139:81–85, 1982.

84. Prinz R.A., Brooks M.H., Churchill R., et al.: Incidental asymptomatic adrenal masses detected by computed tomographic scanning: is operation required? *JAMA* 248:701–704, 1982.

85. Copeland P.M.: The incidentally discovered adrenal mass. *Ann. Intern. Med.* 98:940–945, 1983.

86. Lewinsky B.S., Grigor K.M., Symington T., et al.: The clinical and pathologic features of "non-hor-monal" adrenocortical tumors: report of twenty new cases and review of the literature. *Cancer* 33:778–790, 1974.

87. Bertagna C., Orth D.N.: Clinical and laboratory findings and results of therapy in 58 patients with adrenocortical tumors admitted to a single medical center (1951 to 1978). *Am. J. Med.* 71:855–875, 1981.

88. Didolkar M.S., Bescher R.A., Elias E.G., et al.: Natural history of adrenal cortical carcinoma: a clinico-pathologic study of 42 patients. *Cancer* 47:2153–2161, 1981.

89. Huvos A.G., Hajdu S.I., Brasfield R.D., et al.: Adrenal cortical carcinoma: clinicopathologic study of 34 cases. *Cancer* 25:354–361, 1970.

90. St. John Sutton M.G., Sheps S.G., Lie J.T.: Prevalence of clinically unsuspected pheochromocytoma: review of a 50-year autopsy series. *Mayo Clin. Proc.* 56:354–360, 1981.

91. Engelman K.: Criteria for diagnosis of pheochromocytoma, pp. 1304–1308, in Sjoerdsma A. (moderator): Pheochromocytoma: current concepts of diagnosis and treatment. *Ann. Intern. Med.* 65:1302–1326, 1966.

92. Crout J.R., Sjoerdsma A.: Turnover and metabolism of catecholamines in patients with phaeochromocytoma *J. Clin. Invest.* 43:94–102, 1964.

93. Katz R.L., Patel S., Mackay B., et al.: Fine needle aspiration cytology of the adrenal gland. *Acta Cytol.* (Baltimore) 28:269–282, 1984.

94. Spain D.M., Weinsaft P.: Solitary adrenal cortical adenoma in elderly female. *Arch. Pathol.* 78:231–233, 1964.

95. Russell R.P., Masi A.T., Richter E.D.: Adrenal cortical adenomas and hypertension: a clinical pathologic analysis of 690 cases with matched controls and a review of the literature. *Medicine* (Baltimore) 52:211–225, 1972.

96. Hedeland H., Ostberg G., Hokfelt B.: On the prevalence of adrenocortical adenomas in an autopsy material in relation to hypertension and diabetes. *Acta Med. Scand.* 184:211–214, 1968.

97. Kokko J.P., Brown T.C., Berman M.M.: Adrenal adenoma and hypertension. *Lancet* 1:468–470, 1967.

98. Casola G., Nicolet V., vanSonnenberg E., et al.: Unsuspected pheochromocytoma: risk of blood-pressure alterations during percutaneous adrenal biopsy. *Radiology* 15:733–735, 1986.

99. Mitnick J.S., Bosniak M.A., Megibow A.J., et al.: Non-functioning adrenal adenomas discovered incidentally on computed tomography. *Radiology* 148:495–499, 1983.

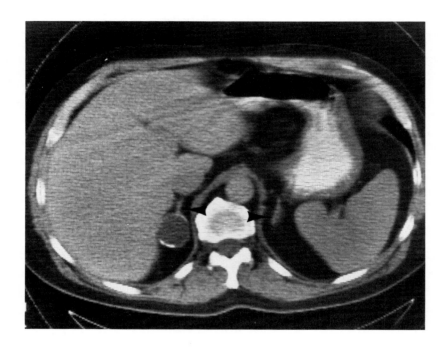

FIG 7–1.

Nonfunctional right adenoma with calcified wall. The male patient in this case was treated at 62 years of age for transitional cell carcinoma of the bladder and adenocarcinoma of the prostate. Eight years later, there was no evidence of disease recurrence.

This CT study of the abdomen was done three years after surgery and shows a solid nodule with calcified wall in the right adrenal gland. Note that a small part of the right adrenal is of normal appearance and that the entire left adrenal gland is normal *(arrowheads)*. Based on the normal adrenal hormone profile, calcification in the adrenal nodule, and a lack of any evidence of metastasis, the presumptive diagnosis was benign nonfunctioning adrenal adenoma, and the management strategy chosen was follow-up alone. Five years later, there was no significant change in the appearance of the nodule on CT, and the patient remained without symptoms. The patient's adrenal hormone profile also remained normal. The most likely diagnosis in this case is a benign, nonfunctional calcified adenoma of the right adrenal.

A

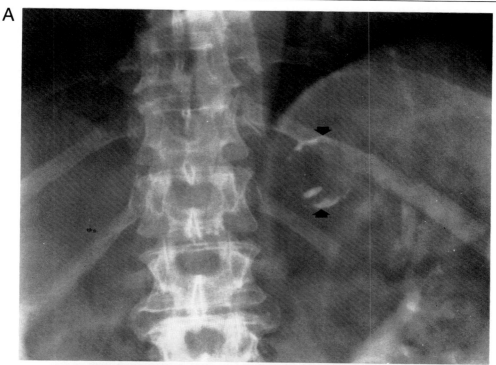

B

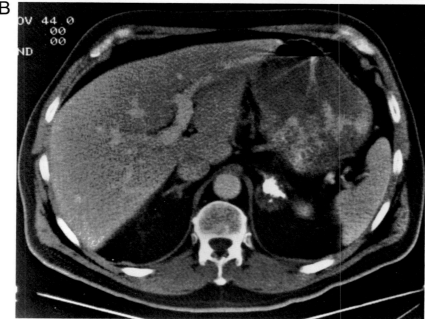

FIG 7–2.

Calcified nonfunctional left adenoma. A 61-year-old man was found to have transitional cell carcinoma of the bladder and total cystectomy was performed.

A, a pyelogram shows left paraspinal curvilinear and circular calcification *(arrows).*

B, the CT scan shows the calcification to be within the wall and also inside the enlarged left adrenal nodule. Because a film obtained four years previously showed calcific densities at the same location, biopsy was thought to be unnecessary. The patient's hormonal profile was normal. A presumptive diagnosis of calcified nonfunctional adenoma of the left adrenal was made. A repeat CT scan eight months later showed no change.

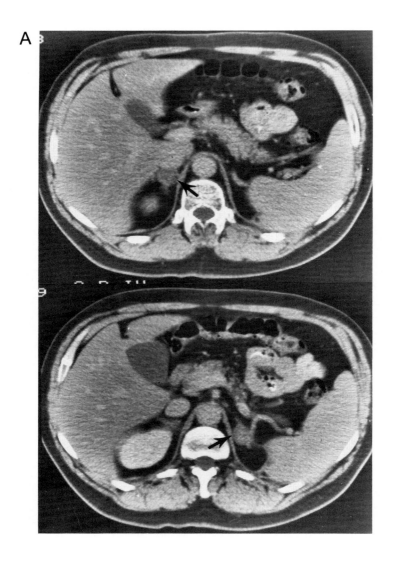

FIG 7–3.
Nonfunctional bilateral adenoma. Malignant melanoma was diagnosed in a 62-year-old woman who had three years previously had cloacogenic carcinoma of the rectum. Abdominal CT was part of the melanoma workup, and bilateral adrenal nodules were discovered.

A, the adrenal nodules are well circumscribed, both measuring approximately 3 × 2 cm. The top CT scan shows the right adrenal nodule and the bottom image the left adrenal nodule *(arrows).* It is not unusual to see a normal portion of a gland on the next image, as in the bottom image where a portion of the normal right adrenal gland is seen. This example emphasizes the importance of examining the entire gland in search for abnormality.

B

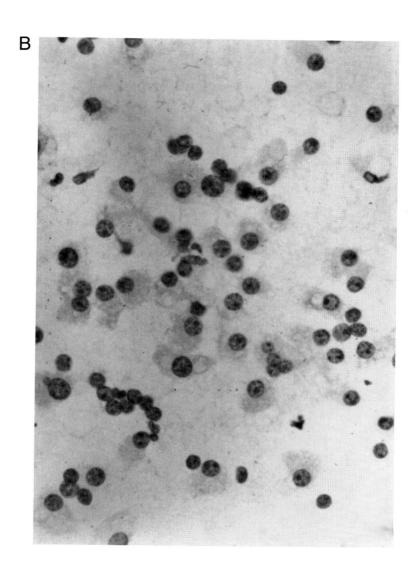

B, because of the high incidence of adrenal metastases from melanoma, percutaneous biopsy of the right adrenal nodule was performed using a 21-gauge Chiba needle. Loose clusters of adrenal cortical cells with typical homogeneous bland naked nuclei are seen. This appearance is characteristic of benign adenoma. (From Katz R.L., Shir- khoda A.: Diagnostic approach to incidental adrenal nodules in the cancer patient: results of a clinical, radiologic, and fine-needle aspiration study. *Cancer* 55:1995–2000, 1985. Reproduced with permission.)

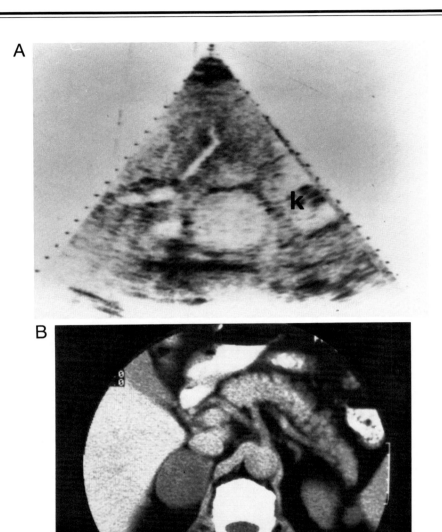

FIG 7–4.
Nonfunctional adenoma (two cases).

   A through **C,** a 64-year-old man with a ten-year history of controlled (120/74 mm Hg) hypertension was evaluated because of upper abdominal discomfort.

   An abdominal sonogram **(A)** made to rule out any abnormality in the pancreas or biliary system reveals an incidental right suprarenal mass on this slightly oblique sagittal view. The mass is seen as homogeneous and hypoechoic without any definite areas of calcification. The upper right renal pole *(k)* is seen caudal to the mass. A CT scan **(B)** of the abdomen confirms the location of the mass within the right adrenal gland. The mass is homogeneous; its attenuation value ranged from 36 to 42 Hounsfield units, and it measured 5 cm anteroposteriorly and 4 cm transversely. No other abnormality was noted. The patient's endocrine profile was negative for pheochromocytoma or any other hyperfunctional adrenal tumor such as carcinoma or functional adenoma. However, because of its large size and the continued abdominal discomfort, the mass was excised.

   At surgery, a 5 × 6 × 4 cm right adrenal mass **(C)** was discovered; it was subsequently proved to be a benign adenoma. This is one of the largest benign adenomas that my colleagues and I have seen (see also Color Plate 31).

   D, another patient, a 60-year-old man with history of adenocarcinoma of the lung, was discovered to have a 2-cm left adrenal nodule on CT (not shown). On T_2-weighted MR image (TR/TE, 2,000/80), the signal intensity of the mass *(arrows)* is similar to that of the liver. A percutaneous biopsy proved this to represent a benign adenoma.

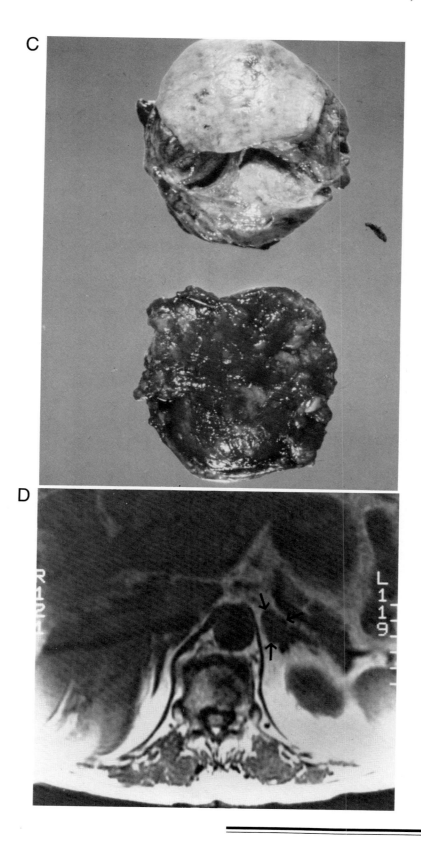

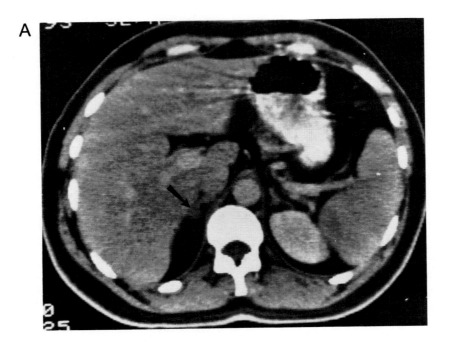

FIG 7–5.
Right aldosteronoma. A 32-year-old man was followed at M. D. Anderson Hospital for sarcoma of the right clavicle. He was found to be hypertensive and hypokalemic. **A,** an abdominal CT scan shows a 1-cm nodule *(arrow)* in the right adrenal gland.

B

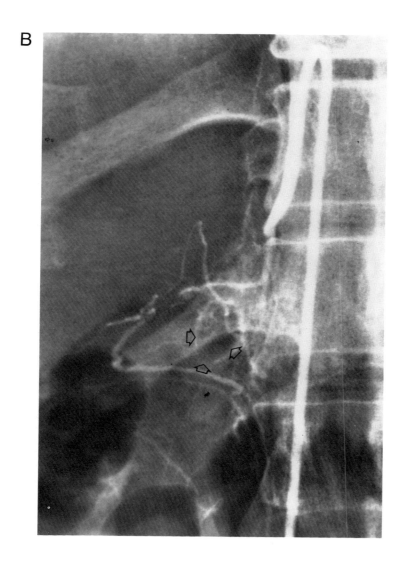

B, venography reveals a small avascular mass *(arrows)* in the adrenal. Venous sampling from the right adrenal vein showed markedly increased aldosterone and cortisol levels.

The patient eventually had right adrenalectomy, and the diagnosis of aldosteronoma was proved.

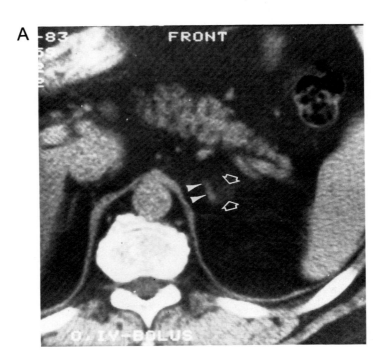

FIG 7–6.

Left aldosteronoma. A 25-year-old man with hypertension was found to have hypokalemia (serum potassium, 2.89 mEq/L) and low serum renin levels.

A, overlapping CT images of fine collimation were obtained and this one shows a small nodule coming off the lateral limb of the left adrenal gland *(arrows)*. The nodule has a lower attenuation value than does the adjacent normal adrenal limb *(arrowheads)*. With the patient's clinical history, a diagnosis of aldosteronoma was suggested, and selective venous sampling from the left adrenal vein proved the high level of aldosterone.

B

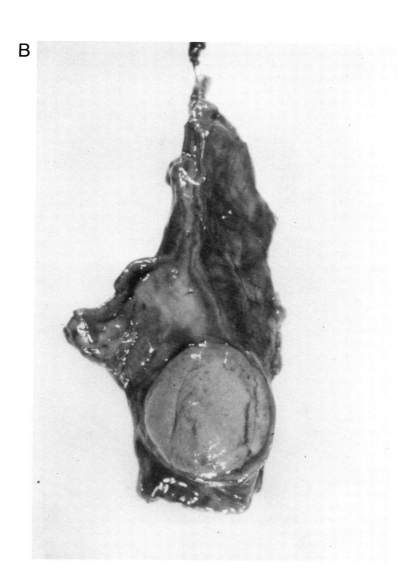

B, surgical specimen from left adrenalectomy shows an 11-mm, well-defined adenoma originating in the lateral limb of the adrenal gland (see also Color Plate 32). (From Shirkhoda A.: Current diagnostic approach to adrenal abnormalities. *J. Comput. Tomogr.* 8:277–285, 1984. Reproduced with permission.)

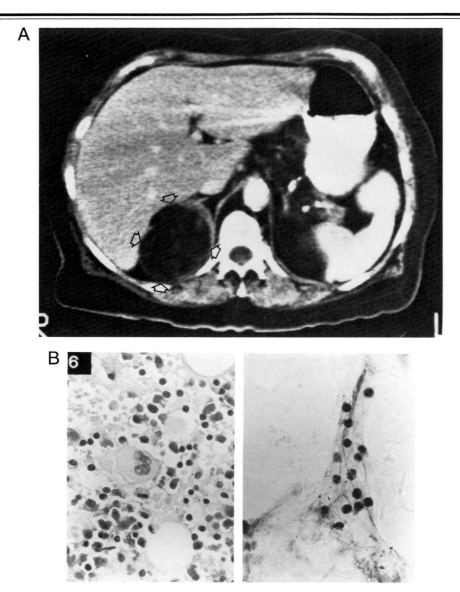

FIG 7–7.

Myelolipoma (two cases).

A and **B,** this 65-year-old hypertensive woman was having cholecystosonography (sonogram not available), and a mass was discovered in the upper pole of the right kidney. The mass reportedly extended to the liver.

To further delineate the mass, a CT scan was obtained **(A)**. It shows a 5.5 × 6.5 cm smooth ovoid mass in the right suprarenal region *(arrows)*. The mass has predominantly a fatty density, and it was thought that it had compressed the upper pole of the right kidney. Differential diagnosis at this point included primary adrenal tumor such as myelolipoma or possibly a renal angiomyolipoma. The renal angiogram was normal, and a percutaneous biopsy was done.

In material taken by percutaneous aspiration **(B)**, there is a mixture of fat and hematopoietic cells consistent with adrenal myelolipoma. This patient has been followed by CT for three years without any changes in the appearance of

the mass. At this point, the diagnosis of myelolipoma stands firm.

C and **D,** another patient, a 33-year-old man, was found to have a right upper quadrant mass on routine physical examination. A tomogram **(C)** from an intravenous pyelogram shows the mass to be well defined *(arrows)* with nonhomogeneous density compressing the right kidney. The CT scan **(D)** reveals the tumor with a mixture of fat and higher-attenuation soft tissue densities above the right kidney. The coronal reconstruction view *(right image)* clearly shows separation of the mass from the kidney.

Angiography further proved separation of the mass and the kidney, and at surgery a well-encapsulated tumor originating in the right adrenal gland was discovered. The pathologic diagnosis was myelolipoma. (**C** and **D** courtesy of Ruppert David, M.D., Department of Radiology, Baylor College of Medicine, Houston, Tex.)

C

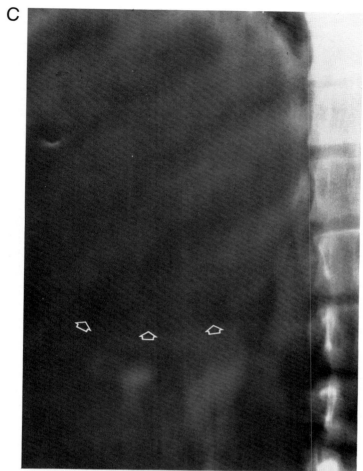

D

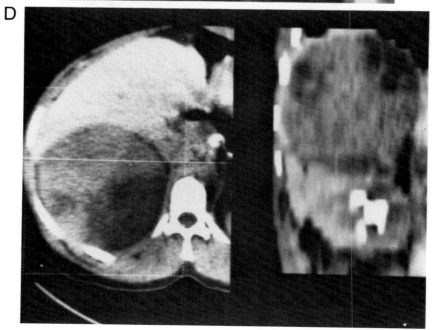

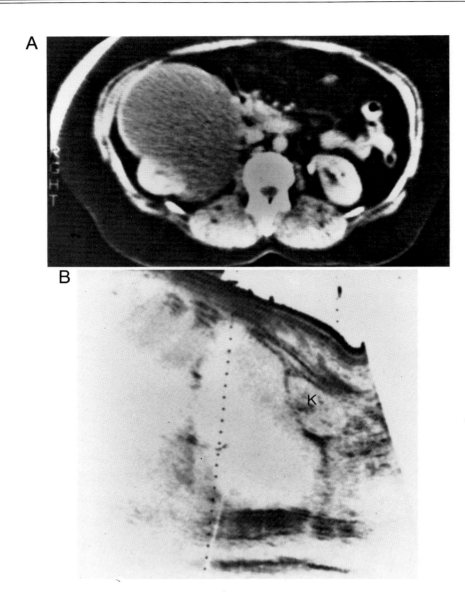

FIG 7–8.
Adrenal cyst (multiple cases).

A and **B,** a 48-year-old woman presented with a palpable mass in the right upper quadrant. She had no other symptoms.

The CT scan **(A)** shows a thick-walled cystic mass adjacent to the right kidney. The mass appears to originate in that kidney at this level, but appeared to be separate from it in another level.

Parasagittal static sonogram **(B)** shows the cystic mass clearly separate from the right kidney *(K)* and within the adrenal gland. This image was used to guide cyst aspiration, which revealed a thick yellow fluid with normal cytology.

C, large left adrenal cyst in a different patient who pre-

sented with a palpable left abdominal mass. Intravenous urogram shows a very large, partially calcified adrenal mass causing inferior displacement of the left kidney. The mass was aspirated under ultrasound guidance, resulting in clear fluid with normal cytology.

D, small right adrenal cyst. Parasagittal real-time ultrasound of the right adrenal in a patient who was followed for possible metastatic breast carcinoma. A 2 × 2 cm anechoic mass with increased through-transmission is seen in the area of the right adrenal *(arrowheads).* It had the same size and shape one year before and most probably represents an adrenal cyst. Notice elevation of the inferior vena cava *(IVC)* and the junction of the right renal vein *(arrow).*

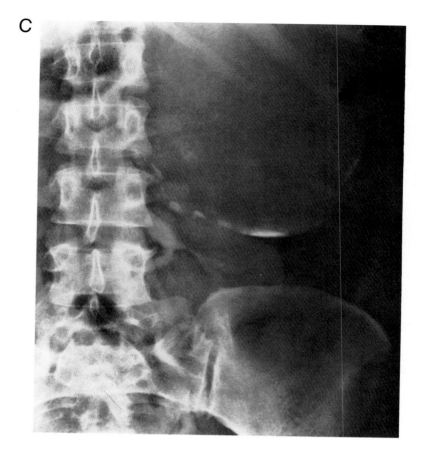

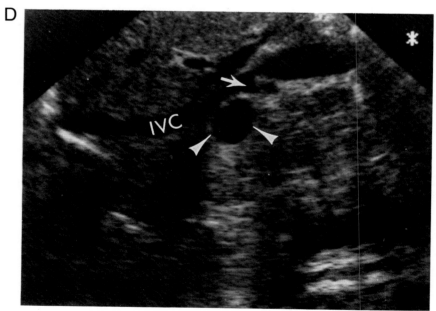

A

B

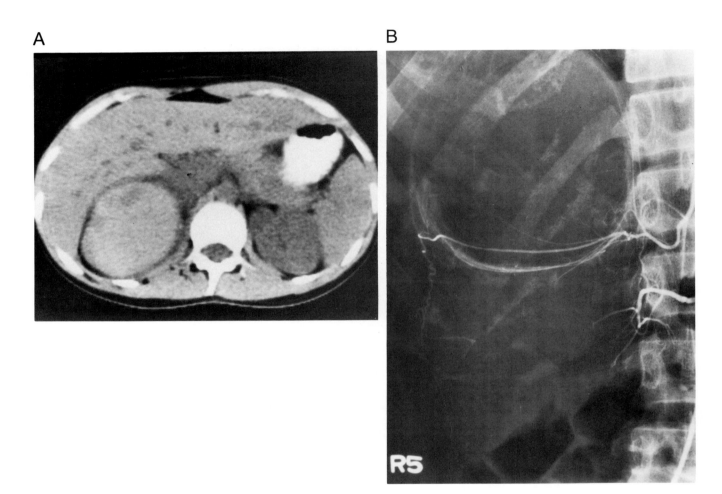

FIG 7–9.

Adrenal hemorrhage (two cases).

A through **C,** a 25-year-old woman developed sharp pain in the right upper quadrant. The pain was spontaneous and became constant.

Initial unenhanced CT scan **(A)** made two days after the onset of pain shows a large mass with a high attenuation value in the region of the right adrenal gland. The mass has a few areas of low density. Adrenal hemorrhage was strongly suspected and arteriography was done to rule out any underlying neoplasm.

Selective right adrenal arteriogram **(B)** shows an avas-cular tumor displacing and stretching the adrenal arteries. No tumor neovascularity is seen.

Two weeks after the initial CT, repeat unenhanced CT scan **(C)** shows loss of density, primarily in the periphery of the mass in a rim shape *(arrows),* supporting the initial diagnosis of hematoma. Follow-up ultrasound studies revealed gradual reduction in the size of the mass.

D, parasagittal sonogram (prone position) of a 16-day-old infant with palpable abdominal mass. The right kidney *(K)* and the hemorrhage in the adrenal gland *(arrows)* are seen. Notice the probable serum level *(arrowheads)* within the hemorrhagic mass.

C

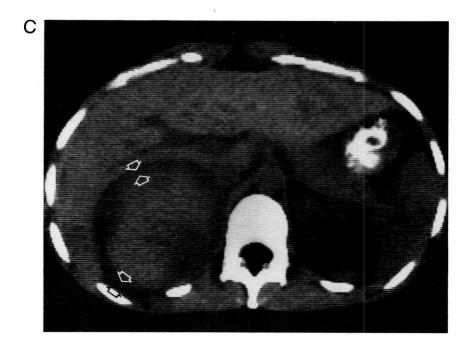

D

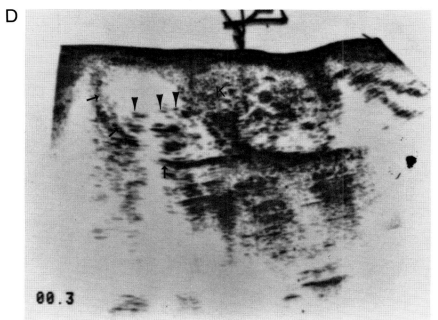

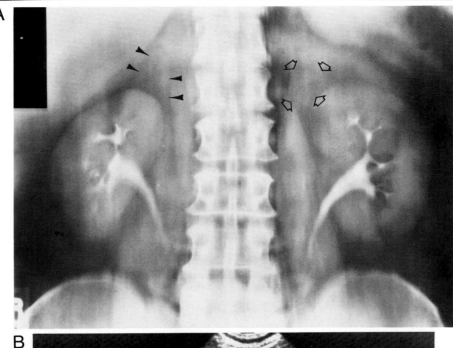

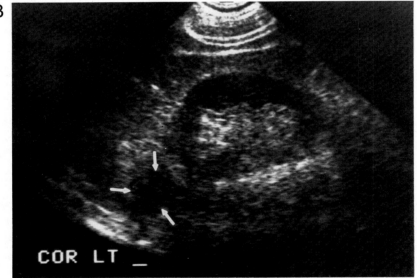

FIG 7–10.

Left pheochromocytoma. A 55-year-old obese man with long-standing hypertension presented with abdominal and back pain and underwent an extensive workup.

A, the nephrotomogram shows a mass in the left adrenal fossa replacing the normal fat in that region *(arrows)*. Observe the normal linear soft tissue densities in the contralateral side, which represent the normal limbs of the right adrenal gland *(arrowheads)*.

B, the coronal sonogram of the left kidney shows a hypoechoic mass in the superior and medial aspect of the left kidney *(arrows)*.

C, abdominal CT shows a 2.5-cm nodule posterior to the pancreas *(p)* and within the left adrenal gland *(arrows)*. A small portion of the adrenal appears to be uninvolved by the tumor *(arrowhead)*. Repeated measurements of urinary catecholamines yielded the readings of 512, 492, and 522 mg/24 hr (normal, 0–280 mg/24 hr). The vanillylmandelic acid assay showed readings of 12, 10, and 9 mg/24 hr (normal, 1–8 mg/24 hr).

With the history of long-standing hypertension, discovery of left adrenal mass, and abnormal laboratory test results, the diagnosis of pheochromocytoma of the left adrenal gland was clear and was proved at surgery. (**C** from Dodd G.D.: The radiologic features of multiple endocrine neoplasia types IIA and IIB. *Semin. Roentgenol.* 20:64–90, 1985. Reproduced with permission.)

D, surgical specimen shows a 2.5-cm nodule within the excised fat, proved histologically to represent a pheochromocytoma (see also Color Plate 33).

C

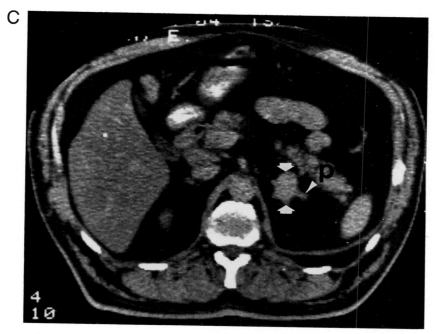

D

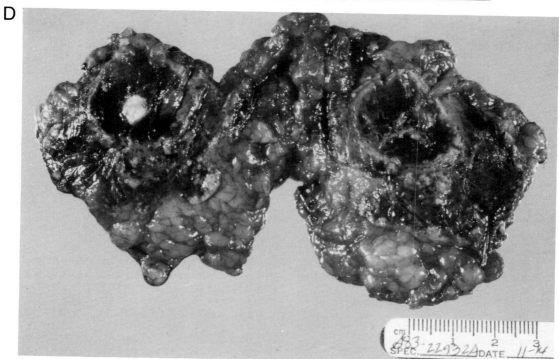

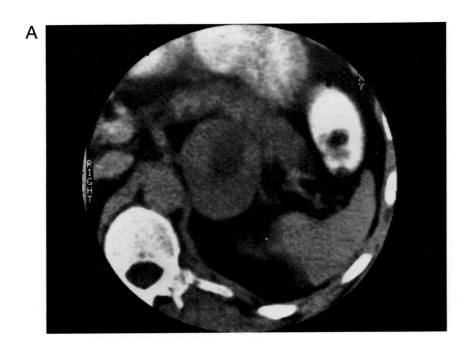

FIG 7–11.

Left pheochromocytoma (two cases).

A and **B,** a 59-year-old man with a diagnosis of bladder carcinoma underwent abdominal and pelvic CT for evaluation of the extent of the malignancy. The CT showed an invasive bladder tumor and a retroperitoneal mass.

A, a 6-cm mass was discovered within the left adrenal gland, displacing the pancreas anteriorly. The mass is well encapsulated and centrally has low density. The patient's blood pressure was 140/90 mm Hg. It was considered possible, although unlikely, that the CT image represented a solitary adrenal metastasis from the bladder neoplasm. Because the patient's blood pressure bordered on being high, his urinary vanillylmandelic acid level was evaluated and was found to be 10 mg/24 hr (normal, 1–8 mg/24 hr).

B, selective left inferior phrenic arteriogram demonstrates a very vascular tumor, consistent with the diagnosis of pheochromocytoma.

At the time of exploration, the left adrenal mass was palpated, and the patient developed severe hypertension, which was immediately corrected by phentolamine. Adrenalectomy was carried out without delay, and the patient's blood pressure normalized. Pathologic diagnosis of the mass was a 7 × 6 cm, well-encapsulated pheochromocytoma.

C, this nonfunctional left pheochromocytoma *(arrow)* in a patient with malignant melanoma was reportedly called metastatic melanoma on percutaneous aspiration biopsy. However, since the mass did not respond to interferon therapy and the patient was otherwise free of disease, it was excised and the diagnosis of pheochromocytoma was established histologically. Because of the presence of pigments, the cytologic differentiation could have been a difficult one.

B

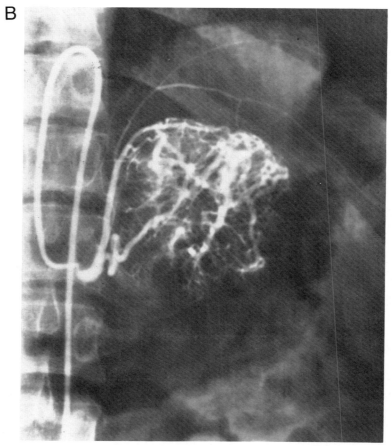

C

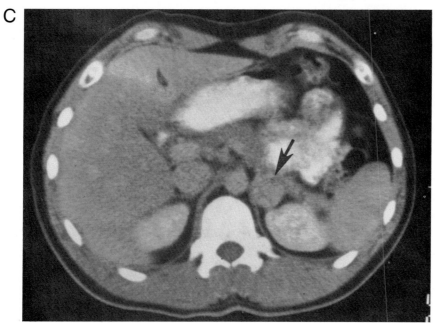

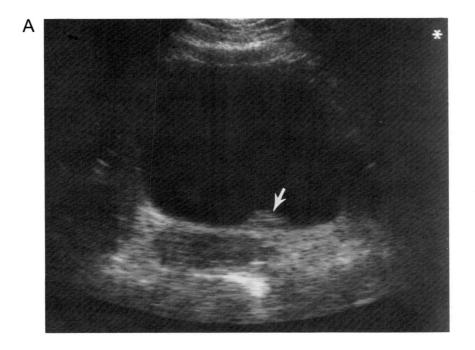

FIG 7–12.
Malignant and multicentric pheochromocytoma. A 42-year-old woman with a 20-year history of hypertension presented with irregular and heavy menses.

A, because there was a palpable mass on vaginal examination, a pelvic sonogram was done. It shows a bladder tumor *(arrow).*

B

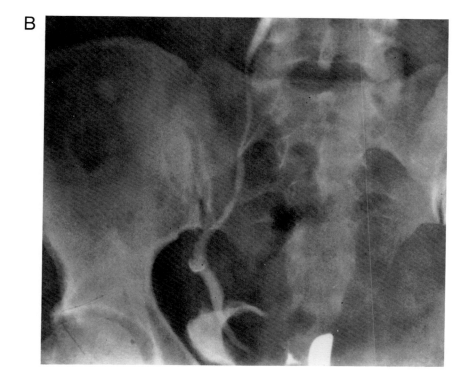

B, a retrograde pyelogram shows patency of the left ureter, with the mass projecting within the bladder lumen. Biopsy suggested the diagnosis of paraganglioma. (*Continued.*)

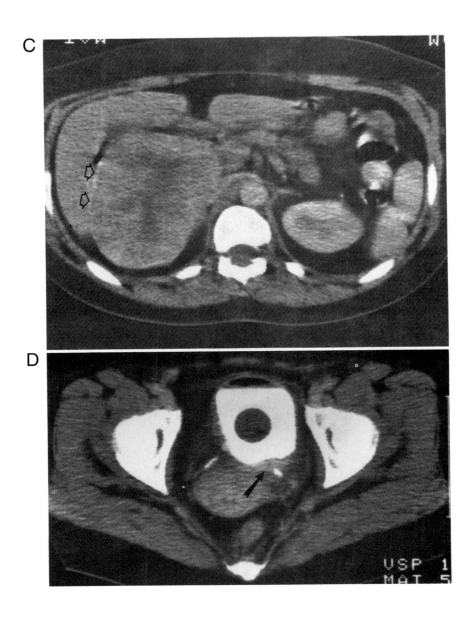

FIG 7–12 (cont.).
C and **D,** an abdominal and pelvic CT scan shows a large right suprarenal tumor. The mass is well encapsulated and has central low density. On several images, there was calcification of the wall *(arrows)*. The pelvic CT scan shows the bladder wall mass *(arrow)* adjacent to the opacified distal left ureter.
    E, the condition of the right kidney and liver was assessed with ultrasound. On this longitudinal sonogram, the echogenic mass with central hypoechoic regions is seen clearly separate from the right kidney and liver. Needle aspiration resulted in hemorrhage, necessitating transfusion.

The pathology report on biopsy material was nondiagnostic; however, because of the long-standing hypertension and probable vascular nature of the adrenal mass, pheochromocytoma was suspected.
    F, total-body ^{131}I-MIBG scanning was done in search of other sites of tumor. This scan shows significant uptake in the region of the right adrenal mass.
    At surgery, a very vascular right adrenal and left bladder sidewall mass was excised. The adrenal mass proved to be malignant pheochromocytoma, and the pelvic mass was a benign pheochromocytoma.

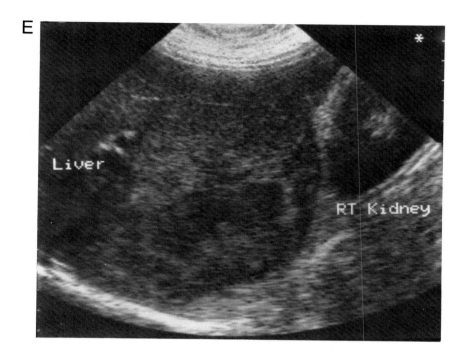

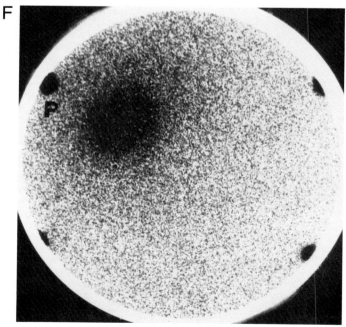

A

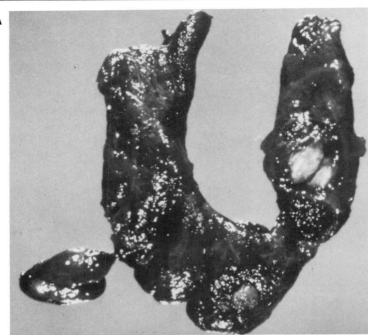

B

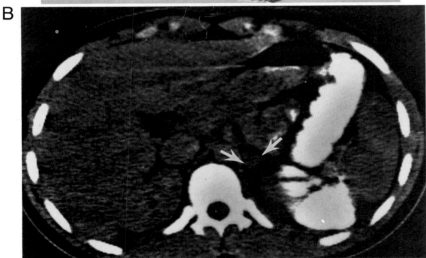

FIG 7–13.

Left pheochromocytoma (MEN type IIA syndrome). A 22-year-old man with hypercalcemia and medullary carcinoma of the thyroid had total thyroidectomy five years ago.

A, at the time of surgery, it was found that he also had parathyroid adenoma, which was treated by subtotal parathyroidectomy, the specimen from which is shown. Diagnosis of MEN type II syndrome was postulated (see also Color Plate 34).

B, this abdominal CT scan, along with endocrine profile, was obtained before surgery in search for pheochromocytoma. Both were reported normal.

C, after five years, the patient remained mildly hypertensive. Further workup included a follow-up abdominal CT, which shows a left adrenal mass. The patient was also found to have high levels of vanillylmandelic acid, metanephrine, and catecholamines in the urine.

Retrospective analysis of the original CT scan taken five years before suggests the presence of a nodule in the left adrenal gland (*arrows* in **B**). On the recent CT scan, the nodule has enlarged, measures approximately 3 cm in diameter, and shows areas of necrosis.

D, posterior view of radionuclide ^{131}I-MIBG scan shows increased radionuclide uptake in the left adrenal nodule (*arrows*), supporting the clinical diagnosis of pheochromocytoma.

At surgery, a 3.5-cm mass and two smaller nodules were found in the left adrenal gland, and the diagnosis of multifocal pheochromocytoma was made. Also, the right adrenal gland was noted to be hyperplastic. The patient underwent bilateral adrenalectomy. The pathology report was pheochromocytoma of the left adrenal and bilateral nodular medullary hyperplasia.

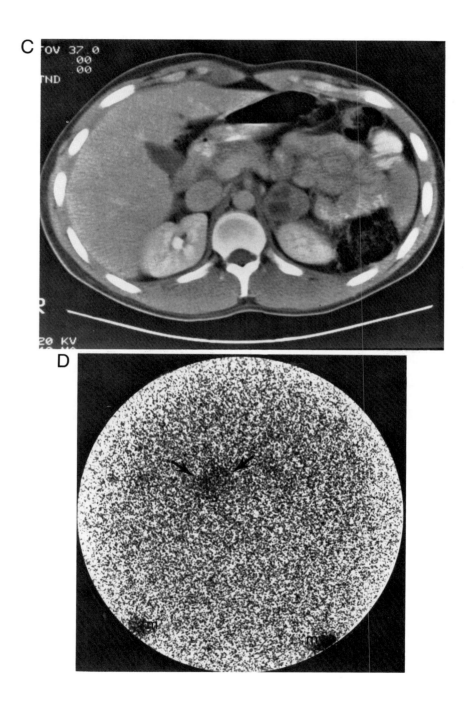

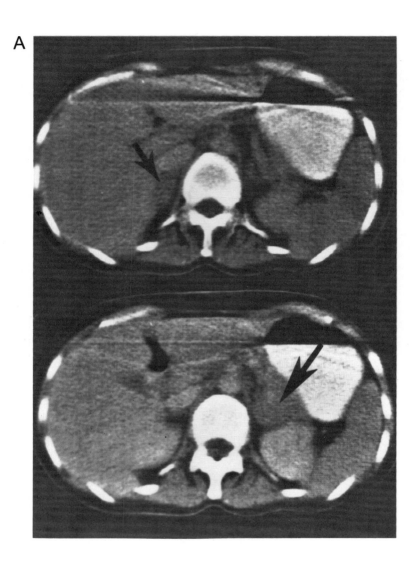

FIG 7–14.
Bilateral pheochromocytoma (MEN type II syndrome). A 21-year-old normotensive woman was diagnosed as having medullary carcinoma of the thyroid and underwent total thyroidectomy. Fifteen years later, she developed neck metastases, which were excised, and then she was followed annually. Eighteen years after thyroidectomy, she reported tachycardia, perspiration, and pulsatile headache. Urinary levels of vanillylmandelic acid, metanephrine, and catecholamines were elevated.

A, abdominal CT scan shows bilateral adrenal nodules, the left larger than the right *(arrows)*. Two months after this scan, the patient underwent bilateral adrenalectomy, and the diagnosis of bilateral pheochromocytoma was established.

This case is, in fact, one of MEN type II syndrome in which there were 18 years between the diagnoses of medullary carcinoma of the thyroid and of pheochromocytoma. Absence of any parathyroid abnormality suggests the diagnosis of MEN type IIB syndrome; however, there was no documented mucosal neuroma.

B, open mouth of a patient with MEN type IIB syndrome and ganglioneuromatosis of the tongue.

C, the marfanoid habitus in MEN type IIB syndrome. Notice the disproportionate length of the limbs in comparison with the remainder of the body. The musculature is wasted, the abdomen protuberant, and the lips thickened. (**B** and **C** from Dodd G.D.: The radiologic features of multiple endocrine neoplasia types IIA and IIB. *Semin. Roentgenol.* 20:64–90, 1985. Reproduced with permission.)

B

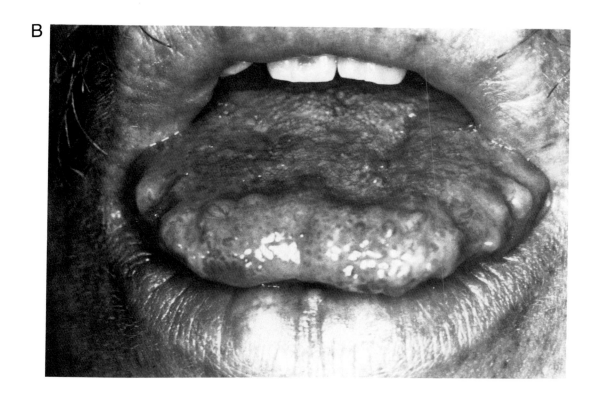

C

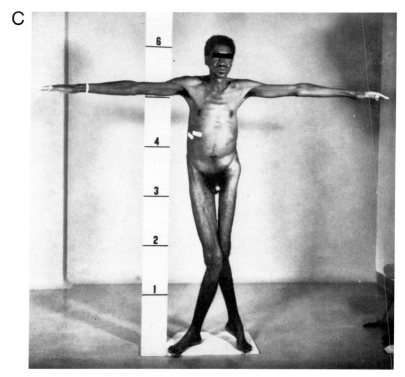

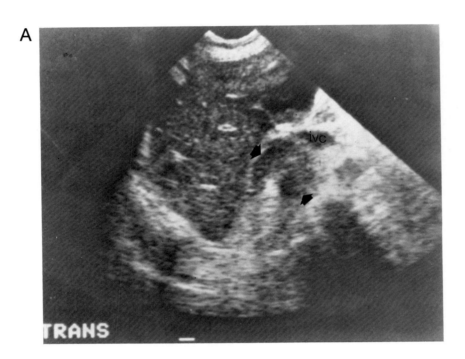

FIG 7–15.
Bilateral adrenal metastases from breast carcinoma. A 56-year-old woman who had been treated ten years before for breast cancer presented with a nodule in the right axilla and right groin. Biopsy showed adenocarcinoma. Total workup was done, including abdominal ultrasound and CT.

A, the ultrasound showed bilaterally enlarged adrenal glands, strongly suggesting metastases. Although the inverted V shape of the right adrenal is preserved on this sector scan, the organ is markedly thickened because of tumor infiltration *(arrows)*. The inferior vena cava *(IVC)* is displaced anteriorly by the large adrenal.

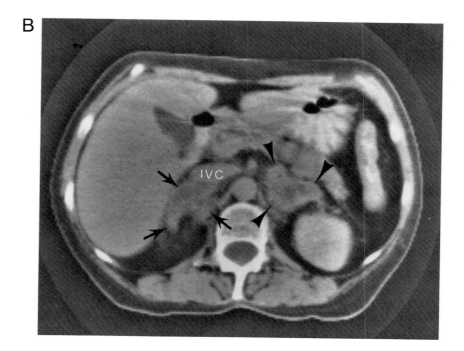

B, on CT scan, the very large adrenal glands are seen with areas of low density. The triangular (*arrowheads,* in the left) and V-shaped (*arrows,* in the right) preservation of the adrenals is better seen here. The inferior vena cava (*IVC*) is displaced anteriorly by the right adrenal metastasis. There was no clinical evidence of adrenal insufficiency. The patient underwent chemotherapy but died nine months later of sepsis. The diagnosis of metastases was proved at autopsy.

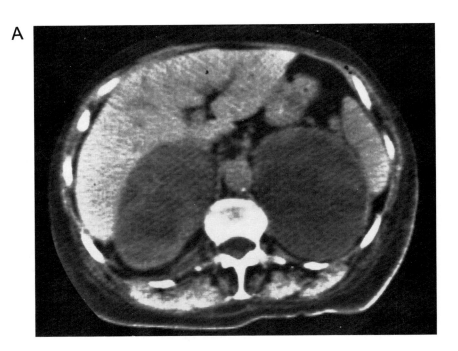

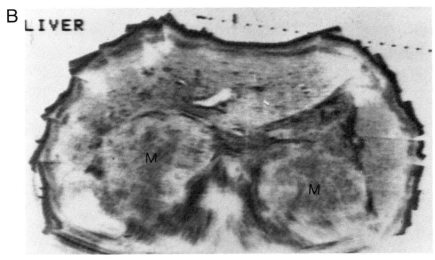

FIG 7–16.
"Headlight" metastases (multiple cases).

A, a 62-year-old woman with breast carcinoma developed metastases and was referred to M. D. Anderson Hospital for chemotherapy. Review of the pathology slides of primary disease revealed carcinoma with sarcomatoid metaplasia.

Abdominal CT shows that both adrenal glands are very large. This finding, which has been described as the "headlight" sign, is consistent with metastases to the adrenal glands.

B, transverse sonogram in a 47-year-old man with malignant melanoma shows bilateral adrenal metastases *(M)* presenting as the headlight sign.

C, the right metastasis (of headlight metastases) in another melanoma patient is seen on this sagittal sonogram to cause elevation of the inferior vena cava *(open arrows).*

D, the fourth case of headlight metastases in another melanoma patient is shown on this enhanced CT image. Narrow window is used to illustrate the solid and cystic compartments of the well-encapsulated bilateral metastases.

C

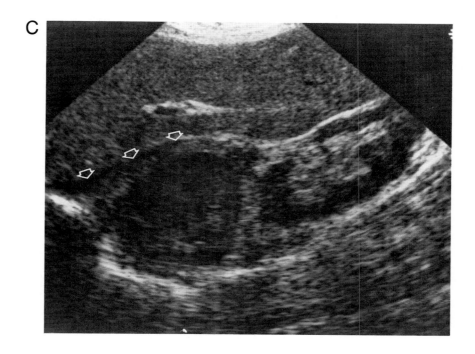

D

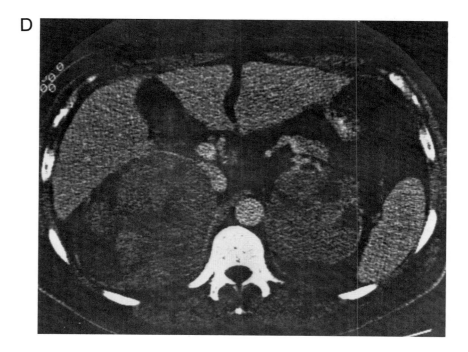

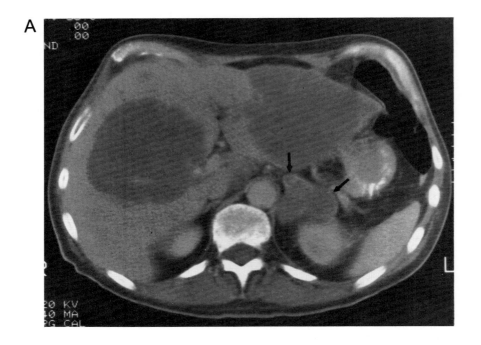

FIG 7–17.
Left adrenal metastasis with tumor extension into renal vein. A 42-year-old woman with a known diagnosis of malignant melanoma underwent abdominal CT because of hepato-megaly.

A, this CT scan shows a large triangular metastasis *(arrows)* in the left adrenal gland. The right adrenal is normal, and there are multiple liver metastases.

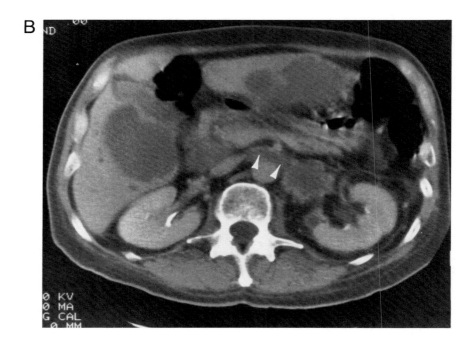

B, at 20 mm below the image in **A,** the inferior part of the left adrenal mass is seen to involve the proximal left renal vein and extend more medially toward the inferior vena cava *(arrowheads).*

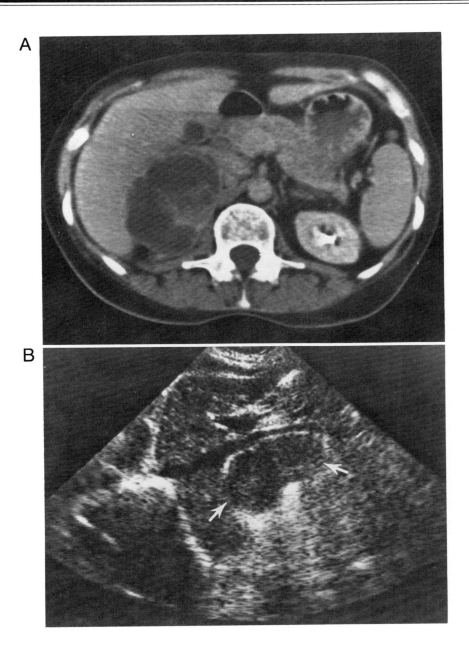

FIG 7–18.
Regression of right adrenal metastases from lung cancer. A 56-year-old woman with a diagnosis of large cell differentiated bronchogenic carcinoma underwent CT of the chest and upper abdomen.

A, upper abdominal CT reveals a large mass in the right adrenal fossa. Because the mass could not be distinguished from the right kidney, an abdominal ultrasound was done.

B, the parasagittal sonogram shows a well-defined suprarenal mass *(arrows)* and normal kidney (not seen here) and liver. Notice that the retrocaval adrenal mass has displaced the inferior vena cava anteriorly. No tumor is seen within the inferior vena cava.

C, ultrasound-guided percutaneous aspiration proved the diagnosis of adenocarcinoma metastases from lung.

D, the patient underwent chemotherapy. The chest radiograph and repeat abdominal CT scan eight months after the first CT revealed that the lung tumor is remarkably smaller and that there is marked shrinkage of the right adrenal metastases.

C

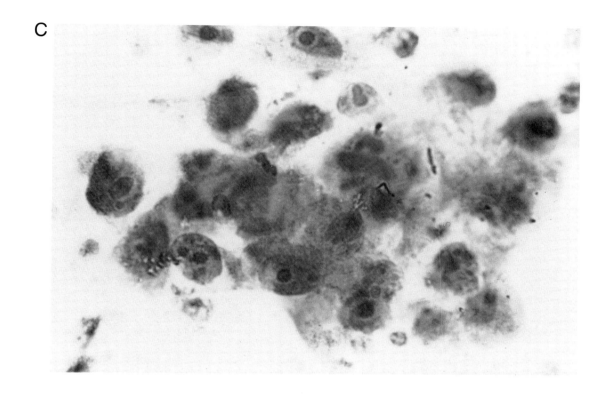

D

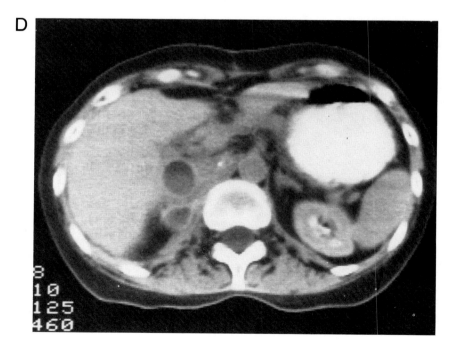

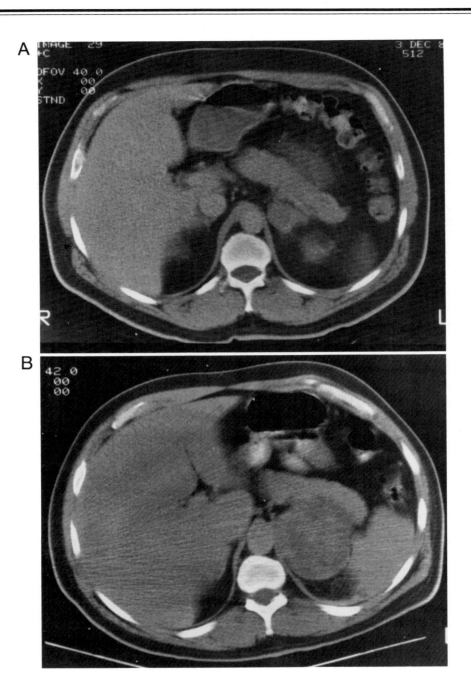

FIG 7–19.
Growing left adrenal metastasis from lung cancer. A 47-year-old man with a diagnosis of squamous cell carcinoma of the lung underwent abdominal CT.

A, a small nodule is seen in the left adrenal gland. A percutaneous fine-needle biopsy was performed on the gland, and findings were compatible with adenoma.

B, the patient underwent radiotherapy of lung and chemotherapy for two months, after which he was reevaluated by chest CT that included the upper abdomen. The adrenal mass has significantly grown in the interim, leaving no doubt that the case is one of adrenal metastases. This case is an example of the needle sampling the normal adrenal cortex and not the metastatic deposit. A normal adrenal cytology can mimic adenoma.

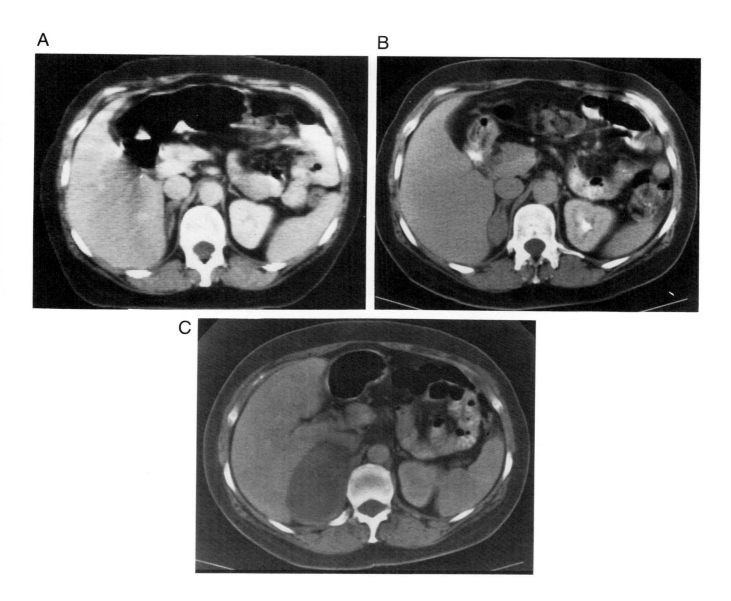

FIG 7–20.
Growing right adrenal metastasis from melanoma. A 33-year-old woman with a diagnosis of malignant melanoma had been receiving chemotherapy for 12 months.

A, the initial CT scan shows the right adrenal gland to be of borderline size. Results were interpreted to be within normal limits, but the patient continued to receive chemotherapy because of pelvic lymphadenopathy.

B, a repeat CT scan five weeks later demonstrates definite metastases to the right adrenal gland. On retrospective analysis the first study shows presence of soft tissue density between the medial and lateral limbs of the adrenal glands. The chemotherapy was continued, and three months later the patient underwent chemoembolization of the right adrenal gland.

C, repeat CT scan 11 months after the study in **A** shows remarkable progression of metastases in the right adrenal. Interestingly, the pelvic lymphadenopathy was stable.

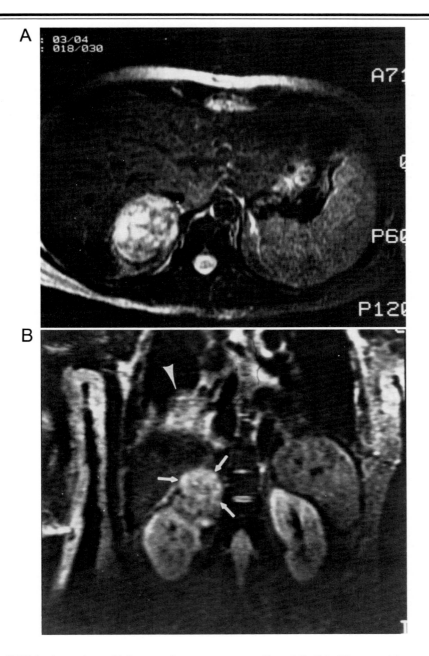

FIG 7–21.

Adrenal metastases (MRI features in multiple cases).

A and **B,** a 49-year-old woman was diagnosed as having right lower lobe bronchogenic carcinoma.

The T$_2$-weighted magnetic resonance images of the upper abdomen in axial **(A)** and coronal **(B)** views (TR/TE, 1,500/70) show a large mass with increased signal intensity in the right adrenal gland *(arrows).* On the coronal image, the right lower lobe primary mass *(arrowhead),* with similar signal intensity, is also evident.

The magnetic resonance findings of a mass showing high signal intensity on T$_2$-weighted images were thought to be characteristic for metastases,[59] which was subsequently proved by biopsy.

C and **D,** this 69-year-old man had left nephrectomy for renal cell carcinoma 20 months ago. At routine CT follow-up, a right adrenal nodule was discovered.

The unenhanced CT scan **(C)** shows a well-defined solid mass *(M)* in the right adrenal gland. A lobulated cyst *(C)* is seen in the upper pole of the right kidney.

The T$_2$-weighted magnetic resonance image (TR/TE, 2,000/80) **(D)** shows the same mass with very high signal intensity *(arrows),* much higher than that of the liver. Notice that an area within the mass displays an even higher signal.

Percutaneous aspiration proved metastatic renal cell carcinoma, and the patient underwent right adrenalectomy. *(Continued.)*

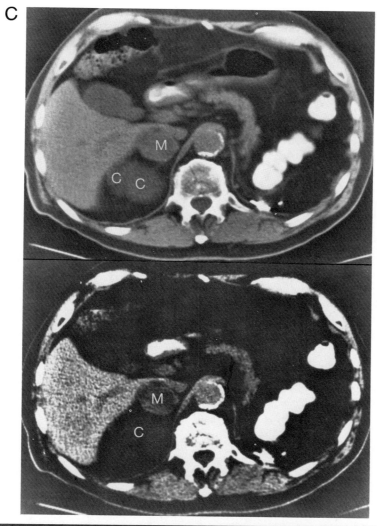

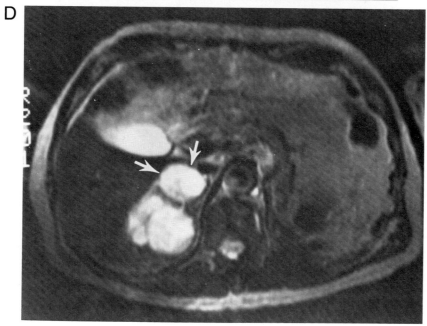

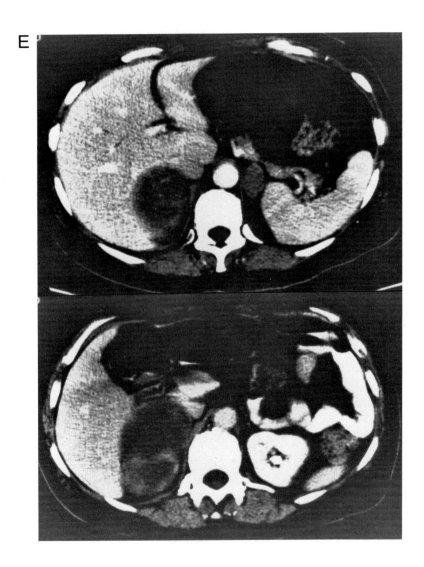

FIG 7–21 (cont.).
E through **G,** a third patient, a 51-year-old woman with known melanoma, presented with abdominal pain. A CT scan **(E)** shows bilateral adrenal masses, with increased density on the right, presumably hemorrhagic metastases. The coronal T$_1$-weighted (TR/TE, 800/25) magnetic reso- nance image **(F)** obtained two months later shows bilateral metastases with right lobulation and probably hemorrhage displaying the high signal intensity. The axial T$_2$-weighted image (TR/TE, 2,000/80) **(G)** shows characteristic increase in the signal intensity of the masses.

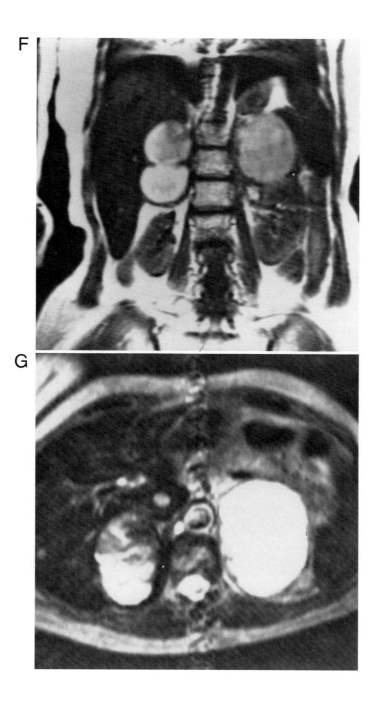

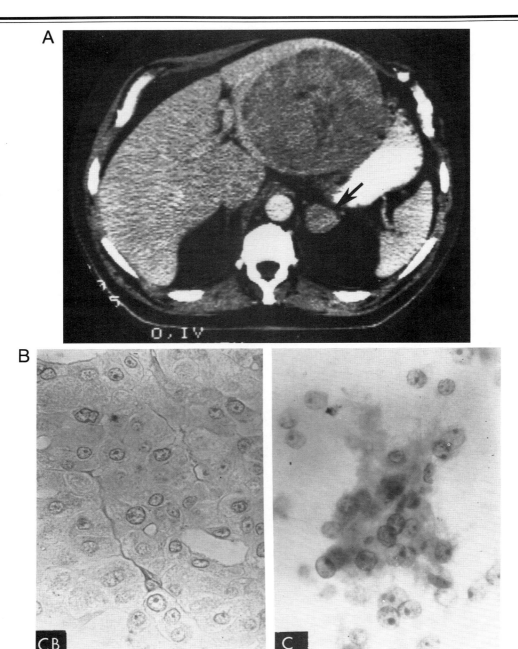

FIG 7–22.

Left adrenal metastasis from hepatoma. A 65-year-old man presented with gradual loss of appetite and weight loss along with a palpable mass in the upper abdomen.

A, abdominal CT scan reveals a large mass within the left lobe of the liver and a 2-cm nodule in the left adrenal gland *(arrow)*. The patient was examined by angiography, and the diagnosis of hepatocellular carcinoma was strongly considered. While the patient was being prepared for left hepatic lobectomy, it was decided to perform a biopsy on the left adrenal mass, since that mass could represent a metastatic lesion.

B, the percutaneous aspiration biopsy proved the adrenal mass to be metastatic hepatocellular carcinoma to the left adrenal gland. The cell block *(CB)* demonstrates a well-formed trabecular arrangement of epithelial cells with cytologic features suggestive of hepatocytes, consistent with hepatoma. The cytologic sample *(C)* shows clusters of polygonal cells with central nuclei and prominent nucleoli with occasional bile pigment, consistent with hepatocellular carcinoma.

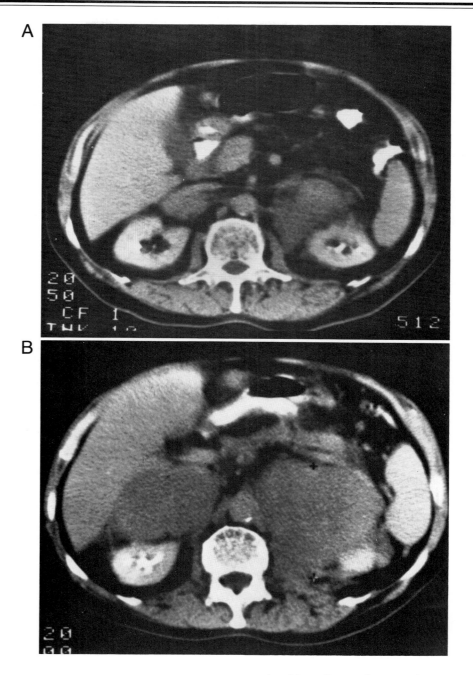

FIG 7–23.
Bilateral small cell carcinoma in adrenals. A 72-year-old man presented with weight loss and upper abdominal pain.

A, abdominal CT scan shows bilateral adrenal masses. No other abnormality was found on CT or other studies. A CT-guided biopsy of the left adrenal mass showed small cell carcinoma. Intensive search for a primary was unsuccessful. Differential diagnosis for a small cell tumor within the adrenal gland would include metastatic oat cell carcinoma, adenoid cystic carcinoma, cloacogenic carcinoma of the rectum, lymphoma, and primary adult neuroblastoma.

B, with the presumptive diagnosis of lymphoma, the patient received chemotherapy. A repeat CT scan in five weeks shows significant enlargement of masses in both adrenals. Further search for a primary failed. The patient died of heart failure, and no autopsy was performed. (Courtesy of Bryan Koons, M.D., Durham County General Hospital, Durham, N.C.)

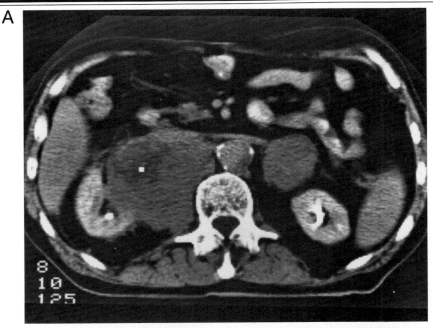

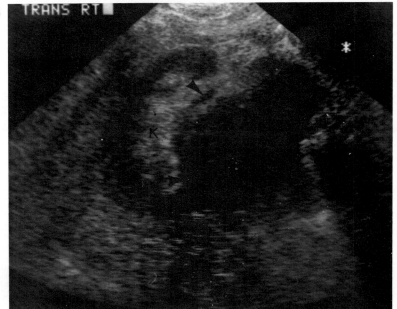

FIG 7–24.

Primary large cell lymphoma of the adrenals. A 74-year-old man who complained of abdominal discomfort and weight loss had a CT examination followed by percutaneous biopsy, both in an outside hospital. A diagnosis of small cell carcinoma was made, but the results of an extensive workup for the primary were normal. He was referred to M. D. Anderson Hospital.

A, abdominal CT reveals bilateral suprarenal masses with the right one not definitely separate from the right kidney. The initial diagnostic considerations included primary right renal cell carcinoma with left adrenal metastasis and bilateral adrenal primary vs. metastatic tumor. No adenopathy was seen.

B, ultrasound was used to see if the mass was separable from the right kidney and also for guided biopsy. On this transverse scan, which corresponds to the CT in **A,** the right kidney *(K)* is displaced laterally by a large, hypoechoic mass. There is a normal plane between the kidney *(arrowheads)* and the mass. Percutaneous biopsy was repeated for cytology, flow cytometry, and evaluation of cell markers, and the diagnosis of large cell lymphoma was established.

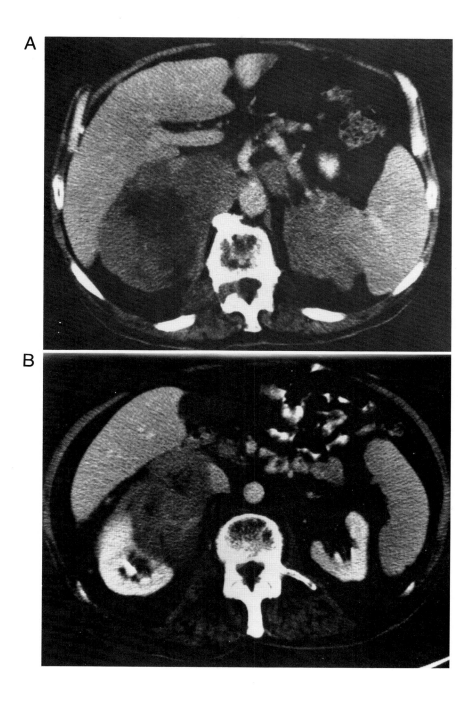

FIG 7–25.
Primary bilateral adrenal lymphoma. A 72-year-old man was known to have neurofibromatosis for many years but recently developed weight loss of about 18 kg (40 lb) over five months. His workup revealed bilateral large adrenal masses, which prompted an evaluation.

A and **B,** a CT scan of the abdomen shows large masses in the region of the adrenal glands with probable right renal infiltration **(B).** The patient's blood pressure was normal, and his endocrine profile was negative for disease. (*Continued.*)

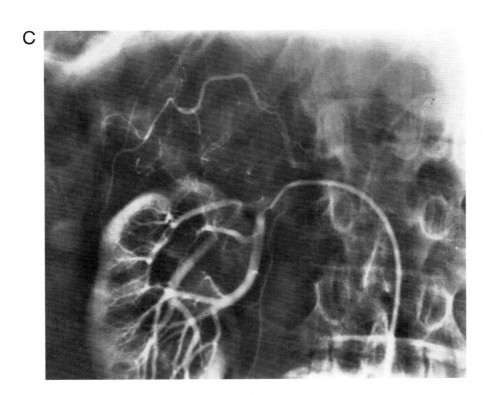

FIG 7–25 (cont.).
C, the renal angiogram shows a normal right kidney with probably a hypovascular tumor of the right adrenal. The left angiogram also showed the same finding. The initial diagnostic considerations included bilateral adrenal neurofibromas or ganglioneuroma, lymphoma, metastases from an unknown primary, and, less likely, bilateral nonfunctional pheochromocytoma or adrenal cortical carcinoma. Percutaneous aspiration cytology of the right adrenal mass suggested lymphoma.

Twenty days later the patient developed massive pneumonia and died. At autopsy, the diagnosis of cutaneous neurofibromas with massive lymphoma replacing both adrenal glands was confirmed.

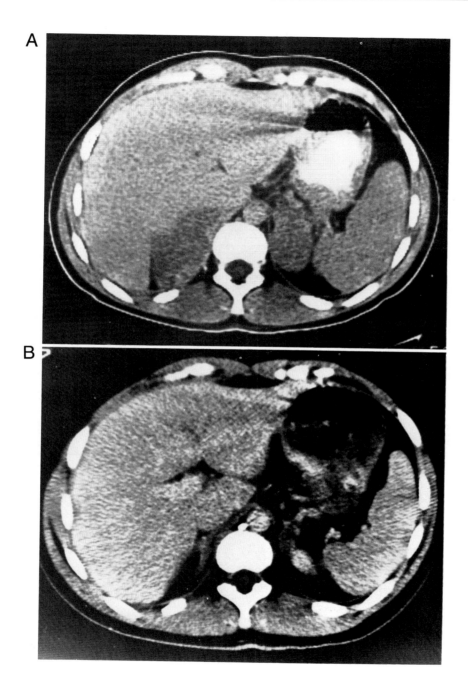

FIG 7–26.

Secondary bilateral adrenal lymphoma. A 28-year-old man presented with progressive adenopathy of submandibular nodes. A diagnosis of lymphoma was established on biopsy.

A, the abdominal CT scan reveals bilateral enlarged adrenal glands, along with mesenteric and retroperitoneal adenopathy. The patient received appropriate chemotherapy for lymphoma.

B, seven weeks after the beginning of treatment, a repeat CT scan shows a remarkable decrease in the size of the adrenals and almost total disappearance of the extensive adenopathy and mesenteric lymphoma.

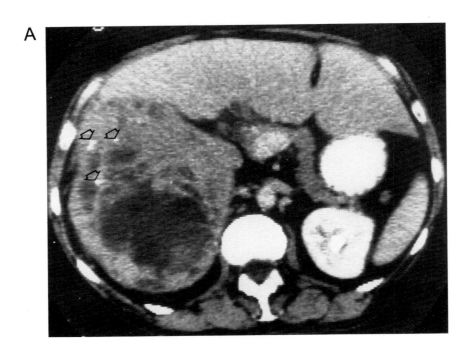

A

FIG 7–27.

Right adrenal leiomyosarcoma. A 59-year-old woman was referred to her local hospital because of an approximately six-month history of intermittent right flank pain, occasional hematuria, and pyuria. On intravenous pyelography, the right kidney was seen to be displaced inferiorly. Because there was a palpable spleen, a liver-spleen scan done reportedly showed a large mass in the right lobe of the liver, along with splenomegaly.

A, a CT scan of the abdomen reveals a large mass separate from the liver in the right upper quadrant, with areas of low density and also areas of calcification *(arrows)*. The right kidney appeared to be displaced inferiorly and laterally and also to be involved by the tumor. The patient's endocrine profile was normal. The most likely diagnosis is nonfunctional adrenal cortical carcinoma.

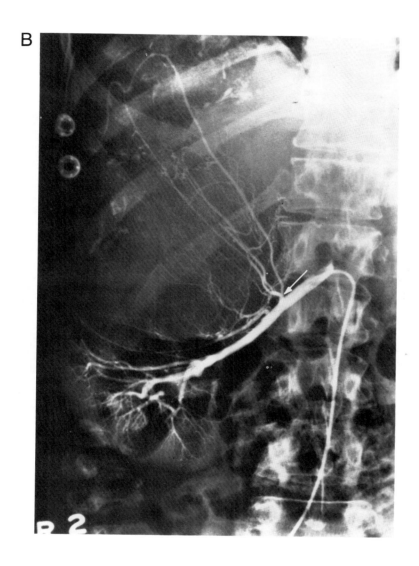

B, selective right renal angiography shows a relatively hypovascular tumor being fed by a fairly large inferior right adrenal artery *(arrow).* Diagnosis of right adrenal neoplasm was confirmed, and percutaneous biopsy proved leiomyosarcoma.

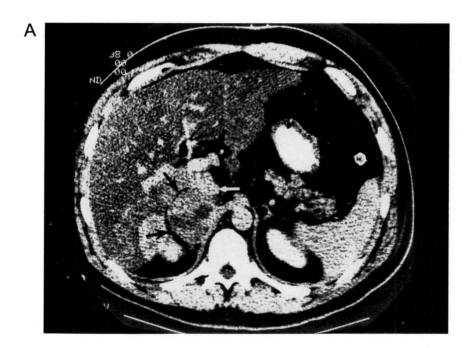

FIG 7–28.
Functional right adrenal cortical carcinoma. A 44-year-old man visited his physician because of a 13.6-kg (30-lb) weight gain in a short time and was found to be hypertensive. For six months he was treated by means of a controlled diet and beta blockers. However, he developed right upper quadrant pain, and a right suprarenal mass was incidentally discovered on a gallbladder sonogram. His endocrine profile was consistent with Cushing's syndrome.

A, the CT scan of the upper abdomen shows a large, well-encapsulated right adrenal mass with areas of low density *(black arrows).* The mass has displaced the inferior vena cava anteriorly *(white arrow).*

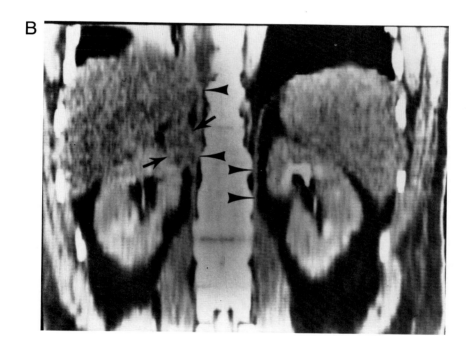

B, a reconstruction image was obtained to confirm the lack of renal invasion. On this farthest posterior, coronally reconstructed image, no definite hepatic or renal invasion is seen. A portion of the tumor *(arrows)* is seen here. It is separate from the crura of the diaphragm *(arrowheads)*.

At surgery, the diagnosis of adrenal cortical carcinoma was proved, and the tumor was entirely excised. The patient underwent postoperative chemotherapy.

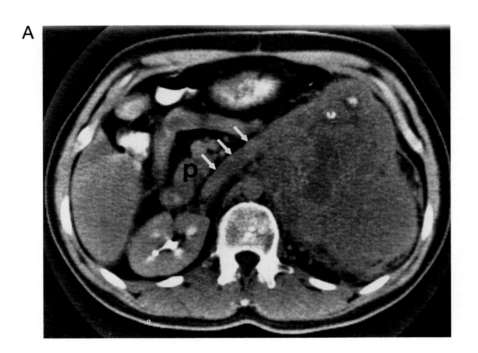

FIG 7–29.

Large nonfunctional left adrenal cortical carcinoma. A 46-year-old man presented with abdominal pressure, nausea, and vomiting. An upper gastrointestinal series showed a retrogastric mass, and endoscopy results were negative for disease. The initial diagnosis was pancreatic neoplasm.

A, a CT scan of the abdomen reveals a large retroperitoneal mass with areas of low density and calcification. The mass displaces the mesenteric vessels and uncinate process of the pancreas *(p)* to the right and extends into the left renal vein *(arrows).* The left kidney (not shown) was displaced inferiorly. Percutaneous biopsy established the diagnosis of adrenal cortical carcinoma.

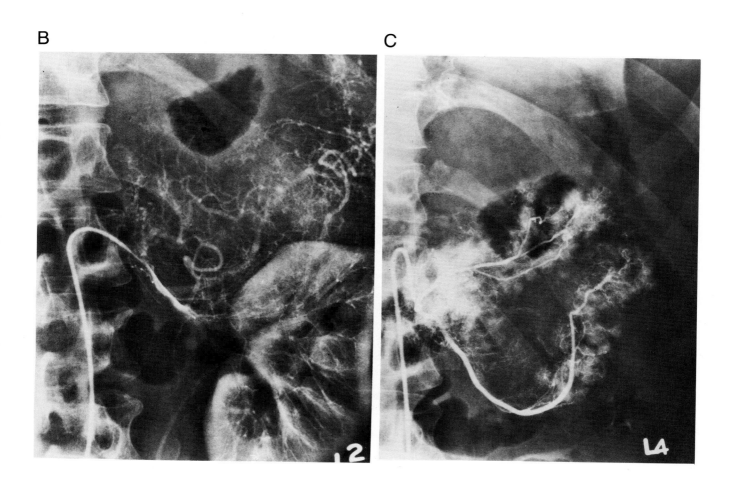

B, a left renal arteriogram shows integrity of the left kidney and tumor vascularity in the suprarenal mass. The mass is very large and moderately vascular with blood supply from the left renal, left superior capsular, and inferior adrenal arteries. There was complete occlusion of the left renal vein, but because of many collaterals, the function of the left kidney was maintained.

C, injection of contrast material into the left middle adrenal arteries shows those arteries to be large and to have abnormal vascularity. This route was used for intraarterial chemotherapy with cisplatin.

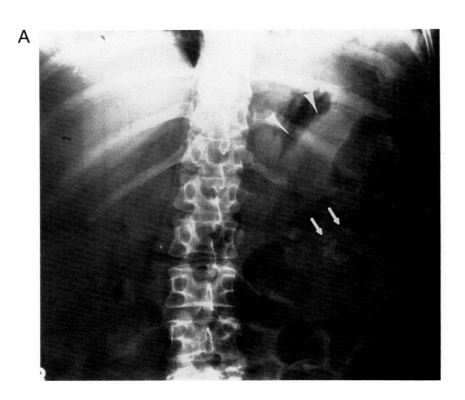

FIG 7–30.

Large functional left adrenal cortical carcinoma. A 34-year-old woman presented with a history of weight gain during the past four years, during which time she was treated for hypertension. In the preceding four months, she had noticed increasing edema in the lower extremities along with abdominal fullness. A mass was palpated on physical examination of the abdomen.

A, the abdominal film shows multiple areas of calcification in the left upper quadrant *(arrows)* with mass effect on gastric air *(arrowheads)*. On intravenous pyelography (not shown), the left kidney was seen to be displaced inferiorly and laterally with its upper pole flattened, making the diagnosis of left adrenal mass most likely. The endocrine profile suggested Cushing's syndrome.

B, the abdominal CT scan, which was made within one week, shows the large, calcified, nonhomogeneous left suprarenal mass displacing the left kidney *(k)* laterally. The mass has directly invaded the left renal vein, extending across the midline to the inferior vena cava *(arrow)*. This invasion was probably responsible for the patient's increasing edema in the lower extremities. In addition, multiple hepatic metastases are seen. Cytology of material aspirated from the primary mass established the diagnosis of adrenal cortical carcinoma.

C, left adrenal angiography, which was done via the left middle adrenal artery, shows the left adrenal tumor with areas of hypervascular blush and neovascularity. Separate injection into the inferior left adrenal artery was also performed. The patient's left middle and inferior adrenal arteries were embolized, and she underwent chemotherapy.

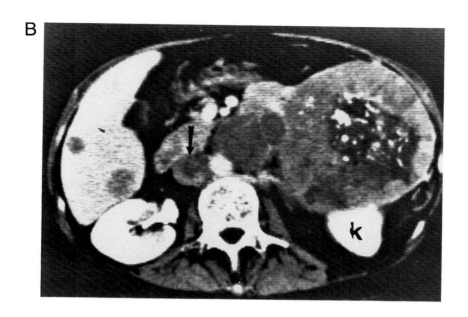

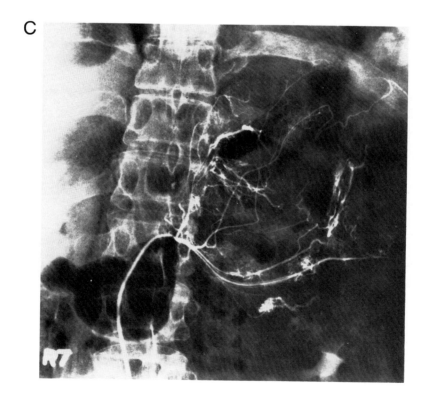

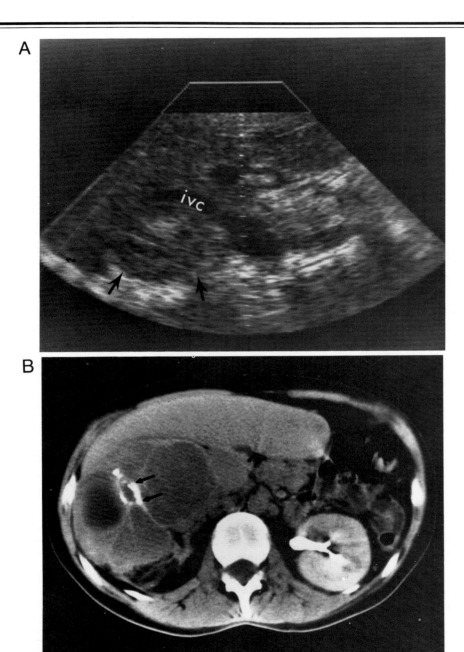

FIG 7–31.

Nonfunctional right adrenal cortical carcinoma. A 45-year-old woman with a two-week history of right upper quadrant pain underwent ultrasound evaluation.

A, the parasagittal sonogram along the inferior vena cava (*ivc*) shows a retrocaval mass *(arrows)* separate from the liver and kidney and located within the right adrenal gland. The inferior vena cava could not be totally evaluated.

B, the CT scan shows a well-defined mass with areas of septation and focal calcification *(arrows)*. The right kidney was normal. The tumor has mainly extended laterally, with slight mass effect on the inferior vena cava.

C, since the inferior vena cava could not be well defined, cavography was done and demonstrated its integrity. On this lateral view, the inferior vena cava is displaced anteriorly by the large retrocaval mass. Attenuation of contrast within the inferior vena cava is due to the mass and slow flow.

Percutaneous biopsy established the diagnosis of adrenal cortical carcinoma. The patient underwent right adrenalectomy and nephrectomy.

D, surgical specimen shows large, well-encapsulated mass with central calcification (see also Color Plate 35).

C

D

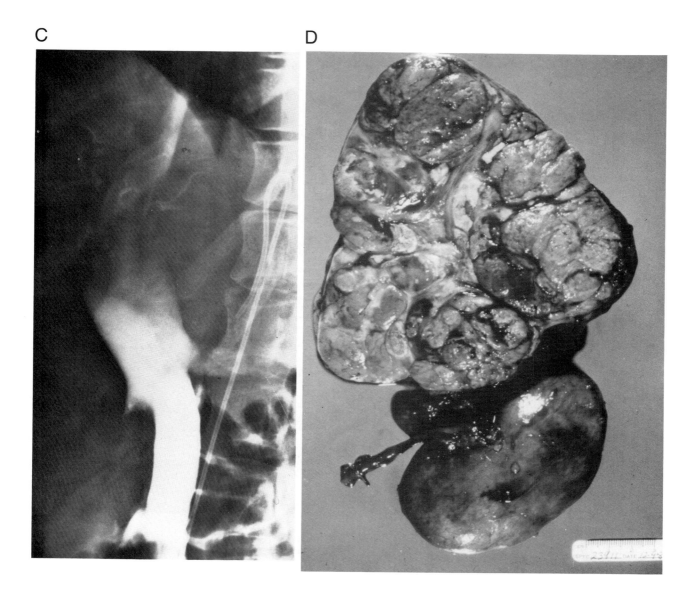

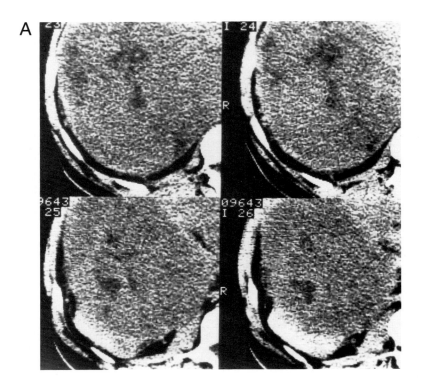

FIG 7–32.
Right adrenal cortical carcinoma with renal invasion. A 50-year-old woman presented with hematuria, and on physical examination a right upper quadrant mass was palpated. Intravenous urography (not shown) suggested primary renal cell carcinoma.

A, on sequential CT a very large mass with areas of low density representing necrosis is seen infiltrating and displacing the right kidney laterally and inferiorly. Most of the upper pole appeared to be involved by tumor.

B, selective right renal arteriogram shows the large inferior right adrenal artery *(arrows)* feeding the hypervascular neoplasm. Tumor parasitization of renal arteries on account of renal infiltration is well seen.

C, inferior venacavogram (lateral view) demonstrates marked anterior displacement of the vein without evidence of tumor invasion.

The patient underwent tumor excision along with right nephrectomy. The diagnosis of adrenal cortical carcinoma with renal invasion was proved.

B

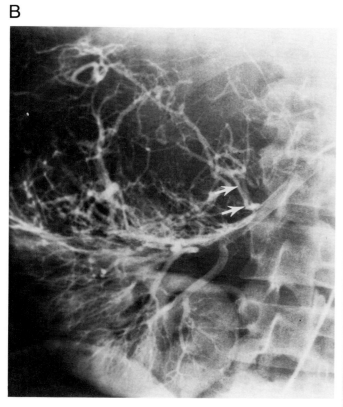

C

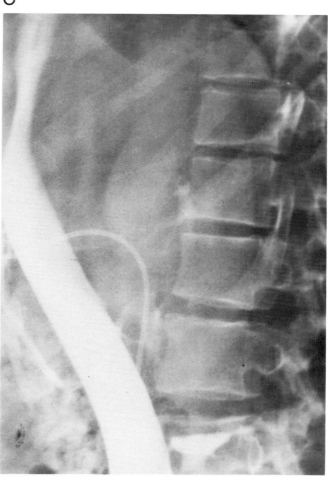

A

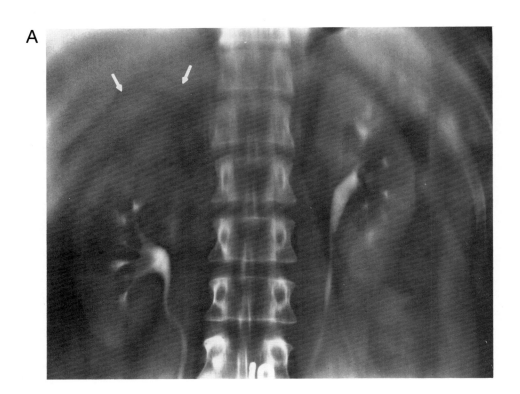

FIG 7–33.
Recurrent right adrenal cortical carcinoma. A 52-year-old man with a history of right adrenal cortical carcinoma resected four years previously developed a nodule in the scar incision. Material aspirated from the nodule was cytologically positive for adrenal cortical carcinoma. The subse-quent routine workup included intravenous urography.

A, the nephrotomogram shows a mass in the region of the right upper pole *(arrows);* the mass could not be separated from the kidney. To determine whether this mass originated in the right kidney or in the adrenal bed, a sonogram was obtained.

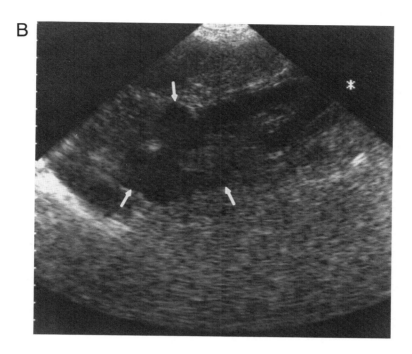

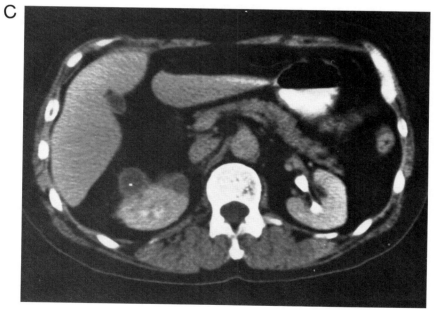

B, the parasagittal sonogram through the right kidney shows an irregularly outlined hypoechoic tumor in the upper pole of the kidney *(arrows).* At this point, it was unclear whether the case was one of a primary renal cell neoplasm, complicated cyst, or, possibly, recurrent adrenal tumor with renal invasion.

C, a CT scan, which was done for guided aspiration biopsy, shows a solid lobulated mass that has infiltrated the upper pole of the right kidney (cursor measures 56 Houns-field units). A CT-guided biopsy proved the mass to be a local recurrence of adrenal cortical carcinoma. The patient did not have any signs or symptoms of endocrine dysfunction or renal abnormality.

The diagnosis of local recurrence of adrenal tumor with renal infiltration in the right suprarenal area and metastasis in the incision was proved at surgery, and the patient underwent resection of the recurrence along with right nephrectomy. *(Continued.)*

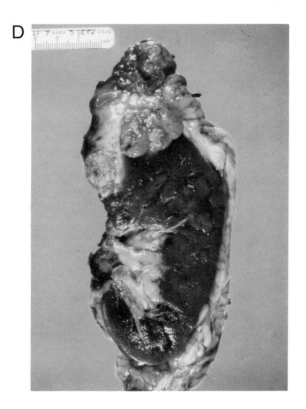

FIG 7–33 (cont.).
  D, surgical specimen shows infiltration of the upper pole of the right kidney by recurrent adrenal cortical carci-noma (see also Color Plate 36).

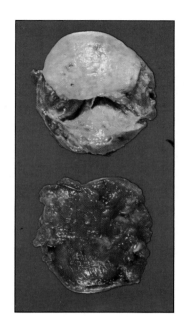

PLATE 31

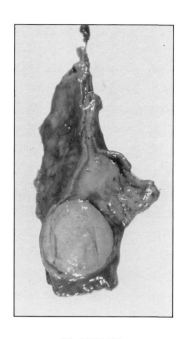

PLATE 32

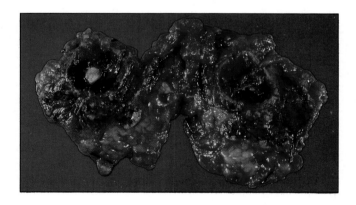

PLATE 33

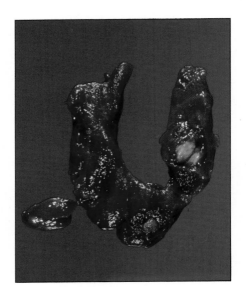

PLATE 34

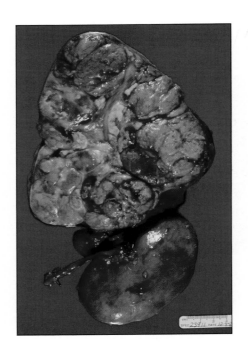

PLATE 35

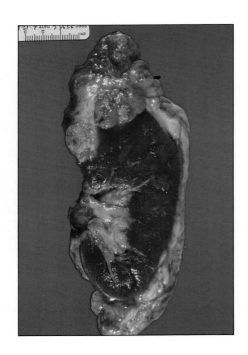

PLATE 36

8

Pediatric Abdominal and Pelvic Neoplasms

Farzin Eftekhari, M.D.

INTEGRATED IMAGING OF MASSES

The purpose of imaging in the management of pediatric abdominal and pelvic tumors is to confirm the presence of a mass, define the organ of origin, determine the internal texture of the mass, and identify invasion of adjacent structures. In addition, imaging serves as a staging procedure. Imaging procedures and the choice of modality vary from one institution to another since no one approach is definitive. Although utilizing a whole set of the older and newer imaging modalities will, of course, increase the accuracy of the diagnosis, the ultimate goal should be the utilization of the minimum number of imaging tests necessary for diagnosis. The achievement of this goal requires the coordinated efforts of radiologists, pediatricians, and surgeons. The radiologic studies performed should take into account the age of the patient and the clinical findings.

In the newborn with abdominal or pelvic mass, because of poor renal function, ultrasound offers information superior to that from urography.[1] For example, if the mass arises from the kidney and is cystic, hydronephrosis or a multicystic kidney is likely, and they can be differentiated by ultrasound supplemented by radionuclide scanning.[2] When the mass arises from the liver, a radionuclide scan will pro-

vide significant information, and it may be diagnostic in hemangioendothelioma.[2, 3] If supplemental information is required in such a case, angiography and perhaps computed tomography (CT) may be performed. In the older infant and young child, ultrasound should probably be the preliminary screening test. Further information, if desired, may be obtained from CT examination.[2]

Although intravenous urography is still being done in many institutions and does indeed provide valuable information about renal function and displacement or obstruction by the mass,[1, 2] it is now believed that CT provides all the necessary data for staging the renal tumor and, if available, should replace urography.[2, 4, 5] Recently published reports on the role of magnetic resonance imaging (MRI) in pediatric tumors[6] appear very promising; this modality may potentially replace all other modalities and consequently become cost effective. Other modalities, such as angiography, lymphangiography, and catheter inferior venacavography, have their indications when the need for more specific information arises.[2, 7]

It is worth emphasizing that maximal diagnostic information should be obtained at minimal cost and with the least trauma, delay, and radiation exposure of the child. It should not be assumed that all of the imaging modalities are complementary.

GENITOURINARY NEOPLASMS

Wilms' Tumor and Other Renal Tumors

Wilms' tumor (Figs 8–1 to 8–10) is the most common abdominal and renal tumor of childhood. It is slightly more common than abdominal neuroblastoma and accounts for 22% of abdominal masses after the newborn period.[2] In neonates and young infants, congenital mesoblastic nephroma (fetal renal hamartoma) is more common.[8] Wilms' tumor has a peak incidence at three years of age.[2] Ninety percent of the tumors occur in children younger than seven years, and 77% occur in children less than five years of age.[9] There is a male predominance. The most common clinical presentation of the tumor is an abdominal mass, although hematuria and hypertension are not uncommon.[8] Associated anomalies include aniridia, hemihypertrophy, and horseshoe kidneys (Fig 8–8).[2, 8–10] It is bilateral in 5% of cases (Figs 8–6 and 8–7), 65% of which are synchronous tumors.[2, 8] Wilms' tumor is histologically a nephrogenic epithelial tumor arising from minute foci of persistent blastemal cells. The tumor has a wide spectrum of histologic pictures, varying from a benign renal blastema (Wilms' tumor in situ) to a highly malignant sarcomatous form. In between lie the ordinary true Wilms' tumors.[8] Wilms' tumor and the so-called variants are classified into favorable and unfavorable histologies, with survivals of 90% and 20% to 30%, respectively.[8, 9]

Interrelated variants of Wilms' tumor include multilocular cystic nephroma, cystic Wilms' tumor, and diffuse nephroblastomatosis (Fig 8–10).[8]

Staging of Wilms' tumors is based on local extent and presence or absence of distant metastases.[8] In stage I, the disease is limited to the kidney and the capsule is intact (Figs 8–1 to 8–4). In stage II, the tumor, still completely excisable, extends beyond the kidney and may infiltrate the renal vein and vena cava but not adjacent organs or nodes (Fig 8–5). In stage III, again a resectable stage, there is nonhematogenous tumor in the abdomen, excluding the liver. In stage IV (Fig 8–9), there are hematogenous metastases, for example, to lungs, liver, brain, or bone. Stage V is defined by bilateral renal involvement. Prognosis depends not only on stage but on the degree of sarcomatous or anaplastic changes. Overall prognosis with surgery and chemotherapy is excellent (80%–90%).[2]

Fetal rhabdomyomatous nephroblastoma (Fig 8–8), which is a predominantly monophasic mesenchymal variant of Wilms' tumor, is not seen in children more than four years of age. Despite its large size, the tumor acts less aggressively and entails a better prognosis than does ordinary Wilms' tumor. Bilateralism occurs in one third of the cases and affects the overall prognosis negatively.[11, 12]

Malignant rhabdoid tumor of the kidney (Fig 8–11), probably not a variant of Wilms' tumor, occurs in younger infants and is one of the most lethal neoplasms of early life. The tumor frequently metastasizes to the brain, but separate primary tumors have been seen in the posterior fossa.[9, 13, 14]

Clear cell sarcoma likewise is a distinct monophasic malignant tumor and tends to metastasize to bone (42%–76%). The survival rate is less than 50%, and the tumor has a tendency to recur locally. Unlike Wilms' tumor, clear cell sarcoma infiltrates the adjacent renal tissue instead of forming a pseudocapsule.[9, 14, 15]

Unlike neuroblastoma, radiologically the Wilms' tumor is a "clean" tumor. A mass is usually seen on the plain film, and there is calcification in 3% to 5% of cases (Figs 8–5 and 8–6).[2, 8]

Urography, which is usually performed through a foot vein to obtain a simultaneous inferior venacavogram, demonstrates an intrarenal mass with marked distortion rather than a displacement of the renal collecting system. In rare cases, an upper pole mass will displace the collecting system downward so that the lesion resembles an adrenal neuroblastoma (Fig 8–2). In 10% of cases, the kidney will not show any function because of either total replacement by the tumor (Fig 8–3) or involvement of the vascular pedicle.[2]

Ultrasound shows a mass that is heterogeneously echogenic and often contains echolucent areas, which suggest necrosis or hemorrhage (Fig 8–4).[2, 8] At times, these areas may develop, or their size and number may increase during chemotherapy (Fig 8–4). Demonstration of the inferior vena cava may be difficult because of severe compression by the tumor.[2]

Computed tomography is considered the optimal modality for diagnosis, staging, and follow-up of Wilms' tumors.[2, 17, 18] It not only defines the renal origin of the tumor but also detects the involvement of the vena cava and regional nodes, status of the opposite kidney, and presence or absence of metastases in the liver and lungs. Tumor necrosis and pseudocapsule are detected more often using CT scans than with sonogram. Computed tomography is also more sensitive in assessing perinephric extension, lymph node involvement, and bilateral tumors.[18] In large, nonresectable tumors, CT is superior to ultrasound for monitoring response to chemotherapy and contemplating possible resection. A Wilms' tumor appears on CT as a low-attenuation mass, arising either centrally or exophytically from the kidney and distorting the collecting system (Figs 8–2 and 8–3).[2, 18] Occasionally, Wilms' tumor will have only a minimal parenchymal component, with the bulk of the tumor seen within the pelvicalyceal system, the so-called botryoid variant.[19] The presence of calcification or fat in the tumor can be easily ascertained (Fig 8–7). Postcontrast scans demonstrate a clear demarcation that probably corresponds to a pseudocapsule of fibrous tissue (Figs 8–2 and 8–3). A crescent-shaped enhancement in the periphery has been reported to be characteristic of Wilms' tumor (Figs 8–2 and 8–3). This appearance corresponds to the compressed residual renal parenchyma. In approximately 5% of patients, the tumor will extend into the renal vein and vena cava. The incidence of calcification as seen on CT is reported to be as high as 13%.[2, 18]

Magnetic resonance imaging has recently been utilized in the workup of Wilms' tumor. The tumor usually shows signal intensities consistent with prolonged T_1 and T_2 relaxation times. Signal intensity is variable because of necrosis and hemorrhage within the tumor.[20]

At present, angiography has limited applications. Inferior venacavography is usually performed in the rare instances in which the vena cava cannot be seen by intravenous urography, ultrasonography, CT, or MRI.[2, 20]

Nephroblastomatosis

Nephroblastomatosis is a well-recognized entity that consists of subcapsular islands of primitive metanephric epithelium. The term nephroblastomatosis typically refers to the diffuse form, whereas the small and localized form is called *nodular renal blastema*. Nephroblastomatosis is closely related to and perhaps a precursor of Wilms' tumor. Because clinical presentation is bilateral nephromegaly before the age of four months, polycystic kidney disease is often erroneously diagnosed.[8, 21, 22]

Radiographically, the patients present with bilaterally enlarged and lobulated kidneys (Fig 8–10). On excretory urography, the involvement is indistinguishable from multiple renal cysts or bilateral renal hamartomas.[21, 22] Ultrasonography establishes the solid nature of the lesions, and contrast-enhanced CT clearly demarcates the nonenhanced nephroblastomatosis from the normally enhancing renal tissue.[16] On angiography, there are multiple subcapsular avascular masses splaying the adjacent vessels.

There is usually no tumor vascularity.[18] On occasion, Wilms' tumor may arise from spontaneously regressing nephroblastomatosis,[21] as in the case presented by Figure 8–10.

Renal Cell Carcinoma

Renal cell carcinoma in children is rare and accounts for 2.3% to 3.8% of all kidney tumors in children.[8, 23–26] It is usually seen in older children, and the peak age at presentation is approximately nine years, in contrast to children with Wilms' tumor, whose peak age of presentation is two to three years. Thirty percent of pediatric patients with renal cell carcinoma present with hematuria, which is more common than in Wilms' tumor. Abdominal or flank pain has been reported in almost 50% of patients. The abdominal mass is smaller than in Wilms' and is palpable in 50% of patients.[25] Renal cell carcinoma is, in fact, a well-differentiated form of Wilms' tumor.[14]

There is a high incidence of calcification within the tumor; calcification is radiographically seen in 25% of patients, which is a higher incidence than in Wilms'.[25] Urographic, sonographic, and CT findings are nonspecific and similar to those in Wilms' (Figs 8–12 and 8–13). Since renal cell carcinoma tends to metastasize to the regional nodes and to the lungs, CT is the modality of choice for assessing the primary and metastatic lesions, either at diagnosis or during follow-up. Surgery is the primary form of therapy, with or without combination radiotherapy and chemotherapy.

Germ Cell Tumors

Germ cell tumors in children derive from the primordial germ cells, which may give rise either to the seminiferous germ cell tumors (dysgerminomas, seminomas, and germinomas) or to embryonal carcinoma. The differentiated type of embryonal carcinoma could develop into either embryonic or extraembryonic forms. The embryonic form includes mature and immature teratomas, and the extraembryonic form includes choriocarcinoma and endodermal sinus tumors.[27]

Teratomas

Teratomas are true congenital neoplasms of germ cell origin and most commonly occur in the ovaries and sacrococcygeal regions.[24, 28, 29] The sacrococcygeal form usually appears before two months of age, in contrast to the ovarian teratomas, which are usually seen in adolescent girls.[29] Teratomas constitute the most common ovarian neoplasms in children. Histologically, they are mature (so-called benign cystic teratoma) in 99% of cases (Fig 8–14) and immature in 1% of cases (Fig 8–15).[27, 30] The sacrococcygeal teratomas may be presented as retrosacral or presacral tumors. Retroperitoneal teratomas account for 2% of teratomas in children and are usually seen as a cystic mass anterior to the kidneys and frequently in the left side (Fig 8–16). Thirty to fifty percent of the retroperitoneal teratomas are presented in the first year of life.[28, 31] Teratomas contain calcifications in 50% to 60% of cases.[2, 28] They may contain hair, bone, fat, and the neural tissues (Figs 8–14 to 8–16). Radiographically, a radiolucent mass containing calcification is usually present. On sonography, teratoma may present as a totally cystic mass with sound transmission (Fig 8–14) or containing solid hyperechoic components (Fig 8–16) representing hair and sebum (dermoid plug).[32] Computed tomography not only delineates the extent of the lesion in the abdomen and pelvis but may also be diagnostic in older children (Fig 8–15).[2]

Endodermal Sinus Tumors

Endodermal sinus tumors or yolk sac tumors were first described by Teilum in 1959 and were initially reported in the ovary and testicle.[33, 34] These tumors, however, are diagnosed with increasing frequency in both gonadal and extragonadal sites, including the vulva, vagina, prostate, sacrococcygeal region, and retroperitoneum.[34–36] Histologically, these tumors are encountered either as a pure form or in combination with other germ cell tumors. In the pediatric age group, 90% are pure lesions. The gonadal primaries frequently metastasize to the retroperitoneal nodes (Fig 8–17). Among the extragonadal primaries, the sacrococcygeal region (Fig 8–18) is the most common site, followed by the vagina (Fig 8–19).[34–36] Clinically, patients with sacrococcygeal lesions may present with buttock mass and difficulty in defecation. Vaginal bleeding is the presenting symptom in the vaginal primaries, which are seen predominantly in infants and are usually located in the posterolateral wall.[34, 36] The α-fetoprotein level is usually elevated and can be used to monitor the response to treatment.[27, 35]

Radiographically, the findings are not specific, and the primary lesion usually appears as a soft tissue mass. Tumors in the sacrococcygeal region usually extend down into the perineum and buttocks and have a tendency to erode the sacrum and coccyx (Fig 8–18).[34] The tumors usually have a high rate of local recurrence and metastasis, typically to the

lungs.[34] Treatment consists of surgical removal, followed by chemotherapy.

Rhabdomyosarcoma of the Genitourinary Tract

Rhabdomyosarcoma (Figs 8–20 to 8–22) is believed to develop from primitive rhabdomyoblasts anywhere in the body, even in the areas where striated muscle is normally not present. Of the three different histologic types (embryonal, pleomorphic, and alveolar soft part), the embryonal is the most common in children.[33, 34] Sarcoma botryoides is a morphological type of embryonal rhabdomyosarcoma presenting as grapelike polypoid masses that usually arise submucosally in hollow organs and protrude into the lumen (Figs 8–20 and 8–22).[33, 35, 37] The genitourinary system is the second most common site of involvement, exceeded by head and neck primaries.[33–35] The bladder is the most common site of genitourinary involvement, and presentation is usually within the first three years of life.[30, 32] At presentation, there may be a solid infiltration of the bladder wall or polypoid masses protruding into the bladder lumen (Fig 8–20). Occasionally, there is a large exophytic mass simulating large ovarian tumor, neuroblastoma, or Ewing's sarcoma. Clinical findings include strangury and obstruction to urination. Hematuria is unusual.[34]

Rarely, the tumor protrudes from the urethra in girls and, if large, may be confused with sarcoma botryoides of the vagina.[34, 37] Rhabdomyosarcoma of the prostate gland (Fig 8–21) typically shows clinical findings of prostatism; there is usually early invasion of the bladder floor and the posterior urethra,[36] with clinical and radiographic findings similar to those in primary bladder rhabdomyosarcoma. Unlike in rhabdomyosarcoma of the bladder, early spread to the regional lymph nodes or distant sites is not uncommon.[34]

Vaginal rhabdomyosarcoma is the most common primary tumor of the vagina and external genitalia in girls.[33–35] The tumor usually arises from the upper third of the anterior vaginal wall and is usually botryoid. The patients usually present with vaginal discharge or bleeding, a vaginal mass, or protrusion of polypoid masses from the vaginal orifice (Fig 8–22).

Occasionally, rhabdomyosarcoma arises from the pelvic floor and perineum and directly invades adjacent bones.[3] Radiographic procedures helpful in assessment include CT, bone scanning, and voiding cystourethrography.[34, 35]

With the advent of chemotherapy, survival has

increased to 60% in all children with rhabdomyosarcoma, and it is even higher in children with genitourinary primaries.[37-41]

ADRENAL AND NEUROGENIC NEOPLASMS

Neuroblastoma and Ganglioneuroma

Neuroblastoma (Figs 8–23 to 8–28) arises from the neurons and is categorized as pure neuroblastoma, ganglioneuroblastoma, or ganglioneuroma according to histologic differentiation.[42, 43]

Neuroblastoma is the third most common childhood neoplasm, following leukemia and brain tumors. It is the second most common solid abdominal tumor in children, exceeded by Wilms' tumor. It originates typically in the adrenal gland and in the sympathetic chain from the neck to the sacrum and, rarely, in the cerebrum, cerebellum, or spinal cord. Fifty-five percent of these tumors occur in the abdomen, two thirds of which originate in the adrenal, and 4% occur in the pelvis. In many cases, the location of the primary remains unknown.[44, 45]

The age at clinical onset of neuroblastoma is two years or younger in 50% of patients, and 75% of patients are less than four years of age.[44] Abdominal neuroblastomas are usually presented as a palpable mass, and on occasion there are peculiar findings such as diarrhea, opsoclonus, ataxia, or symptoms of cord compression.[43] Hypertension as a presenting sign is unusual, although maternal hypertension may be seen because of metastasis of fetal neuroblastoma to the placenta or because of circulating catecholamines.[43] In the staging system introduced by Evans et al.,[43, 46] stage I disease is tumor limited to the organ or structure of origin; stage II is tumor growing out of the primary site but not crossing the midline; stage III is tumor extended across the midline; stage IV is defined by metastasis to the bone, bone marrow, and liver; and stage IV-S is the same as stages I and II except that there are distant metastases but not to bone. This last stage carries a better prognosis than stage IV. Favorable prognostic factors include age less than one year, paraspinal location with extension into the spinal canal, and histologic maturation toward ganglioneuroblastoma or ganglioneuroma.[47-49] Complete surgical excision is the treatment closest to definitive in localized disease.[45] Nonresectable tumors are treated with chemotherapy and then reevaluated for possible surgical resection. Two-year survival is 60% for ages less than one year, 20% for one to two years of age,

and 10% for two to seven years of age.[44, 47, 49] The spontaneous cure rate for neuroblastoma is 5% to 7%, which is higher than for any other childhood tumor.[44]

Ganglioneuromas usually arise from the sympathetic chain and rarely from the adrenal gland, mesentery, alimentary tract, genitourinary system, or nasopharynx.[44] These tumors are incidentally discovered during clinical or radiologic examination (Fig 8–28) or autopsy. If large, they tend to compress the adjacent viscera. Neuroblastomas may mature into the less malignant form of ganglioneuroblastoma or transform to the benign form of ganglioneuroma.[44, 47] The treatment of ganglioneuroma is surgical resection, although complete excision is frequently difficult because of tumor adherence to adjacent structures.

Radiographically, a mass may be evident on plain films. Calcification, seen as cloudlike, punctate, or ringlike areas, is imaged in approximately 32% to 43% of abdominal neuroblastomas (Figs 8–23 to 8–27).[4, 47] Dumbbell-shaped neuroblastomas will frequently erode the pedicle or extend into the extradural space (Fig 8–27).[47-49] Calcification may be evident in the hepatic metastases. On the excretory urogram, the extrarenal origin of the mass is suggested by predominant displacement rather than distortion of the collecting system. When the mass originates from the adrenal gland, the kidney is displaced downward (Fig 8–25); in lesions arising from the sympathetic chains, the kidney is displaced laterally (Fig 8–26), and there may be hydronephrosis caused by compression of the renal pelvis or ureter. Masses arising anterior to the kidney may be overlooked on the excretory urogram.[50] Ultrasound has a limited value in staging and outlining the anatomical boundaries.[4, 51, 52] Typically, it shows a predominantly solid echogenic mass, but cystic areas secondary to necrosis are not uncommon (Fig 8–26).[52] Rarely, an adrenal neuroblastoma is seen at presentation as a cystic mass with occasional low-level echoes.[53, 54] The reasons for hyperechogenic areas in neuroblastoma are not well understood, although they have been related to calcification, hemorrhage, and necrosis. A distinct hyperechoic "lobule" has been described in large neuroblastomas; it corresponded to an aggregate of uniform neuroblastoma cells marginated by reticulin and collagen cells.[55] Ultrasound can be used to detect and monitor liver metastases.[52]

Computed tomography is the most accurate modality in detecting the structure of origin, presence of calcification (sensitivity, 79%), invasion of adjacent organs (liver, kidney, and inferior vena cava), retroperitoneal nodal metastases (Fig 8–26), intraspinal extension (Fig 8–27),[4, 47, 56] and recurrent disease.[57] In one report, intraspinal extension occurred in 7 of 39 cases.[47] Computed tomography is invaluable in stage III neuroblastoma for determining resectability.[56] When the tumor encases the aorta and its major branches, the tumor should be considered unresectable irrespective of its size.[56] The displacement of the great vessels, particularly accompanied by tumor encasement, is an important CT sign for distinguishing neuroblastoma from Wilms' tumor.[58] Although CT is invaluable for staging neuroblastoma, bone metastases can be overlooked. In this regard, bone scan followed by radiography of the involved areas will be helpful.

Magnetic resonance imaging is reported to be useful in defining the tumor boundaries and extension into the kidney and spinal canal.[6, 59] On T_1-weighted sequences, the tumor shows the same signal intensity as the renal medulla and slightly lower intensity than the renal cortex and liver. On T_2-weighted images, the tumor shows increased signal intensity, higher than that of the liver but similar to that of the kidney.

HEPATIC NEOPLASMS

Primary tumors of the liver account for approximately 15% of abdominal tumors in children and are the third most common solid abdominal neoplasm in infants, exceeded by Wilms' tumor and neuroblastoma.[3, 5, 7] Metastatic neuroblastoma is more common than primary malignant hepatic tumor. Approximately two thirds of primary hepatic tumors are malignant.[2, 7] Hepatoblastoma and hepatocarcinoma are the most common malignant primary tumors.

Hepatoblastoma (Figs 8–29 to 8–31) is more common than hepatocarcinoma and occurs within the first three years of life. Usual presenting symptoms are hepatomegaly, fever, anorexia, and weight loss.[2] There is elevation of α-fetoprotein levels.[3, 7, 60] The right lobe of the liver is more commonly involved than the left, and the tumor involves both lobes in approximately 30% to 45% of cases.[2, 60] Hepatocarcinoma occurs in slightly older children, peaking at 4 years of age; however, there is a second peak between 12 and 15 years.[59] There tends to be diffuse involvement of the liver in hepatocarcinoma. The surgical cure rate is 60% for hepatoblastoma and 30% for hepatocarcinoma; without surgery, the mor-

tality rate is 100%.[60]

Radiographically, in hepatic neoplasms, there is hepatomegaly at presentation, with calcification in as many as 25% to 40% of cases.[2, 7] Ultrasonography usually demonstrates an echogenic intrahepatic mass (Figs 8–29 and 8–30). In addition, involvement of the inferior vena cava or portal vein, with cavernous transformation of the portal vein (Fig 8–32), can be demonstrated.[61]

Computed tomography usually shows a solitary or multicentric low-attenuation mass, calcified in one half of cases.[60] The tumor has a lower CT attenuation value than does normal liver, a discrepancy accentuated by administration of contrast material (Figs 8–32 and 8–33).[60] Preoperatively, angiography is mandatory to define the vascular anatomy, anatomical boundaries, and vascular invasion (Fig 8–30).[2, 7] In defining the anatomical boundaries of the tumor, ultrasound, CT, and angiography are complementary.[60]

Vascular tumors of the liver (hemangioma and hemangioendothelioma) are less common than the malignant tumors and account for 10% of primary hepatic tumors in childhood.[7] These tumors are usually detected before the age of six months.[2, 7] Histologic differentiation may at times be difficult, but hemangioendothelioma is more common in the infant, and cavernous hemangioma is more common in the adult. On contrast-enhanced CT, these tumors have a different appearance than hepatoblastoma and become isodense with the rest of the liver.[60] Treatment depends on the extent of the lesion and includes surgical resection or arterial embolization.[2, 3, 5, 7]

Malignant mesenchymal tumors of the liver are extremely rare. They include angiosarcoma, leiomyosarcoma, and fibrosarcoma. Some undifferentiated sarcomas cannot be categorized, and they have been referred to as "embryonal rhabdomyosarcoma," "malignant mesenchymoma," or "embryonal sarcoma." The undifferentiated sarcoma is predominantly a tumor of the pediatric age group, and 51.6% of patients are between six and ten years of age at presentation. An abdominal mass, pain, and elevated temperature are the usual presenting symptoms.[62, 63] Radiologic findings are nonspecific, except to demonstrate a space-occupying lesion of the liver. Ultrasound shows either cystic or solid masses (Fig 8–33). A CT scan usually demonstrates large, well-demarcated intrahepatic cystic areas separated from the adjacent liver by a pseudocapsule. Histologic examination shows undifferentiated sarcoma cells that are near the periphery and surrounded by entrapped, hyperplastic, bile duct–like structures. The prognosis is poor, and the median survival after diagnosis is less than one year.[62, 63]

REFERENCES

1. Dutton R.V., Singleton E.B.: Imaging techniques in pediatric oncology, in Sutow W.W., Fernbach D.J., Vietti T.J. (eds.): *Clinical Pediatric Oncology*, ed. 3. St. Louis, C.V. Mosby Co., 1984, pp. 79–117.
2. Kirks D.R., Merten D.F., Grossmah H., et al.: Diagnostic imaging of pediatric abdominal masses: an overview. *Radiol. Clin. North Am.* 19:527–545, 1981.
3. Miller J.H., Greenspan B.S.: Integrated imaging of hepatic tumors in childhood: Part I. Malignant lesions (primary and metastatic). *Radiology* 154:83–90, 1985.
4. Stark D.D., Moss A.A., Brasch R.C., et al.: Neuroblastoma: diagnostic imaging and staging. *Radiology* 148:101–105, 1983.
5. Amendola M.A., Blane C.E., Amendola B.E., et al.: CT findings in hepatoblastoma. *J. Comput. Assist. Tomogr.* 8:1105–1109, 1984.
6. Dietrich R.B., Kangarloo H., Lenarsky C., et al.: Neuroblastoma: the role of MR imaging. *AJR* 148:937–942, 1987.
7. Wallace S.: Primary liver tumors, in Parker B.R., Castellino R.A. (eds.): *Pediatric Oncologic Radiology*. St. Louis, C.V. Mosby Co., 1977, pp. 301–335.
8. Swischuk L.E.: *Radiology of the Newborn and Young Infant,* ed. 2. Baltimore, Williams & Wilkins Co., 1980, pp. 553–559.
9. Belasco J.B., Chatten J., d'Angio G.J.: Wilms' tumor, in Sutow W.W., Fernbach D.J., Vietti T.J. (eds.): *Clinical Pediatric Oncology*, ed. 3. St. Louis, C.V. Mosby Co., 1984, pp. 588–621.
10. Shashikumar V.L., Somers L.A., Pilling G.P., et al.: Wilms' tumor in the horseshoe kidney. *J. Pediatr. Surg.* 9:185–189, 1974.
11. Gonzalez-Crussi F., Hsueh W., Ugarte N.: Rhabdomyogenesis in renal neoplasia of childhood. *Am. J. Surg. Pathol.* 5:525–532, 1981.
12. Wigger H.J.: Fetal rhabdomyomatous nephroblastoma—a variant of Wilms' tumor. *Hum. Pathol.* 7:613–623, 1976.
13. Fung C.H.K., Gonzalez-Crussi F., Yonan T.N., et al.: "Rhabdoid" Wilms' tumor: an ultrastructural study. *Arch. Pathol. Lab. Med.* 105:521–523, 1981.
14. Beckwith J.B.: Wilms' tumor and other renal tumors of childhood: a selective review from the National Wilms' Tumor Study Pathology Center. *Hum. Pathol.* 14:481–492, 1983.
15. Lamego C.M.B., Zerbini M.C.N.: Bone-metastasizing primary renal tumors in children. *Radiology* 147:449–454, 1983.
16. Fernbach S.K., Feinstein K.A., Donaldson J.S., et al.: Nephroblastomatosis: comparison of CT with US and urography. *Radiology* 166:153–156, 1988.
17. Brasch R.C., Randel S.B., Gould R.G.: Follow-up of

18. Reiman T.A.H., Siegel M.J., Shackelford G.D.: Wilms' tumor in children: abdominal CT and US evaluation. *Radiology* 160:501–505, 1986.
19. Johnson K.M., Horvath L.J., Gaise G., et al.: Wilms' tumor occurring as a botryoid renal pelvicalyceal mass. *Radiology* 163:385–386, 1987.
20. Belt T.G., Cohen M.D., Smith J.A., et al.: MRI of Wilms' tumor: promise as the primary imaging method. *AJR* 146:955–961, 1986.
21. Rosenfield N.S., Shimkin P., Berdon W., et al.: Wilms' tumor arising from spontaneously regressing nephroblastomatosis. *AJR* 135:381–384, 1980.
22. Franken E.A., Yiu-Chiu V., Smith W.L., et al.: Nephroblastomatosis: clinicopathologic significance and imaging characteristics. *AJR* 138:950–952, 1982.
23. Castellanos R.D., Aron B.S., Evans A.T.: Renal adenocarcinoma in children: incidence, therapy and prognosis. *J. Urol.* 111:534–537, 1974.
24. Lynn C.M., Machiz S.: Renal cell carcinoma in children. A report of four cases and a review of literature. *J. Pediatr. Surg.* 8:925–929, 1973.
25. Chan H.S.L., Daneman A., Gribbin M., et al.: Renal cell carcinoma in the first two decades of life. *Pediatr. Radiol.* 13:324–328, 1983.
26. Cassady J.R., Filler R., Jaffe N., et al.: Carcinoma of the kidney in children. *Radiology* 112:691–693, 1974.
27. Copeland L.: Malignant gynecologic tumors in children, in Sutow W.W., Fernbach D.J., Vietti T.J. (eds.): *Clinical Pediatric Oncology*, ed. 3. St. Louis, C.V. Mosby Co., 1984, pp. 744–760.
28. Partlow W.F., Taybi H.: Teratomas in infants and children. *AJR* 112:155–166, 1971.
29. Mahour G.H., Woolley M.M., Trivedi S.N., et al.: Teratomas in infancy and childhood: experience with 81 cases. *Surgery* 76:309–318, 1974.
30. Siegel M.J., McAlister W.H., Shackelford G.D.: Radiographic findings in ovarian teratomas in children. *AJR* 131:613–616, 1978.
31. Anatol T.: Retroperitoneal teratoma in an infant. *West Indian Med. J.* 33:269–271, 1984.
32. Quinn S.F., Erickson S., Black W.C.: Cystic ovarian teratomas: sonographic appearances of the dermoid plug. *Radiology* 155:477–478, 1985.
33. Teilum G.: Endodermal sinus tumor of the ovary and testis. *Cancer* 12:1092–1105, 1959.
34. O'Sullivan P., Daneman A., Chan H.S.L., et al.: Extragonadal endodermal sinus tumors in children: a review of 24 cases. *Pediatr. Radiol.* 13:249–257, 1983.
35. Juckes A.W., Frazer M.M., Dexter D.: Endodermal sinus (yolk sac) tumor in infants and children. *J. Pediatr. Surg.* 14:520–524, 1979.
36. Allyn D.L., Silverberg S.G., Salzberg A.M.: Endodermal sinus tumor of the vagina. *Cancer* 27:1231–1238, 1971.
37. Lee F.A.: Rhabdomyosarcoma, in Parker B.R., Castellino R.A. (eds.): *Pediatric Oncologic Radiology*. St.

Louis, C.V. Mosby Co., 1977, pp. 407–436.

38. Soule E.H., Mahour G.H., Mill S.D., et al.: Soft tissue sarcomas of infants and children: a clinicopathological study of 135 cases. *Mayo Clin. Proc.* 43:313–326, 1968.

39. Pizzo P.A.: Rhabdomyosarcoma and the soft tissue sarcomas, in Levine A.S. (ed.): *Cancer in the Young.* New York, Masson Publishing, 1982, pp. 615–632.

40. Baker M.E., Silverman P.M., Korobkin M.: Computerized tomography of prostatic and bladder rhabdomyosarcomas. *J. Comput. Assist. Tomogr.* 9:780–783, 1985.

41. Raney R.B., Duckett J.W., Donaldson M.H.: Malignant genitourinary tumors, in Sutow W.W., Fernbach D.J., Vietti T.J. (eds.): *Clinical Pediatric Oncology,* ed. 3. St. Louis, C.V. Mosby Co., 1984, pp. 734–736.

42. Gale A.W., Jeliovsky T., Grant A.F., et al.: Neurogenic tumors of the mediastinum. *Ann. Thorac. Surg.* 17:434–443, 1974.

43. Swischuk L.E.: *Radiology of the Newborn and Young Infant,* ed. 2. Baltimore, Williams & Wilkins Co., 1980, pp. 602–608.

44. Friendland G.W., Crowe J.E.: Neuroblastoma and other adrenal neoplasms, in Parker B.R., Castellino R.A. (eds.): *Pediatric Oncologic Radiology.* St. Louis, C.V. Mosby Co., 1977, pp. 267–300.

45. Exelby P.R.: Pediatric oncologic surgery, in Sutow W.W., Fernbach D.J., Vietti T.J. (eds.): *Clinical Pediatric Oncology,* ed. 3. St. Louis, C.V. Mosby Co., 1984, pp. 154–166.

46. Evans A.E., d'Angio G.J., Randolph J.: A proposed staging for children with neuroblastoma. *Cancer* 27:374–378, 1971.

47. Armstrong E.A., Harwood-Nash D.C.F., Ritz C.R., et al.: CT of neuroblastoma and ganglioneuromas in children. *AJR* 139:571–576, 1982.

48. Fagon C.J., Swischuk L.E.: Dumbbell neuroblastoma or ganglioneuroma of the spinal canal. *Am. J. Roentgenol. Radium Ther. Nucl. Med.* 120:453–460, 1974.

49. Evans A.E., Albo V., d'Angio G.J., et al.: Factors influencing survival of children with nonmetastatic neuroblastoma. *Cancer* 38:661–666, 1976.

50. Haller J.D., Berdon W.E., Baker D.H., et al.: Left adrenal neuroblastoma with normal-appearing urogram. *AJR* 129:1051–1055, 1977.

51. Berger D.E., Kuhn J.P., Munschauer R.W.: Computed tomography and ultrasound in the diagnosis and management of neuroblastoma. *Radiology* 128:663–667, 1978.

52. White S.J., Stuck K.J., Blane C.E., et al.: Sonography of neuroblastoma. *AJR* 141:465–468, 1983.

53. Atkinson G.O., Zaatari G.S., Lorenzo R.L., et al.: Cystic neuroblastoma in infants. *AJR* 146:113–117, 1986.

54. Hendry G.M.: Cystic neuroblastoma of the adrenal gland—a potential source of error in ultrasonic diagnosis. *Pediatr. Radiol.* 12:204–206, 1982.

55. Amundson G.M., Trevenen C.L., Mueller D.L., et al.: Neuroblastoma: a specific sonographic tissue pattern. *AJR* 148:943–945, 1987.

56. Boechat M.I., Ortega J., Hoffman A.D., et al.: Computed tomography in stage III neuroblastoma. *AJR* 145:1283–1287, 1985.

57. Stark D.D., Brasch R.C., Moss A.A., et al.: Recurrent neuroblastoma: the role of CT and alternative imaging tests. *Radiology* 148:107–112, 1983.

58. Peretz G.S., Lam A.H.: Distinguishing neuroblastoma from Wilms' tumor by computed tomography. *J. Comput. Assist. Tomogr.* 9:889–893, 1985.

59. Kagan A.R., Steckel R.J.: Diagnostic oncology case study. Retroperitoneal mass with intradural extension: value of MRI in neuroblastoma. *AJR* 146:251–254, 1986.

60. Ternberg J.L., Land V.J.: Tumors of the alimentary tract, in Sutow W.W., Fernbach D.J., Vietti T.J. (eds.): *Clinical Pediatric Oncology,* ed. 3. St. Louis, C.V. Mosby Co., 1984, pp. 775–785.

61. Kauzlaric D., Petrovic M., Barmeir E.: Sonography of cavernous transformation of the portal vein. *AJR* 142:383–384, 1984.

62. Stocker J.T., Ishak K.G.: Undifferentiated (embryonal) sarcoma of the liver: report of 31 cases. *Cancer* 42:336–348, 1978.

63. Ros P.R., Olmsted W.W., Dachman A.H., et al.: Undifferentiated (embryonal) sarcoma of the liver: radiologic-pathologic correlation. *Radiology* 160:141–145, 1986.

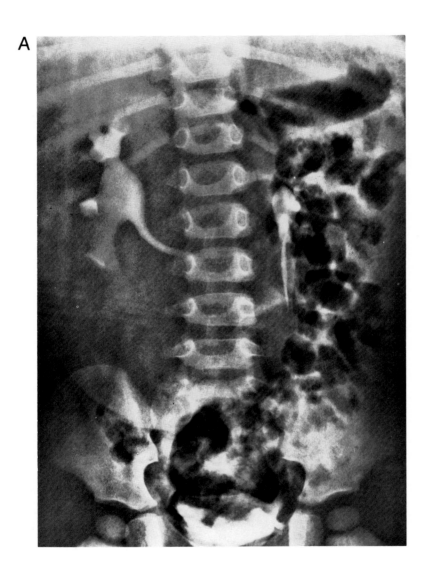

FIG 8–1.
Stage I exophytic Wilms' tumor with compression of adjacent kidney. A 16-month-old girl presented with a six-day history of low-grade fever. A right lower quadrant mass was found on clinical examination.

A, excretory urogram shows large, right lower pole mass extending to the upper pelvis and crossing the midline with compression, minimal distortion, and dilatation of the collecting system. The ureter is stretched and compressed by the tumor.

B and **C,** longitudinal **(B)** and transverse **(C)** views of a sonogram show a heterogeneously echogenic mass *(arrows)* arising from the lower pole and compressing the right kidney *(K)*.

A nephrectomy was performed and a stage I Wilms' tumor of the right lower pole was found to be compressing but not obstructing the collecting system. The patient received chemotherapy postoperatively.

B

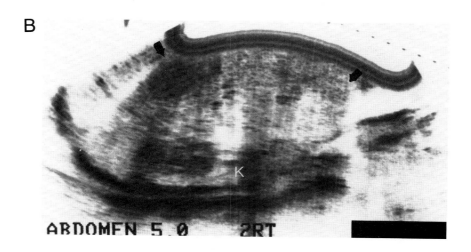

C

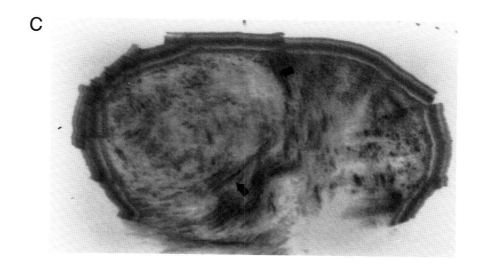

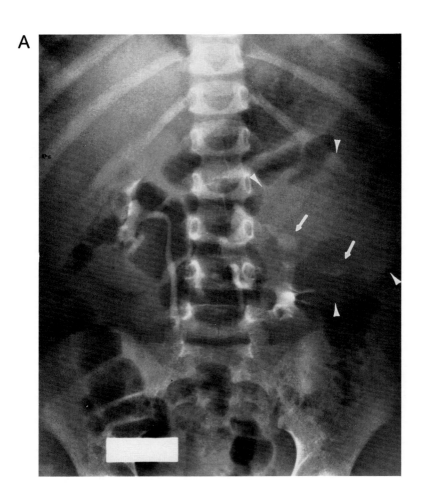

FIG 8–2.
Stage I exophytic Wilms' tumor resembling adrenal neuroblastoma. A five-year-old girl presented to her local physician with fever, loss of appetite, and a palpable abdominal mass.

A, excretory urogram shows a large tumor *(arrowheads)* displacing the left kidney downward, with minimal distortion of the calices *(arrows).*

B, enhanced CT scan shows a large tumor displacing and compressing the adjacent renal tissue anteriorly *(arrowheads).* The tumor shows cystic foci, probably representing necrosis, and also pseudocapular enhancement *(arrows).*

A stage I, partially cystic Wilms' tumor was surgically excised. The tumor was compressing but not invading the renal pelvis. Four firm hilar nodes and the renal vein were free of tumor.

C, anatomical specimen shows a large, lobulated, partly cystic mass replacing most of the left kidney. A rim of normal kidney is seen at the lower pole *(arrows),* corresponding to the crescent sign of compressed renal tissue on CT **(B)** (see also Color Plate 37).

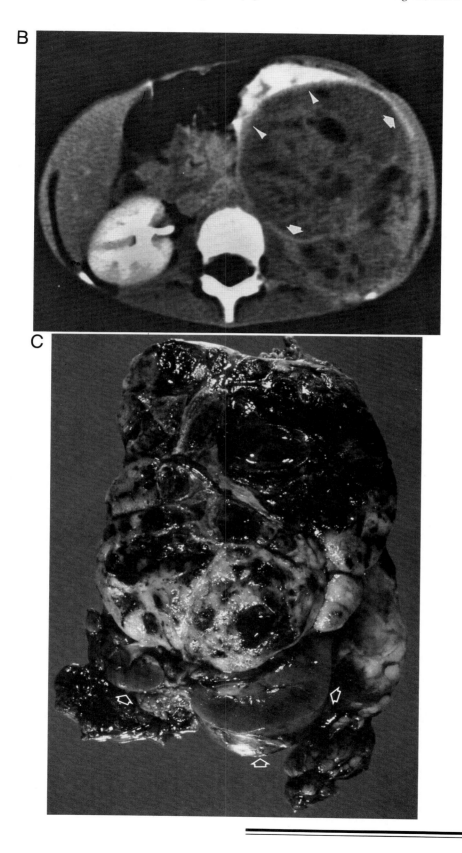

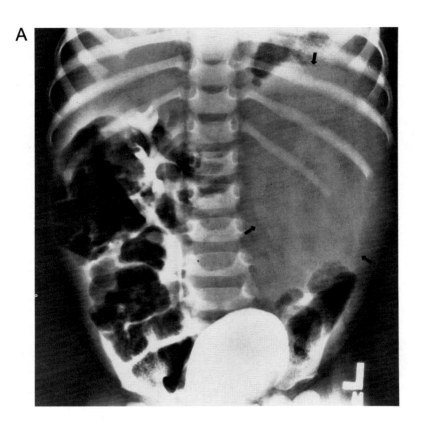

FIG 8–3.
Nonfunctioning kidney replaced by necrotic Wilms' tumor. A girl at age one and one-half years presented with anemia and a nontender, large, firm mass in the left abdomen. She was referred to M. D. Anderson Hospital for excision of the mass.

A, urogram shows a nonfunctioning left kidney, the left flank being occupied by a large soft tissue mass *(arrows)*.

B, a CT scan demonstrates a large, predominantly necrotic mass compressing and obstructing the left renal collecting system *(arrows)*. There is no excretion of the contrast material. The tumor is well encapsulated and contains both solid and necrotic areas.

A stage I Wilms' tumor was removed at surgery. The tumor was almost completely replacing the kidney (95%) and had focally necrotic areas (30%). The mass was obliterating the pelvis and extended into the proximal ureter.

C, cut section of a 14 × 12 cm renal tumor with fish-flesh appearance replacing 95% of the kidney. There are areas of focal hemorrhage and necrosis *(arrows)* (see also Color Plate 38).

Thirteen months later, the patient became comatose following convulsions and was dead on arrival at the hospital. Postmortem examination showed cerebral metastasis.

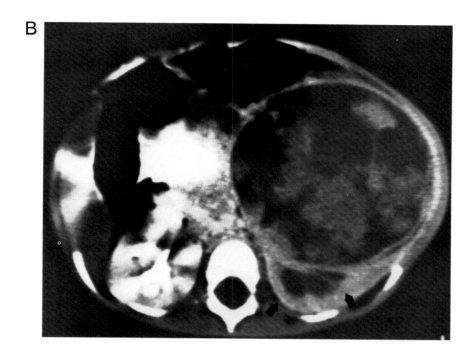

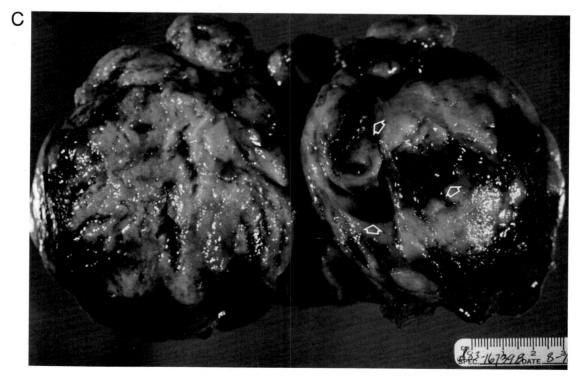

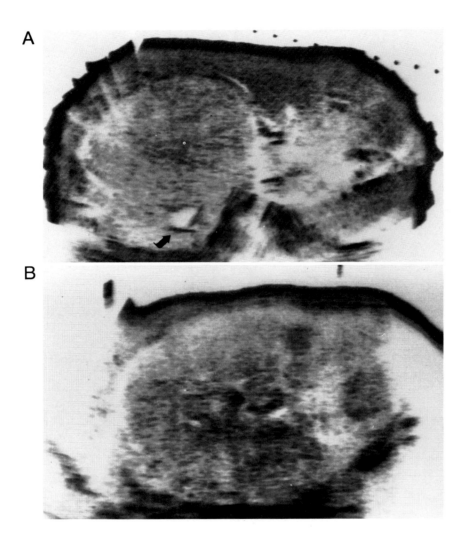

FIG 8–4.

Large Wilms' tumor with increasing necrosis following preoperative chemotherapy. A one-year-old boy developed hematuria, and an abdominal mass was discovered. Wilms' tumor was suspected, and the diagnosis was confirmed at M. D. Anderson Hospital. Because of the very large size of the mass, preoperative chemotherapy was given.

A urogram (not shown) from the referring institution showed a nonfunctioning right kidney.

A and **B,** transverse **(A)** and right sagittal **(B)** sonograms show an echogenic mass with a single echo-free area *(arrow),* suggestive of necrosis, hemorrhage, or a dilated calix. No recognizable renal tissue was seen.

C and **D,** postchemotherapy preoperative transverse **(C)** and right sagittal **(D)** sonograms demonstrate multiple large necrotic foci containing debris *(arrowheads),* indicating response to chemotherapy.

On physical examination, there was no change in the size of the mass after treatment; however, the patient underwent surgery, and a stage I Wilms' tumor was excised. The tumor had almost completely replaced the kidney, leaving only a small rim of compressed renal parenchyma. The tumor was mostly necrotic, with areas of cystic degeneration and focal hemorrhage at the center and near the hilus.

This case illustrates that although the overall size of a seemingly unresectable tumor may not change following chemotherapy, development of cystic areas probably indicates necrosis and, in effect, response to treatment.

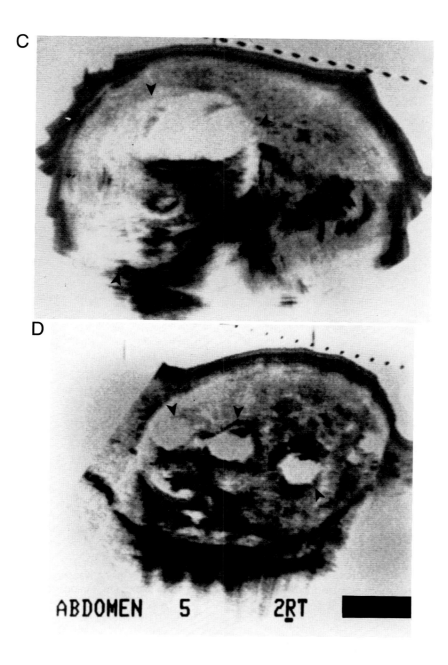

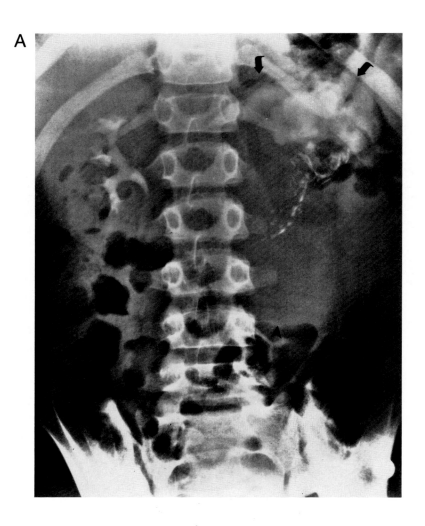

FIG 8–5.
Stage II Wilms' tumor with calcification in the perinephric fat. Difficulty in differentiating intrarenal vs. extrarenal origin. After a fall, a nine-year-old boy was discovered to have a mass that protruded below the left side of his ribs.

A, excretory urogram shows a left flank mass *(arrowheads)* displacing the left kidney superiorly *(tailed arrows)* and obstructing the collecting system. There is dense calcification within the tumor.

B and **C,** longitudinal sonograms 3 and 6 cm to the left of the midline demonstrate a heterogeneous, solid, and well-defined mass anterior to the left kidney. There is an apparent cleavage plane *(open arrow)* between the mass *(M)* and the kidney *(K)* anteriorly, but cleavage is indistinguishable *(closed arrow)* on another plane **(B)**. Notice acoustic shadowing *(S)* arising from the calcified component

of the tumor.

D, a selective left renal angiogram shows compression of the left kidney by a moderately hypervascular mass partially supplied by the renal artery. An aortogram (not shown) demonstrated further blood supply from the first through the third lumbar arteries.

At surgery, a well-circumscribed mass arising from the lower pole of the left kidney was noted; the mass proved to be Wilms' tumor. The tumor involved the perinephric fat, which contained dystrophic calcification. The child was treated with chemotherapy.

On the basis of urography and ultrasound, this mass was interpreted as being extrarenal, and probably a neurogenic tumor. Even the angiogram was not characteristic of an intrarenal tumor. A CT scan or MRI would have been helpful.

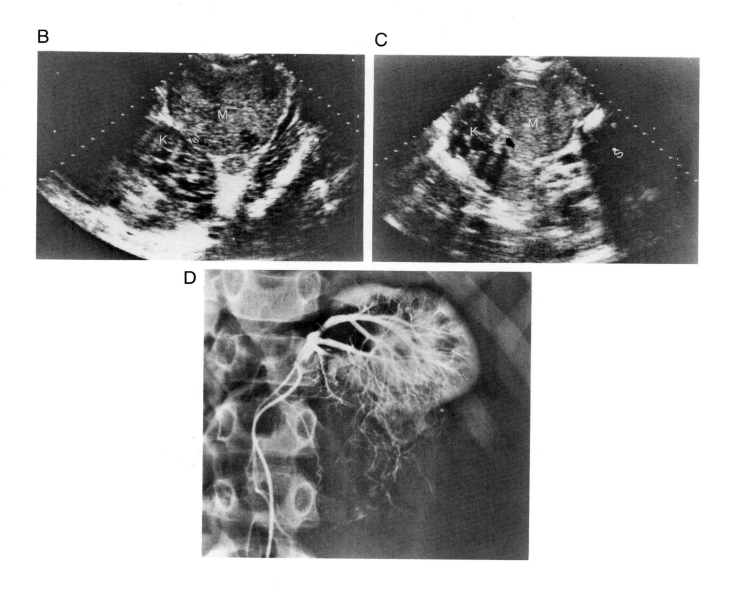

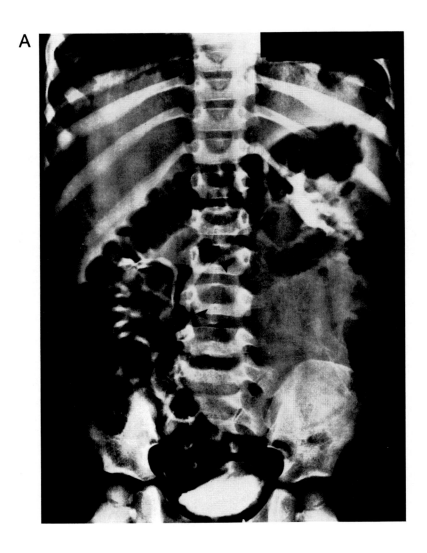

FIG 8–6.
Bilateral metachronous Wilms' tumors with calcification. A two-year-old girl developed fever and chills one week before she was admitted to the hospital. At examination, a mass was discovered in the left lower abdomen.

A, the urogram shows a large, exophytic mass arising from the lower pole of the left kidney and displacing the left ureter across the midline *(arrowheads).* The right kidney was interpreted as normal.

A nephrectomy was performed, and Wilms' tumor was diagnosed. The patient received radiation therapy and chemotherapy.

Approximately four years later, she returned to the hospital with hypertension and a large mass in the abdomen.

B and **C,** plain radiograph **(B)** and urogram **(C)** demonstrate a ringlike calcification *(arrows)* and a large tumor arising from the right kidney. The tumor displaces the ureter medially *(large arrows).*

At surgery, a second primary tumor invading the right renal pedicle was found. A biopsy of the mass proved Wilms' tumor. The patient was treated with chemotherapy but died shortly thereafter.

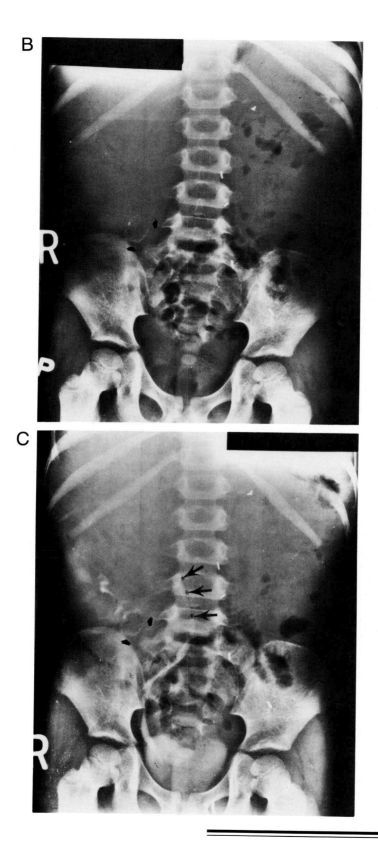

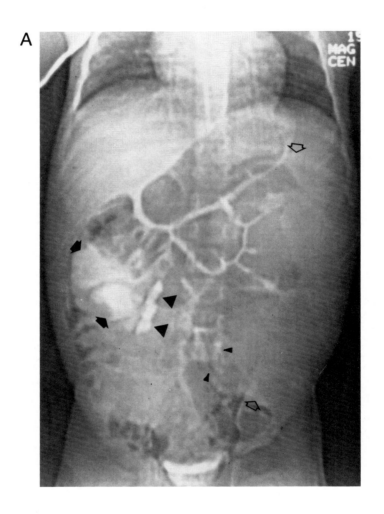

FIG 8–7.
Bilateral synchronous Wilms' tumors. A 14-month-old girl developed fever and vomiting two weeks prior to admission. At this time, a left lower abdominal mass was found and a tumor suspected. Excretory urography (not available) was performed, followed by a CT scan 2 hr later.

A, the preliminary scout for CT scan shows a large mass in the left flank *(open arrows)* and a smaller one in the right. Notice the displaced and distorted calices on the left *(small arrowheads)* and the right lower poles *(large arrowheads);* also note the obstructed right upper pole *(closed arrows)* calices.

B, a CT scan at the level of the midabdomen shows a large mass in the left *(long white arrows)* and an obstructed calix *(short white arrow).* Notice the right-sided large tumor mass containing fat *(open arrow)* and projecting into the dilated collecting system *(closed arrows).*

C, a CT scan at the level of the iliac crests shows the remnant of the left kidney *(black arrows)* and the obstructed calices *(white arrows).*

Laparotomy at the outside institution revealed bilateral Wilms' tumors. The child was then referred to M. D. Anderson Hospital. *(Continued).*

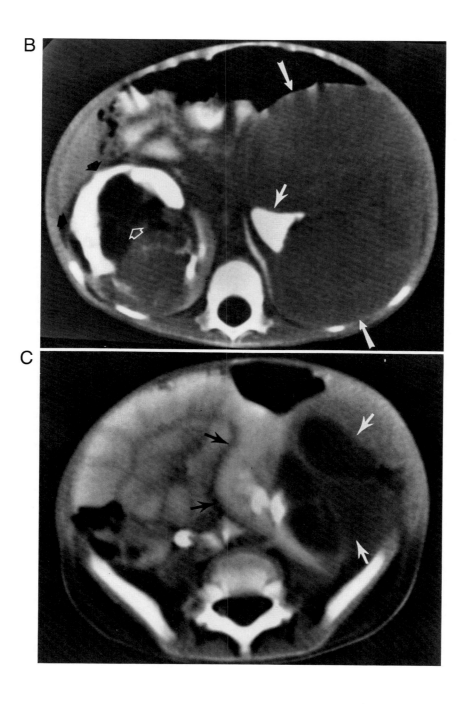

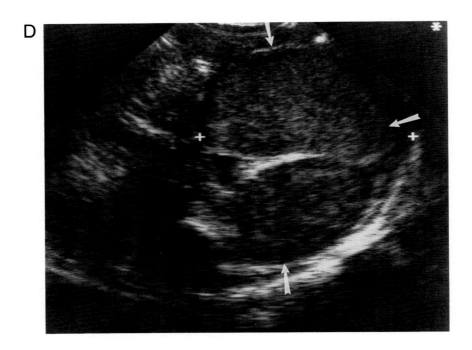

FIG 8–7 (cont.).
D, midabdominal transverse sonogram shows a large solid mass on the left side *(arrows)*. Cystic areas were seen in the lower sections, corresponding to obstructed calices on the CT scan *(white arrows* in **C**).

E, right sagittal sonogram shows polypoid tumor nodules *(closed arrow)* projecting into the dilated collecting system *(open arrows),* corresponding to the CT scan *(closed arrow* in **B**).

The child received chemotherapy for two and one-half months, and follow-up CT scan (not shown) showed slight improvement. Subsequently, the patient underwent total nephrectomy on the left and subtotal (two-thirds) nephrectomy on the right side. The margins of the right kidney were positive for tumor. The tumor extended into both proximal ureters. There were numerous polypoid projections of tumor within the dilated collecting system. Additionally, a small tumor nodule was seen attached to the liver and diaphragm.

E
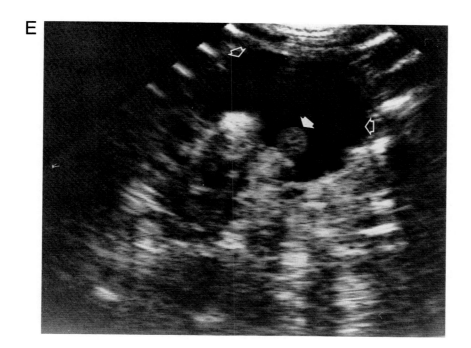

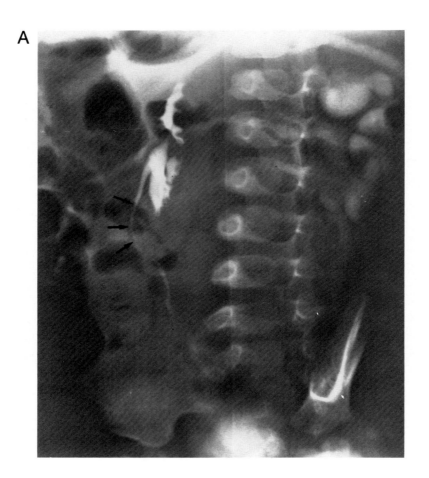

FIG 8–8.
Wilms' tumor, rhabdomyomatous type, arising in horseshoe kidney. A one-year-old boy was referred to M. D. Anderson Hospital with a probable diagnosis of Wilms' tumor. A mass was found on the left side of the abdomen.

A and B, right posterior oblique **(A)** and anteroposterior **(B)** projections from excretory urogram demonstrate a large mass *(arrowheads* in **B***)* arising from and obstructing the left kidney. The tumor crosses the midline. In retrospect, the

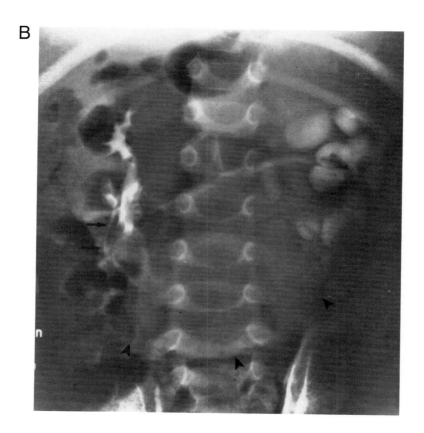

horseshoe kidney is suggested by the malrotated appearance of the right kidney and characteristic course of the right ureter *(arrows)*.

At exploration, a horseshoe kidney was found to harbor a mass in the left lower pole. A nephrectomy was performed at the isthmus. The tumor measured 9 × 9 × 6 cm and was markedly compressing the adjacent renal parenchyma to a thickness of 1 mm. The histology was that of fetal rhabdomyomatous Wilms' tumor.

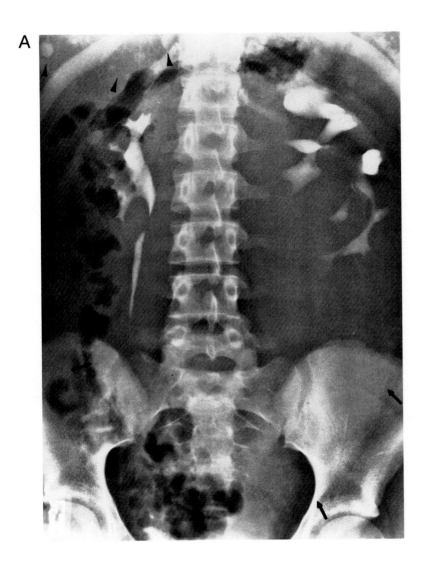

FIG 8–9.
Stage IV metastatic Wilms' tumor in the older child. A 14-year-old girl had a six-month history of abdominal pain and distention as well as early satiety and a decrease in appetite. On physical examination, a large left-sided abdominal mass that extended from the left iliac crest to the left costal margin and crossed the midline was noted. The mass was firm and nontender.

A, excretory urogram shows a huge mass *(arrows),* probably arising from the lower pole of the left kidney, com-

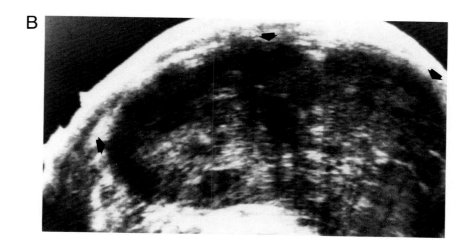

pressing and obstructing the calices. The tumor crosses the midline and displaces the right ureter and the bowel gas. Notice multiple pulmonary metastases *(arrowheads).*

B, transverse lower abdominal sonogram demonstrates a heterogeneous echogenic mass arising from the left side and crossing the midline *(arrows). (Continued).*

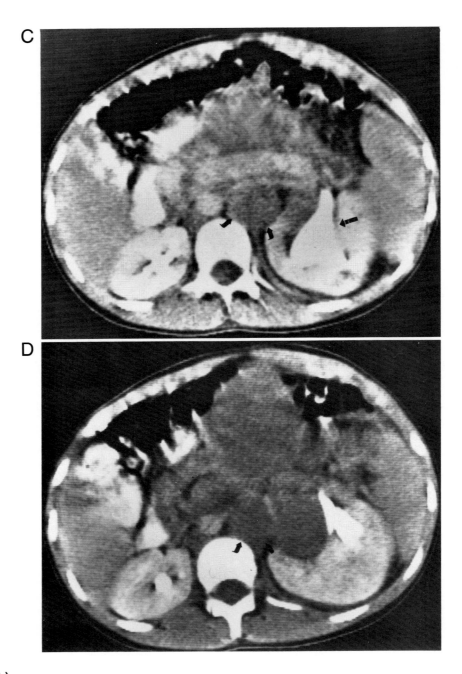

FIG 8–9 (cont.).

C through **E,** on CT, there is a large tumor compressing the pelvicalyceal system and stretching the left ureter *(arrows)*. Notice enhanced septa *(arrowheads* in **E** and **F)** and left paraaortic nodes *(tailed arrows)* displacing the aorta. Also notice the compressed renal parenchyma (crescent sign).

A percutaneous needle biopsy confirmed the diagnosis of Wilms' tumor. The patient received nine courses of vincristine for six weeks. The size of the tumor decreased substantially.

A left nephrectomy was done, and a 21 × 15 × 6 cm mass was removed. There were three perihilar lymph

nodes, ranging from 1 to 2 cm, containing tumor, even though the mass in the lower pole was well encapsulated. The vascular bundle was free of tumor.

F, postchemotherapy surgical specimen shows a glistening, solid intracapsular tumor *(black arrows)* replacing 95% of the left kidney and compressing the adjacent upper pole parenchyma *(white open arrows)* (see also Color Plate 39).

Two weeks postoperatively, the patient developed a nodule in the anterior vaginal wall. The nodule proved to be metastatic Wilms' tumor.

E

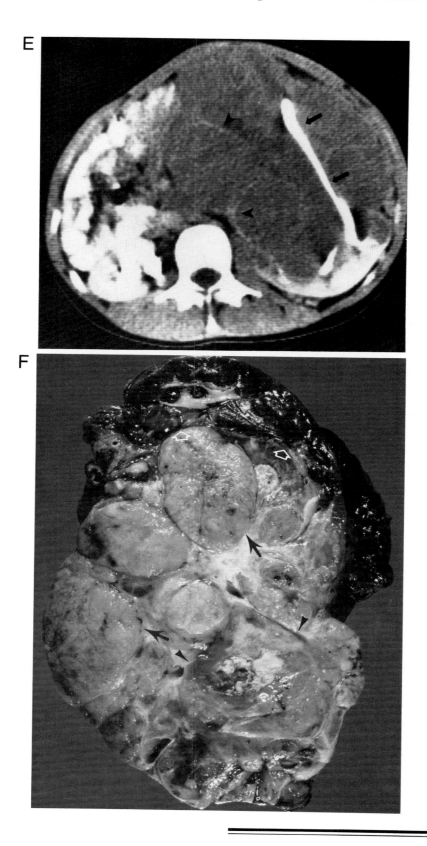

F

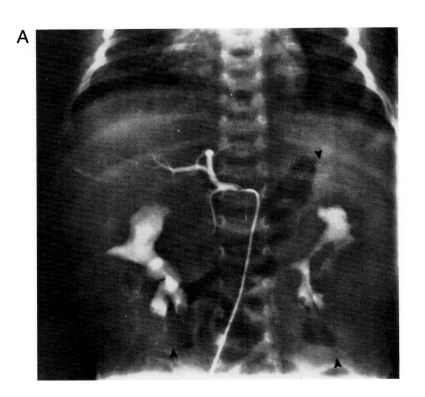

FIG 8–10.
Wilms' tumor arising from regressing nephroblastomatosis. In 1977 a one-month-old boy presented with an enlarged abdomen and palpable kidneys. A urogram and angiogram were obtained and interpreted as adult-type polycystic kidney disease.

A, urogram made during arteriogram shows bilaterally enlarged kidneys *(arrowheads)* with extrinsic pressure on the calices.

B and **C,** selective renal angiograms demonstrate stretching of the vessels around avascular cortical masses *(arrows).*

Three years later, a large left-sided abdominal mass and multiple pulmonary metastases developed. *(Continued.)*

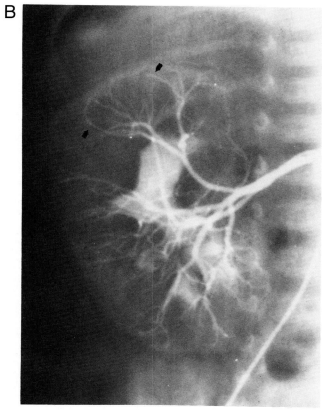

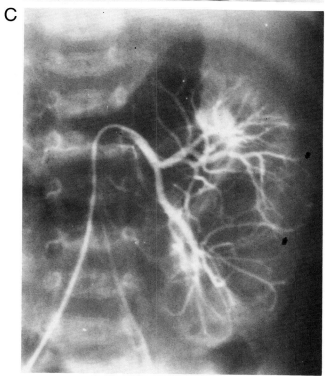

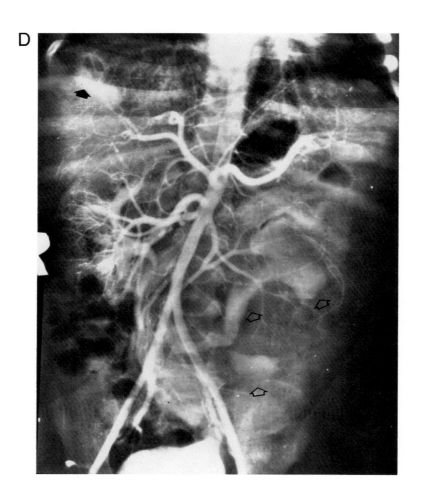

FIG 8–10 (cont.).

D and **E,** aortogram **(D)** and inferior venacavogram **(E)** in 1980 demonstrate the development of a large, hypovascular left renal mass displacing the adjacent vessels. Notice the compressed and distorted collecting system *(open arrows)* and the multiple cavitary pulmonary metastases *(arrows).*

At surgery, a Wilms' tumor was found and nephrectomy performed. No biopsy of the right kidney was done. The child received postoperative radiation therapy and chemotherapy. Lung metastases regressed. Three years later, a radionuclide scan showed defects in the right kidney, and a biopsy was done. The child was then referred to M. D. Anderson Hospital, and an ultrasound of the right kidney was performed.

F, parasagittal right renal sonogram in 1983 shows diffuse distortion of the echo texture and hypoechoic defects within the cortex *(long arrows).*

Review of the outside pathology specimen showed Wilms' tumor in the left kidney with predominant epithelial and blastema cells. Review of the right kidney biopsy specimen showed metanephric blastemas, glomerular immaturity, and cortical cysts.

This case illustrates nephroblastomatosis in an infant, which is frequently misdiagnosed as polycystic kidney. The case was complicated by Wilms' tumor metastatic to the lungs. The infant responded to a combination of surgery, chemotherapy, and radiotherapy and is considered cured.

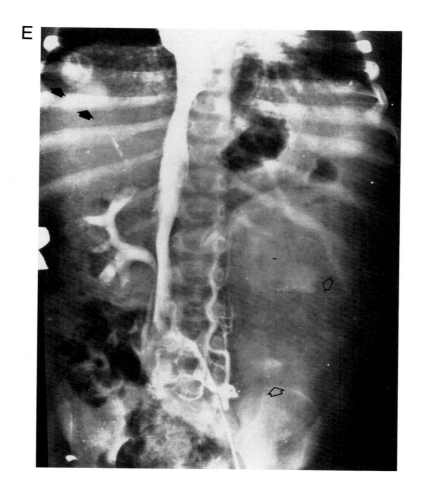

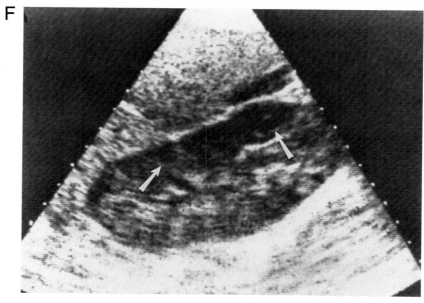

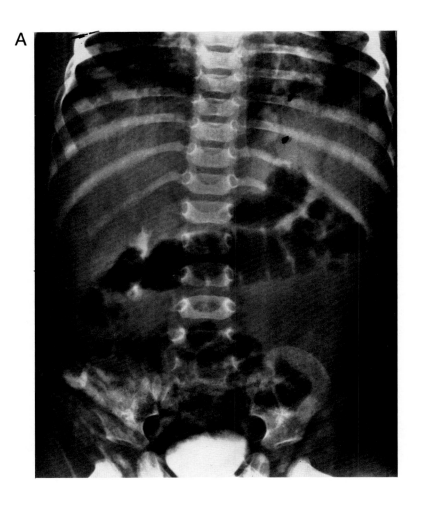

A

FIG 8–11.
Malignant rhabdoid tumor. A 13-month-old boy was seen in another hospital because of nausea, vomiting, low-grade fever, and diarrhea. Subsequently, a left-sided abdominal mass and left-sided facial paralysis were discovered.

A, excretory urogram shows nonfunctioning left kidney and multiple pulmonary metastases *(arrows).*

B, left coronal renal sonogram demonstrates a large hypoechoic mass *(open arrows)* arising from the left kidney *(closed arrows).*

C and **D,** the CT scans show a low-density mass with peripheral enhancement (crescent sign of compressed normal parenchyma) obstructing the opacified calix *(arrow).*

The posterior low-attenuation area *(arrowheads)* probably represents necrosis.

Needle biopsy material from the left renal mass was interpreted as malignant rhabdoid tumor of the kidney. A chest radiograph demonstrated multiple pulmonary metastases. A CT scan of the brain failed to demonstrate metastatic disease; however, cerebral spinal fluid was cytologically positive for malignant cells. A nephrectomy was attempted following chemotherapy, but the procedure had to be canceled because of laryngospasm during anesthesia. The patient subsequently died, and an autopsy could not be performed.

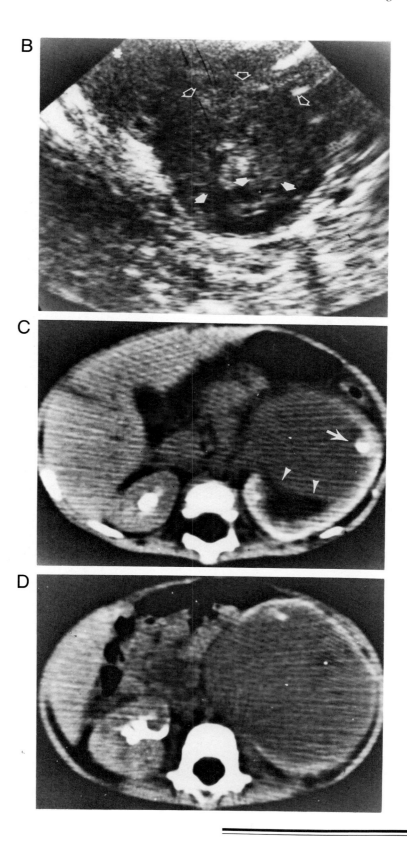

A

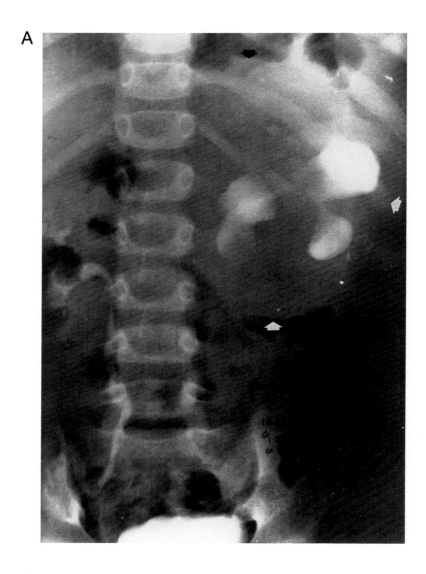

FIG 8–12.
Renal cell carcinoma. A nine-year-old girl presented with a left abdominal mass, and urography was done.

A and **B,** anteroposterior **(A)** and lateral **(B)** views of an excretory urogram show a left intrarenal mass *(arrows)* and distortion and dilatation of the calices. It is impossible to dif-

B

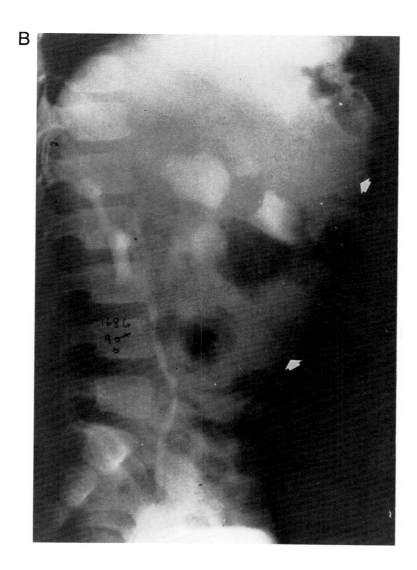

ferentiate renal cell carcinoma from other intrarenal tumors such as Wilms' tumor.

Surgical resection of a large left renal tumor was per-

formed, and a pathologic diagnosis of renal cell carcinoma made.

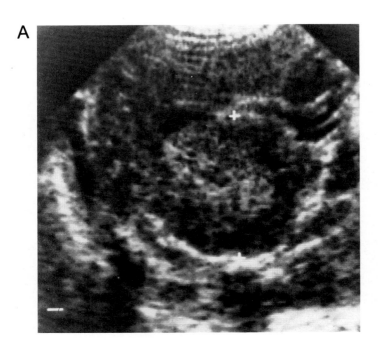

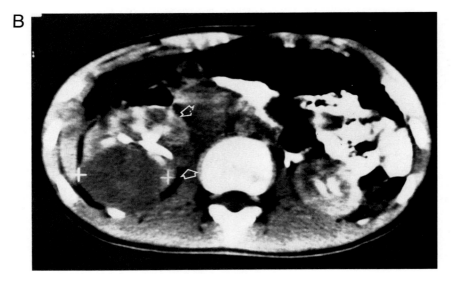

FIG 8–13.

Renal cell carcinoma in the older child with metastases to the cervical spine. A 15-year-old boy was first seen for pain in the left shoulder. He developed neck pain two months later, and a lytic lesion was discovered at C-4. After a further workup that included abdominal ultrasound and CT, he was referred to M. D. Anderson Hospital.

A, transverse sonogram of the right kidney demonstrates an echogenic mass *(cursors)* with a hypoechoic rim.

B, on CT, there is a low-density mass *(cursors)* arising from the posterior aspect of the right kidney, with metastasis to the renal hilus and pericaval nodes *(arrows).*

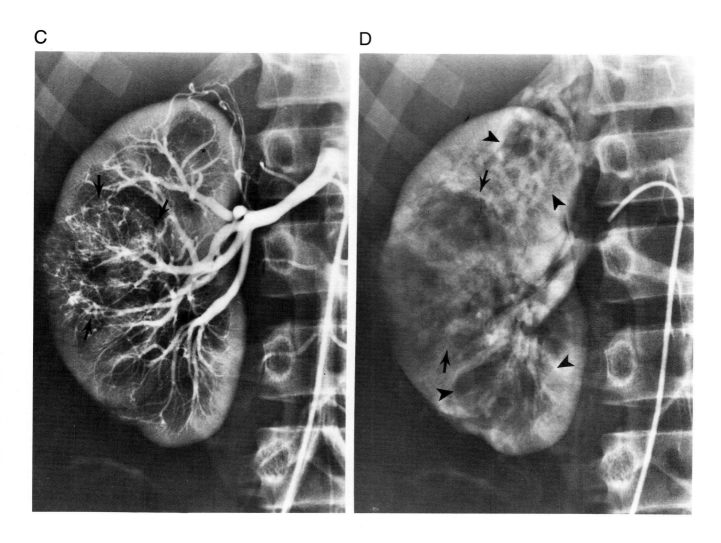

C and **D**, selective right renal angiograms in the arterial **(C)** and venous **(D)** phases showing a hypervascular tumor *(arrows)*. Notice the obstructed upper and lower pole calices *(arrowheads)*.

Ultrasound-guided biopsy of the mass showed renal cell carcinoma. Treatment consisted of irradiation to the neck and embolization of the right renal tumor, followed by chemotherapy. Six months later, the patient died.

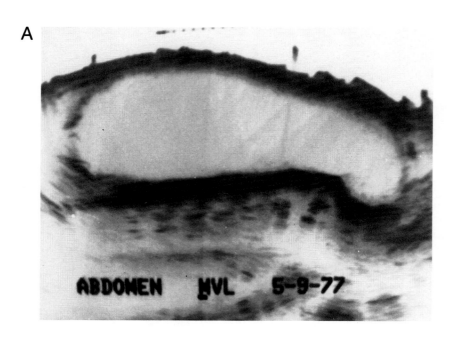

FIG 8–14.
Cystic mature teratoma of the ovary. A 14-year-old girl noticed a "swelling" in her abdomen and also had irregular menses; however, despite the recommendations of the school nurse, she did not consult a physician until ten months later. On referral to M. D. Anderson Hospital, a firm and ill-defined mass was palpated in the abdomen. A uro-gram (not shown) showed partial obstruction of the distal right ureter and hydronephrosis caused by an anterior abdominal mass.

A, sagittal midline sonogram shows a large, pear-shaped anechoic mass with sound transmission that indicates a cystic nature. The mass is arising from the pelvis and extending to the upper abdomen.

B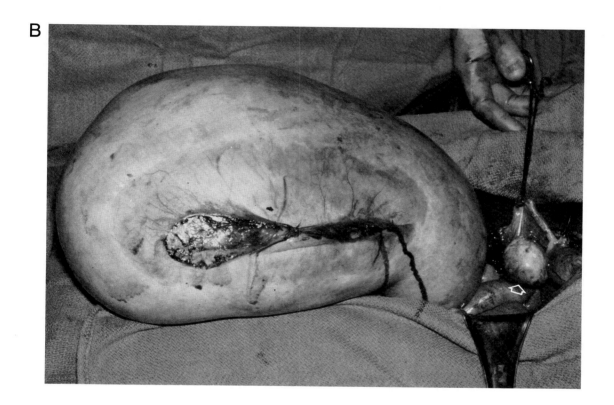

At surgery, a large cystic mass extending from the right adnexa to the xiphoid was discovered. Pathologic diagnosis was cystic mature teratoma.

B, intraoperative photographs of the specimen. Approx-imately 8,000 ml of yellowish, transparent fluid was drained, which contained hair, skin, and bone. Notice corpus luteum cyst of the left ovary *(arrow)* (see also Color Plate 40).

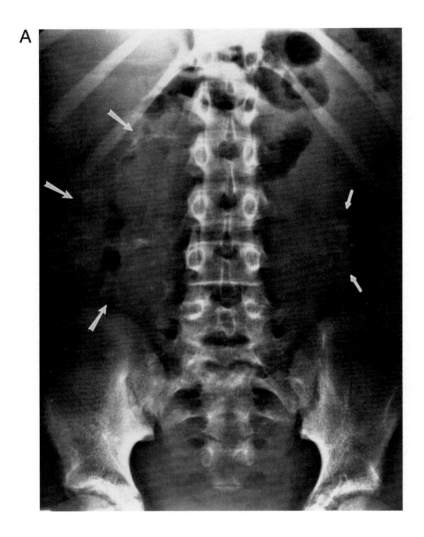

FIG 8–15.
Large calcified immature teratoma of the ovary. An 11-year-old girl had a history of pain, and a palpable large abdominal mass was discovered on physical examination.

A, plain abdominal radiograph shows patchy *(small arrows)* and amorphous *(large arrows)* calcifications scattered throughout the abdomen.

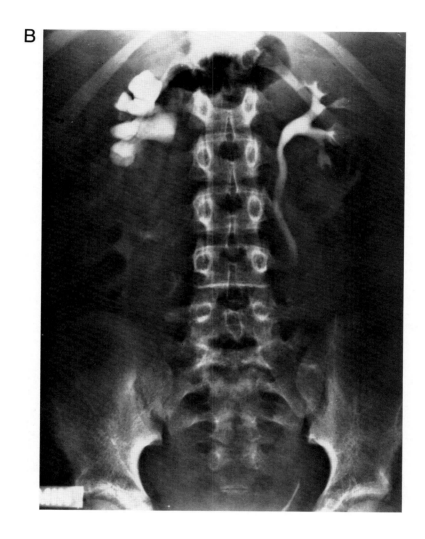

B, urogram demonstrates obstructed right collecting system and mild compression and displacement of the mid- left ureter. *(Continued.)*

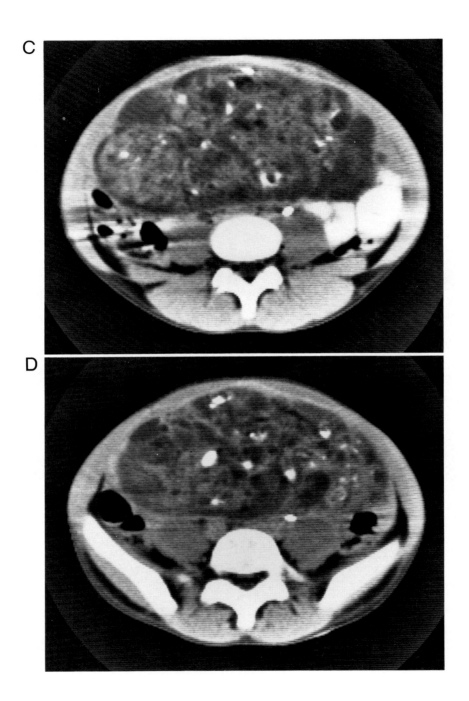

FIG 8–15 (cont.).
C and **D,** upper abdominal **(C)** and pelvic **(D)** CT scans demonstrate a large nonhomogeneous mass consisting of soft tissue, fat, and calcium densities. The mass is displacing the bowel posterolaterally.

At surgery, a large right ovarian mass was removed.

Pathologic examination showed a grade II immature teratoma, with metastases to the lymph nodes. The tumor contained calcifications, ossifications, sebaceous debris, hair, and vesicles. The patient received chemotherapy postoperatively; results of a second-look operation one year later were negative for disease.

E

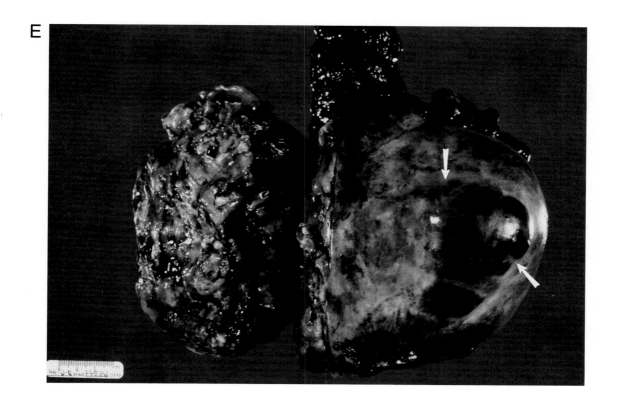

E, surgical specimen shows a solid 8.6 × 16 × 17 cm oval mass *(left)* covered by a glistening, partially translucent membrane. Cut section *(right)* shows a heterogeneous nodular appearance with areas of focal hemorrhage *(arrows)* (see also Color Plate 41).

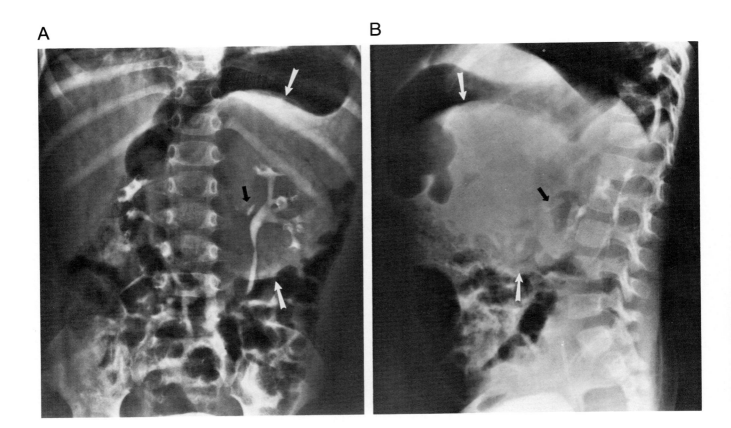

A

B

FIG 8–16.

Cystic mature retroperitoneal teratoma. A woman discovered an abdominal mass in her two-year-old daughter. Except for occasional complaints of abdominal pain, the child had been otherwise without symptoms.

A and **B,** anteroposterior and lateral views of an excretory urogram demonstrate a large extrarenal mass *(white arrows)* with small calcifications *(black arrows)* immersed in a low-density area that probably represents fat.

C, transverse sonogram shows a heterogeneous, complex mass *(arrows)* anterior to the left kidney *(k).* The mass contains hyperechoic elements *(arrowheads)* that probably represent calcification and fat.

At surgery, a large retroperitoneal mass was removed. On histologic examination, it proved to be a mature cystic teratoma containing hair, calcification, and fat.

D, cut section of the 13 × 10 × 7 cm cystic mass with thick capsule containing hair *(arrowheads)* and numerous nodules of sebaceous material *(arrows),* many of which contained calcification (see also Color Plate 42).

C

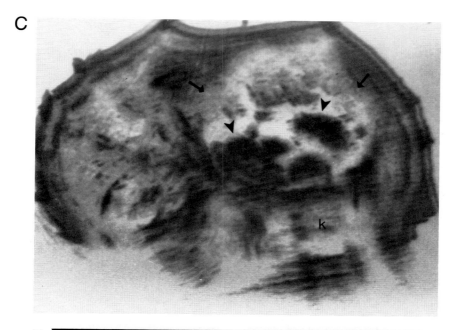

D

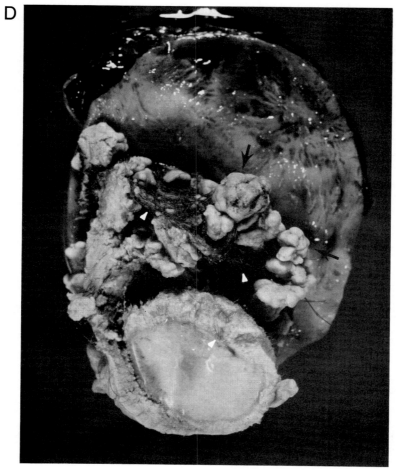

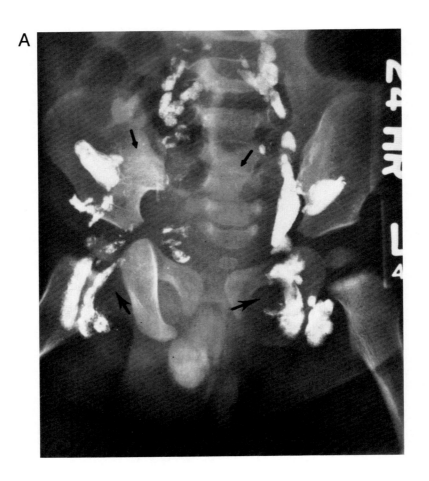

FIG 8–17.
Endodermal sinus tumor of the testicle metastatic to the pelvic nodes. An 18-month-old boy had yolk sac tumor of the testis and underwent a left orchiectomy. On referral to M. D. Anderson Hospital, he had nodal metastases.

A, a 24-hr follow-up film of a bipedal lymphangiogram demonstrates a large nonopacified nodal mass in the right side of the pelvis *(small arrows)* and partial replacement of the right and left inguinal nodes *(large arrows).*

B, excretory urogram subsequent to the lymphangiogram demonstrates a large nodal mass in the right side of the pelvis *(arrows);* the mass compresses the urinary bladder and the opacified nodes.

C, postchemotherapy radiograph of the abdomen shows marked reduction in the size of the pelvic mass and reexpansion of the urinary bladder.

Following chemotherapy, a retroperitoneal node dissection was performed, and no viable tumor was found.

B

C

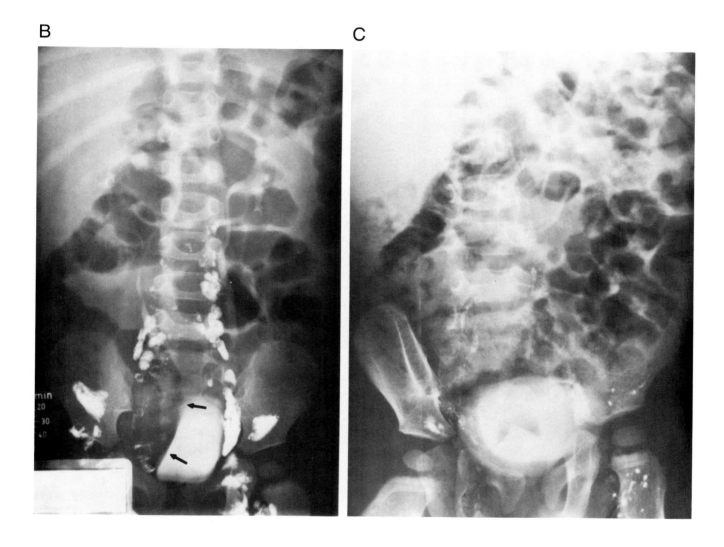

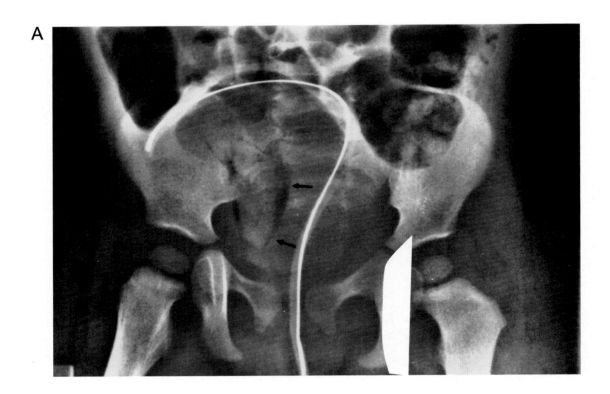

FIG 8–18.

Sacrococcygeal endodermal sinus tumor and mature teratoma (mixed germ cell tumor.) A 13-month-old girl initially presented with a three- to four-week history of difficult, painful, and blood-stained stools and loss of use of both legs. She underwent extensive workup in Saudi Arabia, and a diagnosis of endodermal sinus tumor was established. The

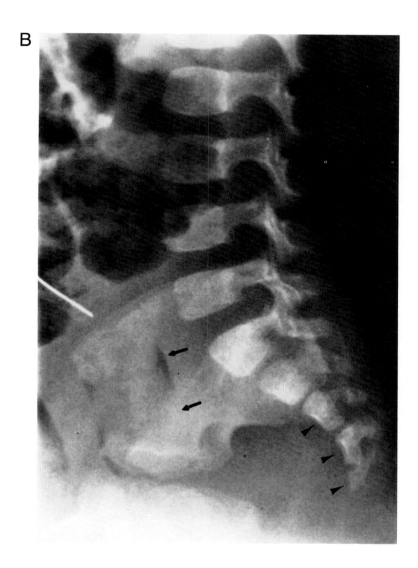

child was then referred to M. D. Anderson Hospital.

A and **B,** frontal **(A)** and lateral **(B)** pelvic radiographs demonstrate displacement of the rectum *(arrows)* to the right and anteriorly, and erosive changes along the anterior margins of the sacral segments *(arrowheads).* Notice the Foley catheter within the displaced urinary bladder. *(Continued.)*

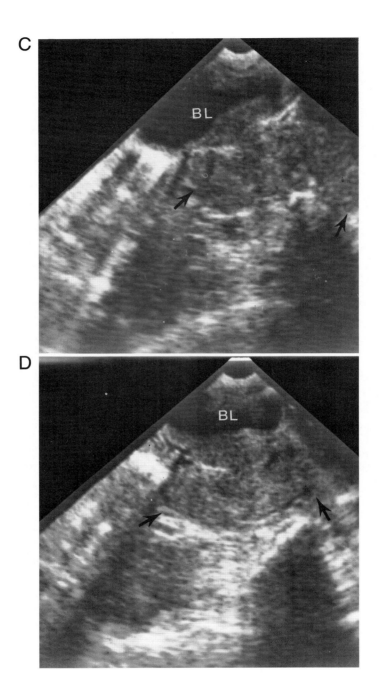

FIG 8–18 (cont.).
C and **D,** pretreatment sagittal **(C)** and transverse **(D)** sonograms demonstrate a large echogenic mass *(arrows)* inferior and posterior to the urinary bladder *(BL).* The mass is displacing and indenting the urinary bladder. The patient received chemotherapy for four months and her α-fetoprotein levels dropped from 318,500 to 131,700 units. Ultrasound (not shown) showed regression of the mass, and CT scan demonstrated residual tumor.

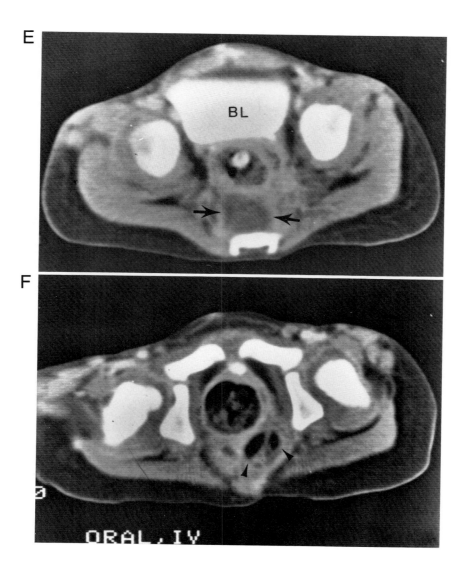

E, postchemotherapy CT scan at the level of the bladder *(BL)* demonstrates residual low-attenuation tumor mass *(arrows)* between the rectum and the sacrum.

F, lower CT section shows the fatty portion *(arrowheads),* presumably representing the teratomatous component of the tumor.

The patient subsequently underwent surgery, and a 4.5-cm soft tissue tumor was removed, as were the coccyx and lower part of the sacrum. Pathologic diagnosis was sacrococcygeal endodermal sinus tumor and mature teratoma. The patient developed metastases to the lungs. These responded to chemotherapy. The tumor recurred in the sacrococcygeal region and the posterior soft tissues, and it became gradually resistant to multiple chemotherapeutic regimens. It was elected to discontinue chemotherapy and keep the patient comfortable during her terminal period.

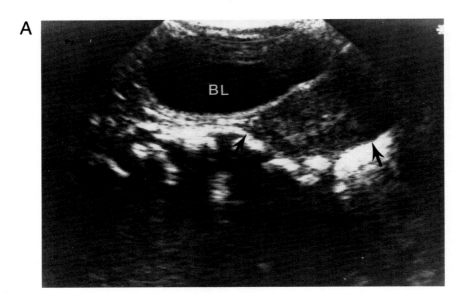

FIG 8–19.

Endodermal sinus tumor of the vagina. An eight-month-old girl had vaginal bleeding and was referred to M. D. Anderson Hospital. The patient underwent a complete pelvic examination under general anesthesia, and a 3 × 4 cm tumor was found in the upper half of the vagina. The tumor encased the cervix and penetrated into the posterior cul-de-sac. A biopsy was done, and pathologic examination confirmed the diagnosis of pure endodermal sinus tumor.

A, midline sagittal sonogram shows an echogenic mass *(arrows)* posterior and inferior to the urinary bladder *(BL)* and occupying the upper vaginal canal.

B, follow-up sagittal sonograms after chemotherapy show complete resolution of the vaginal mass. The patient was treated with chemotherapy, but the tumor recurred locally several months later despite the dramatic initial response *(BL,* bladder).

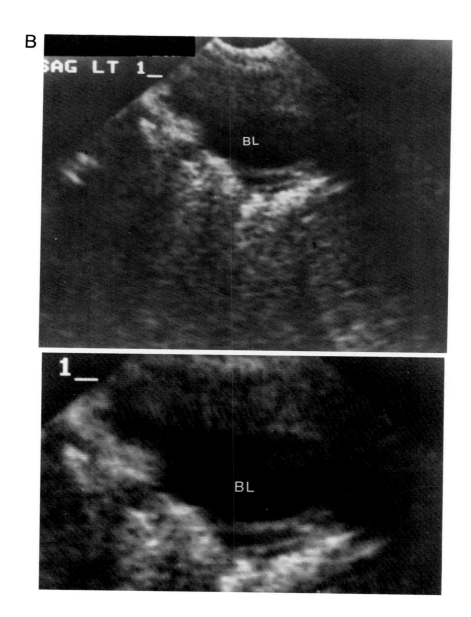

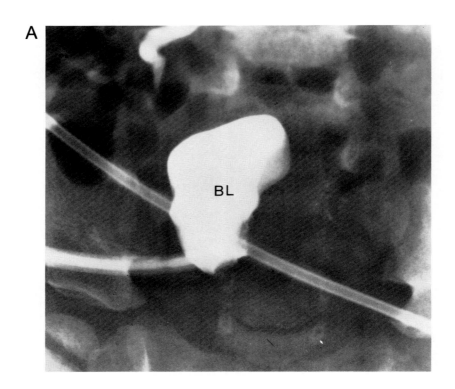

FIG 8–20.
Pelvic rhabdomyosarcoma, probably of bladder origin, with botryoid features. A two-year-old boy was initially evaluated at an outside institution. He had a history of edema in the left leg, a mass in the left lower quadrant, and difficulty with urination.

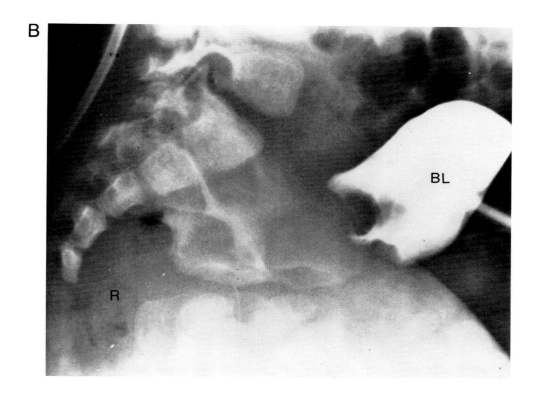

A and **B,** frontal **(A)** and lateral **(B)** cystograms obtained via a suprapubic catheter demonstrate infiltration of the urinary bladder *(BL)* by a large mass arising from the bladder base and projecting into the lumen (botryoid feature). Notice that the rectum *(R)* is displaced posteriorly and there is right ureteral reflux in **A.** *(Continued.)*

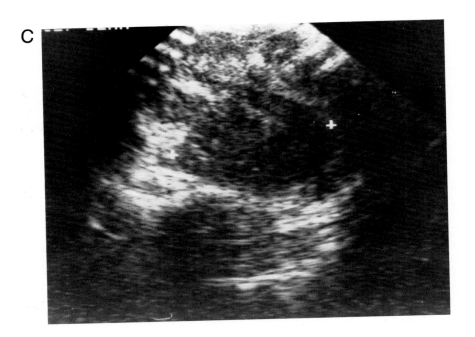

FIG 8–20 (cont.).
C, sagittal sonogram shows a hypoechoic mass *(cursor)* in the floor of the pelvis.

D and **E,** unenhanced CT scans of the pelvis demonstrate a large soft tissue tumor *(arrows)* displacing the urinary bladder *(BL)* and rectum. There is infiltration of the bladder wall.

From these results it was thought likely that the tumor arose from the bladder wall and had both large exophytic **(C–E)** and smaller intraluminal **(B)** components.

Exploratory laparotomy that was done a month later in another hospital showed a pelvic mass obstructing the ureters and compressing the bladder. Pathologic diagnosis was a small, round-cell tumor. A nephrostomy, for bilateral hydronephrosis, was done, and the patient was transferred to M. D. Anderson Hospital. Review of the outside slides showed unclassified small cell malignant neoplasm. Electron microscopy of the bone marrow aspirate demonstrated malignant neoplasm suggestive of metastatic rhabdomyosarcoma. The patient was treated with chemotherapy.

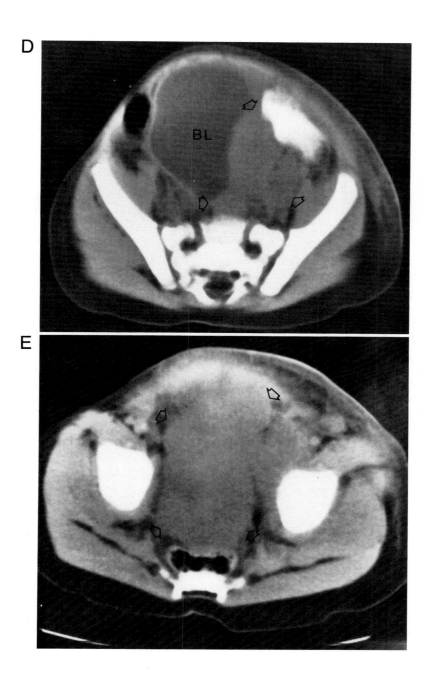

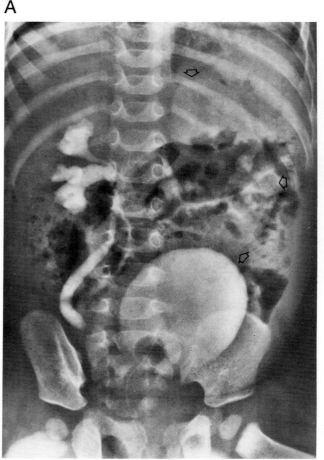

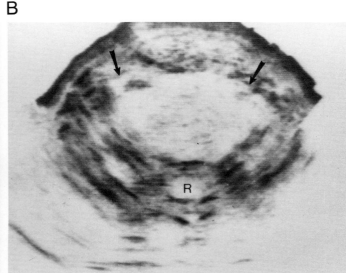

FIG 8–21.

Rhabdomyosarcoma of the prostate. An 11-month-old boy presented with coliclike abdominal pain, and a mass extending to the umbilicus was discovered in the lower abdomen.

A, excretory urogram demonstrates superiorly displaced urinary bladder, right hydronephrosis, and lack of function in the enlarged left kidney *(open arrows)* secondary to ureteral obstruction.

B, axial sonogram of the pelvis shows a hypoechoic mass *(arrows)* anterior to the rectum *(R)*.

C and **D,** these CT scans of the pelvis demonstrate a large mass *(arrows)* arising from the prostate gland and compressing the bladder *(BL)*. There is right inguinal adenopathy and invasion of the perivesical fat *(white arrowheads)* and the right obturator internus muscle *(black arrowheads) (R,* rectum).

Following initial workup, a transrectal biopsy of the prostate demonstrated embryonal rhabdomyosarcoma. The patient was treated with chemotherapy, and there was a good initial response. Approximately 17 months later, metastatic disease developed in the right pelvic-paraaortic nodes in addition to generalized bony metastasis.

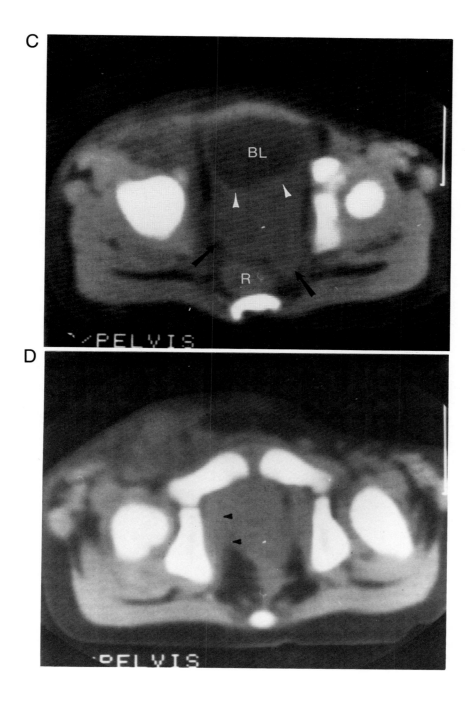

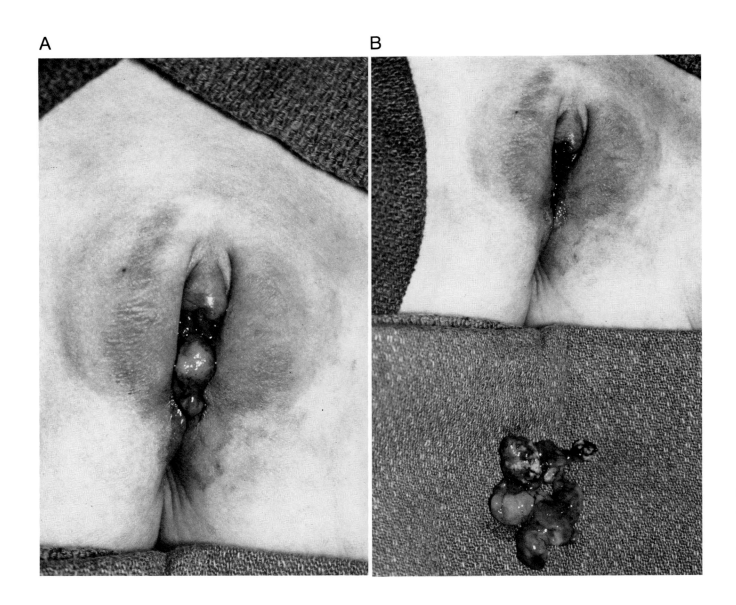

FIG 8–22.
Embryonal rhabdomyosarcoma (sarcoma botryoides) of the vagina. Vaginal bleeding in a 22-month-old girl led her parents to discover "tissue" protruding from her vagina. Because the symptoms disappeared, the couple did not consult a physician until another episode occurred several weeks later. Pathologic examination showed sarcoma botryoides.

A and **B,** clusters of polypoid, grapelike tumors protruding from the vagina **(A).** External view and resected specimen **(B).** (See also Color Plates 43 and 44.)

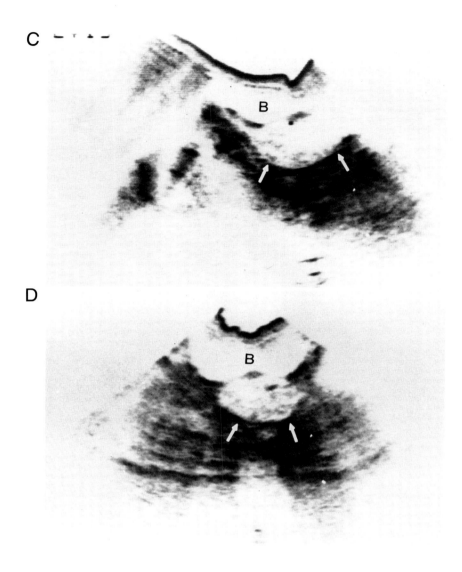

C and **D,** sagittal midline **(C)** and transverse **(D)** sonograms demonstrate a hypoechoic mass *(arrows)* posteroinferior to the urinary bladder *(B).* Botryoid configuration cannot be ascertained from this sonogram.

At M. D. Anderson Hospital, the patient underwent chemotherapy followed by vaginectomy. She was given postoperative chemotherapy and is alive and free of disease five years after diagnosis.

A

B

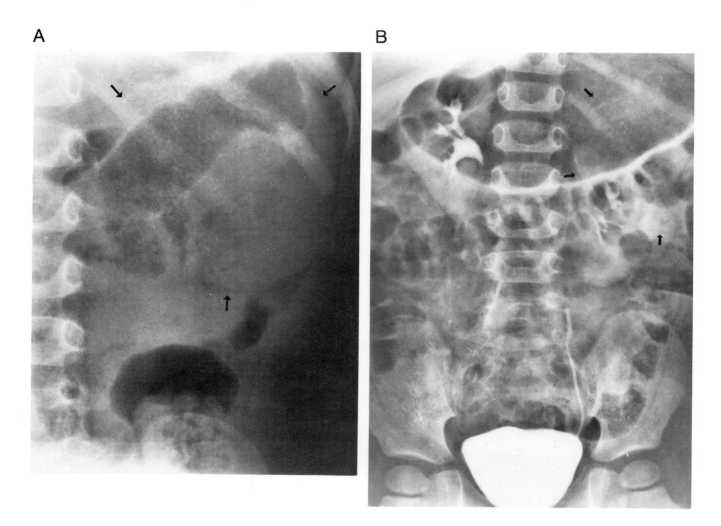

FIG 8–23.
Adrenal ganglioneuroblastoma. A left abdominal mass was detected in this three-year-old girl during routine clinical examination.

A, detailed view of the left upper abdomen shows a large mass containing fine punctate calcifications *(arrows).*

B, excretory urogram shows a large suprarenal mass *(arrows)* compressing and displacing the left kidney downward. Note the medial peripheral enhancement *(arrows).*

On surgical exploration, the mass proved to be a stage I ganglioneuroblastoma of the left adrenal gland. The tumor showed punctate calcification. The patient received postoperative chemotherapy and is free of disease six years after diagnosis.

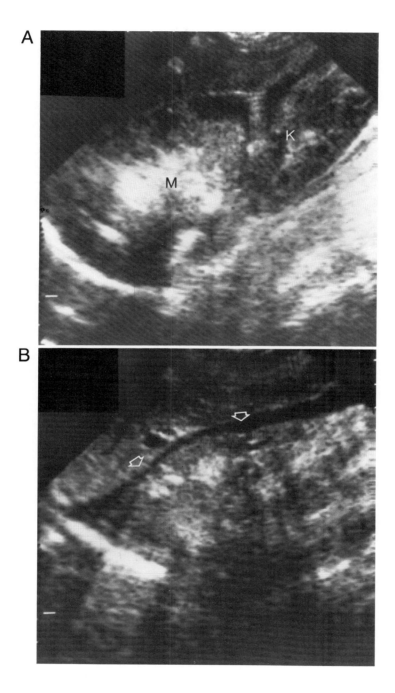

FIG 8–24.

Maturing adrenal neuroblastoma. A five-year-old girl, carrying the diagnosis of right adrenal neuroblastoma, underwent surgical exploration and was treated with chemotherapy at an outside institution.

A and **B,** right parasagittal sonograms show a large, calcified right suprarenal mass *(M)* compressing the kidney *(K)* and elevating the inferior vena cava *(open arrows).* *(Continued.)*

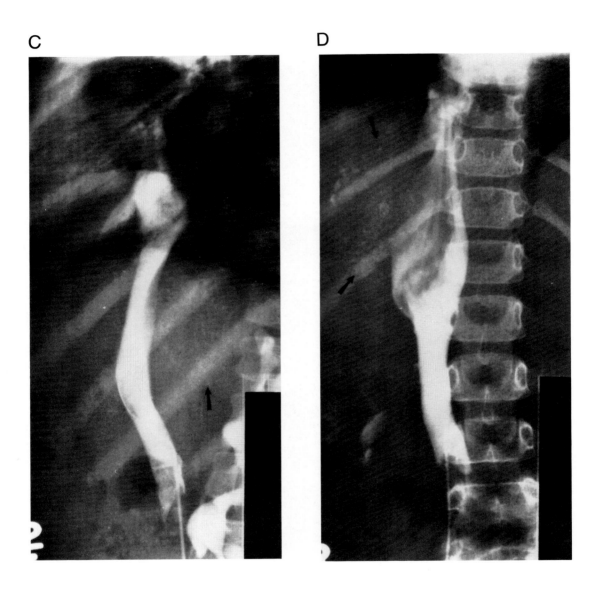

FIG 8–24 (cont.).
C and **D,** oblique and anteroposterior views of inferior venacavogram demonstrate a large, calcified mass *(arrows)* extrinsic to the vena cava.

E and **F,** enhanced CT scans show a large, low-density right adrenal mass *(large arrows);* a densely calcified component extends behind the compressed vena cava *(arrowhead)* and the aorta *(small arrow) (k,* kidney).

At M. D. Anderson Hospital, the patient received additional chemotherapy, but poor response, both clinically and radiographically, led to reexploration and removal of 95% of the tumor. The tumor arose from the right adrenal gland. It extended behind the inferior vena cava and was adherent to the aorta. The tumor also had a separate paraspinal component, thought to represent nodal metastases, both medial and inferior to the right kidney. On final histologic interpretation, no small cell neuroblastic elements were found, and the tumor was classified as ganglioneuroma or, alternatively, maturing neuroblastoma. The patient received radiation therapy and intravenous cisplatin postoperatively. She is currently free of disease three years after diagnosis.

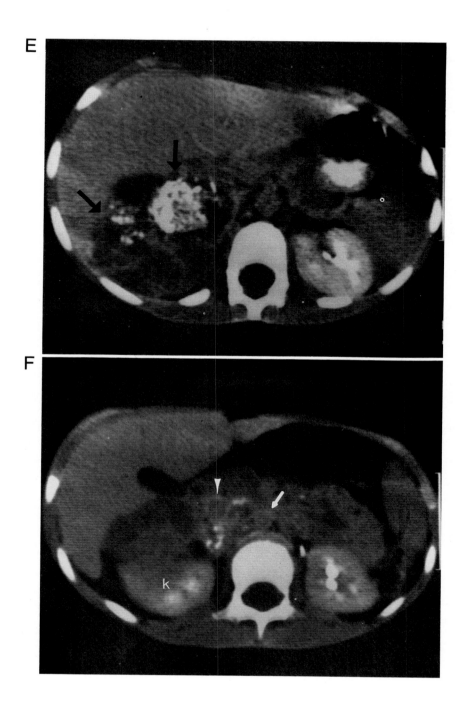

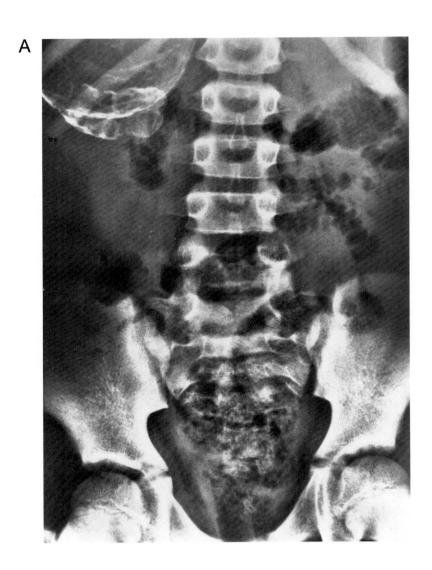

FIG 8–25.
Necrotic adrenal ganglioneuroblastoma. A calcified mass in the right upper quadrant was incidentally discovered on the chest radiograph of a ten-year-old boy who presented with pneumonia.

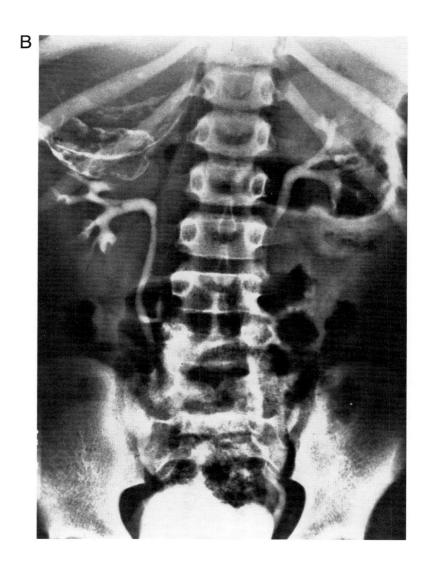

A and **B,** plain abdominal radiograph **(A)** and urogram **(B)** demonstrate a right suprarenal mass with dense, rimlike calcifications. The mass is displacing the renal collecting system downward. *(Continued.)*

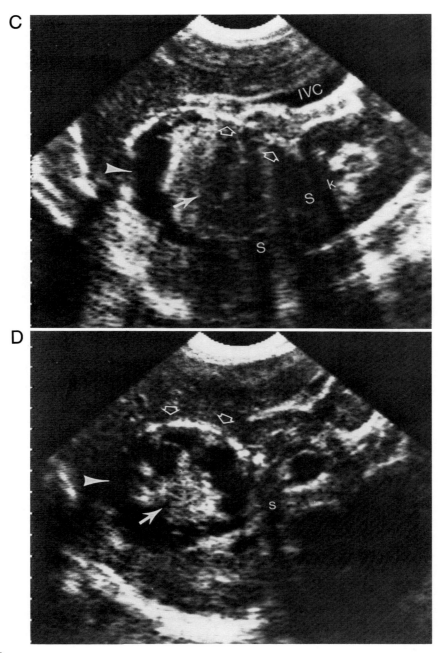

FIG 8–25 (cont.).
C and **D,** right parasagittal **(C)** and transverse **(D)** sonograms demonstrate a complex suprarenal mass containing peripheral calcifications *(open arrows)* and solid *(arrows)* and fluid *(arrowheads)* components. Notice the compressed upper pole of the right kidney *(k) (S,* acoustic shadowing; *IVC,* inferior vena cava).

E, contrast-enhanced CT scan shows a hypodense mass with ringlike peripheral *(arrows)* and cloudlike central *(arrowheads)* calcifications in the right suprarenal region.

At exploration, a 15 × 13 × 5 cm, firm, calcified mass was discovered adherent to the diaphragm, liver, and kidney. The mass was removed, along with the upper pole of

the right kidney.

F, cut section of the mass. The adrenal capsule is thickened and the neoplastic material is brownish, 95% necrotic, and hemorrhagic. Extensive multifocal calcifications were identified in the tumor (not shown) (see also Color Plate 45).

The tumor proved to be a ganglioneuroblastoma of the adrenal gland. There was 95% tumor necrosis, together with good evidence of maturation. A small rim of compressed adrenal gland was present. No tumor was found in the resected portion of the kidney. No chemotherapy was required.

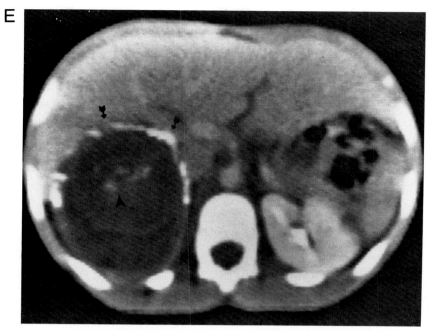

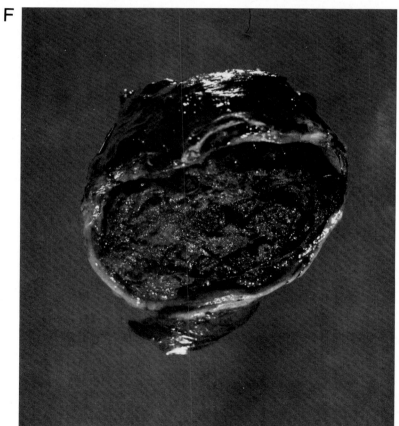

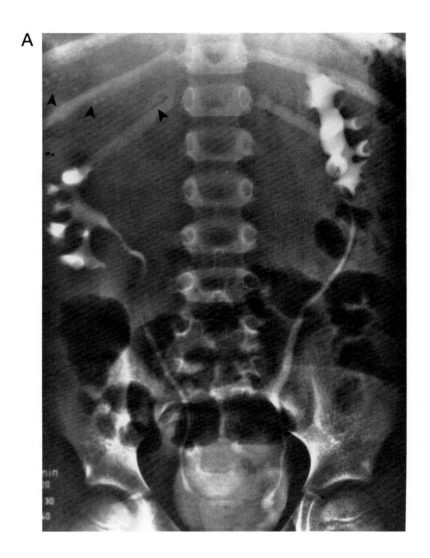

FIG 8–26.

Stage IV adrenal neuroblastoma. A six-year-old boy presented with enlarged cervical nodes, and biopsy of one node showed metastatic neuroblastoma. Subsequent work-up demonstrated a large right adrenal mass with metastasis to the retroperitoneal nodes. There was also bone marrow involvement (stage IV disease).

A, excretory urogram shows extrinsic pressure on the right kidney from a suprarenal mass containing small flecks of calcification *(arrowheads)*. There is also lateral displacement of the left kidney and of both ureters by the enlarged retroperitoneal nodes.

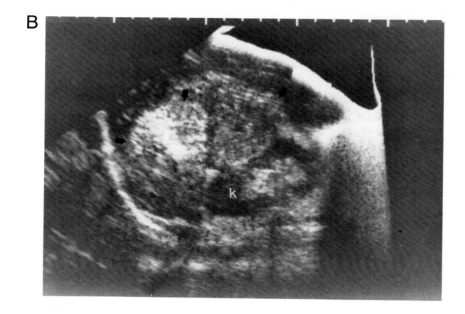

B, right parasagittal sonogram shows a large tumor mass of mixed echogenicity *(arrows)* compressing and dis- placing the right kidney *(k)* downward. *(Continued.)*

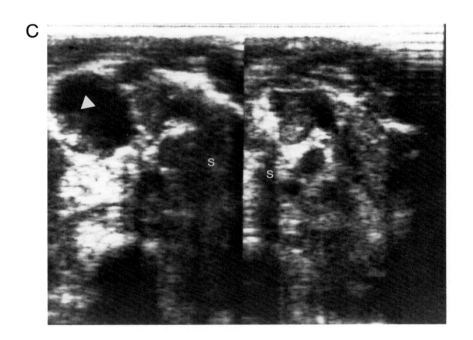

FIG 8–26 (cont.).

C, transverse upper abdominal sonograms show cystic component of the mass *(white arrowhead)* and shadowing *(S)* from the calcified areas.

D, precontrast CT scans demonstrate a large calcified right suprarenal mass *(black arrows)*, calcified nodes *(white arrows)*, and cystic, probably necrotic nodes with mural nodule *(arrowheads)*.

E, postcontrast CT scans show right adrenal mass, probably invading the right kidney *(arrowheads)*.

The patient was treated with chemotherapy, which finally brought the disease under control after one year.

D

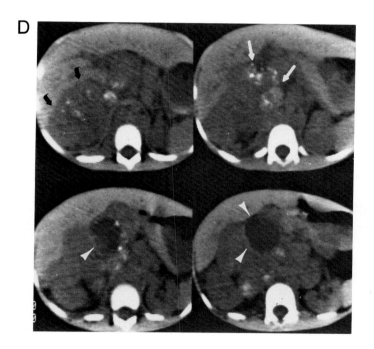

E

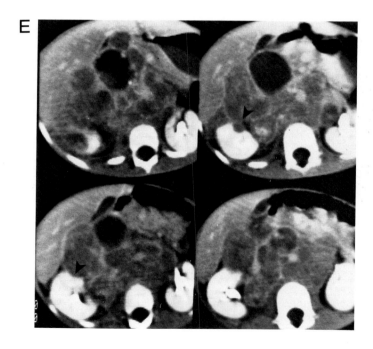

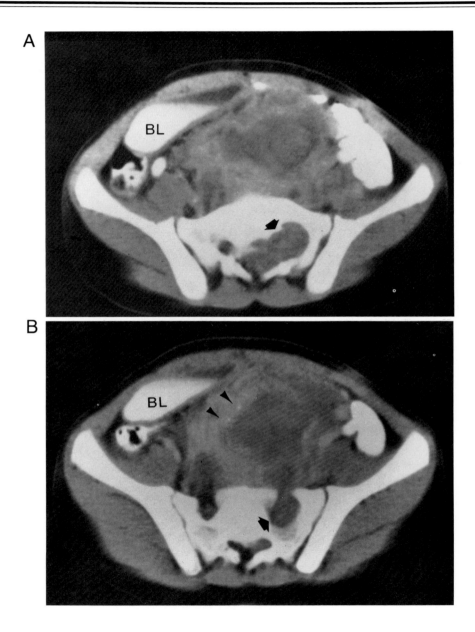

FIG 8–27.
Stage III presacral ganglioneuroblastoma with intraspinal extension. A six-year-old boy was referred to M. D. Anderson Hospital for further evaluation and management of a pelvic mass that had been recently diagnosed. No neurologic deficits other than distended bladder and priapism were noted. Results from a laparotomy performed at the referring institution showed a large pelvic mass extending into the sacral canal. The tumor was considered unresectable, and a biopsy demonstrated 95% ganglioneuroma and approximately 5% neuroblastoma.

A and **B,** contrast-enhanced CT scans of the pelvis demonstrate a large lobulated mass with a small, curvilinear calcification (*arrowheads* in **B**) displacing the bladder *(BL)* and bowel anteriorly. The tumor has enlarged the left sacral foramina and extended into the spinal canal *(arrows)*. A CT metrizamide myelogram (not shown) demonstrated displacement of the dural sac to the right.

The diagnosis was confirmed at M. D. Anderson Hospital, and intraarterial infusion therapy with cisplatin was started; however, this had to be discontinued because of renal failure. Subsequently, the tumor was embolized, but there was no significant response.

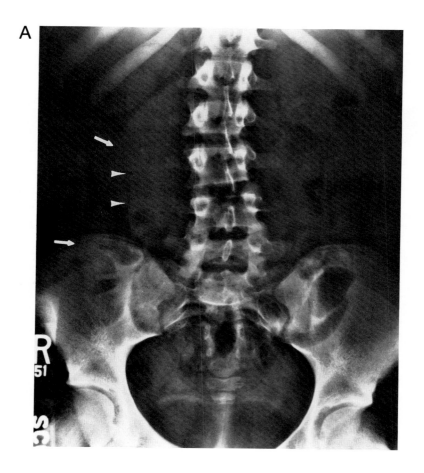

FIG 8–28.

Asymptomatic paraspinal ganglioneuroma. A 15-year-old girl was in good health except for occasional morning pain in the right leg. On a routine physical examination, a right-sided abdominal mass was discovered. A CT scan report-edly showed a large right retroperitoneal mass, and the patient was referred to M. D. Anderson Hospital.

A, plain radiograph shows asymmetric prominence of the right psoas muscle *(white arrows)* and the suggestion of a mass *(white arrowheads). (Continued.)*

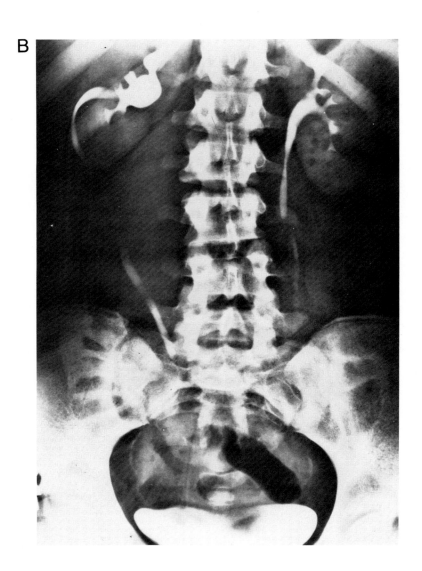

FIG 8–28 (cont.).

B, urogram shows a laterally displaced lower pole of the right kidney and displacement and compression of the right ureter.

C and **D,** right sagittal **(C)** and transverse **(D)** sonograms display a solid, hypoechoic tumor *(black arrow-*

heads) anteromedial to the kidney *(K).*

At surgery, a large, fleshy tumor was found. It arose from the sympathetic chain posteriorly and was embedded in the psoas muscle. Histologic analysis showed a ganglioneuroma in the connective tissue and skeletal muscle.

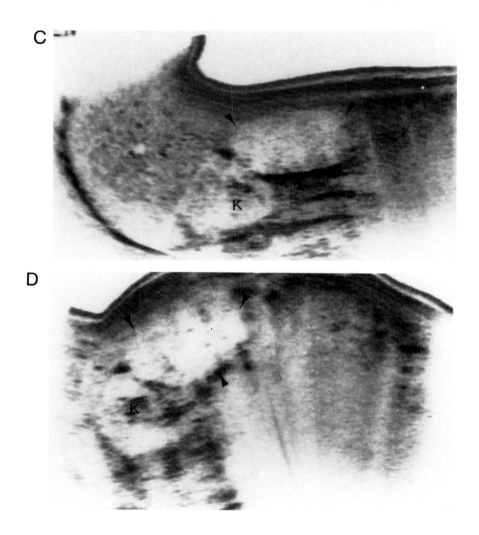

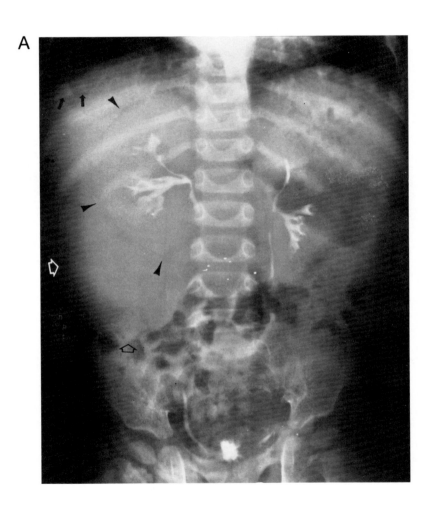

FIG 8–29.

Hepatoblastoma with pulmonary and osseous metastasis. An 18-month-old boy had fever and irritability two weeks prior to hospital admission. A fullness in the abdomen was discovered by the mother and proved to be a mass when examined by the local physician.

A, excretory urogram demonstrates a soft tissue mass *(open arrows)* continuous with the liver and compressing and slightly displacing the right kidney *(arrowheads).* Notice pulmonary metastatic nodules *(small arrows)* in the right side.

B and **C,** right parasagittal **(B)** and transverse **(C)** sonograms demonstrate a highly echogenic hepatic mass compressing the right kidney *(arrows).*

On the patient's referral to M. D. Anderson Hospital, metastatic disease to the lungs and to one dorsal vertebral body was noted. Needle biopsy of the liver showed hepatoblastoma. The α-fetoprotein level was 298,000 units. In view of the poor prognosis, the mother refused to have chemotherapy administered to the child, and he died two months later.

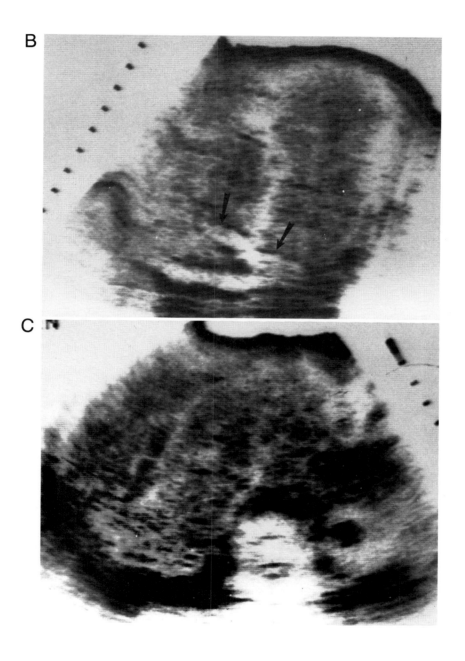

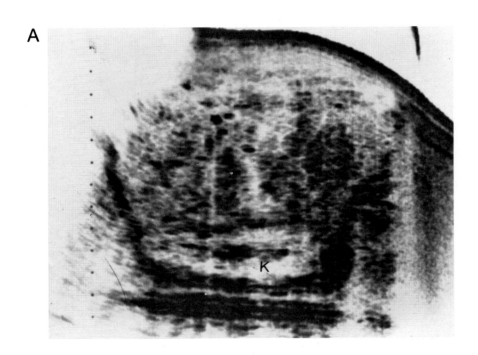

FIG 8–30.
Hepatoblastoma. A 13-month-old boy presented with a large abdominal mass, lethargy, and weight loss of four weeks' duration. On physical examination, the mass was firm, nodular, and fixed. The α-fetoprotein level was normal.

A, right sagittal sonogram shows a posteriorly located hyperechoic mass compressing the right kidney *(K).*

B, right lateral view of a ^{99m}Tc-sulfur colloid scan shows a large defect in the posterior segment of the liver.

C, contrast-enhanced CT scan demonstrates a large, hypodense lesion involving the right lobe and medial segment of the left lobe *(arrows)* of the liver. *(Continued.)*

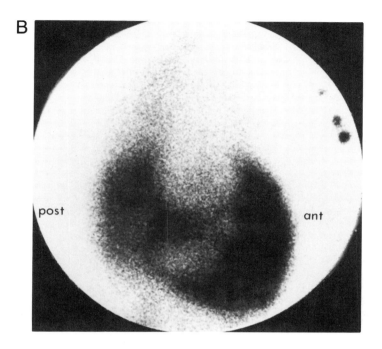

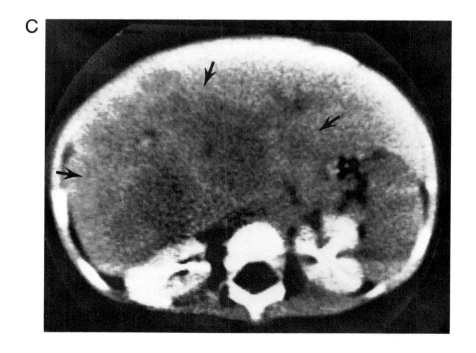

D

E

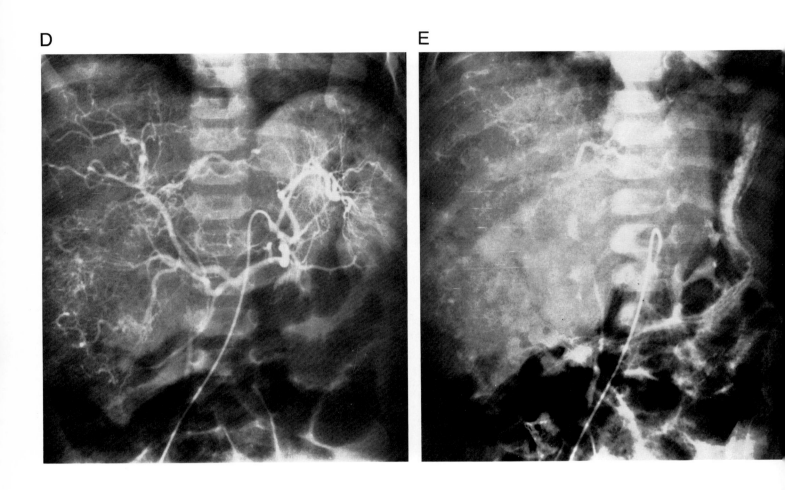

FIG 8–30 (cont.).
D and **E,** celiac angiogram in the arterial **(D)** and venous **(E)** phases shows extensive hepatic involvement by tumor.

At surgery, a primary hepatic tumor was found to oc-cupy the entire medial segment of the left lobe and most of the right lobe. An extended right hepatic lobectomy was per-formed. The pathologic diagnosis was epithelial hepatoblas-toma.

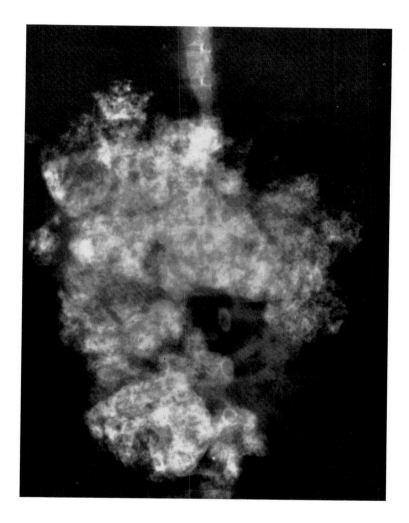

FIG 8–31.

Calcified hepatoblastoma. This two-year-old boy presented with increasing abdominal girth; clinical examination revealed a large, firm abdominal mass.

Plain radiograph of the abdomen demonstrates a huge lobulated and calcified mass. The mass occupies almost the entire abdominal and pelvic cavities.

Biopsy of the mass showed calcified hepatoblastoma. (Courtesy of Dr. Dominique Counet, Institut Gustave Roussy, Villejuif, France.)

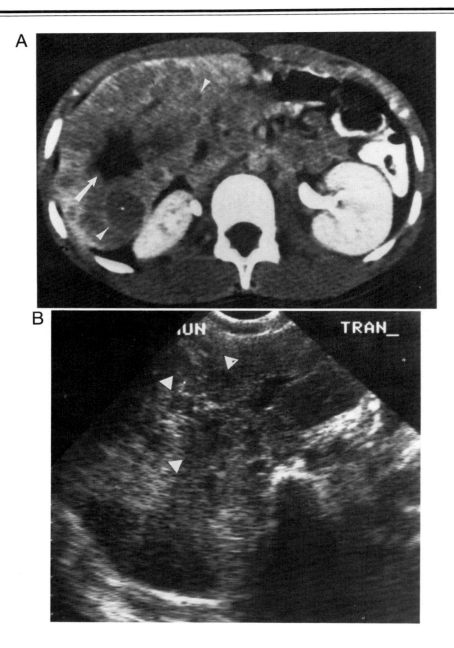

FIG 8–32.
Hepatocellular carcinoma with cavernous transformation of the portal vein and osseous metastasis. A 14-year-old girl presented with an enlarged liver, and workup revealed diffuse involvement of the liver by tumor. She had elevated levels of α-fetoprotein.

A, contrast-enhanced CT scan four months after the initiation of chemotherapy reveals diffuse infiltration of the liver with multiple low-attenuation defects *(arrowheads)* and an area presumed to be necrotic tumor *(arrow)*. The portal vein could not be identified.

B, transverse sonogram of the liver demonstrates multiple hypoechoic defects *(arrowheads)* with diffusely abnormal echo texture.

C, transverse sonogram at the level of the pancreas shows numerous small vessels *(arrows)* anterior to the inferior vena cava *(C)*. The portal vein was not visualized. These findings represent cavernous transformation of the portal vein *(SV,* splenic vein).

D, hepatic angiogram shows a large, hypervascular tumor involving almost the entire liver. The portal vein was not visualized.

A biopsy showed hepatocellular carcinoma. In view of the extent of liver involvement, the patient was treated with chemotherapy. She developed pain in the right groin, and a lytic lesion was subsequently discovered in the right ischium. Biopsy documented metastasis from the liver tumor.

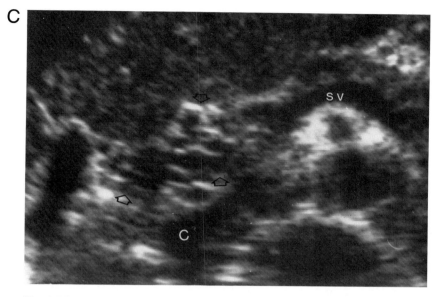

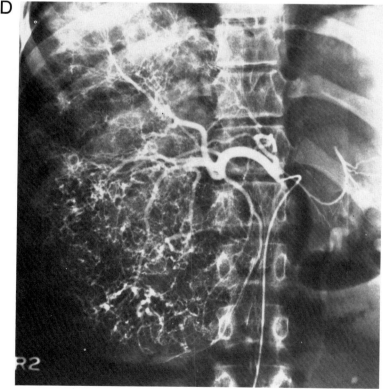

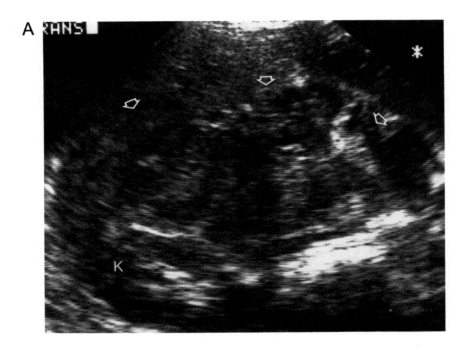

FIG 8–33.
Embryonal mesenchymal sarcoma of the liver. A 13-year-old girl presented at an outside institution with a one-month history of low-grade fever and of subsequent intermittent right-sided abdominal pain. An enlarged liver was discovered on physical examination.

B

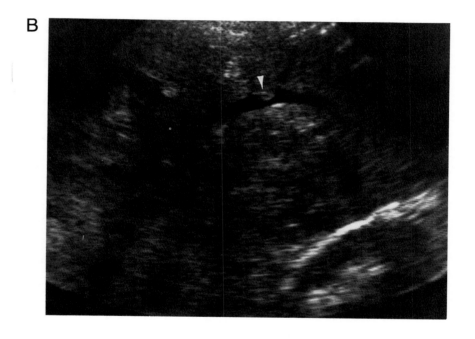

A and **B,** transverse sonogram **(A)** demonstrates a large solid tumor involving the right and the left hepatic lobes *(arrows).* The portal vein was not visualized and was presumed to be infiltrated by the tumor (*K*, kidney). Sagittal sonogram **(B)** demonstrates tumor nodule projecting into the middle hepatic vein *(arrowhead). (Continued.)*

C

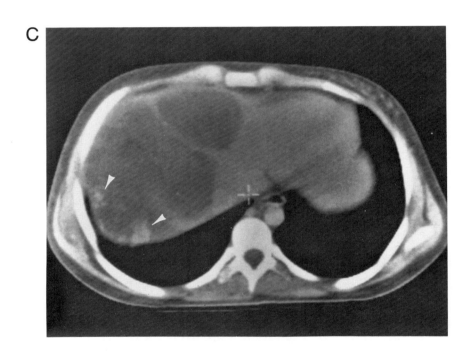

FIG 8–33 (cont.).
C through **E,** contrast-enhanced CT scans demonstrate multiloculated, low-density mass involving the right lobe and medial segment of the left lobe. Notice areas of tumor enhancement *(arrowheads).*

    An ultrasound-guided percutaneous biopsy, as well as a limited laparotomy, failed to demonstrate tumor cells. A standard laparotomy revealed poorly differentiated malignant tumor deep within the mass, consistent with embryonal mesenchymal sarcoma. The patient developed postoperative complications. A transplant of the liver was contemplated, but the patient died before this could be accomplished.

D

E

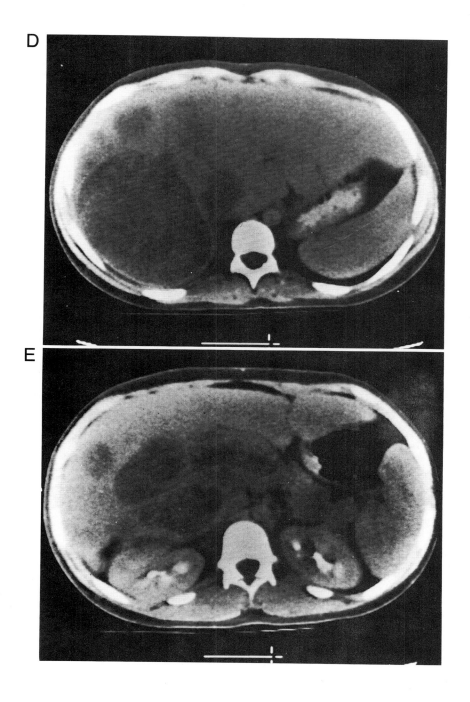

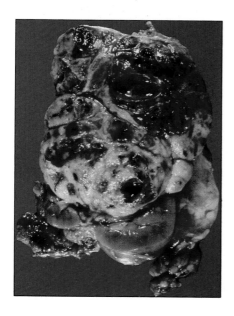

PLATE 37

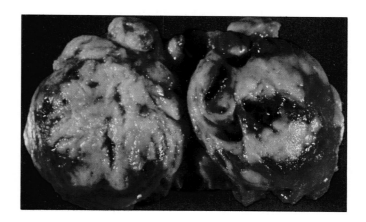

PLATE 38

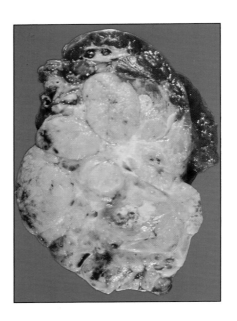

PLATE 39

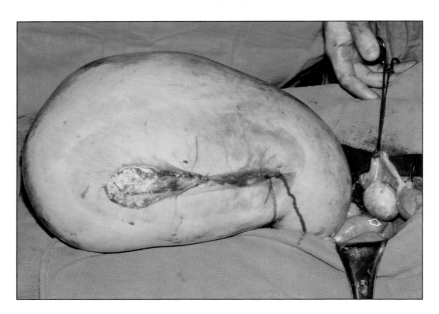

PLATE 40

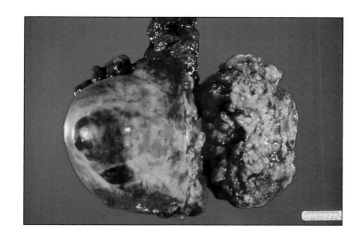

PLATE 41

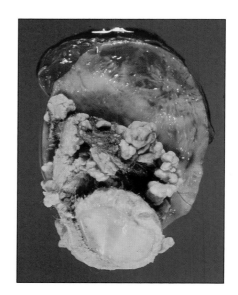

PLATE 42

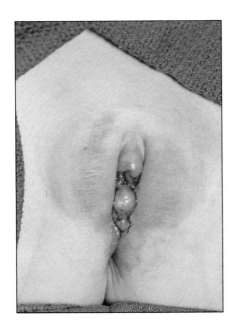

PLATE 43

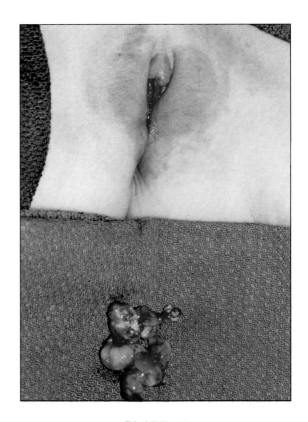

PLATE 44

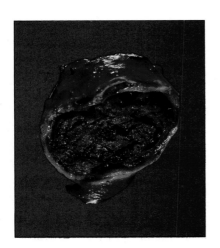

PLATE 45

9

Peritoneal and Extraperitoneal Soft Tissue Neoplasms

Thomas W. Koonce, M.D.

Ali Shirkhoda, M.D.

PERITONEUM

The peritoneum is a thin, glistening sheet of mesenchymally derived cells that lines the abdominal cavity. It is divided into the parietal peritoneum, which lines the walls of the abdominal cavity, and the visceral peritoneum, which covers the intraabdominal organs. The peritoneum participates in a fluid balance within the abdomen, acting both as a secretory and absorptive surface.[1] Additionally, this membranous layer has the capacity to undergo metaplastic changes, forming papillary projections, pseudoacini, squamous nests,[2] and cartilaginous nodules.[3]

Imaging of the peritoneum prior to the advent of computed tomography (CT), ultrasound, and magnetic resonance imaging (MRI) was limited to conventional radiography of the abdomen and various barium examinations of the bowel. These examinations revealed the secondary effects of tumors arising from within the peritoneum, including changes typical of serosal tumor implantation, fixation of small bowel loops secondary to mesenteric involvement, and bowel displacement secondary to the mass effect of a primary tumor. All of these changes

are nonspecific and can be seen with either a primary peritoneal lesion or metastatic tumor implanted within the peritoneum. The sectional imaging modalities, in addition to imaging the secondary effects of the tumor, can more effectively image the primary tumor itself. These modalities have, therefore, become the mainstay of peritoneal tumor detection and follow-up. Further, because of the development of scanning utilizing radiolabeled monoclonal antibodies, nuclear medicine is now emerging in the diagnosis of metastatic disease.[4]

Peritoneal Mesothelioma

Mesothelioma, a rare neoplasm, is by far the most common primary tumor of the peritoneum. In fact, some authors list mesothelioma as the only primary malignant tumor of the peritoneum.[5] It arises from mesenchymally derived cells of the peritoneum, pericardium, or pleura.[6, 7] When present in the abdomen, it is commonly seen in association with pleural mesothelioma or other asbestos-related diseases. There is a high incidence of mesotheliomas among asbestos miners.[8, 9]

The abdomen is the primary site of mesothelioma in 12% to 20% of cases.[8] The peritoneal tumors are associated with a longer and heavier asbestos exposure than tumors of the pleura.[10] There are both malignant and benign forms of mesothelioma. At presentation, the former are typically seen as multiple plaques spreading along the peritoneal surface (Fig 9–1), occasionally with retroperitoneal adenopathy (Fig 9–2). However, the benign variety is usually seen as focal mass.

The CT and sonographic findings in 23 reported cases of peritoneal mesothelioma are summarized in Table 9–1.[11–13] The radiographic findings in this tumor are not specific; they are also seen in diffuse abdominal carcinomatosis, mesothelioma's radiographic homologue. However, there are some findings that can lead one to suspect malignant mesothelioma rather than abdominal carcinomatosis should that distinction be the primary diagnostic consideration. In peritoneal mesothelioma, conventional chest radiography shows changes associated with asbestos exposure in approximately 45% of cases.[13] Computed tomography can increase this percentage by detecting disease not appreciated on the chest radiographs.[12, 13] The volume of ascitic fluid seen in peritoneal mesothelioma tends to be less than that expected for the same degree of peritoneal involvement with abdominal carcinomatosis.[13] Another important sign demonstrated primarily by CT is mesenteric involvement. The CT appearance of mesenteric involvement with mesothelioma has been described as stratified, stellate, or woven (Fig 9–1). Occasionally, with contrast-enhanced CT, the tumor will show a significant degree of enhancement (Figs 9–1 and 9–2). Mesenteric involvement is common with mesothelioma, present in 10 of 12 cases so assessed (Table 9–1), whereas it was seen in only 1 of 27 cases of abdominal carcinomatosis in Levitt et al.'s report.[14] Therefore, the diagnosis of abdominal mesothelioma should be suggested if historical exclusion of other known primary malignancies, particularly ovarian carcinoma, is coupled with some or all of the previously described radiographic signs.

Peritoneal Carcinomatosis

Peritoneal carcinomatosis may occur secondary to direct peritoneal seeding or through hematogenous dissemination by almost any primary lesion. The pathologic, and thus radiologic appearance is extremely variable (Figs 9–3 to 9–8); however, some generalities about tumor types and patterns of spread can be made.

It has been shown that when intraperitoneal seeding occurs, tumor cells follow the normal flow of ascitic fluid, with implantation most likely in dependent areas of pooling.[15] Consequently, there are certain locations that have a greater propensity for involvement, including the pelvis, particularly the pouch of Douglas (50%); the right lower quadrant at the junction of the small bowel mesentery and the mesentery for the ascending colon (40%); the cephalad border of the sigmoid colon (20%); and the right paracolic gutter (20%).[16] Other areas commonly involved are the omentum and the diaphragm, secondary to their functioning as large absorptive surfaces within the abdomen. The site of primary malignancy that most commonly leads to peritoneal seeding in females is the ovary (Figs 9–4,C–D, and 9–6,A); and in males, it is the gastrointestinal tract (Figs 9–3 and 9–4).[17]

One entity, pseudomyxoma peritonei, deserves special attention. It is a form of carcinomatosis in which in addition to the metastatic deposits there is a large amount of mucinous material found in the peritoneal cavity. It is most commonly associated

TABLE 9–1.

Findings by Computed Tomography and Ultrasonography in Peritoneal Mesothelioma

Study	Total No. of Patients	No. of Patients Examined by		Normal Scan	Ascites	Peritoneal Involvement	Mesenteric Involvement	Pleural Involvement
		CT	US*					
Reuter et al.[13]	4	4	4	0/4	4/4	3/4	4/4	3/4
Whitley et al.[12]	8	8	NS†	1/8	7/8	7/8	6/8	4/8
Yeh and Chahinian[11]	11	4	11	0/11	11/11	11/11	NS	NS
TOTAL	23	16	15	1/23	22/23	21/23	10/12	7/12

*US = ultrasound.
†NS = not studied.

with malignant tumors of the ovary and appendix, but rarely it may be seen with tumors of the stomach, urachus, or omphalomesenteric duct.[18, 19] Pseudomyxoma peritonei should not be confused with the benign condition that occurs secondary to intraperitoneal rupture of a cystadenoma of the ovary or appendix.[20] At gross inspection of the abdomen or on CT examination, the findings in these two entities are identical; however, microscopically, there are no malignant cells in the benign, self-limited disease.

The mucinous material in pseudomyxoma peritonei may be free, or it may exist in multiple well-circumscribed nodules or as circumscribed collections. The degree to which any case expresses one or both of these findings determines its radiographic appearance.[21] In the latter, less common presentation, CT shows multiple well-defined, thin-walled nodules with centers of low attenuation (5–20 Hounsfield units) (Fig 9–4,A–B).[22] The findings may be seen with other diseases, the most common differential being multiple pancreatic pseudocysts. However, in the context of typical clinical findings, CT is relatively specific and should lead to a correct diagnosis of pseudomyxoma peritonei.

The more common presentation of free mucinous material with or without demonstrable nodules (Fig 9–4,C–D) may be mistaken for ascitic fluid. Two diagnostically helpful signs found in pseudomyxoma peritonei are (1) scalloping of the liver surface due to serosal implants and (2) septations within the fluid. Scalloping is extremely rare in uncomplicated ascites but is common in pseudomyxoma. However, the latter finding, septations within the fluid, is somewhat less specific; it is seen in several other entities,[23] including complicated ascites. In a recent MRI report of pseudomyxoma peritonei, the signal characteristics of the myxomatous material were deemed different from those of the fluids in pseudocysts or ascites.[24] Thus, MRI may prove in the future to be helpful in the differential diagnosis of these entities.

Hematogenous metastasis presents a somewhat different radiographic appearance than intraperitoneal seeding and, in general, is seen with a different group of neoplasms. A common source is melanoma, which can present as implantation and growth on the serosal surface of the bowel, as submucosal bowel mass (typically on the antimesenteric side), or as metastatic deposits on the parietal peritoneum, the mesentery, or the omentum (Fig 9–5).[14, 25] The melanoma deposits range in number from single to multiple and in size from microscopic to several centimeters. Submucosal melanoma me-

tastases may ulcerate; not only melanoma but Kaposi's sarcoma and lymphoma have a particular propensity for early ulceration and often present as a bull's-eye lesion on a gastrointestinal barium examination. Occasionally, such a metastasis—either submucosal, serosal, or mesenteric—will become large, ulcerate, and communicate with the bowel lumen, so that a large ulcerated mass is seen. Besides melanoma, other primaries (Fig 9–6) commonly metastasizing to the peritoneum hematogenously are breast, lung, and lymphoma. Some consider lymphoma a diffuse multisystem disease, thus not a hematogenously spread entity. When lymphoma involves the peritoneum, it can occur in plaques, spreading along and covering the peritoneal surface. However, this presentation of lymphoma in the abdomen is rare; it most commonly presents in the nodes or the bowel wall.

Statistically, any lesion of the peritoneum should first be considered to represent metastasis. The pattern of spread and the radiologic appearance of the lesion, coupled with a knowledge of the statistical prevalences of the various neoplasms in the different age groups, can be helpful in defining a primary or suggesting a likely differential. This determination can then be used to plan the logical steps of a patient's workup.

RETROPERITONEUM

The retroperitoneum is one of the most challenging areas of the body in terms of clinical, radiologic, and pathologic diagnosis. The variety of neoplasms found here is large, but the overall incidence of any specific neoplasm is very low. These circumstances make it difficult to accumulate a sufficient number of cases to develop reliable statistics. The problem is compounded by the fact that, in general, neoplasms of the retroperitoneum are hard to classify histologically, which leads to disagreement with regard to diagnosis. Sectional imaging allows direct visualization of the retroperitoneum and retroperitoneal structures, thus providing valuable information about tumor location, size, and at times even histology.

Tumors of the major organs of the retroperitoneum (kidneys, adrenal glands, pancreas, great vessels) as well as those of the retroperitoneal portions of the colon and duodenum have been excluded here from the category of retroperitoneal neoplasms.[26] Additionally, primary neoplasms of the retroperitoneal lymph nodes are excluded from this chapter because they are discussed in Chapter 11. The pediatric retroperitoneal neoplasms such as neuroblastoma, ganglioneuroblastoma, ganglioblastoma, rhabdomyosarcoma, and teratoma are described in Chapter 8.

This chapter first examines the major adult malignant retroperitoneal primaries: liposarcoma, malignant fibrous histiocytoma, and leiomyosarcoma. The less common primaries—hemangiopericytoma, extragonadal germ cell neoplasms, neurogenic tumors, and Ewing's sarcoma, chondrosarcoma, and osteosarcoma in the soft tissues—are also illustrated and discussed, as are metastases to the retroperitoneum.

Before a discussion of the tumors that occur within the retroperitoneum can be undertaken, the boundary of this space must be defined. Most agree on its superior border, the diaphragm, and on its anterior border, the posterior parietal peritoneum. Meyers defines the posterior retroperitoneal border as the transverse fascia, allowing a clear and definite margin.[16] Inferiorly, the pelvic brim is considered to separate the retroperitoneum from the pelvis. We shall consider the levator muscles of the pelvic diaphragm as the inferior border of the extraperitoneal space. Laterally, the retroperitoneal margin lacks fascial demarcation. Anatomically, from the posterior pararenal space deep to the transverse fascia, the retroperitoneum potentially communicates with the properitoneal fat. Occasionally, a retroperitoneal tumor will spread into properitoneal fat and present itself as an abdominal wall mass.

A variety of tissues are found within the retroperitoneum. The two most common are loose areolar connective tissue and fat; however, vascular bundles, muscles, nerves, and embryonic rests (particularly of urogenital origin) are also found. Each of these can contribute its own neoplastic variants, which accounts for the large variety of malignant lesions seen (Table 9–2). The absolute incidence of retroperitoneal tumors is small, ranging between 0.1%[27] and 0.5%[29] of all malignancies. Most texts consider liposarcoma followed by leiomyosarcoma as the two most common primaries.[27] However, malignant fibrous histiocytoma may rival them in frequency. In a recent review of 138 patients with a primary retroperitoneal malignant neoplasm seen at M. D. Anderson Hospital, these three were of nearly equal frequency (Table 9–3). The higher frequency of malignant fibrous histiocytoma in this series compared with the older literature reflects a new awareness of and interest in this relatively newly defined pathologic entity.[30, 31]

Overall, tumors of the retroperitoneum have malignant characteristics in 50% to 80% of cases.[32] Additionally, in general, a tumor located in the retroperitoneum will behave more aggressively than the same tumor located elsewhere. This is true even for a benign neoplasm that has apparently been completely excised from this space; there is an increased incidence of recurrence, as well as a tendency for that recurrence to undergo malignant change.[32] Occasionally, benign conditions such as retroperitoneal fibrosis can mimic a malignant neoplasm (Fig 9–9) or adenopathy.[33] Retroperitoneal fibrosis, which in most cases is idiopathic, can result from the consumption of certain types of drugs (e.g., methysergide) or from a leaking aneurysm. At

TABLE 9–2.

Malignant Primary Tumors of the Retroperitoneum*

I. Tumors of mesodermal origin
   Liposarcoma
   Leiomyosarcoma
   Malignant fibrous histiocytoma
   Rhabdomyosarcoma
   Fibrosarcoma
   Vascular tumors: angiosarcoma, lymphangiosarcoma, hemangiopericytoma (B/M)†
   Tumors of mixed type
   Undifferentiated malignant type
II. Tumors of neurogenic origin
   Malignant schwannoma
   Neurofibrosarcoma
   Neuroblastoma, ganglioneuroblastoma (B/M)
   Extraadrenal pheochromocytoma (B/M)
   Paraganglioneuroma (nonsecreting)
   Chemodectoma
   Extraspinal ependymoma
III. Tumors of embryonic remnants
   Seminoma
   Embryonic carcinoma
   Yolk sac tumors
   Choriocarcinoma
   Teratoma (B/M)
   Teratocarcinoma
   Chordoma
   Ectopic ovarian malignant tumors
IV. Miscellaneous tumors
   Carcinoma of heterotopic cortical adrenal tissue
   Tumor with cartilage or bone
   Synoviosarcoma
   Extraskeletal Ewing's sarcoma
   Mesothelioma
   Alveolar soft tissue sarcoma

*Adapted from Rosai J.: *Ackerman's Surgical Pathology*, ed 6. St. Louis, C.V. Mosby Co., 1981, vol. 2; and Reagan M.T., Clowry L.J., Cox J.D., et al.: Radiation therapy in the treatment of malignant fibrous histiocytoma. *Int. J. Radiat. Oncol. Biol. Phys.* 7:311–315, 1981.[28]
†B/M = benign or malignant.

TABLE 9–3.

Tumor Type in 138 Patients With Primary Malignant Tumor of the Retroperitoneum at M. D. Anderson Hospital, 1 January 1981 to 31 August 1984*

Tumor Type	No. of Patients
Liposarcoma	24
Leiomyosarcoma	24
Fibrohistiocytoma	22
Neuroblastoma	15
Unclassified sarcoma	11
Seminoma, pure	8
Unclassified malignant neoplasm	7
Neurofibroma	4
Fibrosarcoma, desmoid	4
Hemangiopericytoma, malignant	3
Malignant embryonal teratoma	3
Ganglioneuroblastoma	3
Nonchromaffin paraganglioma	2
Extragenital choriocarcinoma	2
Embryonal rhabdomyosarcoma	1
Extraskeletal Ewing's sarcoma	1
Adenosquamous carcinoma	1
Embryonal carcinoma	1
Undifferentiated lymphoma, diffuse	1
Embryoma	1
TOTAL	138

*Patient population identified by the Department of Patient Studies, The University of Texas M. D. Anderson Hospital and Tumor Institute, Houston.

TABLE 9–4.

Signs and Symptoms in Patients With Retroperitoneal Masses

I. Vascular[35–38]
  Lower extremity swelling and/or phlebitis
  Pulmonary embolism secondary to thrombosis of inferior vena cava or iliac veins
  Ipsilateral varicocele
  Hemorrhoids
II. Urologic[39]
  Hydronephrosis and flank pain
  Urinary frequency, urgency, and hematuria
  Anuria or uremia
III. Neurologic[40, 41]
  Motor or sphincter changes secondary to involvement of the lumbosacral plexus or spinal cord
  Sympathetic nervous system involvement causing peripheral temperature and sudation differences in the legs
IV. Gastrointestinal[26, 35]
  Hematemesis
  Hematochezia
  Fistula formation
  Obstruction
  Portal hypertension with caput medusae, bleeding, and ascites
  Budd-Chiari syndrome
V. Pulmonary
  Dyspnea secondary to mass effect on the diaphragm
  Hemoptysis secondary to parenchymal metastases
VI. Gynecologic[36]
  Menorrhagia
  Dyspareunia
VII. Endocrine[39, 42]
  Hypertension or sudden death with extraadrenal excreting pheochromocytoma
  Hypoglycemia secondary to an unknown mechanism seen in some mesenchymal tumors; thought to be mediated through an insulinlike substance
  Hypoglycemia seen in some sarcomas
  Gynecomastia and hypoglycemia reported in a case of paraganglioma
VIII. Hemorrhagic[37, 39]
  Acute abdominal pain
  Tenderness
  Hypotension and shock
IX. Other, nonspecific symptoms
  Fever
  Weight loss
  Backache
  Malaise and fatigue

discovery, neoplasms of the retroperitoneum are often quite large.

Not only is the retroperitoneum inaccessible to physical examination, but most retroperitoneal neoplasms produce few early symptoms. When present, symptoms are often vague and nonspecific, sometimes progressing insidiously over months to years. The most common symptom is abdominal pain, and the most common finding is a palpable mass.[27, 34] Many of the signs and symptoms (Table 9–4) are the result of involvement of adjacent structures either by pressure or direct invasion. An exception to the paucity of early symptoms exists in the small group of hormonally active retroperitoneal neoplasms (e.g., secreting paragangliomas). These neoplasms often produce early and relatively specific symptomatology.

Because of these problems with physical examination and symptomatology, diagnostic imaging is the mainstay of detection and follow-up in retroperitoneal masses. A wide variety of imaging procedures can and have been used to evaluate the retroperitoneum, including intravenous pyelography, ultrasonography, angiography, inferior venacavography, upper and lower gastrointestinal studies, CT, and, most recently, MRI. Each of these studies has its place in the evaluation of certain tumor types and in certain anatomical locations. However, of the studies available today, CT appears to be the best choice.

Computed tomography has achieved 100% sensitivity in visualization of retroperitoneal tumors in some series.[34, 43] In certain tumors, mainly fatty or vascular neoplasms, it not only localizes the lesion but to a certain degree also characterizes the tissues.[43] In addition to imaging the primary mass, CT also provides a view of the major intraabdominal organs, particularly the liver, allowing an assessment for distant metastasis. Although the use of MRI in the retroperitoneum is now being assessed, this modality is more expensive than CT and has not yet proved to be more effective. Computed tomography should still be the initial imaging study in a patient with a suspected retroperitoneal mass. Once the information from this examination is obtained, it can be used to dictate which, if any, additional studies are needed.

Liposarcoma

Liposarcoma (Figs 9–10 to 9–16) is reported to be the most common primary tumor of the retroperitoneum.[44] However, the increased awareness and diagnosis of malignant fibrous histiocytoma, which has led to the reclassification of some pleomorphic liposarcomas, may alter these statistics.

Liposarcoma is primarily a tumor of later adult life. In two large series, the median age was in the sixth decade.[45, 46] Cases of liposarcoma in children have been reported, but such a diagnosis should be viewed with suspicion.[45] When these tumors occur in young patients, they tend to behave less aggressively than those of adults.

Outside of the retroperitoneum, the most common site of liposarcoma is the thigh. However, there are interesting differences between these two sites. First, a comparison between the two sites shows a difference of ten years in the average patient age at presentation, with retroperitoneal liposarcomas presenting later. Second, there is an appreciable difference in tumor size, with those of the retroperitoneum being larger. Third, the histologic subtypes of liposarcoma show strong site specificity.

Cases of liposarcoma vary widely in histopathologic structure and clinical activity. Several classifications have been proposed to subdivide liposarcoma. In 1962, Enzinger and Winslow identified and defined four subgroups: well-differentiated (Fig 9–10), pleomorphic (Figs 9–11 and 9–16),[45] myxoid (Fig 9–12), and round cell. The round cell was later reclassified by Evans[46] and a dedifferentiated variety was described (Figs 9–13 to 9–15). The well-differentiated and myxoid subgroups occur mostly in the limbs and yield significantly longer survival times than the pleomorphic and dedifferentiated varieties, which are seen commonly in the retroperitoneum. In Enzinger and Winslow's series, the approximate survival time for a patient with liposarcoma in the retroperitoneum was four years, whereas the patients with a thigh primary survived for an average of nine years.[45]

As previously mentioned, there is a strong correlation between a tumor's histologic subgroup and its clinical activity. This relationship is also shown in the frequency of a tumor's recurrence, its mode of spread, and patient survival time. Following surgery, the well-differentiated and myxoid subgroups recur locally (Fig 9–12) in approximately 50% of cases. When they metastasize (particularly the myxoid variety), there is a propensity to involve the soft tissues, especially in the retroperitoneum. The pleomorphic and dedifferentiated subgroups, on the other hand, behave more aggressively (Figs 9–14 to 9–16). They have a higher incidence of local recurrence and metastasize most commonly to the lungs.

As in most retroperitoneal neoplasms, imaging of retroperitoneal liposarcoma is best done with CT.[43] Ultrasound will show an increased echo pattern in fatty lesions, but it lacks CT's specificity in fat. In large lesions, CT's ability to define all the borders and to develop a picture of the tumor's overall appearance is superior to that of ultrasound.[47, 48] The role of MRI in the imaging of these lesions is under study; some current reports have demonstrated MRI's ability to image and characterize lipomatous lesions.

The CT appearance can at times be specific enough in liposarcoma to challenge and correct a previous histologic diagnosis. Different CT patterns have been described in this tumor, including the solid pattern, the mixed pattern, the pseudocystic pattern, and, finally, the lipomalike liposarcoma. It has even been suggested that the various histologic subgroups could be identified by the CT appearance.[44]

Other fat-containing lesions seen in the retroperitoneum include lipoma (Fig 9–17), angiolipoma, teratoma, lipoplastic lymphadenopathy, dermoid, myelolipoma, angiomyelolipoma, and xanthogranulomatous pyelonephritis. Each of these should be considered in the differential diagnosis of a fatty lesion in the retroperitoneum. However, most can be correctly identified by their tissue of origin, patient age at presentation, and CT or MRI appearance.

In liposarcoma, the radiologist can be particularly helpful in tumor margin identification and thus in preoperative planning. For the surgeon at the operating table and for the pathologist assessing the surgical specimen, tumors with well-differentiated fatty components present particular problems in defining a tumor margin. This is demonstrated in Figure 9–12, a case in which the surgeon failed to recognize the more mature fatty component of the lesion as tumor; therefore, he removed only the more cellular portion, which had exhibited high attenuation on CT. Similarly, in the case Figure 9–13 illustrates, the pathologist before viewing the CT scans considered the open biopsy material as malignant fibrous histiocytoma with normal surrounding fat. The CT findings allowed recognition of the extent of the lesion, and the diagnosis was revised to dedifferentiated liposarcoma with malignant fibrous histiocytoma component. These two cases demonstrate how the radiologist can provide a valuable service not only in the detection of a liposarcoma but also in its diagnosis and the planning of its removal.

Malignant Fibrous Histiocytoma

Malignant fibrous histiocytoma is one of the most commonly occurring sarcomas of middle to late adult life. Since its description in 1964,[49] the number of reported cases has steadily increased. These tumors are found most commonly in the lower extremities (49%), upper extremities (19%), retroperitoneum (16%),[31] and pelvis (Figs 9–18 to 9–21). They are presumed to be of mesenchymal origin; therefore, malignant fibrous histiocytoma has the potential of occurring in any location. Cases have been reported in the lung,[50] kidney,[51] scrotum,[52] vas deferens,[53] heart,[54] aorta,[55] stomach,[56] small intestine,[57] orbit,[58] central nervous system,[59] dura mater,[60] paranasal sinus, nasal cavity, oral cavity, nasopharynx, and soft tissues of the neck.[61]

Malignant fibrous histiocytoma occurs more often in men than in women, at a ratio of as high as 2:1.[30] It may occur at any age but is reported most commonly in individuals over the age of 40. Because of the frequency of the lesion in the older age groups, it has been suggested that any primary malignant tumor found in the soft tissues of an individual 45 years of age or older is most likely malignant fibrous histiocytoma.

This tumor has a highly variable morphological growth pattern that may be described as storiform,

pleomorphic, or fascicular. However, unlike in liposarcoma, subtyping by histologic pattern has not as yet proved to be of clinical value. At times, differentiation between pleomorphic liposarcoma and malignant fibrous histiocytoma can be exceptionally difficult because their pleomorphic histologic patterns are very similar.[31] Additional confusion in the separation of these two tumors occurs because some liposarcomas will dedifferentiate, with sections developing into malignant fibrous histiocytoma.[46]

The prognosis of a patient with a malignant fibrous histiocytoma is related to the location and size of the tumor at the time of diagnosis. When the lesion is found in the retroperitoneum, the prognosis is particularly ominous, with a four-year survival rate of 14%. In Weiss and Enzinger's series of 200 cases (at multiple sites),[31] local recurrence was seen in 44% and metastasis occurred in 42%. The most common site of metastasis was the lung (82%). Metastasis, although relatively common during the clinical course, appears to be a late manifestation. In only one of Weiss and Enzinger's 200 cases did the patient present with metastasis prior to documentation of the primary tumor.

Radiographic manifestations of malignant fibrous histiocytoma include soft tissue masses, usually larger than 5 cm in diameter[31] and, occasionally, peripheral calcifications detected by conventional radiography and by CT. Dorfman and Bhagavan found a mineralized matrix in the pseudocapsule or in the peripheral fibrous septa in cases in which peripheral calcification occurred, the findings so prominent in four of the cases that they considered the possibility of myositis ossificans.[62] On CT examination, regions of low density, presumably secondary to necrosis, are not uncommon (Fig 9–21). In a series of 37 patients reported by Ros et al., areas of low attenuation were identified in 55% of the tumors.[63] It is important to note that a statement concerning previous treatment history was not made in either of the above two series. Our experience and that of others at M. D. Anderson Hospital is that without previous treatment calcification is unusual and that low attenuation within the mass occurs in far fewer than 50% of the cases. Weiss and Enzinger's pathologic series reported hemorrhage with cystic areas (Fig 9–20) in approximately 5% of the cases.[31]

Leiomyosarcoma

Leiomyosarcoma is a malignant tumor of smooth muscle. When these tumors occur in the retroperitoneum, the exact anatomical site of origin is often not established. They are thought to arise from the smooth muscle cells of the blood vessels,[51] the spermatic cord, or the embryonic remnants of the wolffian and müllerian ducts. They can occur in the gastrointestinal tract,[64] kidney,[65] and genitourinary tract,[66, 67] among many other places. The reported incidence of leiomyosarcoma varies, ranging between 11% and 15% of all retroperitoneal malignancies.[68]

The clinical behavior of this tumor is difficult to define. In part this is due to the tumor's relative infrequency and the difficulty of predicting leiomyosarcoma's clinical activity based on its histologic appearance.[51, 64, 69] Prognosis depends on the location of the neoplasm. For example, when the primary site is in the retroperitoneum, the two-year survival is 16%, compared with a 40% survival when the primary lesion is in the stomach.[70, 71] Metastasis is most commonly hematogenous and to the lungs and liver; however, metastases to soft tissues, bone,[67, 70, 72] spleen,[72] lymph nodes, omentum, and mesentery have all been reported.[73] Imaging retroperitoneal leiomyosarcomas is similar to imaging other soft tissue primaries, with CT being the most rewarding approach.

The tumor's usual CT appearance of a low-attenuation area (Fig 9–22) correlates with the pathologic finding of a high incidence of central necrosis. This finding is seen not only in the primary lesions but also in their metastases.[71] When seen, the necrosis can be helpful in differentiating this tumor from other large retroperitoneal masses. Unfortunately, like most findings in radiology (and particularly in the retroperitoneum), this is far from being pathognomonic. Displacement of the small and large bowel on barium studies is very commonly seen (Figs 9–23 and 9–24).

Hemangiopericytoma

Hemangiopericytoma, first described by Stout and Murray in 1942 as a tumor of pericytes,[74] can arise anywhere the capillaries are present. The retroperitoneum has a particularly high incidence of these lesions; approximately one fourth of all hemangiopericytomas occur here.[75, 76] The neoplasm can be either malignant or benign, although histologically this differentiation is often very difficult.[75] Metastatic rates vary from 11% to 20%, and local recurrence rates as high as 50% have been reported.[77] The metastases are mainly hematogenous, to the bones, lungs, and liver. Less frequently, the regional nodes are involved.[75] Five-year survival approxi-

mates 50%; however, it is less when the neoplasm is in the retroperitoneum, where complete excision is often impossible.[78]

These tumors are almost always solitary and are highly vascular at angiography (Fig 9–25).[79] On CT scan, they are seen as a well-defined soft tissue mass that can enhance if bolus contrast material is delivered.

Extragonadal Germ Cell Tumors

Extragonadal germ cell tumors are exceedingly rare. Some authors have questioned the existence of these tumors based on well-documented reports of spontaneous regression of testicular primaries with continued growth of the tumors' metastatic deposits.[80] They believe that the metastatic deposits are misinterpreted as primary lesions. Other reports strongly support the existence of extragonadal germ cell primaries.[81]

A review of 19 cases reported from M. D. Anderson Hospital in 1973 showed all the common histologic types of intragonadal primaries to be found outside the gonads as well (seminoma, choriocarcinoma, malignant teratoma, embryonal carcinoma), and 8 of the 19 occurred in the retroperitoneum.[81]

These tumors may be very large or of smaller size and can display areas of cystic changes (Fig 9–26) on CT scan. The primary tumor could occur in an undescended testis (Fig 9–27); in these cases, the descended testis also has a higher incidence of tumor occurrence.

Neurogenic Tumors

Neurogenic tumors, excluding those of childhood (neuroblastoma, ganglioneuroblastoma, ganglioneuroma), account for only a small percentage of retroperitoneal tumors. They include neurilemomas (Fig 9–28), neurofibromas (Fig 9–29), malignant schwannomas, chordomas, and both chromaffin and nonchromaffin paragangliomas (Figs 9–30 to 9–32).

Neurilemoma is one of the truly encapsulated neoplasms of the body.[27] It occurs most commonly on the flexor surfaces of the extremities and in the head and neck and has almost no malignant potential. Most neurilemomas are well-defined solid tumors, but they often develop cystic areas when they become large (Fig 9–28). The usual cell of origin is Schwann's cell.

Neurofibroma, like neurilemoma, has its origin in Schwann's cells; however, its gross, microscopic, and ultrastructural appearances, as well as its clinical activity, are quite different from those of neurilemoma.[82] Neurofibromas can be solitary (Fig 9–29) or multiple, the latter being known as neurofibromatosis.[83] When neurofibromas grow large and result in diffuse tortuous enlargement of the peripheral nerves, they are then designated as plexiform neurofibromas.[27] Neurofibromas, unlike neurilemomas, have a potential to undergo malignant change to malignant schwannomas.

Malignant schwannomas are thought to be the malignant counterparts of neurofibroma. They may arise from a solitary neurofibroma or in association with von Recklinghausen's disease (neurofibromatosis).[84–86] They may have very slow growth rates but tend to entail a poor prognosis; there are high rates of local recurrence and of distant metastasis, particularly when the primary is located in the retroperitoneum.[85]

Chordoma, a tumor from a remnant of the primitive notochord, most commonly occurs in the sacrum or clivus, but in 5% to 10% of cases it arises from the lumbar or lower thoracic area and can present in the retroperitoneum.[32]

Paraganglioma is a tumor of the neuroepithelial cells that are scattered throughout the body.[87] The largest collection of these cells is in the adrenal medulla. The extraadrenal paragangliomas can be divided into two large groups: the chromaffin (Fig 9–31), associated with clinical evidence of norepinephrine or epinephrine secretions (or both), and the nonchromaffin (Fig 9–30), which are essentially nonfunctioning.[27] They are occasionally multiple (Fig 9–32). Most of the nonchromaffin paragangliomas are found in the head and neck, whereas the chromaffin paragangliomas are most common in the thoracolumbar and paraaortic regions.[88–93] Rarely, a nonchromaffin paraganglioma will present as a retroperitoneal mass. A 1986 review of the English literature showed only 14 reported cases of malignant paraganglioma that occurred in the retroperitoneum.[87]

One rare tumor is extraspinal, extracranial ependymoma, which occurs mostly in the soft tissue, either in the subcutaneous tissue over the coccyx or in the retrorectal space or the broad ligament. When these tumors are in the sacrococcygeal area, they are thought to arise from the extradural filum terminale or the ependymal rests. Those arising at other locations belong to a category of monodermal teratoma. The extracranial ependymomas do metastasize (Fig 9–33), but the length of survival is relatively long.[94]

Extraskeletal Soft Tissue Sarcoma

Ewing's Sarcoma

Extraskeletal Ewing's sarcoma is found in subcutaneous tissue of the trunk and limbs, in the retroperitoneum, in the pelvis, and in paravertebral regions. Pathologically, it cannot be differentiated from the osseous Ewing's sarcoma. The tumor is equally distributed between both sexes and appears ten years later than the osseous type. It metastasizes to the lungs and occasionally to the bones.[95] The primary neoplasm presents as a soft tissue mass (Fig 9–34), which may display areas of necrosis on CT. Occasionally, the tumor infiltrates into the adjacent soft tissue and organs.

Chondrosarcoma

Extraskeletal chondrosarcoma is a rare neoplasm that arises from the soft tissue of the extremities, shoulders, buttocks, and, rarely, pelvis and abdomen. It is unrelated to synovium, cartilage, bone, or tendon sheaths, occurs between the ages of 40 and 70 years, and is less aggressive than the osseous type.[96] It may display areas of calcification but in some cases is seen only as a large soft tissue mass (Fig 9–35) without calcified cartilage. Histologically, extraskeletal chondrosarcoma resembles osseous chondrosarcoma.

Osteosarcoma

Extraskeletal osteosarcoma is an extremely rare tumor that occurs in the lower and upper extremities, trunk, retroperitoneum, and head and neck. The mean age of occurrence is 53 years. Excluded from this entity are the parosteal type and osteosarcoma arising in kidney, breast, or lung.[97] Careful radiologic study is needed to rule out continuity of tumor with bone. Computed tomography and angiography are helpful in revealing the extent, the vascularity, and sometimes the origin of the tumor. Typically, a soft tissue mass with areas of spotty calcification is seen (Fig 9–36) in a patient who has normal liver values but an elevated alkaline phosphatase value.[98] Histologically, extraskeletal osteosarcoma is similar to osseous osteosarcoma, but its five-year survival rate is only 15.6%.

Metastasis to the Retroperitoneum

Metastases in the retroperitoneum are most commonly seen in the lymph nodes. There are very few specific findings that might suggest an organ of origin for metastasis in the retroperitoneum, but germ cell neoplasms of the testis (Figs 9–37 and 9–38) and melanoma (Fig 9–39) deserve special mention.

The lymph drainage of the testis is along the course of the gonadal vein. Thus, the first nodes involved with metastasis are not pelvic but paraaortic: on the left at the level of the renal hilus and on the right at approximately the L-2 to L-3 level. Therefore, in a male patient between 15 and 35 years of age, if large lymph nodes are seen in these areas without other adenopathy or mass, metastatic testicular cancer should be the primary diagnosis. An exception to this lymph drainage pattern occurs when a testicular primary invades the epididymis or when the scrotum is contaminated by invasion or biopsy. In these circumstances, either the pelvic or paraaortic nodes can be the first group of nodes metastatically involved.

Melanoma is another tumor in which a primary diagnosis may be suggested by the pattern of metastasis to the retroperitoneum. When melanoma disseminates, it can involve almost any structure, but in the retroperitoneum it commonly involves the soft tissues, particularly the fat. The metastatic deposits appear as multiple, round soft tissue masses scattered within the retroperitoneal fat.[99] This appearance is somewhat unusual in other tumors and is very suggestive of melanoma.

Also it has been our experience that retroperitoneal nodal metastasis from squamous cell carcinoma (e.g., from the cervix) has a tendency to erode the adjacent bone and act aggressively (Fig 4–29). Aside from these tumors, however, the other lesions that metastasize to the retroperitoneum yield few if any specific radiologic findings.

REFERENCES

1. Robbins S.L.: *Pathologic Basis of Disease.* Philadelphia, W.B. Saunders Co., 1974, p. 980.
2. Crome L.: Squamous metaplasia of the peritoneum. *J. Pathol. Bacteriol.* 62:61–68, 1950.
3. Rosai J.: *Ackerman's Surgical Pathology,* ed. 6. St. Louis, C.V. Mosby Co., 1981, vol. 2, pp. 1482–1483.
4. Engelstad B.L., Spitler L.E., Del Rio M.J., et al.: Phase I immunolymphoscintigraphy with an In-111-labeled antimelanoma monoclonal antibody. *Radiology* 161:419–422, 1986.
5. Moertel C.G.: Peritoneal mesothelioma: current clinical concepts. *Gastroenterology* 63:346–350, 1973.
6. Brenner J., Sordillo P.P., Magill G.B., et al.: Malignant mesothelioma of the pleura: review of 123 patients. *Cancer* 49:2431–2435, 1982.
7. Lerner H.J., Schoenfield D.A., Martin A., et al.: Malignant mesothelioma: the Eastern Cooperative Oncology Group (ECOG) experience. *Cancer* 52:1981–1985, 1985.
8. Wagner J.C., Sleggs C.A., Marchand P.: Diffuse pleural mesothelioma and asbestos exposure in the North Western Cape Province. *Br. J. Ind. Med.* 17:260–271, 1960.
9. Selikoff I.J., Churg J., Hammond E.C.: Relation between exposure to asbestos and mesothelioma. *N. Engl. J. Med.* 272:560–565, 1965.
10. Newhouse M.L., Thompson H.: Mesothelioma of pleura and peritoneum following exposure to asbestos in the London area. *Br. J. Ind. Med.* 22:261–269, 1965.
11. Yeh H.C., Chahinian A.P.: Ultrasonography and computed tomography of peritoneal mesothelioma. *Radiology* 135:705–712, 1980.
12. Whitley N.O., Brenner D.E., Antman K.H., et al.: CT of peritoneal mesothelioma: analysis of eight cases. *AJR* 138:531–535, 1982.
13. Reuter K., Raptopoulos V., Reale F., et al.: Diagnosis of peritoneal mesothelioma: computed tomography, sonography, and fine-needle aspiration biopsy. *AJR* 140:1189–1194, 1983.
14. Levitt R.G., Sagel S.S., Stanley R.J.: Detection of neoplastic involvement of the mesentery and omentum by computed tomography. *AJR* 131:835–838, 1978.
15. Meyers M.A.: Distribution of intra-abdominal malignant seeding: dependency on dynamics of flow of ascitic fluid. *AJR* 119:195–206, 1973.
16. Meyers M.A.: *Dynamic Radiology of the Abdomen: Normal and Pathologic Anatomy,* ed. 2. St. Louis, C.V. Mosby Co., 1981.
17. Buie L.A., Jackman R.J., Vickers P.M.: Extrarectal masses caused by tumors of the recto-uterine or retrovesical space. *JAMA* 117:167–169, 1941.
18. Fernandez R.N., Daly J.M.: Pseudomyxoma peritonei. *Arch. Surg.* 115:409–414, 1980.
19. Limber G.K., King R.E., Silverberg S.G.: Pseudomyxoma peritonei: a report of ten cases. *Ann. Surg.* 178:587–593, 1973.
20. Higa E., Rosai J., Pizzimbone C.A., et al.: Mucosal hyperplasia, mucinous cystadenoma, and mucinous cystadenocarcinoma of the appendix. *Cancer* 32:1525–1541, 1973.
21. Novetsky G.J., Berlin L., Epstein A.J., et al.: Case report. Pseudomyxoma peritonei. *J. Comput. Assist. Tomogr.* 6:398–399, 1982.
22. Rao M.S., Watanabe I.: Pseudomyxoma peritonei: report of an unusual case. *Oncology* 32:21–26, 1975.
23. Seshul M.D., Coulam C.M.: Pseudomyxoma peritonei: computed tomography and sonography. *AJR* 136:803–806, 1981.
24. Weigert F., Lindner P., Rohde U.: Computed tomography and magnetic resonance of pseudomyxoma peritonei. *J. Comput. Assist. Tomogr.* 9:1120–1122, 1985.

25. Goldstein H.M., Beydoum M.R., Dodd G.D.: Radiologic spectrum of melanoma metastatic to the gastrointestinal tract. *AJR* 129:605–612, 1977.

26. Bose B.: Primary malignant retroperitoneal tumours: analysis of 30 cases. *Can. J. Surg.* 22:215–220, 1979.

27. Rosai J.: *Ackerman's Surgical Pathology,* ed. 6. St. Louis, C.V. Mosby Co., 1981, vol. 2.

28. Reagan M.T., Clowry L.J., Cox J.D., et al.: Radiation therapy in the treatment of malignant fibrous histiocytoma. *Int. J. Radiat. Oncol. Biol. Phys.* 7:311–315, 1981.

29. Gullino D., Merlo G.: Anatomia e pathologia tumorale dello spazio sotto-peritoneale. *Minerva Chir.* 15:1061–1080, 1960.

30. Kearney M.M., Soule E.H., Ivins J.C.: Malignant fibrous histiocytoma: a retrospective study of 167 cases. *Cancer* 45:167–178, 1980.

31. Weiss S.W., Enzinger F.M.: Malignant fibrous histiocytoma. An analysis of 200 cases. *Cancer* 41:2250–2266, 1978.

32. Johnson A.H., Searls H.H., Grimes O.F.: Primary retroperitoneal tumors. *Am. J. Surg.* 88:155–161, 1954.

33. Brun B., Laursen K., Sorensen I.N., et al.: CT in retroperitoneal fibrosis. *AJR* 137:535–538, 1981.

34. Kairalouma M.I., Krause-Makitalo B., Pokela R., et al.: Primary retroperitoneal tumours in adults. *Ann. Chir. Gynecol.* 73:313–318, 1984.

35. Duncan R.E., Evans A.T.: Diagnosis of primary retroperitoneal tumors. *J. Urol.* 117:19–23, 1977.

36. Hill E.C.: Retroperitoneal tumors in gynecology. *Am. J. Obstet. Gynecol.* 82:1243–1251, 1961.

37. Filler R.M., Harris S.H., Edwards E.A.: Characteristics of the inferior-cava venogram in retroperitoneal cancer. *N. Engl. J. Med.* 266:1194–1197, 1962.

38. Schoen U.: Budd-Chiari-Syndrom bei retroperitonealem Neurinom. *Dtsch. Med. Wochenschr.* 97:335, 1972.

39. Fouty W.J., Sacher E.C., Cronemiller P.D., et al.: Rare retroperitoneal tumors presenting as acute abdominal conditions requiring operation. *J. Int. Coll. Surg.* 42:233–239, 1964.

40. Wetzel N., Arieff A., Tuncbay E.: Retroperitoneal, lumbar and pelvic malignancies simulating the disc syndrome. *Arch. Surg.* 86:1069, 1961.

41. Brown R.C., Maisey D.N., Day J.L.: Unilateral lumbar sympathectomy due to retroperitoneal tumour (short report). *Br. Med. J. (Clin. Res.)* 1:410, 1978.

42. Dell'Acqua G.B., Sensi S.: Paraneoplastisches endokrines Syndrom bei einem retroperitonealen Paraganglion. *Munch. Med. Wochenschr.* 115:1171–1174, 1973.

43. Pistolesi G.F., Procacci C., Caudana R., et al.: C.T. criteria of the differential diagnosis in primary retroperitoneal masses. *Eur. J. Radiol.* 4:127–138, 1984.

44. Friedman A.C., Hartman D.S., Sherman J., et al.: Computed tomography of abdominal fatty masses. *Radiology* 139:415–429, 1981.

45. Enzinger F.M., Winslow D.J.: Liposarcoma. A study of 103 cases. *Virchows Arch. Pathol. Anat.* 335:367–388, 1962.

46. Evans H.L.: Liposarcoma. A study of 55 cases with a reassessment of its classifications. *Am. J. Surg. Pathol.* 3:507–523, 1979.

47. Cohen W.N., Seidelkmann F.E., Bryan P.J.: Computed tomography of localized adipose deposits presenting as tumor masses. *AJR* 128:1007–1011, 1977.

48. Hunter J.C., Johnston W.H., Genant H.K.: Computed tomography evaluation of fatty tumors of the somatic soft tissues: clinical utility and radiologic-pathologic correlation. *Skeletal Radiol.* 4:79–91, 1979.

49. O'Brien J.E., Stout A.P.: Malignant fibrous xanthomas. *Cancer* 17:1445–1458, 1964.

50. Ozzello C., Stout A.P., Murray A.R.: Cultural characteristics of malignant histiocytomas and fibrous xanthomas. *Cancer* 16:331–334, 1963.

51. Hashimoto H., Tsuneyoshi M., Enjoji M.: Malignant smooth muscle tumors of the retroperitoneum and mesentery: a clinicopathologic analysis of 44 cases. *J. Surg. Oncol.* 28:177–186, 1985.

52. Meares E.M. Jr., Kempson R.L.: Fibrous histiocytoma of the scrotum in an infant. *J. Urol.* 110:130–132, 1973.

53. Farah R.N., Bohne A.W.: Malignant fibrous histiocytoma of spermatic cord. *Urology* 3:782–783, 1974.

54. Shah A.A., Chure A., Sbarbaro J.A., et al.: Malignant fibrous histiocytoma of the heart presented as an atrial myxoma. *Cancer* 42:2466–2471, 1978.

55. Chen K.T.K.: Primary malignant fibrous histiocytoma of the aorta. *Cancer* 48:840–841, 1981.

56. Balfe D.M., Koehler R.E., Karstaedt N., et al.: Computed tomography of gastric neoplasms. *Radiology* 140:431–436, 1981.

57. Sewell R., Levine B.A., Harrison G.K., et al.: Primary malignant fibrous histiocytoma of the intestine: intussusception of a rare neoplasm. *Dis. Colon Rectum* 23:198–201, 1980.

58. Font R.L., Hidayat A.A.: Fibrous histiocytoma of the orbit. A clinicopathologic study of 150 cases. *Hum. Pathol.* 13:199–209, 1982.

59. Gonzalez-Vitale J., Slavin R.E., McQueen J.D.: Radiation-induced intracranial malignant fibrohistiocytoma. *Cancer* 37:2960–2963, 1976.

60. Lam R.M., Colah S.A.: Atypical fibrous histiocytoma with myxoid stroma: a rare tumor lesion arising from dura mater of the brain. *Cancer* 43:237–245, 1979.

61. Blitzer A., Lawson W., Bille H.F.: Malignant fibrous histiocytoma of the head and neck. *Laryngoscope* 87:1477–1499, 1977.

62. Dorfman H.D., Bhagavan B.S.: Malignant fibrous histiocytoma of soft tissue with metaplastic bone and cartilage formation: a new radiologic sign. *Skeletal Radiol.* 8:145–150, 1982.

63. Ros P.R., Viamonte M. Jr., Rywlin A.M.: Malignant fibrous histiocytoma: mesenchymal tumor of ubiquitous origin. *AJR* 142:753–759, 1984.

64. Akinari O.E., Dozoris R.R., Weiland L.H.: Leiomyosarcoma of the small and large bowel. *Cancer* 42:1375–1384, 1978.

65. Shirkhoda A., Lewis E.: Sarcoma and sarcomatoid renal cell carcinoma of the kidneys: CT and angiographic features. *Radiology* 162:353–357, 1987.

66. Bennington J.L., Beckwitz J.B.: Tumors of the kidney, renal pelvis and ureter, in *Atlas of Tumor Pathology.* Washington, D.C., Armed Forces Institute of Pathology, 1975, ser. 2, fasc. 12, p. 213.

67. Camuzz F.A., Block N.L., Charyulu K., et al.: Leiomyosarcoma of prostate gland. *Urology* 18:295–297, 1981.

68. Lofgren L.: Primary retroperitoneal tumours. A histopathological, clinical and follow-up study supplemented by follow-up study of a series from the Finnish Cancer Register. *Ann. Acad. Sci. Fenn.* (A) 129:5–86, 1967.

69. Wile A.G., Evans H.L., Romsdahl M.M.: Leiomyosarcoma of soft tissue: a clinicopathologic study. *Cancer* 48:1022–1032, 1981.

70. Kay S., McNeil D.D.: Leiomyosarcoma of retroperitoneum. *Surg. Gynecol. Obstet.* 129:285–288, 1969.

71. Nauert T.C., Zornoza J., Ordonez N.: Gastric leiomyosarcoma. *AJR* 139:291–297, 1982.

72. Christoffersen J.: Leiomyosarcoma of retroperitoneum. *Surg. Gynecol. Obstet.* 129:285–288, 1969.

73. Ackerman L.V.: Tumors of the retroperitoneum, mesentery and peritoneum, in *Atlas of Tumor Pathology.* Washington, D.C., Armed Forces Institute of Pathology, 1954, sect. 6, fasc. 23 and 24, p. 11.

74. Stout A.P., Murray M.R.: Hemangiopericytoma: a vascular tumor featuring Zimmermann's pericytes. *Ann. Surg.* 116–126, 1942.

75. Felix E.L., Wood D.K., Das Gupta T.K.: Tumors of the retroperitoneum. *Curr. Probl. Cancer* 6:1–47, 1981.

76. Enzinger F.M., Smith B.H.: Hemangiopericytoma. An analysis of 106 cases. *Hum. Pathol.* 7:61–82, 1976.

77. Backwinkel K.D., Diddams J.A.: Hemangiopericytoma. Report of a case and comprehensive review of the literature. *Cancer* 25:896–901, 1970.

78. O'Brien P., Brasfield R.D.: Hemangiopericytoma. *Cancer* 18:249–252, 1965.

79. Angarvall L., Kindblom L.G., Nielsen H.M., et al.: Hemangiopericytoma. A clinicopathologic, angiographic and microangiographic study. *Cancer* 42:2412–2427, 1978.

80. Prather L.J., Gardiner W.R., Frerichs J.B.: Regression and maturation of primary testicular tumors with progressive growth of metastases. A report of six new cases and a review of the literature. *Stanford Med. Bull.* 12:12, 1954.

81. Johnson D.E., Lanier J.P., Mountain C.F., et al.: Extragonadal germ cell tumors. *Surgery* 73:85–90, 1973.

82. Stout A.P.: Neurofibroma and neurilemoma. *Clin. Proc.* 5:1–12, 1946.

83. Crowe F.W., Schull W.J., Neel J.V.: A Clinical, Pathological, and Genetic Study of Multiple Neurofibromatosis. American Lecture Series, no. 281. Springfield, Ill., Charles C Thomas, Publisher, 1956.

84. D'Agostino A.N., Soule E.H., Miller R.H.: Sarcomas of the peripheral nerves and somatic soft tissues associated with multiple neurofibromatosis (von Recklinghausen's disease). *Cancer* 16:1015–1027, 1963.

85. White H.R. Jr.: Survival in malignant schwannoma. An 18-year study. *Cancer* 27:720–729, 1971.

86. Woodruff J.M.: Peripheral nerve tumors showing glandular differentiation (glandular schwannomas). *Cancer* 37:2399–2413, 1976.

87. Mikhail R.A., Moore J.B., Reed D.N., et al.: Malignant retroperitoneal paragangliomas. *J. Surg. Oncol.* 32:32–36, 1986.

88. Farr H.W.: Carotid body tumors. A 30 year experience at Memorial Hospital. *Am. J. Surg.* 114:614–619, 1967.

89. Glenn F., Gray G.F.: Functional tumors of the organ of Zuckerkandl. *Ann. Surg.* 9:578–585, 1976.

90. Olson J.R., Abell M.R.: Nonfunctional, nonchromaffin paragangliomas of the retroperitoneum. *Cancer* 23:1358–1367, 1969.

91. Smith W.T., Hughes B., Ermocilla R.: Chemodectoma of the pineal region, with observations of the pineal body and chemoreceptor tissue. *J. Pathol. Bacteriol.* 92:69–76, 1966.

92. Kepes J.J., Zacharias D.L.: Gangliocytic paragangliomas of the duodenum. Report of two cases with light and electron microscopy examination. *Cancer* 27:61–70, 1971.

93. Taylor H.B., Helwig E.B.: Benign nonchromaffin paragangliomas of the duodenum. *Virchows Arch. Pathol. Anat.* 335:356–366, 1962.

94. Bell D.A., Woodruff J.M., Scully R.E.: Ependymoma of the broad ligament. A report of two cases. *Am. J. Surg. Pathol.* 8:203–209, 1984.

95. Soule E.H., Newton W. Jr, Moon T.E., et al.: Extraskeletal Ewing's sarcoma: a preliminary review of 26 cases encountered in the Intergroup Rhabdomyosarcoma Study. *Cancer* 42:259–265, 1978.

96. Smith M.T., Farinacci C.J., Carpenter H.A.., et al.: Extraskeletal myxoid chondrosarcoma: a clinicopathological study. *Cancer* 37:821–827, 1976.

97. Rao U., Cheng A., Didolkar M.S.: Extraosseous osteogenic sarcoma: clinicopathological study of eight cases and review of literature. *Cancer* 41:1488–1496, 1978.

98. Das Gupta T.K., Hadju S.I., Foote F.W. Jr.: Extraosseous osteogenic sarcoma. *Ann. Surg.* 168:1011–1022, 1968.

99. Shirkhoda A.: Computed tomography of perirenal metastases. *J. Comput. Assist. Tomogr.* 10:435–438, 1986.

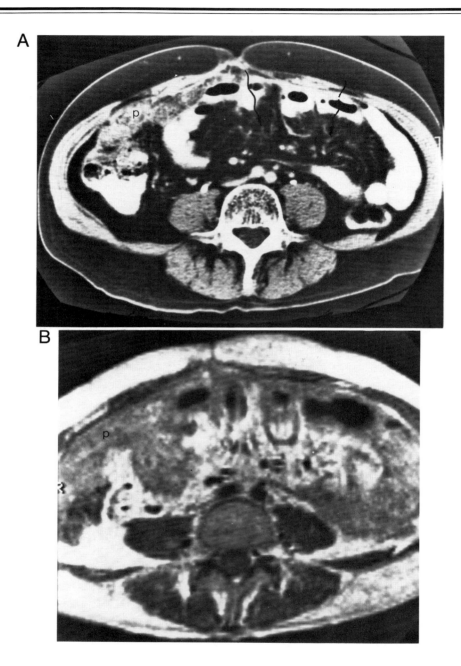

FIG 9–1.
Peritoneal mesothelioma (two cases).

A through **D,** a 54-year-old man with a two-year history of vague abdominal pain, intermittent fever, and nausea was admitted to his local hospital, where he underwent an extensive workup.

Lower abdominal CT and magnetic resonance images are paired (**A** with **C,** and **B** with **D**) for comparison. In the anterior peritoneum, there is plaquelike soft tissue density *(P)* with intermediate signal intensity on T$_2$-weighted magnetic resonance images. The stratified *(curved arrows)* and nodular *(open arrows)* areas probably represent neoplastic infiltrate within the mesenteric fat.

With a clinical diagnosis of cholelithiasis and chronic cholecystitis, the patient underwent cholecystectomy. At surgery, a diffuse, fibrotic chronic peritonitis with inflamed omentum and a mildly inflamed gallbladder were discovered. The surgeon also described the intraperitoneal organs as loosely adherent to each other. At pathology, the gallbladder showed stones and changes of chronic cholecystitis, and the omental biopsies revealed mesothelioma of the peritoneum. The patient was referred to M. D. Anderson Hospital for chemotherapy. *(Continued.)*

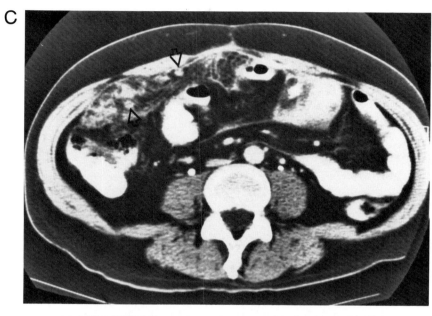

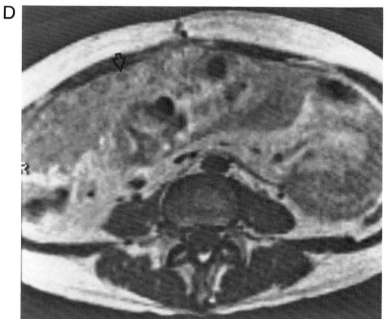

E

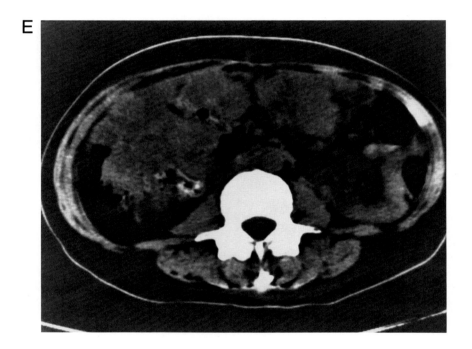

FIG 9–1 (cont.).
E and **F,** another patient, a 36-year-old woman with a one-year history of vague abdominal pain, was found to have a palpable mass in the right flank. Small bowel barium exam-ination showed displacement without invasion. Computed tomography scans before **(E)** and after **(F)** intravenous con-trast show a large, nonhomogeneous mass in the right

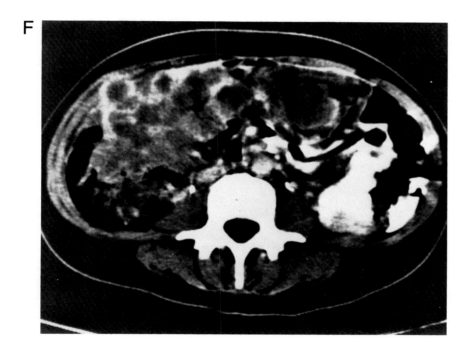

F

lower quadrant with significant enhancement. Laparotomy was done in the region of the tumor and revealed a mass involving the lymph nodes and spreading over almost the entire peritoneal cavity. The pathologic diagnosis of the open-biopsy specimen was consistent with sarcomatoid mesothelioma. The patient received chemotherapy, and her disease was under control at one-year follow-up.

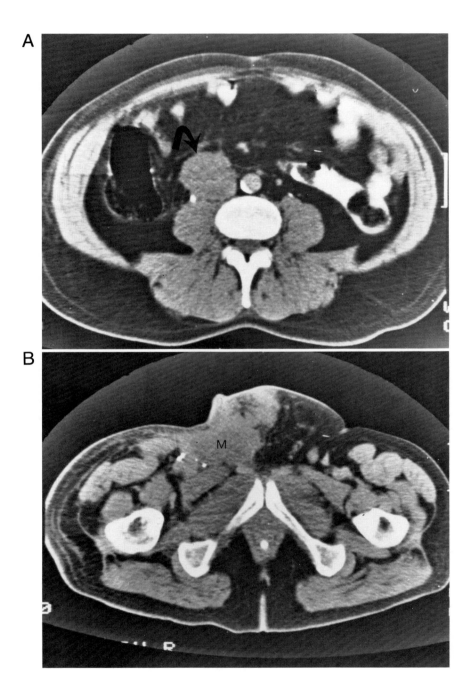

FIG 9–2.
Mesothelioma of tunica vaginalis. A 58-year-old man with right scrotal enlargement underwent a right inguinal orchiectomy. The pathologic diagnosis was mesothelioma of the tunica vaginalis testis. One month later, he underwent a right pelvic node and groin dissection with hemiscrotomy. In three months he presented with subcutaneous nodules and a mass. Biopsy of the latter proved recurrent mesothelioma, and the patient was referred to M. D. Anderson Hospital.

A and **B,** the CT scans at the time of recurrence show the patient's right groin area with the multiple tumor nodules *(M)* and retroperitoneal adenopathy *(curved arrow).*

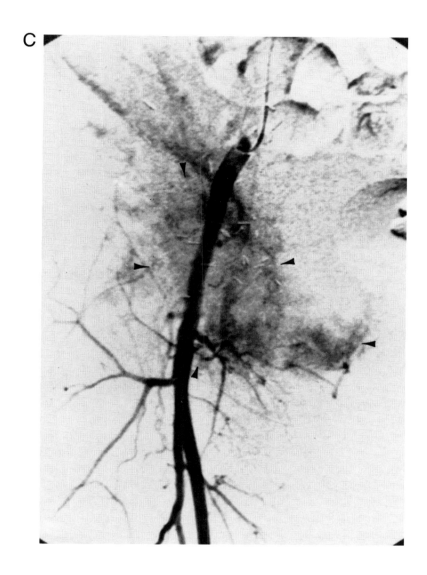

C, a common femoral artery angiogram shows tumor staining in the area of disease recurrence *(arrowheads)*. The catheter was left in this position for intraarterial chemo-therapy. Following one month of intraarterial treatment coupled with systemic chemotherapy, complete resolution of the tumor was seen. *(Continued.)*

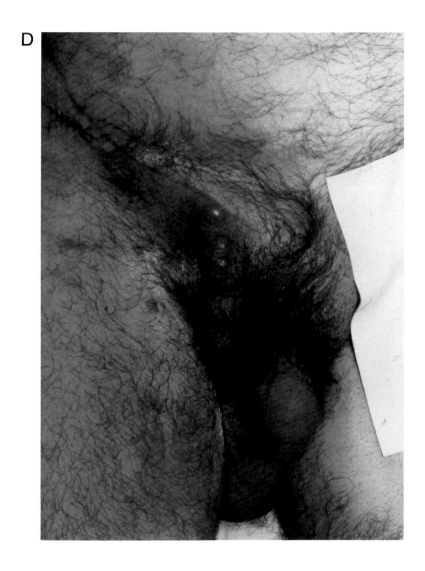

Fig 9-2 (cont.).
D and E, at the time of recurrence **(D),** inguinal masses are seen. Following a month of therapy **(E),** the complete disappearance of tumor nodules is seen.

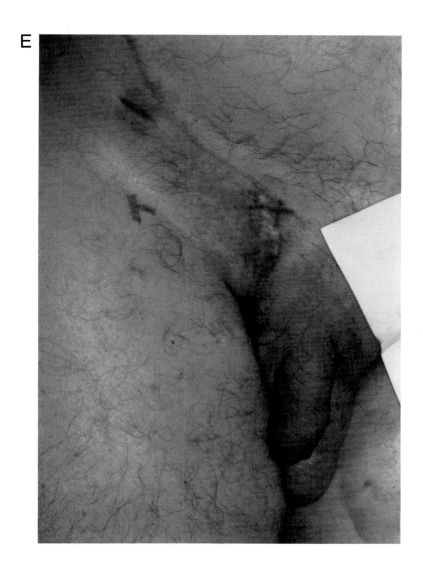

The response rate to chemotherapy in mesothelioma is very low. This case illustrates an exceptional response with combined intraarterial and systemic chemotherapy.

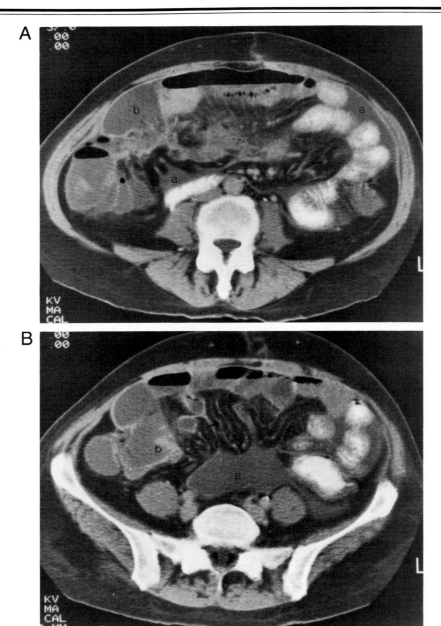

FIG 9–3.

Peritoneal carcinomatosis (two cases).

A and **B,** a 48-year-old man had colon resection for carcinoma. Two years later, ascites developed, and a CT scan was obtained.

These CT images through the abdomen and pelvis reveal multiple dilated loops of bowel *(b),* ascites *(a),* and peritoneal soft tissue striations *(straight arrows).* The patient subsequently died, and diffuse peritoneal carcinomatosis was found at autopsy.

This case demonstrates a stratified mesenteric appearance seen on CT in peritoneal carcinomatosis. This appearance is more frequent in peritoneal mesothelioma than in abdominal carcinomatosis; however, abdominal carcinoma-

tosis is by far the more frequent etiology of this CT observation because of its much higher overall incidence.

C and **D,** this patient with history of resected liposarcoma of the thigh underwent routine follow-up by CT study.

Pelvic CT images **(C)** show a well-defined mass *(arrow)* anterior to the left iliopsoas muscles. There was a questionable soft tissue density *(open arrows)* in the midpelvis. However, unopacified bowel loops were the other consideration.

T$_2$-weighted magnetic resonance image (TR/TE, 2,000/80) **(D)** shows both masses seen on CT to display high signal intensity. These were later proved to represent metastatic sarcoma. Areas of peritoneal metastasis are also seen *(arrows).*

C

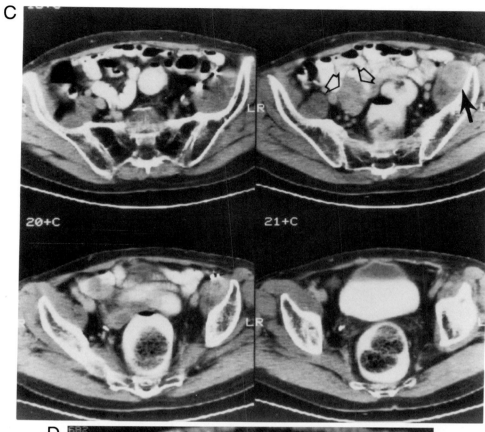

D

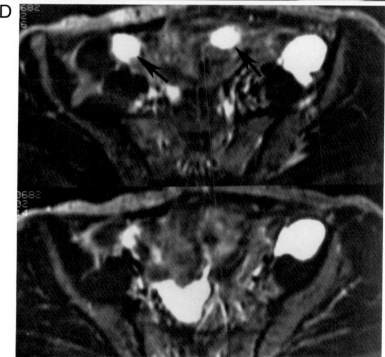

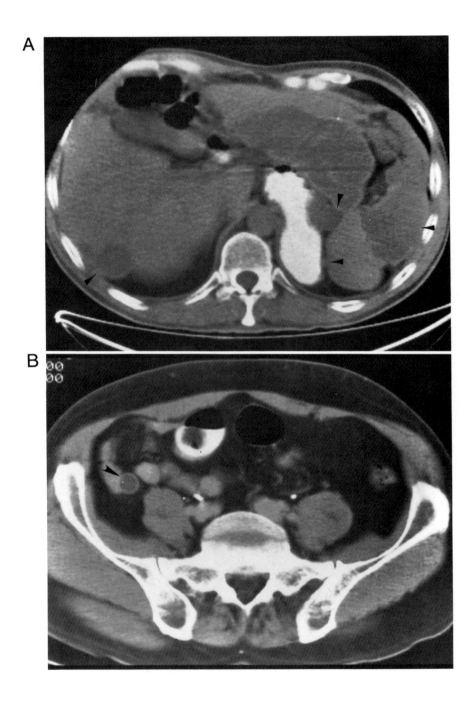

FIG 9–4.

Pseudomyxoma peritonei (two cases).

A and **B,** a 47-year-old man who had a mucinous adenocarcinoma of the appendix removed two years ago presented with abdominal distension and bloating. A CT examination was performed, followed by exploratory laparotomy.

The CT scans show multiple intraabdominal peritoneal implants appearing as thin-walled cystic structures with homogeneous low attenuation *(arrowheads).*

This multicystic appearance is a less common CT presentation of pseudomyxoma peritonei than the ascites-like appearance seen in **C** and **D.**

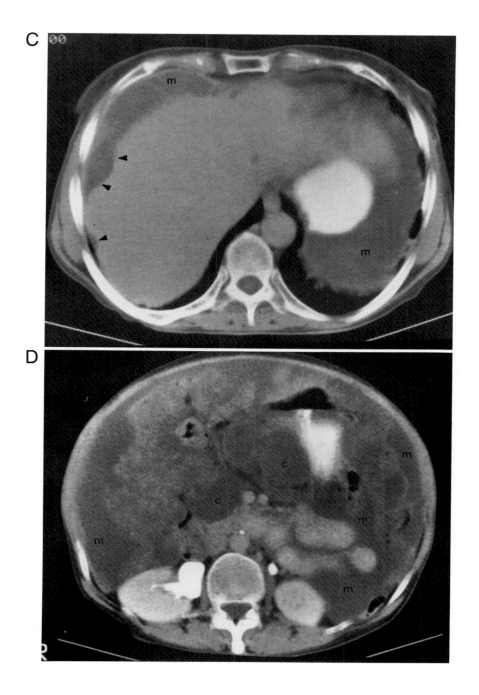

C and **D,** in another case, a 38-year-old woman with previous total abdominal hysterectomy and salpingo-oophorectomy for ovarian mucinous adenocarcinoma developed abdominal distension. The CT scans show scalloping *(arrowheads)* at the liver surface, intraperitoneal mucinous material *(m),* and cystic areas within the fluid *(c),* all consistent with the diagnosis of pseudomyxoma peritonei.

This second case demonstrates the more common appearance of pseudomyxoma peritonei, namely, a large amount of mucinous fluid within the abdomen. Hepatic scalloping is a helpful differential sign.

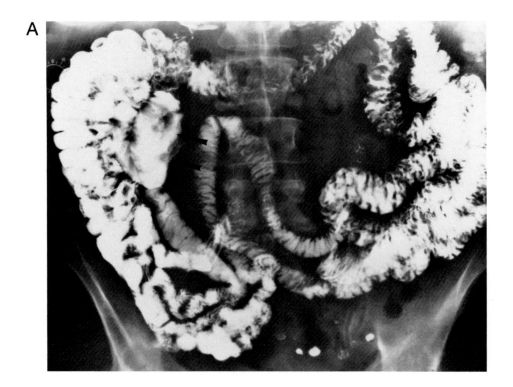

FIG 9–5.
Intraperitoneal metastases from melanoma (two cases). Both of these patients with a known history of melanoma presented with vague abdominal pain. One had blood in the stool, and the other had anemia.

A, a single radiograph from a small bowel study demonstrates a large ulcerated mass in the right side of the abdomen *(arrows)*. The large extraluminal barium collection in an ulcerated mass suggests a diagnosis of melanoma or leiomyosarcoma.

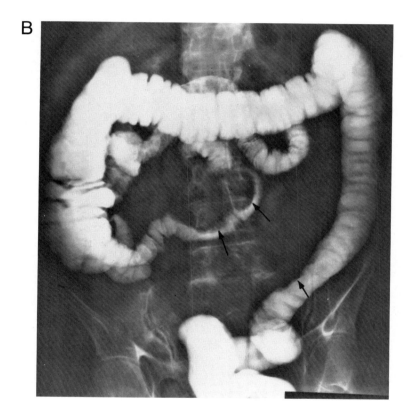

B, a film from a barium enema examination of another patient demonstrates several serosal metastatic implants *(arrows).*

The second film shows two of the common sites for tumor implantation and growth secondary to intraperitoneal seeding: the superior border of the sigmoid colon, and the junction of the small bowel mesentery and the cecum.

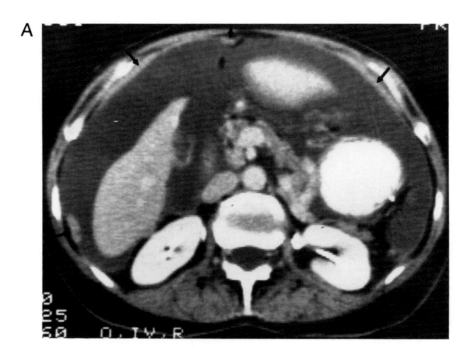

FIG 9–6.

Plaquelike peritoneal metastases and implants (multiple cases).

A, a 74-year-old woman with the diagnosis of left ovarian carcinoma and metastases to the sigmoid colon and omentum had a left salpingo-oophorectomy, partial sigmoidectomy, and total omentectomy. Three months after surgery, while receiving chemotherapy, she presented with loss of appetite, increasing abdominal girth, and problems with bowel movement. A CT scan shows diffuse peritoneal implants *(arrows)* and extensive ascites.

B, this 29-year-old woman presented with left hip pain and a 2.3-kg (5-lb) weight loss. The pain was originally attributed to a muscle pulled while playing tennis. Pelvic ex-

amination disclosed a mass. A CT scan reveals extensive tumor implantation along the peritoneum, with a large amount of ascites. Notice that there is no scalloping of the liver like that demonstrated in the pseudomyxoma peritonei. A limited laparotomy proved the diagnosis of soft tissue Ewing's sarcoma of the uterus metastatic to the omentum and peritoneal surface. The patient received chemotherapy and radiation therapy but died two years later.

C, this 35-year-old woman with previously diagnosed carcinoma of the colon presented with increasing abdominal girth. The transverse sonogram reveals multiple metastatic peritoneal implants *(arrows)* and a large amount of ascites. On other images, there were omental metastases.

B

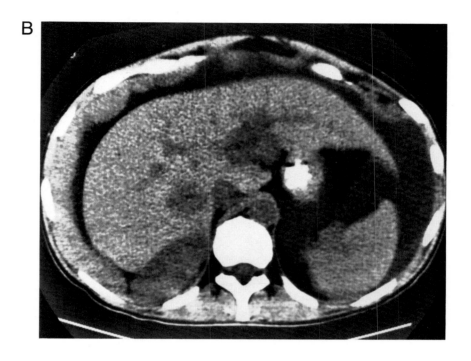

C

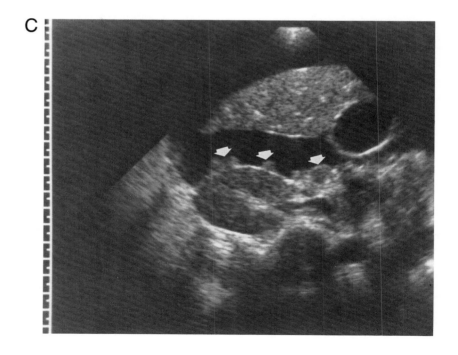

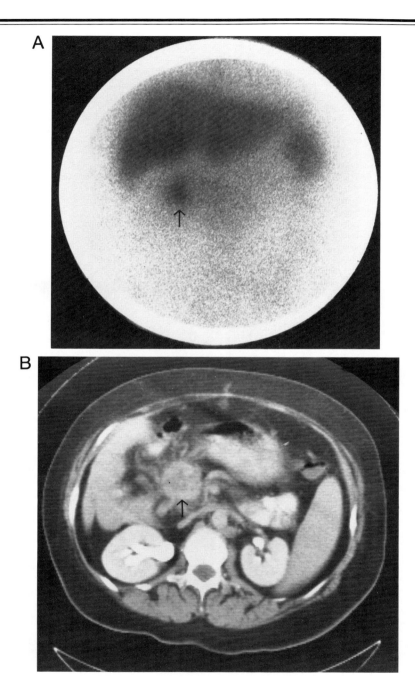

FIG 9–7.

Colon carcinoma metastatic to peritoneum. A 54-year-old woman with a history of colon carcinoma treated by surgery and chemotherapy presented with an elevated level of serum carcinoembryonic antigen (CEA). Nuclear imaging utilizing radiolabeled monoclonal antibody to colonic CEA was performed.

A, a film from monoclonal antibody imaging of the mid-abdomen shows normal uptake in the liver and spleen but an area of abnormal uptake projecting in the right flank *(ar-*

row).

B, a midabdominal CT image demonstrates that the abnormality seen on the monoclonal antibody study is an enlarged parapancreatic node *(arrow).* Biopsy of the node proved metastatic colon carcinoma.

This case demonstrates that monoclonal antibody imaging can be helpful in diagnosing metastatic disease. The technique as it improves is becoming an important part of patient evaluation.

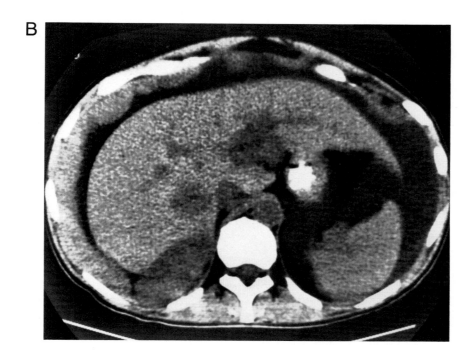

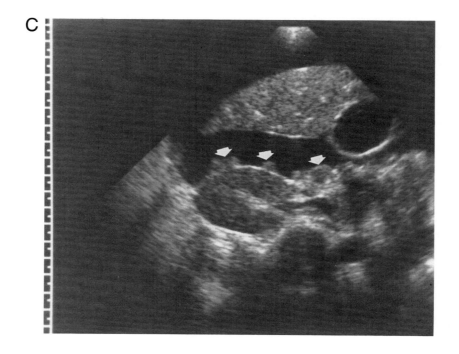

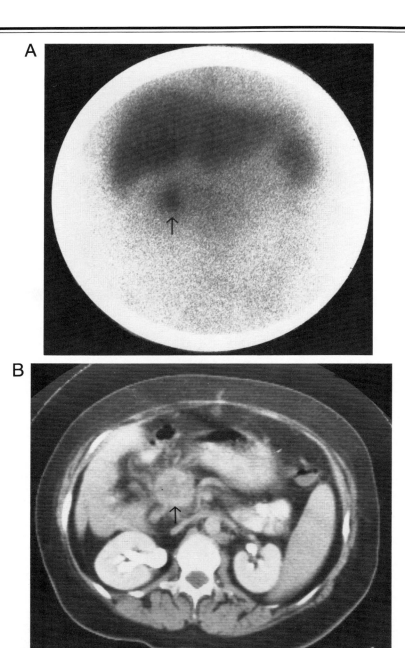

FIG 9–7.
Colon carcinoma metastatic to peritoneum. A 54-year-old woman with a history of colon carcinoma treated by surgery and chemotherapy presented with an elevated level of serum carcinoembryonic antigen (CEA). Nuclear imaging utilizing radiolabeled monoclonal antibody to colonic CEA was performed.

A, a film from monoclonal antibody imaging of the mid-abdomen shows normal uptake in the liver and spleen but an area of abnormal uptake projecting in the right flank *(ar-*

row).

B, a midabdominal CT image demonstrates that the abnormality seen on the monoclonal antibody study is an enlarged parapancreatic node *(arrow).* Biopsy of the node proved metastatic colon carcinoma.

This case demonstrates that monoclonal antibody imaging can be helpful in diagnosing metastatic disease. The technique as it improves is becoming an important part of patient evaluation.

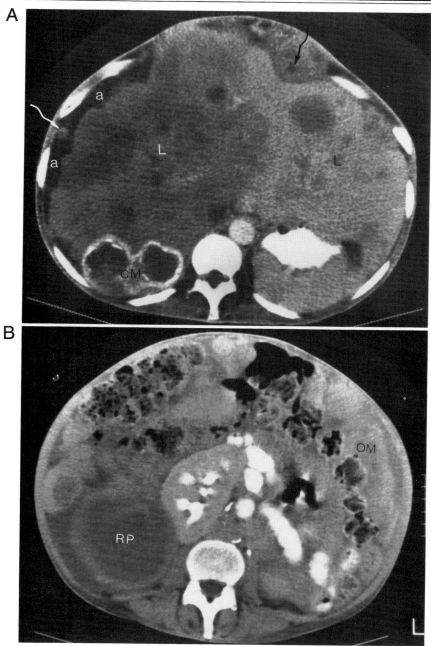

FIG 9–8.
Adenocystic carcinoma of the palate metastatic to peritoneum.

A 44-year-old woman had a right maxillectomy 12 years ago for adenocystic carcinoma of the submucosal soft tissues of the palate. She remained disease free until she presented with an abdominal mass.

A and **B,** computed tomographic images through the abdomen show peritoneal implants *(curved arrows)*, liver metastases *(L)*, ascites *(a)*, and calcified *(CM)* and cystic *(RP)* retroperitoneal metastases. The right kidney is displaced, and there are also serosal and omental tumor implants *(OM)*.

An exploratory laparotomy was performed, and the patient was found to have diffuse abdominal carcinomatosis with hepatic metastasis. The pathology was metastatic adenocystic carcinoma. This case demonstrates that almost any primary tumor can metastasize to the peritoneum or retroperitoneum. A history of a prior tumor must never be overlooked when a differential for an abdominal mass is being developed.

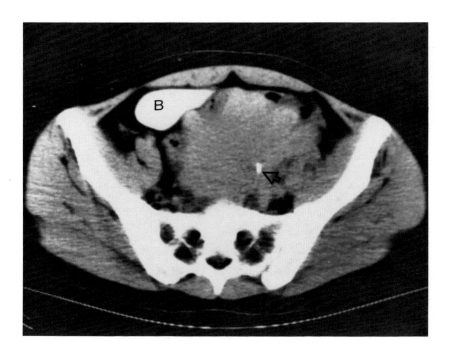

FIG 9–9.
Retroperitoneal fibrosis. This 32-year-old man presented with left flank pain, and intravenous urography showed left distal ureteral obstruction, bladder deviation, and left hydronephrosis.

The CT scan shows a large mass with irregular borders. The mass infiltrates between the bladder *(B)* and distal left ureter *(arrow);* it extended superiorly to the level of the aortic bifurcation.

Percutaneous needle biopsy was nondiagnostic and open biopsy was performed. The tumor was found to be densely sclerotic tissue surrounding the left ureter and involving the colon, with adhesion of mesentery and bowel. Because the tumor was inoperable, a colostomy was done. The biopsy results were consistent with retroperitoneal fibrosis.

A

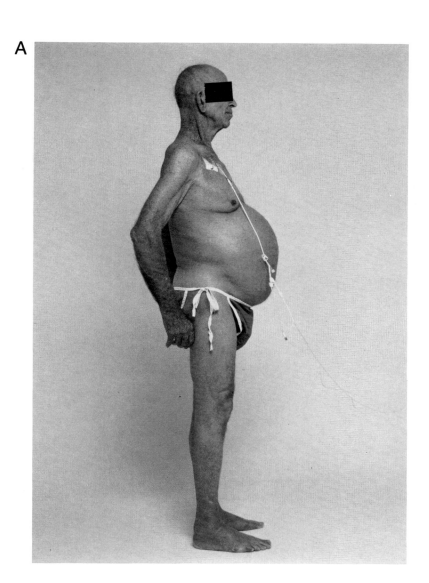

FIG 9–10.
Well-differentiated liposarcoma. A 64-year-old man presented complaining of early satiety. On questioning, the patient revealed a 13.6-kg (30-lb) weight loss and increasing abdominal girth over the last 18 months. Physical examination revealed a 20 × 15 cm mobile mass in the midabdomen. An upper gastrointestinal and barium enema examination demonstrated bowel displacement without signs of invasion.

A, the lateral view of the patient shows a very large abdomen (see also Color Plate 46). *(Continued.)*

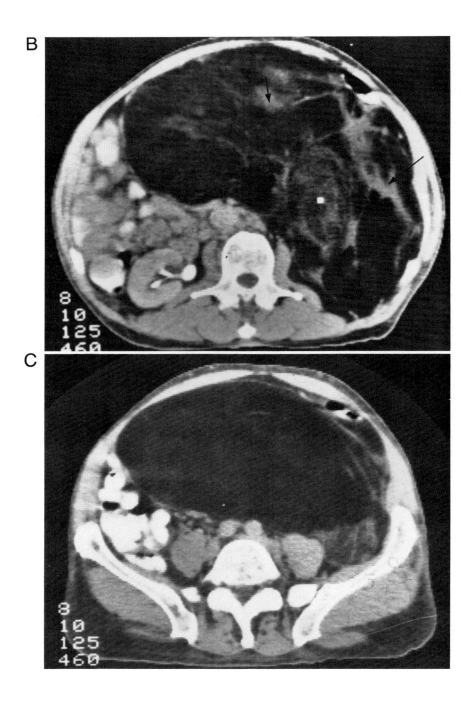

FIG 9–10 (cont.).
B and **C,** these CT scans through the midabdomen **(B)** and upper pelvis **(C)** show the large, predominantly fatty tumor with internal irregular areas of higher-density tissue *(arrows).* Needle biopsy suggested well-differentiated liposarcoma.

D

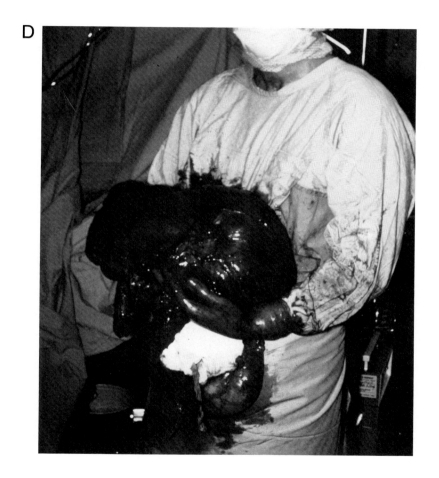

D, at surgery, a 42 × 37 × 30 cm nonencapsulated fatty mass was discovered and excised (see also Color Plate 47).

Postoperatively, the patient did well and at latest follow-up was two years out from his operation without evidence of disease.

This case shows how large a retroperitoneal soft tissue tumor, such as a liposarcoma, can become prior to any significant symptomatology. The CT findings in this case—a large, mainly fatty tumor with internal high densities—are rather classic for well-differentiated liposarcoma.

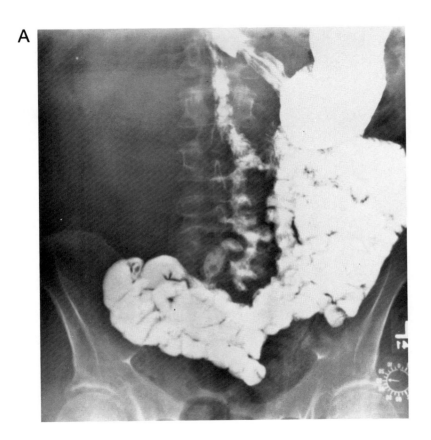

A

FIG 9–11.
Well-differentiated and pleomorphic liposarcoma. A 54-year-old man presented complaining of right flank pain. Physical examination revealed a palpable right abdominal mass.

A, a film from gastrointestinal barium study shows dis-placement of the bowel, with the second portion of the duo-denum being displaced to the midline. The visualized por-tions of the jejunum and ileum are also displaced to the left and inferiorly. There is no evidence of tumor invasion of the bowel.

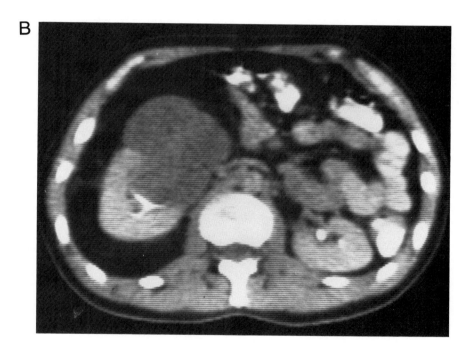

B, axial CT image through the midpole of the kidneys shows two different abnormal soft tissue densities in the right side of the abdomen. The one in the right renal hilus is almost of muscle density; the other, which surrounds the kidney, is completely of fat density. Note elevation of the right kidney with respect to the left by the fatty component of the tumor.

At surgery, a 22 × 13 × 15 cm retroperitoneal mass was removed. It was surrounded by a thin, fibrous capsule and had two histologic components. The first, which made up most of the tumor, was a very well differentiated liposarcoma. The second, more pleomorphic component corresponded to the central areas in the renal hilus. The tumor was seen to infiltrate to or originate in the fat of the renal pelvis and capsule but did not invade the renal parenchyma or ureter.

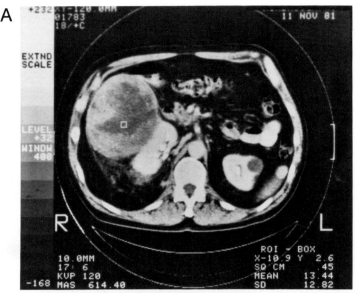

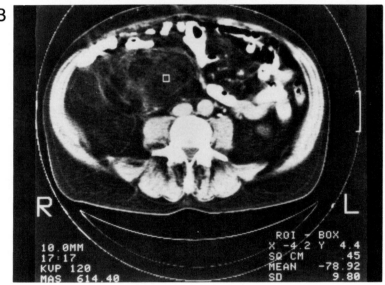

FIG 9–12.
Myxoid and well-differentiated liposarcoma. This 76-year-old man had experienced gradual-onset malaise over two years. He underwent a CT examination of the abdomen. Barium gastrointestinal studies from one year ago reportedly were normal.

A and **B,** a biphasic mass is seen on the CT images. The lower portion of the mass (−78 Hounsfield units) is near normal fat density; the upper portion (13–74 Hounsfield units) is closer to muscle density. The mass is displacing the bowel and right kidney. It contains striated areas of increased density, creating a septated appearance.

At laparotomy, the high-density part of the mass was recognized as tumor and excised. The histologic diagnosis was myxoid liposarcoma. The patient then underwent radia-

tion therapy with 5,000 cGy delivered in 33 treatments over 55 days.

C and **D,** follow-up CT scans demonstrate that, although the high-density mass has been removed, the lower-density well-differentiated component continues to be present and has slightly grown in size. The right kidney is farther displaced.

The patient was referred to M. D. Anderson Hospital for further therapy. A second operation was contemplated, but it was not attempted because of multiple medical problems encountered from the first operation. Chemotherapy was initiated, and four years later the patient is alive with disease. This case points out how difficult it can be to define the tumor margins in a large fatty lesion comprising areas of varying differentiation.

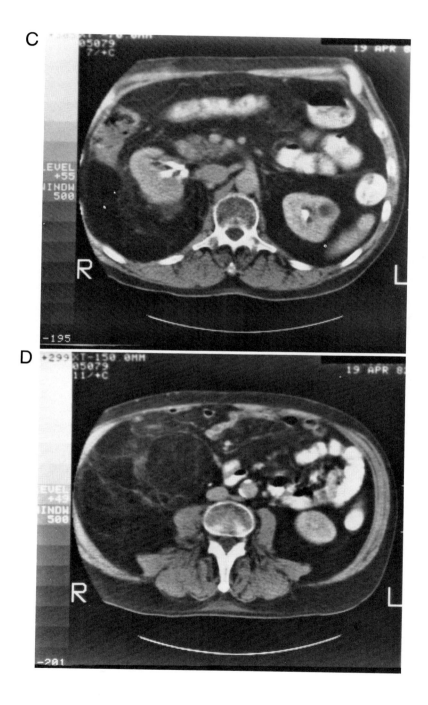

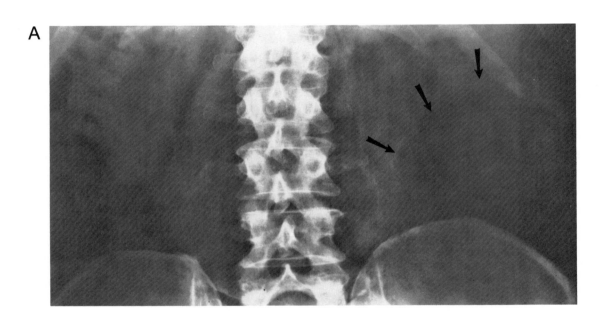

FIG 9–13.

Dedifferentiated liposarcoma. A 50-year-old man presented with back pain and on physical examination was found to have a mass in the abdomen.

A, a plain film of the abdomen shows a radiolucent mass *(arrows)* in the left abdomen.

B and **C,** these CT scans reveal a large tumor with two different densities. The high-attenuation portion of the tumor surrounds the aorta and the inferior vena cava and displaces the right kidney laterally. The low-density portion, which represents the more differentiated part of the tumor, is seen in the left half of the abdomen. It displaces the left kidney *(K)* down to the pelvis.

An incisional biopsy yielded an initial diagnosis of malignant fibrous histiocytoma in adipose tissue. The final pathologic report on the surgical specimen was grade 3 sarcoma with components of fibrosarcoma, neurogenic sarcoma, and fibrous histiocytoma. The case was then referred to M. D. Anderson Hospital, where it was reviewed by a senior pathologist. By review of the CT scan plus the microscopic material, the diagnosis of dedifferentiated liposarcoma was made.

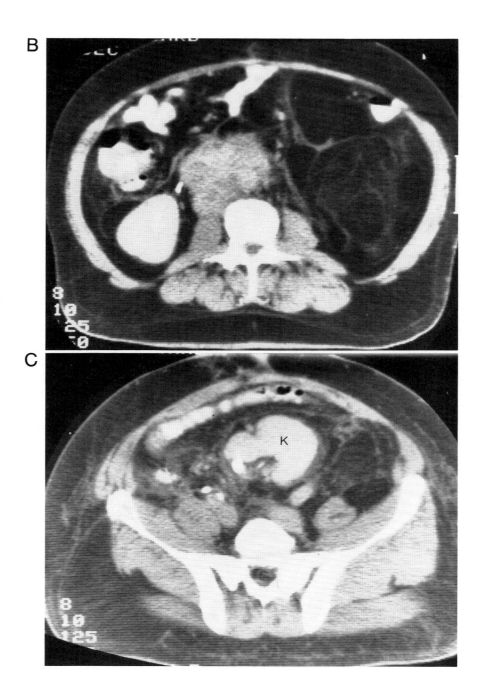

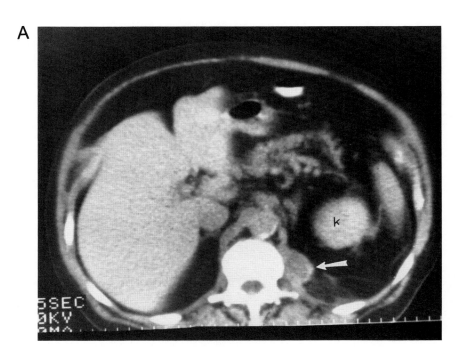

FIG 9–14.
Dedifferentiated liposarcoma with recurrence. A 68-year-old man with a four-year history of abdominal pain and hospitalizations for cholecystitis and deep venous thrombosis re-presented with an unrelieved feeling of abdominal fullness. A CT examination was done.

A, a CT scan through the midabdomen demonstrates anterior displacement of the left kidney *(k)* with striations of the posterior perirenal fat. In addition, a nodular higher-attenuation component is seen *(arrow)* adjacent to the left crus.

B, a lower image shows the varying CT appearance of the tumor. In the left perirenal space, the fat is of nearly normal density; however, again there are abnormal striations. In the midline, the mass is of higher attenuation *(arrowheads).*

Needle biopsy of the midline mass resulted in a diagnosis of liposarcoma. At surgery, a 3,500-g, 26 × 29 × 11 cm mass was excised. Included in the excised specimen were the left kidney and left colon. Histologically, most of the tumor was well-differentiated liposarcoma, except in the paraspinal area, where a dedifferentiated component was seen. The patient was given chemotherapy, and CT was repeated eight months later.

C, a CT image eight months after surgery and chemotherapy shows the recurrent liposarcoma along the left paraspinal area. Only the dedifferentiated component was present at the time of second surgery.

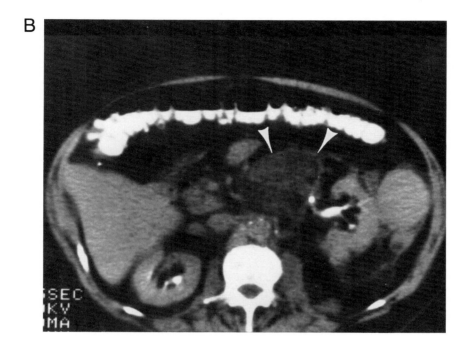

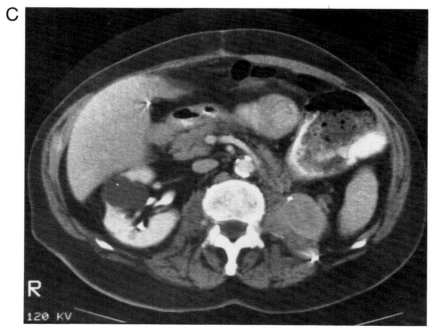

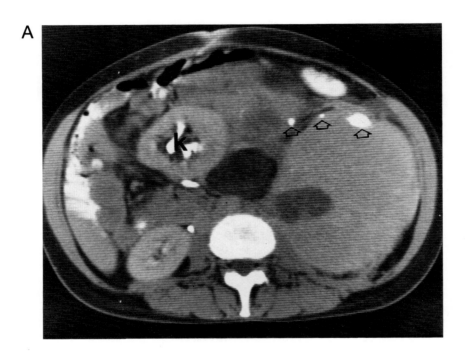

FIG 9–15.
Dedifferentiated liposarcoma that recurred as osteosarcoma.

    This 53-year-old woman presented with a three-month history of progressive abdominal enlargement and generalized malaise. A CT examination was done.

    A, midabdominal CT image demonstrates a very large mass with mixed attenuation and areas of calcification *(ar-*

rows). Note the marked displacement of the left kidney *(k).*

    Biopsy proved liposarcoma and the patient received two courses of chemotherapy, followed by excision of a 4,550-g, 26 × 20 × 15 cm mass along with the left kidney. The pathologic diagnosis was dedifferentiated liposarcoma. Chemotherapy was continued for two years, until the patient presented with a high serum alkaline phosphatase value. Reevaluation included an abdominal CT examination.

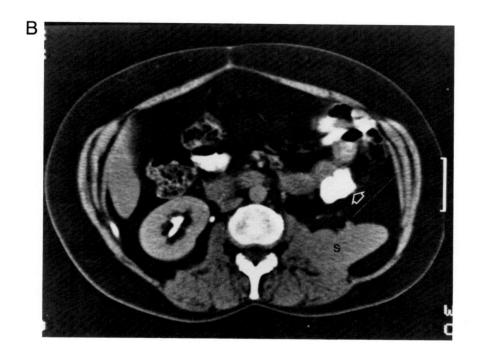

B, this CT scan shows evidence of the left nephrectomy; it was otherwise reported normal. Spleen *(s)* is seen in the left renal fossa.

For four months, the elevated serum alkaline phosphatase value persisted; a bone scan was obtained in an attempt to determine its etiology. *(Continued.)*

C

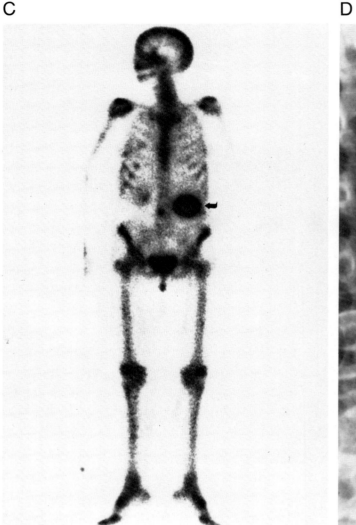

D

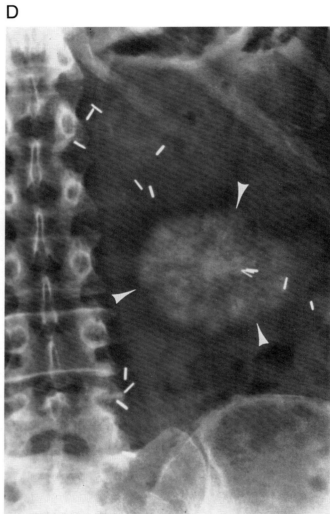

FIG 9–15 (cont.).
C, anterior view of radionuclide bone scan reveals significant concentration of the radiopharmaceutical in the left flank *(arrow).* The nuclear physician, without knowing there had been left nephrectomy, thought this represented an obstructed left kidney. A plain abdominal film and CT scan were obtained.

D, plain film of the abdomen demonstrates a large, ossified mass with linear densities, similar to the sunburst appearance *(arrowheads).*

E, the CT scan shows a very large, ossified mass in the left flank. Retrospectively, the mass is easily seen on the CT scan of four months before *(arrow in* **B***)*. There has been marked growth of the mass.

Biopsy proved recurrent liposarcoma with osteoid matrix suggesting osteosarcomatous degeneration. The recurrent tumor was excised, and the patient received chemotherapy.

F and **G,** a follow-up abdominal film **(F)** in eight months shows multiple ossified nodules throughout the peritoneum *(arrows).* These were neither present on previous films nor seen at surgery. They pick up bone-scanning agent **(G)** and presumably represent peritoneal osteosarcomatosis.

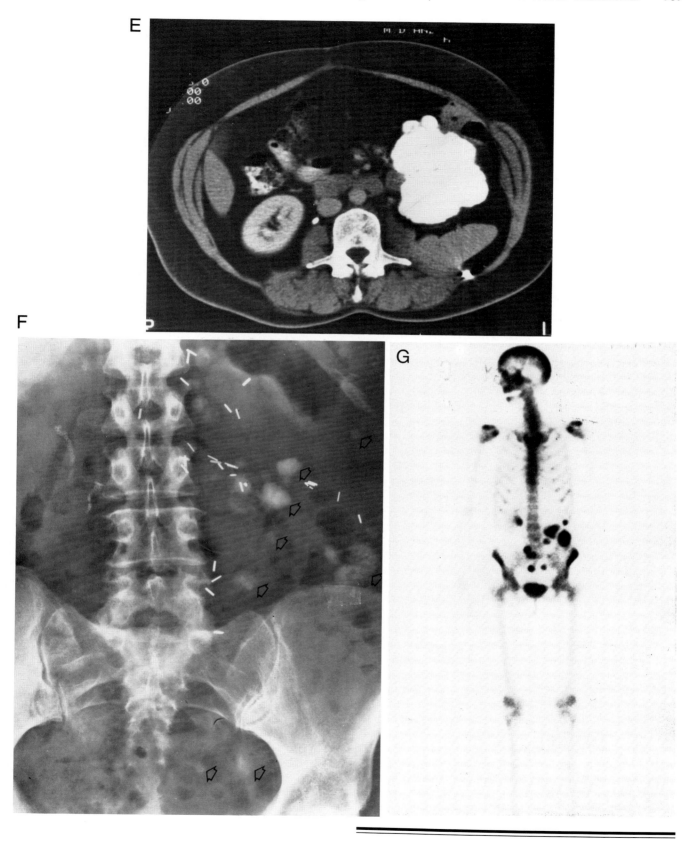

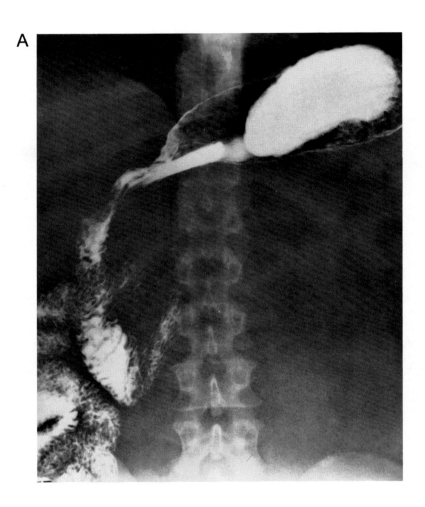

FIG 9–16.
Pleomorphic liposarcoma with recurrence. This 38-year-old man had been in good health, but for one month he had noticed early satiety and some increase in abdominal girth. Physical examination revealed a palpable mass, and upper gastrointestinal barium study and CT were done, followed by angiography and surgery.

A, frontal view from the upper gastrointestinal examination shows superior displacement of the stomach with lateral displacement of the duodenum and jejunum. No evidence of bowel invasion is seen.

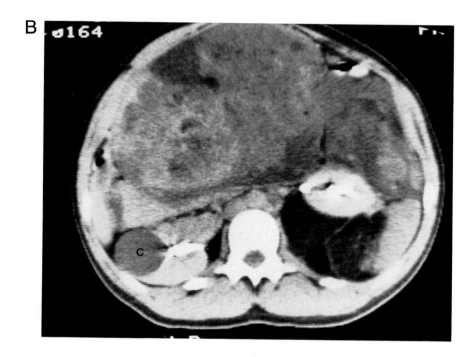

B, a CT scan at midabdominal level shows a large mass with marked nonhomogeneity ranging from fat in the left posterior perirenal space to near muscle density in the midabdomen. The mass extends from the left retroperitoneal space to the right lateral abdominal wall. Incidentally, there is a right renal cortical cyst *(C). (Continued.)*

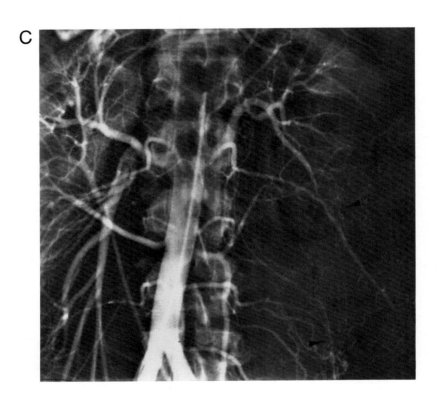

FIG 9–16 (cont.).
C and **D**, early **(C)** and late **(D)** films from a midline aortogram show marked displacement of the mesenteric vessels
by a hypovascular mass. Several irregular tumor vessels
are noted on the films *(arrowheads).* This lesion is slightly
more vascular than the typical liposarcoma.

Surgical exploration revealed two distinct masses, each
about 12 × 12 cm. Because of the extent of the lesions,
biopsies only were taken, and the patient was referred to
M.D. Anderson Hospital. He was treated with five courses
of chemotherapy, without significant response. Surgery was
performed, with all gross evidence of disease removed.

Maintenance chemotherapy was continued for the next two
and one-half years, when a repeat CT scan was obtained.

E, this CT scan two and one-half years following the
primary surgery shows recurrent disease in the left perirenal
area with anterior displacement of the kidney. Note that
there are three phases to the recurrent mass: one (−100
Hounsfield units) of near fat density *(cursor),* a second of
slightly higher attenuation *(curved arrow),* and a third near
muscle attenuation anterior and lateral to the kidney *(open
arrows).* The patient underwent a second operation. The
specimen had components of well-differentiated and dedifferentiated liposarcoma.

D

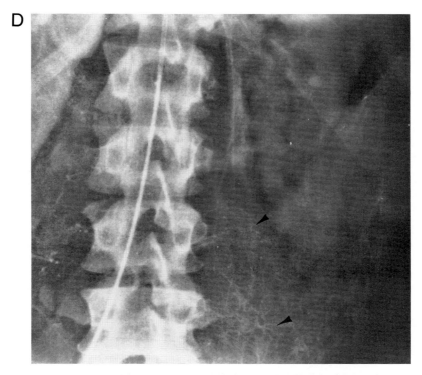

E

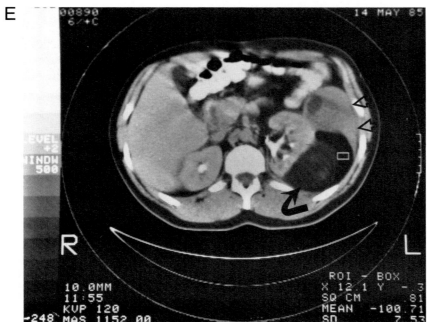

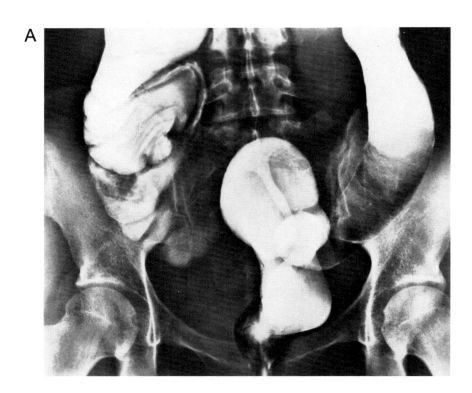

A

FIG 9–17.
Lipoma. A 38-year-old woman with a four-year history of right hip and right leg pain was found on pelvic examination to have a mass in the right presacral region. Additionally, an area of paresthesia was identified in the right thigh.

A, an anteroposterior film from a barium enema examination shows displacement of the rectum to the left with intact mucosa.

B and **C,** axial CT images through the lower pelvis demonstrate that the fatty tumor extends from within the pelvis, where it displaces the rectum, through the sciatic notch, to involve the gluteus medius muscles of the right buttock *(arrows)*.

The pure, homogeneous fat density demonstrated by CT in this case is typical of a benign lipoma. This appearance should be kept in mind when looking at liposarcomas. We have seen some well-differentiated liposarcomas in which there were areas of a density identical to that seen in benign lipoma; however, other areas would demonstrate streaking with higher-density septations or masses.

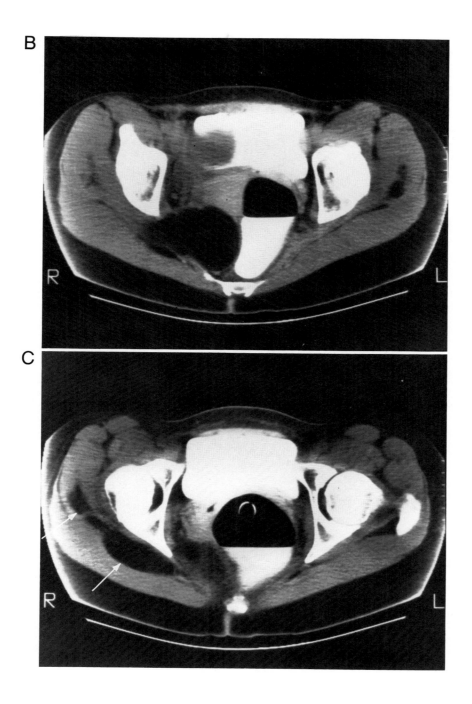

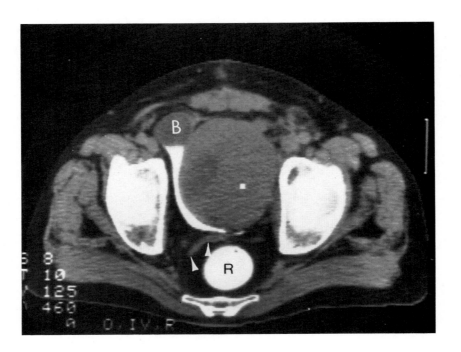

FIG 9–18.
Pelvic malignant fibrous histiocytoma. A 61-year-old man presented with pelvic pressure that had increased over a four-month period and that had resulted in urinary and fecal frequency. Physical examination suggested a pelvic mass, and a CT scan was obtained.

A CT image through the midpelvis reveals a large, well-demarcated mass displacing the partially opacified bladder *(B)* to the right. The attenuation value of the mass was mixed (20–50 Hounsfield units) but predominantly in the muscle density range. Prostate, rectum *(R),* and seminal vesicles *(arrowheads)* were normal.

A laparotomy and incisional biopsy of the mass followed, resulting in severe bleeding that required a 10-unit transfusion at the time of surgery. Pathologic diagnosis was malignant fibrous histiocytoma, and no attempt was made at further removal of the tumor. Treatment was by chemotherapy.

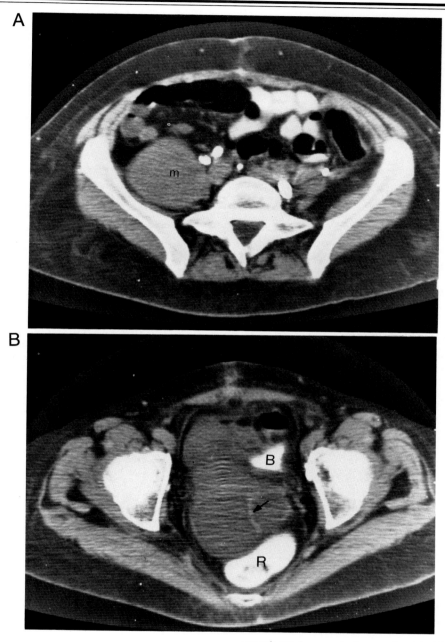

FIG 9–19.

Pelvic malignant fibrous histiocytoma. A 53-year-old woman presented with a five-month history of fever, abdominal pain, and weight loss. She had a history of hysterectomy for uterine fibroids. At another institution, her conventional radiologic examinations were normal. A CT scan was subsequently obtained, and the patient was then referred to M. D. Anderson Hospital.

A, a CT image in the midpelvis demonstrates a large, well-marginated mass *(m)* in the right iliac fossa. Percutaneous biopsy of this mass established the diagnosis of malignant fibrous histiocytoma.

B, a CT image in the lower pelvis shows another well-marginated mass between the bladder *(B)* and the rectum *(R)*. Areas of mixed density are seen within this mass, suggesting that there is some necrosis or hemorrhage. Additionally, there is evidence of a septation *(arrow)* within the mass.

Surgery confirmed the CT appearance of two separate masses within the pelvis, one measuring 7 × 10 cm along the right pelvis and one measuring 8 × 10 cm in the lower midline. Although these two masses could represent a primary **(B)** and its metastasis **(A),** their similar sizes, different densities, and the clinical lack of other metastatic disease make two separate primaries most likely.

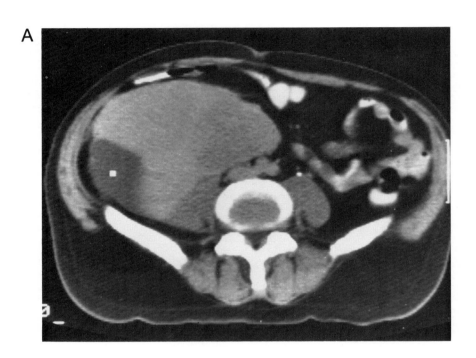

FIG 9–20.
Pelvic and retroperitoneal malignant fibrous histiocytoma. This 68-year-old man noticed a palpable mass in the right lower quadrant. He underwent CT examination, followed by biopsy, angiography, and surgery.

A, a CT image in the lower abdomen and upper pelvis reveals a large mass abutting the right psoas muscle. With the exception of a cystic area *(cursor)* with low attenuation (10–20 Hounsfield units), the mass is similar in density to the musculature. Percutaneous biopsy of the retroperitoneal mass showed malignant spindle cells, but the tumor type could not be specified.

B and **C,** angiographic films following injection of the right third **(B)** and fourth **(C)** lumbar arteries show a hypervascular mass with neovascularity and an early draining vein *(large arrows)*. The right kidney is elevated by the large retroperitoneal mass *(open arrows),* and the right ureter is stretched medially *(arrowheads)*.

The patient subsequently had resection for the retroperitoneal mass, and the diagnosis of malignant fibrous histiocytoma was made. He received chemotherapy and has been followed and has remained without evidence of disease for 18 months. Like most mesenchymal tumors, malignant fibrous histiocytoma exhibits a range of vascularity, this case being more vascular than most.

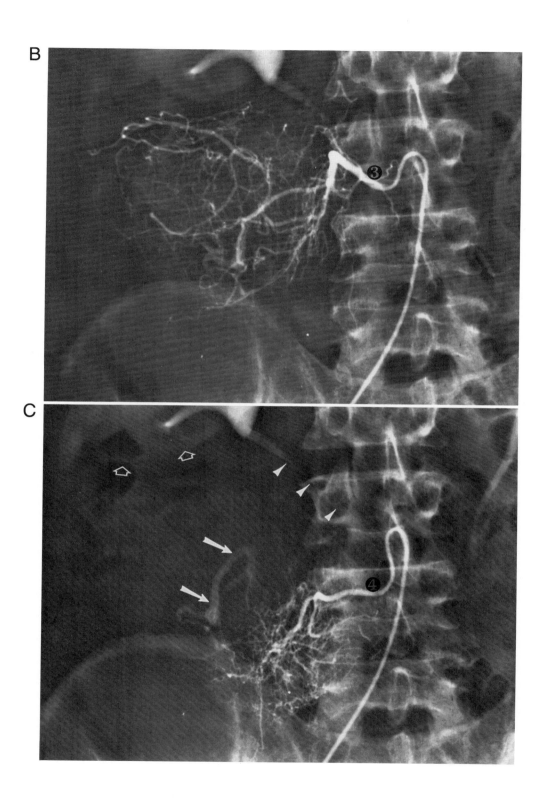

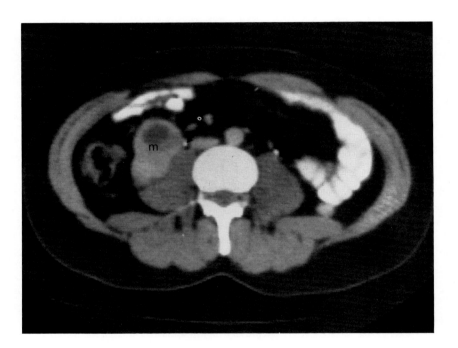

FIG 9–21.
Retroperitoneal malignant fibrous histiocytoma. A 41-year-old man presented with a urinary tract infection, and the intravenous pyelogram showed medial displacement of the right ureter. A CT examination was recommended.

The enhanced CT image reveals a well-circumscribed mass *(m)*, with partial enhancement and with an area of necrosis, abutting the right psoas muscle. The right ureter *(arrow)* is slightly displaced medially. With the central low density and mass enhancement, one should consider leiomyosarcoma in the differential diagnosis.

Surgical exploration revealed a 5 × 5 cm tumor, which was excised with clear margins. Pathologic diagnosis was malignant fibrous histiocytoma. There was no evidence of disease at the latest follow-up of 14 months.

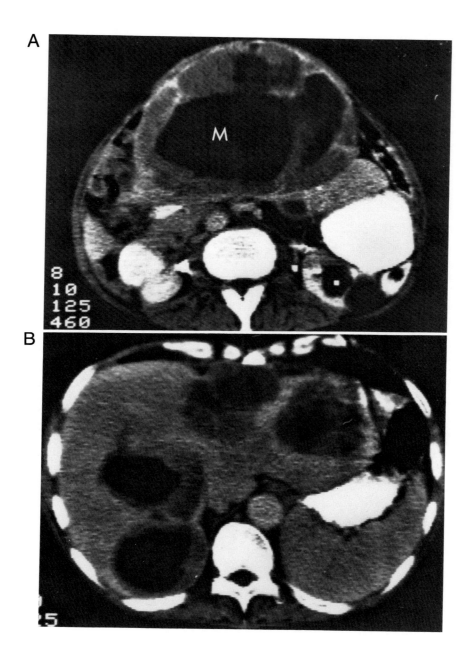

FIG 9–22.

Primary and metastatic leiomyosarcoma (three cases).

A and **B,** this 39-year-old woman presented with anemia and a large, palpable abdominal mass. On CT scan, there is a large mass *(M)* in the midabdomen with areas of low attenuation. In addition, there are multiple lesions with similar characteristics in the liver **(B),** representing metastases. The low-attenuation areas represent necrosis, which is rather typical for primary and metastatic leiomyosarcoma. *(Continued.)*

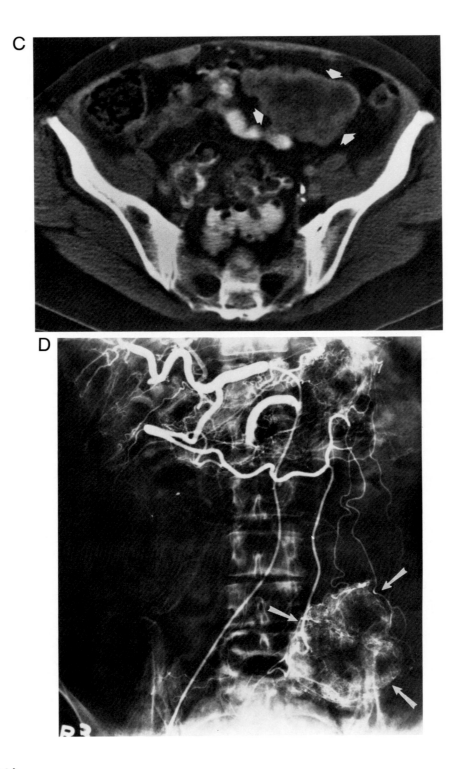

FIG 9–22 (cont.).
C through **E,** this 47-year-old man presented with anorexia and hepatomegaly. A mass was palpable in the left lower quadrant. The CT scan **(C)** demonstrates a mass with a central low density and peripheral enhancement *(white arrows)* in the left lower quadrant. The hepatic artery angiogram **(D)** demonstrates large omental branches from the

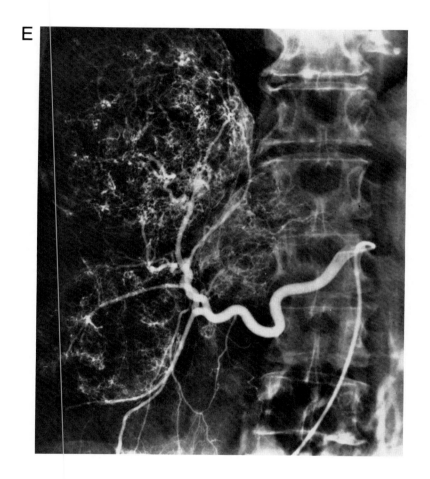

gastroepiploic artery feeding the hypervascular mass in the left lower quadrant *(arrows)*. A selective injection into the replaced right hepatic artery **(E)** demonstrates hypervascu- lar metastatic leiomyosarcoma in the liver. Percutaneous biopsy of the pelvic mass proved the diagnosis of leiomyosarcoma. *(Continued.)*

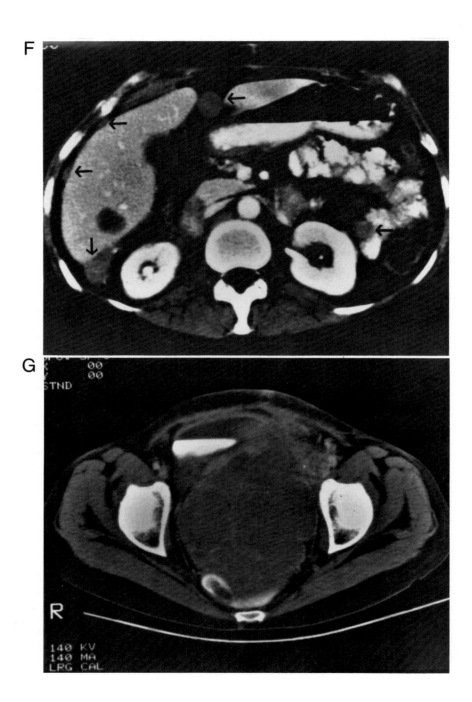

FIG 9–22 (cont.).
F and **G,** this 53-year-old man had a 3-cm leiomyosarcoma excised from the small bowel one year ago and now presented with vague abdominal pain. A pelvic mass was palpable. The abdominal CT image **(F)** shows liver metastases, as well as multiple subcapsular and peritoneal metastatic seeding of leiomyosarcoma *(arrows).* The pelvic CT scan **(G)** shows nonhomogeneous soft tissue mass in the pouch of Douglas; biopsy of this mass proved metastatic leiomyosarcoma. The pouch of Douglas is a common site of intraperitoneal tumor implantation and growth secondary to neoplastic seeding within the peritoneal cavity.

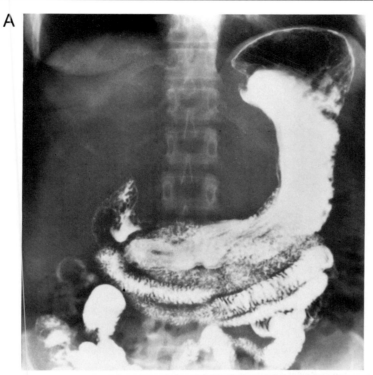

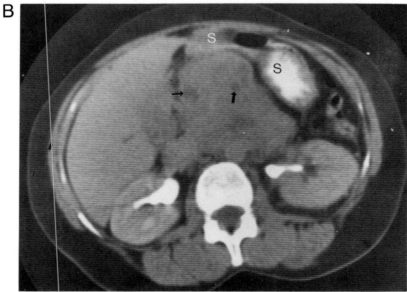

FIG 9–23.

Retroperitoneal leiomyosarcoma. This 59-year-old woman had epigastric pain with meals and noticed a mass in her upper abdomen. An upper gastrointestinal examination and CT were performed.

A, film from the upper gastrointestinal examination demonstrates a soft tissue mass effect on the gastric lesser curvature.

B, a midabdominal CT scan shows a poorly marginated mass with areas of low density *(arrows)* displacing the stomach *(S)* and the pancreas. The mass extends to the porta hepatis and to the periaortic and pericaval regions. The findings were suggestive of leiomyosarcoma, which was proved by needle aspiration biopsy.

Three years after diagnosis, the patient is still undergoing treatment with chemotherapy.

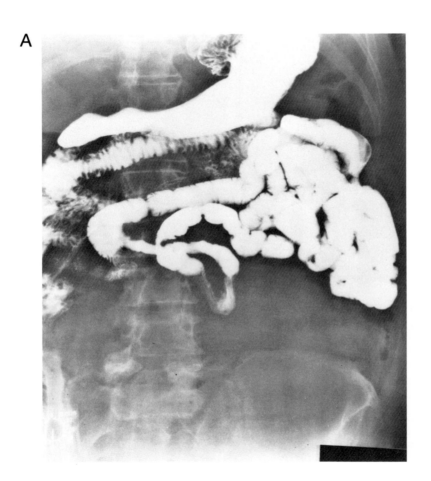

FIG 9–24.
Large retroperitoneal leiomyosarcoma. This 53-year-old woman presented because of abdominal pain and post-menopausal bleeding. Dilatation and curettage results were negative for disease. The pain continued, and five months later a large abdominal mass was palpated. An upper gastrointestinal examination and abdominal CT studies were performed.

A and **B,** single films from upper gastrointestinal **(A)** and barium enema **(B)** examinations demonstrate displacement and compression of the bowel. No evidence of wall invasion is seen.

C, this CT scan reveals a large, relatively well margin-ated intraabdominal and pelvic soft tissue mass. The mass is relatively homogeneous and lacks the low-density necrotic areas commonly seen in leiomyosarcoma.

At exploratory laparotomy, a very large retroperitoneal mass was seen to extend from 5 cm below the xiphoid into the pelvis. The lesion was extremely vascular, and biopsy resulted in 1,000-ml blood loss. The pathologic diagnosis was leiomyosarcoma. Chemotherapy yielded no response, and the patient died five months after diagnosis.

B

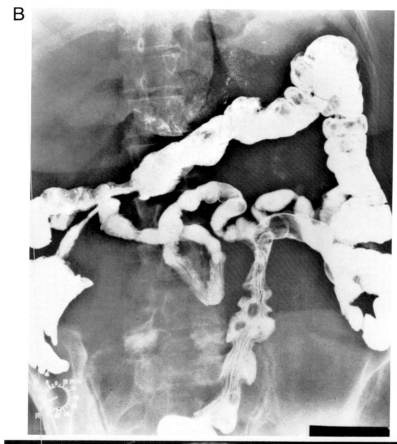

C

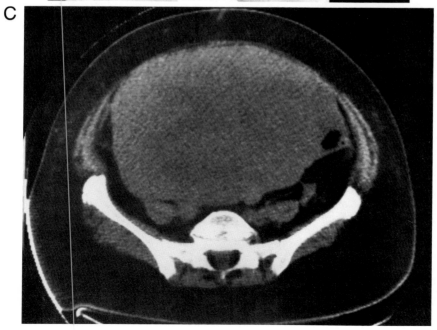

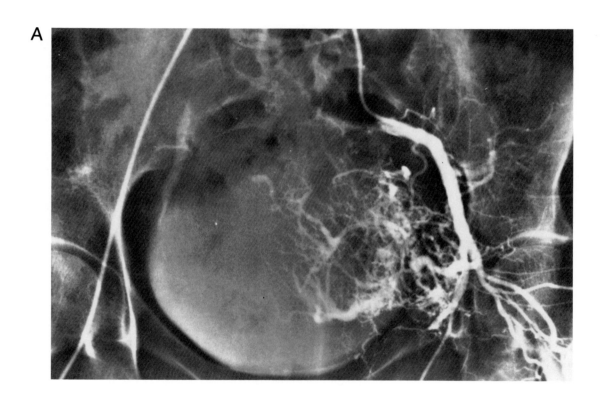

FIG 9–25.
Pelvic hemangiopericytoma (two cases).

A, a 39-year-old woman presented with pelvic pain and dysuria, and a left pelvic mass was palpated on physical examination. The mass was solid on ultrasound, and angiography was done before surgery. The angiogram made by left internal iliac artery injection demonstrates a large, hypervascular mass with areas of neovascularity. This intensively vascular angiographic finding is fairly characteristic of hemangiopericytoma, which in this case was proved at surgery.

B

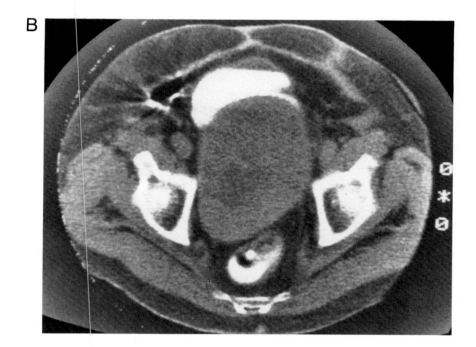

Three months after surgery, recurrence was demonstrated on physical examination and by angiography. The tumor failed to respond to chemotherapy, so it was treated with external radiation. The patient was followed for five years without evidence of disease, but seven years after the surgery she developed lung, liver, and bone metastases.

B, computed tomographic image of a hemangiopericytoma of the pelvis in a 70-year-old man. This well-defined homogeneous mass was discovered on routine prostate examination. It was excised and the bed treated by irradiation. The patient subsequently developed lung metastases and died.

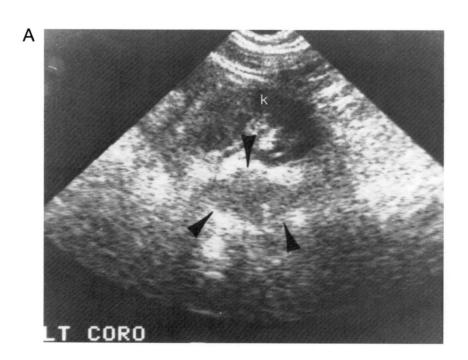

FIG 9–26.

Extragonadal retroperitoneal seminoma. A 38-year-old man with several episodes of left flank pain underwent intravenous pyelography, which reportedly showed lateral deviation of the left ureter. His physical examination and testicular sonogram were normal. Abdominal ultrasound and then CT were done.

A, oblique sonogram through the left flank demonstrates a hypoechoic mass *(arrowheads)* anterior and medial to the left kidney *(k)*.

B, midabdominal CT image reveals a homogeneous soft tissue mass *(M)* abutting the aorta and the left psoas muscle. Biopsy established the diagnosis of seminoma, and the patient underwent chemotherapy.

C, this CT image taken during the patient's treatment course demonstrates internal attenuation changes as well as reduction in the size of the mass. Subsequent exploration revealed a pure seminoma with areas of necrosis.

During treatment of nonseminomatous germ cell tumors, the tumor mass, whether the primary lesion or a metastatic deposit, often becomes cystic (see Fig 9–37). On rebiopsy, such an area will often show maturation to benign cystic teratoma. The low-density changes seen in this case, a pure seminoma, were considered secondary to tumor necrosis.

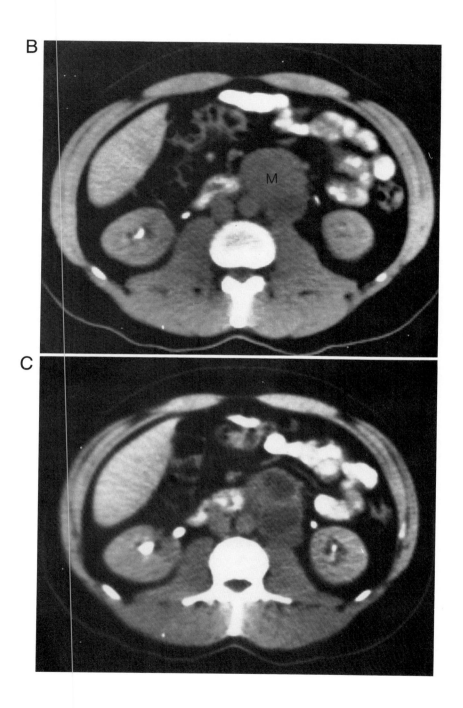

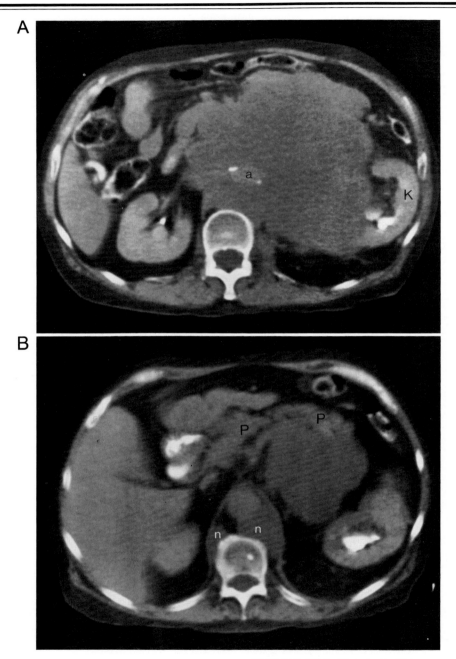

FIG 9–27.
Retroperitoneal seminoma in an undescended testis. This 57-year-old man presented with abdominal pain and a palpable midabdominal mass. The left testis was absent. Left orchiopexy had been done when the patient was six years old, but, according to the history, the left testis had immediately ascended back into the abdomen.

A, on midabdominal CT image, there is a huge retroperitoneal mass encircling the aorta *(a)* and displacing the left kidney *(K)* laterally.

B, slightly higher in the abdomen, one can see retrocrural nodal metastases *(n)* and anterior displacement of the pancreas *(P)* by the mass. This group of nodes is commonly involved in testicular primaries.

Biopsy of the large mass was positive for pure seminoma. Chemotherapy was begun; however, the patient suffered a myocardial infarction and died. At autopsy, a 20 × 20 × 15 cm retroperitoneal tumor mass was identified. The left testis was not found but was thought most likely to be the source of the large retroperitoneal tumor.

This case demonstrates the well-known increased risk for a primary neoplasm in an undescended testis. It is less well known that the opposite testis, although descended, is also at increased risk for neoplasm.

A

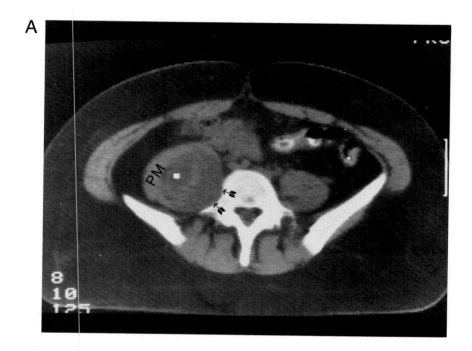

FIG 9–28.

Neurilemoma (two cases).

A, a 35-year-old woman with a two-week delay in menstruation was found on sonography to have a high, right-sided pelvic mass. The CT shows the mass to be well defined, with areas of nonhomogeneous density adjacent to the right psoas muscle. The psoas muscle *(PM)* appears to drape on to the mass. The tumor has been present for a long time, as it has caused a concavity in the adjacent vertebral body *(arrows)*. The patient underwent resection of an encapsulated neurilemoma.

Neurilemoma is a benign tumor; however, it may be difficult to histologically differentiate from a low-grade neurofibrosarcoma. *(Continued.)*

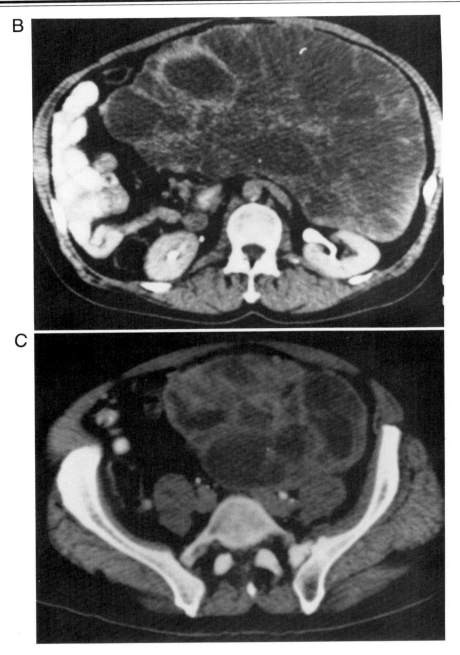

FIG 9–28 (cont.).

B through **E**, a 55-year-old man reported increasing abdominal girth of at least two years' duration. In his hometown, he had exploratory laparotomy; a huge, multilobulated intraabdominal tumor was sampled by biopsy but not removed. Biopsy material was confusing as to whether the mass was a benign or malignant mesenchymal tumor. The patient was referred to M. D. Anderson Hospital, where the diagnosis of benign neurilemoma was made from the biopsy material. Computed tomography was performed, followed by angiography and surgery.

The CT images through the midabdomen **(B** and **C)** show a large, well-defined, nonhomogeneous multiseptated mass extending down into the midpelvis. No infiltration into the adjacent organs or bowel is seen.

The superior mesenteric artery angiogram **(D)** demonstrates the mass to be hypovascular. There is displacement of the vessels but no evidence of encasement. Some small, tortuous vascularities are seen *(arrows)*.

The surgical specimen **(E)** shows a lobulated, compartmentalized appearance, which correlates with the CT images. The histologic diagnosis was benign neurilemoma (see also Color Plate 48).

D

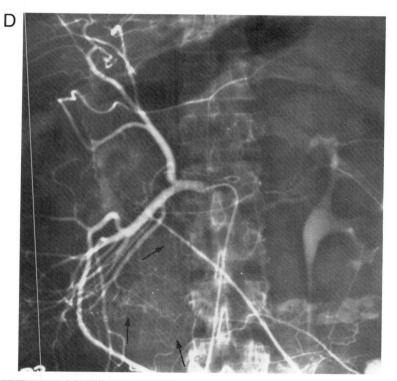

E

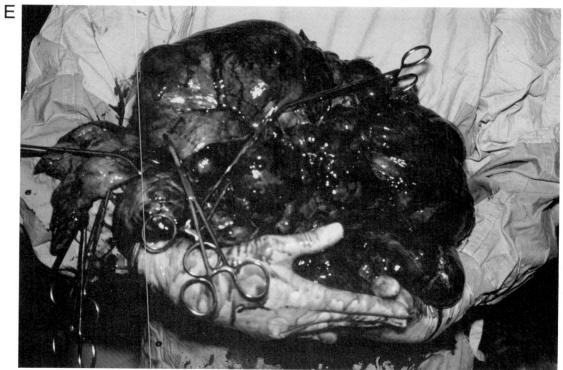

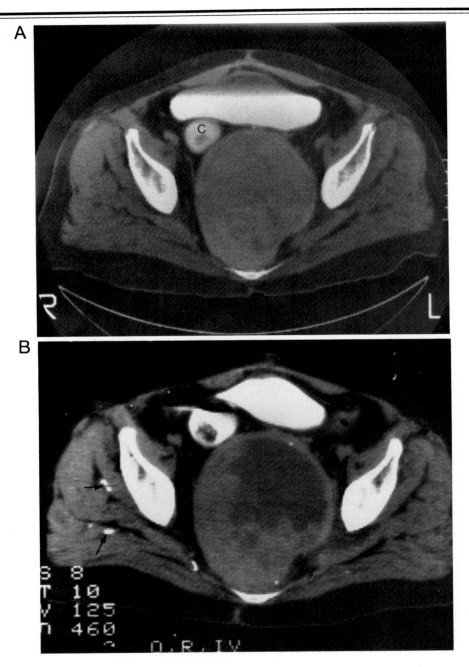

FIG 9–29.
Pelvic neurofibroma. A 59-year-old woman presented with an anal fissure. Pelvic examination revealed a large pelvic mass, and a CT scan was obtained.

A, the CT image of the pelvis shows a large, encapsulated mass within the pelvis. The mass abuts the sacrum and displaces the colon *(C)* anteriorly and to the right side.

At exploratory laparotomy, the tumor was fixed to the sacrum, and biopsy specimens were obtained. With the diagnosis of neurofibroma, the patient was referred to M. D. Anderson Hospital. She underwent five courses of systemic and three courses of intraarterial chemotherapy, without significant change in tumor size or appearance. The patient was then treated with three courses of internal iliac artery embolization.

B, a CT scan following three courses of embolic therapy shows significant internal density changes within the mass. Areas of low density represent necrosis as the result of infarction. Some Ivalon particles are identified in the periphery of the mass and within the right buttock *(arrows)*.

At reexploration, the neurofibroma was removed.

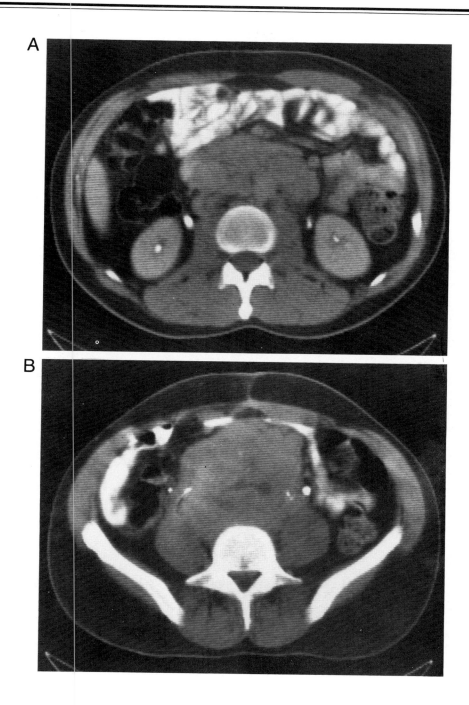

FIG 9–30.
Nonchromaffin paraganglioma. A 45-year-old man presented with a palpable abdominal mass. He was otherwise without symptoms.

A and **B,** there is a conglomerate mass in the midabdomen and upper pelvis obliterating the psoas and the aorta. In the upper pelvis, the mass displays central low density, probably necrosis. The ureters are deviated laterally.

Surgery revealed a 15 × 16 cm mass proven pathologically to be nonchromaffin paraganglioma. Postoperative treatment was by chemotherapy, and there was no evidence of disease as of four years of follow-up.

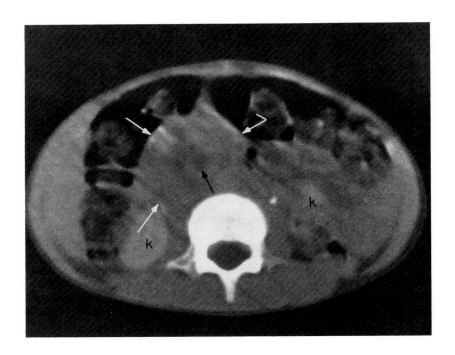

FIG 9–31.

Malignant chromaffin paraganglioma (extraadrenal pheo-chromocytoma). An 11-year-old boy presented with a four-year history of dizziness, fainting, tachycardia, and occasional abdominal pain. During a severe episode of abdominal pain, he was operated on with the diagnosis of acute appendicitis. Because of the normal appendix, the operation was converted into an exploratory laparotomy, and a large retroperitoneal mass was discovered. The mass was extremely vascular, and problems with bleeding and acute hypertension were encountered on the attempted biopsy. The operation was terminated, and the patient transferred to M. D. Anderson Hospital.

At presentation, the patient's blood pressure was 150/94 mm Hg, and there was a palpable mass in the midabdomen. The patient's catecholamine and vanillylmandelic acid values were markedly elevated. An abdominal CT scan was obtained.

The CT image demonstrates a large mass *(white arrows)* in the retroperitoneum and a low-density area *(black rows)*

arrow) within the inferior vena cava. The lower pole of each kidney is seen *(k)*. With a clinical and CT diagnosis of extraadrenal pheochromocytoma, the patient went to surgery.

During surgery, a metastatic nodule was seen within the inferior vena cava and removed along with the primary neoplasm. Postoperative chemotherapy was administered, and the patient was followed for four years, when a follow-up chest radiograph revealed two pulmonary nodules. These were removed, and the histologic findings in both nodules were identical to those in the patient's retroperitoneal primary malignant chromaffin paraganglioma.

In paragangliomas, it is extremely difficult to predict by histology the malignant potential of a primary lesion. Interestingly, in this case, the primary lesion seemed by histology to be benign, and there was no evidence of vascular invasion in the lesion itself; however, this tumor was obviously malignant, because a tumor nodule was removed from the inferior vena cava and later the tumor recurred within the chest.

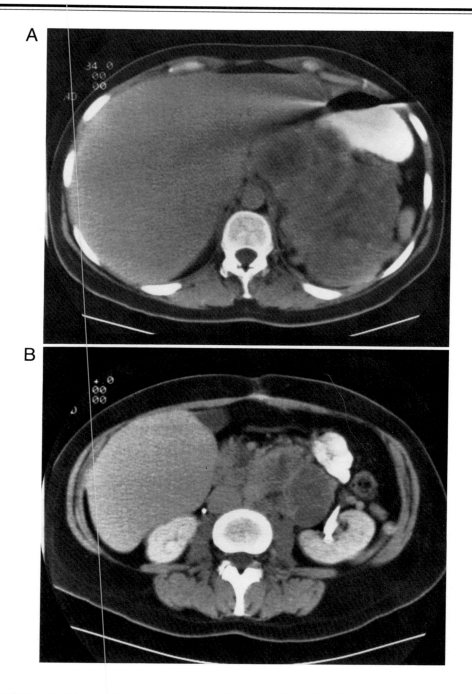

FIG 9–32.
Multiple paraganglioma. A 34-year-old woman presented with right upper quadrant pain and a palpable abdominal mass.

A and **B,** the CT images show a large, multilobular mass in the periaortic area. The mass contains multiple areas of low attenuation and superiorly extends to the level of the pancreas and the esophagogastric junction.

At exploratory laparotomy, the mass was seen to ex-
tend from the diaphragm to the aortic bifurcation. The lesion was very vascular, and the histologic diagnosis was paraganglioma.

One year later, the patient developed a neck mass on the left side, posterior to the left lobe of the thyroid. This was proved to represent a second paraganglioma. The patient has been undergoing chemotherapy since diagnosis of the abdominal paraganglioma.

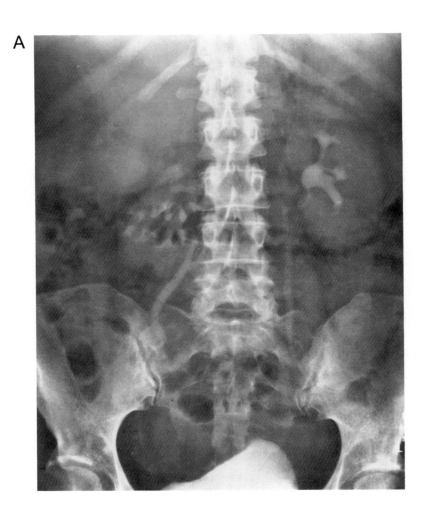

A

FIG 9–33.
Abdominal metastatic ependymoma. A 53-year-old woman presented 13 years after an exploratory laparotomy and excision of an undifferentiated tumor, probably a mesothelioma or ependymoma. Recently, during assessment because of episodes of postmenopausal bleeding, a pelvic mass was discovered on physical examination.

A, on the intravenous pyelogram, there are two soft tissue masses, one in the right pelvis and one in the right upper quadrant. The latter has displaced the right kidney inferiorly.

B, these CT images reveal multiple soft tissue masses with areas of necrosis. The masses extend throughout the right side of the abdomen, some having the appearance of peritoneal seeding. There is evidence of liver metastasis, but the right kidney is normal.

On surgical exploration, a 10 × 10 cm mass was discovered in the cul-de-sac. It incorporated the uterus and right ovary and was removed. Massive peritoneal seeding and liver metastases were also seen. The histologic diagnosis of the surgical specimen was extraneuroaxial ependymoma in the rectosigmoid region with peritoneal metastases. The patient chose to receive postoperative chemotherapy. Her status has been stable in the three years of follow-up.

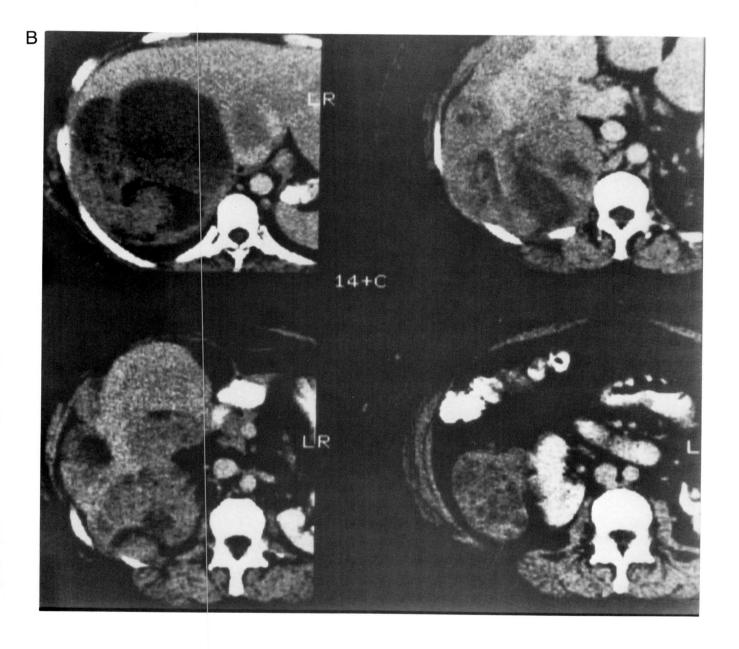

A

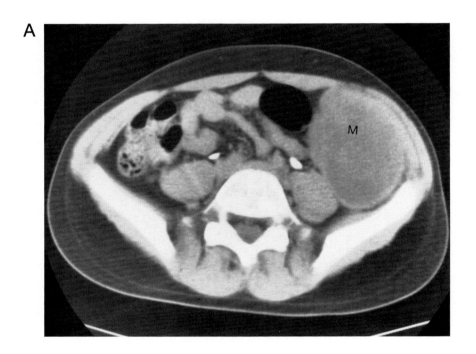

FIG 9–34.
Soft tissue Ewing's sarcoma. A 12-year-old boy who had left lower quadrant blunt trauma two months ago noted swelling and pain in the area. His routine workup was normal, but the mass in the left lower quadrant became larger and over the next four weeks more painful. A CT scan was obtained, followed by ultrasound, angiography, and biopsy.

A, the CT scan demonstrates a large, relatively homogeneous soft tissue mass *(M)* just anterior to the left psoas and iliacus muscles. It cannot be separated from the ante-rior abdominal wall.

B, sagittal sonogram shows the mass *(M)* and the left iliac wing *(IW)*. The solid tumor is shown not to be of bony origin.

C, selective angiographic study of the tumor blood supply from the external iliac artery demonstrates the mass to be moderately vascular and to have areas of blush *(arrows)*.

Open biopsy established the diagnosis of soft tissue Ewing's sarcoma.

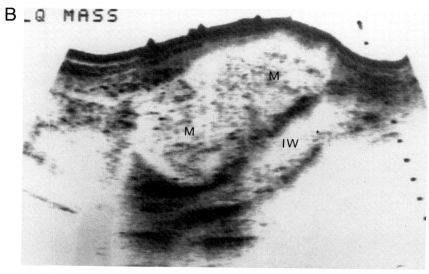

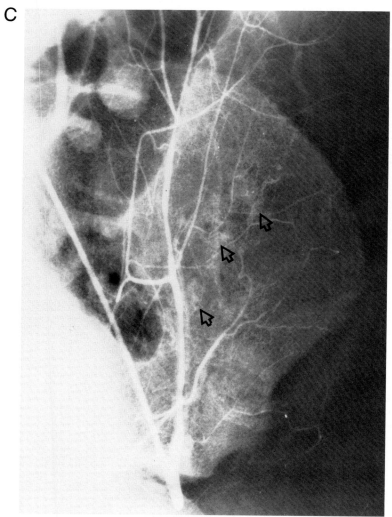

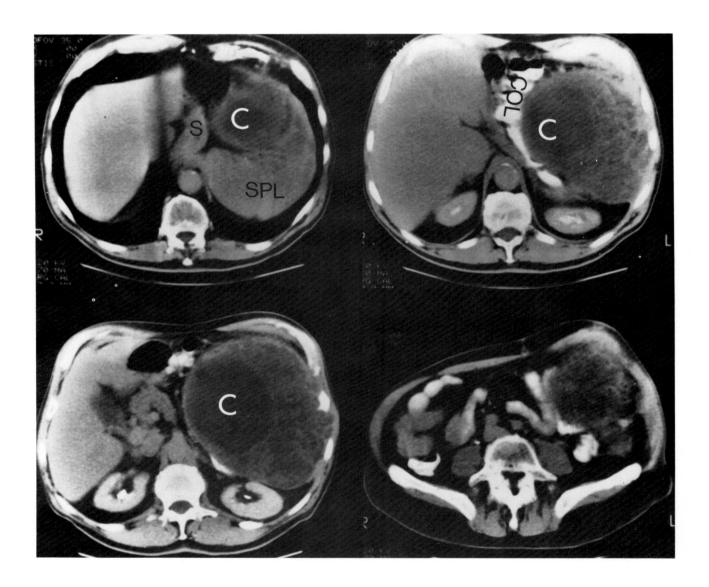

FIG 9–35.
Intraabdominal soft tissue chondrosarcoma. This 81-year-old man with a history of a 44-kg (20-lb) weight loss was found to have a left upper quadrant abdominal mass.

The CT images show a large, partially cystic *(C)* mass in the left side of the abdomen, extending from the diaphragm to the upper pelvis. The mass is well encapsulated, with the lateral margins being blended into the abdominal wall. It has displaced the stomach *(S)* and colon *(COL)* me-

dially and the spleen *(SPL)* posteriorly. As was also seen on barium study of the gastrointestinal tract, no bowel invasion was present.

A percutaneous biopsy was done and the diagnosis of grade 1 chondrosarcoma established. The patient received several courses of chemotherapy, followed by radiotherapy. One-year follow-up showed slight progression in the size of the mass. The patient declined surgery.

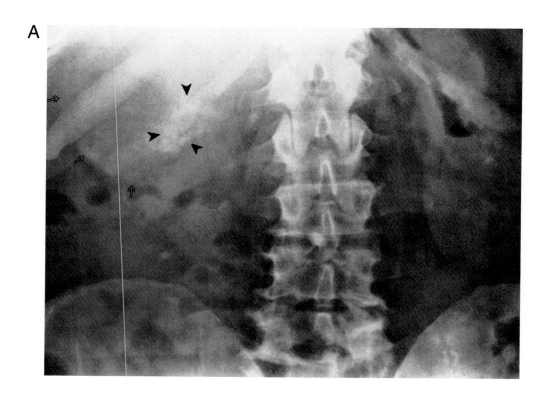

FIG 9–36.
Retroperitoneal soft tissue osteosarcoma. This 53-year-old man had routine chest radiography, and a calcified mass was discovered in the right upper quadrant. The patient was completely without symptoms.

A, the early film from intravenous pyelography shows the mass *(arrows),* which has multiple areas of calcification *(arrowheads),* to be adjacent to the upper pole of the right kidney. *(Continued.)*

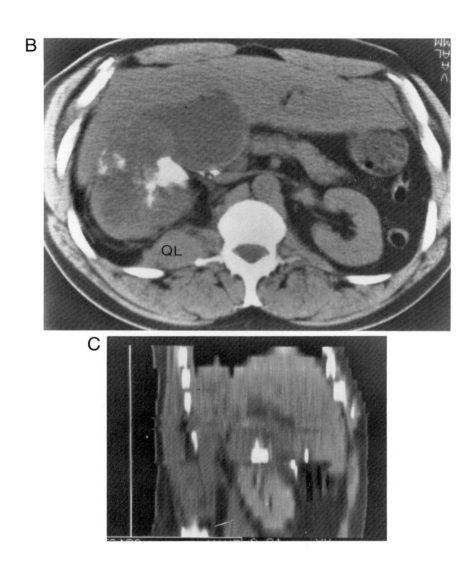

FIG 9–36 (cont.).
B, the axial CT scan shows the cystic and solid compartments of the mass along with calcifications. There is involvement of the right quadratus lumborum muscle *(QL).*

   C, parasagittal reconstruction of CT images reveals separation of the mass from the right kidney. There was evidence of direct infiltration into the right quadratus lum-

borum muscle. On angiography, the major blood supply to the mass was noted to be from the right inferior adrenal artery, and the origin of the mass was thought to be in the adrenal gland. A percutaneous biopsy was done and the diagnosis of extraskeletal retroperitoneal osteosarcoma established.

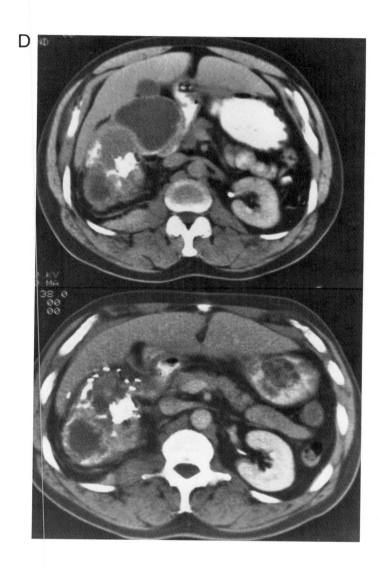

D, CT images after several courses of intraarterial chemotherapy show increasing calcification within the tumor. This was followed by tumor excision. A 10 × 10 cm mass was removed, along with the right adrenal gland. Diagnosis of a necrotic osteosarcoma was confirmed; the adrenal gland was normal. One year after surgery, the patient was without symptoms of the disease.

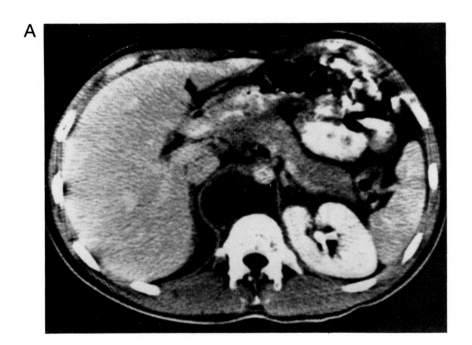

FIG 9–37.
Thoracoabdominal metastatic teratoma. This 24-year-old man had a history of testicular teratocarcinoma with mixed embryonal component, for which he had orchiectomy six months prior to this admission. At the time of orchiectomy, he had mediastinal and retroperitoneal adenopathy, for which he received chemotherapy. His metastases responded to chemotherapy; however, on the follow-up radiograph and CT scan, it was difficult to tell whether the residual malignant tumor had converted to a mature teratoma or

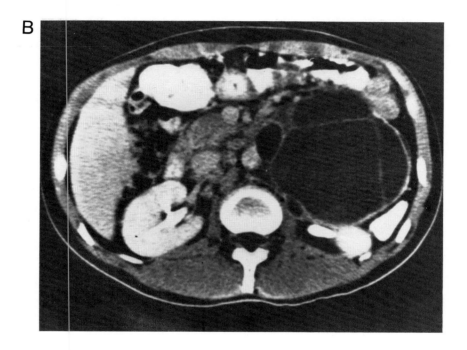

just undergone cystic changes.

Eight months after orchiectomy, he presented with a palpable abdominal mass and underwent CT examination.

A and **B,** the CT scans of the abdomen demonstrate cystic masses with septations behind the crura of dia-

phragm and in the left retroperitoneum.

A thoracoabdominal lymph node dissection was performed, and the pathologic diagnosis of a mature teratoma made.

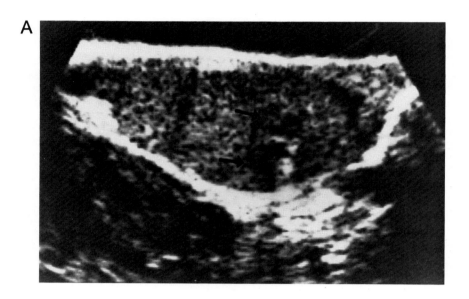

FIG 9–38.
Embryonal cell carcinoma of testis with retroperitoneal metastasis. A 29-year-old man presented with abdominal fullness, and the CT scan revealed a retroperitoneal mass. Biopsy proved the mass to be embryonal cell carcinoma. Physical examination of the testes was normal, but ultrasound showed a 1.2-cm focal abnormality of the left testis, probably representing occult primary. This finding did not change after six months of systemic chemotherapy, and an orchiectomy was done.

A, a sagittal ultrasonographic view of the left testis shows the tumor mass *(arrows)* within the lower pole.

B, the bisected pathologic specimen of the left testis shows the focal abnormality detected at ultrasound *(arrowheads).*

C, enhanced CT scan demonstrates the large retroperitoneal masses *(top image)* extending along both sides of the aorta.

At pathology, there was no evidence of tumor in the abnormal area seen in the lower pole of the left testis; however, this is in keeping with a response of the testicular primary to preoperative chemotherapy. Nine months into the therapy (three months after orchiectomy), the patient had a complete response, with chemical markers returning to normal values and regression of the retroperitoneal mass *(bottom image* in **C**).

This case demonstrates that a patient may present with only a large retroperitoneal mass clinically apparent yet have a clinically occult testicular primary. Ultrasonography has proved its utility in detecting these occult testicular lesions.

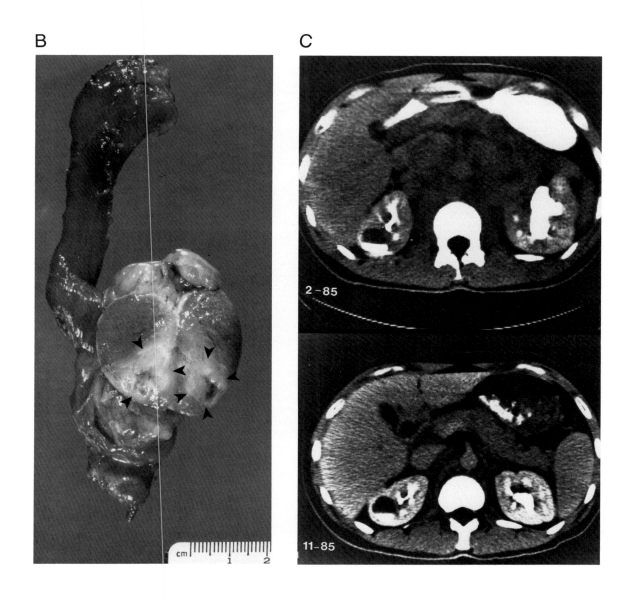

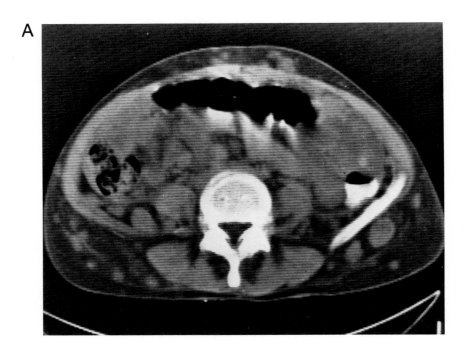

FIG 9–39.
Metastatic melanoma to the retroperitoneum (multiple cases).

A through **C,** three cases of fairly typical advanced metastatic melanoma are illustrated. Notice that there are many subcutaneous nodules **(A)** in addition to mesenteric, hepatic **(B),** and retroperitoneal **(B** and **C)** metastases. When metastasis occurs, there is a particular propensity in the retroperitoneum for the nodules to involve the perirenal space (*arrows* in **C**).

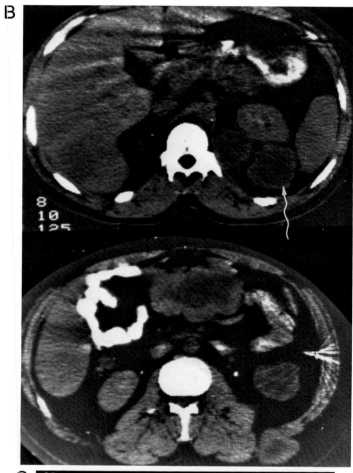

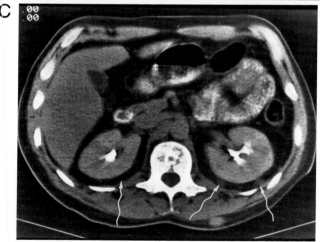

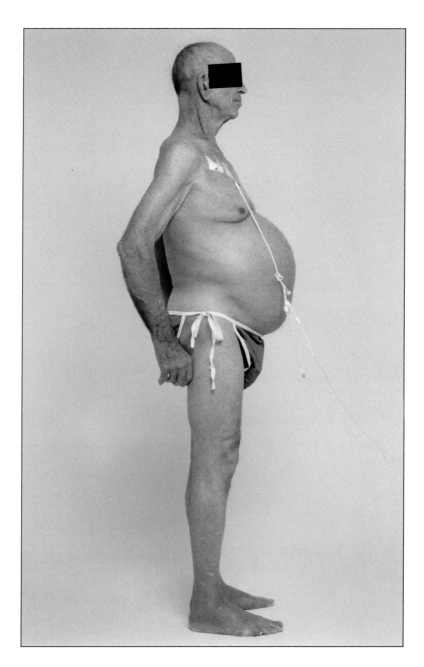

PLATE 46

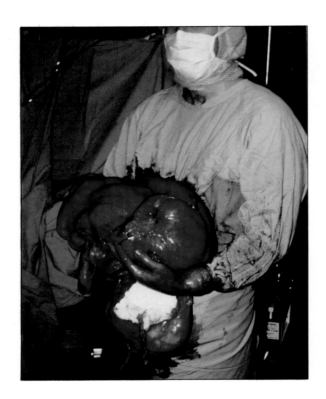

PLATE 47

PLATE 48

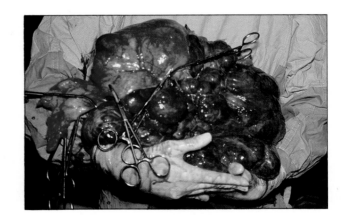

10

Pelvic and Abdominal Musculoskeletal Neoplasms

Ali Shirkhoda, M.D.

Marvin H. Chasen, M.D.

John E. Madewell, M.D.

Neoplasms originating in osseous and muscular structures of the abdomen and pelvis are common. In a series reported by Dahlin, 694 of 6,221 primary bone tumors (11%) originated in the pelvis and were most often malignant, at a ratio of 4:1.[1]

There is a wide spectrum of oncological conditions that involve the musculoskeletal structures within the abdomen and pelvis. These can be classified according to the organ of involvement.

This chapter discusses and illustrates the neoplastic conditions of the bones and soft tissues of the pelvis, spine, and abdominal wall. At the end, neoplasms of the thoracoabdominal junction and difficulties in imaging this area are discussed.

PRIMARY MALIGNANT BONE TUMORS

Primary bone tumors, excluding multiple myeloma, account for only 0.5% of all human malignancies.[2] Approximately 11% of primary bone tumors are located within the pelvis, and 80% of these are malignant. Conventional radiography and tomography are usually adequate for the initial study and frequently provide a specific diagnosis. How-

ever, when tumor location and extent are sought, and the tumor's effect on adjacent soft tissues, neurovascular bundles, and organs needs to be determined, computed tomography (CT) and magnetic resonance imaging (MRI) are most helpful. Occasionally, primary bone tumors of the pelvis arise superficially; in these cases, the radiograph may show the bone to be normal and not demonstrate the soft tissue mass. In addition, lesions may be missed by conventional means in areas, such as the spine, pelvis, and thoracic wall, difficult to image by those means. In these cases, CT and MRI are ideally suited to lesion detection. In fact, if a bone tumor is suspected and cannot be detected by conventional means, CT or MRI studies should be considered.[3–5]

Chondrosarcoma

Chondrosarcoma accounts for more than 25% of primary osseous malignancies within the pelvis. It frequently originates in the innominate bone and acetabular region (Figs 10–1 and 10–2) and occasionally arises from the sacrum (Fig 10–3). The tumor often occurs in the third to seventh decades of life and is more frequent in men than in women.[1] Origin is in a preexisting osteochondroma in approximately 10% of cases (Fig 10–4), and the tumor may also arise from an enchondroma (Fig 10–5). Nearly 10% of typical low-grade chondrosarcomas will give rise to a highly aggressive anaplastic sarcoma, either fibrosarcoma or osteosarcoma.[6] Initial symptoms are generally mild and insidious in onset. A long clinical evolution is characteristic. The tumor usually manifests extensive lytic bone destruction with poor margination, and a soft tissue mass is typically seen. Typical of cartilaginous lesions, chondrosarcomas may have discrete, punctate, and irregular ringlike matrix calcifications (see Fig 10–2). Without typical calcification, radiologic differentiation of chondrosarcoma from other malignant tumors may be difficult.

Chondrosarcoma is radioresistant and is often treated by radical resection.[7] Computed tomography in these patients is instrumental in determining the extent and resectability of disease and in selecting and designing the surgical procedure. After treatment, changes that might suggest recurrence can probably be detected earlier on CT (Fig 10–6).

Osteosarcoma

Osteosarcoma is the osseous malignancy most frequently seen in the pediatric age group and accounts for 20% of all primary sarcomas of bone.[8] The amount of osteoid produced by the neoplastic cells is variable, resulting in different radiologic patterns from lytic and mixed to blastic types of osteosarcoma. Predominance of cartilaginous, osteoid, fibrous, or vascular elements results in subdivisions such as chondroblastic (Fig 10–7), osteoblastic (Fig 10–8), fibroblastic, and telangiectatic (Fig 10–9) osteosarcoma. The last group can be easily mistaken for aneurysmal bone cyst or even benign giant cell tumor, and nearly one third of the patients in this group will have pathologic fractures.[9] Almost 90% of osteosarcomas in the pelvis occur in the innominate bone.

The pelvis is a common site for Paget's disease, and osteosarcoma may arise from this condition and complicate it.[10] Osteosarcoma may also occur in the pelvis following radiation therapy (Fig 10–10).[11] Osteosarcoma is rare in the spine (Fig 10–11).

Radiographically, the tumor may either be osteolytic or osteoblastic, but frequently it has a mixed appearance. It is associated with destruction of the cortex and medullary portion of the bone and with a soft tissue mass.

In osteosarcoma, as in chondrosarcoma, CT is helpful in determining the extent of tumor.[12] Staging of the disease has improved considerably with the use of thoracic CT. Since most of these patients receive intraarterial chemotherapy prior to any radical surgery, in addition to conventional films, CT is helpful in evaluating the response to treatment (Fig 10–12).[13]

Ewing's Sarcoma

Ewing's sarcoma is a very malignant neoplasm that most often occurs between the ages of 5 and 15 years, although occurrence in the fourth decade of life and beyond has been reported.[14] Approximately 25% of these tumors are within the osseous pelvis (Figs 10–13 to 10–17). The spine is frequently involved by Ewing's sarcoma metastatic from other sites but is an infrequent site of primary involvement (Fig 10–18). A review of 1,020 cases from the literature yielded a 3.5% incidence of primary spinal Ewing's sarcoma, although that figure dropped to 0.9% when the sacrum was excluded.[15, 16] Like osteosarcomas, these tumors are lytic, blastic, or a mixture of both. In most cases, they show a very irregular, permeative type of destruction and very poor margination (Fig 10–13). They are often associated with a large soft tissue mass (Figs 10–14 to 10–16) that does not contain matrix mineralization. It should be noted that occasionally there are few or no radiographically demonstrable changes, and subtle tumor effects in the medullary canal and soft tissue components are best seen on CT scan (Fig 10–16).[17] These subtle changes are even better demonstrated by MRI.

Improved treatment techniques have raised the overall five-year survival in Ewing's sarcoma from 15% to around 50%. But the prognosis in pelvic Ewing's sarcoma is worse, with five-year survival still at about 10%.[7]

Lymphoma

About one half of patients who have osseous lymphoma also have the disease elsewhere in the body. About 20% of skeletal lymphomas arise in the pelvis, and these account for 10% of malignant bony tumors in the pelvis. In these patients, a lymphangiogram or CT study is essential to exclude retroperitoneal nodal disease. Although it can involve any bone, skeletal lymphoma is more common in the axial skeleton. While bone involvement is a sign of advanced disease, it appears early in nearly 20% of Hodgkin's patients.[18]

Radiologically, osseous lymphoma in the pelvis

is very similar to Ewing's sarcoma; unless the patient's age is known (the former tumor occurs in older patients), it is difficult to differentiate the two. Pelvic lymphomas are rare before the age of ten years. They are lytic, sclerotic, or, quite often, a mixture of lytic and reactive sclerosis (Fig 10–19).[19, 20] When there is also extraskeletal lymphoma, the bony lesions may be multiple. Occasionally, there are numerous areas of lysis scattered throughout the skeleton, which may make a specific radiographic diagnosis difficult (Fig 10–20). In these patients, CT scan will be essential for detecting the osseous abnormality.

Chordoma

Except for multiple myeloma (see later discussion), chordoma is the most common primary sacral neoplasm. It arises along the path of the primitive notochord and has a predilection for the upper and lower ends of the spinal column. Therefore, it is limited in the pelvis to the sacrum.[21, 22] Patients are generally more than 30 years of age, and the tumor is three times more common in males.

Characteristically, chordoma is a midline, destructive lesion with poor margination, containing either calcific deposits or bony fragments in about 50% of the cases (Figs 10–21 and 10–22). However, the consistency of the tumor varies from solid to an almost liquid mucoid tissue. Occasionally, the chordoma arises superficially, so that the sacrum is radiographically normal and the tumor is essentially a soft tissue mass. In these patients, and also in those cases in which the lesions may be totally obscured by overlying bowel gas, CT scanning is essential for preoperative diagnosis of the primary lesion and evaluation of possible metastasis for surgical planning (Fig 10–22). Magnetic resonance imaging has great potential in these patients because it provides sagittal images and can determine the extent of sacral vertebral involvement[23] as well as invasion of the adjacent muscles (Fig 10–23). The growth of the tumor is very slow; metastases (Fig 10–22) are uncommon. Treatment is radical resection. Recurrences are not uncommon and usually occur within the soft tissue. In detecting postoperative disease recurrence, especially that in soft tissue, MRI is of great value (Fig 10–24).

Myeloma and Plasmacytoma

If one accepts multiple myeloma as a primary bone tumor, it should then be listed as the most common primary osseous neoplasm. Most myelomas and plasmacytomas arise in the axial skeleton, with the pelvis among the most common sites (Figs 10–25 and 10–26). They typically involve the bone marrow and are usually multicentric. This tumor is strikingly more common in blacks, in whom it accounts for 7.2% of all cancers, compared with 1.1% of cancers in whites.[24, 25] The disease is rare in patients less than 50 years of age, and 70% of the patients are male.

Radiographically, myelomas and plasmacytomas are single or multiple small, lytic lesions in the trabecular bone, with later involvement of the cortex. In cases of plasmacytoma, there is usually an expansile bony lesion with residual trabeculae (Fig 10–25). Very rarely, the tumor is seen as a sclerotic lesion (Fig 10–26). However, this appearance is seen more frequently after treatment (Figs 10–27 and 10–28). In two major series, 75% and 79% of the patients had radiographically demonstrable skeletal lesions.[26, 27] It is not unusual to see a false-negative radionuclide bone scan. The radionuclide image may be positive before the radiograph shows evidence of myeloma but may subsequently revert to normal in the presence of an abnormal radiograph.[28] Also, when the disease is diffuse, the radiograph may show only nonspecific demineralization.[29] Computed tomography scan may not be needed when there is an abnormal radiograph, but, even in these patients, an associated soft tissue mass and adenopathy are easily discovered on CT (Fig 10–28). In patients in whom radiographs are normal and there is clinical diagnosis of multiple myeloma, CT often provides significant information that directly affects the therapeutic decisions; this modality should, in particular, be considered in such cases when there is bone pain.[30] In cases of solitary plasmacytoma, the disease may be associated with a large soft tissue mass; CT scan in these patients is of particular help.[31]

Angiosarcoma

Angiosarcoma includes the two primary vascular bone sarcomas: hemangioendothelioma and hemangiopericytoma.[32] The first is more common in bone (Fig 10–29), and the second occurs mostly in soft tissue. Hemangioendothelioma may be present as a solitary bone lesion or as multicentric bone lesions; the latter entail a more favorable prognosis. Radiographic findings are nonspecific in solitary hemangioendothelioma; the lesion can resemble metastasis, myeloma, and such other lytic lesions as aneurysmal bone cyst.

Paget's Disease

Paget's disease usually occurs in people over the age of 50. It is characterized by osteosclerotic resorption of bone and simultaneous overgrowth of new bony spicules that are poorly calcified and irregular. The most common locations are the spine, sacrum, femur, cranium, sternum, pelvis, tibia, and jaws. Paget's sarcoma occurs in approximately 0.15% of patients with Paget's disease; however, it is thought to arise in up to 10% of patients with very extensive disease. Sarcoma is the most serious complication of Paget's disease, since 70% of patients are dead within one year. Osteosarcoma is the most common type, but fibrosarcoma and anaplastic sarcoma can occur.[33] Giant cell tumor arises rarely in pagetoid bone and may be benign or malignant (Fig 10–30).[34] The malignant giant cell tumor is quite aggressive and rapidly fatal, behaving like the usual Paget's sarcoma.[34] However, the benign type is not as aggressive as those developing in bone and affected by Paget's disease. The prognosis is good in this type of tumor.[35] If a giant cell tumor develops, CT will show destructive changes along with a soft tissue mass.[36] Biopsy should be done to differentiate this finding from sarcomatous changes.

PRIMARY BENIGN BONE TUMORS

Primary benign osseous tumors of the pelvis and spine may be chondrogenic, osteogenic, or fibrogenic. They may also originate in vascular, neurogenic, or lipogenic elements within the bone.[37] However, only about 2% of all bone tumors in the pelvis are benign. Conventional radiography and tomography are essential in the evaluation of these patients. When the lesion is located in an anatomically complex region such as the acetabulum, cross-sectional imaging becomes essential for diagnosis.

Osteochondroma

Osteochondroma, which is the most common benign bone tumor, is rare in the pelvis and usually occurs in the metaphyseal region of long bones. Radiologically, the periosteal surface and the cortex of the tumor are contiguous with the underlying bone, as is the medullary cavity. The cauliflower shape of the tumor, with the cartilaginous matrix, and lack of a significant soft tissue mass are helpful signs for making the diagnosis (Fig 10–31). Less than 1% of these tumors become malignant.

Enchondroma

Enchondroma is a lesion of mature hyaline cartilage and can occur at any age and in any bone. It appears as a well-marginated lytic lesion, often with stippled calcification (Fig 10–5). Pathologic fracture, scalloping, or lytic areas in a mineralized lesion are suspicious for malignancy.

Chondroblastoma

Chondroblastoma is usually seen as a well-defined, lucent lesion in the epiphysis of a long bone in the immature skeleton. However, in adults it may occur in unusual sites such as the innominate bone or scapula.

Osteoid Osteoma

Osteoid osteoma is commonly seen as a sclerotic lesion with a nidus in the proximal femur. It is also a common tumor in the spine (Fig 10–32), where it may clinically mimic lumbar disk disease.

Osteoblastoma

Osteoblastomas are also common in the spine. They are usually expansile, and about one half are partially mineralized (Fig 10–33).[38]

Hemangioma

Hemangiomas are the most common spinal benign vascular bone tumor. They occur more frequently in females (Fig 10–34). The spectrum of symptoms can range from asymptomatic to symptoms of cord compression.[32]

Giant Cell Tumors

Giant cell tumors make up about 60% of benign sacral lesions and are seen more frequently in females.[39] Radiologically, they are characterized by lytic lesions with ill- or well-defined margins and occasionally a soft tissue mass is seen (Figs 10–35 and 10–36). This tumor almost always presents as an isolated neoplasm, and its differentiation from aneurysmal bone cyst (Fig 10–37), metastases, plasmacytoma, or chordoma may be difficult. It has been associated with Paget's disease (Fig 10–30).[34, 35] Giant cell tumors can be benign or malignant, the latter quite aggressive and usually fatal and the former entailing a very good prognosis. Treatment is surgery and occasionally radiation therapy. However, there is a chance of postirradiation sarcoma in nearly 20% of the patients. More recently, these tumors have been treated with arterial embolization with good response.[40] In these cases, there will be a gradual increase in the density of tumor, resulting in tumoral calcification (Fig 10–36).

OSSEOUS METASTASES

Metastases to the skeleton account for approximately 65% of all malignant bone tumors in adults.[2] Depending on the primary neoplasm, the lesions are lytic (Fig 10–38), blastic, or a mixture of both (Fig 10–39), and they can be single or multiple. Lytic osseous lesions are commonly seen in patients with lung, kidney, thyroid, and breast carcinoma and in those with melanoma. The blastic metastases are mostly noted in prostatic and gastrointestinal malignancies. The spectrum of differential diagnosis will significantly vary depending on the age of the patient and whether there is a single bone lesion or multiple bone lesions.

Radionuclide bone scan remains the leading diagnostic modality for screening a cancer patient to rule out skeletal metastasis. However, to increase the specificity of an abnormal finding on scintigraphy, correlative radiographs should be obtained. Since occasionally the osseous metastasis is associated with a soft tissue mass, CT or MRI is helpful to demonstrate the extent of the mass (see Fig 10–38), especially when the mass is in the neighborhood of a major neurovascular bundle.

PRIMARY SOFT TISSUE NEOPLASMS

The soft tissue neoplasms can be simply classified, in accordance with guidelines established by Enzinger, on the basis of histologic type (Table 10–1).[41] The common benign tumors are fibroma, lipoma, leiomyoma, hemangioma, and lymphangioma. The most common primary malignant soft tissue neoplasms are malignant fibrous histiocytoma, liposarcoma, clear cell sarcoma, and epithelioid sarcoma. The other malignant tumors include soft tissue Ewing's sarcoma, leiomyosarcoma, synovial sarcoma, and soft tissue osteosarcoma. Early diagnosis of these neoplasms is of utmost importance since most of them are aggressive and tend to have early metastases.

Depending on the histology, size, location, and stage of the tumor, the survival rate varies. A five-year survival rate of 64% was reported for malignant fibrous histiocytoma,[42] and a ten-year survival rate of 11% was reported for synovial sarcoma.[43] Radical local excision is often the treatment of choice, and there is good evidence to indicate that the nature and adequacy of surgery have a strong influence on local recurrence rates and on the development of metastases.[44–46]

Soft tissue neoplasms are often difficult to identify by conventional radiologic techniques, mainly because the inherent density of these tumors may be similar to that of adjacent normal tissue. Furthermore, in certain anatomically complex areas of the body, such as the pelvis, paraspinal region, and abdominal wall, these tumors are rather difficult to evaluate by routine radiography

TABLE 10–1.

Histologic Classification of Soft Tissue Tumors*

Histologic Classification	Example(s)
Fibrous tissue	Fibroma, fibrosarcoma
Fibrohistiocytic	Fibrous histiocytoma, malignant fibrous histiocytoma
Adipose tissue	Lipoma, angiolipoma, myelolipoma, liposarcoma
Muscle tissue	Leiomyoma, leiomyosarcoma
Blood vessel	Hemangioma, hemangiosarcoma
Lymph vessel	Lymphangioma, lymphangiosarcoma
Synovial tissue	Synovial sarcoma
Mesothelial tissue	Mesothelioma
Peripheral nerve	Neuroma, neurofibroma, malignant schwannoma
Autonomic ganglia	Ganglioneuroma, neuroblastoma
Paraganglionic structure	Paraganglioma
Cartilage and bone-forming tissues	Extraskeletal osteoma and osteosarcoma, soft tissue chondrosarcoma

*Adapted from Enzinger F.M., Weiss S.W.: *Soft Tissue Tumors*. St. Louis, C.V. Mosby Co., 1983, pp. 5–7.

because of overlying bowel and other structures.

Sonography, CT, and MRI offer a noninvasive approach to the diagnosis of soft tissue neoplasms. Ultrasonography is capable of detecting the size, depth, and extent of these tumors. Because of differences in acoustic impedance, this modality can determine the internal consistency of the lesion. The differentiation of cystic, solid, and complex masses can usually be made, depending on the location and size of the lesion.[47] The size and extent of the lesion are very important in those patients who are to undergo follow-up radiation therapy or chemotherapy. Sonography cannot distinguish a malignant from a benign neoplasm inasmuch as either can be anechoic or seen as a complex mass.[48, 49] Because of the density differences between fat and soft tissue on CT, this modality allows separation of muscle and fascial plane and provides a cross-sectional image of normal and abnormal tissues. A problem arises with CT when a tumor that is small or that is isodense compared with normal structures is to be imaged in an anatomical setting of insufficient fat. Detailed knowledge of soft tissue anatomy allows precision in the confirmation, localization, and characterization of abnormal processes.

In soft tissue neoplasms, CT is more than 90% accurate in the prediction of resectability and in the detection of recurrent tumor.[50] Caution must be exercised, however, when one is attempting to differentiate benign from malignant tumors solely on the basis of CT appearance, because the CT characteristics usually seen with benign tumors are occasionally present with malignant tumors, and vice versa. However, the CT appearance is occasionally so distinctive that a specific diagnosis can be suggested. Weekes et al. studied 84 patients with soft tissue neoplasms and reported that CT was able to demonstrate the lesion or lesions in each case and to provide adequate anatomical definition in most of the cases.[3] Histology was often difficult to predict from CT images, but the authors were able to differentiate benign from malignant lesions in 88% of patients. Correct histologic prediction may be possible in cases of lipoma, hemangioma, and sometimes liposarcoma. Computed tomography may be helpful in the evaluation of adjacent bony invasion by primary soft tissue tumors, although this invasion happens very infrequently. In fact, even in very large and aggressive soft tissue neoplasms the adjacent bone usually remains intact.[3] When there is bony destruction, the origin of the lesion may be within the bone, with the soft tissue involvement representing extension.

Magnetic resonance is able to demonstrate soft tissue neoplasms with a superior contrast resolution and the flexibility of multiplanar imaging.[51] The former results from differences in proton density and in T_1 and T_2 relaxation times. Whereas fat, muscles, tendons, ligaments, nerves, and blood vessels each have different MRI characteristics, the benign tumors—with the exception of desmoids, hemangiomas, and a condition such as arteriovenous malformation—have fairly characteristic features. They are usually homogeneous and well marginated, with increased signal intensity on T_2-weighted images (white) and decreased on T_1-weighted images (dark).[5] Most malignant soft tissue tumors are nonhomogeneous, with mixed signal intensity on both T_1- and T_2-weighted images. This appearance may be secondary to tumor necrosis, calcification, or a particular type of tumor matrix (osteoid, fibrous, or cartilaginous). However, adipose tissue or fat-containing neoplasms, because of the high content of mobile protons as well as short T_1 and T_2 relaxation times, are characterized by high signal intensity. As a result, they appear white on both T_1- and T_2-weighted images.[52]

For these reasons, MRI is becoming more important in the workup of patients with soft tissue tumors. It has been reported to be equal or superior to CT in distinguishing tumors from normal soft tissue.[53] With CT, the density of a soft tissue mass is often similar to that of muscle; therefore, in addition to the use of iodine, careful comparison with the opposite sites is necessary, and proper window width and level must be applied to see the lesion. However, the incidence of defining the anatomical extent of a neoplasm is higher with MRI because of greater soft tissue contrast and the capability of multiplanar imaging.[51] Fluid might be suspected in a lesion with very long T_1 and T_2 relaxation times. Such lesions therefore appear relatively dark on T_1-weighted images and become substantially brighter on T_2-weighted images. Most of the soft tissue neoplasms, particularly the malignant ones, because of edema and a mixed tissue structure will display an intermediate signal intensity that will be different on T_1- and T_2-weighted images.[54] It has become clearly understood that the T_1 and T_2 relaxation times are prolonged in neoplastic tissue.[29]

Following are brief descriptions of the common malignant and benign primary soft tissue neoplasms.

Malignant Fibrous Histiocytoma

Malignant fibrous histiocytoma is a high-grade bone (Fig 10–40) and soft tissue (Fig 10–41) neoplasm that metastasizes quickly.[55] It is probably the most common soft tissue sarcoma in older patients. A primary bone malignant fibrous histiocytoma usually presents as a lytic lesion, sometimes with lymph node metastasis. In cases of primary tumor in soft tissue, most of the imaging modalities can be used for evaluation, although ultrasound is probably the fastest method of identifying the size of a superficially located mass (Fig 10–41).[4] Magnetic resonance imaging has been advocated in the evaluation of soft tissue tumors; it can demonstrate with clarity the local extent of the neoplasm and the internal structure of the mass and, by means of different signal intensities, display different tissue components.[52]

Lipoma

The most common benign soft tissue tumor is lipoma, which frequently occurs in the shoulders, neck, and extremities. Lipomas also may be seen in the pelvis (Fig 10–42). They are usually well-defined, encapsulated tumors with uniform low density.[56]

Liposarcoma

Liposarcomas usually show a heterogeneous density on CT. However, the density and CT appearance in these tumors depend on the degree of differentiation. Those that are poorly differentiated are between water and fat density.[56] This tumor is widely discussed in Chapter 9.

Fibrosarcoma

Like liposarcomas, fibrosarcomas show a heterogeneous pattern on CT. They are difficult to differentiate from other sarcomas or even from such benign conditions as hemorrhage or infection (Fig 10–43).

Rhabdomyosarcoma

Rhabdomyosarcomas follow liposarcomas and fibrosarcomas in order of frequency in soft tissue. Apart from embryonal botryoid rhabdomyosarcomas, these tumors are found primarily in the extremities. Necrosis, hemorrhage, and cystic transformation can be the predominant features of the tumor in the form that occurs in adults. Rhabdomy-

osarcomas can be localized or have a very aggressive and infiltrative appearance on CT and MRI (Fig 10–44).

Hemangioma

Hemangiomas are not infrequent within the soft tissue or muscle (Fig 10–45). There are capillary and cavernous types, which may be calcified.

Soft Tissue Ewing's Sarcoma

Soft tissue Ewing's sarcomas present a fairly uniform histologic picture that is indistinguishable from that of osseous Ewing's sarcomas. They are friable tumors, commonly with areas of necrosis, cystic formation, and hemorrhage. The mean age of patients is about 25 years, and the tumors grow very quickly,[37] often without bony abnormality. There are bony changes in almost 10% of cases, with periosteal reaction, cortical thickening, erosion, or simply increased density of the adjacent bone. In most cases, CT will show the tumor mass, the relation of the mass to adjacent organs, and changes following treatment.[38] These tumors have a propensity to metastasize to lungs and bones.

Neurofibroma

Neurofibromas are usually seen along the distribution of major neurovascular bundles in the paraspinal area, retroperitoneum, pelvis, and subcutaneous region and can be associated with bony lesions (Fig 10–46). In the pelvis or spine, they can be associated with enlargement of the neural foramina (Fig 10–47),[57] thickening of the nerve roots,[58] thecal sac ectasia, and vertebral deformity (Fig 10–48). If the tumor is predominantly subcutaneous, or when it has caused lymphatic obstruction, it will be associated with elephantiasis (Fig 10–49).[59]

Neurogenic Sarcoma

The neurogenic sarcoma may originate in either the fibroblastic elements of the nerve sheath (neurofibrosarcoma) or the Schwann's cell (malignant schwannoma or malignant neurilemoma). The pathologic determination of this origin is difficult. The tumor may present as a mass, which in some cases invades adjacent bone or soft tissue (Fig 10–50). The radiologic differentiation of presacral neurogenic sarcoma from chordoma is difficult (Figs 10–51 and 10–52).

Extraskeletal Chondrosarcoma

Extraskeletal chondrosarcomas are either myxoid or mesenchymal in type; the latter are highly malignant, occur in younger patients, and in most cases produce metastases. Myxoid extraskeletal chondrosarcomas occur mostly in the extremities, whereas those of mesenchymal type are commonly seen in the head and neck[60] and less frequently in the thighs. The mesenchymal type may be associated with calcification or bone formation on radiography. As in other types of soft tissue sarcoma, CT and MRI are helpful in assessing the extent of tumor and in evaluating response to therapy (Fig 10–53).

Hemangiopericytoma

Hemangiopericytoma is primarily a tumor of adult life; it is rare in children. The growth is very slow, and the tumor is usually large at diagnosis. There is some association with hypoglycemia.[61] Hemangiopericytomas are very hypervascular and commonly occur in the lower extremities and pelvis.[62] Radiologically, they present as a soft tissue mass, infrequently with areas of calcification, and often on angiography or radionuclide flow study they are very vascular (Fig 10–54).

SOFT TISSUE METASTASES

Direct soft tissue extension of malignancy is more common than metastases. However, we have seen soft tissue and muscle metastases from such primaries as colon, kidney, breast, ovary, and bladder neoplasms (Fig 10–55).

DIAPHRAGM: COMPLEXITIES AT THE THORACOABDOMINAL JUNCTION

The diaphragm is the main muscle of respiration and the transitional interface from thorax to the abdomen (thoracoabdominal junction). It is basically a central tendon (a crescentic aponeurosis) with muscular insertions arising from the sternal, costal, and lumbar regions.[63]

Transdiaphragmatic pathways exist between the abdomen and thorax for the spread of disease (benign and malignant), but actual primary tumor involvement of the diaphragm is rare.[64] Routine radiographic studies can provide useful data in the

evaluation of the thoracoabdominal junction, but in many cases this region is totally obscured on such images (Fig 10–56). Therefore, CT demonstration of the diaphragm may be crucial in defining the thoracoabdominal junction. However, transaxial analysis of this junction by CT can be a difficult task.

Normal Computed Tomography Anatomy at the Thoracoabdominal Junction

The dome-shaped hemidiaphragm on CT is seen in cross-section as a series of enlarging concentric circles or ovals as one proceeds caudally. At the thoracoabdominal junction, structures within the circle or oval are intraabdominal (subphrenic) and those outside are within the thorax.[65] Direct observation of a hemidiaphragm as an interface or stripe depends on the difference in contrast between what is peripheral or central to that hemidiaphragm. In normal cases, observation of an interface or stripe usually depends on the presence of air peripheral to the hemidiaphragm and fat central to the hemidiaphragm (i.e., within the abdomen) (Fig 10–57).

Abnormal Computed Tomography Anatomy at the Thoracoabdominal Junction

In disease states that produce pleural effusion or effusions, ascites (or a subphrenic abscess), or both, locating the diaphragm and distinguishing pleural fluid from ascites can become very difficult, and a number of useful signs have been proposed for such evaluations (i.e., diaphragm, interface, bare areas, and displaced crus signs).[65–68] However, no single sign is reliable in all cases, and combinations of these signs may be necessary in certain cases (Figs 10–58 to 10–60). Little attention has been paid to an additional sign, namely, bare area of the spleen, that can be very valuable in evaluating the left hemidiaphragm in the presence of effusion, ascites, or a left subphrenic abscess (Figs 10–60 and 10–61).[69]

Volume loss within the lower lobes is common in the presence of pleural fluid (see Fig 10–59). With large effusions, aspects of other lobes may also exhibit volume loss (Fig 10–62). The role of the inferior pulmonary ligament as a tether of the lower lobe to the mediastinum and hemidiaphragm is paramount in understanding patterns of lower lobe volume loss (Fig 10–62).[70] Subpulmonic effusions in conjunction with lower lobe volume loss can mimic the diaphragm and lead to the incorrect localization of a disease process.[71, 72] Understanding the relationship of the inferior pulmonary ligament to the lower lobe and diaphragm, together with careful evaluation of images cranial and caudal to the questionable region, often resolves the problem (Figs 10–63 and 10–64).

Ultrasound Versus Computed Tomography Re-formations

Pathologic processes at the thoracoabdominal junction not resolved by routine techniques can be evaluated by CT or ultrasound. Some authors hold that ultrasound is the most useful technique for localizing disease at the right thoracoabdominal junction because it can directly image the diaphragm in a sagittal plane (Fig 10–65).[73] However, comparable evaluation of the left junction is often unsuccessful, and CT evaluation is required. Other authors have successfully evaluated many such complexities with only transaxial CT imaging.[65] If sufficient transaxial CT images are available, re-formation analysis (coronal, sagittal, or oblique) may be perfectly adequate in defining a thoracoabdominal complexity without resorting to ultrasound (Fig 10–66).[74] Combined CT and ultrasound evaluations should be performed only when absolutely necessary.

Tumor Analysis at the Thoracoabdominal Junction

Complexities at the thoracoabdominal junction due primarily to pleural fluid, ascites, or both were previously discussed. Complex tumor analysis may be far more extensive, involving large aspects of the chest wall extending from high in the thorax to the thoracoabdominal junction (Fig 10–67). Anterior tumor involvement at the junction may actually invade through the tissues of the anterior abdominal wall (Fig 10–68). Tumor recurrence within the thorax may invade through the diaphragm and involve the abdomen or originate within the abdomen and invade into or through the diaphragm (Figs 10–69 and 10–70). Primary tumors of the diaphragm are rare, but some tumors (e.g., mesothelioma) appear to utilize the diaphragm as one of the serosal surfaces by which the tumor extends and invades (Fig 10–71).

REFERENCES

1. Dahlin D.C.: *Bone Tumors: General Aspects and Data on 6,221 Cases*, ed. 3. Springfield, Ill., Charles C Thomas, Publisher, 1978.
2. del Regato J.A., Spjut H.J. (eds.): *Ackerman and del Regato's Cancer: Diagnosis, Treatment and Prognosis*, ed. 5. St. Louis, C.V. Mosby Co., 1977.
3. Weekes R.G., McLeod R.A., Reiman H.M., et al.: CT of soft-tissue neoplasms. *AJR* 144:355–360, 1985.
4. Yiu-Chiu V.S., Chiu L.C.: Complementary values of ultrasound and computed tomography in the evaluation of musculoskeletal masses. *RadioGraphics* 3:46–81, 1981.
5. Berquist T.H.: Bone and soft tissue tumors, in Berquist T.H., Ehman R.L., Richardson M.L. (eds.): *Magnetic Resonance of the Musculoskeletal System*. New York, Raven Press, 1987, pp. 85–108.
6. Dahlin D.C., Beabout J.W.: Dedifferentiation of low-grade chondrosarcomas. *Cancer* 28:461–466, 1971.
7. Sim F.H. (ed.): *Diagnosis and Treatment of Bone Tumors: A Team Approach*. Mayo Clinic Monograph. Thorofare, N.J., Slack, 1983.
8. Spjut H.J., Fechner R.C., Ackerman L.V.: Tumors of bone and cartilage, in *Atlas of Tumor Pathology*. Washington, D.C., Armed Forces Institute of Pathology, 1971, ser. 2, fasc. 5, suppl.
9. Huvos A.G., Rosen G., Bretsky S.S., et al.: Telangiectatic osteogenic sarcoma: a clinicopathologic study of 124 patients. *Cancer* 49:1679–1689, 1982.
10. Greditzer H.G. III, McLeod R.A., Unni K.K., et al.: Bone sarcomas in Paget disease. *Radiology* 146: 327–333, 1983.
11. Weatherby R.P., Dahlin D.C., Ivins J.C.: Postradiation sarcoma of bone: review of 78 Mayo Clinic cases. *Mayo Clin. Proc.* 56:294–306, 1981.
12. deSantos L.A., Bernardino M.E., Murray J.A.: Computed tomography in the evaluation of osteosarcoma: experience with 25 cases. *AJR* 132:535–540, 1979.
13. Shirkhoda A., Jaffe N., Wallace S., et al.: Computed tomography of osteosarcoma after intraarterial chemotherapy. *AJR* 144:95–99, 1985.
14. Lavallee G., Lemarbre L., Bouchard R., et al.: Ewing's sarcoma in adults. *J. Can. Assoc. Radiol.* 30: 223–227, 1979.
15. Whitehouse G.H., Griffiths G.J.: Roentgenologic aspects of spinal involvement by primary and metastatic Ewing's tumor. *J. Can. Assoc. Radiol.* 27:290–297, 1976.
16. Pilepich M.V., Vietti T.J., Nesbit M.E., et al.: Ewing's sarcoma of the vertebral column. *Int. J. Radiat. Oncol. Biol. Phys.* 7:27–31, 1979.
17. Ginaldi S., deSantos L.A.: Computed tomography in the evaluation of small round cell tumors of bone. *Radiology* 134:441–446, 1980.
18. Braunstein E.M.: Hodgkin disease of bone: radiographic correlation with the histological classification. *Radiology* 137:643–646, 1980.
19. Pear B.L.: Skeletal manifestations of the lymphomas and leukemias. *Semin. Roentgenol.* 9:229–240, 1974.
20. Vieta J.O., Friedell H.L., Craver L.F.: A survey of Hodgkin's disease and lymphosarcoma in bone. *Radiology* 39:1–14, 1942.
21. Firooznia H., Pinto R.S., Lin J.P., et al.: Chordoma: radiologic evaluation of 20 cases. *AJR* 127:797–805, 1976.

22. Utne J.R., Pugh D.G.: The roentgenologic aspects of chordoma. *AJR* 74:593–608, 1955.

23. Rosenthal D.I., Scott J.A., Mankin H.J., et al.: Sacrococcygeal chordoma: magnetic resonance imaging and computed tomography. *AJR* 145:143–147, 1985.

24. Axtell L.M., Hyers M.H.: Contrasts in survival of black and white cancer patients 1960–1973. *JNCI* 60:1209–1215, 1978.

25. Young J.L. Jr., Asire A.J., Pollack E.S.: *SEER Program: Cancer Incidence and Mortality in the United States, 1973–1976.* DHEW publication no. (NIH)78–1837. Bethesda, Md., National Cancer Institute, 1978.

26. Kyle R.A.: Multiple myeloma: a review of 869 cases. *Mayo Clinic Proc.* 50:29–40, 1975.

27. Gompels B.M., Votaw M.L., Martel W.: Correlation of radiological manifestations of multiple myeloma with immunoglobulin abnormalities and prognosis. *Radiology* 104:509–514, 1972.

28. Zimmer W.D., Berquist T.H., McLeod R.A., et al.: Magnetic resonance imaging of bone tumors. Comparison with CT. *Radiology* 155:709–718, 1985.

29. Wahner H.W., Kyle R.A., Beabout J.W.: Scintigraphic evaluation of the skeleton in multiple myeloma. *Mayo Clin. Proc.* 55:739–746, 1980.

30. Schreiman J.S., McLeod R.A., Kyle R.A., et al.: Multiple myeloma: evaluation by CT. *Radiology* 154:483–486, 1985.

31. Woodruff R.K., Whittle J.M., Malpas J.S.: Solitary plasmacytoma. I: Extramedullary soft tissue plasmacytoma. *Cancer* 43:2340–2343, 1979.

32. Unni K.K., Ivins J.C., Beabout J.W., et al.: Hemangioma, hemangiopericytoma, and hemangioendothelioma (angiosarcoma) of bone. *Cancer* 27:1403–1414, 1971.

33. Greenfield G.B.: *Radiology of Bone Diseases,* ed. 3. Philadelphia, J.B. Lippincott Co., 1980, pp. 108–123, 533–558.

34. Hutter R.V.P., Foote F.W., Frazell E.L., et al.: Giant cell tumors complicating Paget's disease of bone. *Cancer* 16:1044–1056, 1963.

35. Schwajowica F., Slullitel I.: Giant cell tumor associated with Paget's disease of bone. *J. Bone Joint Surg. (Am.)* 48:1340–1348, 1966.

36. Francis R., Lewis E.: CT demonstration of giant cell tumor complicating Paget disease. *J. Comput. Assist. Tomogr.* 7:917–918, 1983.

37. Sim F.H., Unni K.K., Wold L.E., et al.: Benign bone tumors, in Sim F.H. (ed.): *Diagnosis and Treatment of Bone Tumors: A Team Approach.* Mayo Clinic Monograph. Thorofare, N.J., Slack, 1983, pp. 109–151.

38. Marsh B.W., Bonfiglio M., Brady L.P., et al.: Benign osteoblastoma: range of manifestations. *J. Bone Joint Surg. (Am.)* 57:1–9, 1975.

39. Campanacci M., Giunti A., Olmi R.: Giant cell tumors of bone: a study of 209 cases with long-term follow up in 130. *Ital. J. Orthop. Traumatol.* 1:249–277, 1975.

40. Eftekhari F., Wallace S., Chuang V.P., et al.: Intraarterial management of giant-cell tumors of the spine in children. *Pediatr. Radiol.* 12:289–293, 1982.

41. Enzinger F.M., Weiss S.W.: *Soft Tissue Tumors.* St. Louis, C.V. Mosby Co., 1983, pp. 5–7.

42. Soule E.H., Enriquez P.: Atypical fibrous histiocytoma, malignant fibrous histiocytoma, malignant histiocytoma, and epithelioid sarcoma: a comparative study of 65 tumors. *Cancer* 30:128–143, 1972.

43. Cadman N.L., Soule E.H., Kelly P.J.: Synovial sarcoma: an analysis of 134 tumors. *Cancer* 18:613–627, 1965.

44. Martin R.G., Butler J.J., Albores-Saavedra J.: Soft tissue tumors: surgical treatment and results, in *Tumors of Bone and Soft Tissue.* Chicago, Year Book Medical Publishers, 1965, pp. 333–347.

45. Shiu M.H., Castro E.B., Hajdu S.I., et al.: Surgical treatment of 297 soft tissue sarcomas of the lower extremity. *Ann. Surg.* 182:597–602, 1975.

46. Simon M.A., Enneking W.F.: The management of soft-tissue sarcomas of the extremities. *J. Bone Joint Surg. (Am.)* 58:317–327, 1976.

47. Lindell M.M., Wallace S.: Soft tissue tumors of the appendicular skeleton, in Bragg D.G., Rubin P., Youker J.E. (eds.): *Oncologic Imaging.* New York, Pergamon Press, 1985, pp. 587–627.

48. Goldberg B.B.: Ultrasound evaluation of superficial masses. *Journal of Clinical Ultrasound* 3:91–94, 1975.

49. Hayama I., Fukuma H., Masuda S., et al.: Ultrasonic tomography of tumors in the soft tissue and bone [meeting abstract]. *Nippon Seikeigeka Gakkai Zasshi* 67 (special), 1977.

50. Golding S.J., Husband J.E.: The role of computed tomography in the management of soft tissue sarcomas. *Br. J. Radiol.* 55:740–747, 1982.

51. Weekes R.G., Berquist T.H., McLeod R.A., et al.: Magnetic resonance imaging of soft tissue tumors: comparison with CT. *Magn. Reson. Imaging* 3:345–352, 1985.

52. Reiser M., Rupp N., Heller H.J., et al.: MR-tomography in the diagnosis of malignant soft-tissue tumours. *Eur. J. Radiol.* 4:288–293, 1984.

53. Hudson T.M., Hamlin D.J., Enneking W.F., et al.: Magnetic resonance imaging of bone and soft tissue tumors: early experience in 31 patients compared to CT. *Skeletal Radiol.* 13:134–146, 1985.

54. Moon K.L., Genant H.K., Helms C.A., et al.: Musculoskeletal applications of nuclear magnetic resonance. *Radiology* 147:161–171, 1983.

55. Dahlin D.C., Unni K.K., Matsuno T.: Malignant (fibrous) histiocytoma of bone—fact or fancy? *Cancer* 39:1508–1516, 1977.

56. Hunter J.C., Johnston W.H., Genant H.K.: Computed tomography evaluation of fatty tumors of the somatic soft tissues: clinical utility and radiologic-pathologic correlation. *Skeletal Radiol.* 4:79–91, 1979.

57. Shirkhoda A., Brashear H.E.R., Zelenik M.E., et al.:

Sacral abnormalities—computed tomography versus conventional radiography. *CT* 8:41–51, 1984.

58. Daneman A., Mancer K., Sonley M.: CT appearance of thickened nerves in neurofibromatosis. *AJR* 141:899–900, 1983.

59. Holbert B.L., Lamki L.M., Holbert J.M.: Uptake of bone scanning agent in neurofibromatosis. *Clin. Nucl. Med.* 12:66–67, 1987.

60. Guccion J.G., Font R.L., Enzinger F.M., et al.: Extraskeletal mesenchymal chondrosarcoma. *Arch. Pathol.* 15:336–340, 1973.

61. Bommer G., Altenaehr F., Kuehnau J. Jr., et al.: Ultrastructure of hemangiopericytoma associated with paraneoplastic hypoglycemia. *Zeitschrift fuer Krebforschung und Klinische Onkologie* 85:231–241, 1976.

62. Enzinger F.M., Smith B.H.: Hemangiopericytoma. An analysis of 106 cases. *Hum. Pathol.* 7:61–82, 1976.

63. Romanes G.J. (ed.) *Cunningham's Textbook of Anatomy,* ed. 12. New York, Oxford University Press, 1981, pp. 352–354.

64. Naidich D.P., Zerhouni E.A., Siegelman S.S.: The diaphragm, in Naidich D.P., Zerhouni E.A., Siegelman S.S. (eds.): *Computed Tomography of the Thorax.* New York, Raven Press, 1984, pp. 305–314.

65. Alexander E.S., Proto A.V., Clark R.A.: CT differentiation of subphrenic abscess and pleural effusion. *AJR* 140:47–51, 1983.

66. Teplick J.G., Teplick S.K., Goodman L., et al.: The interface sign: a computed tomographic sign for distinguishing pleural and intra-abdominal fluid. *Radiology* 144:359–362, 1982.

67. Griffin D.J., Gross B.H., McCracken S., et al.: Observations on CT differentiation of pleural and peritoneal fluid. *J. Comput. Assist. Tomogr.* 8:24–28, 1984.

68. Dwyer A.: The displaced crus: a sign for distinguishing between pleural fluid and ascites on computed tomography. *J. Comput. Assist. Tomogr.* 2:598–599, 1978.

69. Vibhakar S.D., Bellon B.M.: The bare area of the spleen: a constant feature of the ascitic abdomen. *AJR* 141:953–955, 1984.

70. Rost R.C., Proto A.V.: Inferior pulmonary ligament: computed tomographic appearance. *Radiology* 148:479–483, 1983.

71. Proto A.V., Rost R.C.: CT of the thorax: pitfalls in interpretation. *RadioGraphics* 5:792–796, 1985.

72. Federle M.P., Mark A.S., Guillaumin E.S.: CT of subpulmonic pleural effusions and atelectasis: criteria for differentiation from subphrenic fluid. *AJR* 146:685–689, 1986.

73. Bedi D.G., Fagan C.J., Hayden C.K.: The opaque right hemithorax: identifying the diaphragm with ultrasound. *Tex. Med.* 81:37–42, 1985.

74. Foley W.D., Lawson T.L., Berland L.L., et al.: Reformatted coronal display of upper abdominal computed tomography: comparison with ultrasonography. *J. Comput. Assist. Tomogr.* 5:496–502, 1981.

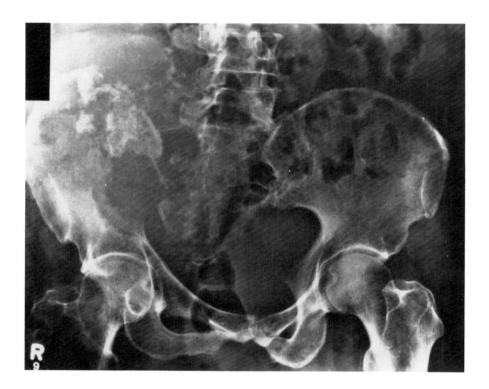

FIG 10–1.

Iliac chondrosarcoma. This 49-year-old man presented with a large mass in the right lower abdomen and pelvis. A mass was first noted approximately seven years ago in the right hip area, but during the last year it has enlarged and made him uncomfortable. He saw a physician, and after biopsy the diagnosis of chondrosarcoma was established.

The pelvic radiograph, obtained just after the patient sought medical attention, shows remarkable destruction of the right iliac wing, including the sacrum and fifth lumbar vertebra; a large soft tissue mass extends above the iliac crest into the lower abdomen. The mass has areas of discrete punctate and flocculate calcification. The deformity of the pelvis is related to loss of sacroiliac joint integration by tumor destruction and superior subluxation of the right pelvis.

Chondrosarcoma is the most likely diagnosis with these findings, especially with this calcification pattern. Occasionally, metastasis, particularly in mucinous adenocarcinoma and prostatic carcinoma, shows spotty calcification. Multiple myeloma with amyloid formation and bone lesions in primary amyloidosis can also calcify with a spotty pattern similar to that in this case.

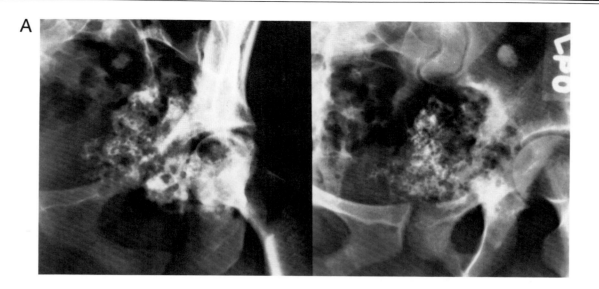

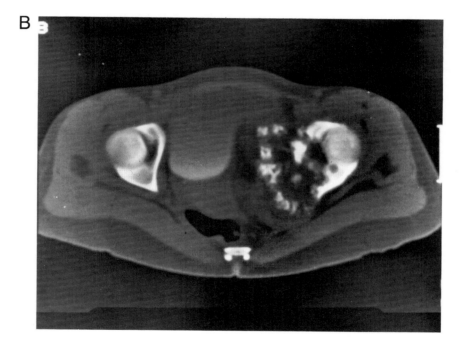

FIG 10–2.

Acetabular chondrosarcoma. This 28-year-old woman presented with gradual-onset pain in the left hip. A mass was palpated on vaginal examination.

A, the oblique view of the left hip shows destruction of the medial acetabulum, and a soft tissue mass containing areas of curvilinear, or rings and arcs of, calcification. This signifies mature chondroid matrix with enchondral bone formation.

B, the CT scan demonstrates the extent of the soft tissue mass and bony destruction. The cartilaginous rings and arcs of calcification are again seen. Other pelvic organs, including the bladder, uterus, and rectum, are displaced by the mass.

This pattern of rings and arcs of calcification is typical for chondroid lesions. Since there is such a large soft tissue nonmineralized component in this location, chondrosarcoma is the most likely diagnosis. Rarely, osteochondromas occur at this site with this same pattern.

Percutaneous biopsy findings were consistent with chondrosarcoma.

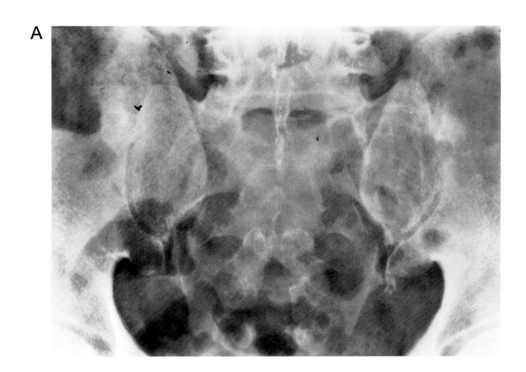

FIG 10–3.
Sacral chondrosarcoma. This 56-year-old man presented with dull left hip pain that radiated to the left leg and that was associated with numbness of the left big toe. Myelography for disk disease was normal.

A, this pelvic film was initially reported as normal. Evaluation of the sacrum is indeed difficult in this image because of overlying intestinal contents. However, the left sacroiliac joint is minimally widened inferiorly and shows punctate calcification, and an ill-defined destruction of the left middle and lower sacrum and ilium can be noted.

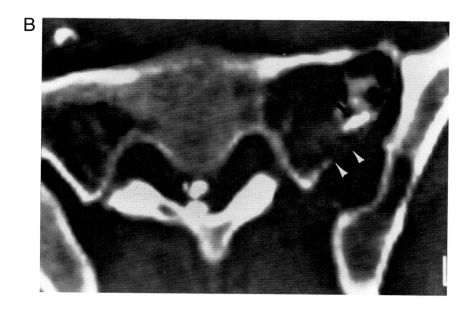

B, pelvic CT shows that within the upper left sacral ala there is a destructive lesion that contains calcification *(arrow).* Also, there is thinning of the adjacent cortical bone *(arrowheads),* widening of the sacroiliac joint, and lysis in the adjacent ilium.

With the calcification and extent of lesion shown on CT, one should first consider chondrosarcoma with metastasis, chondroblastic osteosarcoma, and amyloid formation, the last the least likely (see Fig 10–1). With the joint widening and bony destruction on both sides of the joint, as shown on the CT scan, one could consider soft tissue tumors arising in the joint or adjacent soft tissue. Such lesions could represent synovial sarcoma or other soft tissue sarcomas that sometimes calcify.

In this case chondrosarcoma was diagnosed on percutaneous biopsy. Treatment was irradiation.

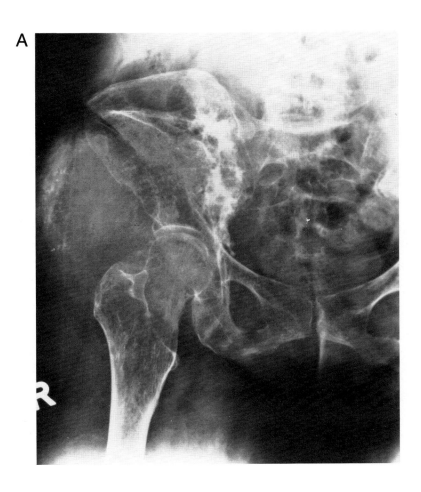

FIG 10–4.
Malignant chondrosarcomatous transformation within an osteochondroma. This 56-year-old woman with congenital
multiple exostosis had asymptomatic osteochondroma of
the iliac bones, pubis, right ulna, and proximal and distal
femurs, among other bones. When the patient was 54, a
tender mass was noted in the right pelvis, and this area was
explored. Chondrosarcoma was diagnosed. After surgery,
the disease was well controlled by local irradiation. However, two years later the patient noted an enlarging mass
and radiographs showed involvement of the proximal femur.

A, on the plain film, there is a large mass that involves
the proximal femur and right iliac wing and that extends laterally into the adjacent muscles. It shows spotty calcifica-

tion. Proximal femoral widening and other smaller exostoses
are noted in the pubic bones. The large sclerotic area in the
region of the sacroiliac joint is from prior treatment.

B and **C,** CT scans reveal complete destruction of the
right anterior acetabulum and a large mass with areas of
calcification. The mass extends both medially **(B)** and laterally **(C)** within the pelvis. Both the sacrum and right iliac
wing are partially destroyed. The patient underwent extensive tumor resection.

D, incidentally, the benign osteochondromas of the
proximal tibia and distal femur are seen in the same lower
extremity. There is also marked soft tissue wasting consistent with the chronic dysfunction and poor utilization of the
extremity.

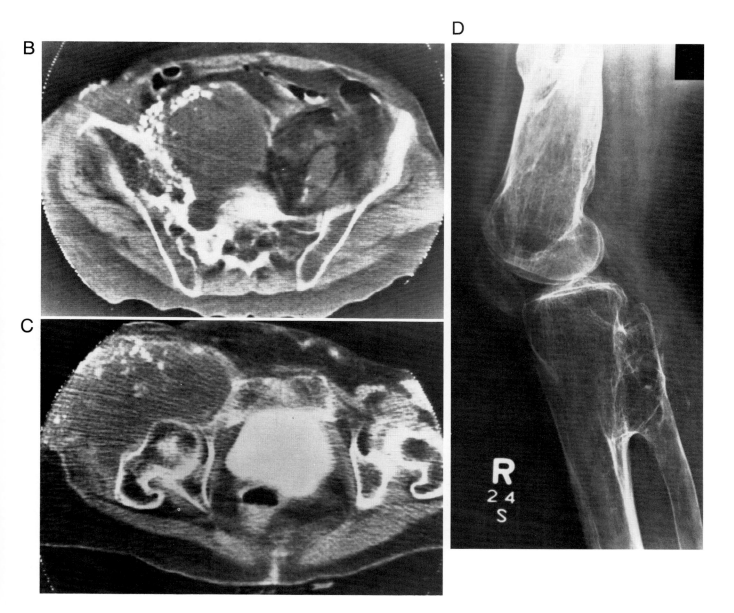

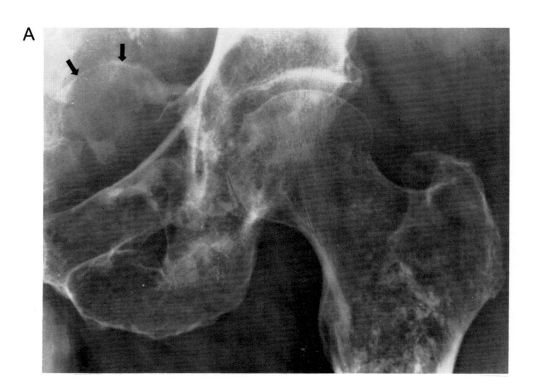

FIG 10–5.
Malignant chondrosarcomatous transformation of enchondroma. This 65-year-old man with an established diagnosis of Ollier's disease (multiple enchondromas, or enchondromatosis) involving both extremities and the pelvis presented with increasing pain of the left hip and a limp of the lower left extremity.

A and **B,** the pelvic radiograph **(A)** shows expansion of the lesion *(arrows)* with a soft tissue mass compared with a film **(B)** made one year previously. Enchondroma in the proximal left femur is seen with typical chondroid calcification.

C, the CT scan demonstrates a soft tissue mass *(arrows)* destroying the posterior left acetabulum. The mass shows areas of calcification and projects in the pelvis so that the bladder and rectum are displaced.

Given the known diagnosis of multiple enchondromas, the presence of a lesion with cortical breakout, soft tissue mass, and calcification makes one consider chondrosarcoma until proved otherwise.

Percutaneous biopsy confirmed the diagnosis of chondrosarcoma, which was due to malignant transformation of a benign enchondroma. Treatment was by internal hemipelvectomy.

B

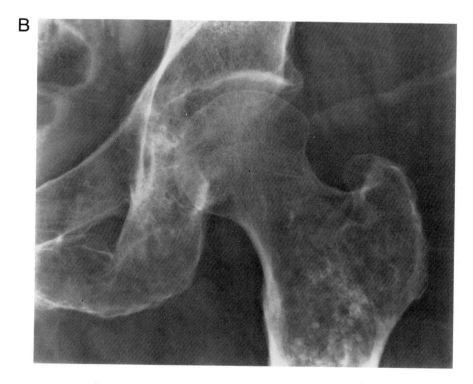

C

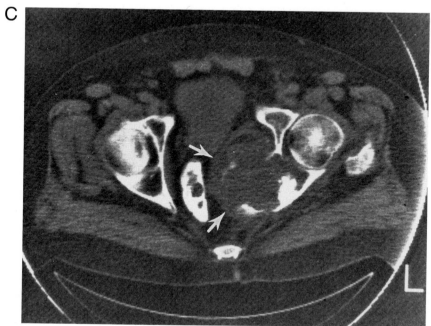

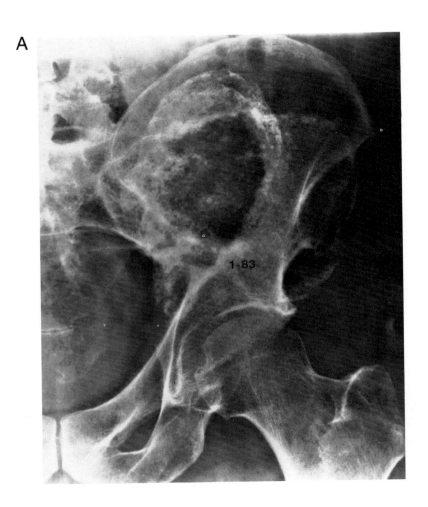

FIG 10–6.
Pelvic chondrosarcoma with recurrence. This 47-year-old man presented initially six years ago with a six-month history of low back pain radiating to his left lower extremity.

A, the pelvic radiograph demonstrates bony destruction along with punctate or spotty calcification, suggestive of chondrosarcoma. Chondrosarcoma was proved by biopsy, but because the sacroiliac joint was involved, the patient was not considered a candidate for hemipelvectomy and instead received radiotherapy.

B, postirradiation film (four months later) shows pro-gressive calcification and margination, both of which evidence healing.

C, three years later, the patient experienced new pain in the area. The pelvic radiographs showed destruction of the left superior pelvic rim. Computed tomography demonstrates a partially calcified lesion, and new soft tissue density in the posterior aspect of the left buttock. The posterior margin of the original lesion is disrupted, with tumor extending into the soft tissue.

At this time, biopsy proved local recurrence, and the patient underwent chemotherapy.

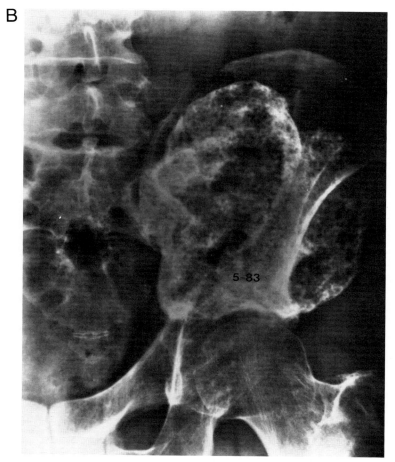

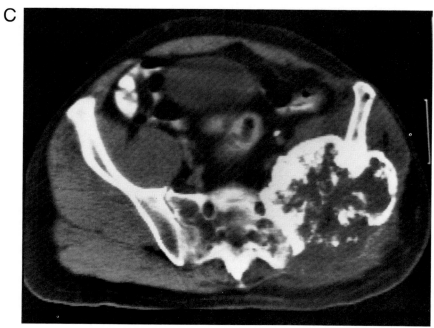

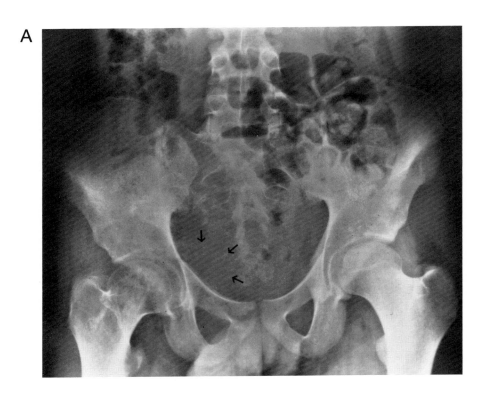

FIG 10–7.
Chondroblastic osteosarcoma (two cases).

A through **C,** an 18-year-old man presented with an eight-month history of right leg pain associated with weakness. A physical therapist ordered roentgenography. The pelvic film **(A)** shows soft tissue calcification *(arrows),* focal bone loss in the acetabular area with reflex osteoporosis of the proximal femur, and periosteal reaction in the right pubic ramus and ischium. Biopsy proved chondroblastic osteosarcoma.

B, the arteriogram (right internal iliac artery injection),
which was obtained before intraarterial chemotherapy, shows areas of blush and neovascularity *(arrows).*

C, the CT-angiogram was done by injection of contrast into the right obturator artery. It reveals extension of the enhancing mass to the adjacent structures and the presence of collaterals.

After several courses of chemotherapy and radiotherapy, the tumor mass was well under control, with significant shrinkage. Surgery was not considered because of extension of tumor into the sacroiliac joint and sacrum. *(Continued.)*

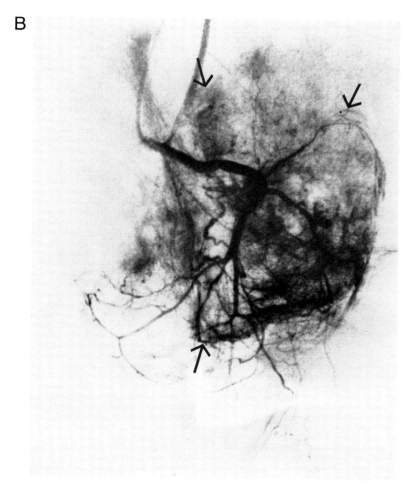

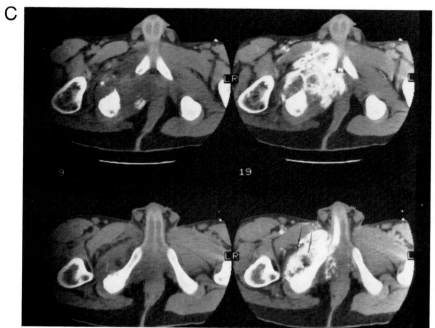

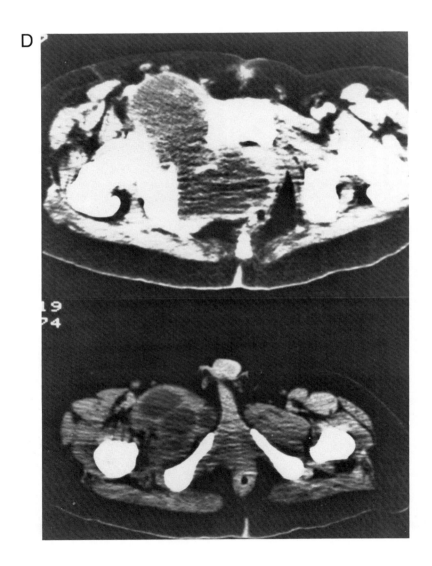

FIG 10–7 (cont.).
D, in another patient, a 36-year-old man who presented with gradual swelling of the right groin, a pelvic CT scan shows a large soft tissue mass that herniates posteriorly into the ischiorectal fossa and anteriorly into the inguinal area. The radiograph showed partial destruction of the right superior pubic ramus. Percutaneous biopsy results were compatible with chondroblastic osteosarcoma.

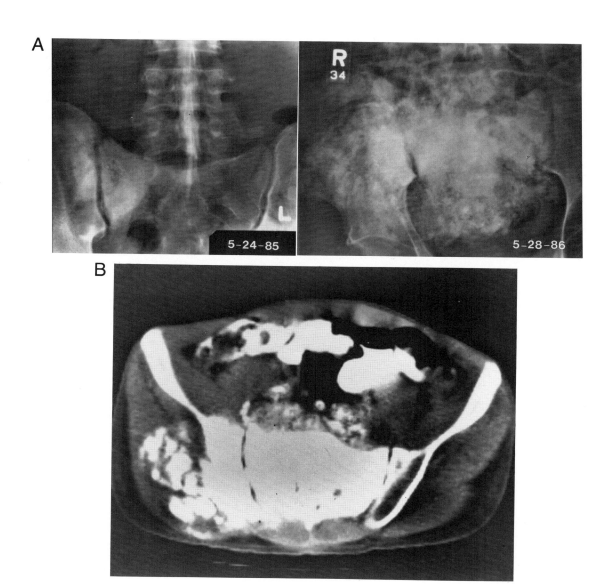

FIG 10–8.
Osteoblastic osteosarcoma of the sacrum. This 27-year-old man presented with a few weeks' history of low back pain radiating to the left leg and associated with a limp.

A, a sclerotic lesion of the right sacrum and adjacent iliac bone was discovered. With diffuse homogeneous bony sclerosis, an osteosarcoma is most likely. Occasionally, blastic metastasis can simulate a primary osteosarcoma, but it is very unlikely in this age group. A biopsy was performed and osteosarcoma diagnosed. The pelvic film made one year later, during the chemotherapy regimen, shows significant progression of disease, with enlargement of the soft tissue mass and more tumor mineralization.

B, a CT scan after chemotherapy shows involvement of the entire sacrum. The lesion crosses the right sacroiliac joint and extends into the adjacent muscles and soft tissues.

A

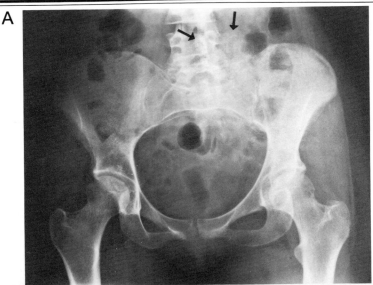

B

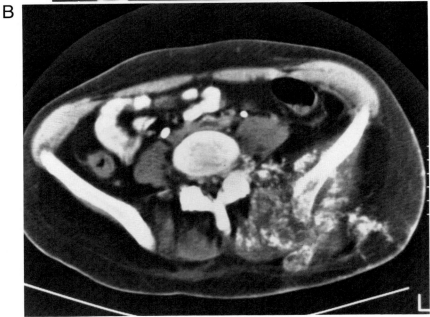

FIG 10–9.

Telangiectatic osteosarcoma of the iliac wing. A 21-year-old woman presented with gradual-onset pain in the left side of the pelvis and left lower extremity. A mass was palpable in the left buttock on physical examination.

A, a pelvic radiograph shows a sclerotic left iliac wing associated with a soft tissue mass, which contains calcification, and an ill-defined left border of the sacrum. The calcific mass extends along the left side of the L-5 vertebral body *(arrows)*.

B and **C,** computed tomography demonstrates partial destruction of the ilium and sacrum, along with a large soft tissue mass with calcification. The mass extends predominantly outside of the pelvis and invades the gluteal muscles. It infiltrates into the left sacroiliac joint and anteriorly into the pelvis, involving the left iliacus muscle *(arrowheads).* Su-

periorly, the mass extended into the posterior paraspinal muscles and into the left neural foramen of L-5/S-1.

With the aggressive bone destruction and soft tissue mass, a malignant primary bone tumor is most likely. This matrix calcification is somewhat punctate with areas of confluence. The pattern can be seen in osteosarcoma but is not specific and may also be seen in chondrosarcoma, chondroblastic osteosarcoma, and rarely even metastasis. A biopsy was done and osteosarcoma established.

D, the angiogram shows a very vascular tumor with extensive neovascularity. The tumor extends beyond the pelvis in many directions. The patient did have pulmonary metastases.

Treatment was intraarterial chemotherapy and radiation therapy, followed by intravenous chemotherapy.

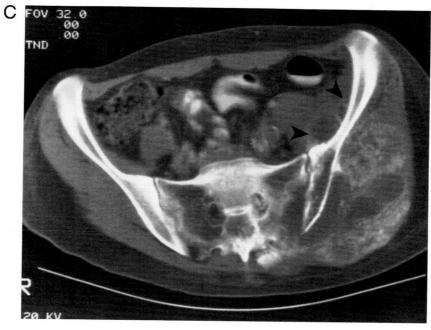

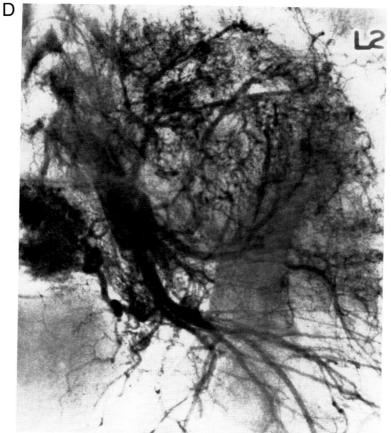

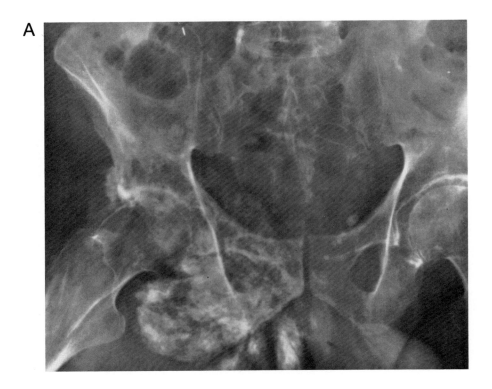

FIG 10–10.

Postirradiation osteosarcoma. This 72-year-old man had been treated for prostatic carcinoma with surgery and radiation therapy eight years ago. Recently, he developed grad-ual-onset pain and weakness in the right lower extremity.

A, a pelvic radiograph shows destruction and sclerotic changes of the right ischium, pubis, and acetabulum, and an associated soft tissue mass.

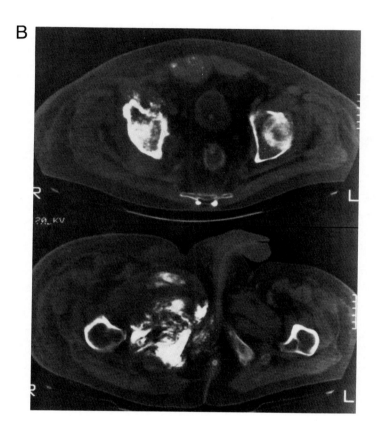

B, a CT scan demonstrates the extent of bony destruction and soft tissue infiltration. The tumor was also seen to invade the right hip joint.

This is an aggressive tumor with extensive calcified matrix. The matrix pattern has confluent clouds, suggesting osteoid elements, as well as punctate areas, suggesting chondroid elements. Thus, we could consider either osteosarcoma or chondrosarcoma with this pattern. It would be unlikely for a malignant fibrous histiocytoma to have this much calcified matrix, so, with the history, a postirradiation osteosarcoma is most likely.

Fluoroscopically guided percutaneous biopsy established the diagnosis of osteosarcoma. With the history of prior radiotherapy, this tumor was presumed to be secondary to radiation therapy.

A

B

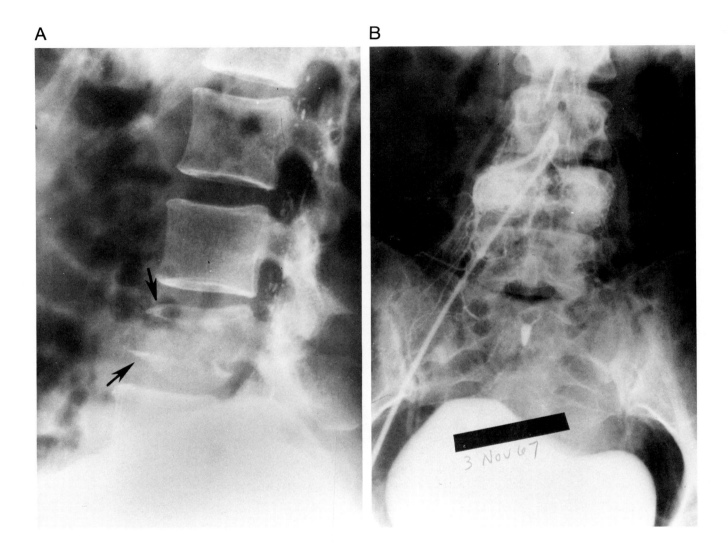

FIG 10–11.
Vertebral osteosarcoma (multiple cases).

A and **B,** this man presented with low back pain. The lateral plain film **(A)** shows lytic destruction of the fourth lumbar vertebra *(arrows),* with partial lysis of the pedicles. A pathologic compression fracture has also occurred. Contrast material from prior myelography is seen. The angiogram **(B)** demonstrates the hypervascular nature of the osteosarcoma, which is confined mostly to the L-4 vertebra.

C, this male patient presented with leg weakness and low back pain that radiated into his legs. A plain film of the abdomen shows a mixed lesion of the fourth lumbar vertebra *(arrowheads),* with lysis and blastic patterns. The vertebra is compressed mostly on the right side, with cortical destruction and tumor (osteosarcoma) breakout into the right paraspinal area.

D, this 25-year-old woman complained of midback pain with tingling into the left side of the chest and abdomen. The radiograph shows a blastic lesion of the ninth thoracic vertebra, with soft tissue extension producing bulging of the left paraspinal stripe and tumor spreading laterally into the left side. Biopsy proved osteosarcoma.

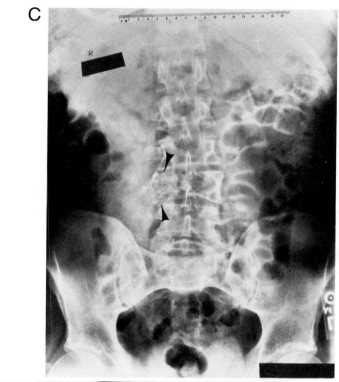

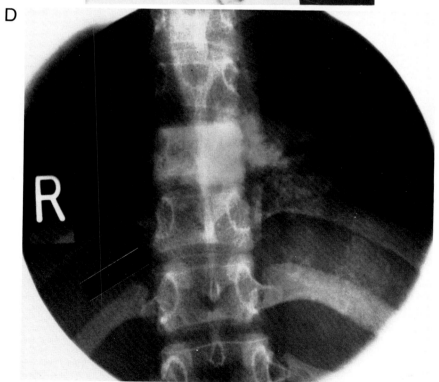

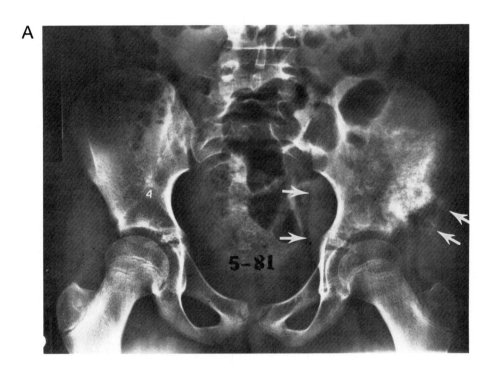

FIG 10–12.
Recurrent osteosarcoma of iliac wing. An 11-year-old girl presented with a painful left hip and a limp, and a left iliac wing osteosarcoma was diagnosed by biopsy.

A, the initial radiograph demonstrates osteosarcoma involving the left iliac wing and associated with a large soft tissue mass *(arrows).* Osteoid mineralization was seen in the ilium and soft tissue extension.

The patient underwent several intravenous and intraar-terial chemotherapy regimens, which included methotrexate and cisplatin.

B and **C,** four months later, a radiograph of the pelvis **(B)** shows increased calcification in the sclerotic lesion associated with reduction and mineralization of the soft tissue mass. At this time, a CT scan of the pelvis **(C)** reveals a well-marginated shell of calcification without associated soft tissue mass. The patient experienced no symptoms for more than one year. *(Continued.)*

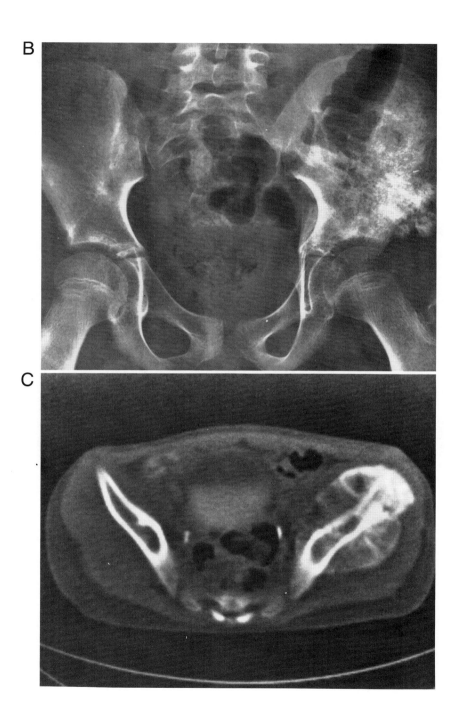

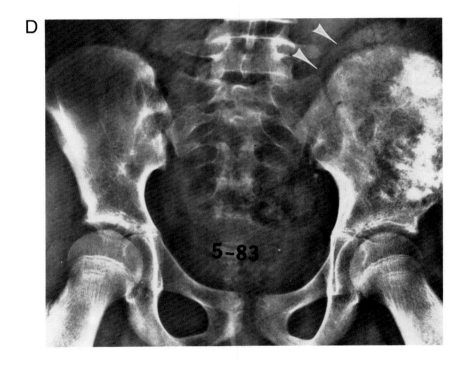

FIG 10–12 (cont.).
D and **E,** two years after the initial presentation, a pelvic radiograph **(D)** shows an additional soft tissue mass projecting above the left iliac crest *(arrowheads).* A CT scan of the pelvis from this time **(E)** demonstrates an enlarging soft tissue mass and destruction of the previously noted shell.

E

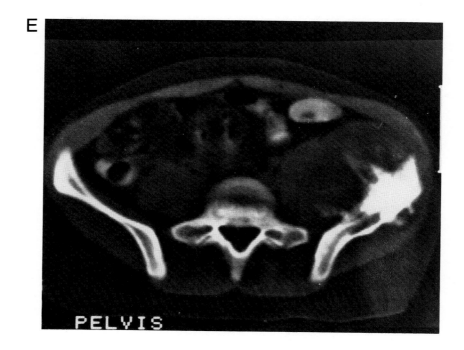

PELVIS

There is increasing density in additional soft tissue mass. The biopsy proved recurrent osteosarcoma. (From Shirkhoda A., Jaffe N., Wallace S., et al.: Computed tomography of osteosarcoma after intraarterial chemotherapy. *AJR* 144:95–99, 1985. Reproduced with permission.)

A

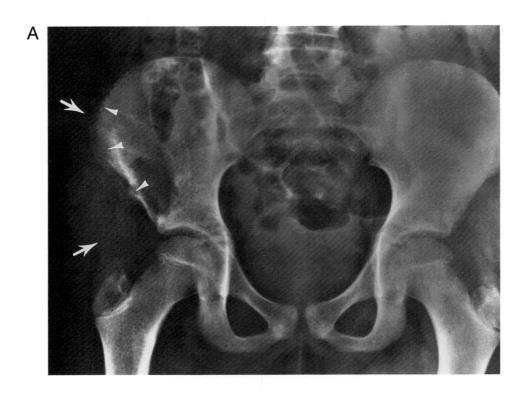

FIG 10–13.
Ewing's sarcoma. This 10-year-old girl developed right hip pain one month prior to presentation; in the interim, she had acquired a limp.

A, her pain was controlled by analgesics at home, but because of the limp, a radiograph was obtained. It shows "moth-eaten" lytic and sclerotic changes in the right iliac wing associated with a soft tissue mass *(arrows).* The lateral border of the right iliac wing is markedly irregular *(arrowheads)* and destroyed.

B, a CT scan shows destruction of the iliac wing with a large soft tissue mass predominantly extending posteriorly and laterally, involving the right gluteal muscles.

Given this lytic lesion characterized by aggressive

moth-eaten destruction and a large soft tissue mass, the age of the patient, and the flat bone location, Ewing's sarcoma is most likely. However, other focal lytic metastases can be similar in appearance. Also, leukemia may on occasion present with focal aggressive bone destruction like this pattern.

Biopsy was done and the diagnosis of Ewing's sarcoma established. The patient was admitted for treatment.

C, eight months after intraarterial and intravenous chemotherapy, a repeat CT scan shows complete disappearance of the soft tissue mass, along with reparative changes in the iliac wing. This response was considered an excellent one, and follow-up one year later showed no evidence of recurrence.

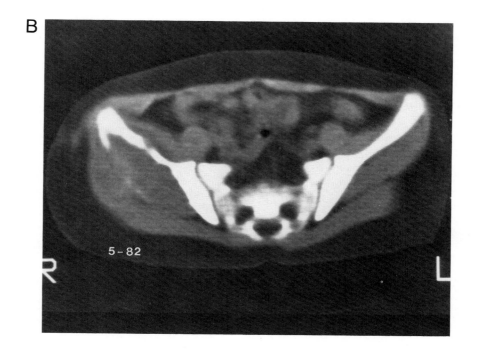

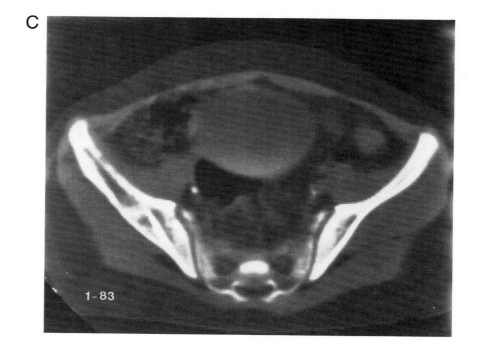

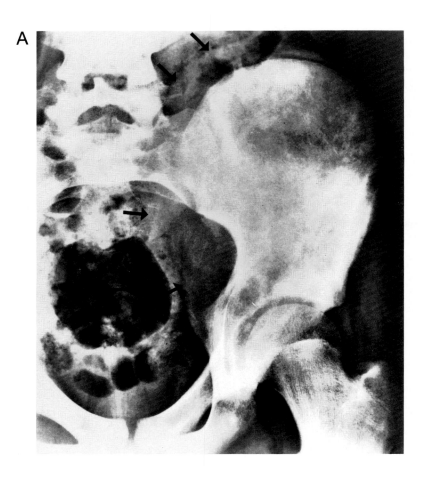

FIG 10–14.
Iliac wing Ewing's sarcoma with posttherapy change (two cases).

A through **C,** a 15-year-old boy who presented with gradual-onset pain in the left pelvis was discovered on plain radiography to have a sclerotic lesion. The radiograph of the left pelvis **(A)** shows the sclerotic lesion to involve the iliac wing and to be associated with a soft tissue mass that protrudes both medially and superiorly beyond the bone *(arrows)*.

B, the pelvic CT scan shows a very large soft tissue mass with areas of increased density and irregularity of the adjacent bony cortex. The mass extends both laterally and medially beyond the left iliac wing. Other images showed the sunburst appearance. The medial aspect of the lesion has two components: centrally, there is a calcific rim *(ar-rows)* with destruction (between *arrows*), which probably represents earlier growth of the tumor; about this is an adjacent soft tissue mass in the periphery, which represents the most recent tumor growth.

Percutaneous biopsy of the pelvic lesion yielded a diagnosis of Ewing's sarcoma. Pulmonary metastases were also demonstrated at this time. The patient received chemotherapy and six weeks of external radiotherapy. The pain decreased significantly.

C, a follow-up CT scan after treatment shows a well-defined lesion with a remarkable increase in the amount of calcification. Also, the soft tissue mass has significantly decreased in size.

The radiologic findings, along with the patient's clinical response, favored the decision of continued chemotherapy. *(Continued.)*

B

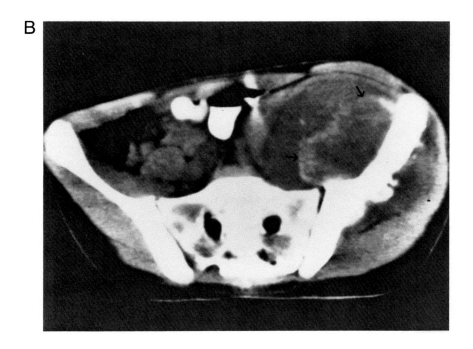

C

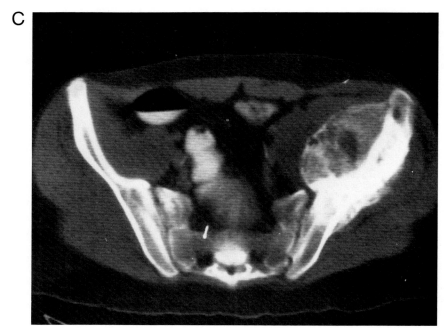

D

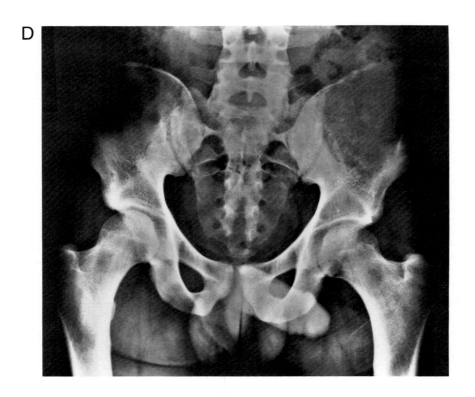

E

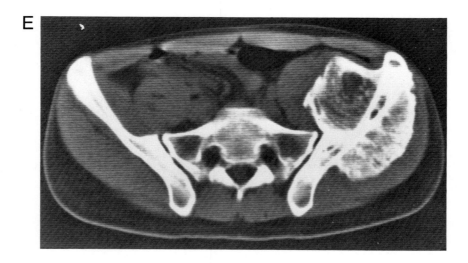

FIG 10–14 (cont.).
D and **E**, in a different patient, also with Ewing's sarcoma of the left iliac wing, a prechemotherapy pelvic film **(D)** shows a lytic lesion and a soft tissue mass. A posttherapy CT scan **(E)** demonstrates development of massive calcification, which is a sign of healing.

A

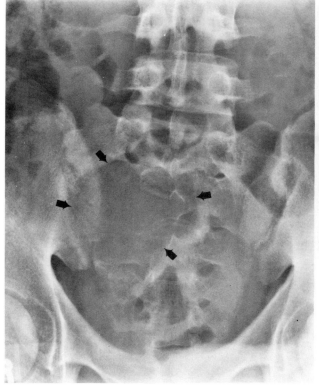

B

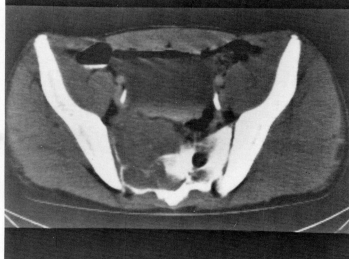

FIG 10–15.
Sacral Ewing's sarcoma. This 16-year-old boy presented with low back pain and pain radiating to the right lower extremity after a football injury. Radiologic workup was undertaken to rule out herniated disk.

A, on a pelvic radiograph, a large lytic lesion *(arrows)* is seen in the right side of the sacrum.

B, a CT scan shows a large lytic sacral lesion with extension into the right sacroiliac joint and an associated soft tissue mass projecting anteriorly.

These images show an aggressive lytic sacral lesion with soft tissue extension and no matrix calcification. This pattern can certainly be seen in Ewing's sarcoma. However, other tumors, such as giant cell tumor, lytic metastasis, leukemia, neurofibrosarcoma, and nonmineralizing chondrosarcoma, may show a similar pattern. Chordoma can have this pattern, but it and giant cell tumor usually occur in an older age group.

A percutaneous biopsy established the diagnosis of Ewing's sarcoma, and the patient underwent chemotherapy.

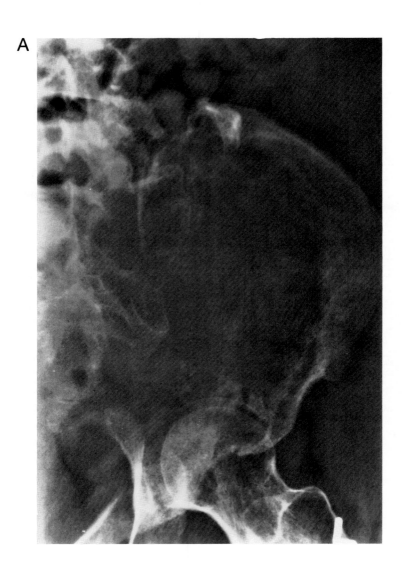

FIG 10–16.
Iliac and sacral Ewing's sarcoma. This 27-year-old woman for more than four months and during the latter part of a pregnancy noticed gradual pain and swelling in the left buttock. Percutaneous biopsy was done, and the diagnosis of undifferentiated sarcoma made. At the time of cesarean section, she had open biopsy, and Ewing's sarcoma was diagnosed.

A, a plain film of the left pelvis shows extensive destruction of the left iliac wing and disease involvement of the sacroiliac joint and adjacent sacrum. Disuse atrophy of the proximal femur is seen.

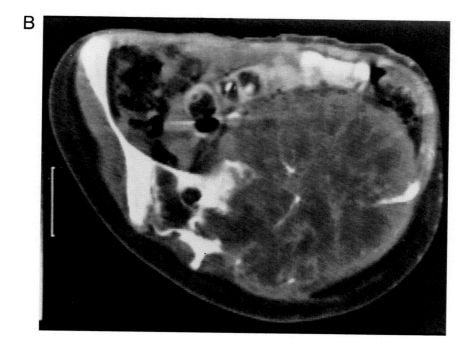

B, a CT scan shows a large soft tissue mass with residual bony trabecula replacing most of the left iliac wing and left sacrum.

These studies were done after cesarean section. Treatment was embolization and chemotherapy.

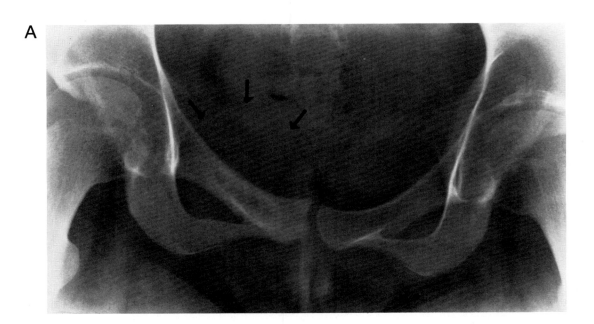

FIG 10–17.

Ewing's sarcoma of the pubis. This 17-year-old girl with a five-day history of sharp radiating right pubic pain underwent radiologic examination.

A, a mixed blastic and lytic lesion is seen in the right pubic ramus; there is an associated soft tissue mass *(arrows)*.

B, the soft tissue mass is better defined on the CT scan.

With the mixed sclerotic and aggressive lytic pattern plus the soft tissue mass, a malignant tumor is most likely. This is a common pattern in Ewing's sarcoma; however, poorly differentiated osteosarcoma, lymphoma, and chondrosarcoma may also show similar patterns.

A biopsy proved the diagnosis of Ewing's sarcoma.

C, four months later, after the patient has received chemotherapy, the radiograph shows increased sclerosis compatible with reparative changes. The soft tissue mass has decreased in size.

B

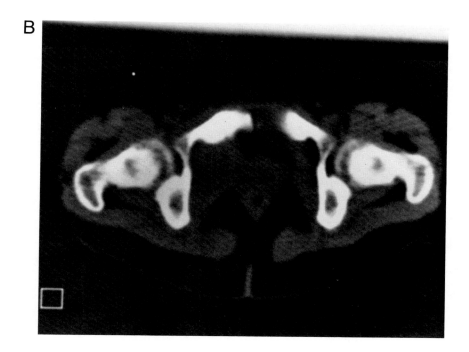

C

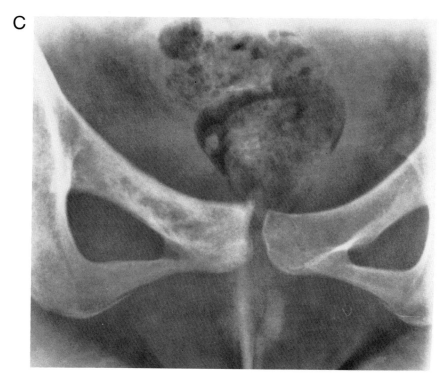

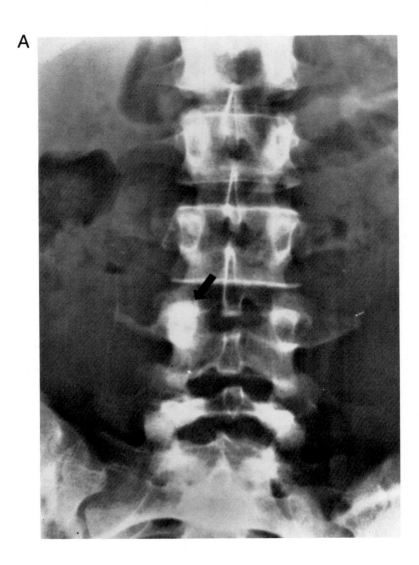

A

FIG 10–18.

Vertebral Ewing's sarcoma. This 16-year-old girl presented to her local physician because of back pain. Radiographic studies were done, followed by CT.

A, the lumbar spine film shows sclerotic changes of the right pedicle of L-4 *(arrows),* with partial destruction of the right transverse process of L-4. There is also a soft tissue mass.

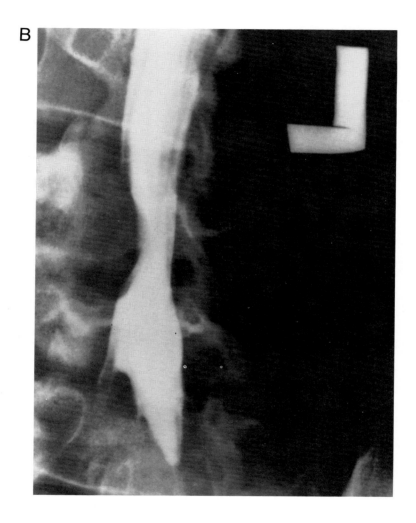

B, the oblique view of a lumbar myelogram shows a right lateral epidural soft tissue mass at the L-4 level, with destruction of the inferior articular facet. *(Continued.)*

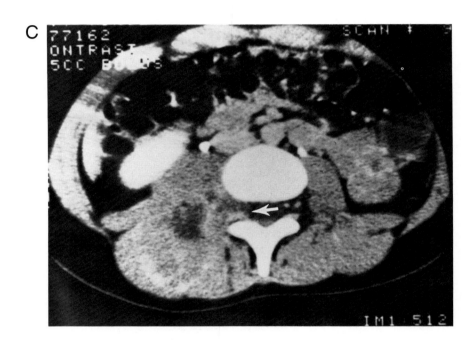

FIG 10–18 (cont.).
C and **D,** the CT reveals a large mass involving the right paraspinal muscles and extending into the epidural space *(open arrow)* via the neural foramen *(white arrow).*

A sclerotic pedicle presents many diagnostic possibilities, such as osteoid osteoma, blastic metastasis, Ewing's sarcoma, lymphoma, stress fracture, osteoblastoma, and such congenital causes as a hypoplastic or absent pedicle on the opposite side. This case has aggressive bony destruction of the transverse process and pars interarticularis and a large soft tissue mass, which imply a malignant pro-cess. Given the extradural mass and neural foramin involvement, even neurofibrosarcoma could be considered. However, in this age group, along with the findings of primary bone involvement and the soft tissue extension, Ewing's sarcoma is most likely.

A biopsy was done, and the diagnosis of Ewing's sarcoma was established. The patient had an L-3 through L-5 laminectomy and then was referred for further treatment.

E, two and one-half months later, after the patient had received five courses of chemotherapy, a CT scan shows resolution of the soft tissue mass.

D

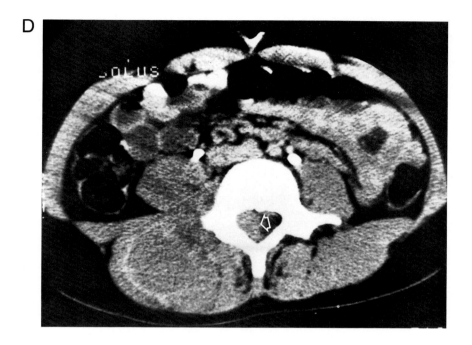

E

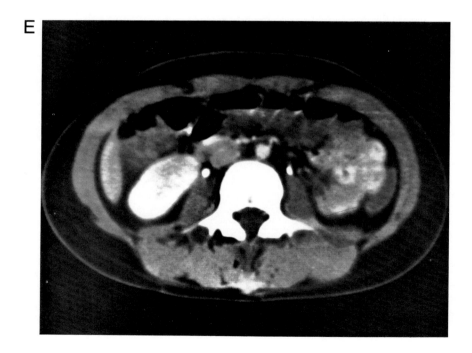

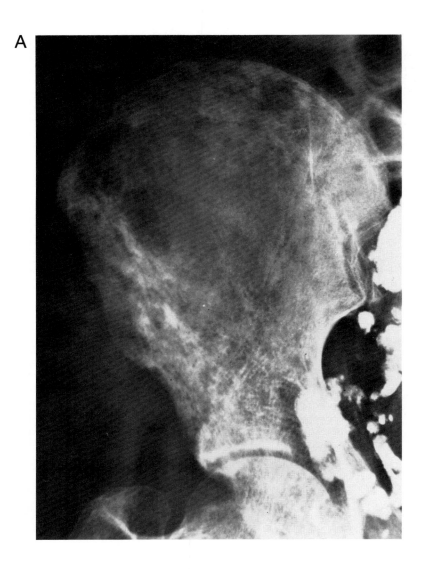

A

FIG 10–19.
Bone lymphoma (multiple cases).

A, a 37-year-old man presented with pain in the right iliac area. The original pelvic radiographs and all other examinations were normal, and the patient was treated for a possible herniated disk. This follow-up film from seven months after presentation, during that treatment, shows lytic and sclerotic lesions in the right iliac wing. Biopsy proved this involvement to represent histiocytic lymphoma. At this time, a lymphangiogram was normal, and no primary site of lymphoma was found.

B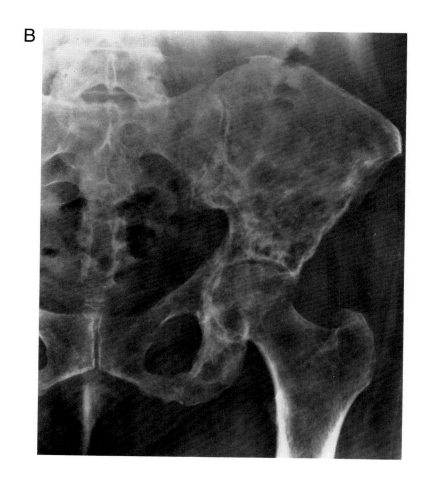

B, this 53-year-old woman presented with a painful left hip. This radiograph shows extensive lytic and sclerotic changes thought to represent metastases. Workup for a primary tumor was negative. Bone marrow biopsy from the left ilium showed histiocytic lymphoma, for which the patient underwent chemotherapy. *(Continued.)*

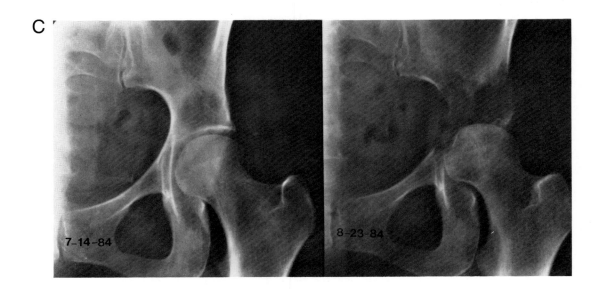

C

7-14-84

8-23-84

FIG 10–19 (cont.).

C, this 45-year-old woman, who presented with fever of unknown origin, developed left hip pain. The radiograph from this time *(left)* shows a suggested lytic lesion. The remainder of the bones were normal radiographically, but bone scan (not shown) revealed additional lesions in the spine, humerus, and femur. With the diagnosis of osseous metastases, biopsy of the left acetabulum was consistent with a large cell lymphoma. No adenopathy was discovered on abdominal and pelvic CT. A radiograph from five weeks later *(right)* demonstrates progressive destruction.

D and **E,** a 16-year-old boy with a seven-week history of increasing back pain had a severe compression deformity of the L-3 vertebra **(D),** with a posterior component detached into the spinal canal. Four sequential CT images through the disk and vertebra **(E)** demonstrate compressed and fractured L-3 and detachment of the posterior fragments into the spinal canal. There is a moderate degree of spinal stenosis, which is most severe on the right side *(open arrow).* Percutaneous biopsy of L-3 established the diagnosis of large cell lymphoma.

Lymphoma of bone shows a variety of patterns, including bony destruction with either a lytic, blastic, or mixed pattern. The mixed pattern (illustrated in **A** and **B**) is the most common.

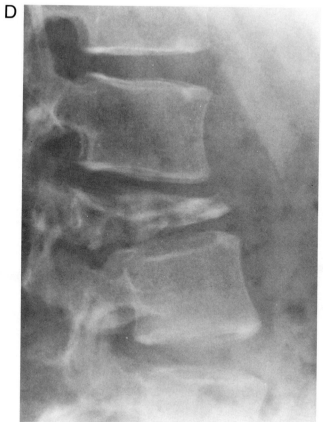

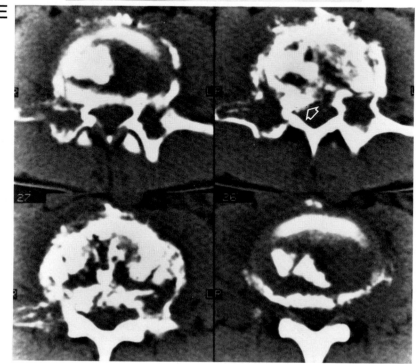

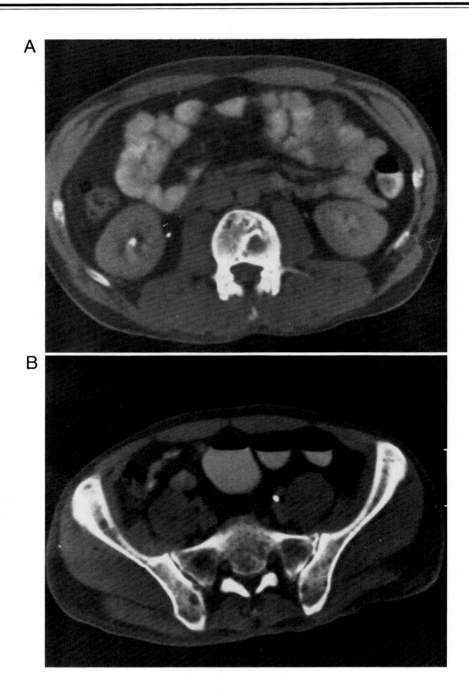

FIG 10–20.
Diffuse lymphocytic lymphoma. A 34-year-old man presented with back pain. The lumbar spine radiograph (not shown) revealed erosive changes of the second lumbar vertebra, which was also the only abnormal area on radionuclide bone scan. Percutaneous biopsy of L-2 established the diagnosis of lymphocytic lymphoma.

A and **B,** abdominal and pelvic CT scans were done for staging. Partial destruction of L-2 was again seen. In addition, there are numerous radiolucent lesions seen throughout the pelvic bones and spine.

C and **D,** the pelvic radiograph **(C)** and the radionuclide bone scan **(D)** of the pelvis were interpreted as normal.

This patient has multiple lytic bone lesions, a finding most commonly seen in skeletal metastasis or multiple myeloma. This pattern is known to occur in lymphoma but is much less common than metastasis.

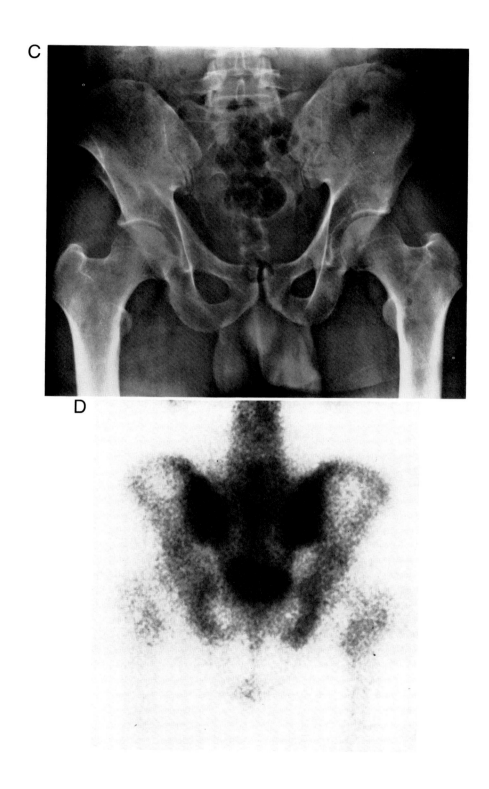

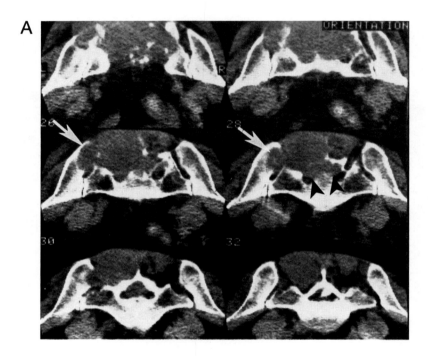

FIG 10–21.

Sacral chordoma. This 47-year-old woman presented with gradual-onset weakness in the left lower extremity associated with mild urinary and severe fecal incontinence. A large mass was palpated on rectal examination. On plain film (not shown), there was evidence of soft tissue density in the pelvis, with partial destruction of the sacrum seen through the shadows of the bowel gas.

A, the CT scan was made with the patient prone because she was unable to lie on her back. On the axial images, there is extensive bony destruction of all segments of the sacrum except S-1. Soft tissue extension into the right sacroiliac joint *(arrows)* is seen, as is superior extension into the first sacral neural foramina *(arrowheads).* Soft tissue contains boney fragments.

B

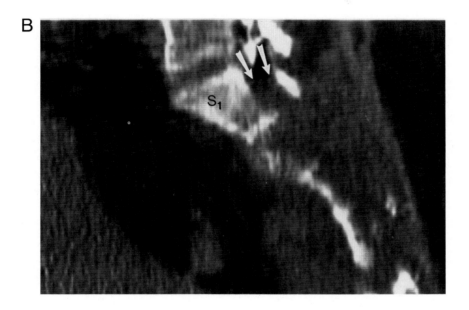

B, on the sagittal reconstruction CT scan, which was obtained from 3-mm-interval axial images, there is superior extension of the tumor mass into the spinal canal *(arrows)* and partial destruction of the first sacral vertebra *(S1).* The posterior extent and anterior extent of the soft tissue mass are better delineated on the reconstructed sagittal image.

With this large area of aggressive lytic destruction that crosses into the ilium and extends both anteriorly and (mostly) posteriorly, chordoma is certainly possible. Primary bone tumors to include in the differential diagnosis are chondrosarcoma, osteosarcoma, and even an aggressive osteoblastoma. Metastasis from a hematogenous route or even drop metastasis is possible. Occasionally, neurofibrosarcoma has this pattern, arising independently or with neurofibromatosis.

Percutaneous biopsy proved the diagnosis of chordoma in this case, and the patient underwent surgery.

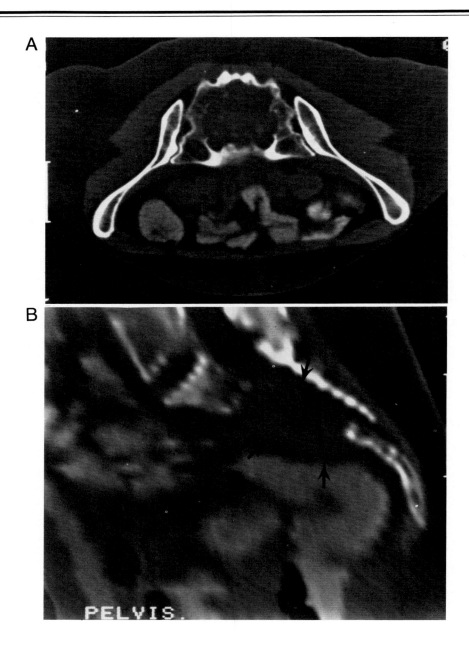

FIG 10–22.
Sacral chordoma with liver metastasis. This 33-year-old woman presented with low back pain, and a conventional radiograph (not shown) demonstrated a lytic lesion in the sacrum. She had no known primary malignancy and her routine workup, except for the liver function tests, was normal.

A, a pelvic CT scan shows destruction of the middle and lower sacrum. The lesion is lytic with aggressive pattern and has small areas of mineralization. This can be seen in chordoma but is also seen in chondrosarcoma, which cannot be excluded in this case without biopsy. A biopsy was performed and chordoma established.

B, to assess the integrity of the first sacral vertebra, a parasagittal midline reconstruction image was obtained. This image demonstrates significant destruction of S-2 through S-5 *(arrows)*, with minimal erosion of the inferior and posterior portion of S-1.

C, abdominal CT was performed because of abnormal liver function values. This scan demonstrates a hepatic lesion. Biopsy proved the lesion to represent metastasis from the primary sacral chordoma.

D, an angiogram reveals a moderately vascular sacral tumor. The tumor was embolized, and the patient received intraarterial infusion chemotherapy. A hepatic angiogram showed a single metastasis to be hypervascular, and that metastasis was embolized.

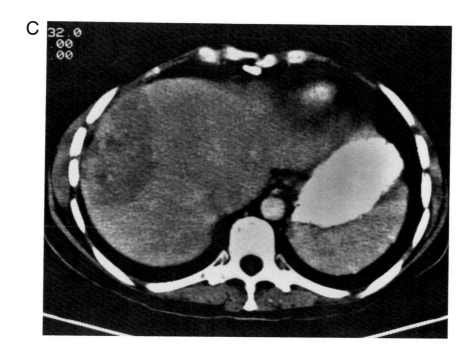

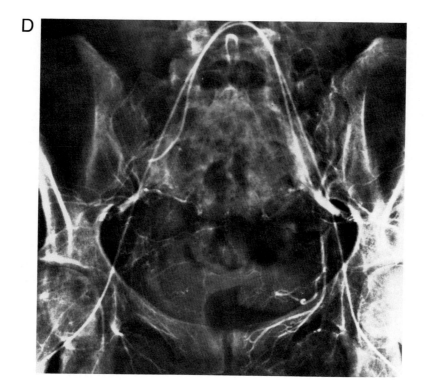

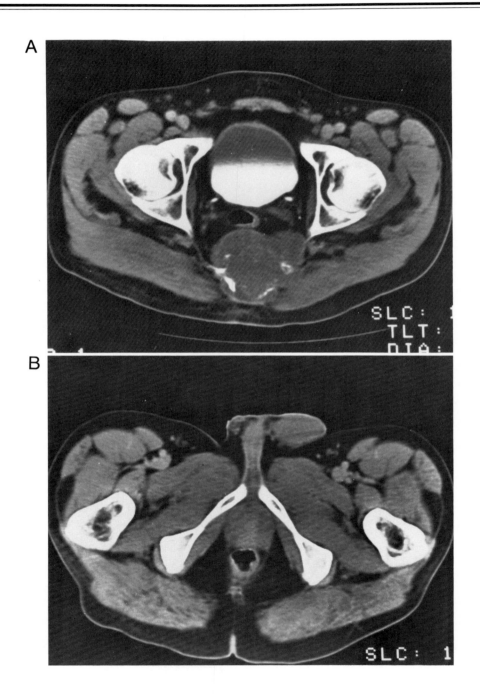

FIG 10–23.
Chordoma with muscle invasion. This 42-year-old man had a history of sacrococcygeal pain for one year, which had been conservatively managed. In the past month, the pain had become worse. The rectal examination disclosed a mass, which was seen on pelvic radiography (not shown) to be associated with sacral destruction.

A and **B,** a pelvic CT scan **(A)** shows destruction of the lower sacrum and presence of a large soft tissue mass. Per-cutaneous biopsy established the diagnosis of chordoma. The lower pelvic CT image **(B)** shows normal rectum and gluteal muscles.

C and **D,** the T_2-weighted magnetic resonance images (TR/TE, 2,000/80) show the mass as an intense signal, evidence of invasion into the right gluteus maximus muscle *(arrows).* This invasion could not be appreciated on corresponding CT images **A** and **B.** *(Continued.)*

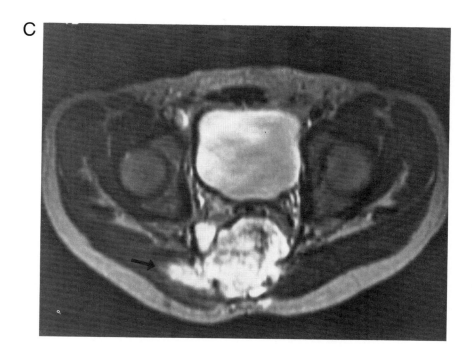

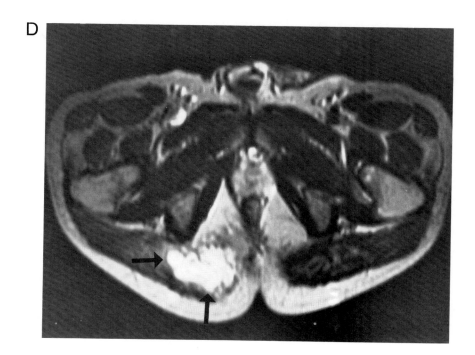

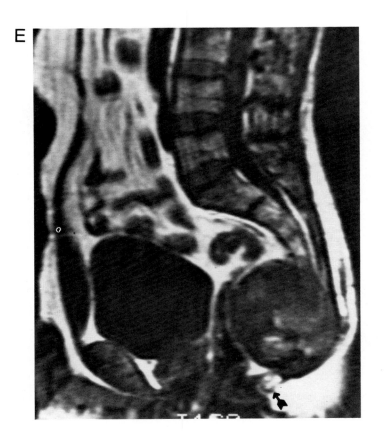

FIG 10–23 (cont.).
E, a sagittal T₁-weighted magnetic resonance image (TR/ TE, 600/25) shows well-defined borders of the tumor with involvement of the distal sacrum and proximal coccyx. The tip of the coccyx is seen to be intact *(arrow)*. The mass has variable signal intensities.

The tumor was surgically excised, with preservation of the first three sacral vertebrae.

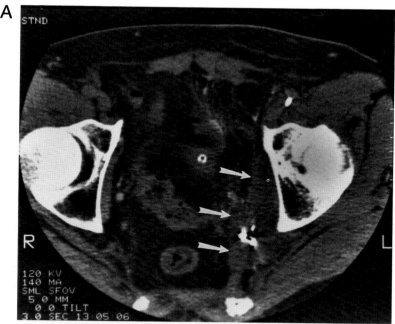

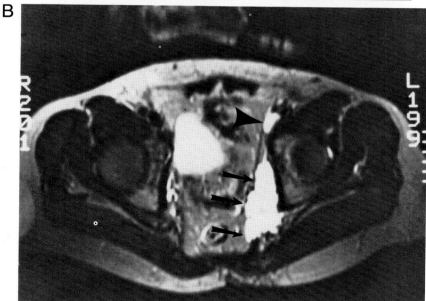

FIG 10–24.

Recurrent chordoma. This 56-year-old man had had a sacral chordoma excised two years ago and now returned with pain radiating to the left leg.

A, a pelvic CT scan shows increased soft tissue density *(arrows)* medial to the left internal obturator muscle and extending into the sacrosciatic notch. There are a few surgical clips in the area. Persistent fibrosis vs. recurrent tumor could not be differentiated.

B, a T$_2$-weighted magnetic resonance image (TR/TE, 2,000/80) displays a mass with high signal intensity *(arrows)*, which excludes fibrosis and makes recurrent tumor most likely. In addition, a node with similar signal intensity *(arrowhead)* is seen in the left external iliac region.

Percutaneous biopsy of the mass proved recurrent chordoma with probable metastasis to the iliac node.

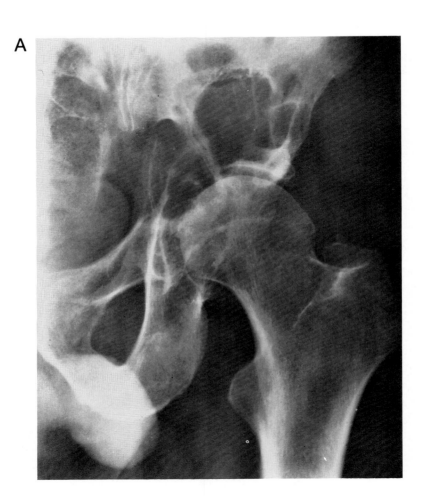

FIG 10–25.

Pelvic plasmacytoma. This 67-year-old man presented with a two-month history of left hip pain.

A, the anterior view of the left hip shows a large, expansile lytic lesion of the acetabulum. The lesion has predominantly sclerotic borders. No other bony lesions were seen, making a diagnosis of metastases less likely.

B and **C,** a pelvic CT scan **(B)** and a coronally reconstructed CT image **(C)** of the left hip show the small soft tissue mass along with destruction of the acetabular roof.

This large, well-defined lytic lesion with expansion presents many differential possibilities. Plasmacytoma is certainly high on the list, but metastasis, especially from renal cell carcinoma or thyroid carcinoma, should be considered. Primary cartilage tumor (enchondroma or chondrosarcoma), chondromyxoid fibroma, and giant cell tumor (except this patient is older than would be expected) can be considered.

A percutaneous biopsy established the diagnosis of plasmacytoma.

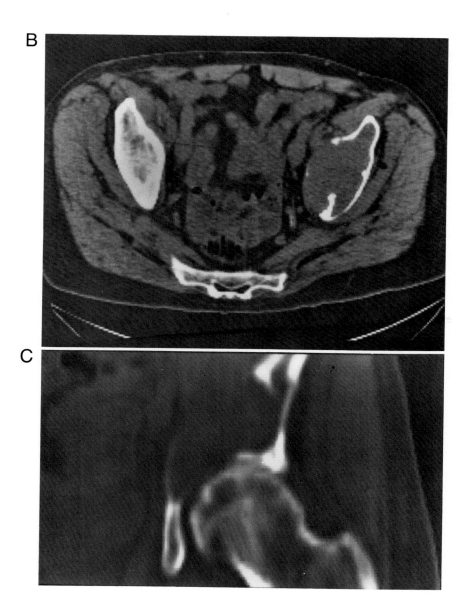

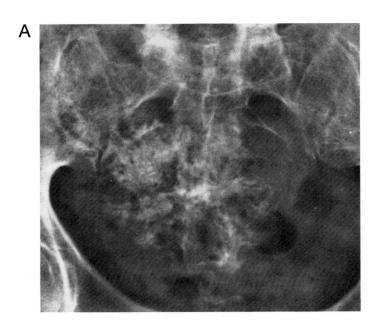

A

FIG 10–26.
Sacral sclerotic plasmacytoma. In this 70-year-old woman with an eight-month history of lower extremity numbness, rectal examination suggested an indurated presacral mass.

A and **B,** the anterior pelvic film **(A)** shows a large, sclerotic sacral lesion with areas of spotty calcification. The lateral view of the sacrum **(B)** shows the longitudinal extent of the tumor. There is no dominant soft tissue mass.

C, a CT scan shows a minimal soft tissue mass anteriorly and sacral foraminal encroachment. With this calcification pattern the initial, preoperative diagnosis included such cartilaginous lesions as chondrosarcoma and chondroblastic osteosarcoma. Rarely, a chordoma or plasmacytoma with amyloid formation would be considered.

Percutaneous biopsy established the diagnosis of plasmacytoma, and the patient received local radiation therapy.

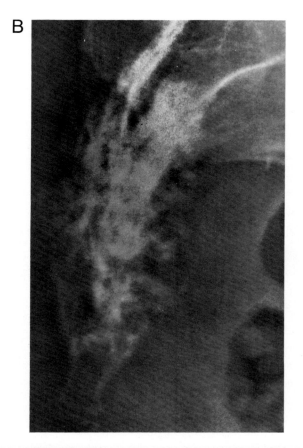

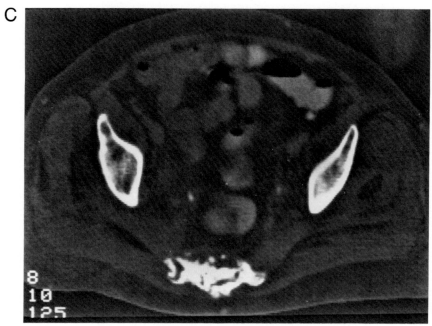

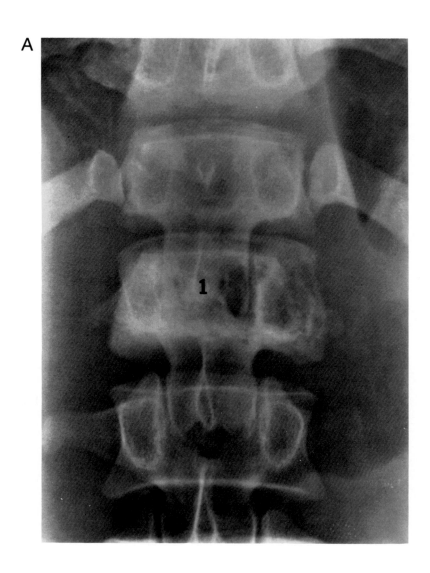

FIG 10–27.
Vertebral plasmacytoma. A 29-year-old man had an injury to his back two weeks ago while playing basketball. Because of the stiffness, radiographic films were obtained.

A, on the anterior view, there is a mixed sclerotic and lytic lesion seen in L-1. Sclerosis involves predominantly the right side, whereas the left is lytic with an associated paraspinal mass. The disk spaces are intact.

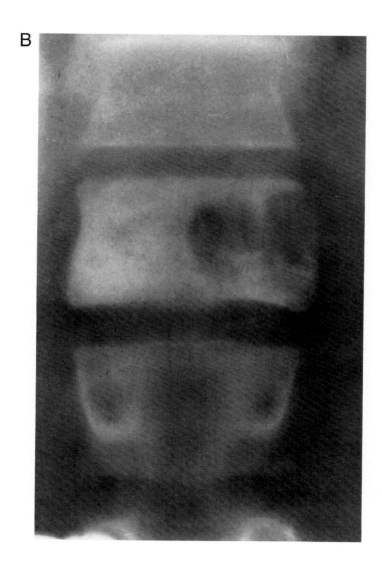

B, the anterior tomogram reveals involvement of the entire L-1 vertebra, predominantly by sclerotic changes. The lytic lesion is confined to a portion of the left side. Because of the mixed pattern of the lesion, the differential diagnosis would include lymphoma, metastasis, and even a primary osteosarcoma of the vertebra (this last occurs rarely).

Percutaneous biopsy revealed well-differentiated plasma cells compatible with the diagnosis of plasmacytoma. The patient underwent radiation therapy.

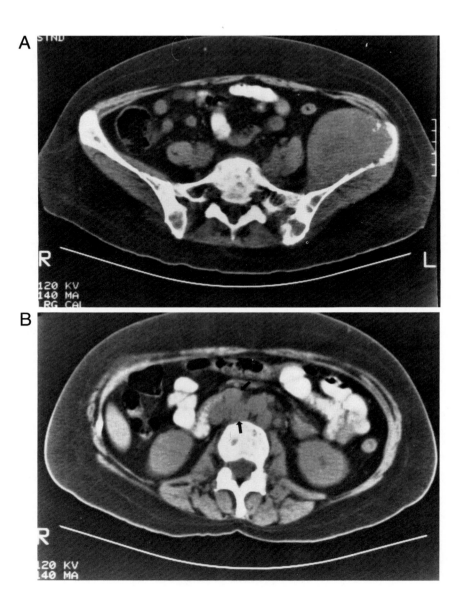

FIG 10–28.
Multiple myeloma and plasmacytoma. A 39-year-old woman presented with back pain. Radiographs showed multiple osteolytic lesions in the pelvis and spine, proved by biopsy to be multiple myeloma. The bone marrow showed 60% plasma cells. A palpable mass in the pelvis made abdominal and pelvic CT necessary.

A, the CT scan of the pelvis shows a large soft tissue mass in the left iliac fossa. The mass involves the left iliacus muscle and destroys the left iliac wing; it was proved to represent myeloma. In addition, there are multiple other skeletal lytic lesions.

B, the abdominal image reveals diffuse retroperitoneal adenopathy *(arrows)* involving the paraaortic and interaortic caval chains.

The patient received appropriate chemotherapy, but it was complicated by systemic candidiasis. Five months after the initial study, she was readmitted for evaluation. Her bone marrow had nearly 100% plasma cells.

C, the repeat CT of the abdomen and pelvis shows stable multiple osseous lytic lesions with partial resolution of the soft tissue mass, along with increased calcification in the left iliac fossa. In addition, there was a decrease in the retroperitoneal adenopathy.

D, the plain films corresponding to the CT scans in **A** (1) and **C** (2) show the initial lytic lesion (1) and posttherapy sclerosis (2).

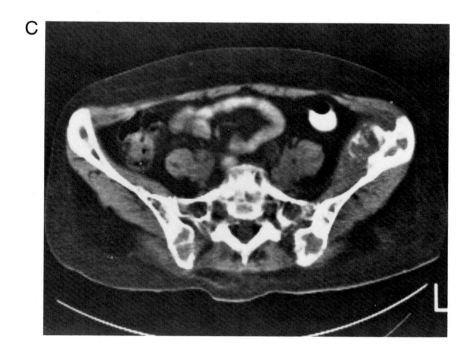

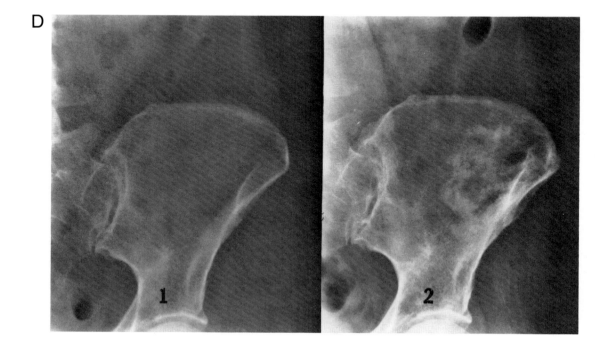

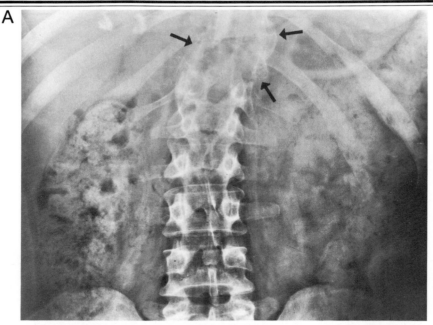

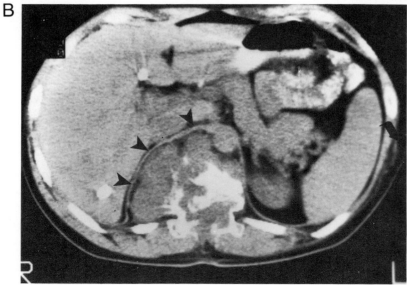

FIG 10–29.
Hemangioendothelioma. This 29-year-old man with a history of multiple fibrous dysplasia and fractures of the humerus and hip presented with back pain and severe lower extremity weakness.

A, the radiograph demonstrates deformity in the region of the thoracolumbar junction, with destruction of the 12th thoracic vertebra *(arrows).* A myelogram showed a complete block at this level.

B, a CT scan shows destruction of the 12th thoracic vertebra associated with a large soft tissue mass. The extraskeletal mass extends mostly to the right, causing elevation of the right crus *(arrowheads)* and aorta. The spinal canal is filled with tumor.

The pattern is that of aggressive bony destruction with a large soft tissue mass and no matrix mineralization. Metastasis and myeloma (plasmacytoma) would have to be the first considerations. Occasionally, primary bone and disk tumors such as chondrosarcoma, osteosarcoma, and even chordoma can produce this pattern. Infection such as tuberculous spondylitis may cause extensive destruction; however, destruction is usually not this localized and tends to produce more bony reaction and sclerosis.

The patient underwent internal spinal stabilization, during which a biopsy was obtained. The diagnosis of hemangioendothelioma was made. During follow-up, the patient developed bilateral pulmonary metastases and eventually died.

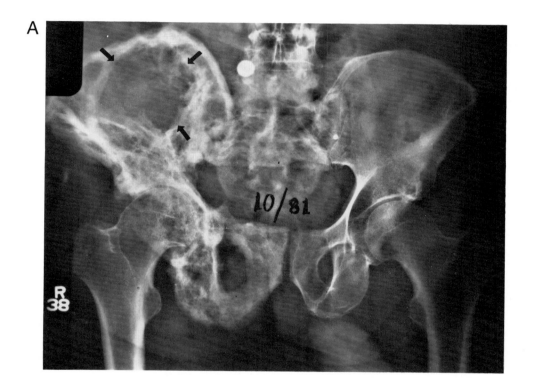

FIG 10–30.
Paget's disease and giant cell tumor. This 72-year-old man had known Paget's disease of the pelvis for the last 35 years.

The plain radiograph of the pelvis taken four years ago (not shown) demonstrated marked thickening of the iliac bone and iliopubic ramus, typical of Paget's disease of the entire right pelvis. However, recently, because of a new onset of pain and swelling of the right lower extremity, another radiograph was made, followed by pelvic CT.

A, on the pelvic film, no significant changes were seen in the extensive sclerotic areas of the lower ilium, sacrum, and L-5 vertebra. The right iliac wing, however, shows a large lytic area *(arrows). (Continued.)*

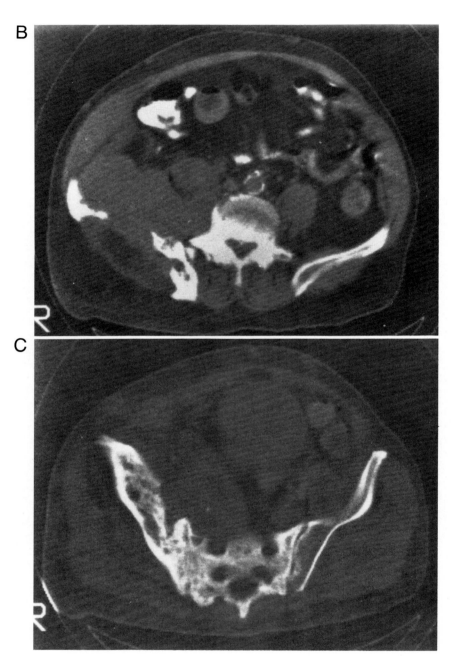

FIG 10–30 (cont.).
B and **C,** unenhanced CT scan shows sclerosis and destruction of the anterior sacrum and right ilium. These changes are associated with a large soft tissue mass. The mass extends into the gluteal muscles posteriorly and iliopsoas muscles anteriorly.

Large focal destruction in the right ilium strongly suggests a secondary lesion in Paget's disease. Such a finding could represent a giant cell tumor; however, other lesions would also have to be considered, such as lytic osteosarcoma, chondrosarcoma, fibrosarcoma, and even (although these would be rare) metastasis, myeloma, or osteomyelitis superimposed on Paget's bone.

A needle biopsy of the lytic area was done, and a diagnosis of giant cell tumor was made.

The patient responded to chemotherapy and underwent embolization one year later. However, two years later, because of pain and an enlarging mass, a second course of chemotherapy followed by embolization had to be performed.

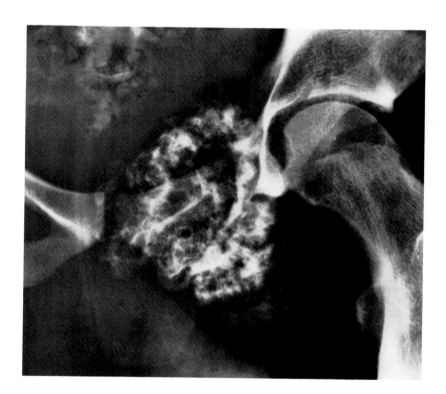

FIG 10–31.
Osteochondroma. This 19-year-old man presented with a urinary tract infection. A mass was palpable on rectal examination.

The pelvic film discloses a large cartilaginous mass that involves the left symphysis and ischium. The mass fills the obturator foramen. The lesion is typical for a cartilage tumor, and the most likely diagnosis is a cauliflower-shaped osteochondroma, but sarcomatous degeneration cannot be ruled out. The typical matrix mineralization with stipples, punctate calcification, and rings and arcs is well demonstrated. The lesion must be removed; even if it is an osteosarcoma now, in this central location it has the potential for transformation to a secondary chondrosarcoma.

Biopsy established the diagnosis of the benign cartilaginous lesion, which was totally excised. Eleven years' follow-up showed no evidence of recurrent tumor.

A

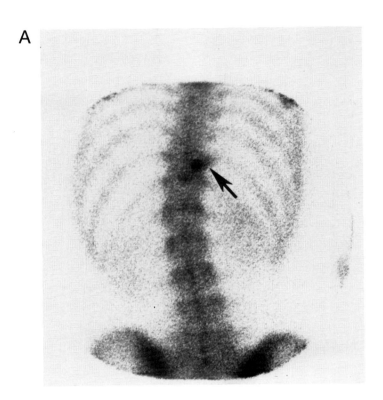

FIG 10–32.
Vertebral osteoid osteoma. This 21-year-old man presented with back pain with splinting of body movement toward the right side.

A, posterior view from a bone scan shows scoliosis with increased activity in the right pedicle of the 11th thoracic vertebrae *(arrow).*

B, anteroposterior tomogram demonstrates the sclerotic right pedicle of T-11 with an ill-defined inferior rim and adjacent focal sclerotic lesion *(arrow).*

C, the CT scans in the axial and coronal planes demonstrate the sclerotic lesion *(arrows);* the nidus is consistent with a diagnosis of osteoid osteoma.

B

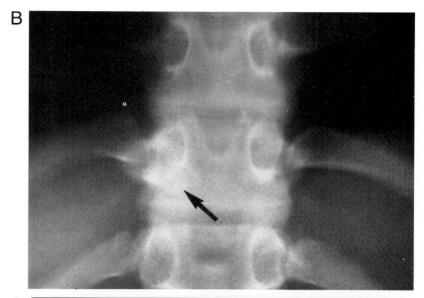

C

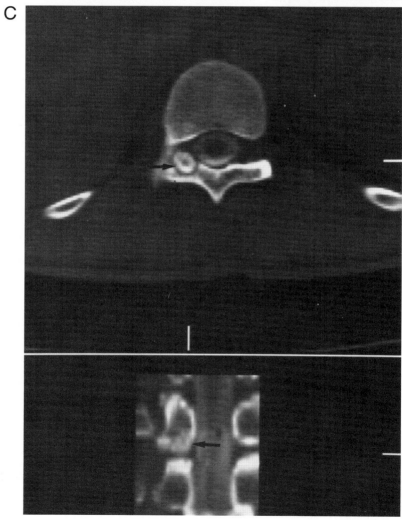

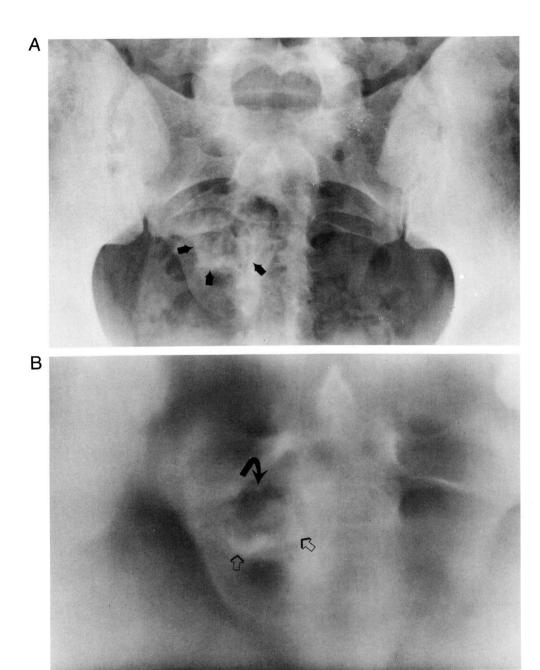

FIG 10–33.
Sacral osteoblastoma. This 24-year-old man in excellent health presented with gradual-onset pain in the right sacral area. This pain had persisted for nearly four years, but pelvic films were reportedly normal. Eventually, pelvic tomograms were obtained.

A, the anterior view of the sacrum shows that the right midsacrum is denser than the left, which finding was attributed to overlying bowel gas. However, close observation suggests an area of sclerotic changes *(arrows)*, probably at the S-3 and S-4 level.

B, an anterior sacral tomogram shows a well-defined sclerotic lesion in the middle and lower right sacrum *(open arrows)*. The adjacent neural foramen *(curved arrow)* is partially obliterated.

Needle biopsy showed osteoblastic proliferation with differential diagnosis of osteoblastoma, osteosarcoma, or reactive osteoblastic proliferation. Open biopsy established the diagnosis of osteoblastoma, and the area from S-2 to S-5 was excised.

A

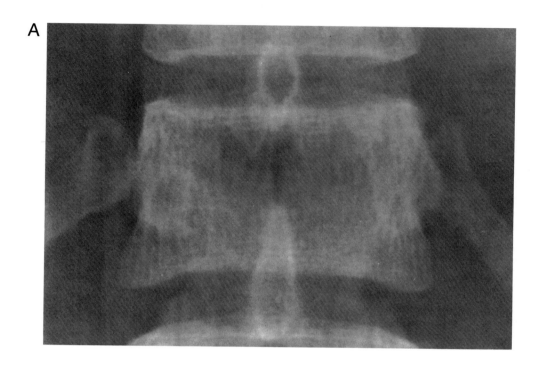

B

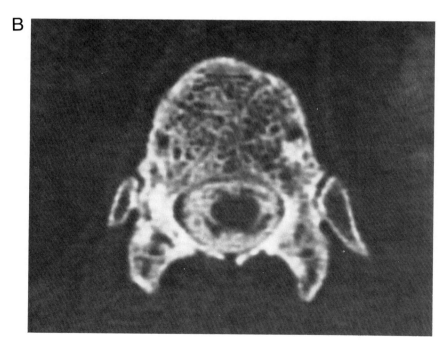

FIG 10–34.
Vertebral hemangioma. A 41-year-old woman with back pain underwent workup because of possible disk disease.

A, the frontal view of the T-12 vertebra shows increased vertical trabeculation within the bone. The vertebra is of normal size.

B, a CT scan after myelography with water-soluble contrast material shows the prominent bony trabeculae. No disk herniation was discovered.

This is a classic pattern for hemangioma.

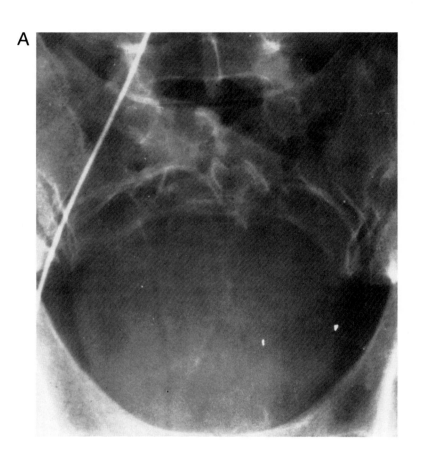

A

FIG 10–35.
Giant cell tumor of the sacrum. This 38-year-old man with a six-month history of low back pain underwent radiographic examination of the pelvis and lumbosacral spine.

A, destruction of the lower sacrum is shown on this plain radiograph, and a CT scan of the pelvis was done. This cone-down view is the scout for angiography and shows a catheter in the right iliac artery.

B, sequential CT images show destruction of the sacrum from S-2 to S-5. There is an associated large soft tissue mass. Also, the coccyx could not be identified. This lytic lesion with a large soft tissue component has fairly sharp margins on the CT scan. Giant cell tumor is the favored diagnosis in this age group and with this pattern. However, other lesions could be considered, such as chordoma, chondrosarcoma, neurofibrosarcoma, and even well-marginated metastasis from such primaries as renal cell carcinoma and thyroid carcinoma.

Biopsy was done and the findings interpreted as chordoma. The patient was referred for treatment.

The outside pathologic slides were reviewed and interpreted by the pathologist at M. D. Anderson Hospital, and the diagnosis of giant cell tumor was established. The patient underwent angiography and embolization.

C, the left iliac angiogram shows a hypervascular tumor of the sacrum. The tumor is primarily being supplied from internal iliac arteries. The patient underwent three courses of bilateral internal iliac embolization at four-month intervals, each of which was tolerated well. Three follow-ups at six-month intervals showed continuous healing that involved increasing sclerosis.

B

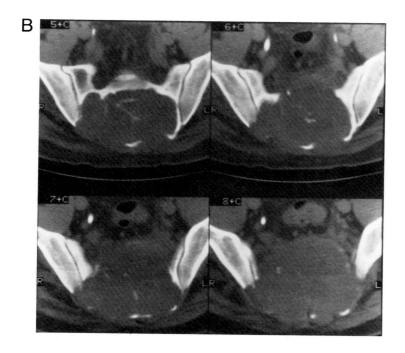

C

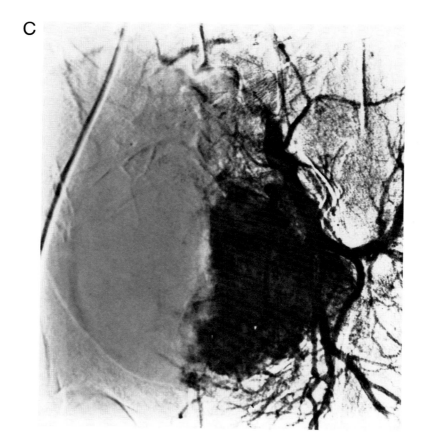

A

B

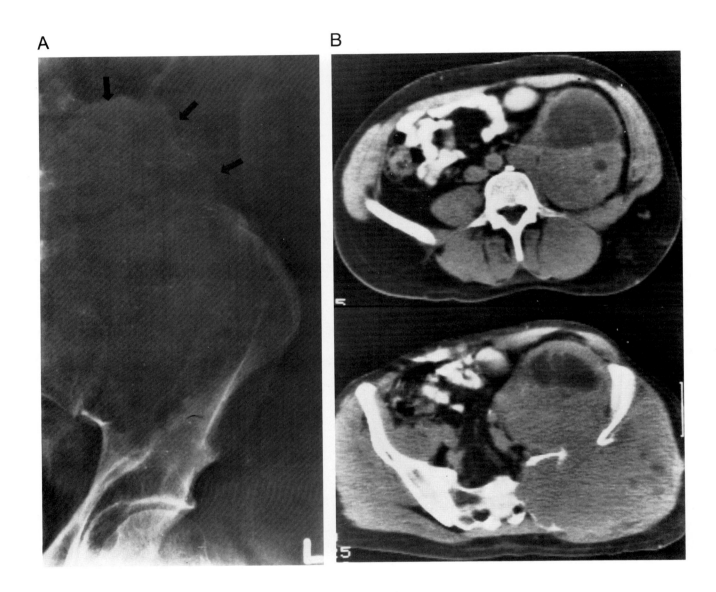

FIG 10–36.
Giant cell tumor of the iliac bone. This 35-year-old man had left flank and lower extremity pain for nearly one year. An abdominal mass was palpated on physical examination, and radiologic studies were requested.

A, there is a very large, aggressive, ill-defined lytic lesion destroying the left iliac wing and sacrum and associated with a large soft tissue mass *(arrows).* The mass extends superiorly to the level of the third lumbar vertebra. The differential diagnosis includes nonmineralized chondrosarcoma, Ewing's sarcoma, plasmacytoma, and giant cell tumor.

B, computed tomography scans reveal that most of the left iliac wing, left sacroiliac joint, and left half of the sacrum

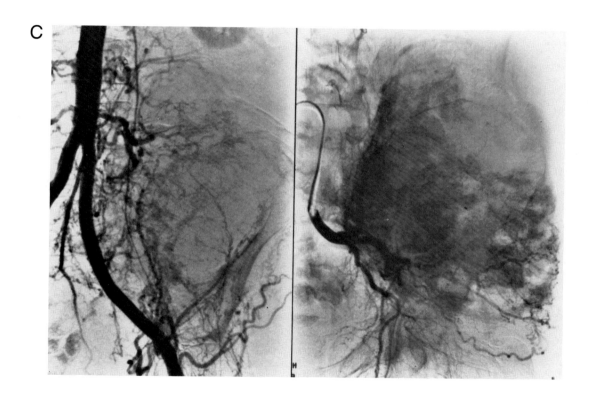

are destroyed. The large soft tissue mass, which contains areas of low density that probably represent necrosis, extends into the adjacent muscles. Percutaneous biopsy confirmed the diagnosis of giant cell tumor, so embolization and chemotherapy were considered.

C, an aortogram and a selective left internal iliac arteriogram reveal the mass to be hypervascular with areas of neovascularity. The left fourth and fifth lumbar arteries were embolized, and the catheter was left in the left internal iliac artery for infusion chemotherapy.

Two months later, the left internal iliac artery was also embolized, and the follow-up CT scans showed progressive calcification about the soft tissue mass. *(Continued.)*

D

E

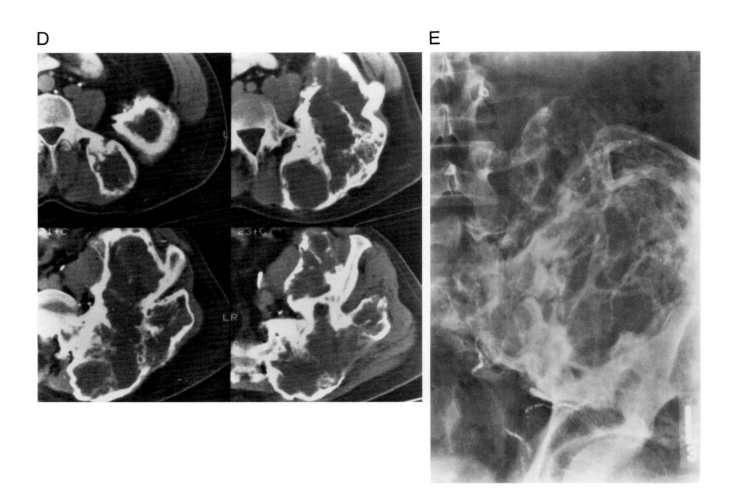

FIG 10–36 (cont.).
D, these CT images were obtained three years later and show complete calcification about the lesion.

E, the corresponding pelvic film from the three-year follow-up visit shows calcified, healed lesion.

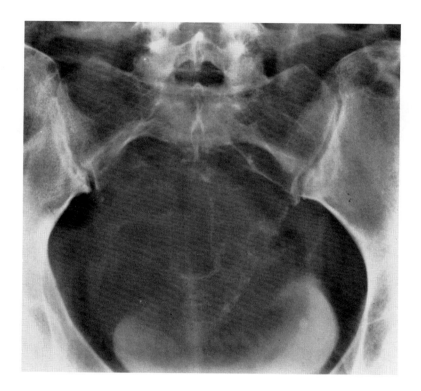

FIG 10–37.
Aneurysmal bone cyst of sacrum. This 30-year-old woman had been having intermittent muscular pain over the sacrum for two years.

Anterior view of the sacrum from an intravenous pyelogram shows a large, expansile lytic lesion that involves most of the lower sacrum. There is a smooth mass effect on the dome of the opacified bladder from the uterus.

This is a nonspecific pattern and can certainly be seen in other diseases such as giant cell tumor, chordoma, chondroid lesion (enchondroma and chondrosarcoma), osteoblastoma, and, occasionally, well-marginated metastasis.

Reportedly, this patient was operated on, the surgery followed by 4,000 cGy of radiation therapy. The pathologic slides were reviewed, and the diagnosis of aneurysmal bone cyst was established.

A

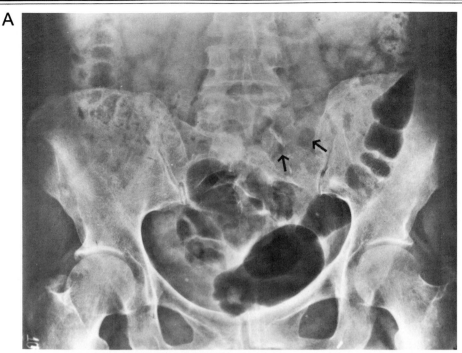

B

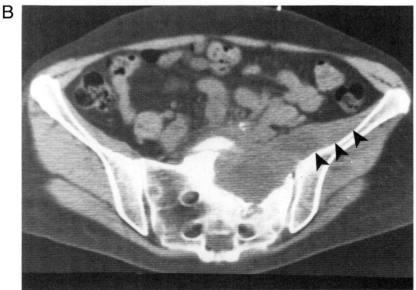

FIG 10–38.
Sacral and iliac metastasis (three cases).

A and **B,** this 43-year-old woman had squamous cell carcinoma of the cervix treated by irradiation seven years ago. The pelvic film **(A)** suggests destruction of the left upper sacral ala *(arrows).*

A CT scan **(B)** shows destruction of S-1 and part of S-2, along with a soft tissue mass *(arrowheads)* extending to and involving the left iliacus muscle.

A percutaneous biopsy proved recurrent squamous cell carcinoma of the cervix. Intraarterial chemotherapy was given.

C and **D,** this 34-year-old man had a parietal meningioma resected nine years ago. He now has a one-year history of right hip pain. The pelvic film **(C)** shows a right iliac lytic lesion extending into sacroiliac joint as seen on CT **(D).** Both primary bone tumor (e.g., aneurysmal bone cyst, plasmacytoma, possible giant cell tumor) and metastasis were diagnostic possibilities.

An aspiration biopsy showed malignant spindle cell neoplasm consistent with metastatic meningeal sarcoma. There was no evidence of intracranial recurrence. Treatment was intraarterial chemotherapy and external irradiation. *(Continued.)*

C

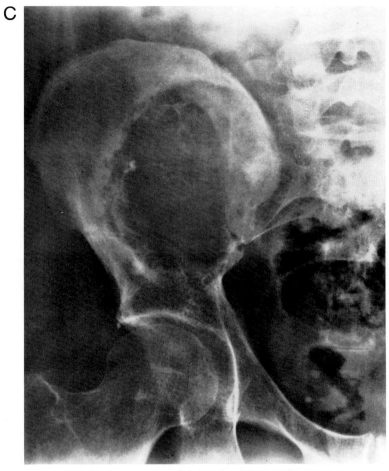

D

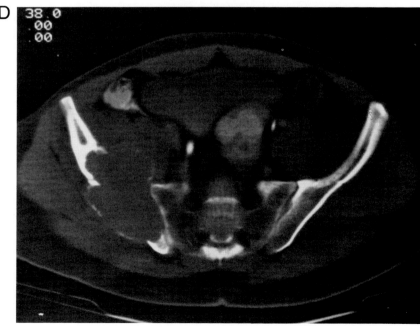

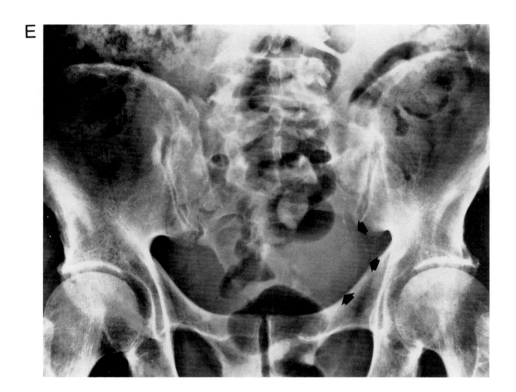

FIG 10–38 (cont.).

E through **G,** this 55-year-old man presented with a three-month history of left buttock pain. A pelvic film **(E)** shows a soft tissue mass *(arrows),* with sacral destruction. A posterior-view bone scan **(F)** suggests a focal area of photon deficiency *(arrowheads).* Axial magnetic resonance images **(G)** using T_2 first-echo *(top,* TR/TE, 2,000/40) and second-echo *(bottom,* TR/TE, 2,000/80) sequences show a large soft tissue mass with nonhomogeneous signal intensity. Biopsy proved squamous cell carcinoma; the source was later discovered from bronchial washing.

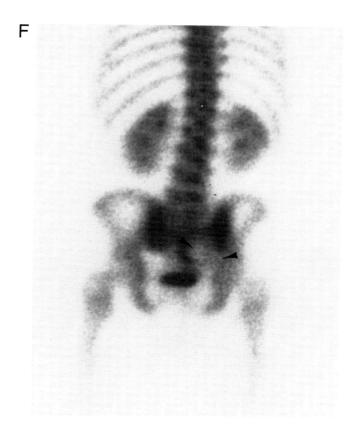

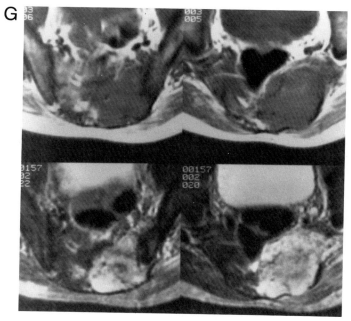

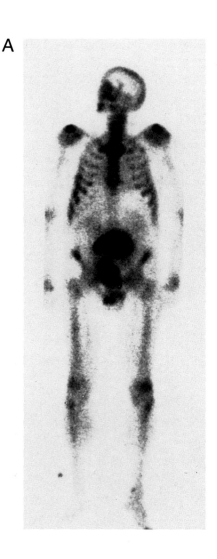

FIG 10–39.
Vertebral metastasis. This 72-year-old man had an adenocarcinoma of the prostate diagnosed five years ago, at
which time it was also found that he had metastatic disease
in the sacrum. He underwent bilateral orchiectomy and received radiation therapy. Five years later, the patient presented with progressive low back pain.

A, a radionuclide bone scan demonstrates a new area
of intense uptake in the lower lumbar spine.

B and **C,** frontal and lateral radiographs show a large
destructive and sclerotic lesion involving the L-4 vertebra. A
significant calcified soft tissue mass displaces the abdominal aorta anteriorly *(arrowheads)*. Given the history of irradiation, the possibility of osteosarcoma was raised.

D, a CT scan was done to evaluate the extent of the
disease. It shows a calcified mass infiltrating the psoas
muscles. The mass is confined to the anterior aspect of the
lower lumbar spine, not extending into the spinal canal.

Percutaneous biopsy proved the tumor to be adenocarcinoma similar to the primary prostatic neoplasm.

B

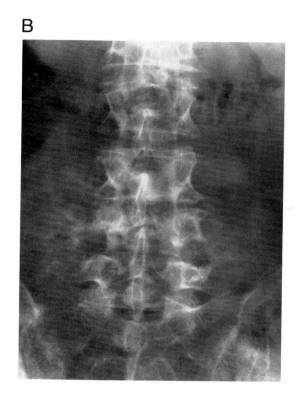

C

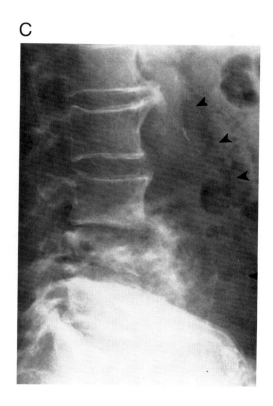

D

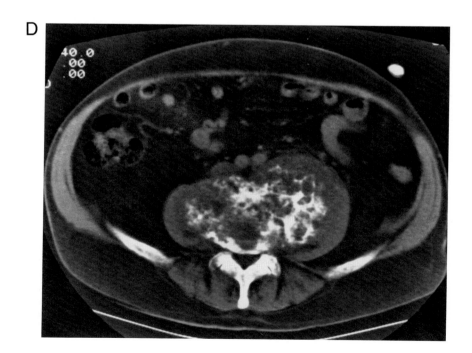

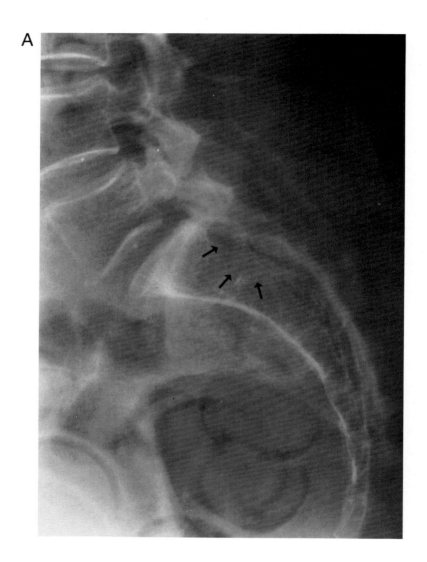

FIG 10–40.
Osseous malignant fibrous histiocytoma (two cases).

A and **B,** this 70-year-old woman with low back pain radiating to the right toe was thought to have disk disease. A lateral sacral view **(A)** suggests destruction of S-1 and S-2 *(arrows),* and therefore a CT scan **(B)** was done. There is a lytic lesion in the right side of the sacrum involving the adjacent posterior ilium. Differential diagnosis included metastasis, myeloma, neurogenic tumor, and possibly primary

bone neoplasm. A fluoroscopically guided biopsy proved the diagnosis of malignant fibrous histiocytoma.

C, this 64-year-old man with a right limp was discovered to have a palpable mass in the right hip area. On this film, there is destruction of the lateral right ilium and of the right acetabulum, along with a very large soft tissue mass *(arrows).* Percutaneous biopsy established the diagnosis of malignant fibrous histiocytoma.

B

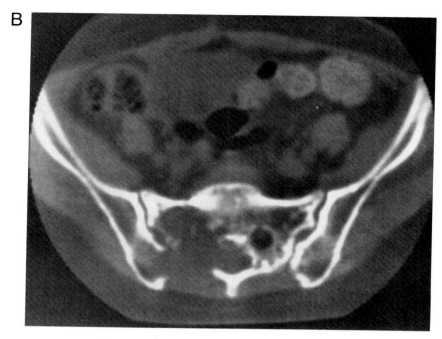

C

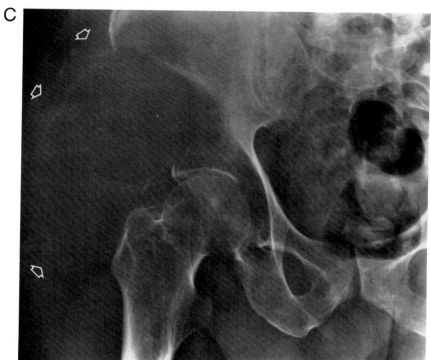

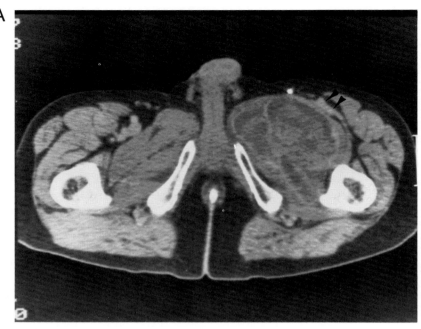

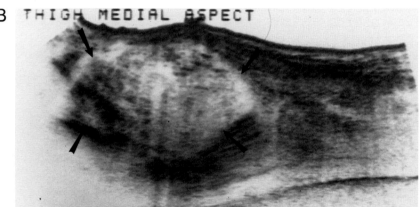

FIG 10–41.

Soft tissue malignant fibrous histiocytoma (two cases).

A and **B,** a 53-year-old man noticed pain in his left groin and two months later found a lump there. He sought medical attention, and a biopsy was done.

The CT scan **(A)** shows a large, well-encapsulated mass in the proximal anterior left groin and thigh. The mass starts from the level of the symphysis pubis and extends approximately 12 cm caudally. It has areas of necrosis and displaces and infiltrates the adjacent muscle groups, without bony invasion. The femoral vessels *(arrowheads)* are draped on the mass. There is a clip from previous biopsy.

Ultrasonography **(B)** was performed to better delineate the craniocaudal extension of the mass and thus to provide a mass size for reference use in evaluating the response to chemotherapy. The tumor is well marginated *(arrows)* and displays a nonhomogeneous echo pattern internally.

The patient completed preoperative chemotherapy and then underwent hemipelvectomy. The final diagnosis was

the same as initial biopsy findings, namely, consistent with malignant fibrous histiocytoma.

C and **D,** this 39-year-old woman with previous history of two primary malignancies, breast and cervix, presented with lower extremity paralysis. Myelogram showed T-11 block, and with the diagnosis of metastasis, laminectomy was done. Pathologic diagnosis was myxoid malignant fibrous histiocytoma.

CT scan **(C)** shows a soft tissue mass in the left paraspinal region elevating the left crus of the diaphragm. It could not be determined whether or not the mass extends to the epidural space.

Axial T_1-weighted *(top,* TR/TE, 700/25) and T_2-weighted *(bottom,* TR/TE, 2,000/80) pulse-sequence images **(D)** were obtained showing a mass with heterogeneous signal intensity infiltrating into the left neural foramen and to the posterior epidural space *(arrowheads).* The cord *(arrow)* is displaced to the right side.

C

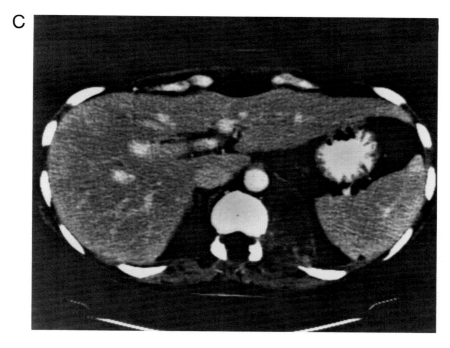

D

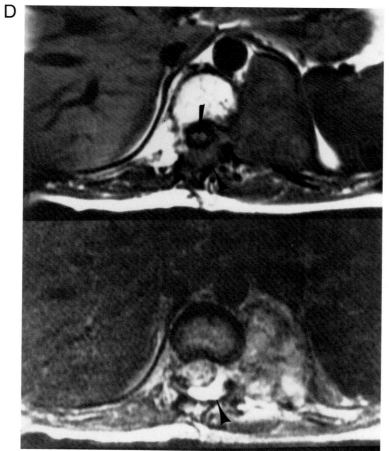

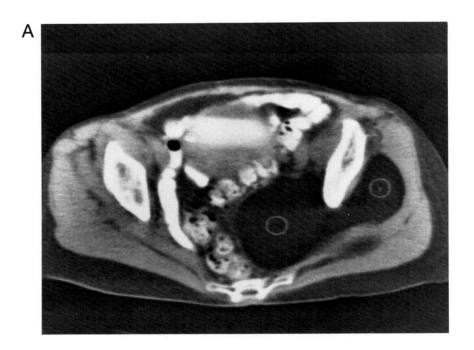

FIG 10–42.

Pelvic lipoma (two cases).

A, this 74-year-old woman with chronic constipation was found on rectal examination to have a pelvic mass, and a CT scan was requested. A large fatty tumor displacing the rectosigmoid colon to the right side is seen within the pelvis. The mass herniates through the sacrosciatic foramen and extends to the lateral surface of the iliac bone. The two cursors measure the density of the mass as ranging from −70 to −90 Hounsfield units. Percutaneous biopsy proved the mass to represent benign lipoma.

Occasionally in well-differentiated and myxoid liposarcoma of the soft tissue, there is demonstrable fat; however, it is usually nonhomogeneous with other elements of higher density.

B and **C,** axial and coronal magnetic resonance images in another patient with pelvic lipoma show a mass with typical high signal intensity by T_1-weighted pulse sequence. Herniation of the tumor through the sacrosciatic notch is seen *(arrows),* similar to the case in **A.**

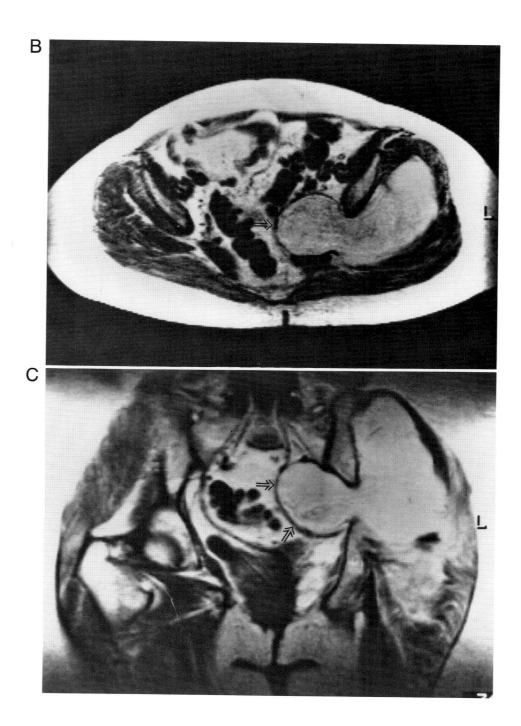

A

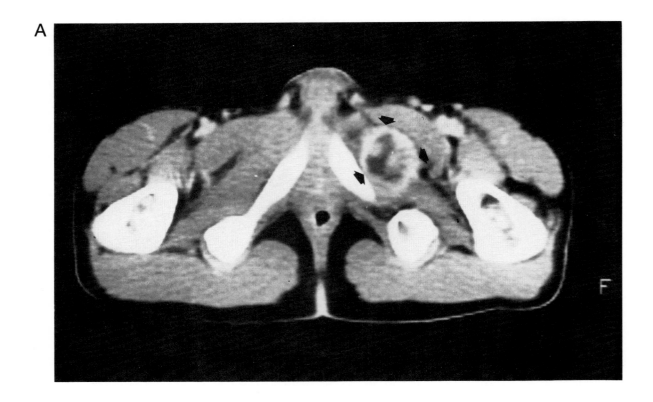

FIG 10–43.
Fibrosarcoma of obturator muscle. A 14-year-old boy presented with left inguinal pain and swelling. A mass was palpable on physical examination.

A, contrast-enhanced CT was performed. The scan shows a heterogeneous mass with peripheral enhancement; the mass involves the external obturator muscle *(arrows).*

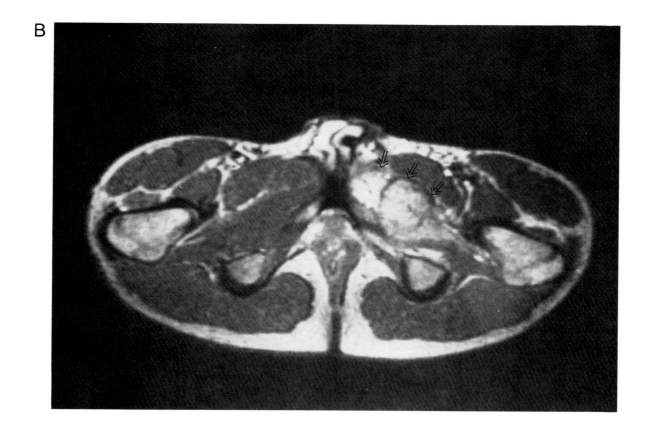

B

B, the magnetic resonance image of the primary tumor, made with a T_2-weighted pulse sequence (TR/TE, 2,000/40), shows a mass with very high signal intensity *(arrows)*, distinct from the surrounding muscles. Notice the medial extension of the tumor within the muscle.

Biopsy established the diagnosis of fibrosarcoma. (Courtesy of Dr. Dominique Counet, Institut Gustave Roussy, Villejuif, France.)

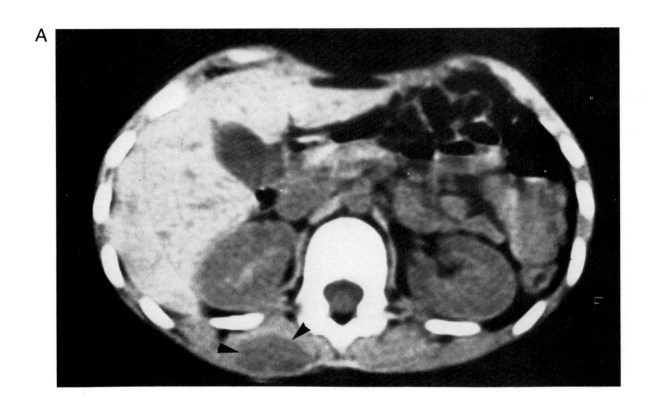

FIG 10–44.

Rhabdomyosarcoma (paraspinal and pelvic, two cases).

A through **C,** a 12-year-old girl was found to have a dorsolumbar rhabdomyosarcoma, which was surgically resected. During follow-up, it was discovered that there was a local palpable mass. The unenhanced CT scan **(A)** shows a low-density lesion *(arrowheads)* involving the right longissimus dorsi muscle.

B, following bolus intravenous administration of con-

trast material, there is a marked enhancement of the mass in a relatively heterogeneous manner *(arrow).*

C, the T_2-weighted magnetic resonance image using first echo (TR/TE, 2,000/40) shows a mass with a very high signal intensity due to long T_2.

A biopsy of the mass proved residual rhabdomyosarcoma. (**A** through **C** courtesy of Dr. Dominique Counet, Institut Gustave Roussy, Villejuif, France.) *(Continued.)*

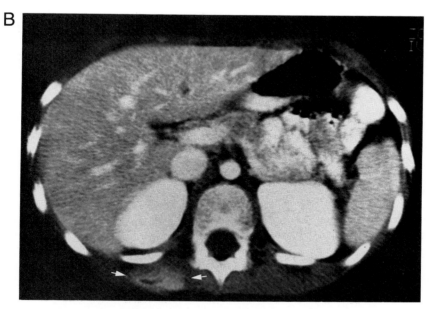

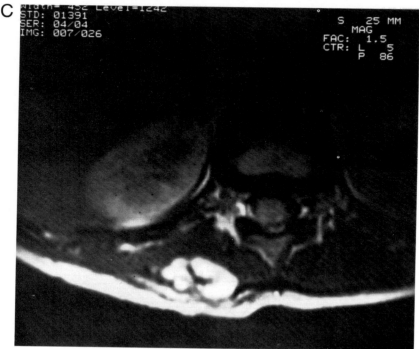

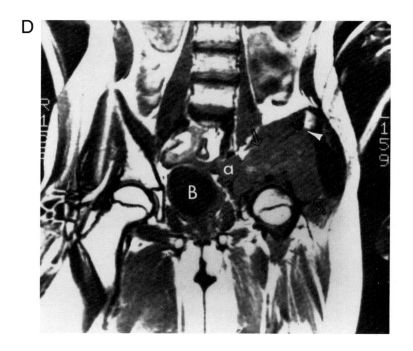

FIG 10–44 (cont.).
D and **E,** in another patient, a 13-year-old girl with pelvic rhabdomyosarcoma, the T$_1$-weighted coronal magnetic res-onance images show a large pelvic soft tissue mass her-niating through the left sacrosciatic notch *(arrows).* The iliac wings *(IW)* are seen, along with a large portion of the tumor

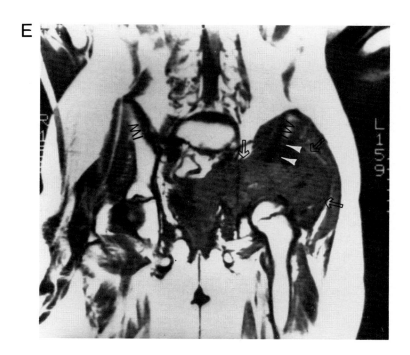

outside of the pelvis and displacing but not invading the muscles. The tumor almost encircles the iliac bone with adenopathy *(a)*, and there is probable tumor within the marrow *(arrowheads)*. The left acetabular joint is intact. The urinary bladder *(B)* is displaced to the right.

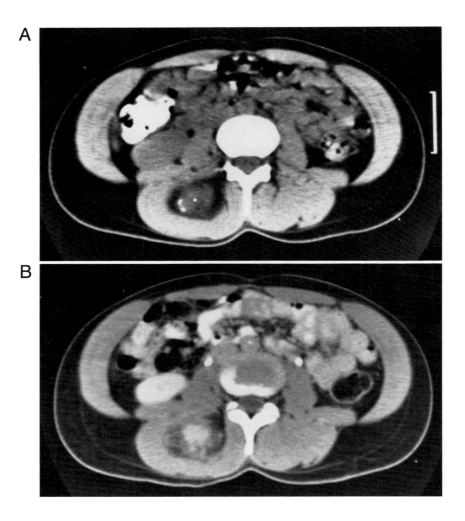

FIG 10–45.
Intramuscular hemangioma. This 24-year-old woman had episodes of right lower lumbar pain for about four years. Recently, because of a fall, she underwent radiologic workup that included CT and angiography.

A, the unenhanced CT scan shows a well-circum- scribed mass in the right paraspinal muscle. The mass includes areas of calcification.

B, the CT scan made after contrast injection shows significant enhancement of the mass, suggesting a diagnosis of a vascular tumor such as hemangioma.

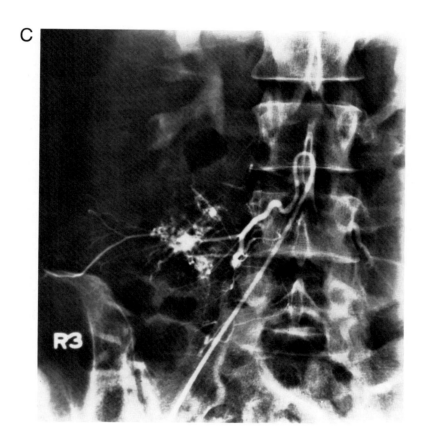

C, an angiogram, made on selective injection into the fourth right lumbar artery, shows a vascular mass.

Surgery proved the diagnosis of intramuscular hemangioma.

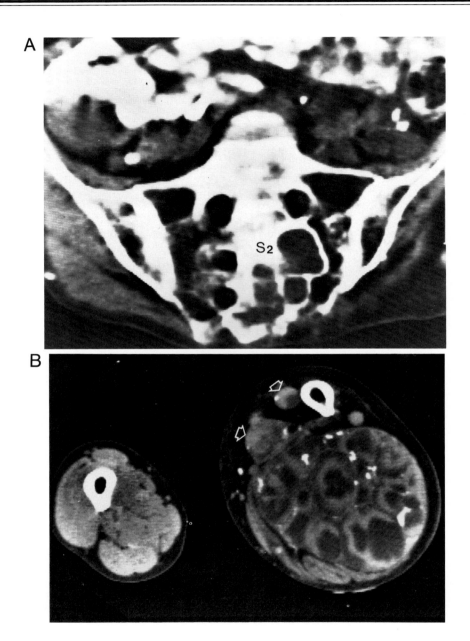

FIG 10–46.
Neurofibromatosis (two cases).

A and **B,** this 43-year-old woman had neurofibromatosis for many years and treatment had been conservative. However, because of recent constant pain in the lower extremities, particularly in the left side where a large mass was known to be, she underwent CT examination of the pelvis and thighs. This CT scan of the sacrum **(A)** demonstrates widening of the sacral foramina due to multiple neurofibromas. In this direct coronal image, involvement of the left second sacral nerve root *(S2)* is better seen.

B, a partially calcified, large neurofibroma, associated with significant muscle atrophy, is seen in the left thigh. On this image, at least three neurofibromas are seen, two smaller ones *(open arrows)* in the anteromedial aspect of the thigh and the much bigger one in the posterior aspect. The atrophic muscles are displaced posteriorly and medially.

To rule out the possibility of sarcomatous degeneration, multiple percutaneous biopsies were obtained from several regions of the mass, proving benign neurofibroma. The patient also had multiple cutaneous neurofibromas on her back.

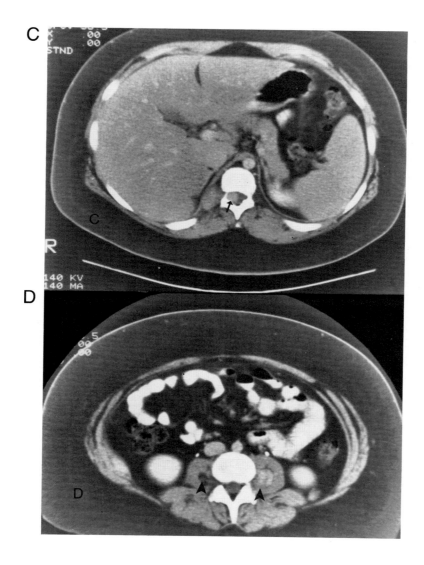

C and **D,** in another patient, who had cutaneous pigmentations (cafe au lait spots), abdominal CT scans demonstrate multiple paraspinal neurofibromas. On the top image, part of a dumbbell-shaped lesion is seen in the left neural foramen, with the smaller portion *(arrow)* located in the epidural space. The bottom image shows the neurofibromas *(arrowheads)* deep within the psoas muscles. The patient also had sacral nerve neurofibromas without bony abnormality.

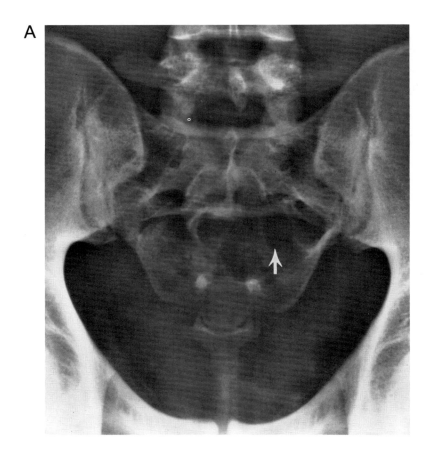

FIG 10–47.
Presacral schwannoma. This 22-year-old man presented with a five-month history of low back pain and right hip pain. Recently, he experienced difficulty in urinating.

A, anterior view of the sacrum reveals a poorly defined lytic lesion in the center and left side of the sacrum at the S-3 level. Notice enlargement of the neural foramen *(arrow).*

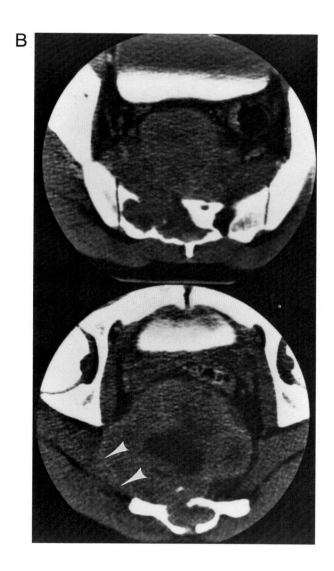

B, two CT images show the large necrotic soft tissue mass with destruction of the sacrum and widening of the neural foramen. The well-defined large soft tissue mass projects anteriorly behind the bladder. The plane between the mass and adjacent right piriform muscle *(arrowheads)* cannot be delineated. *(Continued.)*

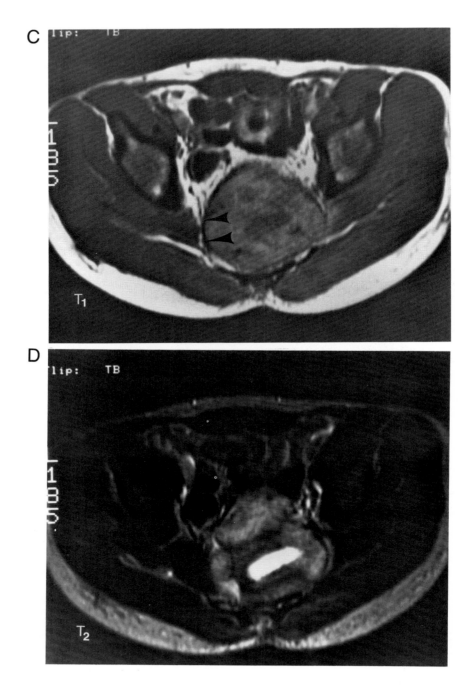

FIG 10–47 (cont.).
C and **D,** the T$_1$-weighted (TR/TE, 800/25) and T$_2$-weighted (TR/TE, 2,000/80) axial images show the mass to yield intermediate signal intensity, and there is no evidence of invasion of adjacent muscle (*arrowheads* in T$_1$ image). Central fluid due to necrosis is seen as an area of high signal intensity on the T$_2$-weighted image.

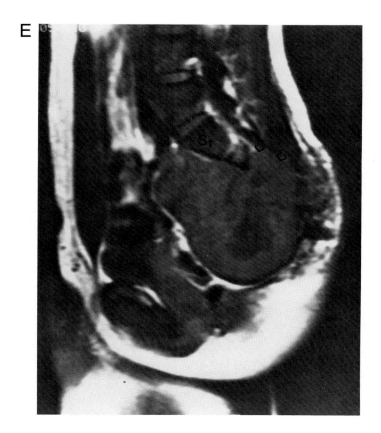

E, on the T_1-weighted sagittal magnetic resonance image (TR/TE, 600/25), the mass is seen to extend posteriorly into the spinal canal *(open arrows)*. The S-1 vertebra is intact, and there is no evidence of invasion of adjacent bowel.

Biopsy established the diagnosis of schwannoma, and the patient underwent transsacral retrorectal resection.

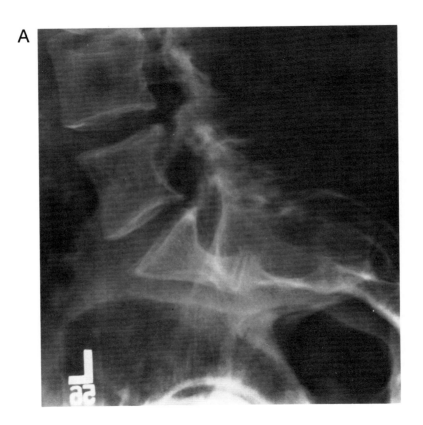

FIG 10–48.
Neurofibromatosis with vertebral deformity. This 32-year-old man with known neurofibromatosis was evaluated for possible neurofibrosarcoma. However, multiple biopsies of his plexiform neurofibromas failed to show malignancy.

A through **C,** lateral view of lower lumbar spine **(A)** shows posterior scalloping of L-4, L-5, and S-1 vertebrae. The lateral myelogram **(B)** proves the presence of dural ectasia. The midline sagittal T$_1$-weighted (TR/TE, 800/25) magnetic resonance image **(C)** shows the scalloping and ectasia of dura mater. *(Continued.)*

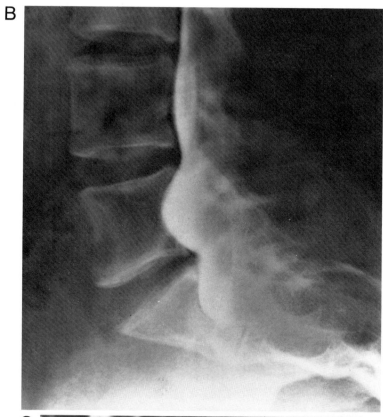

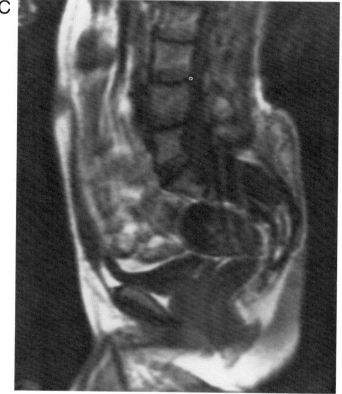

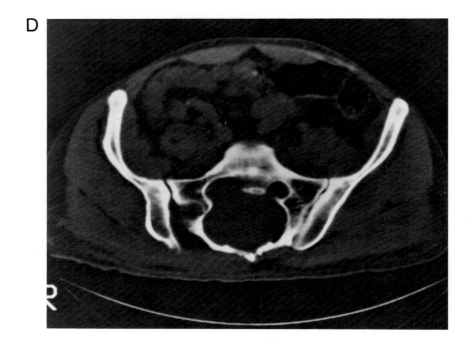

FIG 10–48 (cont.).
D through **F,** chronically expanded distal spinal canal is seen on CT **(D);** a scan made after contrast injection shows occupation by a large cerebrospinal fluid-filled thecal sac **(E).** Presence of ectatic cerebrospinal fluid-filled thecal sac can also be proved noninvasively by T_2-weighted (TR/TE, 2,000/80) magnetic resonance image **(F).**

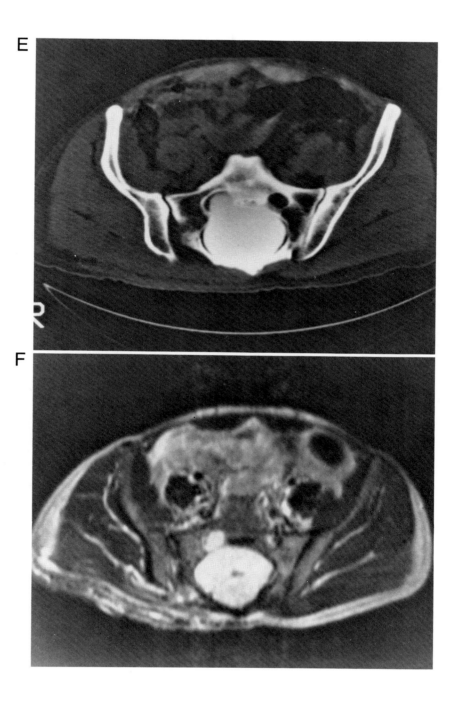

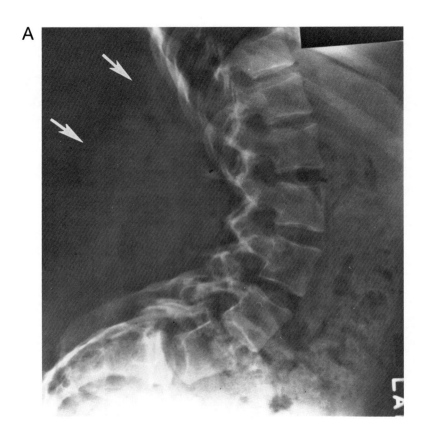

FIG 10–49.

Neurofibromatosis. This 32-year-old black woman had a known diagnosis of neurofibromatosis and elephantiasis neurofibromatosa for many years. She had undergone multiple previous operations for removal of cutaneous neurofibromas.

A, the lateral lumbar spine view shows increased lordosis with large soft tissue masses of the back *(arrows).*

B and **C,** the CT scans reveal a large soft tissue mass involving the subcutaneous fat of the back. There is evidence of left iliac wing erosion *(arrows).* The biopsy of this area showed multiple neurofibromas with prominent melanin pigmentation and extensive involvement of fibroadipose tissue, but no malignancy. *(Continued.)*

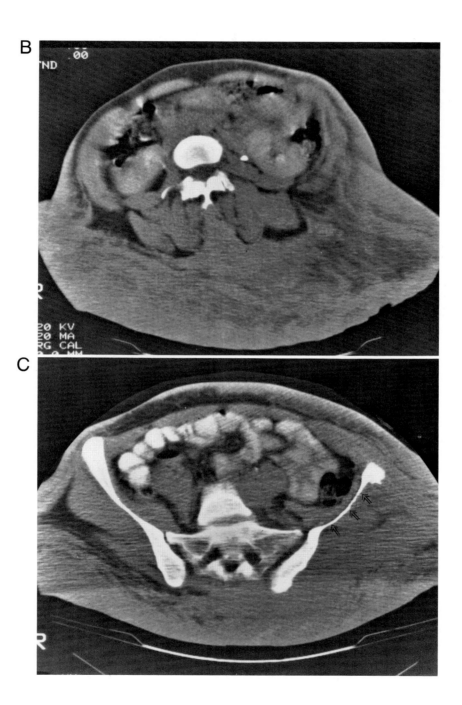

D

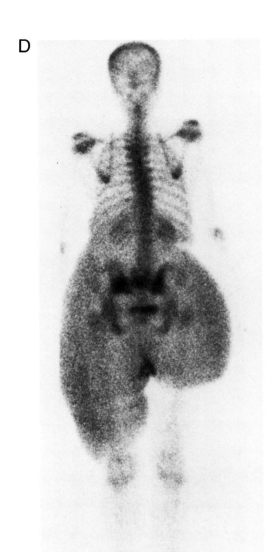

E

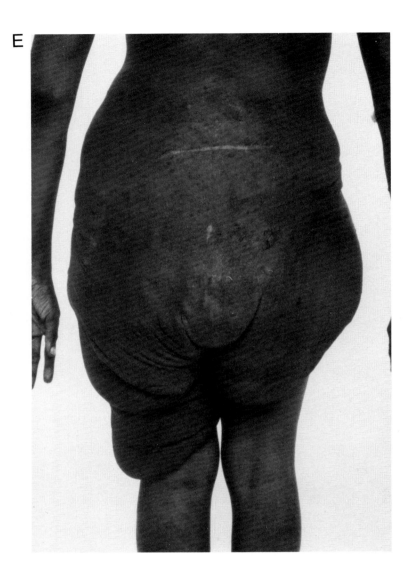

FIG 10–49 (cont.).
D, the posterior-view bone scan made with technetium 99m–labeled methylen diphosphonate shows marked uptake within the abnormal subcutaneous soft tissue masses of the back and proximal thighs. (**C** and **D** from Holbert B.L., Lamki L.M., Holbert J.M.: Uptake of bone scanning agent in neurofibromatosis. *J. Clin. Nucl. Med.* 12:66–67, 1987. Reproduced with permission.)

E, the posterior view of the patient shows the typical appearance of elephantiasis neurofibromatosa (see also Color Plate 49).

A

B

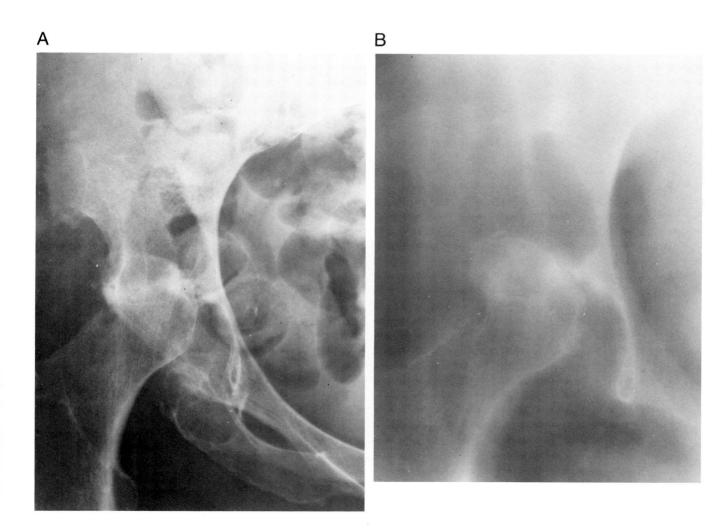

FIG 10–50.

Neurofibrosarcoma. A 43-year-old woman presented with gradual-onset right hip pain and a limp.

A, right hip film shows subluxation of the femoral head, with lytic lesions involving the acetabulum.

B, the tomogram suggests involvement of the ilium by the destructive process.

Percutaneous biopsy yielded a diagnosis of synovial sarcoma. The patient was referred to M. D. Anderson Hospital, where she underwent hemipelvectomy. The final pathologic diagnosis was a soft tissue myxoid neurofibrosarcoma of left hip with bone and muscle involvement.

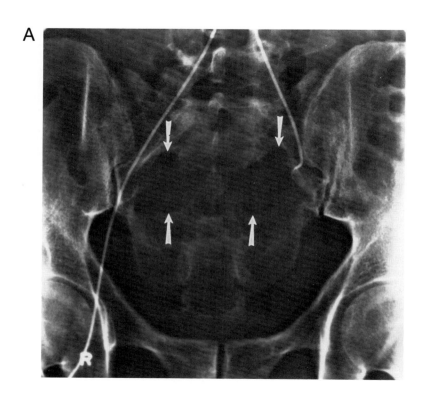

FIG 10–51.

Sacral neurofibrosarcoma. This 42-year-old man with intermittent low back pain for three years developed radiculopathy in the left lower extremity. In the past four months, the pain frequency increased, and the patient complained of urinary hesitancy and frequency and difficulty with the urinary stream. A mass was palpated on rectal examination.

A, the preangiography pelvic film shows a lytic lesion in the sacrum, along with widening of the sacral neural foramina *(arrows).* A bone scan (not shown) revealed a corresponding "cold" area.

B

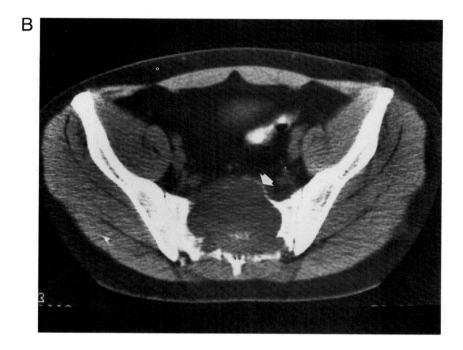

B, a pelvic CT scan was obtained and shows a large soft tissue mass with extensive destruction of the sacrum. The mass is projecting anteriorly with a rim of cortical bone *(arrow).*

With a differential diagnosis of chordoma, giant cell tu-mor, or neurofibroma, a further evaluation, by MRI of the pelvis, of the craniocaudal extent of this mass and of involvement of the sacral vertebral bodies was recommended. *(Continued.)*

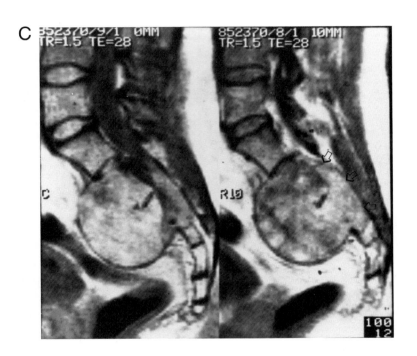

FIG 10–51 (cont.).
C and **D,** both proton-density (TR/TE, 1,500/28) **(C)** and T₁-weighted (TR/TE, 500/28) **(D)** magnetic resonance images were obtained and show a well-encapsulated mass destroying S-2 through S-4, with extension posteriorly into the sacral canal *(arrows)*. The previously noted anterior extension is also seen. The contents of the mass have relatively long T_1 and T_2 relaxation times. The rectum *(R)* and bladder *(BL)* are not involved by the tumor.

Percutaneous biopsy was done using a posterior approach, and the diagnosis of neurofibrosarcoma was established.

E, an angiogram shows the mass to be somewhat hypervascular. Angiography was followed by three sessions of embolization as a preoperative procedure. The tumor was eventually excised.

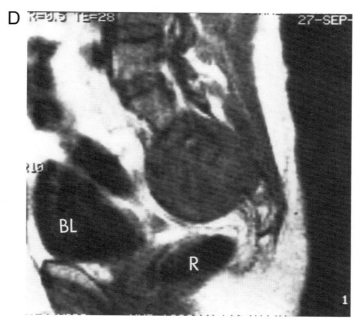

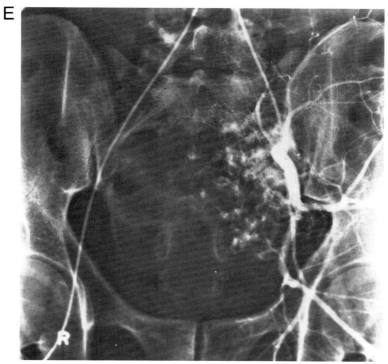

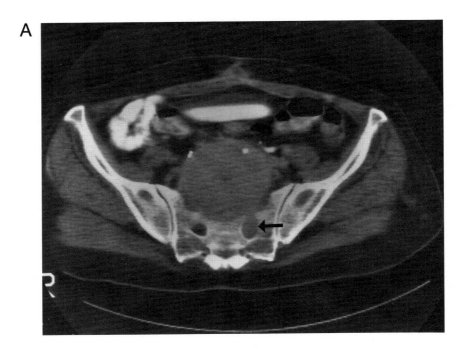

FIG 10–52.
Presacral neurofibrosarcoma. This 59-year-old woman sought medical care because of constant lower back pain and severe pain during defecation. Physical examination revealed a minimally tender large and hard mass arising from deep in the pelvis directly posterior to the vaginal cuff. No bony abnormality was seen on the radiograph, and the barium enema examination and intravenous pyelogram showed a mass effect on the colon and bladder.

A and **B,** the CT scan shows a large, well-encapsulated

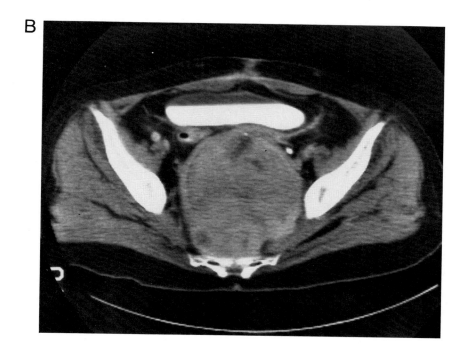

nonhomogeneous mass in the presacral space, displacing the rectum and bladder anteriorly. The left fourth neural foramen is slightly widened (*arrow* in **A**).

The initial diagnosis was a gynecologic tumor, and exploration was done. But the wedge biopsy showed neurofibrosarcoma, and it was found to be inoperable. The patient was referred to M. D. Anderson Hospital, where she received several courses of chemotherapy. The tumor responded to treatment, and 14 months later the mass was completely excised.

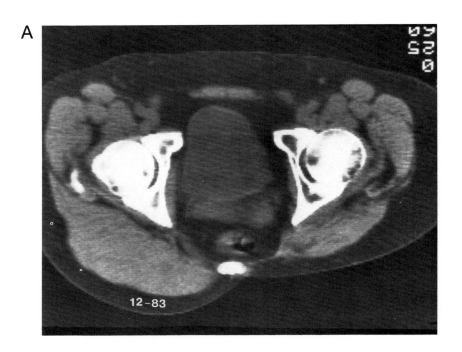

FIG 10–53.
Soft tissue chondrosarcoma. This 28-year-old man was found at the age of 16 to have a malignant histiocytic lymphoma arising from the right buttock. Treatment was irradiation. However, it was discovered 11 years later that the tumor had undergone transformation to a postirradiation pleomorphic sarcoma with metastases, and surgery and chemotherapy were given.

A, this postsurgical unenhanced CT scan, made with the patient in a prone position, shows no evidence of residual neoplasm. There was also no evidence of metastatic disease.

B, fourteen months later, the patient presented with pulmonary metastases, and an enhanced CT scan reveals local recurrence of the tumor. The recurrent neoplasm displays some degree of contrast enhancement, but there is no calcification.

C, the proton-density coronal magnetic resonance images (TR/TE, 1,500/28) show a well-circumscribed, encapsulated mass within the gluteal muscles. The mass displays intermediate signal intensity. No invasion of adjacent bladder or rectum was seen.

The patient underwent resection for the mass, and a diagnosis of chondrosarcoma in the skeletal muscle and fibrous tissue was made.

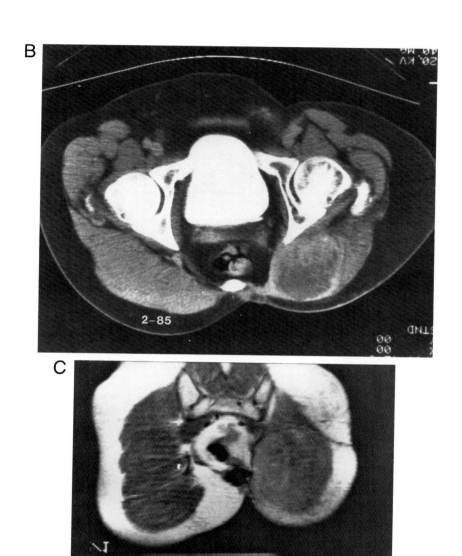

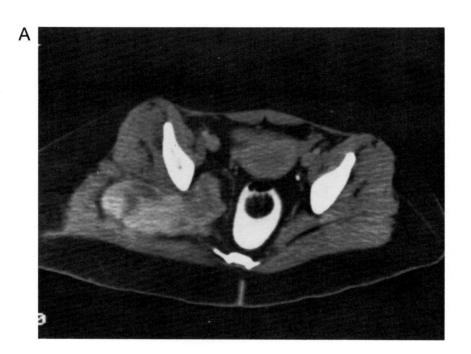

FIG 10–54.
Soft tissue hemangiopericytoma. This 21-year-old woman was found to have a right pelvic mass when she sought a routine Papanicolaou smear examination. Her workup included a pelvic CT scan.

A, a large enhancing mass is seen in the right gluteal region, extending into the sacroiliac notch. On this axial midpelvic image, most of the mass is outside of the pelvis, displacing the gluteus maximus and medius muscles laterally and posteriorly. The right piriform muscle is probably infiltrated, and the rectum is slightly displaced to the left side by the intrapelvic component of the mass.

B

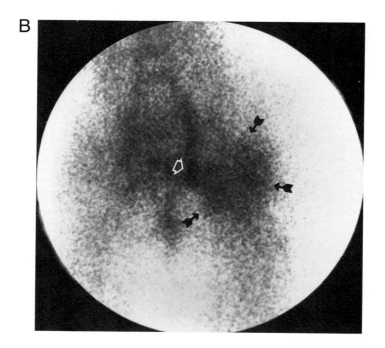

B, a posterior radionuclide flow study was performed by using ^{99m}Tc-labeled methylen diphosphonate as part of bone scan. This image shows a very hypervascular lesion in the region of the right hip *(arrows).* Notice the medial extension of the mass within the pelvis *(open arrow).* The bone scan was otherwise normal.

The patient had a transgluteal biopsy in her hometown, and the diagnosis of mesenchymal tumor was made. However, even after the slides were reviewed by several pathologists, it could not be decided whether the tumor was benign or malignant. The patient was referred to M. D. Anderson Hospital, where surgical exploration was eventually done. The tumor was completely excised through the gluteal incision, and the final pathologic diagnosis was hemangiopericytoma.

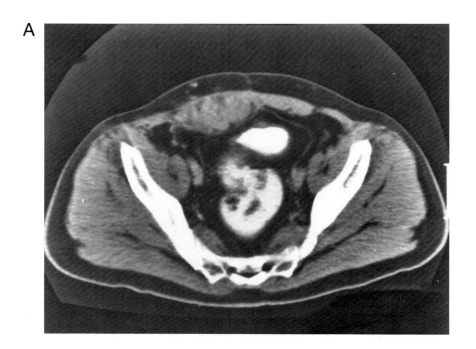

FIG 10–55.
Muscular and soft tissue metastases (multiple cases).

A, this 48-year-old man had a right nephrectomy seven years ago because of renal cell carcinoma. He developed localized abdominal tenderness and on CT a mass was discovered within the right rectus abdominis muscle. Biopsy and then local resection proved metastatic renal cell carcinoma.

B and **C,** in another patient, a 35-year-old man with a diagnosis of transitional cell carcinoma of the bladder, the original CT scan **(B)** shows a bladder tumor in the left side *(arrows)* and the normal rectus muscles. Six months later **(C),** during which period the patient received chemotherapy, the bladder tumor is stable but there are bilateral metastases *(open arrows)* in rectus abdominis muscles. *(Continued.)*

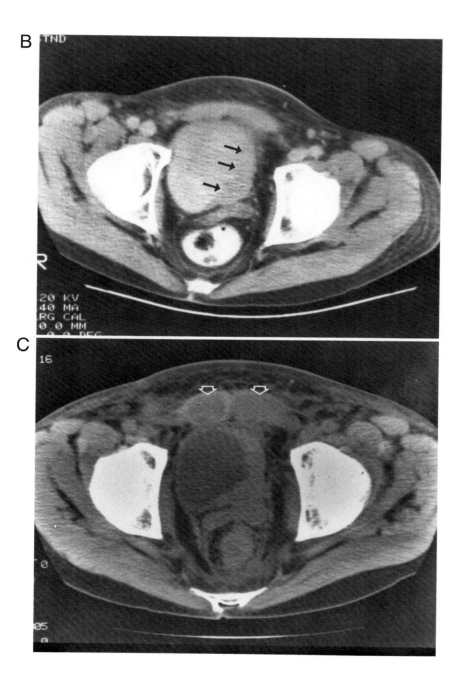

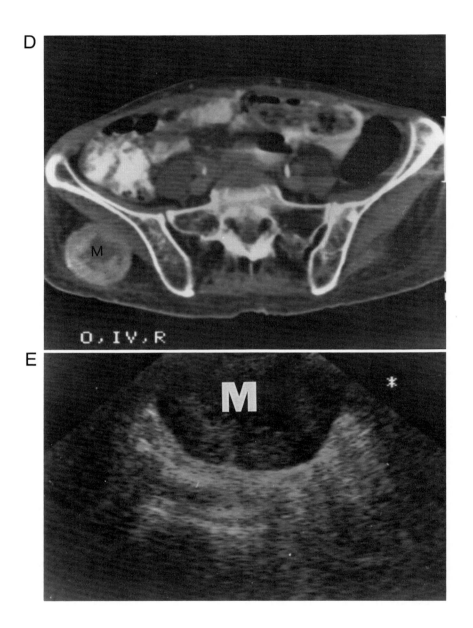

FIG 10–55 (cont.).
D and **E,** this 60-year-old woman 15 years ago had leiomyosarcoma excised from her wrist. She developed metastatic lesions in the abdomen and soft tissues **(D).** While she was receiving chemotherapy, the subcutaneous lesions were followed by sonography **(E)** to determine response to treatment. The metastatic mass *(M)* in the buttock is within the subcutaneous fat **(D),** as seen both on sonogram and CT scan.

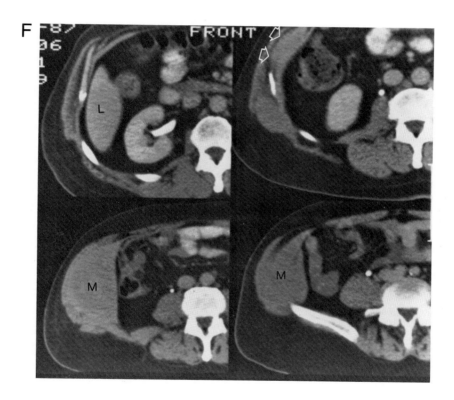

F, this 59-year-old man with previously treated diffuse large cell lymphoma presented with a subcutaneous nodule in the leg and a right flank mass. The CT scan shows an infiltrative mass in the right lateral abdominal wall *(arrows),* starting just below the lower edge of the liver *(L).* The mass *(M)* extends into the upper iliac fossa. Biopsy proved recurrent large cell lymphoma.

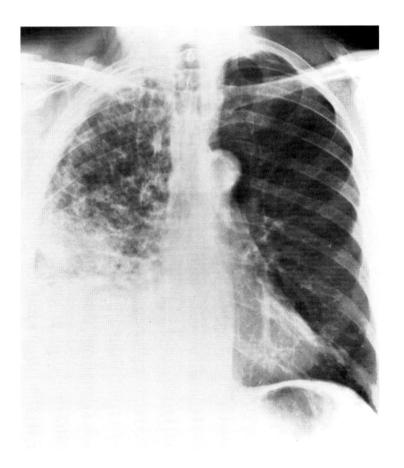

FIG 10–56.
Obscured thoracoabdominal junction. There is complete obscuration of the right thoracoabdominal junction on this posteroanterior radiograph. The parenchymal disease is evident, but further evaluation in the juxtadiaphragmatic region is impossible.

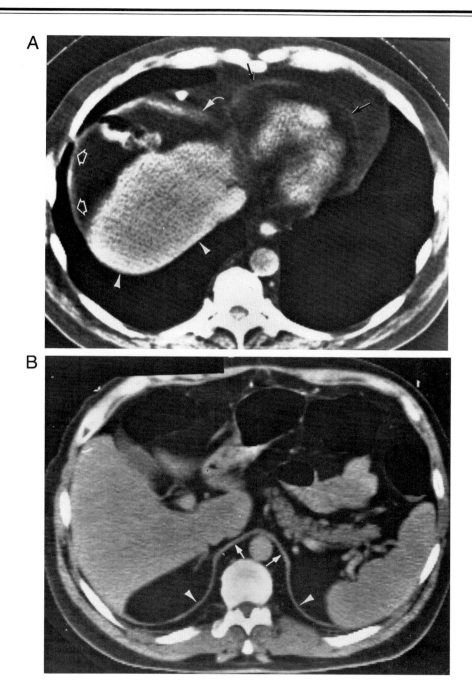

FIG 10–57.
Normal CT anatomy (two cases).

 A, the CT image is at the level of the right thoracoabdominal junction. A right diaphragmatic interface is formed by peripheral lung and liver *(arrowheads);* a diaphragmatic stripe is formed by peripheral lung and intraabdominal fat *(open arrows).* Note the pericardium at this level *(arrows),* and the transition from mediastinal fat to the anterior aspect of the right hemidiaphragm *(curved white arrow).*

 B, a CT scan in another patient demonstrates a normal transition between the diaphragmatic crura *(arrows)* and more posteromedial aspects of the diaphragm *(arrowheads).* The abundant intraabdominal fat (in Gerota's space) and extrapleural paraspinal fat provide the contrast for the stripe presentation of the diaphragm.

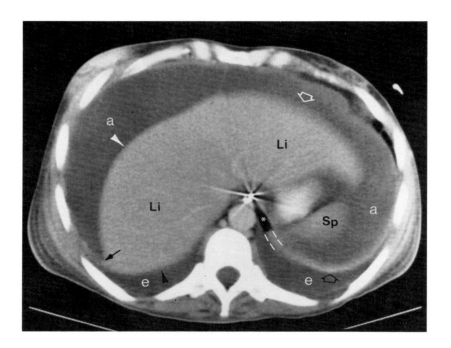

FIG 10–58.
Thoracoabdominal complexity. This CT scan at the level of the thoracoabdominal junction demonstrates a right posterior (peripheral) pleural effusion *(e),* forming a blurred interface (interface sign) with the diaphragm *(black arrowhead).* On the left, a stripe (diaphragm sign) is formed by peripheral pleural effusion *(e)* and intraabdominal ascites *(a) (open black arrow).* Some of this stripe may represent compressed lung *(dotted lines),* which is contiguous with more anteromedial aerated lung *(asterisk).* The spleen *(Sp)* at this level is surrounded by ascites, but the coronary ligament (bare area of the liver sign) restricts the posterior location of the ascites on the right *(arrow).* Note the sharper interface formed by the ascites and liver *(Li)*[66] on the right *(white arrowhead)* but the equivalent of a blurred interface sign on the left *(open white arrow).* The interface sign is due to volume averaging in transaxial planes and can occur on both sides of the diaphragm.

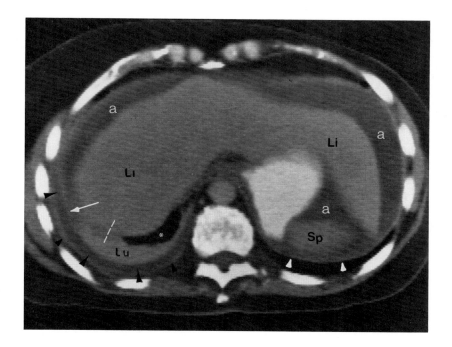

FIG 10–59.
Thoracoabdominal complexity. The transition from thorax to abdomen on this CT image is easy to appreciate on the left, but much more difficult on the right. Peripheral air within the left lower lobe and intraabdominal ascites *(a)* outline a faint left diaphragm stripe (diaphragm sign) *(white arrowheads).* On the right, the combination of parietal pleura *(small black arrowheads)*, pleural effusion *(large black arrowheads)*, compressed lung *(Lu)*, aerated lung *(asterisk)*, and ascites *(a)* presents a complex thoracoabdominal junction. Without the demonstration of a portion of the coronary ligament *(white arrow)*, the parietal pleura could be confused with a diaphragm stripe, the pleural effusion with ascites, the compressed lung with liver *(Li)*, and the aerated lung with part of a subphrenic abscess. Note how the similar contrast between the liver and compressed lung, along with the volume averaging across the transition between the two *(dotted line)*, contributes to this thoracoabdominal complexity *(Sp, spleen).*

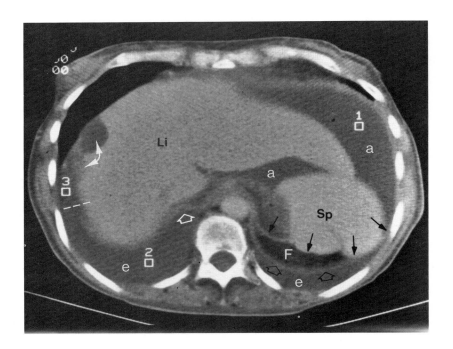

FIG 10–60.
Thoracoabdominal complexity. The bare area of the spleen *(Sp)*[69] *(black arrows)* is illustrated on this CT scan of a patient with ovarian cancer. This bare area prevents the left-sided ascites *(a)* from flowing posterior to the spleen in much the same manner as the bare area of the liver. The fat *(F)* in the superior aspect of Gerota's space provides excellent contrast for demonstrating the diaphragm *(open black arrows)* in the presence of peripheral pleural effusion *(e)*. Note the displaced crus sign[67] on the right *(open white arrow)*. Also note the presence of liver metastases *(curved double arrow)* and poor definition of the interface between the liver *(Li)* and right-sided pleural effusion *(e)* due to malignant serosal implants *(dotted line)*.

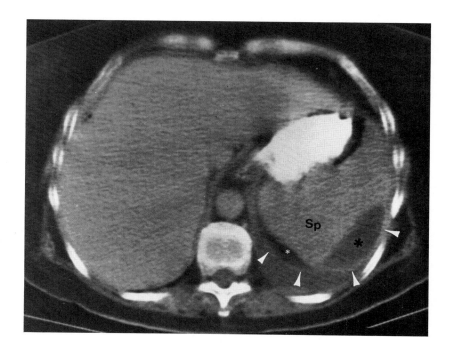

FIG 10–61.
Thoracoabdominal complexity. This CT scan at the level of the left thoracoabdominal junction illustrates the value of the bare area of the spleen. Fat in the superior aspect of Ge-rota's space *(white asterisk)* contributes to the observation of the left hemidiaphragm *(arrowheads)* in the presence of a pleural effusion. This helps isolate the fluid collection *(black asterisk)* as being subdiaphragmatic in location.

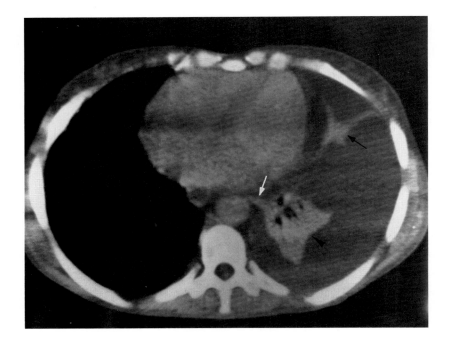

FIG 10–62.
Volume loss, inferior pulmonary ligament, and subpulmonic effusion. This CT scan demonstrates compressive volume loss within the lower lobe *(arrowhead)*. In addition, there is loss of volume within the lingula *(black arrow)*. Note how the lower lobe is tethered to the mediastinum by the inferior pulmonary ligament *(white arrow).*[69]

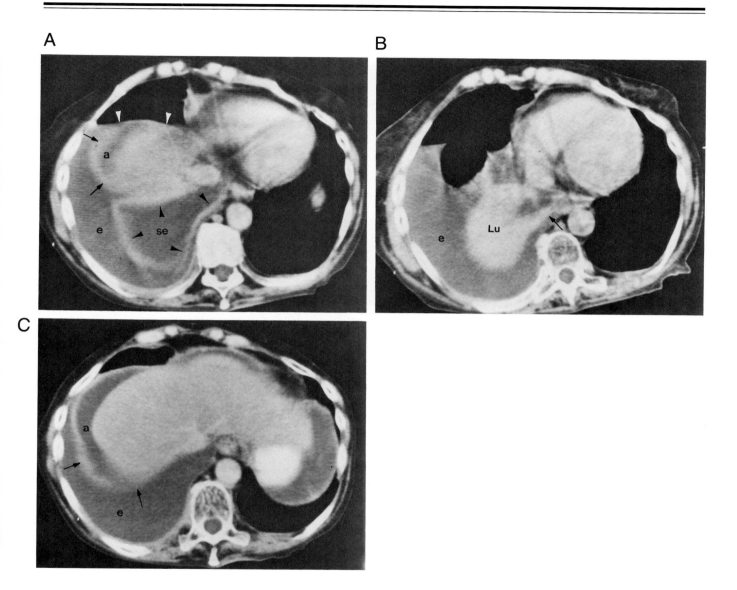

FIG 10–63.
Pseudodiaphragm and subpulmonic effusion.

A, a pseudodiaphragm *(black arrowheads)* is produced by the periphery of compressed lower lobe outlined as a stripe by peripheral effusion *(e)* and subpulmonic effusion *(se).* The actual diaphragm is demonstrated anteriorly as an interface *(white arrowheads)* and more laterally as a broad stripe *(arrows)* outlined by peripheral pleural effusion and central intraabdominal ascites *(a).* Note that this patient has a high coronary ligament relative to the dome of the diaphragm.

B, an image immediately cranial to **A** verifies the compressed lung *(Lu)* floating in the effusion *(e).* Note how the compressed lower lobe is tethered to the mediastinum by the inferior pulmonary ligament at the expected location *(arrow).*[70]

C, an image immediately caudal to **A** verifies that only pleural effusion *(e)* exists at a level below the pseudodiaphragm of **A.** The actual diaphragm *(arrows)* is again outlined by the peripheral effusion and central ascites *(a).* Note that the ascites is more prominent at this lower level, as is the arc of the diaphragm (compare with **A**). Also note the bare area of the liver (coronary ligament) at this level *(right arrow).* (From Proto A.V., Rost R.C.: CT of the thorax: pitfalls in interpretation. *RadioGraphics* 5:792–796, 1985. Reproduced with permission.)

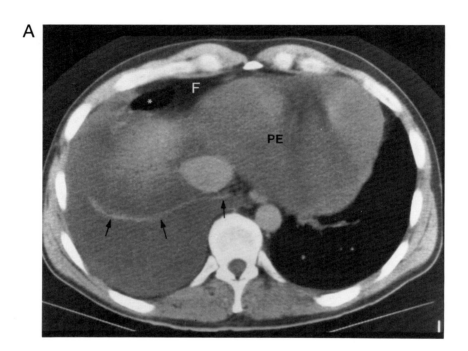

FIG 10–64.

Pseudodiaphragm.

A, a pseudodiaphragm *(arrows)* is produced by compressed lung floating in pleural effusion. Effusion anterior to this stripe combined with aerated lung *(asterisk)* could mimic a subphrenic process. Note the medial aspect of this stripe in the expected position of the inferior pulmonary ligament tether to the mediastinum *(right arrow).* This tether should not be confused with a displaced crus sign (see Fig 10–58). This provides a clue to the lung origin of this pseudodiaphragm. The presence of fat *(F)* in the anterior paracardiac aspect of the mediastinum also contributes to the transition from thorax to abdomen. This patient also has a large pericardial effusion at the level of the diaphragmatic aspect of the pericardium *(PE).*

B, an image immediately cranial to **A** demonstrates air bronchograms within the compressed lung tissue *(arrows).* This verifies that the stripe in **A** is not the right hemidiaphragm.

C, an image immediately caudal to **A** shows the interface of pleural effusion with the true diaphragm (interface sign) *(arrowheads).* Again note the pericardial effusion *(PE).* This and the preceding figure illustrate the need for careful evaluation of images above and below the thoracoabdominal junction to avoid errors in interpretation.

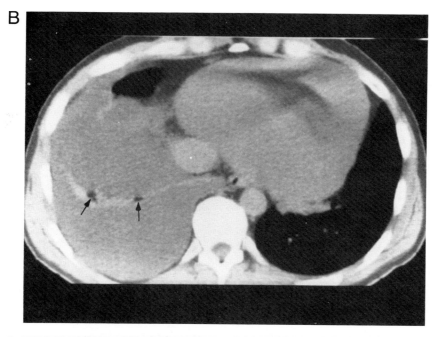

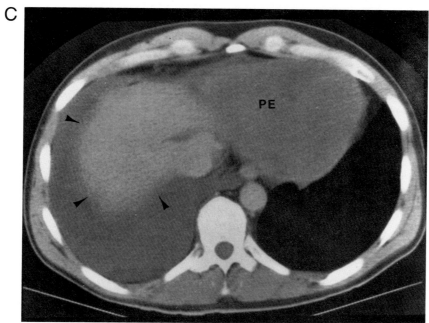

A

B

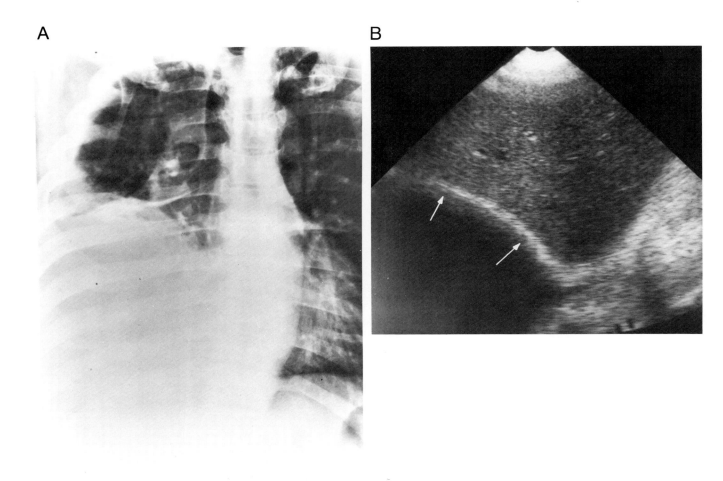

FIG 10–65.
Ultrasound at the thoracoabdominal junction.

A, this right decubitus chest radiograph fails to define the thoracoabdominal junction or separate mass from loculated fluid.

B, a longitudinal ultrasound image easily defines the inverted right hemidiaphragm *(arrows)*. The echoes just above the diaphragm represent tumor tissue in this patient with biopsy-proved mesothelioma *(arrowheads)*. The opacity in **A** was a combination of loculated effusion and tumor tissue.

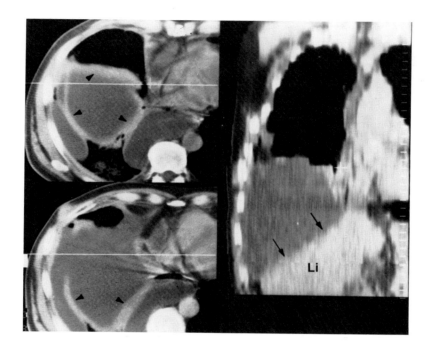

FIG 10–66.
Computed tomography re-formation at the thoracoabdominal junction. The coronal CT re-formation in this patient demonstrates inversion of the right hemidiaphragm *(arrows).* The diaphragm is not seen as a stripe (no difference in contrast), but its position can be inferred from the caudal displacement of the liver *(Li).* The transaxial images show the large loculated effusion surrounding islands of compressed lung tissue *(arrowheads).* Note that aerated lung rather than fluid *(upper image)* occupies the posterior hemithorax, confirming the loculated state of the fluid. The coronal re-formation was computer generated from the transaxial images without additional exposure or cost to the patient.

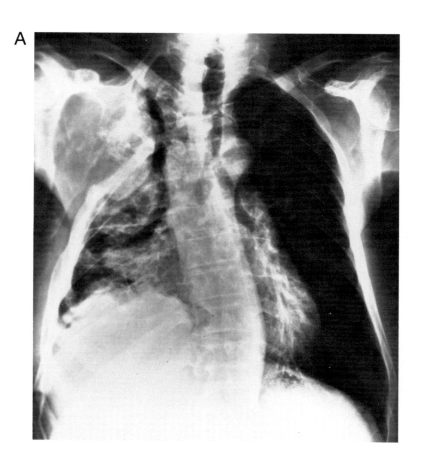

A

FIG 10–67.

Thoracoabdominal chondrosarcoma. This 60-year-old man with multiple exostoses had several benign osteochondromas removed from his right second through fourth ribs 25 years ago. Five years ago, he had a recurrent lesion, which was found to be chondrosarcoma. A second recurrence was discovered most recently, for which he was to have a third surgery.

A, the present chest radiograph shows marked deformity of the right thoracic cage, with evidence of previous surgery and extensive calcified tumor recurrence originating in the region of the prior surgery.

B, the CT scan at the level of the aortic arch demonstrates large soft tissue masses with areas of popcorn-type calcification (see Fig 10–1), characteristic for the presence of chondroid matrix in this malignant neoplasm.

C, a sagittal re-formation at the thoracoabdominal junction shows extension of the disease into the pleural cavity with tumor filling the posterior costophrenic gutter and causing anterior displacement of the liver *(Li) (arrows)* and inferior displacement of the right kidney *(arrowhead)*. Recurrent chondrosarcoma was found at surgery.

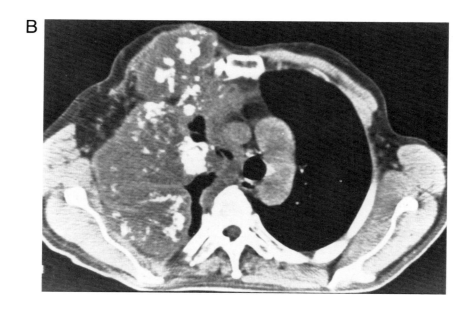

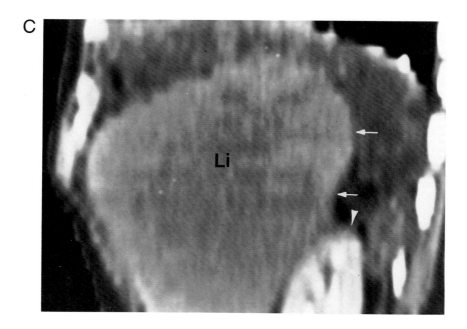

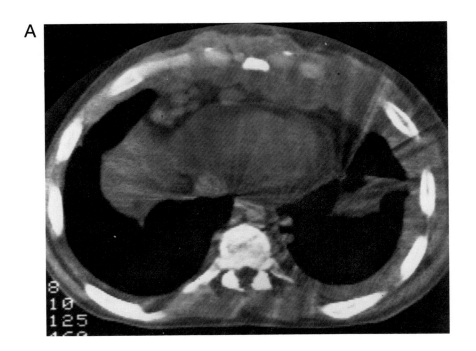

FIG 10–68.

Thoracoabdominal lymphoma. This 24-year-old man had a known history of nodular sclerosing Hodgkin's disease, for which he had been treated during the last three years. He now presented with recurrent disease involving the mediastinum and lower abdominal wall at the thoracoabdominal junction.

A and **B,** the CT scans demonstrate extensive lymphomatous involvement of the anterior abdominal wall, extending superiorly into the chest wall. There are multiple enlarged nodes in the anterior paradiaphragmatic region. Some pleural effusion is present, as are two nodules in the left lung.

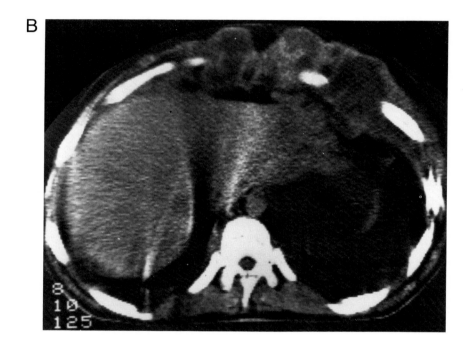

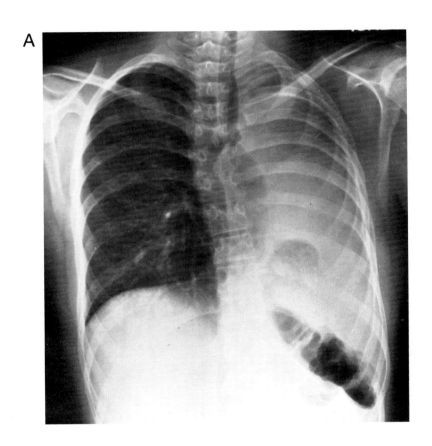

FIG 10–69.

Thoracoabdominal recurrent teratocarcinoma. This 17-year-old boy had a prior pneumonectomy because of extensive involvement of the left hemithorax by teratocarcinoma. He now presented with evidence of recurrent disease in the soft tissue of the lower anterior thoracoabdominal wall.

A, the routine radiograph shows the prior pneumonec-tomy but provides no additional data on possible tumor recurrence within the thorax or abdomen.

B and **C,** the CT scans demonstrate extensive tumor recurrence in the postpneumonectomy space, with spread into and through the diaphragm. There is extension of tumor into the abdomen *(asterisks)* and the soft tissues of the thoracoabdominal wall *(arrows).*

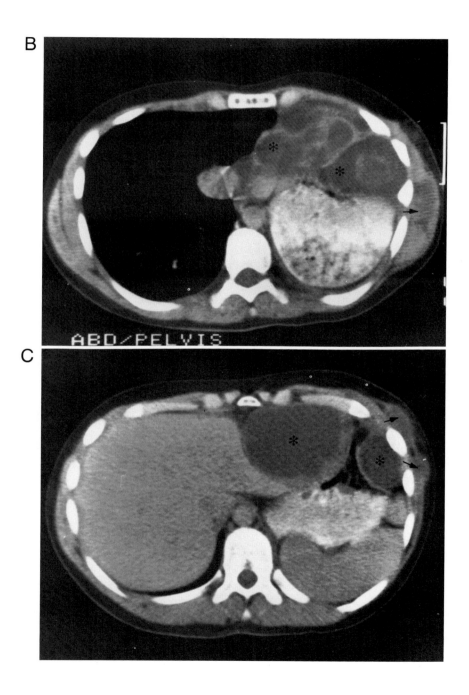

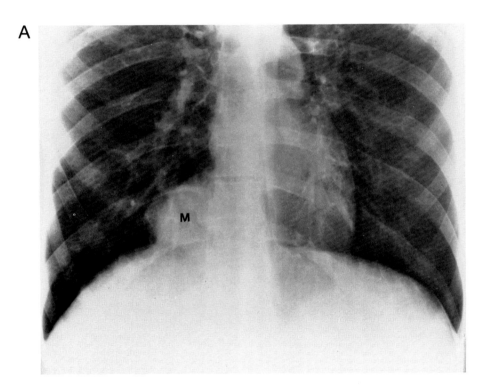

FIG 10–70.
Hepatoma infiltrating the diaphragm. A 21-year-old man presented with a three-month history of weight loss, fatigue, and right upper quadrant pain. Physical examination revealed hepatomegaly.

A, a chest radiograph demonstrates a large right cardiophrenic mass *(M).*

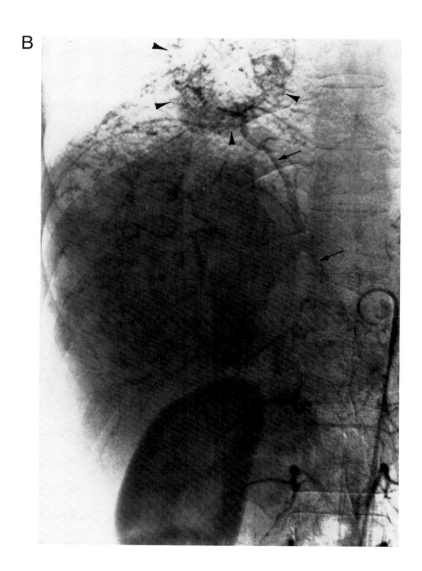

B, a subsequent hepatic arteriogram shows extensive involvement of the liver by a hepatoma (biopsy proved), with tumor extension into the diaphragm *(arrowheads).* Note the inferior phrenic artery supply to this mass *(arrows).*

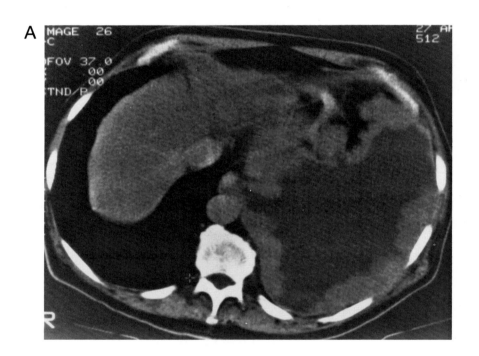

FIG 10–71.
Mesothelioma, with diaphragmatic invasion (two cases).

A and **B,** this 67-year-old man with a known diagnosis of left pleural mesothelioma had thoracic CT for reevaluation. This CT image **(A)** shows extensive involvement of the left hemithorax by mesothelioma. The combined tumor tissue and fluid displace mediastinal structures. Additional transaxial images (not shown) failed to demonstrate the thoracoabdominal junction, and inversion of the diaphragm was suspected.

B, a coronal re-formation confirms the massive involvement of the left hemithorax and easily demonstrates inversion of the diaphragm. Note the tumor masses about the superior surface of the inverted diaphragm *(arrows).*

C, a CT analysis on a different patient with mesothelioma shows how this lesion progresses from the diaphragmatic surface to invade the right crus of the diaphragm *(arrowheads).*

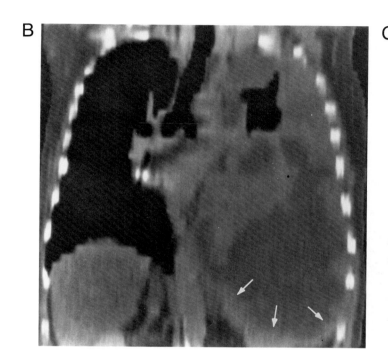

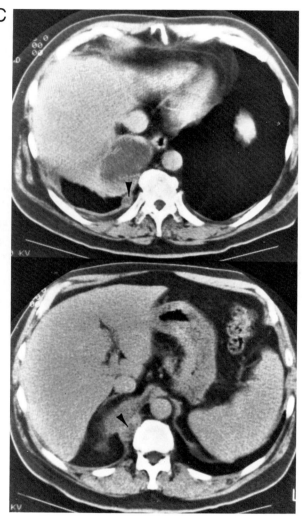

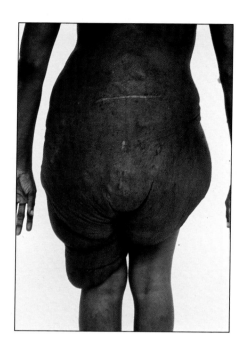

PLATE 49

11

Abdominal and Pelvic Imaging of Lymphomas and Leukemias

Luceil B. North, M.D.

In lymphoma and leukemia, abdominal and pelvic imaging is primarily used to evaluate the lymph nodes. However, the presentation of non-Hodgkin's lymphoma is often extranodal, and there may or may not be regional or diffuse adenopathy.

Untreated Hodgkin's disease and non-Hodgkin's lymphoma differ in distribution of involvement, so imaging workup is tailored to predicted sites of disease. Hodgkin's disease tends to occur with contiguity (Fig 11–1)[1, 2] in the retroperitoneal, common iliac, and external iliac nodes. In non-Hodgkin's lymphoma, on the other hand, the intraabdominal nodes are frequently involved in addition to the retroperitoneal and pelvic nodes, and lesions of solid organs and the gastrointestinal tract are common. Recurrent lymphoma may occur in any site.

Hodgkin's disease is typically first seen in early stages, with neck and mediastinal adenopathy, but 20% to 40% of patients with supradiaphragmatic presentation prove to have disease in the abdomen (Figs 11–2 and 11–3). Patients with relapsed Hodgkin's disease may have involvement of any nodal or extranodal site, and a non-Hodgkin's lymphoma pattern may be simulated (Fig 11–4). Patients with non-Hodgkin's lymphoma often present with intraabdominal disease with nodal or extranodal disease (Figs 11–5 to 11–7).[3, 4] In leukemia, there may be nodal enlargement, hepatosplenomegaly, or infil-tration of such solid organs as the kidneys, uterus, ovaries, or testes.

Lymphangiography and computed tomography (CT) are routinely used for the basic staging of abdominal disease. Other modalities used for staging in selected patients include ultrasonography, gastrointestinal barium studies, and nuclear imaging. Magnetic resonance imaging (MRI) has not yet proved to be beneficial in nodal evaluation or to offer significant information unavailable by CT.

Ultrasonography has proved to be very useful in leukemia for the evaluation of such solid organs as the kidneys, uterus, ovaries, and testes. In lymphoma and leukemia patients with soft tissue masses, it is used to outline extent of disease and the relationship of masses to the skeleton.[5–7]

Nuclear imaging of the liver and spleen has frequently been performed but is of limited usefulness.[8, 9] Gallium scanning has been used to detect active disease, but the results are nonspecific and dependent on histopathology.[10–14] Its greatest utility is in assessing for activity in residual masses and for relapse in previously treated areas.[15–19] A number of comparative studies to determine efficiency have been done among the various imaging modalities.[20–26]

Whether to use lymphangiography or CT as the initial study in lymphoma depends on the type of lymphoma, the availability of appropriate equipment, and the experience and expertise of the radiologists. It may also depend on whether or not staging laparotomy is performed routinely.

In Hodgkin's disease, lymphangiography can be used as the primary or sole staging method since nodal enlargement is typically retroperitoneal and pelvic. There are descriptions of technique and nodal patterns in the literature,[27–29] and the technique has a high degree of accuracy.[30–33] The procedure can be done at any age and may be repeated as needed. If the lower limb lymphangiogram shows abnormal nodes in the abdomen and pelvis, further staging may be unnecessary. Fewer than 5% of Hodgkin's patients with normal lymphangiographic results will have mesenteric nodal disease at laparotomy.[21, 30] Approximately 30% with a normal lymphangiogram will have disease in the spleen or the celiac or portal nodes, but usually those foci are too small to be detected by currently available imaging methods (Fig 11–8).[31, 34, 35] In conjunction with CT, some contrast agents, such as ethiodized oil emulsion 13 (EOE-13),[36] have been shown to enhance detectability of lesions in the spleen and liver, but these are not yet generally available. Liver-spleen nuclear scanning has been largely disappointing in patients with Hodgkin's disease, serving mainly to indicate size of the organs (Fig 11–9). The usefulness of MRI in detecting lesions not detectable by ultrasonography or CT has not been established.

In non-Hodgkin's lymphoma, CT is probably the most efficacious single modality for primary staging of the abdomen and pelvis.[21, 30, 34, 37] Patients with non-Hodgkin's lymphoma frequently have enlarged nodes in the abdomen outside of the lymphangiogram-imaged area, and extranodal sites of disease are common (Figs 11–10 to 11–29).[38, 39] In patients in whom CT results are normal, lymphangiography may detect disease in normal-sized or slightly enlarged lymph nodes. Not only the presence of disease but whether that disease is bulky or extensive is significant for therapy planning and prognosis.[40]

In patients with leukemia, abdominal and pelvic imaging is done mainly to evaluate for adenopathy and for liver and spleen enlargement (Fig 11–30).[41–45] There may be extranodal disease, either because of leukemic infiltration or as the lymphoma counterpart of the disease (e.g., chronic lymphocytic leukemia and lymphocytic lymphoma [Figs 11–31 to 11–35] and myelocytic leukemia and granulocytic sarcoma [Figs 11–36 and 11–37]). Lymphangiography detects retroperitoneal and pelvic nodes and has been useful in staging.[48] If knowledge of the extent of disease is essential for management, CT is the imaging modality of choice. In acute leukemias, extranodal involvement is common, and the kidney and spleen are the solid organs most commonly involved (Fig 11–38).[49, 50] Ovary (Fig 6–14) and testis (Fig 5–39) are frequent sites of disease in children, especially in cases of relapse.[51–53] Ultrasonography may be quite helpful in following patients for solid organ involvement (Fig 11–39). Lesions of bone may be associated with soft tissue masses presenting in the abdomen or pelvis.[54]

Lymphangiography has some definite advantages over other imaging modalities. Because nodal architecture is outlined, subtle changes can be detected even in small nodes. An experienced lymphangiographer can usually differentiate between enlarged nodes due to hyperplasia and the abnormal nodes of lymphoma. Contrast-filled nodes can often be followed for months with a single abdominal radiograph, and subtle changes in size or shape may be detected before changes are seen by CT (Fig 11–40). Lymphangiography may be used in patients of any age and repeated as necessary.

On the other hand, lymphangiography is time-consuming and requires that the radiologist have considerable experience and expertise in performing the procedure and interpreting the findings. General anesthesia is usually necessary in the very young.[55] The examination is typically limited to visualization of femoral, inguinal, external iliac, common iliac, and retroperitoneal nodes to the level of L-2, although occasionally other nodes may fill with contrast via collateral lymphatics. Whereas CT will be positive for nodal disease in only a few Hodgkin's patients in whom lymphangiographic results are normal, patients with non-Hodgkin's lymphoma frequently have other nodal or extranodal disease.

In some centers, CT has completely replaced lymphangiography, largely because of its more complete nodal and extranodal imaging in the abdomen and pelvis.[39] Abdominal and pelvic masses and nodal enlargement outside of the lymphangiographically defined area are imaged, including high paraaortic (above the level of L-2) and retrocrural nodes, as well as intraabdominal nodes in the gastrohepatic ligament, parapancreatic area, porta hepatis, and celiac axis, and about the splenic hilus.[56] At M. D. Anderson Hospital, we have found that lymphangiography and CT are complementary in many instances and that the latter is not necessarily a substitute for the former. Enlarged nodes detected by CT may be shown by lymphangiography to be due to hyperplasia or to aggregation of small nodes. If both procedures are to be used, it is helpful to begin with lymphangiography, because the opacified nodes serve as markers on CT examination.

The disadvantages of CT include the expense for frequent repeated studies, the discomfort to the patient, and the inability to detect early nodal relapses, which can be readily detected by visualization of contrast-filled nodes on a single abdominal radiograph as a lymphangiographic follow-up (Figs 11–30 and 11–35).[57]

REFERENCES

1. Kaplan H.S.: *Hodgkin's Disease*, ed. 2. Cambridge, Mass., Harvard University Press, 1980, pp. 96–98.
2. Kadin M.E., Glatstein E., Dorfman R.F.: Clinicopathologic studies of 117 untreated patients subjected to laparotomy for the staging of Hodgkin's disease. *Cancer* 27:1277–1294, 1970.
3. Heifetz L.J., Fuller L.M., Rodgers R.W., et al.: Laparotomy findings in lymphangiogram-staged I and II non-Hodgkin's lymphomas. *Cancer* 45:2778–2786, 1980.
4. Goffinet D.R., Warnke R., Dunnick N.R., et al.: Clinical and surgical (laparotomy) evaluation of patients with non-Hodgkin's lymphomas. *Cancer Treat. Rep.* 61:981–992, 1977.
5. Strauss S., Libson E., Schwartz E., et al.: Renal sonography in American Burkitt lymphoma. *AJR* 146:549–552, 1986.
6. Shirkhoda A., Staab E.V., Mittelstaedt C.A.: Renal lymphoma imaged by ultrasound and gallium-67. *Radiology* 137:175–180, 1980.
7. Goh T.S., LeQuesne G.W., Wong K.Y.: Severe infiltration of the kidneys with ultrasonic abnormalities in acute lymphoblastic leukemia. *Am. J. Dis. Child.* 132:1204–1205, 1978.
8. Lipton M.J., DeNardo G.L., Silverman S., et al.: Evaluation of the liver and spleen in Hodgkin's disease—I. The value of hepatic scintigraphy. *Am. J. Med.* 52:356–361, 1972.
9. Silverman S., DeNardo G.L., Glatstein E., et al.: Evaluation of the liver and spleen in Hodgkin's disease—II. The value of splenic scintigraphy. *Am. J. Med.* 52:362–366, 1972.
10. Anderson K.C., Leonard R.C.F., Canellos G.P., et al.: High-dose gallium imaging in lymphoma. *Am. J. Med.* 75:327–331, 1983.
11. Silberstein E.B.: The role of tumor-imaging radiopharmaceuticals. *Am. J. Med.* 60:226–237, 1976.
12. Richman S.D., Appelbaum F., Levenson S.M., et al.: [67]Ga radionuclide imaging in Burkitt's lymphoma. *Radiology* 117:639–645, 1975.
13. Adler S., Parthasarathy K.L., Bakshi S.P., et al.: Gallium-67-citrate scanning for the localization and staging of lymphomas. *J. Nucl. Med.* 16:255–260, 1975.
14. Edwards C.L., Hayes R.L.: Scanning malignant neo-
15. Brown M.L., O'Donnell J.B., Thrall J.H., et al.: Gallium-67 scintigraphy in untreated and treated non-Hodgkin's lymphomas. *J. Nucl. Med.* 19:875–879, 1978.
16. Turner D.A., Fordham E.W., Ali A., et al.: Gallium-67 imaging in the management of Hodgkin's disease and other malignant lymphomas. *Semin. Nucl. Med.* 8:205–218, 1978.
17. Levi J.A., O'Connell M.J., Linell W., et al.: Role of [67]gallium citrate scanning in the management of non-Hodgkin's lymphoma. *Cancer* 36:1690–1701, 1975.
18. Henkin R.E., Polcyn R.E., Quinn J.L.: Scanning treated Hodgkin's disease with ^{67}Ga citrate. *Radiology* 110:151–154, 1974.
19. Glass R.B.J., Fernbach S.K., Conway J.J., et al.: Gallium scintigraphy in American Burkitt lymphoma—accurate assessment of tumor load and prognosis. *AJR* 145:671–676, 1985.
20. Bruneton J.-N., Schneider M. (eds.): *Radiology of Lymphomas*. New York, Springer-Verlag, 1986, pp. 60–69.
21. Castellino R.A., Marglin S.I.: Imaging of abdominal and pelvic lymph nodes—lymphography or computed tomography? *Invest. Radiol.* 17:433–443, 1982.
22. Ichiya Y., Oshiumi Y., Kamoi I., et al.: [67]Ga scanning and upper gastrointestinal series of gastric lymphomas. *Radiology* 142:187–192, 1982.
23. Cohen M.D., Siddiqui A., Weetman R., et al.: Hodgkin disease and non-Hodgkin lymphomas in children—utilization of radiological modalities. *Radiology* 158:499–505, 1986.
24. Zornosa J., Ginaldi S.: Computed tomography in hepatic lymphoma. *Radiology* 138:405–410, 1981.
25. Cabanillas F., Zornosa J., Haynie T.P., et al.: Comparison of lymphangiograms and gallium scans in the non-Hodgkin's lymphomas. *Cancer* 39:85–88, 1976.
26. Seabold J.E., Votaw M.L., Keyes J.W., et al.: Gallium citrate ^{67}Ga scanning—clinical usefulness in lymphoma patients. *Arch. Intern. Med.* 136:1370–1374, 1976.
27. Clouse M.E.: Lymphoma of abdomen and retroperitoneum, in Clouse M.E., Wallace S. (eds.): *Lymphatic Imaging*, ed. 2. Baltimore, Williams & Wilkins Co., 1985, pp. 264–289.
28. Wallace S., Jackson L., Schaffer B., et al.: Lymphangiograms—their diagnostic and therapeutic potential. *Radiology* 76:179–199, 1961.
29. Jing B.S., McGraw J.P.: Lymphangiography in diagnosis and management of malignant lymphomas. *Cancer* 19:565–572, 1966.
30. Marglin S.I., Castellino R.A.: Noninvasive evaluation of newly diagnosed lymphomas. *Appl. Radiol.* 14:79–84, 1985.
31. Castellino R.A., Hoppe R.T., Blank N., et al.: Computed tomography, lymphography, and staging laparotomy—correlations in initial staging of Hodgkin disease. *AJR* 143:37–41, 1984.
32. Marglin S., Castellino R.: Lymphographic accuracy in

plasms with gallium 67. *JAMA* 212:1182–1190, 1970.

632 consecutive, previously untreated cases of Hodgkin disease and non-Hodgkin lymphoma. *Radiology* 140:351–353, 1981.

33. Kademian M.T., Wirtanen G.W.: Accuracy of bipedal lymphography in Hodgkin's disease. *AJR* 129: 1041–1042, 1977.

34. North L.B., Wallace S.: Initial staging of lymphoma using chest and abdominal radiographic techniques, in Ford R.J. Jr., Fuller L.M., Hagemeister F.B. (eds.): *Hodgkin's Disease and Non-Hodgkin's Lymphoma: New Perspectives in Immunopathology, Diagnosis, and Treatment.* UT M.D. Anderson Clinical Conference on Cancer. New York, Raven Press, 1984, vol. 27, pp. 51–66.

35. Vlasak M.C., Martin R.G., Fuller L.M., et al.: Clinical staging of Hodgkin's disease—results of staging laparotomy. *Cancer Bull.* 35:209–214, 1983.

36. Thomas J.L., Bernardino M.E., Vermess M., et al.: EOE-13 in the detection of hepatosplenic lymphoma. *Radiology* 145:629–634, 1982.

37. Castellino R.A.: Imaging techniques for extent determination of Hodgkin's disease and non-Hodgkin's lymphoma. *Prog. Clin. Biol. Res.* 132D:365–372, 1983.

38. Glazer H.S., Lee J.K.T., Balfe D.M., et al.: Non-Hodgkin lymphoma—computed tomographic demonstration of unusual extranodal involvement. *CRC Crit. Rev. Diagn. Imaging* 18:1–28, 1982.

39. Lee J.K.T., Balfe D.M.: Computed tomography evaluation of lymphoma patients. *Radiology* 149:211–217, 1983.

40. Jagannath S., Velasquez W.S., Tucker S.L., et al.: Tumor burden assessment and its implication for a prognostic model in advanced diffuse large-cell lymphomas. *J. Clin. Oncol.* 4:859–865, 1986.

41. Geoffray A., Shirkhoda A., Wallace S.: Abdominal and pelvic computed tomography in leukemic patients. *J. Comput. Assist. Tomogr.* 8:857–860, 1984.

42. Schrier S.L.: The leukemias and the myeloproliferative disorders, in Rubenstein E., Federman D.D. (eds.): *Scientific American Medicine.* New York, Scientific American, 1984, pp. 1–22.

43. Liepman M.K.: The chronic leukemias. *Med. Clin. North Am.* 64:705–727, 1980.

44. Miller D.R.: Acute lymphoblastic leukemia. *Pediatr. Clin. North Am.* 27:269–291, 1980.

45. Rundles R.W., Moore J.O.: Chronic lymphocytic leukemia. *Cancer* 42:941–945, 1978.

46. Meis J.M., Butler J.J., Osborne B.M., et al.: Granulocytic sarcoma in nonleukemic patients. *Cancer* 58:2697–2709, 1986.

47. Sowers J.J., Moody D.M., Naidich T.P., et al.: Radiographic features of granulocytic sarcoma (chloroma). *J. Comput. Assist. Tomogr.* 3:226–233, 1979.

48. Grellet J., Curet P., Laemmel M.G., et al.: Correlation between lymphographic grouping and anatomic and clinical stages in chronic lymphoid leukemia. *AJR* 133:797–803, 1979.

49. Sutow W.W., Fernbach D.J., Vietti T.J.: *Clinical Pediatric Oncology,* ed. 3. St. Louis, C.V. Mosby Co., 1984.

50. Araki T.: Leukemic involvement of the kidney in children: CT features. *J. Comput. Assist. Tomogr.* 6:781–784, 1982.

51. Shirkhoda A., Eftekhari F., Frankel L.S., et al.: Diagnosis of leukemic relapse in the pelvic soft tissues of juvenile females. *JCU* 14:191–195, 1986.

52. Rayor R.A., Scheible W., Brock W.A., et al.: High-resolution ultrasonography in the diagnosis of testicular relapse in patients with acute lymphoblastic leukemia. *J. Urol.* 128:602–603, 1982.

53. Chessells J.M.: Acute lymphoblastic leukemia. *Semin. Hematol.* 19:155–171, 1982.

54. Belasco J.B., Bryan J.H., McMillan C.W.: Acute promyelocytic leukemia presenting as a pelvic mass. *Med. Pediatr. Oncol.* 4:289–295, 1982.

55. Castellino R.A., Bellani F.F., Gasparini M., et al.: Radiographic findings in previously untreated children with non-Hodgkin's lymphoma. *Radiology* 117:657–663, 1975.

56. Ellert J., Kreel L.: The role of computed tomography in the initial staging and subsequent management of the lymphomas. *J. Comput. Assist. Tomogr.* 4:368–391, 1980.

57. Pera A., Capek M., Shirkhoda A.: Lymphangiography and CT in the follow-up of patients with lymphoma. *Radiology* 164:631–633, 1987.

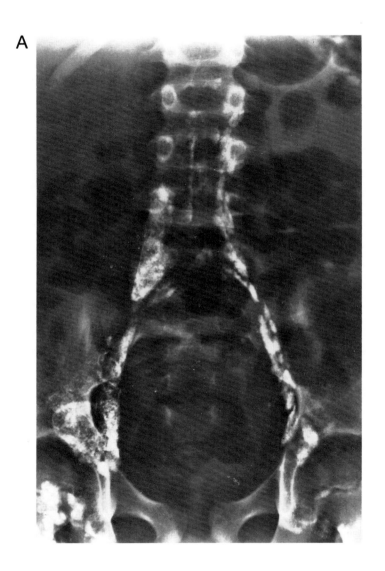

FIG 11–1.
Hodgkin's disease, nodular sclerosing type. A five-year-old boy presented with a knot in his right groin.

   A through **C,** frontal **(A)** and oblique **(B** and **C)** lymphangiograms show foamy, enlarged nodes with defects on the right *(arrows).* The nodes on the left are normal. Oblique views are necessary to display the nodes adequately. *(Continued.)*

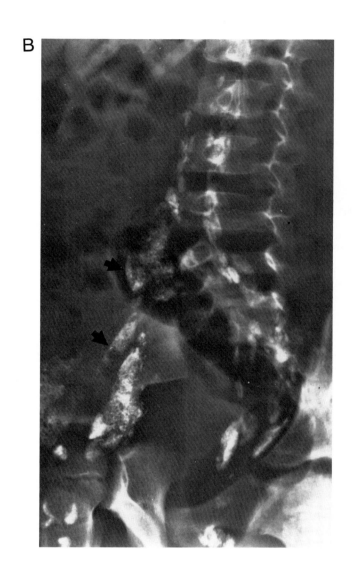

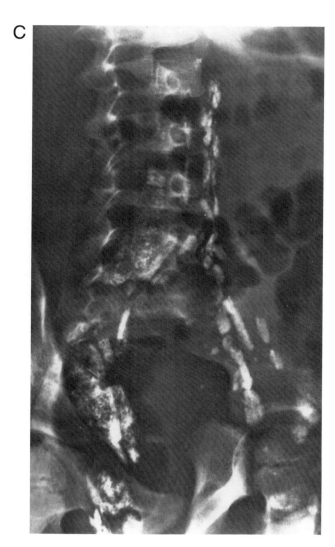

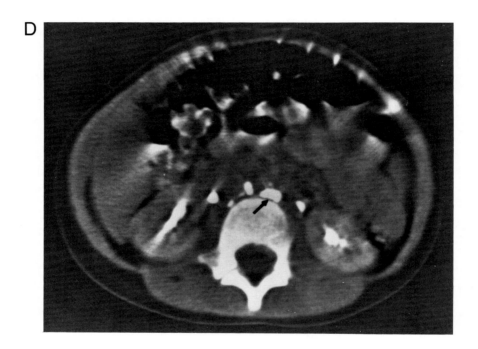

FIG 11–1 (cont.).
   D and **E,** because of the lack of fat, these CT images are difficult to interpret even with contrast material in the lymph nodes. At both levels, the erroneous impression that the nodes on the left are enlarged *(arrow)* is given. The effect occurs because multiple lymph nodes are clustered.
   It is not unusual for nodal involvement to be unilateral

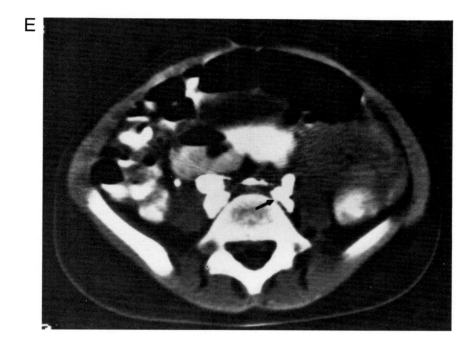

in early stages of Hodgkin's disease, but involvement is typically contiguous. In spite of the apparent left nodal enlargement on CT, the lymphangiograms clearly show those nodes to be normal in size and configuration.

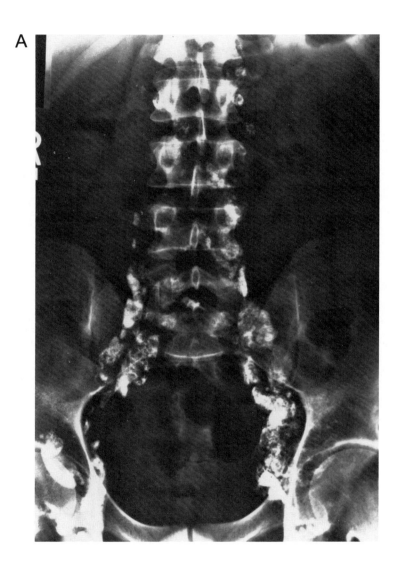

FIG 11–2.
Hodgkin's disease, nodular sclerosing type. A 33-year-old man had a one-year history of weight loss, drenching night sweats, generalized pruritus, and inguinal adenopathy that had been waxing and waning.

A, the lymphangiogram shows abnormal lymph nodes in the paraaortic, bilateral common iliac, and left external iliac regions.

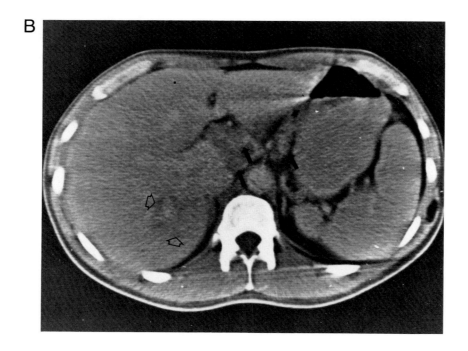

B, a CT scan shows enlarged nodes *(arrows)* in the gastrohepatic and portal areas. Also, there is an area of low density *(open arrows)* in the liver, but the spleen is normal. *(Continued.)*

C

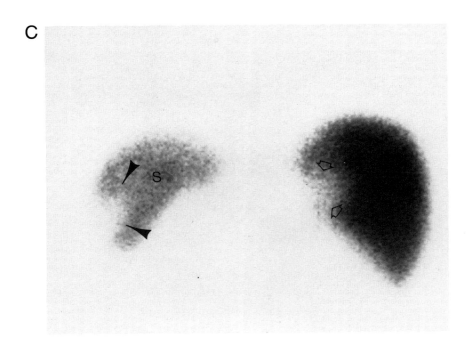

FIG 11–2 (cont.).
  C, posterior view of the liver-spleen scan shows diffuse decreased uptake along with a large defect in the lateral aspect of the spleen *(arrowheads).* The liver involvement is also seen on nuclear study *(open arrows).*
  D and **E,** coronal sonogram of the spleen **(D)** shows an area of nonhomogeneous echogenicity in the spleen *(arrowheads).* The midline transverse scan **(E)** shows the enlarged nodes *(N)* in the porta hepatis.
  Patients with systemic complaints are more likely to have intraabdominal disease than are those who have no symptoms.

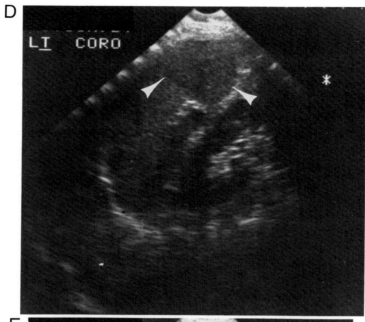

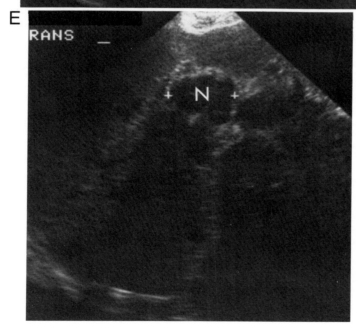

A

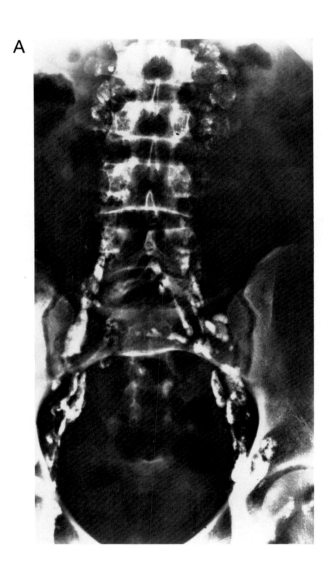

FIG 11–3.
Hodgkin's disease, lymphocyte-predominance type. A 20-year-old man who presented with abdominal pain, nausea, and vomiting had CT examination followed by lymphangiography.

A, a lymphangiogram shows enlarged lymph nodes with abnormal architecture, particularly in the paraaortic, common iliac, and left external iliac areas.

B, a CT scan shows large nodal masses involving the celiac and portal nodes *(arrows)*. There are multiple defects

in the spleen *(S)*, and there is probable involvement of the left kidney *(K)*.

C, two months later, a radiograph of the abdomen shows the lymph nodes to be markedly decreased in size and to have essentially normal architecture, except for those in the upper paraaortic areas *(arrows)*.

Six months later, following therapy, the only abnormal finding of a staging laparotomy was a single focus of lymphoma in the spleen.

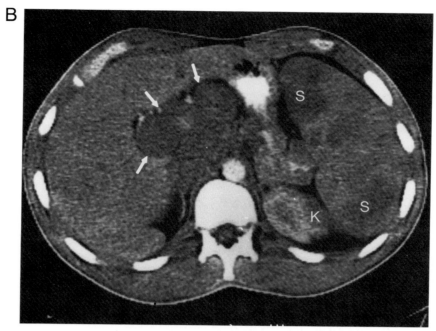

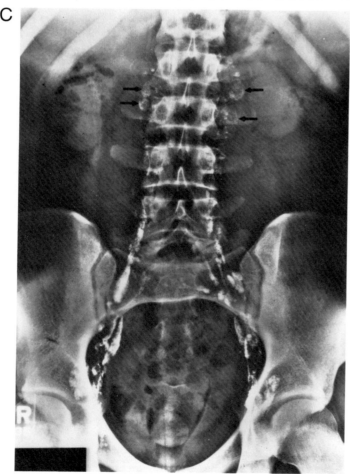

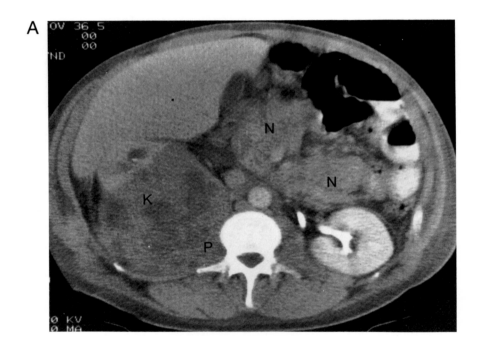

FIG 11–4.

Hodgkin's disease, nodular sclerosing type. A 30-year-old man presented with one of the several relapses of Hodgkin's disease that he had since diagnosis five years previously.

A, computed tomography through the kidneys shows masses involving the mesenteric nodes *(N)*, the right kidney *(K)*, and psoas muscle *(P)*.

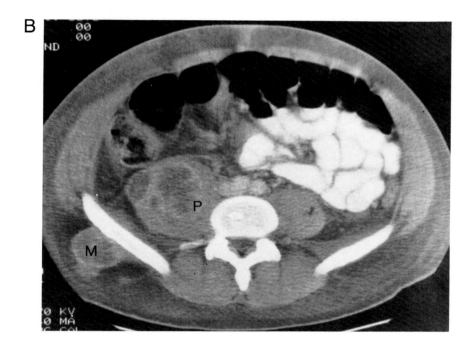

B, an image obtained at the level of the iliac crest shows the inferior extent of the mass, which involves the psoas muscle *(P)*. There was also a mass posterior to the right iliac crest *(M)*.

Soft tissue involvement by Hodgkin's disease is seen only in the advanced stages of disease and is far more common in the non-Hodgkin's lymphomas, particularly in large cell lymphoma.

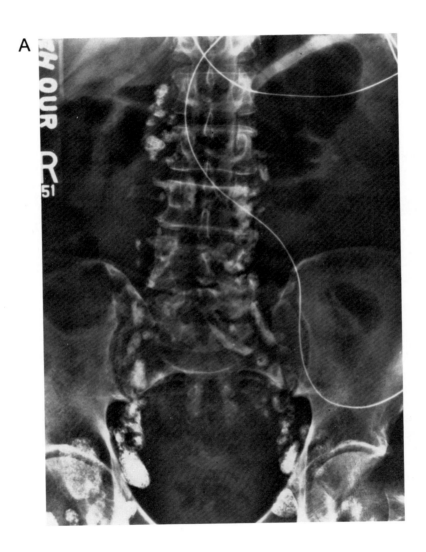

FIG 11–5.
Nodular large cell lymphoma. A 67-year-old man presented with a large cervical mass. A biopsy was performed, and diagnosis of nodular large cell lymphoma was made.

A, the original lymphangiogram is normal.

B, a repeat lymphangiogram one year later shows diffuse enlargement of all the lymph nodes and abnormal nodal architecture.

C, one month later, following chemotherapy, an abdominal radiograph shows the lymph nodes to have considerably decreased in size, although they remain larger than on the initial imaging.

During the course of the disease, the lymph nodes were noted to wax and wane in size with the timing of the various chemotherapy courses.

B

C

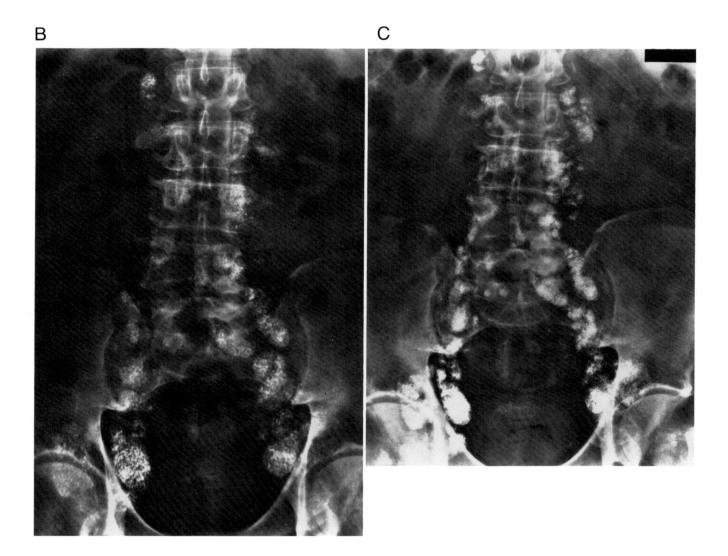

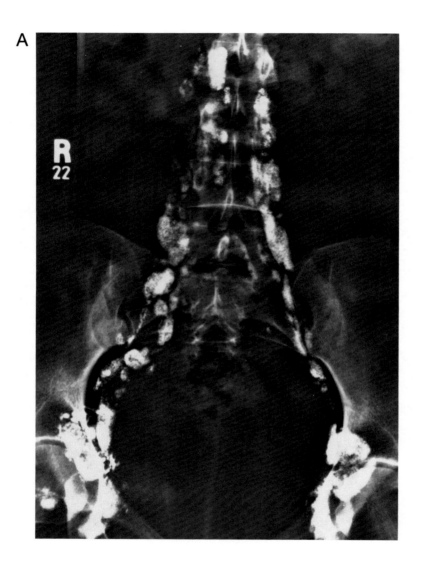

FIG 11–6.

Diffuse large cell lymphoma. In a 37-year-old woman, diffuse large cell lymphoma was diagnosed by biopsy of a subcutaneous tissue mass just proximal to the elbow in the left arm.

A, a lymphangiogram shows somewhat enlarged lymph nodes with normal architecture and was interpreted as showing only hyperplastic nodes.

B, a CT scan done before lymphangiography shows an enlarged right common iliac lymph node *(arrow)* at the level of the iliac crests. The interpretation of the CT scan would be positive for lymphoma.

C, a CT scan at the level of the hip joints, where several enlarged hyperplastic lymph nodes were seen by lymphangiography, shows no adenopathy. The only enlarged lymph node detected by CT was that shown in **B.**

Lymphangiography is especially useful in evaluating nodal architecture and for distinguishing between enlarged nodes and clustered smaller nodes.

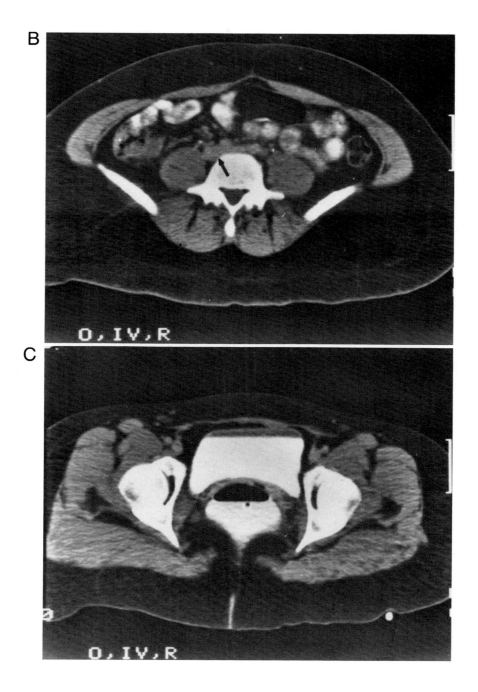

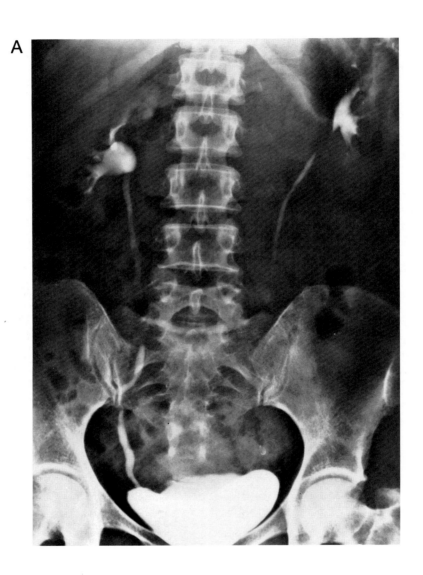

FIG 11–7.

Diffuse large cell lymphoma. A 56-year-old woman with enlarged left supraclavicular lymph nodes showed a large, left upper quadrant mass on physical examination. The mass was thought to be separate from the spleen.

A, an intravenous pyelogram shows lateral displacement of the left kidney and proximal ureter by a large left paraspinal mass.

B, the lymphatic phase of the lymphangiogram shows the flow toward the large, abnormal nodes in the left upper quadrant corresponding to the mass seen on the intravenous pyelogram.

C, a supine radiograph of the abdomen taken 24 hr later for the nodal phase shows not only the mass *(M)* in the left upper quadrant, but massively enlarged lymph nodes in the left midabdomen *(arrows)*. There is incomplete emptying of the lymphatic channels on account of obstruction by tumor.

Before other modalities were available, intravenous pyelography was used to indirectly outline nodal masses by visualizing displacement of the kidneys, ureters, or bladder. But masses have to be quite large or strategically located before they will displace surrounding structures.

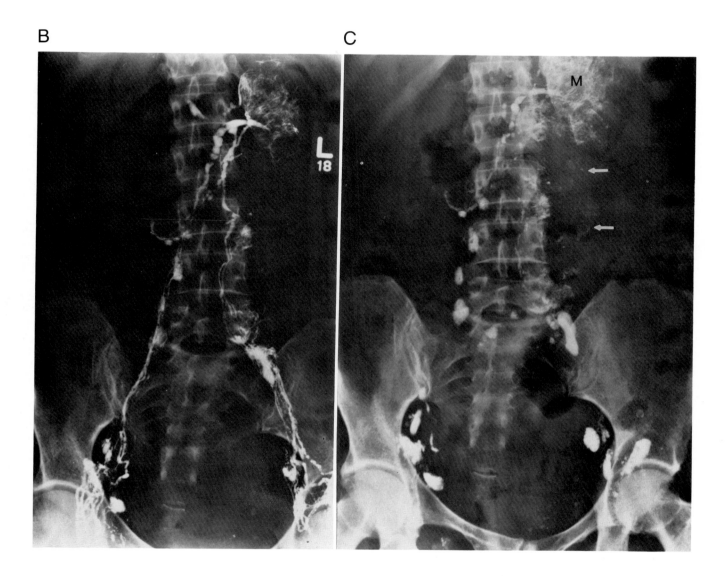

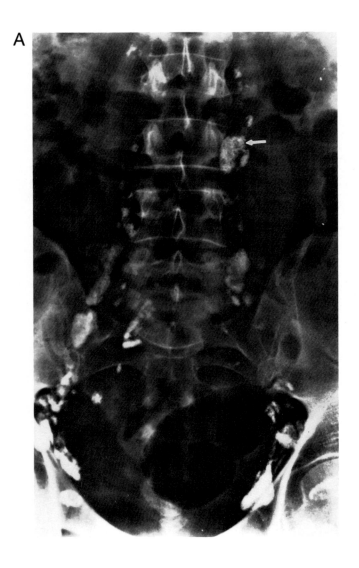

FIG 11–8.
Hodgkin's disease, mixed-cellularity type. This 34-year-old man presented with an enlarged cervical node, on which a biopsy was performed. Then he underwent radiologic workup.

A, a lymphangiogram shows abnormal lymph nodes *(arrow)* in the paraaortic area. Laparotomy confirmed involvement of the paraaortic nodes, but lymphoma was also found in the spleen and in the lymph nodes in the region of the common duct and celiac axis.

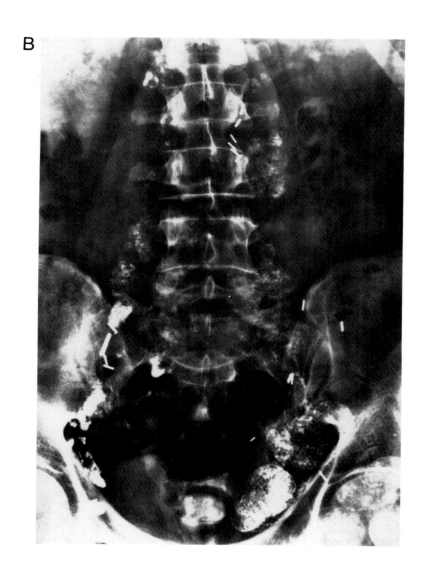

B, the patient received chemotherapy and was lost to follow-up for eight years. He returned with a large mass in the left groin, and a repeat lymphangiogram shows diffuse enlargement and abnormal architecture of the pelvic and retroperitoneal lymph nodes.

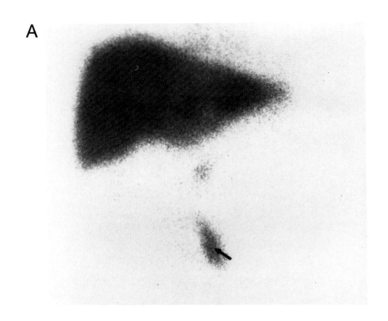

A

FIG 11–9.
Diffuse large cell lymphoma. An 83-year-old man was admitted with abdominal and right groin masses.

   A, the anterior view of the liver-spleen technetium 99m–sulfur colloid nuclear scan shows nonvisualization of the spleen in the left upper quadrant. An area of activity in the lower midabdomen *(arrow)* was thought to be the displaced spleen secondary to a large abdominal mass.

   B and **C,** computed tomography shows a large necrotic mass *(S)* in the left abdomen. The mass was presumed to represent spleen, since the spleen was not otherwise seen. The left kidney *(K)* is somewhat displaced and rotated because of the large mass. The low-density area in the kidney is fat in the renal pelvis, which is seen in an unusual plane because of the displacement.

   In retrospect, the nuclear scan actually shows an enlarged spleen almost totally replaced by tumor, with only a small rim of functioning tissue remaining, represented by the area of uptake. Necrotic or low-density areas are not uncommon in untreated lymphomas in any location.

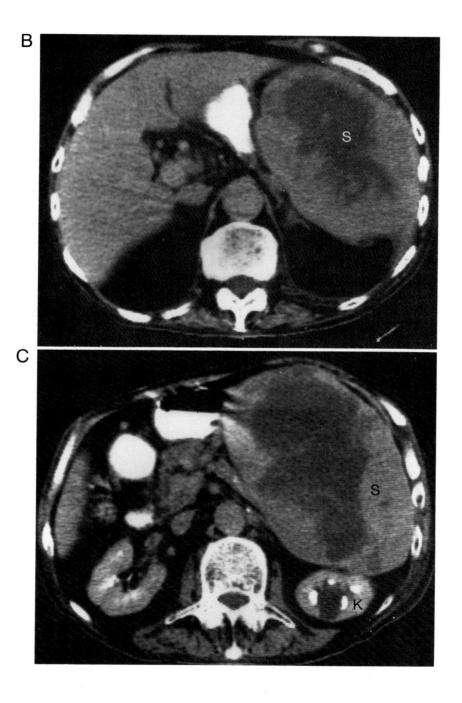

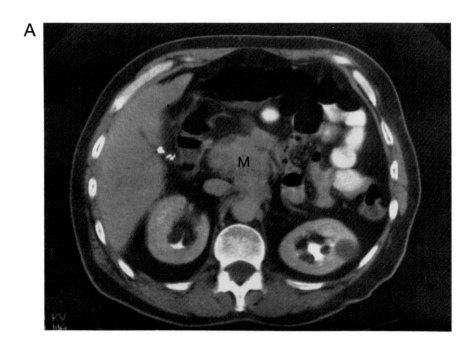

FIG 11–10.
Diffuse large cell lymphoma. A 73-year-old man presented with a six-week history of abdominal pain. The CT results were thought to most likely represent carcinoma of the pancreas, but needle biopsy of the mass showed lymphoma.

A, computed tomography through the kidneys shows a mass *(M)* in the region of the celiac axis and head of the pancreas. The low-density area in the left kidney is a simple cyst.

B

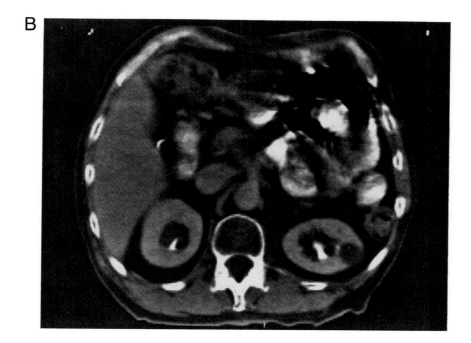

B, a CT scan 14 months later, following chemotherapy, shows resolution of the adenopathy with minimal soft tissue thickening.

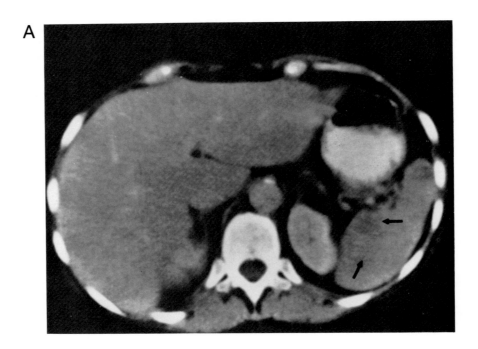

FIG 11–11.
Nodular mixed cell and large cell lymphoma. A 62-year-old woman had for two years been undergoing treatment for nodular mixed lymphoma. She presented with severe left upper abdominal pain.

A, CT shows no enlargement of the spleen, but multiple focal defects are evident *(arrows).* The liver is considered normal at this time. At splenectomy, large cell lymphoma was diagnosed.

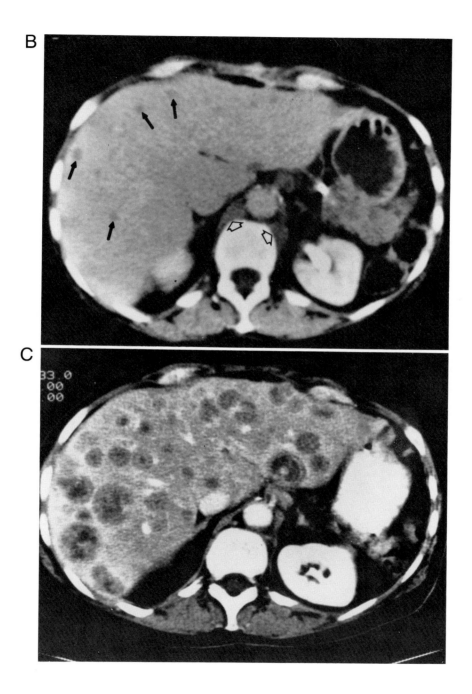

B, a CT scan made seven weeks later, while the patient was receiving therapy, shows multiple low-density areas *(arrows)* in the liver that were not present previously and that were presumed to also represent large cell lymphoma. Notice that retrocrural adenopathy *(open arrows)* has developed.

C, two months later, CT shows that the disease in the liver has progressed in spite of chemotherapy.

Transformation to a more aggressive histopathology is common in lymphoma.

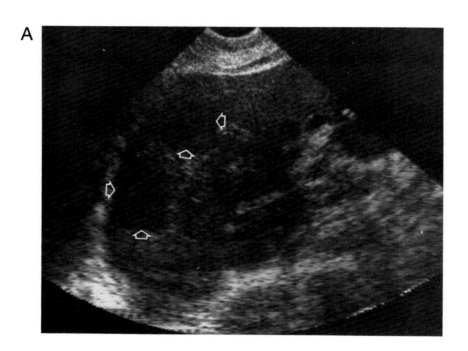

FIG 11–12.
Nodular poorly differentiated large cell lymphoma of the liver. A 62-year-old woman had pain and discomfort in the right upper quadrant for four months. An enlarged liver was found clinically.

A, a transverse sonogram of the liver shows marked distortion of the normal echogenicity of the liver, including hypoechoic areas *(arrows)*. The left lobe is normal.

B, a CT scan shows marked abnormality of the right lobe of the liver, including large low-density areas.

C, a celiac angiogram demonstrates a large hypovas-cular mass displacing the segmental branches of the right hepatic artery. Some tumor vascularity is present at the periphery of the mass.

A liver biopsy at exploratory laparotomy showed areas of both nodular poorly differentiated lymphoma and large cell lymphoma. This was the only site of lymphoma found at laparotomy.

Occasionally, two different cell types are identified in a single biopsy site, as in this patient. This is justification for multiple biopsies, particularly if the tumor is not responding as expected.

B

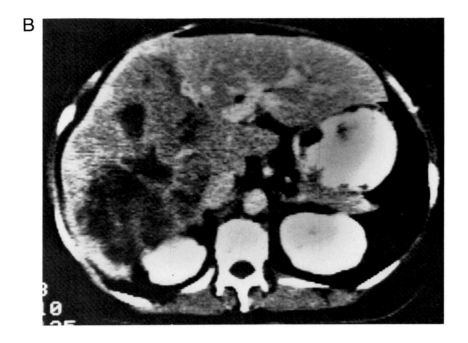

C

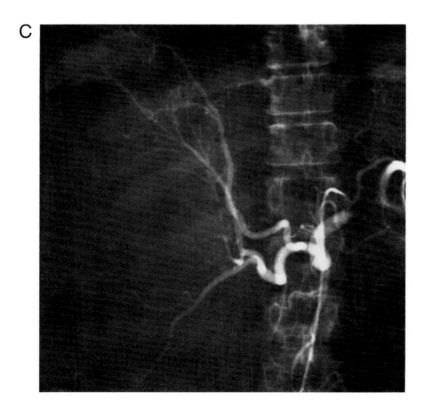

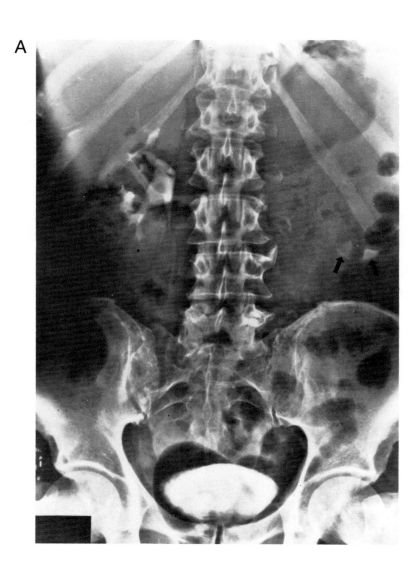

FIG 11–13.

Diffuse large cell lymphoma. A 55-year-old man, who had been treated for lymphoma for one year, had recent onset of hematuria.

A, an intravenous pyelogram shows no left renal out-line. Displaced calices in the left flank *(arrows)* are the only evidence of function of the kidney.

B, computed tomography through the kidneys shows a large mass occupying most of the left kidney, with only a rim of functioning cortex seen laterally *(arrows).* The mass extends to the midline and involves the retroperitoneal nodes *(N).*

C, a selective left renal arteriogram shows elongation of the left renal artery and a mass with moderate to low vascularity in the upper pole.

It would be difficult to say whether the mass originated in the retroperitoneal nodes and extended into the kidney or was primary in the kidney. However, there was other nodal disease, including extensive mesenteric adenopathy. The kidneys are frequently involved in non-Hodgkin's lympho-mas.

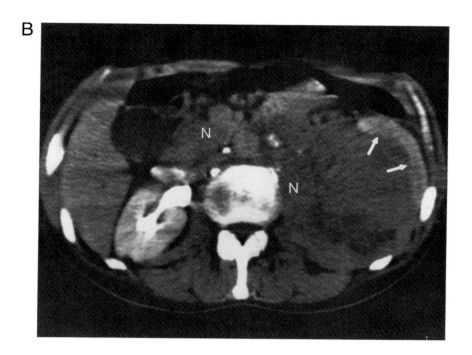

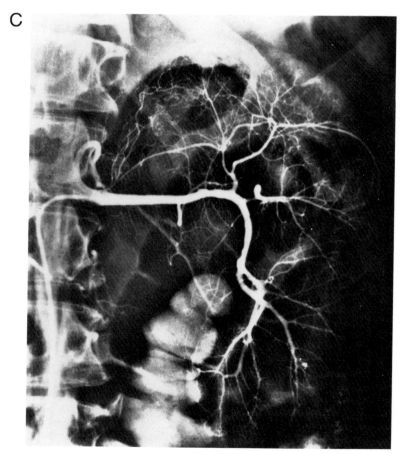

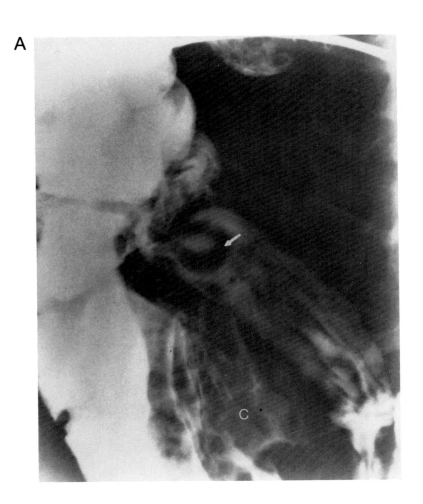

FIG 11–14.
Large cell lymphoma. A 66-year-old woman had masses in the left breast and right submandibular area and had vague gastrointestinal complaints. Ductal carcinoma was found in the breast lesion. Needle biopsy of the submandibular mass was suggestive of large cell lymphoma.

A, a small bowel follow-through shows a mass *(arrow)* in the region of the ileocecal valve and extrinsic compression of the cecum *(C)* and distal ileum. The filling defect seen just proximal to the ileocecal valve is similar to the lesions that were noted in the stomach and represents submucosal involvement by lymphoma.

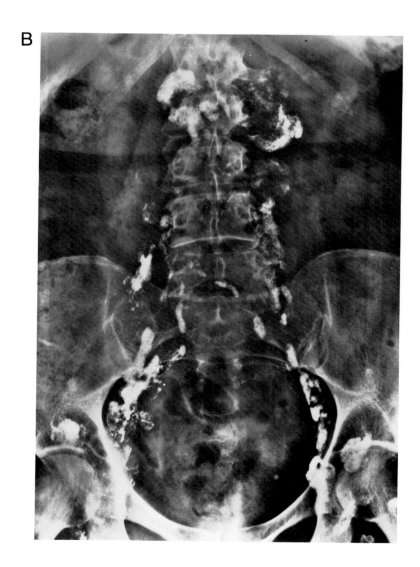

B, a lymphangiogram shows enlarged and distorted nodes in the paraaortic and right external iliac areas.

Biopsy of the stomach at endoscopy confirmed the diagnosis of diffuse large cell lymphoma (see Fig 1–16).

A

B

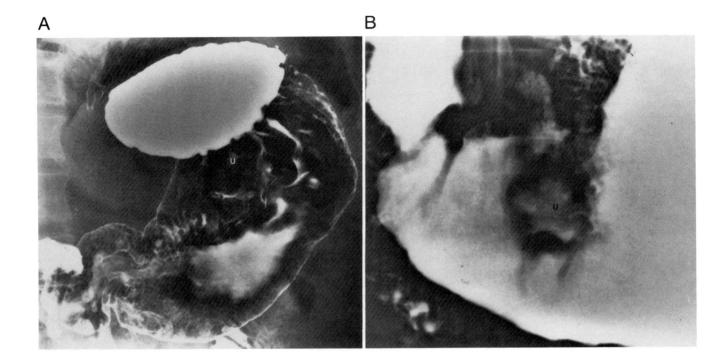

FIG 11–15.
Diffuse large cell lymphoma. A 74-year-old man presented with a six-month history of regurgitation and of finding the taste of red meat unpleasant. There were no other symptoms. Endoscopy revealed stomach ulcer, which was ultimately proved to be due to diffuse large cell lymphoma.

A and **B,** an image from an upper gastrointestinal series shows thickening and irregularity of the gastric folds,

with an area of ulceration *(U)* in the upper portion of the stomach and also in the antrum.

C and **D,** the images from small bowel follow-through show lesions involving the cecum *(c)* and distal ileum *(arrows).*

The distortion of the structures indicates direct tumor involvement rather than extrinsic compression and is characteristic of gastrointestinal lymphoma.

C

D

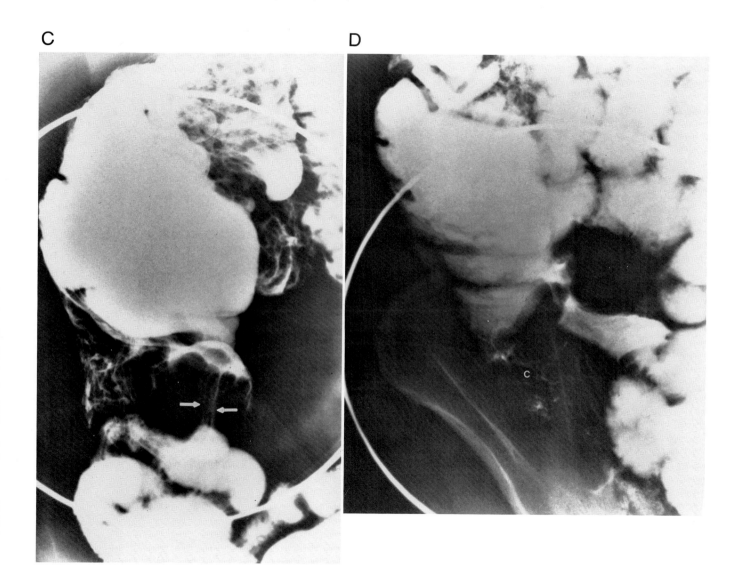

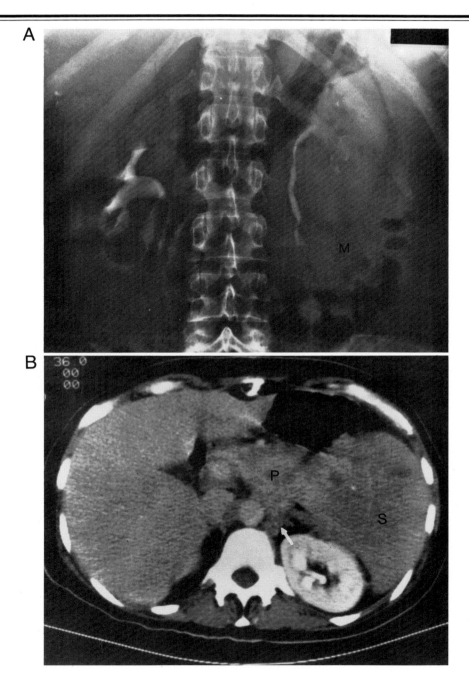

FIG 11–16.
Large cell lymphoma. A 56-year-old woman presented with a four-month history of upper gastrointestinal discomfort and low-grade fever.

A, an intravenous pyelogram shows a mass *(M)* in the left side of the abdomen, adjacent to the left kidney.

B, a CT scan shows a mass involving the spleen *(S)* and the tail of the pancreas *(P)* with loss of definition of the planes. There is also evidence of retroperitoneal adenopathy *(arrow)*.

C, an image from the upper gastrointestinal series shows an extrinsic mass along the lesser curvature of the stomach *(arrows)*.

D, an image from the small bowel follow-through shows extrinsic mass along a portion of the small bowel at the level of the sacroiliac joint *(arrow)*.

Laparotomy was performed with a presumptive diagnosis of carcinoma of the pancreas. The tumor involved the lower pole of the spleen, splenic flexure of the colon, greater curvature and fundus of the stomach, and tail of the pancreas, with fixation to the retroperitoneum. There was also retroperitoneal lymphadenopathy. The biopsy specimen showed large cell lymphoma.

C

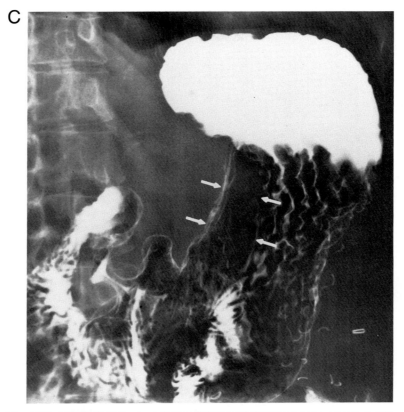

D

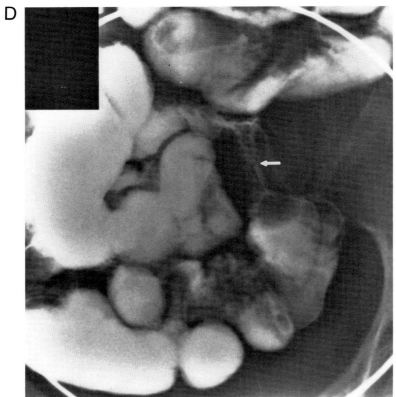

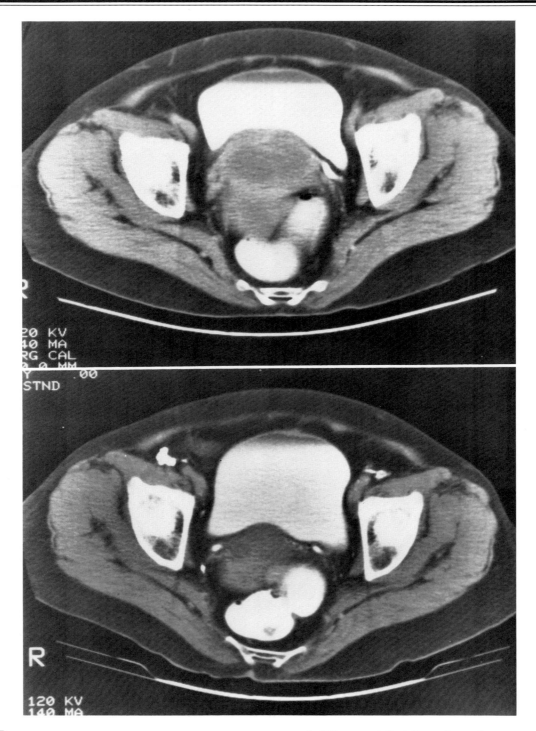

FIG 11–17.
Large cell uterine lymphoma. This 64-year-old woman had postmenopausal bleeding for ten days. A diagnosis of large cell lymphoma was made at the time of uterine curettage and cervical biopsy. No other disease was found.

A CT scan at that time showed a mass with multiple low-density areas involving the uterus *(upper image).*

A follow-up examination two months following chemotherapy showed regression of the uterine mass *(lower image).*

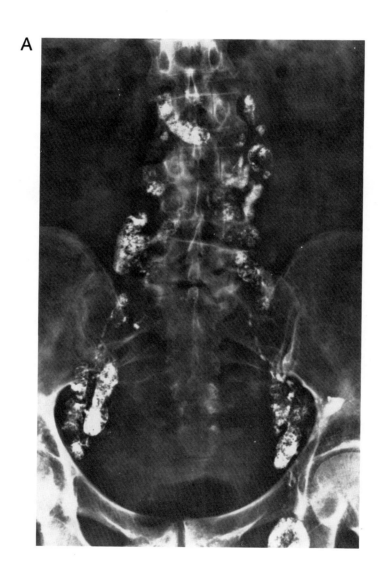

FIG 11–18.
Diffuse large cell lymphoma. A 78-year-old woman had a diagnosis of lymphoma established by biopsy of a right inguinal mass. The woman had previously had a hysterectomy. **A,** a lymphangiogram shows all the pelvic and retroperitoneal lymph nodes to be enlarged and to have abnormal architecture. (*Continued.*)

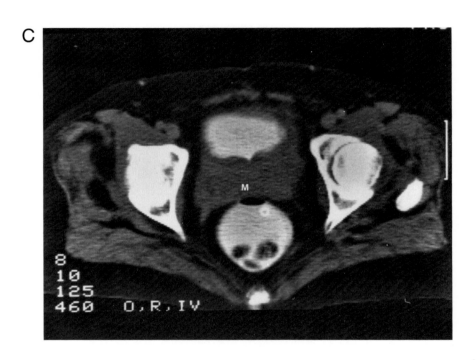

FIG 11–18 (cont.).

B, CT of the pelvis just prior to lymphangiography shows a soft tissue mass *(M)* in the cul-de-sac that is in the usual position of the cervix between the bladder and rectum.

C, following chemotherapy, a radiograph of the abdomen nine months later shows that the lymph nodes have returned to normal size and configuration.

D, CT at that time shows the soft tissue mass to have resolved.

Appropriate clinical information is vital since the pelvic mass could be erroneously interpreted as related to the uterus.

C

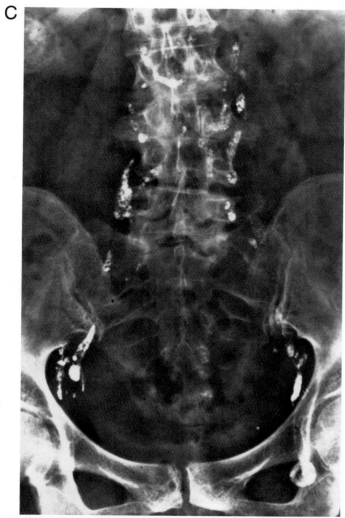

D

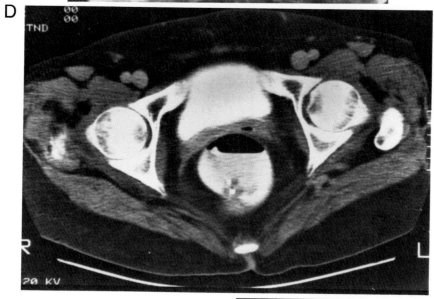

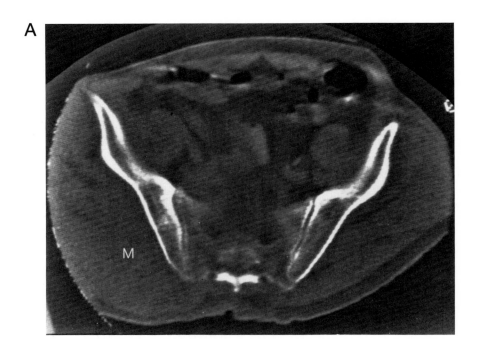

FIG 11–19.
Diffuse large cell lymphoma. A 75-year-old man presented with a growing mass in the right buttock. Biopsy of the mass showed diffuse large cell lymphoma.

A, a CT scan through the pelvis shows the large mass *(M)* in the right buttock. This was the only evidence of lymphoma.

B, five months later, after chemotherapy, CT shows complete resolution of the mass with some residual atrophic changes in the muscles.

C, two years later, CT of the upper abdomen shows relapse of lymphoma involving the retrocrural nodes *(arrow)* and the right paraspinal area *(P).* At that time, these findings were the only evidence of active lymphoma.

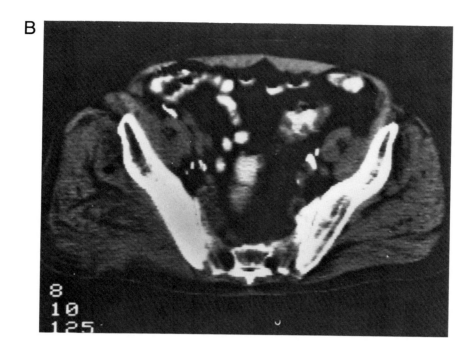

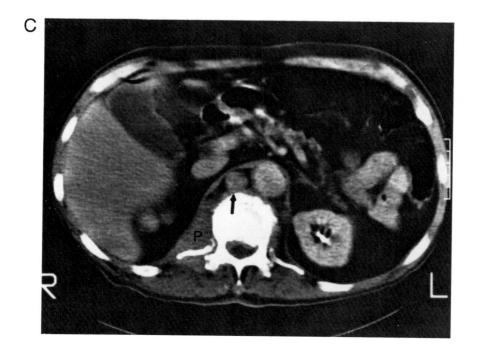

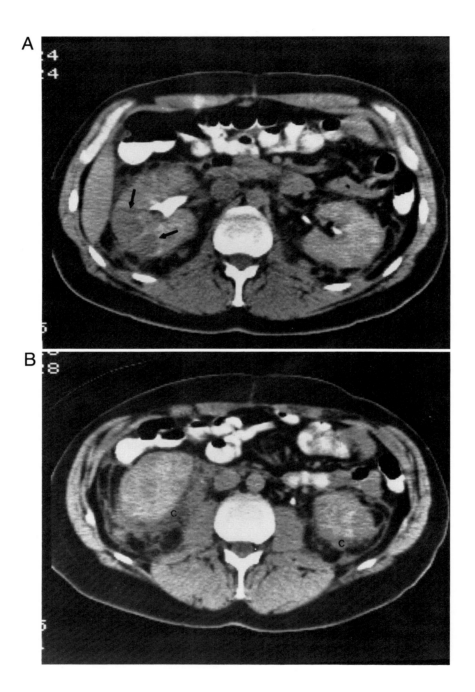

FIG 11–20.
Diffuse large cell lymphoma. A 37-year-old man had received chemotherapy for one year for diffuse large cell lymphoma. A large abdominal mass had decreased in size, but subsequently a new focus of disease developed in the thigh.

A and **B,** CT shows that there were also solid masses *(arrows)* in the kidneys, as well as marked irregularity of the renal capsules *(C).*

Renal involvement is not uncommon in non-Hodgkin's lymphomas.

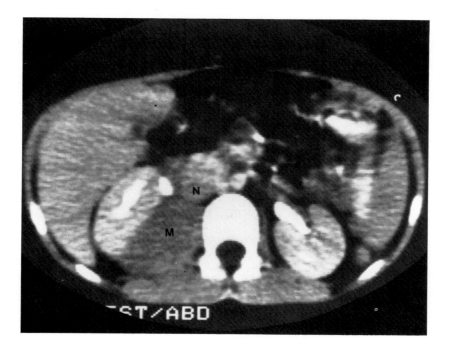

FIG 11–21.

Burkitt's lymphoma. A nine-year-old boy had been treated for four months for Burkitt's lymphoma involving the abdomen, pleural spaces, and bone marrow. Computed tomography shows tumor *(M)* on the right involving the kidney and the psoas and quadratus lumborum muscles. A retrocaval nodal mass *(N)* is also present.

American Burkitt's lymphoma is seen in young patients and predominantly involves intraabdominal nodes and organs.

A

B

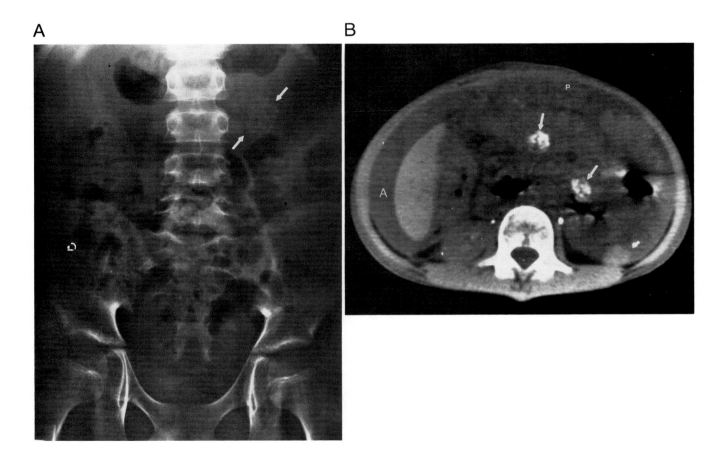

FIG 11–22.
Burkitt's lymphoma. A ten-year-old boy was seen for an abdominal mass sampled by biopsy at surgical exploration. At that time he also had extensive retroperitoneal adenopathy. There was prompt response to chemotherapy, but ten months later a repeat exploratory laparotomy showed tumor involvement of the pancreas, bowel, and much of the abdominal cavity.

A, a radiograph of the abdomen at the time of repeat laparotomy shows calcification in nodes in the left upper quadrant *(arrows)*.

B, a CT scan of the abdomen at the same time shows areas of calcification *(arrows)*, ascites *(A)*, and extensive peritoneal disease along the abdominal wall *(P)* and mesentery, and also surrounding the retroperitoneal structures.

Although calcification is more commonly seen in treated mediastinal nodes of Hodgkin's disease, it can be seen in any lymphoma in any location following treatment by radiation therapy, chemotherapy, or a combination of the two modalities.

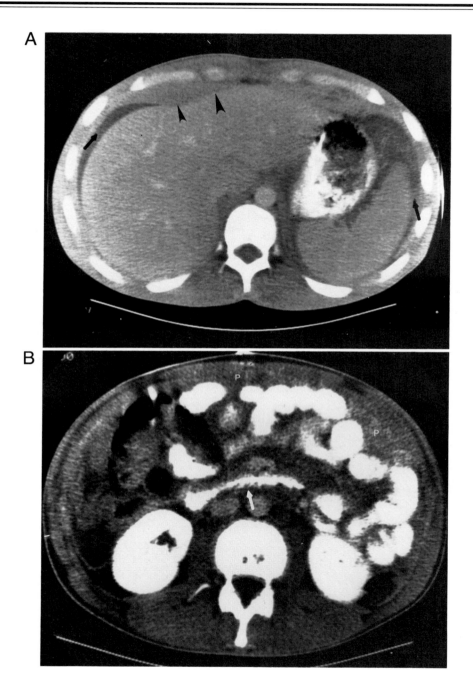

FIG 11–23.
Burkitt's lymphoma. A 17-year-old boy had abdominal pain, weight loss, and night sweats. A large retroperitoneal mass, which was classified as a small cell tumor, was found at laparotomy. Three months later, the patient presented with a large pleural effusion and a mass in the lower abdomen. A diagnosis of Burkitt's lymphoma was made on biopsy of the latter.

A, a CT scan of the upper abdomen shows ascites *(arrow)* around the liver and spleen along with thickening of the peritoneum *(arrowheads)*.

B, a CT scan through the kidneys shows diffuse intraabdominal disease in the bowel wall and peritoneal cavity *(P)*. The transverse duodenum seen anterior to the great vessels is encased in tumor *(arrow)*.

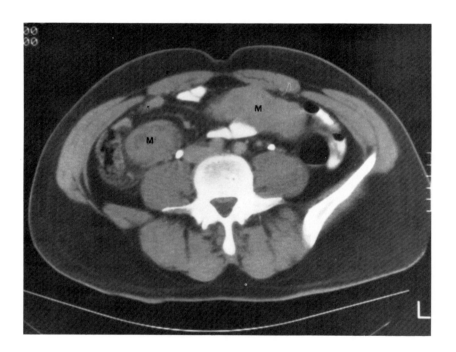

FIG 11–24.
Nodular mixed lymphoma. This CT scan is from a 30-year-old man with nodular mixed lymphoma diagnosed two years previously by biopsy of a left axillary lymph node and treated by chemotherapy. Computed tomography at the time of diagnosis showed paraaortic adenopathy. Follow-up CT through the level of the iliac crest shows two mesenteric masses *(M)*. No retroperitoneal or pelvic adenopathy was identified.

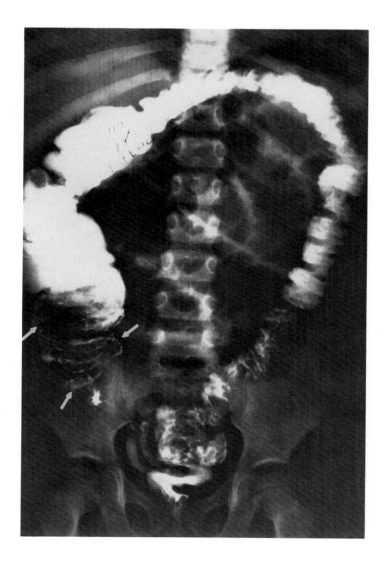

FIG 11–25.
Unclassified lymphoma. A seven-year-old girl had had abdominal pain and discomfort with hyperactive bowel sounds for one and one-half months.

A barium enema shows typical appearance of intussus-ception involving the cecum *(arrows)*. At laparotomy, lymphoma of unknown type was found in the distal ileum.

Any type of tumor involving the distal ileum or at the ileocecal valve can present as intussusception in either children or adults.

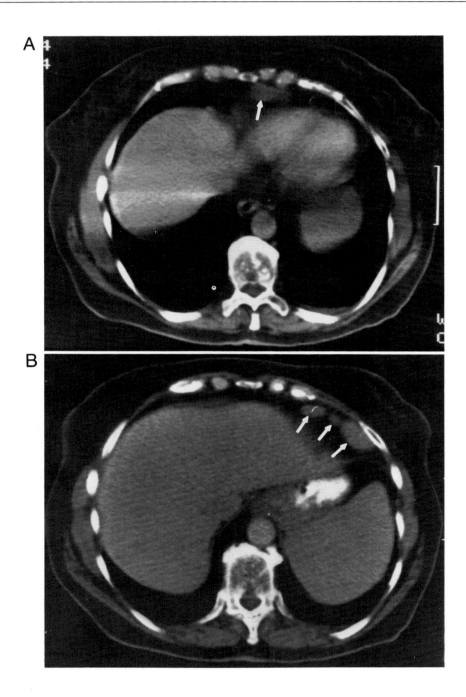

FIG 11–26.
Nodular poorly differentiated lymphocytic lymphoma. A 70-year-old woman had been seen for a painless enlargement of lymph nodes in both groins three years prior to the current examination.

A and **B,** the CT scans show splenomegaly and multiple enlarged lymph nodes, including diaphragmatic nodes *(arrows).*

Enlargement of diaphragmatic nodes is frequently seen in both Hodgkin's and non-Hodgkin's lymphomas. Identification of such involvement is essential if radiation therapy is planned, since these nodes might lie outside either a chest or abdominal portal.

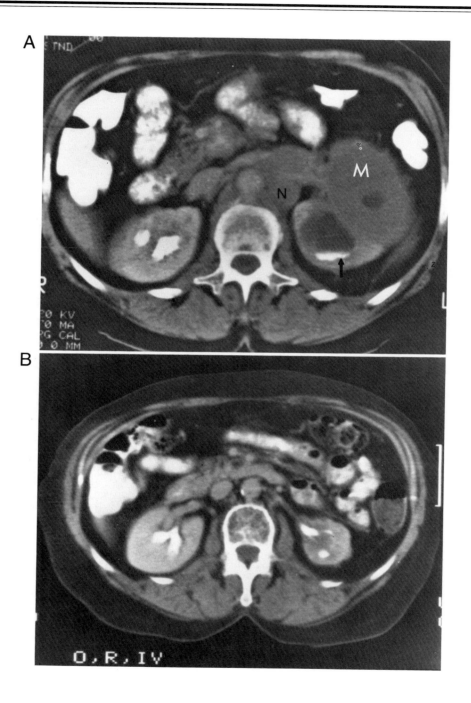

FIG 11-27.

Nodular poorly differentiated lymphocytic lymphoma. A 66-year-old woman presented with chest pain and right pleural effusion. Biopsy of a small submandibular lymph node yielded the diagnosis of lymphoma. During abdominal imaging procedures, it was noted that the left upper urinary tract was obstructed.

A, a CT scan shows a large right renal mass *(M)* as-sociated with involvement of the left retroperitoneal lymph nodes *(N)*. There is obstruction of the renal pelvis and dila-tation of a calix that is partially filled with contrast material *(arrow)*.

B, a CT scan made 18 months later shows total reso-lution of the mass following chemotherapy, leaving a func-tioning, hypoplastic kidney.

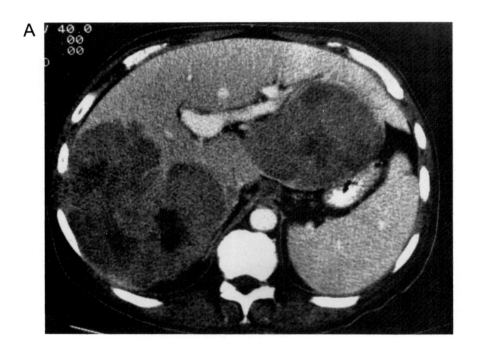

FIG 11–28.
Nodular poorly differentiated lymphocytic lymphoma and large cell lymphoma. A 56-year-old man was initially known to have nodular poorly differentiated lymphocytic lymphoma by biopsy of a supraclavicular lymph node. A biopsy of a lesion that developed in the femur a year later showed large cell lymphoma. One year after that, the patient developed dyspnea and hepatosplenomegaly.

A through **C,** all three CT images show that more than 50% of the liver is replaced by tumor. A large lesion involving the left kidney is seen in **C.** There is also extensive adenopathy, including of the peripancreatic *(P)* and retroperitoneal nodes *(R),* as shown in **B** and **C.** In spite of the extensive tumor, no abnormality was detected in the spleen.

The distribution of non-Hodgkin's lymphomas is not predictable. In Hodgkin's disease, splenic foci of disease would be expected in a patient with liver involvement.

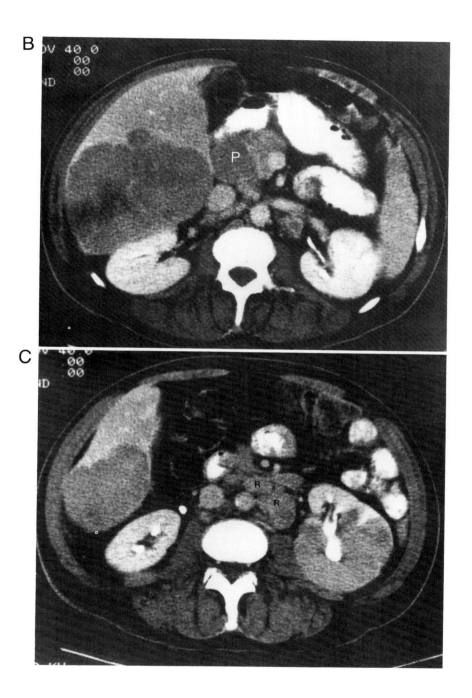

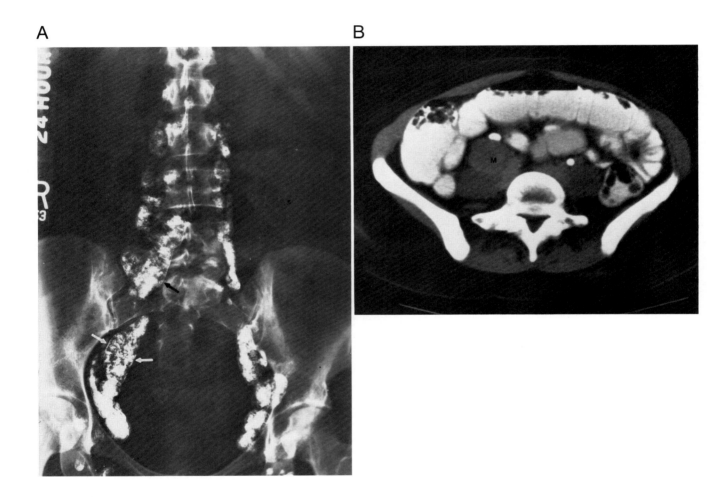

FIG 11–29.

Poorly differentiated lymphocytic lymphoma. A 32-year-old woman presented with an enlarged node in the left axilla. There were no abdominal complaints.

A, a lymphangiogram shows, particularly on the right, enlarged lymph nodes with markedly abnormal architecture.

B, a CT scan prior to lymphangiography shows a mass *(M)* between the right psoas muscle and right ureter, corresponding to enlarged nodes in the right external iliac and common iliac areas seen in **A** *(arrows).*

Regardless of the absence of localized abdominal or systemic complaints and regardless of disease site, all patients with lymphoma should be assessed for abdominal disease.

A
B

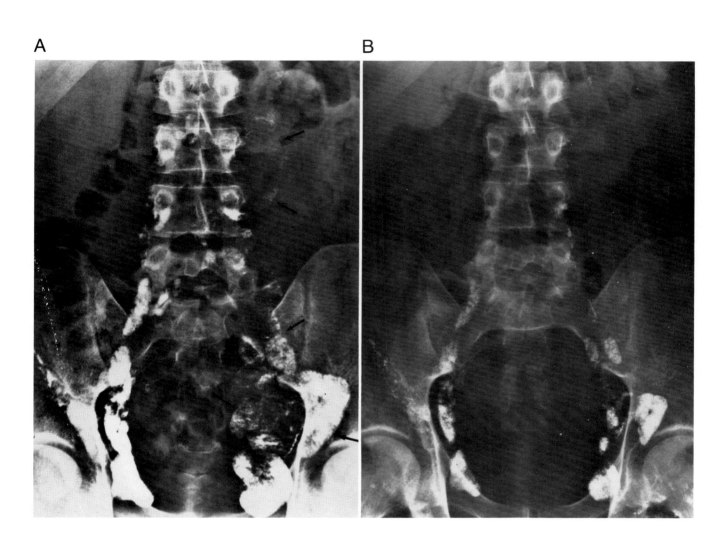

FIG 11–30.
Chronic myelocytic leukemia. A 28-year-old man was known to have had chronic myelocytic leukemia for two years.

A, the initial lymphangiogram shows massively enlarged nodes in the periaortic and left iliac areas *(arrows).*

B, one month following chemotherapy, a radiograph of the abdomen shows the lymph nodes to have become nearly normal in size.

In spite of the rapid response shown here, the patient died after a short interval. At autopsy there were leukemic infiltrates in the liver, retroperitoneal nodes, bone marrow, lungs, heart, kidneys, adrenal glands, leptomeninges, and brain.

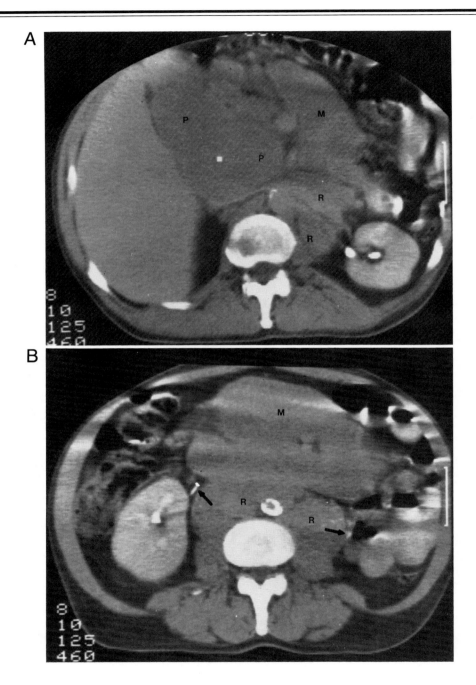

FIG 11–31.
Chronic lymphocytic leukemia and lymphocytic lymphoma. A 51-year-old man had had chronic lymphocytic leukemia for three years and had undergone splenectomy. Despite therapy, disease was progressive.

A, abdominal CT shows a conglomerate of enlarged nodes in the retroperitoneum *(R)* and massive enlargement of portal, peripancreatic *(P),* and mesenteric *(M)* nodes.

B, at the renal level, the ureters *(arrows)* are displaced by large retroperitoneal masses *(R).* Massive enlargement of mesenteric nodes *(M)* is also seen at this level.

C, in the pelvis, large lymph nodes *(N)* deform the urinary bladder. The ureters *(arrows)* are not obstructed in spite of the massive adenopathy.

D, a pelvic lymphangiogram shows the massively enlarged lymph nodes with foamy appearance that produce the deformity of the urinary bladder.

Masses from the leukemias and lymphomas tend to displace rather than obstruct, as opposed to carcinomas, which tend to invade and obstruct early in their course. This difference holds true in all areas of the body.

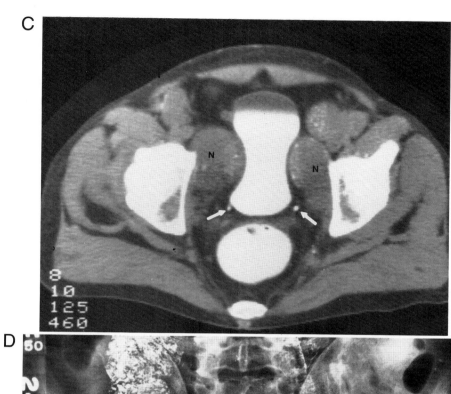

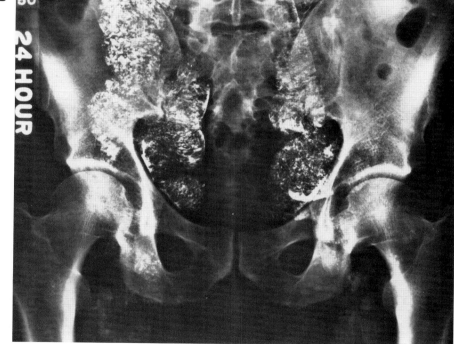

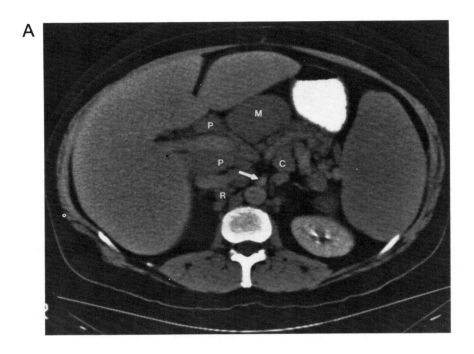

FIG 11–32.
Chronic lymphocytic leukemia and lymphocytic lymphoma.
A 52-year-old man who had had chronic lymphocytic leukemia for one year developed progressive abdominal discomfort, loss of appetite, night sweats, excessive fatigue, and, finally, symptoms of peritonitis. Exploratory laparotomy showed a perforated sigmoid diverticulum, and an intraoperative biopsy of enlarged mesenteric lymph nodes revealed lymphocytic lymphoma. There was also lymphoma in the sigmoid diverticulum.

A, a CT scan of the abdomen at the level of the celiac artery *(arrow)* shows extensive adenopathy involving the retroperitoneal *(R),* celiac *(C),* and portal *(P)* nodes, as well as a mesenteric mass *(M).* The celiac artery and its branches *(arrow)* are entrapped within the nodes.

B, a CT scan through the level of the gallbladder shows the retroperitoneal *(R)* and mesenteric *(M)* nodal masses. There is a loop of bowel *(arrows)* entrapped by the masses.

C, the transverse sonogram of the upper abdomen demonstrates multiple nodes around the celiac artery and its major branches *(arrows).* This is almost at the same level as **A.**

Although the adenopathy is extensive, the nodes maintain a somewhat discrete pattern, as contrasted with the example in Fig 11–31, in which the nodes form a conglomerate mass. Both patterns of adenopathy are seen in leukemia and lymphoma, but the conglomerate pattern is more common in lymphoma.

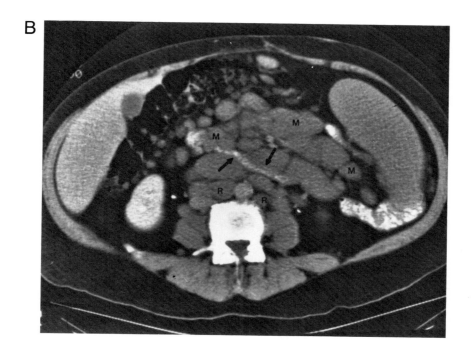

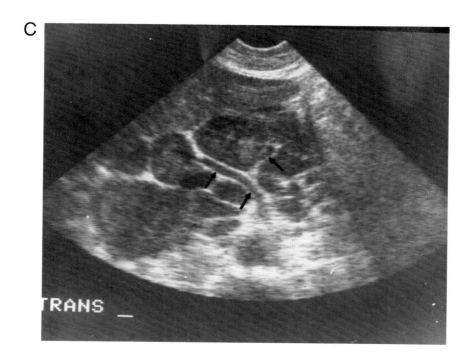

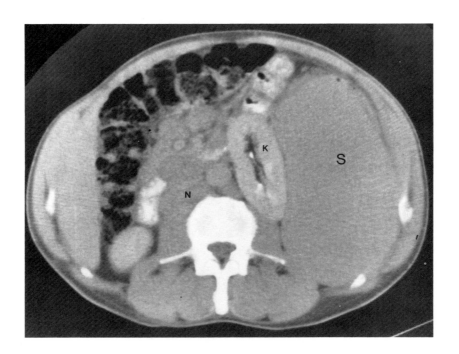

FIG 11–33.
Chronic lymphocytic leukemia and lymphocytic lymphoma. A 63-year-old man with chronic lymphocytic leukemia had been diagnosed 13 years previously. A bone marrow biopsy had shown lymphocytic lymphoma in the marrow one year prior to the current examination; at that time, the patient had also received radiotherapy for lymphocytic infiltration in the left vocal cord and in the base of the tongue.

Computed tomography shows a massively enlarged spleen *(S),* as well as retroperitoneal adenopathy *(N).* Although the left kidney *(K)* is displaced and flattened by the spleen, there is no evidence of renal infiltration or obstruction.

A massively enlarged spleen is common in lymphocytic leukemia and lymphocytic lymphomas.

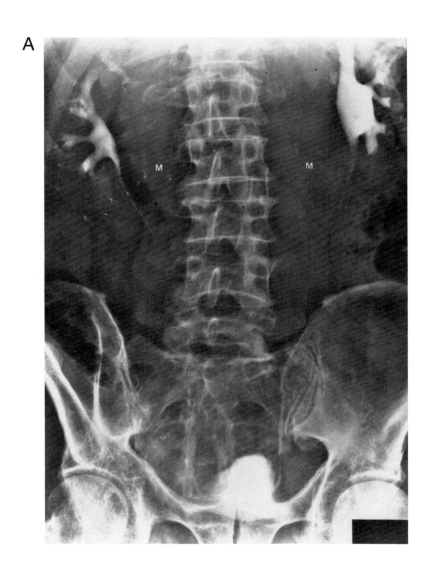

FIG 11–34.
Chronic lymphocytic leukemia and well-differentiated lymphocytic lymphoma. A 74-year-old man had had chronic lymphocytic leukemia and well-differentiated lymphocytic lymphoma for three years.

A, an intravenous pyelogram shows displacement of both kidneys and proximal ureters, indicative of retroperitoneal masses *(M). (Continued.)*

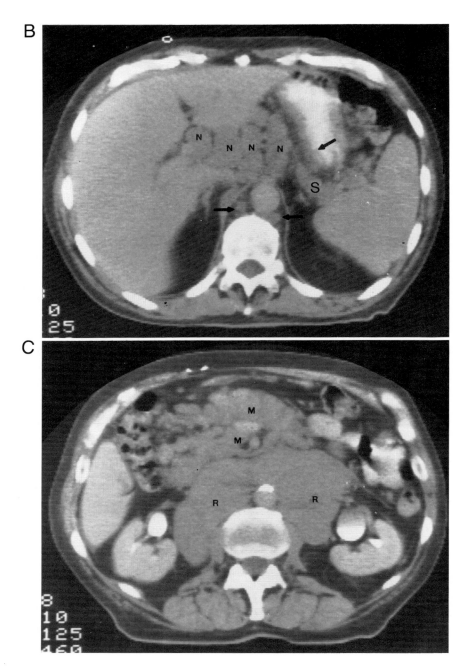

FIG 11–34 (cont.).

B, a CT scan through the upper abdomen shows enlarged nodes in the portahepatic, gastrohepatic, and celiac regions *(N),* as well as in the splenic hilus *(S).* Retrocrural adenopathy is also present *(arrows).*

C, CT through the midkidney level shows massive retroperitoneal adenopathy *(R)* that displaces both kidneys, as well as mesenteric adenopathy *(M).*

D, at the sacroiliac joints, enlarged lymph nodes are seen in the internal and external iliac regions *(N),* with the large lymph nodes on the right displacing the right ureter *(arrow)* medially.

E, massively enlarged lymph nodes *(N)* compress and deform the urinary bladder.

Patients with chronic lymphocytic leukemia and lymphocytic lymphoma tend to have the most striking nodal enlargement, and involvement may extend to all the nodal groups, as in this patient. Although the intravenous pyelogram shows enlarged nodes displacing the proximal upper urinary tract as well as deforming the right side of the urinary bladder, it does not reflect the numerous other enlarged nodes.

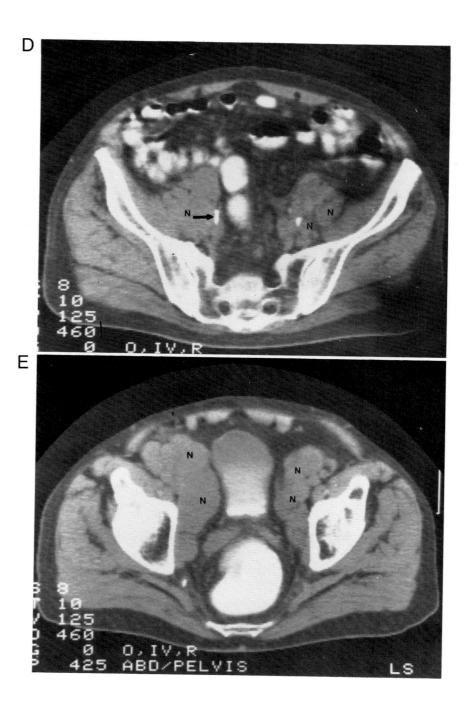

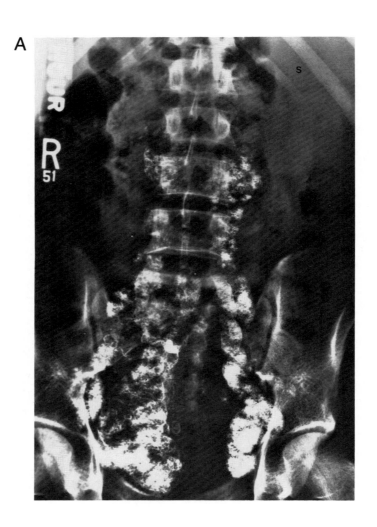

FIG 11–35.
Chronic lymphocytic leukemia and well-differentiated lymphoma. This 29-year-old man had chronic lymphocytic leukemia and well-differentiated lymphoma with hepatosplenomegaly and generalized adenopathy.

A, lymphangiogram shows generalized nodal enlargement. The massively enlarged lymph nodes in the right side of the pelvis correlate well with CT scans obtained at the same time. Note that the spleen *(S)* is also enlarged.

B, a CT scan of the upper abdomen shows hepatosplenomegaly and gastrohepatic adenopathy. The contrast-filled stomach *(arrows)* is squeezed between the enlarged liver *(L)*, gastrohepatic nodes *(N)*, and spleen *(S)*.

C, at the level of L-1, the markedly enlarged spleen *(S)* on the left and nodal masses on the right displace the kidneys. There is extensive retroperitoneal adenopathy *(N)*. The lymph nodes usually do not opacify by lymphangiography above the level of L-2 *(L,* liver). *(Continued.)*

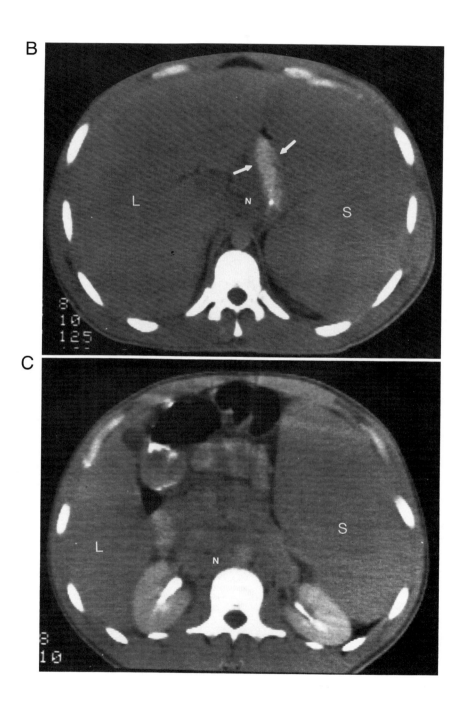

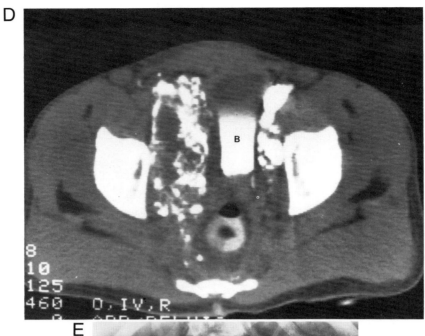

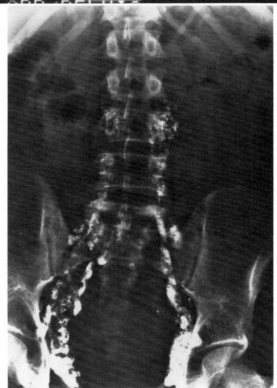

FIG 11–35 (cont.).

D, at the level of the hip joints, massively enlarged external iliac nodes on the right displace and deform the urinary bladder *(B).*

E, two months later, the radiograph of the abdomen shows marked decrease in size of the lymph nodes as well as decrease in size of the spleen.

The radiographic features in this case are typical of the findings of acute lymphocytic leukemia and lymphocytic lymphoma. The patient's age is atypical in that this is generally a disease of older individuals.

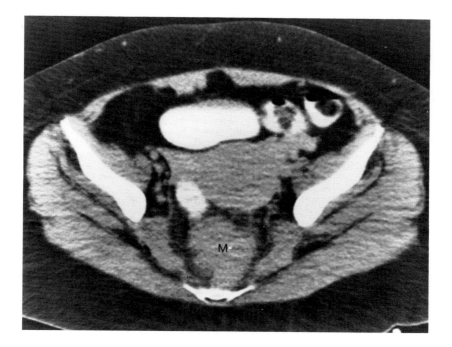

FIG 11–36.
Acute myelocytic leukemia and granulocytic sarcoma (chloroma). A 47-year-old woman with a two-year history of acute myelocytic leukemia presented with a two-week history of numbness in the right buttock spreading to the right perineal area.

Pelvic CT shows a presacral mass *(M)*. Needle biopsy of the mass showed granulocytic sarcoma.

Granulocytic sarcoma is an extramedullary solid tumor expression of myelocytic leukemia. These tumors may have a greenish color and are then called chloromas.

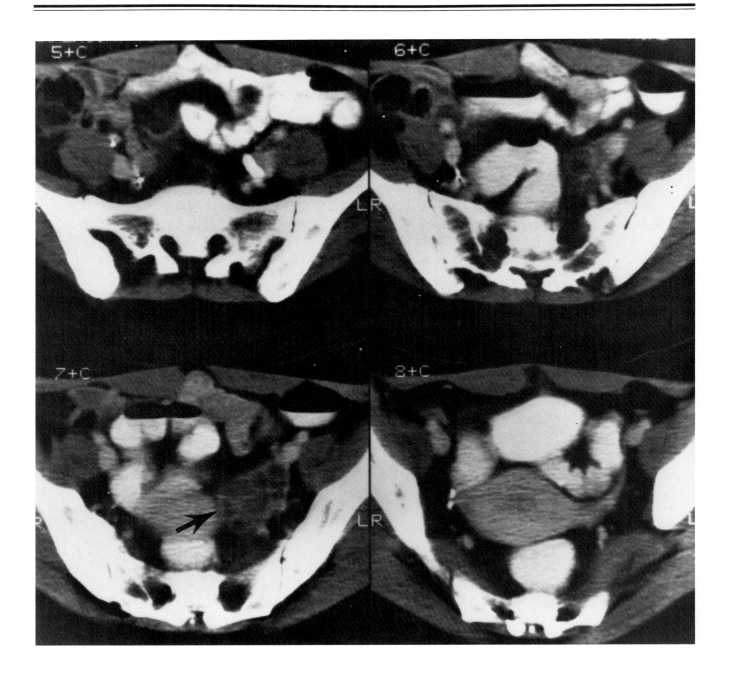

FIG 11–37.
Granulocytic sarcoma (chloroma). A 26-year-old woman developed symptoms of urinary tract disease and on pelvic examination was found to have a mass in the left side of the pelvis.

Pelvic CT images show a cystic-appearing mass *(arrow)* in the region of the left ovary.

At surgery, an 11.5 × 11 × 9 cm solid mass that involved the left ovary was removed. Microscopic examination showed the mass to be a granulocytic sarcoma (chloroma). At that time and at latest follow-up one year later she had no evidence of leukemia, and her bone marrow remained normal.

Granulocytic sarcoma occasionally occurs in patients who do not have leukemia at the time of diagnosis. Leukemia may occur shortly afterward or may not occur over an extended period of follow-up.[46, 47]

A

B

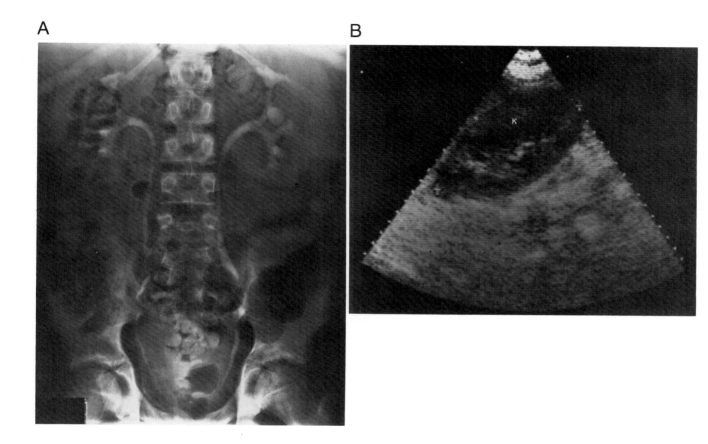

FIG 11–38.

Acute lymphocytic leukemia (renal infiltration). A 13-year-old boy presented with a severe nosebleed. Enlarged liver and spleen were clinically noted. A bone marrow examination established the diagnosis of acute lymphocytic leukemia.

A, although there were no renal symptoms, an intravenous pyelogram was made as part of the clinical staging. The kidneys are enlarged, in keeping with leukemic infiltra-tion. There is also an enlarged spleen.

B, a sonogram of the kidneys shows bilateral renal enlargement. The right kidney *(K),* as seen on this sagittal view, measures 14.4 × 9.2 × 4.4 cm. The left kidney was also enlarged, measuring 13.8 × 7.6 × 7.6 cm. There is a slight change in the normal architecture of the kidney, but no local lesion can be identified. The pattern is presumably due to diffuse leukemic infiltrate.

A

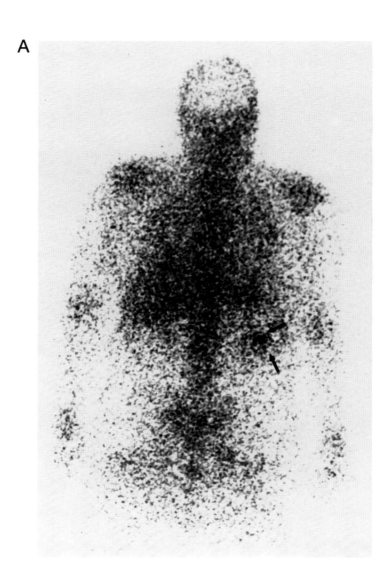

FIG 11–39.
Chronic myelogenous leukemia. This is a 64-year-old man with a white blood cell count of more than 100,000/μL, a markedly enlarged spleen, and pain in the left upper quadrant. He subsequently had a splenectomy.

A, four years following the original diagnosis, a gallium scan with anterior view shows a focal area of increased uptake in the left upper quadrant *(arrows)*. There is normal distribution of gallium in the liver and bones.

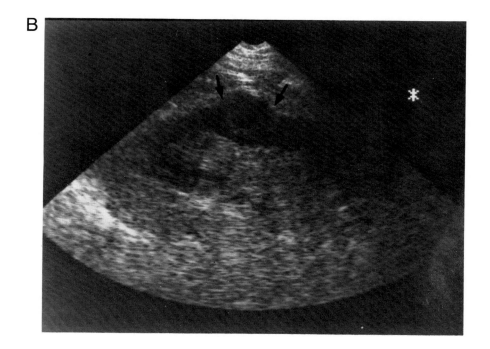

B, a longitudinal sonogram of the left kidney shows a hypoechoic mass in the lateral aspect of the kidney *(arrows),* corresponding to abnormal gallium uptake. Because there was no evidence of renal infection, this was presumed to represent localized infiltration of the kidney by leukemia.

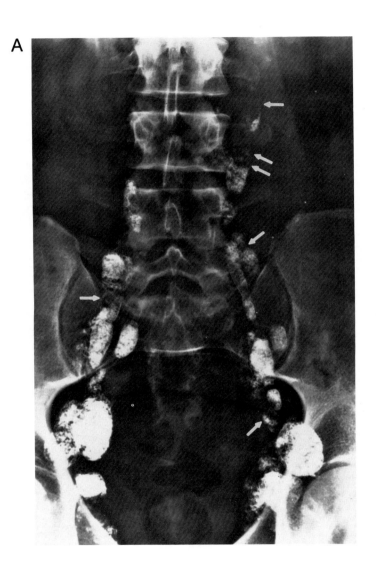

FIG 11–40.
Nodular poorly differentiated lymphoma. A 42-year-old man with nodular poorly differentiated lymphoma developed a new cervical mass one month before these images were made.

A, a lymphangiogram shows all opacified lymph nodes to be abnormal, with enlargement and irregular distribution of contrast material within the nodes. Many of the nodes are partially replaced by tumor *(arrows).*

B and C, some nodes *(arrows)* are visible by CT of the abdomen, but these are certainly much less impressive than by lymphangiography.

D, the only really enlarged lymph nodes *(N)* seen by CT are in the pelvis.

Lymphangiography far more graphically illustrates the extent of disease in lymph nodes than does CT. Since treatment strategy might be altered according to the extent of disease, assessment of nodes by CT alone may not be adequate for treatment planning.

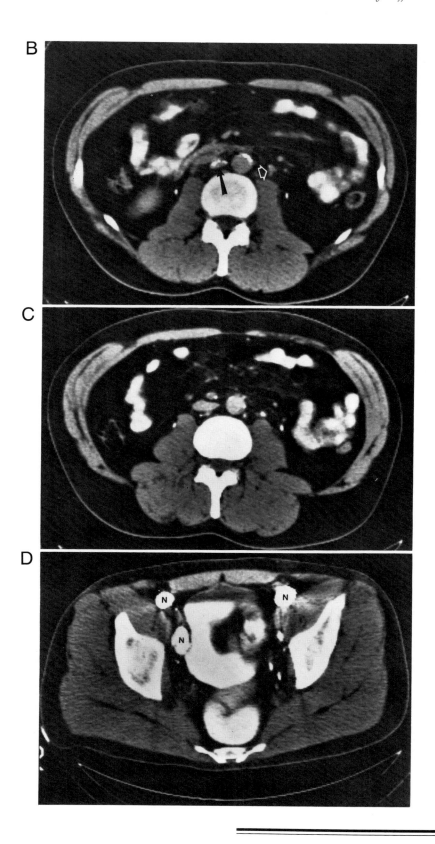

12

Magnetic Resonance Imaging in Abdominal and Pelvic Oncology

Anthony R. Lupetin, M.D.

Magnetic resonance imaging (MRI) is a rapidly evolving new imaging technology that has already assumed a primary role in the diagnosis of most disorders of the central nervous system. Diagnostic radiologists and other scientists worldwide are continuing to collect more data to determine the future of this method in evaluating other parts of the body. This chapter is designed to provide an introduction to the diagnostic abilities of MRI in evaluating the abdomen, retroperitoneum, and pelvis in oncology patients. It is targeted primarily for physicians whose interests lie in the field of cross-sectional imaging. However, I believe that all diagnostic radiologists and medical professionals who deal with oncology patients will find this presentation interesting and useful to their practices.

A detailed discussion of the physical principles of MRI is beyond the scope of this chapter. Therefore, it is presumed that the reader is familiar with the basics[1] before reviewing this work. A complete list of references related to the field of oncology and body MRI is included at the end of the text.

The MRI studies presented in this chapter were performed on the Siemens Magnetom, a liquid nitrogen– and helium-cooled, 0.5-tesla (0.5-T) superconducting magnet.

In the work presented here, only spin-echo pulse sequences were utilized to image the abdomen, retroperitoneum, and pelvis. In most cases,

both T_1- and T_2-weighted pulse sequences were utilized to evaluate the pathology at hand. The T_1-weighted pulse sequences almost always consisted of repetition times (TRs) of between 0.3 and 0.7 sec with echo times (TEs) of 35 or 70 msec. Five to seven T_1 images can be obtained in 5 min or less. The T_2-weighted pulse sequences almost always consisted of TRs of 1.5 to 2.1 sec and TEs ranging from 35 to 120 msec. Seven to nine images are obtained in approximately 18 min with these T_2 studies. In almost all cases, a 1-cm slice thickness was utilized. With a 256 by 256 pixel matrix, a maximum resolution of 2 mm is obtainable when the body coil is used as the transmitting and receiving coil.

One of the major advantages of MRI is the ability to obtain direct coronal and sagittal images. In the body MRI protocols, axial sections are usually obtained first. Most images displayed in this chapter are in the axial plane since that view is the most useful for comparing MRI with computed tomography (CT). However, in approximately 50% of the body MRI studies here, coronal or sagittal images were obtained to better demonstrate a particular pathologic abnormality.

It is often confusing for the beginner to remember the signal intensities that occur in normal and pathologic tissue on T_1 and T_2 scans. In general, on T_1-weighted scans, tissues with a short T_1 relaxation time (e.g., fat) generate an intense signal and therefore appear white on MRI films photographed with standard gray-scale values. Tissues with a long T_1 value on T_1-weighted scans (e.g., fluid in a renal cyst or urine in the bladder) generate a low signal intensity and therefore appear dark gray on the films. Those tissues with intermediate T_1 relaxation times (e.g., muscle) generate a midrange signal intensity and so will appear light gray on MRI films using a T_1-weighted technique.

This situation is reversed on T_2-weighted scans. A tissue with a short T_2 value generates a low signal intensity and therefore appears dark gray on MRI films. A tissue with a long T_2 relaxation time (urine in the bladder) generates a high signal intensity and therefore appears white on MRI films using a T_2-weighted technique. If the tissue has an intermediate-range T_2 relaxation time, it will generate a midrange intensity and appear light gray on MRI films using a T_2-weighted technique.

Blood flowing at normal intracorporeal velocities does not generate an MRI signal because of the flow-void phenomenon, and it therefore is seen as a black region on MRI films. Bowel gas and cortical bone also do not generate MRI signals and therefore also appear as black regions.

The 0.5-T magnet utilized was operated at field strengths of 0.352 and 0.5 T. Some of the simple rules that follow may not apply to images made at higher field strengths. These rules will be helpful primarily in the interpretation of the images displayed in this chapter.

1. Fat demonstrates a high signal intensity on the T_1- and T_2-weighted pulse sequences utilized herein.

2. A variety of midrange signal intensities are observed in all intraabdominal and pelvic organs, lymph nodes, and muscular structures on T_1-weighted images.

3. When one moves from T_1- to T_2-weighted scans, there is an increase in signal intensity in normal spleen, kidneys, adrenal glands, pancreas, and lymph nodes. Signal intensity increases to a much lesser degree in liver, possibly because of iron stores in this organ.

4. Corticomedullary differentiation is routinely observed on T_1-weighted studies (renal cortex more intense than renal medulla) but is not well visualized on T_2-weighted studies.

5. Differences in T_2 relaxation times of intrauterine tissue layers allow separation of endometrium from myometrium on T_2-weighted images.

6. Air-filled bowel loops demonstrate a low intraluminal signal intensity. If fluid is present within the lumen of a loop of bowel, it demonstrates a low signal intensity on T_1-weighted images and a high signal intensity on T_2-weighted images. When peristaltic artifacts are minimal, the gut wall can be separated from adjacent peritoneal fat.

7. Blood flowing at normal velocity demonstrates a very low signal intensity or no signal. Intraluminal thrombus demonstrates a high signal intensity on T_1-weighted images; that intensity decreases to some degree on T_2-weighted images. This pattern is useful in separating thrombus from pathologic causes of increased intraluminal signal intensity; in the latter case, there tends to be a relative increase in signal intensity on T_2 scans.

8. Unconcentrated bile in the gallbladder demonstrates low signal intensity on T_1 scans and high intensity on T_2 scans. Concentrated bile demonstrates high signal intensity on both T_1- and T_2-weighted images.

An orally administered MRI-specific contrast agent for general use in gastrointestinal imaging is not yet available. This has hindered intraabdominal diagnosis in regions where bowel loops lie adjacent to important anatomical structures. In general, the best MR images in the body are obtained where anatomy is relatively fixed (i.e., not subject to respiratory or peristaltic motion), as in the pelvis, retroperitoneum, and paraspinal areas. In this regard, the most difficult areas to image are the peridiaphragmatic structures, the region along the anterior abdominal wall, and the intestinal tract. Glucagon may be utilized as an agent to reduce peristaltic artifacts generated on MRI studies.[2]

A useful respiratory gating mechanism or software technique for eliminating respiratory artifacts is also not yet available. By using T_1-weighted pulse sequences with short TRs and TEs, one can overcome some of the respiratory artifacts seen in the peridiaphragmatic and anterior abdominal wall region. The use of TRs below 0.5 sec combined with TEs at or below 15 msec and respiratory gating can eliminate almost all of the respiration-induced artifacts that might be present on body MRI studies.

ABDOMEN

Liver

Normal liver parenchyma demonstrates a homogeneous midrange signal intensity on T_1- and T_2-weighted MR images obtained with currently available spin-echo pulse sequences (Fig 12–1). The average T_1 and T_2 relaxation times of normal liver have been measured: T_1, 533 msec (SD $\pm$ 136; range, 228–956 msec); T_2, 56 msec (SD $\pm$ 8; range, 38–112 msec).[3–5] Vascular structures within the liver, including the hepatic veins, portal veins, hepatic arteries, and inferior vena cava, are consistently visualized because of the flow-void phenomenon.[6,7] Periportal, perihepatic, and falciform fissure fat defines the borders and interstices of the liver and structures within the porta hepatis.[8–11] A low signal intensity has been observed along the surface of the liver and is secondary to a chemical-shift artifact and not the liver capsule.[12] Normal intrahepatic biliary ducts are not usually visualized with MRI.[9–11]

At present, conventional spin-echo and inversion-recovery MRI is considered equal to CT in the ability to detect focal intrahepatic abnormalities.[5, 13–15] This situation may improve with the advent of a successful respiratory gating technique or the ability to perform short TR/TE pulse sequences[16] or phase-contrast MRI.[17] Various MRI contrast agents, including liver-specific forms, are also being developed and may further improve the modality's ability to detect focal liver disease,[18, 19] although successful hepatic contrast enhancement depends on optimization of MRI pulse sequences.[20] It has been shown that primary or secondary focal hepatic malignant lesions have T_1 and T_2 relaxation times longer than those for normal liver.[4, 5, 9, 13, 21–23] This fact translates into a visible signal intensity difference between neoplasm and normal liver on MRI studies, with the degree of contrast differentiation depending on the selection of the appropriate MRI pulse sequence.[24–27]

In general, on T_1-weighted MRI studies, hepatic neoplasm demonstrates a lower signal intensity than adjacent liver (Figs 12–2 and 12–3).[16, 21] For several years, commercially available MRI devices did not have the ability to obtain heavily T_1-weighted studies (TRs $<$ 0.5 sec, TEs $<$ 20 msec), making the detection of hepatic metastatic disease on the basis of T_1 relaxation time differences difficult. Recently, Stark et al. have pioneered the use of pulse sequences with shorter TRs and TEs in intermediate field strength and have markedly improved the conspicuity of hepatic metastatic lesions on T_1-weighted studies.[16] These newer T_1 sequences can be performed in a shorter period of time and with a noticeable decrease in respiratory and peristaltic artifact on the MR image.

On T_2-weighted pulse sequences, focal malignant hepatic disease demonstrates a higher signal intensity than adjacent normal liver parenchyma (Figs 12–4 and 12–5). Until recently, T_2-weighted pulse sequences were the technique of choice in screening the liver for focal metastatic disease.[21] However, in an intermediate field strength the availability of T_1-weighted pulse sequences with short TRs and TEs has obviated the need for T_2 studies when screening the liver for metastases because T_2 scans utilize a longer measuring time, provide a poorer signal to noise ratio, and are more subject to respiratory and peristaltic artifacts than T_1-weighted studies.[16]

After much initial enthusiasm,[8, 9] it has been recognized that MRI cannot at present be utilized in most cases to diagnose a specific intrahepatic malignancy on the basis of a characteristic T_1 or T_2 relaxation time.[5, 13, 21] It has been reported that a spectrum of T_1 and T_2 relaxation times can be observed in a group of similar intrahepatic neoplasms in different patients or in multiple neoplasms of the same type or different types in the same patient.[5, 13, 21] However, many authors have stated that conventional spin-echo MRI has the ability to distinguish benign focal hepatic disease such as hepatic cyst or hemangioma from hepatic malignancy such as hepatoma or metastatic disease.[21, 28–31]

It is obvious from the MRI literature and from the personal experience of myself and my colleagues that MRI is an extremely sensitive technique in the detection of hepatic hemangioma (Figs 12–6 and 12–7). The diagnostic sensitivity of MRI in the detection of hemangioma is secondary to the extremely prolonged T_2 relaxation time of hemangioma in relation to normal liver parenchyma and solid hepatic primary or metastatic tumor.[28–31] Although MRI can reliably separate hepatic hemangioma from metastases and most other primary tumors, occasionally necrotic metastatic lesions will also display a very long T_2 relaxation time (Fig 12–8). In fact, the measured T_2 values of the lesions in Figure 12–8 were longer than those of many of the hemangiomas reported in the MRI literature.[28–31] It is interesting that hepatic metastases secondary to adenocarcinoma of the stomach and endometrium have been reported to display T_2 values equal to those of hemangioma.[28, 30] Because of these reports, further clinical research must be performed to determine whether MRI can reliably separate hemangioma from all forms of hepatic metastatic disease or only from metastatic deposits of certain primary neoplasms.

Colleagues and I have found MRI useful in evaluating surface hepatic metastatic disease from ovarian neoplasm (Fig 12–5) and in evaluating intrahepatic inferior vena caval compression by metastatic disease within the liver (Fig 12–9). Magnetic resonance imaging has not been found to be better than other imaging modalities in the evaluation of leukemic or lymphomatous infiltration of the liver.[32]

Magnetic resonance imaging is useful in the detection of primary hepatocellular carcinoma, particularly in those lesions greater than 2 cm in diameter.[22, 23] It will detect the characteristic fibrous capsule of hepatoma twice as frequently as CT and therefore will more often allow a specific diagnosis.[23] This modality is also sensitive in detecting the areas of steatosis that occur in hepatoma but not in other common focal hepatic lesions.[23] On both T_1- and T_2-weighted studies, it may also provide a specific diagnosis of focal nodular hyperplasia by demonstrating the characteristic central scar (Fig 12–10).

Magnetic resonance imaging has proved to be variably useful in evaluating diffuse hepatic disease (Figs 12–9 and 12–11). Hepatic cirrhosis and diffuse fatty liver may not be visible on MR images obtained with conventional spin-echo techniques unless the findings are severe and focal in nature.[8, 9, 33–35] However, spin-echo MRI can suggest the presence of diffuse hepatocellular disease by demonstrating collateral portal venous channels such as a recanalized umbilical vein.[36] Proton spectroscopic imaging (chemical-shift imaging) allows detection of lesser degrees of focal or diffuse fatty infiltration of the liver.[37–40] This technique may prove to be useful in the detection of focal metastatic lesions in the patient with fatty liver.[41]

Magnetic resonance imaging is also useful in the detection of disease states that cause increased iron or copper deposition in the liver.[42, 43] The paramagnetic effect of locally increased iron or copper stores extremely decreases T_2 relaxation in liver parenchyma and moderately decreases T_1, causing a generalized decrease in hepatic signal intensity, predominantly secondary to the effect on T_2 relaxation.[42] In my experience, metastatic lesions or focal lesions from infectious disease are probably better visualized in patients with hepatic metal-deposition states because of the large difference in signal intensity between the pathologic lesion and the metal-containing liver (Fig 12–11).

In general, MRI has not been shown to be an effective method for diagnosing primary neoplasms of the gallbladder or biliary tree.[44] Dilated intrahepatic and extrahepatic biliary ducts may appear isointense with adjacent liver parenchyma on a particular pulse sequence; therefore, it is recommended that a multisequence study be performed when the

biliary tree is evaluated.[44] Colleagues and I have encountered one case in which T_2-weighted scans did demonstrate the porta hepatis involvement of a cholangiocarcinoma (Fig 12–12). We have also found MRI useful in demonstrating metastatic masses in the porta hepatis and their effect on the adjacent portal vein and inferior vena cava (Fig 12–13).

Spleen

The normal spleen demonstrates a homogeneous signal intensity and is routinely well visualized with MRI. In contrast to the liver, the spleen demonstrates a somewhat higher signal intensity on T_2-weighted images than on T_1-weighted images.[45] Intrasplenic vascular structures are better visualized with MRI in comparison with other imaging modalities.[6] Splenic size is particularly well documented on sagittal or coronal MRI scans.[46]

Few references to the abnormal spleen are present in the MRI literature. Kressel et al. studied five patients with splenomegaly due to various causes and found lymphomatous and leukemic infiltration to cause focal regions of decreased signal intensity on T_1-weighted studies.[47]

Colleagues and I have studied splenic metastatic disease in several patients and have noted that, in comparison with normal splenic parenchyma, these lesions display a relatively lower signal intensity on T_1-weighted images and a higher signal intensity on T_2-weighted studies. In this regard, the appearance of splenic metastatic disease is similar to that of hepatic metastatic disease on both T_1- and T_2-weighted studies (Fig 12–14).

As in the liver, the generalized decreased signal intensity observed in the spleen in metal-deposition diseases is caused mainly by the T_2 effect of the increased intrasplenic metal concentration (Fig 12–15).[42, 43, 48] In this situation, if there are coexisting abnormalities such as microabscesses in the spleen, they will be seen as bright spots on T_2-weighted scans (Fig 12–11).

Magnetic resonance imaging provides routinely excellent visualization of the splenic vein on axial images[6] without administration of intravenous contrast medium, and it can be utilized to detect splenic vein thrombosis (Fig 12–16) induced by a paraneoplastic syndrome or adjacent tumor.

General Abdomen

The use of MRI in the detection of primary malignancies of the gastrointestinal tract has been limited by the lack of a commercially available MRI-specific oral contrast agent and routinely poor definition of bowel structures because of respiratory and peristaltic artifacts. The stomach is the structure best evaluated with MRI at the present time, because perigastric fat and intraluminal gas will, in most cases, provide sharp definition of the gastric wall and allow detection of neoplastic thickening. In the stomach, adenocarcinoma (Fig 12–17), lymphoma, and leiomyosarcoma (Fig 12–18) can be diagnosed by MRI on the basis of morphological changes. In my experience, MRI has been successful in demonstrating perigastric adenopathy and hepatic metastatic disease secondary to all forms of gastric neoplasia, although it may fail to detect the calcifications of leiomyosarcoma.

There is no specific role for MRI at present in the staging of primary neoplasms of the large and small bowels, although the modality can be utilized to demonstrate invasion of large intraabdominal vascular channels by these neoplasms (Fig 12–19). Magnetic resonance imaging can demonstrate focal mesenteric metastases from intraabdominal or extraabdominal primary malignancies (Fig 12–20).

This modality is useful in oncology patients for studying diaphragmatic abnormalities, whether they are due to hematogenous metastatic disease (Fig 12–21) or direct neoplastic invasion (Fig 12–22). In particular, coronal and sagittal images allow a precise definition of normal and pathologic diaphragmatic anatomy (Fig 12–22).

RETROPERITONEUM

Kidneys

The MRI appearance of the normal kidney is dependent on the pulse sequence utilized. On inversion-recovery and T_1-weighted spin-echo studies, the longer T_1 relaxation time of renal medulla (570–800 msec) in comparison with renal cortex (390–600 msec) allows routine corticomedullary differentiation, with the renal medulla displaying a lower signal intensity than adjacent renal cortical structures. On T_2-weighted studies at 0.5 T, the kidney demonstrates a relatively homogeneous appearance, with little evidence of corticomedullary differentiation. The signal intensity of the normal kidney, in comparison with surrounding anatomical structures, is greater on T_2- than on T_1-weighted studies.

The borders of the kidney and the extent of the renal sinus are sharply defined on MRI studies by the high signal intensity of fat in these regions. The

flow-void phenomenon allows the precise definition of renal arterial and venous branches. The collapsed or urine-filled renal collecting system can be identified by its low signal intensity on T_1, which contrasts with adjacent renal sinus fat. The renal capsule cannot be identified as a separate structure, although routine definition of the anterior and posterior limbs of Gerota's fascia is available, allowing separation of the retroperitoneum into the perirenal and pararenal compartments.[49–52]

Magnetic resonance imaging has been found useful in the diagnosis and staging of renal neoplasms.[53–56] Hricak et al. have documented the prolongation of mean T_1 and T_2 relaxation times of renal carcinoma in comparison with those of normal renal parenchyma.[53] The T_1 and T_2 relaxation times of primary renal neoplasms should be higher than those of ipsilateral normal renal parenchyma, psoas muscle, and retroperitoneal fat.[53] However, despite measured differences between tumor and normal renal parenchyma, the wide range of T_1 and T_2 values in a given renal neoplasm may occasionally produce masses that are visually isointense with renal parenchyma on either T_1- or T_2-weighted scans, or on both.[53] Leung et al. have demonstrated greater enhancement of renal tumors on MRI in comparison with contrast-enhanced CT after intravenous injection of gadolinium-labeled diethylenetriamine pentaacetic acid (DTPA).[49]

Magnetic resonance imaging has several specific advantages over other imaging modalities in staging primary renal neoplasms (Fig 12–23). The course and caliber of important renal and perirenal vascular structures can be demonstrated without administration of intravenous contrast medium.[54] With the use of a multiecho pulse sequence, it is possible to detect intraluminal thrombus formation in the renal vein or inferior vena cava (Figs 12–24 and 12–25) and to confidently separate this abnormality from flow-related causes of increased intraluminal signal intensity.[54, 57, 58] Compared with other imaging modalities, the improved resolution of retroperitoneal and renal hilar vascular anatomy by MRI allows a more confident diagnosis of adenopathy in the perirenal space and retroperitoneum.[54] Direct invasion of adjacent lipomatous and muscular structures by primary renal neoplasm or distant metastases (Fig 12–26) is also well demonstrated with MRI.[54] The relative inability of MRI to detect calcification in renal masses is a negative aspect of the modality (Figs 12–27 and 12–28).

Magnetic resonance imaging can reliably separate renal cysts from solid tumor.[53, 59] Compared with malignant renal neoplasms, simple renal cysts demonstrate a lower signal intensity on T_1-weighted studies and higher intensity on T_2-weighted studies.[53, 59] Hemorrhagic renal cyst, frequently observed in patients with polycystic kidney syndrome, will display a signal intensity much higher than renal neoplasm on T_1-weighted studies.[49]

Transitional cell carcinoma of the renal pelvis may be detectable only on the basis of replacement of renal sinus fat by a mass with different signal intensity (Fig 12–29). In the experience of my colleagues and myself, and also in that of others,[49] the signal intensity of urothelioma has been identical to that of normal renal parenchyma on T_1- and T_2-weighted studies. Renal or perirenal lymphoma may demonstrate an intensity similar to that of normal renal parenchyma on T_1- and T_2-weighted studies, so that diagnosis must be by morphological criteria (Figs 12–30 and 12–31). Since retroperitoneal fat and lymphoma may be isointense on T_2 scans (Fig 12–31), the use of T_1 scans to define the extrarenal extent of renal and perirenal lymphoma is recommended. A specific diagnosis of angiomyolipoma can be obtained with MRI because of the predominantly fatty nature of these lesions (producing a high signal intensity on T_1-weighted MRI studies).[49]

Magnetic resonance imaging is a sensitive technique in the detection of hydronephrosis without the administration of intravenous contrast medium.[49, 60] Loss of corticomedullary differentiation in hydronephrotic kidneys on T_1-weighted studies may be a sign of renal failure (specific to MRI) and indicate the need for such therapeutic action as percutaneous nephrostomy.[49] In the oncology patient, in addition to axial scans, coronal and sagittal images may become useful in demonstrating the obstructing retroperitoneal mass, the level of ureteral obstruction, the proximal hydroureter, and hydronephrosis.

Adrenal Glands

Magnetic resonance imaging reliably identifies both adrenal glands in axial and coronal planes.[61] The normal adrenal gland demonstrates a signal intensity similar to that of adjacent liver on T_1- and T_2-weighted scans.[61, 62] Adrenal corticomedullary differentiation has been described, with the medulla appearing less intense than cortex on T_1-weighted studies.[61, 62] The small size and unusual configuration of the normal adrenal gland have prevented accurate determination of T_1 and T_2 relaxation times. Utilization of a surface coil in T_1-weighted studies of the adrenal gland reportedly improves resolution of this organ by a threefold increase in the signal to noise ratio.[63]

There is considerable promise for MRI in characterizing the nature of focal adrenal masses.[64–66] Nonfunctioning adrenal adenomas are common in the general population and therefore frequently encountered in oncology patients. It is possible to reliably separate the nonfunctioning adrenal adenoma from other solid nonadenomatous adrenal lesions with MRI by both qualitative (visual) and quantitative (calculated T_1 and T_2 values and intensity ratio) criteria.[66] Adenomas visually appear hypointense in comparison with normal hepatic parenchyma on T_1- and T_2-weighted studies, with the effect more obvious on T_1-weighted MRI examinations (Fig 12–32).

Adrenal metastases (Fig 12–33), adrenal cortical carcinoma (Fig 12–34), pheochromocytoma (Fig 12–35), neuroblastoma, and adrenal lymphoma all appear hyperintense in comparison with normal liver parenchyma on T_2-weighted studies and are therefore separable from benign adenoma.[64–67] Adrenal myelolipoma and hemorrhage demonstrate relative hyperintensity in comparison with the liver on T_1-weighted studies and are also separable from adenoma.[64–66] In general, nonfunctioning adrenal adenomas demonstrate a homogeneous low signal intensity on T_1 and T_2, as opposed to the heterogeneous appearance of metastatic lesions and primary carcinomas as seen on T_2-weighted images.[66]

Magnetic resonance imaging has been utilized in diagnosis, staging, and prediction of tumor resectability in patients with neuroblastoma and can demonstrate changes in tumor size and intensity in response to chemotherapy and radiation treatment.[68, 69] In the presence of primary adrenal carcinoma (Fig 12–34), pheochromocytoma (Fig 12–35), or neuroblastoma, MRI can reliably stage the tumor in terms of invasion of adjacent fatty and muscular structures.[67–69] Formation of tumor thrombus with extension into the inferior vena cava can also be demonstrated.[58]

Pancreas

Until now, MR imaging of the pancreas has been limited by the lack of a commercially available oral contrast agent and degradation of the pancreatic MR image due to respiratory and peristaltic artifacts intrinsic to abdominal MRI scans. Recently, the advent of commercially available T_1-weighted pulse sequences with short TRs and TEs has led to better visualization of the pancreas because of an improved signal to noise ratio and lessening of respiratory and peristaltic artifacts.[16] The application of surface-coil technology to MR imaging of the pancreas also may lead to better routine visualization of this organ.[70] The normal pancreas demonstrates a homogeneous midrange signal intensity on T_1- and T_2-weighted scans.[45] The T_1 and T_2 relaxation times of the normal pancreas have been calculated: T_1, 448 ± 131 msec; T_2, 52 ± 6 msec.[71, 72] Typically, the head, body, tail, and uncinate process of the pancreas demonstrate an identical signal intensity (Fig 12–1). The normal pancreatic duct is not routinely visualized with MRI at present.[73] However, an advantage of MRI over other imaging techniques is the superior visualization of peripancreatic vascular structures, which sharply delineate pancreatic borders in most cases.[6]

Pancreatic carcinoma can be detected with MRI on the basis of morphological criteria alone or by a signal intensity difference from normal pancreatic tissue.[70–72] In my experience, pancreatic adenocarcinoma demonstrates the same or a slightly lower signal intensity than adjacent normal pancreatic tissue on T_1-weighted studies but a higher signal intensity when T_2-weighted sequences are utilized (Fig 12–36). Tumor-induced pancreatic duct dilatation, peripancreatic fat plane tumor invasion, adenopathy, pseudocyst, phlegmon, ascites, and hepatic metastases may all be demonstrated with MRI.[70–72] In identifying invasion of peripancreatic vascular structures by pancreatic neoplasm, MRI is superior to other modalities.[70, 71] Pancreatic calcifications are not well visualized with MRI, however.[70–72]

Magnetic resonance imaging has been described as a useful technique in identifying pancreatic islet cell tumors and other functioning pancreatic lesions.[70] Colleagues and I have found it a useful modality in arriving at a specific diagnosis of cystadenoma or cystadenocarcinoma of the pancreas based on the characteristic T_1 and T_2 appearances of the cystic regions of these tumors (Fig 12–37). We have also studied one case of giant cell sarcoma of the pancreas (which is a rare lesion) that demonstrated a signal intensity on T_1- and T_2-weighted studies similar to that of pancreatic adenocarcinoma (Fig 12–38).

General Retroperitoneum

Normal retroperitoneal lymph nodes can occasionally be visualized with MRI and demonstrate a homogeneous midrange signal intensity on T_1-weighted studies and a relative increase in signal intensity on T_2-weighted examinations.[74–78] This modality is superior to others in providing diagnostic contrast between adenopathy and adjacent vascular structures (which show low signal intensity) (Fig 12–39) and retroperitoneal fat (which shows high signal intensity) without the administration of contrast medium.[74–76]

It is possible at present to obtain T_1 and T_2 relaxation measurements only from normal lymph nodes with diameters greater than 10 mm.[74] A generalized increase in the T_1 and T_2 values of malignant lymph nodes in comparison with normal lymph nodes has been demonstrated.[74, 76] However, a significant overlap of T_1 and T_2 values between normal, inflammatory, and malignant adenopathy has been encountered, preventing specific diagnosis by quantitative data.[74, 76] In detecting lymphadenopathy by the usual CT morphological criteria, MRI is probably as accurate as CT scanning (Fig 12–40).[75–78]

The MRI appearance of primary retroperitoneal neoplasms in the adult population has been described.[79] The modality is useful in demonstrating the extent of the lesion and the involvement of adjacent vascular and muscular structures (Fig 12–41). Liposarcoma demonstrates a significantly higher signal intensity on T_1-weighted images in comparison with other primary retroperitoneal tumors (Fig 12–42). Primary retroperitoneal leiomyosarcoma, neurofibrosarcoma (Fig 12–43), lymphoma (Figs 12–40 and 12–44), and fibrous histiocytoma demonstrate similar signal intensities on T_1- and T_2-weighted studies. Lymphangioma, a benign cystic disorder, can be differentiated from solid tumors by its low signal intensity on T_1-weighted studies, which is characteristic of fluid-filled structures (Fig 12–41). In a series of 15 patients with benign and malignant paraspinal neurogenic tumors, MRI in each case accurately determined the presence or absence of extradural extension via neural foramen or vertebral body erosion (Fig 12–43).[80]

When an abnormality of the inferior vena cava is suspected in an oncology patient, MRI can be utilized as the initial screening study.[81] A complete set of T_1-weighted axial and sagittal sections of the inferior vena cava can now be obtained in less than 8 min and will reliably demonstrate the course and caliber of this structure (Fig 12–45). It has been found that MRI is superior to contrast-enhanced CT in identifying the cause and level of obstruction or narrowing of the inferior vena cava in a patient with lower extremity edema.[81] In staging the inferior vena cava involvement by renal, adrenal, or retroperitoneal neoplasm, MRI has been found to be equal to contrast-enhanced CT, although the MRI study is performed without subjecting the patient to intravenous contrast medium or ionizing radiation.

Magnetic resonance imaging has also been found useful in demonstrating primary and secondary neoplastic abnormalities of the iliopsoas muscle (Figs 12–46 and 12–47).[82]

PELVIS

Female Pelvis

Because of the lack of significant respiratory artifacts in the pelvic region, MRI can generally provide superb definition of the anatomy of the female genital tract in axial, coronal, and sagittal planes. Sagittal plane sections in particular can reliably demonstrate cephalocaudally oriented fat planes separating the urinary bladder and rectum from the vagina, cervix, and uterus.[83–87]

The uterus is best demonstrated on sagittal MRI sections. Because the endometrium and myometrium yield similar long T_1 values, the uterus displays a homogeneous midrange signal intensity on T_1-weighted images, with poor differentiation of uterine tissue layers (Fig 12–48,A).[83] On T_2-weighted images, the high signal intensity of the endometrium allows visual separation from the myometrium, which displays a higher intensity in the miduterus (Fig 12–48). The endometrial and myometrial layers are separated on T_2 images by a low-intensity zone that may represent the stratum basale of endometrium[83] or, in fact, be part of myometrial tissue.[88] Uterine size, position, and volume can be determined with MRI, and cyclic endometrial changes due to menstruation can be documented by observing changes in the thickness of the intrauterine high-intensity zone on T_2-weighted studies.[83]

The anterior and posterior cervical lips are routinely demonstrated by MRI; T_2 scans optimally separate cervical signal intensity (low) from that of the myometrium (midrange). A high signal intensity is observed in the vagina and cervical canal on T_1- and T_2-weighted studies and is likely related to proteinaceous mucous secretions.[83]

The ovaries will demonstrate a homogeneous midrange signal intensity on T_1 images and increase in signal intensity on T_2 studies (Fig 12–49), often revealing the low-intensity tunica albuginea peripherally. The round ligaments, broad ligaments, and other adnexal supportive structures will also demonstrate a low signal intensity on T_1- and T_2-weighted images secondary to their fibrous nature (Fig 12–48). Magnetic resonance imaging also

sharply defines pelvic fat and muscular and bony pelvic sidewall anatomy.[83–87]

Magnetic resonance imaging is a sensitive detector of intrauterine pathology as small as 1 cm.[86–92] It will characterize uterine leiomyoma free of degenerative changes by a homogeneous low signal intensity mass on T_1- and T_2-weighted studies and can predict the mucosal, submucosal, or serosal origin of these tumors (Fig 12–50). Leiomyoma displaying hyaline, myxomatous, or fatty degeneration will display a nonhomogeneous higher signal intensity on MRI studies.[90] It may be possible to predict sarcomatous degeneration of large leiomyomas when tumor vessels are identified within the mass by MRI (Fig 12–51).

Several reports have described the use of MRI in the diagnosis and staging of endometrial carcinoma, although the number of cases is small.[86, 88, 91, 92] Despite the ability of MRI to separate myometrium and endometrium on T_2 studies, it has not been convincingly proved that MRI can accurately demonstrate the depth of myometrial invasion by endometrial carcinoma, which is the key factor in evaluating stage I lesions. The modality is able to demonstrate cervical invasion and indicate a stage II lesion or obstruction of the endocervical os that results in hematometra (Fig 12–52). It is certainly useful in detecting stage III and IV lesions, which extend outside the uterus to invade the parametrium, pelvic fat, gut, urinary bladder, or pelvic sidewall.[86, 88, 91, 92]

Undoubtedly, MRI plays a significant role in staging cervical carcinoma.[86, 88, 91, 92] At present, it cannot differentiate between normal cervix and stage I carcinoma on the basis of a signal intensity difference, although we have demonstrated hematometra secondary to cervical canal occlusion by a stage I lesion (Fig 12–53). T_2 studies can possibly demonstrate uterine invasion (stage IIA) by cervical carcinoma when the normal triple-intensity pattern of the uterus is replaced by tumor, which tends to display a midrange signal intensity (Fig 12–54). Extension of tumor into the pericervical fat (stage IIA) or parametrium (stage IIB) is easily discernible, as is pelvic sidewall invasion (stage III) (Fig 12–55) and vesical and rectal involvement (stage IV) (Fig 12–56).

Magnetic resonance imaging is useful in the diagnosis and staging of primary benign and malignant ovarian neoplasms, although degree of malignancy cannot be predicted by T_1 and T_2 values.[91–93] Sagittal MRI sections display large pelviabdominal masses of ovarian origin and characterize cystic, stromal, or hemorrhagic portions by specific signal intensity (Fig 12–57). Magnetic resonance imaging can demonstrate capsule thickness, internal septation, and ascites but usually will not depict calcification. According to Weigert et al., it is not possible to differentiate ascites from pseudomyxoma peritonei (Fig 12–58).[94]

Magnetic resonance imaging can demonstrate the unilateral (stage IA) or bilateral (stage IB) origin of stage I carcinoma of the ovary and can depict ascites, although an assessment of capsule integrity (stage IC) is currently not possible. The modality is accurate in demonstrating uterine (stage IIA), parametrial (stage IIB), pelvic sidewall (stage IIB), or intraabdominal (stage III) spread of ovarian neoplasm. On MRI, Krukenberg's tumor of the ovary (Fig 12–59) has an appearance identical to that of primary ovarian tumors.

Magnetic resonance imaging has the ability to provide a narrow differential diagnosis when a solitary extrauterine pelvic mass is detected.[95] A cystic pelvic mass has the least specific appearance, with a low signal intensity on the T_1 scan and high intensity on the T_2 scan. In this situation, the differential diagnosis includes mucinous and serous cystadenoma and cystadenocarcinoma (Figs 12–60 and 12–61), benign cystic teratoma and ovarian thecoma (Fig 12–62), paraovarian cyst, and follicular cyst. A lesion characterized by a homogeneous high signal intensity on a T_1 scan usually represents benign cystic teratoma, endometrioma, or hemorrhagic ovarian cyst. Benign cystic teratoma can be specifically diagnosed on T_1 or T_2 scans when foci of low signal intensity, which indicate areas of bone genesis, are observed. Its specific diagnosis is also indicated on T_1 scans when a lesion displays three separate internal signal intensities representing areas of fat (high intensity), fluid (midrange intensity), and bone (low intensity) (Fig 12–63). Ovarian fibroma demonstrates a low signal intensity on T_1 and T_2 images because of its fibrous content, again allowing a specific diagnosis (Fig 12–64).

Male Pelvis

As in the female pelvis, MRI of the male pelvis can provide superb images in three planes because of the lack of significant respiratory and peristaltic artifacts. The normal prostate gland demonstrates a homogeneous low signal intensity on T_1-weighted studies (Fig 12–65), with a marked increase in intensity on T_2-weighted pulse sequences.[96–98] The prostatic capsule is not routinely visualized but has been demonstrated in vitro as a low-intensity structure on T_1-weighted studies.[99] Magnetic resonance imaging

does not clearly characterize the peripheral and central zones of the prostate gland by differences in signal intensity, although Denonvilliers' fascia and the verumontanum can be observed in vivo.[98] The course of the prostatic urethra can be well identified after insertion of a Foley catheter (Fig 12–66). A periprostatic rim on T_2-weighted studies was initially described by Poon et al.[98] and was ascribed to the periprostatic venous plexus. Ling et al.[99] have identified periprostatic veins as a low signal intensity on T_2 studies and suggest that the high-intensity region described by Poon et al. actually represents a portion of the prostate gland and not periprostatic tissue or veins. All authors agree that MRI provides precise definition of the prostatic borders because of differences in signal intensity between the prostate gland and the pelvic fat and that the prostate gland can be reliably separated from adjacent structures such as the pelvic floor musculature, symphysis pubis, seminal vesicles, urinary bladder, and rectum.[96–99]

Normal seminal vesicles are routinely visualized with MRI. They demonstrate a signal intensity similar to that of the prostate gland on T_1-weighted studies and are relatively brighter than the prostate gland on heavily T_2-weighted studies.[96–98] Pelvic fat fills the seminal vesicle angle and separates the seminal vesicles from the adjacent prostate gland, rectum, and urinary bladder. Magnetic resonance imaging will routinely delineate the corpora cavernosa of the penis at their ischial attachment sites and on T_2-weighted studies will depict low-intensity fascial septa separating the brighter corpora cavernosa and corpora spongiosa.[96] The flow-void phenomenon will identify the internal spermatic vessels in the inguinal canal and separate them from high-intensity fat and the midrange signal intensity of the ductus deferens.

After much initial enthusiasm,[96, 98] it is currently believed that, although MRI can readily demonstrate derangement in the normal architecture of the prostate gland, it cannot reliably distinguish between prostatic carcinoma (Fig 12–67) and benign prostatic hypertrophy (Fig 12–68).[99, 100] When the currently available T_1-weighted pulse sequences are utilized, regions of acute or chronic prostatitis, benign prostatic hypertrophy, and prostatic carcinoma usually demonstrate a signal intensity similar to that of normal prostatic parenchyma.[96–101] However, it is recognized that T_2-weighted sequences, although nonspecific, will best identify regions of prostatic abnormality on an anatomical basis[99] and may localize an occult neoplasm not obvious by other techniques.[101] At present, it is believed that benign prostatic hypertrophy characteristically produces a generalized nodular prostatomegaly with a nonhomogeneous signal intensity on T_2-weighted images, with occasional areas of lower signal intensity observable. Unfortunately, prostatic carcinoma in most cases demonstrates a similar appearance, although neoplasm more often produces a homogeneous increase in signal intensity on T_2-weighted studies.[99]

Despite the inability of MRI to specifically diagnose prostatic malignancy, it appears that the modality is useful in staging known prostatic carcinoma.[97–100, 102] The total number of reported patients with prostatic carcinoma staged with MRI is small, but there is a consensus that spread of prostatic malignancy into the periprostatic fat can be defined with MRI, with tumor extension demonstrating a lower signal intensity than adjacent pelvic fat on T_1 and T_2 studies.[97–100, 102] At present, MRI can correctly identify stage C prostatic carcinoma by demonstrating extracapsular extension into the fat within the seminal vesicle angle (stage C1) or actual invasion of the seminal vesicles (stage C2) (Fig 12–67). In this regard, sagittal images are most useful in evaluating the relationship of prostatic tumor to fat of the seminal vesicle angle, because the fat plane is oriented mainly along the cephalocaudal axis. At present, MRI is probably equal to other imaging modalities in the detection of pelvic adenopathy, bony metastatic disease, and other findings indicating stage D prostatic carcinoma. It is not clear if MRI will aid in the workup of lesions confined by the prostatic capsule (stages A and B). Magnets with greater field strengths may allow extremely T_2-weighted studies to be performed that will precisely demonstrate the volume of prostatic gland involved by tumor and therefore aid in separating stage A1 from stage A2 and stage B1 from stage B2 lesions, wherein the amount of prostatic gland involved is the key factor.

Bladder and Miscellaneous Pelvic Masses

Magnetic resonance imaging is a sensitive technique in demonstrating the location of pelvic adenopathy (Fig 12–69) and in studying vascular and lymphatic lesions (Fig 12–70), as well as demonstrating primary neoplasms that arise from the muscular and bony pelvic sidewall. As with retroperitoneal adenopathy,[74–78] MRI precisely separates large pelvic lymph nodes from adjacent fatty and vascular structures in a way similar to or better than other imaging modalities. The relative signal intensity of pelvic adenopathy will be higher on T_2-weighted studies (Fig

12–69). As with primary lymphomatous masses arising in other anatomical regions, the borders of pelvic lesions of this type are better defined on T_1-weighted studies. This is due to similarities in signal intensity between lymphoma and pelvic fat on currently available T_2-weighted pulse sequences at 0.5 T (Fig 12–71).

In primary osseous tumors of the pelvis such as lymphoma (Fig 12–72) and Ewing's sarcoma (Fig 12–73), MRI provides superb delineation. The potential of MRI in staging benign and malignant paraspinal neurogenic tumors has been described.[80] When lesions of this type arise in the perisacral region, MRI can accurately detect the degree of involvement of the sacrum, lumbosacral plexus, or epidural spinal canal (Fig 12–74).

At present, MRI may be the imaging procedure of choice for studying the sacrum on account of its ability to obtain direct sagittal sections. Metastatic deposits and such primary sacral tumors as plasmacytoma (Fig 12–75) demonstrate a relatively low signal intensity and contrast sharply with the high signal intensity of bone marrow within the sacrum and the adjacent retrorectal and retrosacral fat planes. This visually striking difference in signal intensity allows sharp definition of the intraosseous and soft tissue borders of such lesions (Fig 12–75).[103]

Magnetic resonance imaging has been shown to be useful in the detection and staging of primary malignancies of the urinary bladder, with consistent depiction of lesions larger than 1.5 cm in diameter.[104–107] Fisher et al. have correlated MR image findings and the tumor-node-metastasis (TNM) classification of bladder carcinomas.[105] It is obvious in my colleagues' and my experience that MRI can be utilized to demonstrate the findings in stage T3 and T4 lesions—when tumor has extended into the deep muscle layer (stage T3A), into the perivesical fat (stage T3B), into adjacent pelvic organs (stage T4A), or into the pelvic sidewall (stage T4B). However, Fisher et al. further suggest that MRI may be useful in staging lesions confined to the bladder wall (stages T1 and T2),[105] although few cases of this type have been described in the literature.

It does appear that extension of bladder tumor within the bladder wall is best documented on T_2-weighted studies (Fig 12–76),[105] whereas invasion of the perivesical fat, pelvic organs, or pelvic sidewall is better delineated on T_1-weighted examinations.[105] Sagittal and coronal sections are very often useful in demonstrating superiorly or inferiorly directed tumor extensions.

Clinically manifest abnormalities related to the

urachus are rare. Colleagues and I have studied two cases of primary urachal masses, one a cyst and one due to adenocarcinoma. With the urinary bladder distended, the extent of the urachal mass in the space of Retzius can be well demonstrated (Fig 12–77). On T_1-weighted studies, there is a much higher signal intensity in the presence of urachal neoplasm than in uncomplicated cysts.

REFERENCES

1. Newton T.H., Potts D.G.: *Advanced Imaging Techniques.* San Anselmo, Calif., Clavadel Press, 1983.
2. Weinreb J.C., Maravilla K.R., Redman H.C., et al.: Improved MR imaging of the upper abdomen with glucagon and gas. *J. Comput. Assist. Tomogr.* 8: 835–838, 1984.
3. Bernardino M.E., Small W., Goldstein J., et al.: Multiple NMR T2 relaxation values in human liver tissue. *AJR* 141:1203–1208, 1983.
4. Borkowski G.P., Buonocore E., George C.R., et al.: Nuclear magnetic resonance (NMR) imaging in the evaluation of the liver: a preliminary experience. *J. Comput. Assist. Tomogr.* 7:768–774, 1983.
5. Moss A.A., Goldberg H.I., Stark D.D., et al.: Hepatic tumors: magnetic resonance and CT appearance. *Radiology* 150:141–147, 1984.
6. Higgins C.B., Goldberg H.I., Hricak H., et al.: Nuclear magnetic resonance imaging of vasculature of abdominal viscera: normal and pathological features. *AJR* 140:1217–1225, 1983.
7. Fisher M.R., Wall S.D., Hricak H., et al.: Hepatic vascular anatomy on magnetic resonance imaging. *AJR* 144:739–746, 1985.
8. Doyle F.H., Pennock J.M., Banks L.M., et al.: Nuclear magnetic resonance imaging of the liver: initial experience. *AJR* 138:193–200, 1982.
9. Smith F.W., Mallard J.R., Reid N., et al.: Nuclear magnetic resonance tomographic imaging in liver disease. *Lancet* 1:963–966, 1981.
10. Davis P.L., Moss A.A., Goldberg H.I., et al.: Nuclear magnetic resonance imaging of the liver and pancreas. *RadioGraphics* (special edition), January 1984.
11. Haaga J.R.: Magnetic resonance imaging of the liver. *Radiol. Clin. North Am.* 22:879–890, 1984.
12. Weinreb J.C., Brateman L., Babcock E.E., et al.: Chemical shift artifact in clinical magnetic resonance images at 0.35 T. *AJR* 145:183–185, 1985.
13. Heiken J.P., Lee J.K.T., Glazer H.S., et al.: Hepatic metastases studied with MR and CT. *Radiology* 156:423–427, 1985.
14. Kerlan R.K., Hricak H., Gross B.H., et al.: Nuclear magnetic resonance and computed tomographic angiography in the detection of hepatic metastases. *J. Clin. Gastroenterol.* 5:461–464, 1983.
15. Bydder G., Young I.R.: MR imaging of the liver using short T1 inversion recovery sequences. *J. Comput. Assist. Tomogr.* 9:1084–1089, 1985.
16. Stark D.D., Wittenberg J., Edelman R.R., et al.: Detection of hepatic metastases: analysis of pulse sequence performance in MR imaging. *Radiology* 159:365–370, 1986.
17. Stark D.D., Wittenberg J., Middleton M.S., et al.: Liver metastases: detection by phase-contrast MR imaging. *Radiology* 158:327–332, 1986.
18. Saini S., Stark D.D., Ferrucci J.T., et al.: Particulate iron oxide (magnetite): a reticuloendothelial system-specific liver MR contrast agent. Paper presented at the Society of Magnetic Resonance Imaging meeting, Philadelphia, March 1986.
19. Saini S., Ferrucci J.T., Stark D.D., et al.: Gadolinium-DTPA-enhanced MRI of liver cancer using rapid scanning techniques. Paper presented at the Society of Magnetic Resonance Imaging meeting, Philadelphia, March 1986.
20. Greif W.L., Buxton R.B., Lauffer R.B., et al.: Pulse sequence optimization for MR imaging using a paramagnetic hepatobiliary contrast agent. *Radiology* 157:461–466, 1985.
21. Ohtomo K., Itai Y., Furui S., et al.: Hepatic tumors: differentiation by transverse relaxation time (T2) of magnetic resonance imaging. *Radiology* 155:421–423, 1985.
22. Vermes M., Leung A.W.L., Bydder G.M., et al.: MR imaging of the liver in primary hepatocellular carcinoma. *J. Comput. Assist. Tomogr.* 9:749–754, 1985.
23. Ebara M., Ohto M., Watanabe Y., et al.: Diagnosis of small hepatocellular carcinoma: correlation of MR imaging and tumor histologic studies. *Radiology* 159:371–377, 1986.
24. Hendrick R.E., Nelson T.R., Hendee W.R.: Optimizing tissue contrast in magnetic resonance imaging. *Magn. Reson. Imaging* 2:193–204, 1984.
25. Wehrli F.W., MacFall J.R., Glover J.H., et al.: The dependence of nuclear magnetic resonance (NMR) image contrast on intrinsic and pulse sequence timing parameters. *Magn. Reson. Imaging* 2:3–16, 1984.
26. Perman W.H., Hilal S.K., Simon H.E., et al.: Contrast manipulation in NMR imaging. *Magn. Reson. Imaging* 2:23–32, 1984.
27. Schmidt H.C., Tscholakoff D., Hricak H., et al.: MR imaging contrast and relaxation times of solid tumors in the chest, abdomen and pelvis. *J. Comput. Assist. Tomogr.* 9:738–748, 1985.
28. Stark D.D., Felder R.C., Wittenberg J., et al.: Magnetic resonance imaging of cavernous hemangioma of the liver: tissue-specific characterization. *AJR* 145:213–222, 1985.
29. Glazer G.M., Aisen A.M., Francis I.R., et al.: Hepatic cavernous hemangioma: magnetic resonance imaging. *Radiology* 155:417–420, 1985.
30. Itai Y., Ohtomo K., Furui S., et al.: Noninvasive diagnosis of small cavernous hemangioma of the liver: advantage of MRI. *AJR* 145:1195–1197, 1985.

31. Sigal R., Lanir A., Atlan H., et al.: Nuclear magnetic resonance imaging of liver hemangiomas. *J. Nucl. Med.* 26:1117–1122, 1985.

32. Weinreb J.C., Brateman L., Maravilla K.R.: Magnetic resonance imaging of hepatic lymphoma. *AJR* 143:1211–1214, 1984.

33. Wenker J.C., Baker M.K., Ellis J.H., et al.: Focal fatty infiltration of the liver: demonstration by magnetic resonance imaging. *AJR* 143:573–574, 1984.

34. Stark D.D., Bass N.M., Moss A.A., et al.: Nuclear magnetic resonance imaging of experimentally induced liver disease. *Radiology* 148:743–751, 1983.

35. Stark D.D., Goldberg H.I., Moss A.A., et al.: Chronic liver disease evaluation by magnetic resonance. *Radiology* 150:149–151, 1984.

36. Weinreb J.C., Hodges S., Garcia R.: Magnetic resonance imaging of patent umbilical veins. *AJR* 144:747–748, 1985.

37. Dixon W.T.: Simple proton spectroscopic imaging. *Radiology* 153:189–194, 1984.

38. Lee J.K.T., Dixon W.T., Ling D., et al.: Fatty infiltration of the liver: demonstration by proton spectroscopic imaging. Preliminary observations. *Radiology* 153:195–201, 1984.

39. Rosen B.R., Carter E.A., Pykett I.L., et al.: Proton chemical shift imaging: an evaluation of its clinical potential using an *in vivo* fatty liver model. *Radiology* 154:469–472, 1985.

40. Pykett I.L., Rosen B.R.: Nuclear magnetic resonance: *in vivo* proton chemical shift imaging. *Radiology* 149:197–201, 1983.

41. Lee J.K.T., Heiken J.P., Dixon W.T.: Detection of hepatic metastases by proton spectroscopic imaging. Work in progress. *Radiology* 156:429–433, 1985.

42. Stark D.D., Mosley M.E., Bacon B.R., et al.: Magnetic resonance imaging and spectroscopy of hepatic iron overload. *Radiology* 154:137–142, 1985.

43. Brasch R.C., Wesbey G.E., Gooding C.A., et al.: Magnetic resonance imaging of transfusional hemosiderosis complicating thalassemia major. *Radiology* 150:767–771, 1984.

44. Dooms G.C., Fisher M.R., Higgins C.B., et al.: MR imaging of the dilated biliary tract. *Radiology* 158:337–341, 1986.

45. Ehman R.L., Kjos B.O., Hricak H., et al.: Relative intensity of abdominal organs on MR imaging. *J. Comput. Assist. Tomogr.* 9:315–319, 1985.

46. Kressel H.Y., Axel L., Glover G., et al.: Coronal nuclear magnetic resonance (NMR) imaging of the abdomen at 0.5 tesla. *J. Comput. Assist. Tomogr.* 8:29–31, 1984.

47. Kressel H.Y., Axel L., Thickman D.I., et al.: NMR imaging of the abdomen at 0.12 T: initial experience with a resistive magnet. *AJR* 141:1179–1186, 1983.

48. Runge V.M., Clanton J.A., Smith F.W., et al.: Nuclear magnetic resonance of iron and copper disease states. *AJR* 141:943–948, 1983.

49. Leung A.W.L., Bydder G.M., Steiner R.E., et al.: Magnetic resonance imaging of the kidneys. *AJR* 143:1215–1227, 1984.

50. Hricak H., Crooks L.E., Sheldon P., et al.: Nuclear magnetic resonance imaging of the kidney. *Radiology* 146:425–432, 1983.

51. Smith F.W., Reid A., Mallard J.R., et al.: Nuclear magnetic resonance tomography imaging in renal disease. *Diagn. Imaging* 51:209–213, 1982.

52. LiPuma J.P.: Magnetic resonance imaging of the kidney. *Radiol. Clin. North Am.* 22:925–941, 1984.

53. Hricak H., Williams R.D., Moon K.L. Jr., et al.: Nuclear magnetic resonance imaging of the kidney: renal masses. *Radiology* 147:765–772, 1983.

54. Hricak H., Demas B.E., Williams R.D., et al.: Magnetic resonance imaging in the diagnosis and staging of renal and perirenal neoplasms. *Radiology* 154:709–715, 1985.

55. Choyke P.L., Kressel H.Y., Pollack H.M., et al.: Focal renal masses: magnetic resonance imaging. *Radiology* 152:471–478, 1984.

56. Kulkarni M.V., Shaff M.I., Sandler M.P., et al.: Evaluation of renal masses by MR imaging. *J. Comput. Assist. Tomogr.* 8:861–865, 1984.

57. Kaufman L., Crooks L.E., Sheldon P.E., et al.: Evaluation of MRI imaging for detection and quantification of obstructions in vessels. *Invest. Radiol.* 17:554–560, 1982.

58. Amparo E.G., Hricak H., Higgins C.B., et al.: MR evaluation of venous thrombosis and other venous abnormalities associated with neoplasms. *Radiology* 153:168–172, 1984.

59. Smith F.W., Hutchison J.M.S., Mallard J.R., et al.: Renal cyst or tumor? Differentiation by whole body NMRI. *Diagn. Imaging* 1:61–65, 1981.

60. Thickman D.I., Kundel H.L., Biery D., et al.: MRI evaluation of hydronephrosis in the dog. *Radiology* 152:113–117, 1984.

61. Schultz C.L., Haaga J.R., Fletcher B.D., et al.: Magnetic resonance imaging of the adrenal glands. *AJR* 143:1235–1240, 1984.

62. Moon K.L. Jr., Hricak H., Crooks L.E., et al.: Nuclear magnetic resonance imaging of the adrenal gland: a preliminary report. *Radiology* 147:155–160, 1983.

63. White E.M., Edelman R.R., Stark D.D., et al.: Surface coil MR imaging of abdominal viscera: II. The adrenal glands. *Radiology* 157:431–436, 1985.

64. Reineg J.W., Doppman J.L., Dwyer A.J., et al.: Adrenal masses differentiated by MR. *Radiology* 158:81–84, 1986.

65. Reineg J.W., Doppman J.L., Dwyer A.J., et al.: MRI distinction between adrenal adenomas and metastases. *J. Comput. Assist. Tomogr.* 9:898–901, 1985.

66. Glazer G.M., Woolsey E.J., Borrello J., et al.: Adrenal tissue characterization using MR imaging. *Radiology* 158:73–79, 1986.

67. Fink I.J., Reineg J.W., Dwyer A.J., et al.: MR imaging of pheochromocytomas. *J. Comput. Assist. Tomogr.* 9:454–458, 1985.

68. Cohen M.D., Weetman R., Provisor A., et al.: Magnetic resonance imaging of neuroblastoma with a 0.15-T magnet. *AJR* 143:1241–1248, 1984.

69. Fletcher B.D., Kopiwoda S.Y., Strandjord S.E., et al.: Abdominal neuroblastoma: magnetic resonance imaging and tissue characterization. *Radiology* 155:699–703, 1985.

70. Simeone J.F., Edelman R.R., Stark D.D., et al.: Surface coil MRI imaging of the abdominal viscera: III. The pancreas. *Radiology* 157:437–442, 1985.

71. Stark D.D., Moss A.A., Goldberg H.I., et al.: Magnetic resonance and CT of the normal and diseased pancreas: a comparative study. *Radiology* 150: 153–162, 1984.

72. Smith F.W., Reid A., Hutchinson J.M.S., et al.: Nuclear magnetic resonance imaging of the pancreas. *Radiology* 142:677–680, 1982.

73. Haaga J.R.: Magnetic resonance imaging of the pancreas. *Radiol. Clin. North Am.* 22:869–877, 1984.

74. Dooms G.C., Hricak H., Mosley M.E., et al.: Characterization of lymphadenopathy by magnetic resonance relaxation times: preliminary results. *Radiology* 155:691–697, 1985.

75. Dooms G.C., Hricak H., Crooks L.E., et al.: MRI of the lymph nodes: demonstration of lymph nodes by MRI in comparison with CT. *Radiology* 153:719–728, 1984.

76. Lee J.K.T., Heiken J.P., Ling D., et al.: Magnetic resonance imaging of abdominal and pelvic lymphadenopathy. *Radiology* 153:181–188, 1984.

77. Lawson T.L., Foley W.D., Thorsen M.K., et al.: MRI of discrete and conglomerate retroperitoneal lymph node masses. *RadioGraphics* 5:471–482, 1985.

78. Ellis J.H., Bies J.R., Kopecky K.K., et al.: Comparison of NMR and CT imaging in the evaluation of metastatic retroperitoneal lymphadenopathy from testicular carcinoma. *J. Comput. Assist. Tomogr.* 8:709–719, 1984.

79. Dooms G.C., Hricak H., Sollitto R.A., et al.: Lipomatous tumors and tumors with fatty component: MR imaging potential and comparison of MR and CT results. *Radiology* 157:479–483, 1985.

80. Lupetin A.R., Rothfuss W.R., Deeb Z., et al.: Magnetic resonance evaluation of the paraspinal neurogenic tumor. Paper presented at the Society for Magnetic Resonance Imaging meeting, Philadelphia, March 1986.

81. Lupetin A.R., Beckman I., Dash N., et al.: Magnetic resonance evaluation of the inferior vena cava. Paper presented at the American Roentgen Ray Society meeting, Washington, D.C., April 1986.

82. Weinreb J.C., Cohen J.M., Maravilla K.R.: Iliopsoas muscles: MR study of normal anatomy and disease. *Radiology* 156:435–440, 1985.

83. Hricak H., Alpers C., Crooks L.E., et al.: Magnetic resonance imaging of the female pelvis: initial experience. *AJR* 141:1119–1128, 1983.

84. Snoep G.: Magnetic resonance imaging of the normal female pelvis. *Diagn. Imag. Clin. Med.* 54:57–63, 1985.

85. Bryan P.J., Butler H.E., LiPuma J.P., et al.: NMR scanning of the pelvis: initial experience with a 0.3 T system. *AJR* 141:1111–1118, 1983.

86. Butler H.E., Bryan P.J., LiPuma J.P., et al.: Magnetic resonance imaging of the abnormal female pelvis. *AJR* 143:1259–1266, 1984.

87. Bryan P.J., Butler H.E., LiPuma J.P., et al.: Magnetic resonance imaging of the pelvis. *Radiol. Clin. North Am.* 22:897–915, 1984.

88. Lee J.K.T., Gersell D.J., Balfe D.M.: The uterus: in vitro MR-anatomic correlation in normal and abnormal specimens. *Radiology* 157:175–179, 1985.

89. Hamlin D.J., Pettersson H., Fitzsimmons J., et al.: MR imaging of uterine leiomyomas and their complications. *J. Comput. Assist. Tomogr.* 9:902–907, 1985.

90. Hricak H., Tscholakoff D., Heinrich S.L., et al.: Uterine leiomyomas: correlation of MR, histopathologic finding and symptoms. *Radiology* 158:385–391, 1986.

91. Bies J.R., Ellis J.H., Kopecky K.K., et al.: Assessment of primary gynecologic malignancies: comparison of 0.15-T resistive MRI with CT. *AJR* 143: 1249–1257, 1984.

92. Hricak H., Lacey C., Schriock E., et al.: Gynecologic masses: value of magnetic resonance imaging. *Am. J. Gynecol.* 1:31–37, 1985.

93. Hamlin D.J., Fitzsimmons J.R., Pettersson H., et al.: Magnetic resonance imaging of the pelvis. Evaluation of ovarian masses at 0.15 T. *AJR* 145:585–590, 1985.

94. Weigert F., Lindner P., Rohde U.: Computed tomography and magnetic resonance of pseudomyxoma peritonei. *J. Comput. Assist. Tomogr.* 9: 1120–1122, 1985.

95. Lupetin A.R.: The focal pelvic mass. A comparative study of 50 cases evaluated with ultrasound/CT/MRI. Paper presented at the Society of Magnetic Resonance in Medicine meeting, London, September 1985.

96. Hricak H., Williams R.D., Spring D.B., et al.: Anatomy and pathology of the male pelvis by magnetic resonance imaging. *AJR* 141:1101–1110, 1983.

97. Bryan P.J., Butler H.E., Nelson A.D., et al.: Magnetic resonance imaging of the prostate. *AJR* 146:543–548, 1986.

98. Poon P.Y., McCallum R.W., Henkelman M.M., et al.: Magnetic resonance imaging of the prostate. *Radiology* 154:143–149, 1985.

99. Ling D., Lee J.K.T., Heiken J.P., et al.: Prostatic carcinoma and benign prostatic hyperplasia: inability of MR imaging to distinguish between the two diseases. *Radiology* 158:103–107, 1986.

100. Buonocore E., Hesemann C., Pavlicek W., et al.: Clinical and *in vitro* magnetic resonance imaging of prostatic carcinoma. *AJR* 143:1267–1272, 1984.

101. Herman S.D., Friedman A.C., Radecki P.D., et al.:

Incidental prostatic carcinoma detected by MRI and diagnosed by MRI/CT-guided biopsy. *AJR* 146: 351–352, 1986.

102. Steyn J.H., Smith F.W.: Nuclear magnetic resonance imaging of the prostate. *Br. J. Urol.* 54:726–728, 1982.

103. Rosenthal D.I., Scott J.A., Mankin H.J., et al.: Sacrococcygeal chordoma: magnetic resonance imaging and computed tomography. *AJR* 145:143–147, 1985.

104. Fisher M.R., Hricak H., Crooks L.E.: Urinary bladder MR imaging. Part I. Normal and benign conditions. *Radiology* 157:467–470, 1985.

105. Fisher M.R., Hricak H., Tanagho E.A.: Urinary bladder MR imaging. Part II. Neoplasms. *Radiology* 157:471–477, 1985.

106. Demas B.E., Hricak H., Williams R.D.: Magnetic resonance imaging in the evaluation of urologic malignancies. *Semin. Urol.* 3:27–33, 1985.

107. Resnik M.I.: Nuclear magnetic resonance imaging of bladder cancer. *Prog. Clin. Biol. Res.* 162(A):225–265, 1984.

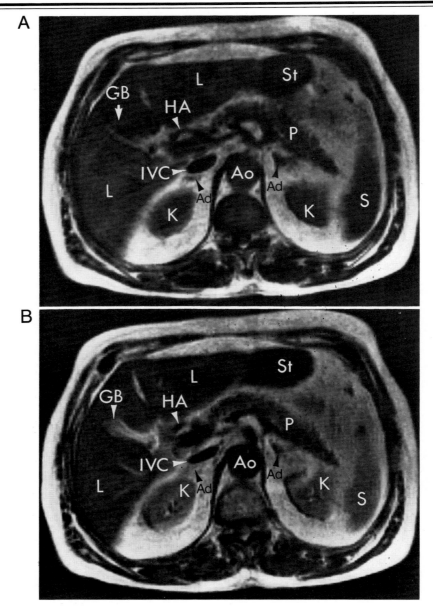

FIG 12–1.
Normal abdominal anatomy on MRI.

A, T$_1$-weighted axial scan (TR, 0.5 sec; TE, 35 msec): Liver *(L)*, spleen *(S)*, and pancreas *(P)* normally demonstrate a homogeneous midrange signal intensity on T$_1$-weighted scans. The high signal intensity of intraabdominal fat allows organ delineation. The stomach *(St)* can be identified by a very low signal intensity due to intraluminal gas. Blood vessels (aorta, inferior vena cava, hepatic artery) demonstrate a low signal intensity because of flow-void phenomenon induced by rapidly flowing blood. The gallbladder *(GB)*, because of the presence of unconcentrated intraluminal bile, demonstrates a low signal intensity on T$_1$-weighted scans. If bile is concentrated, a higher signal intensity is observed on T$_1$-weighted scans. Precise definition of the adrenal gland *(Ad)* and kidney border *(K)* is allowed by retroperitoneal fat *(Ao,* aorta; *HA,* hepatic artery; *IVC,* inferior vena cava).

B, T$_2$-weighted axial scan (TR, 2.1 sec; TE, 70 msec): Relative to T$_1$-weighted scans, signal intensity increases for the spleen *(S)* and kidney *(K)* on T$_2$-weighted scans. The pancreas *(P)* and liver *(L)* normally demonstrate a persistent midrange signal intensity on T$_2$-weighted scans. Signal intensity increases on T$_2$-weighted scans for unconcentrated bile within the gallbladder *(GB)* because of its fluid content (long T$_2$ value). Concentrated bile demonstrates a high signal intensity on both T$_1$- and T$_2$-weighted scans because of its fat content *(Ad,* adrenal gland; *Ao,* aorta; *HA,* hepatic artery; *IVC,* inferior vena cava; *St,* stomach).

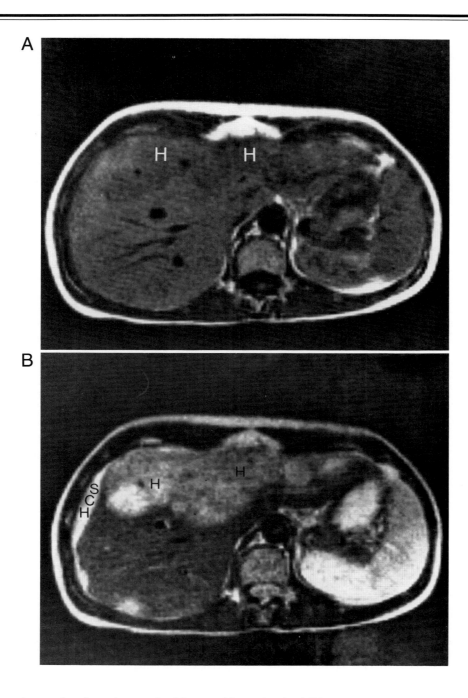

FIG 12–2.

Hepatoma with subcapsular hematoma. A 60-year-old woman with a history of hepatic cirrhosis and recent weight loss was evaluated with MRI to exclude hepatoma.

A, T_1-weighted axial scan (TR, 0.7 sec; TE, 35 msec): The scan demonstrates an ill-defined area of decreased signal intensity in the left lobe of the liver, defining the location of a left hepatic hepatoma *(H)*. Definition of the hepatoma by contrast difference from normal liver is poor, and a subcapsular hematoma from previous CT-guided biopsy is not clearly visible.

B, T_2-weighted axial scan (TR, 2.1 sec; TE, 35 msec): The left hepatic hepatoma *(H)* is better visualized on this T_2-weighted scan because of the relatively long T_2 relaxation time characteristic of hepatoma and most hepatic tumors. Now visible is the right lateral and posterior hepatic subcapsular hematoma *(SCH)* secondary to previous CT-guided biopsy. The hematoma is relatively fresh, which accounts for its low signal intensity on the T_1-weighted scan.

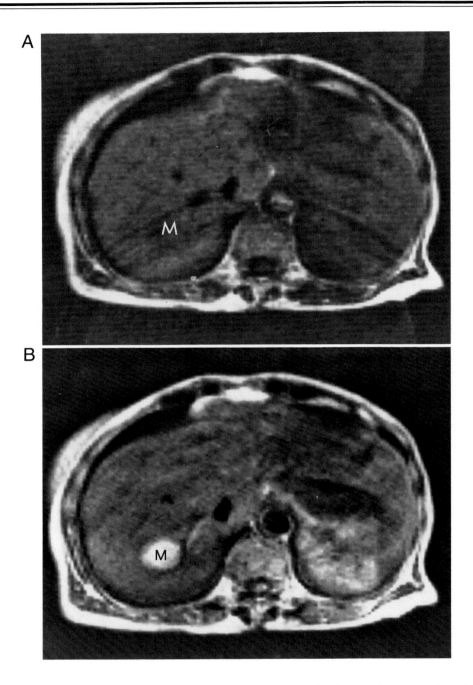

FIG 12–3.
Hepatic metastasis from adenocarcinoma of the colon. A 50-year-old man with previously diagnosed hepatic metastatic disease from colon carcinoma underwent an MRI study.

A, T_1-weighted axial scan (TR, 0.3 sec; TE, 35 msec): A solitary right hepatic lesion *(M)* is discovered on this study. Hepatic metastatic lesions from gastrointestinal adenocarcinomas typically demonstrate a low signal intensity on T_1-weighted scans because of a relatively long T_1 relaxation time.

B, T_2-weighted axial scan (TR, 1.5 sec; TE, 41 msec): Metastatic lesion from adenocarcinoma of the gastrointestinal tract typically demonstrates a high signal intensity on T_2-weighted scans because of long T_2 relaxation time. In our experience, metastatic lesions from most gastrointestinal primary tumors are best visualized on a contrast basis on T_2-weighted scans *(M,* metastasis).

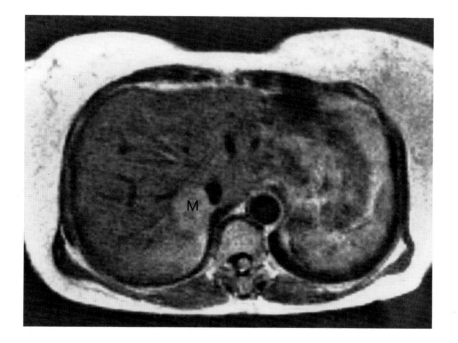

FIG 12–4.
Hepatic metastasis from adenocarcinoma of the colon. T_2-weighted axial scan (TR, 2.1 sec; TE, 35 msec): A T_2-weighted MRI scan demonstrates a metastatic lesion *(M)* in the right lobe of the liver; the lesion was not noted on CT scans. At present, CT and MRI are considered equally effective in detecting hepatic metastatic lesions, with an occasional case encountered in which MRI demonstrates a lesion not visible on CT.

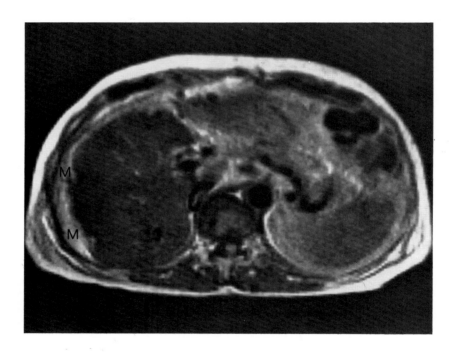

FIG 12–5.
Hepatic surface metastasis from ovarian carcinoma. This is a 70-year-old woman with previously diagnosed mucinous ovarian adenocarcinoma. T_2-weighted axial scan (TR, 1.5 sec; TE, 40 msec): Metastatic hepatic surface implants from ovarian carcinoma can be well delineated with MRI utilizing T_2-weighted scans. The extensive involvement of the right anterior and lateral hepatic surface that can be noted on this T_2 scan was not visible on a previous CT study (*M*, metastasis).

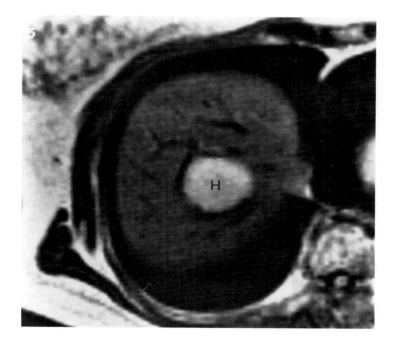

FIG 12–6.

Hepatic hemangioma. T_2-weighted axial scan (TR, 2.1 sec; TE, 70 msec): An 18-year-old woman undergoing sonographic evaluation for right upper quadrant pain was found to have a hyperechoic liver lesion. A hepatic hemangioma *(H)* is seen with a prolonged T_2 relaxation time and demonstrates a very high signal intensity. In most cases, hemangioma can be separated from hepatic metastatic disease based on this property, although totally cystic metastases or those from gastrointestinal leiomyosarcomas can also demonstrate this appearance. The lesion in this case was discovered incidentally by ultrasound.

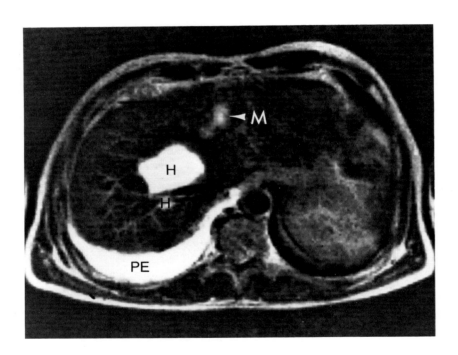

FIG 12–7.
Coexisting hepatic hemangioma and metastasis. T$_2$-weighted axial scan (TR, 2.1 sec; TE, 70 msec): In a 59-year-old man with bronchogenic carcinoma and left hepatic metastatic disease *(M)*, note the markedly higher signal intensity displayed by the hepatic hemangioma *(H)* in the right lobe in comparison with the lower signal intensity observed in the metastatic lesion of the left lobe. In most cases, MRI has the potential to separate hemangioma from solid metastatic disease. A right pleural effusion *(PE)* is also present.

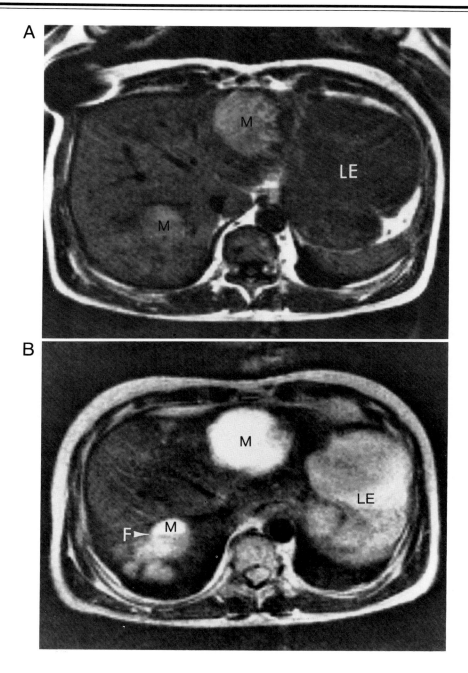

FIG 12–8.
Hepatic metastasis from gastric leiomyosarcoma. The patient is a 60-year-old man with proved gastric leiomyosarcoma.

A, T_1-weighted axial scan (TR, 0.5 sec; TE, 35 msec): A high signal intensity in hepatic metastatic disease from gastric leiomyosarcoma is seen on T_1-weighted scans. This appearance has not been observed in other forms of hepatic metastatic disease. It may relate to necrosis or the vascular nature of these deposits. In this case, a high signal intensity is observed in left and right hepatic metastatic lesions *(M),* which contrasts with the lower signal intensity of the primary gastric tumor (*LE,* gastric leiomyosarcoma).

B, T_2-weighted axial scan (TR, 2.1 sec; TE, 70 msec): It has been suggested that MRI can separate hemangioma from hepatic metastatic disease based on the prolonged T_2 relaxation time of hemangioma. Colleagues and I have found this to be true in most cases, although totally necrotic metastatic lesions or those from leiomyosarcoma can have T_2 relaxation times equal to or longer than hemangioma, as in this case. Magnetic resonance imaging can demonstrate fluid levels within necrotic metastases, as here in the right hepatic lesion. The signal intensity for the gastric leiomyosarcoma *(LE)* increased on this T_2-weighted scan (*M,* metastasis; *F,* fluid level).

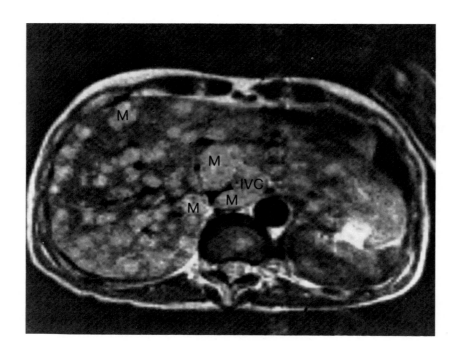

FIG 12–9.
Diffuse hepatic metastases compressing the inferior vena cava. This is a 52-year-old man with a history of colon carcinoma and liver metastasis. T_2-weighted axial scan (TR, 2.1 sec; TE, 70 msec): In evaluation of the inferior vena cava, MRI has become the procedure of choice. Diffuse hepatic metastatic disease is noted on this T_2 scan, which additionally delineates marked compression of the inferior vena cava *(arrowhead, IVC)* by three pericaval metastases *(M)*.

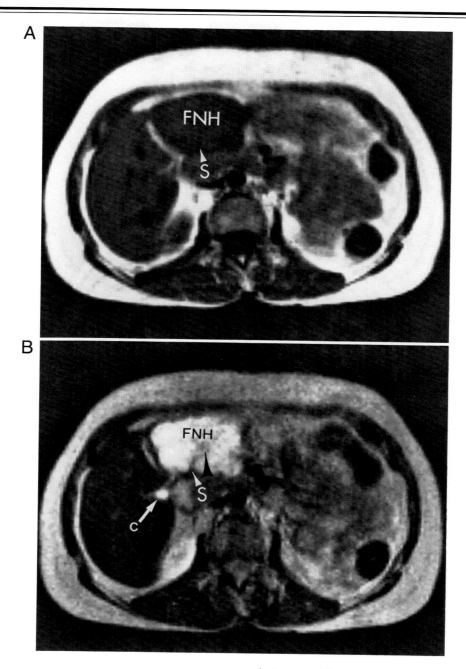

FIG 12–10.
Focal nodular hyperplasia. This is a 32-year-old woman with a ten-year history of ingestion of oral contraceptives.

A, T₁-weighted axial scan (TR, 0.5 sec; TE, 35 msec): Focal nodular hyperplasia *(FNH)* of the liver, a benign condition, can demonstrate a signal intensity on T₁- and T₂-weighted scans similar to that observed in hepatic metastatic lesions. Occasionally, as in this case, a central low-intensity scar *(S* and *arrowheads)* can be demonstrated, which allows specific characterization of this lesion. Note the overall similar signal intensity of focal nodular hyperpla-sia to normal liver on this T₁ scan with a subtle low-intensity scar in its center and posterior aspect.

B, T₂-weighted axial scan (TR, 1.5 sec; TE, 76 msec): The marked increase in signal intensity observed in focal nodular hyperplasia on T₂ scans can mimic the appearance of hemangioma or hepatic metastatic disease. There remains subtle definition of an internal scar *(S),* which helps to characterize this lesion. Note the small hepatic cyst *(C);* the cyst demonstrates a characteristic high signal intensity. This lesion was not noted on the T₁ scan *(FNH,* focal nodular hyperplasia).

A

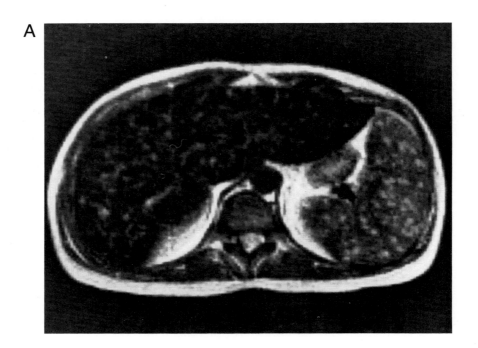

FIG 12–11.
Miliary hepatosplenic aspergillosis in lymphoma.

A, T$_2$-weighted axial scan (TR, 2.1 sec; TE, 70 msec): As in the case of this 22-year-old woman with Hodgkin's lymphoma, MRI can provide important information in the workup of the immune-compromised patient. An MRI study was performed to demonstrate transfusion hemosiderosis. The hemosiderosis induced a diffuse low signal intensity in the liver and spleen because of the deposition of ferric iron in the reticuloendothelial system. Multiple, diffuse, punctate foci of high signal intensity were observed incidentally in the liver and spleen of this patient on the MRI study. The foci were shown by CT-guided biopsy to represent miliary aspergillosis.

B, contrast-enhanced CT scan shows multiple low-density lesions in the liver, spleen, and kidneys, compatible with microabscesses.

C, sagittal sonographic section of spleen demonstrates hypoechoic spleen microabscesses.

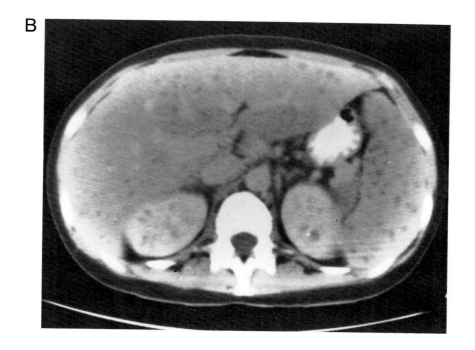

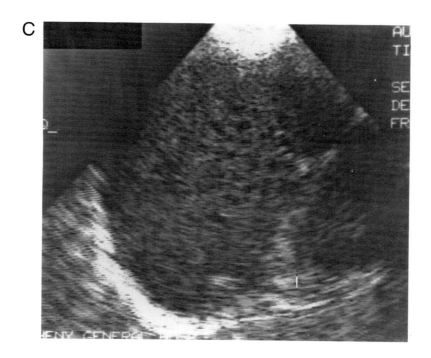

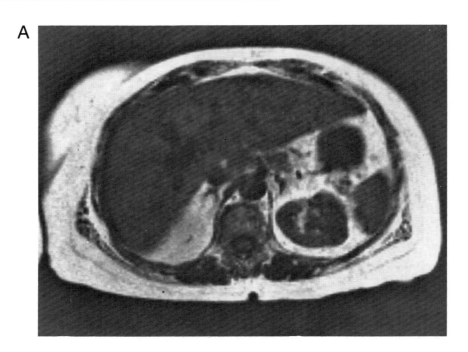

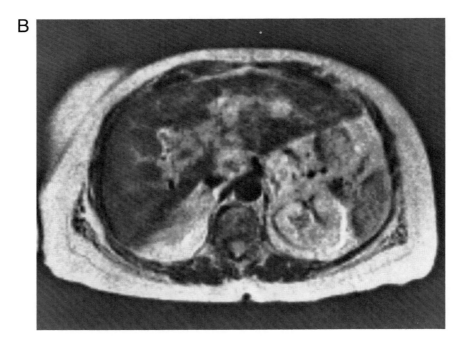

FIG 12–12.
Cholangiocarcinoma with spread into the porta hepatis. This is a 62-year-old man with known biliary duct carcinoma.

A, T₁-weighted axial scan (TR, 0.5 sec; TE, 35 msec): The image does not show significant abnormality.

B, T₂-weighted axial scan (TR, 2.1 sec; TE, 70 msec):

In comparison with **A,** note the high intensity of the metastatic disease within the radicles of the porta hepatis on this T₂-weighted scan. In some cases, MRI is useful in demonstrating the spread of primary tumors of the biliary tree along the pathways of the porta hepatis. Metastatic cholangiocarcinoma was found at surgery.

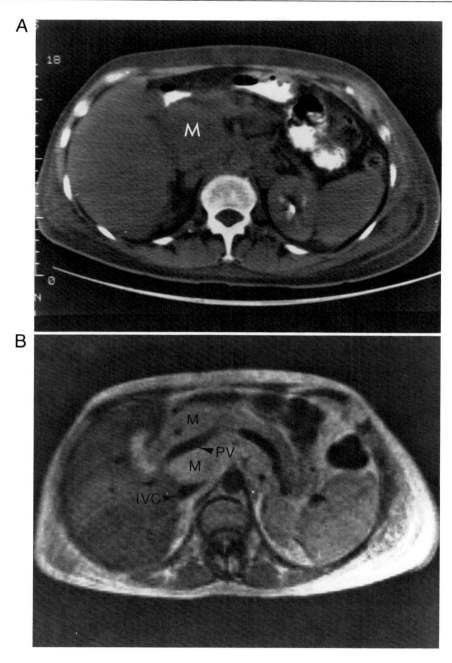

FIG 12–13.
Porta hepatis metastasis from breast carcinoma. In a 42-year-old woman with breast carcinoma and rapid onset of lower extremity edema, evidence of compression of the inferior vena cava was sought.

A, a mass *(M)* in the porta hepatis was demonstrated by CT, although the exact relation of the mass to the vena cava and other vascular structures could not be delineated *(M,* metastasis).

B, T_2-weighted axial scan (TR, 2.1 sec; TE, 70 msec):

Magnetic resonance imaging provides precise definition of the metastatic mass in the porta hepatis because the relatively long T_2 value of the mass contrasts with the lower intensity of normal liver. Note encasement of the portal vein *(PV)* and compression of the inferior vena cava *(IVC)* by the mass *(M),* information not available on the previous CT study. I currently prefer MRI for evaluating relationships of tumor to adjacent vascular structures, as the scans can be obtained without intravenous administration of contrast medium.

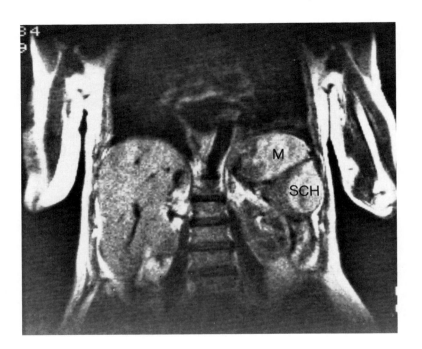

FIG 12–14.
Splenic metastatic disease. T_1 coronal scan (TR, 0.5 sec; TE, 30 msec): In a 54-year-old man, metastatic disease to the spleen from a pancreatic carcinoma induced significant intrasplenic and subcapsular hematoma that necessitated splenectomy. At surgery, the larger, medial region with intense MR signal *(M)* represented a hemorrhagic metastatic lesion, and the more inferolateral, less intense lesion *(SCH)* represented subcapsular hematoma.

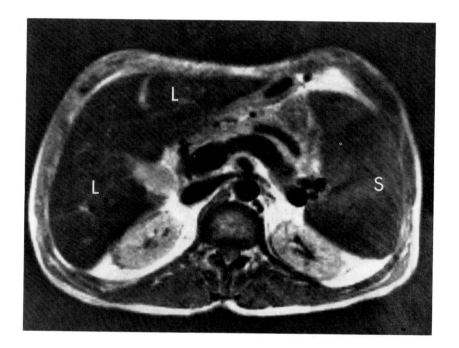

FIG 12–15.

Myelofibrosis. T_2-weighted axial scan (TR, 2.1 sec; TE, 70 msec): This 50-year-old man developed myelofibrosis as a complication of myeloid metaplasia. Magnetic resonance imaging can be utilized to demonstrate the degree of splenomegaly in patients with myelofibrosis, a common final pathway of many hematologic disorders. The increased ferric iron stores in the spleen and liver in this disorder will induce a very low signal intensity in the liver and spleen. This decrease in signal intensity due to iron deposition has been found to be related mainly to T_2 effects and thus will be more obvious on T_2-weighted scans, as in this case (*S,* spleen; *L,* liver).

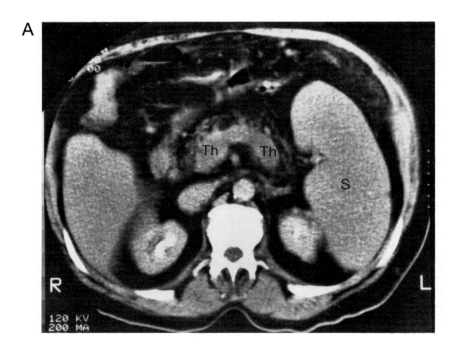

FIG 12–16.
Splenic vein thrombosis in myelofibrosis.

A, enhanced CT: Splenic vein thrombosis is an uncommon but recognized manifestation of myelofibrosis. Computed tomography suggested a filling defect in the splenic vein consistent with thrombus in a 48-year-old man with myelofibrosis. Splenomegaly was also observed (*Th,* thrombus; *S,* spleen).

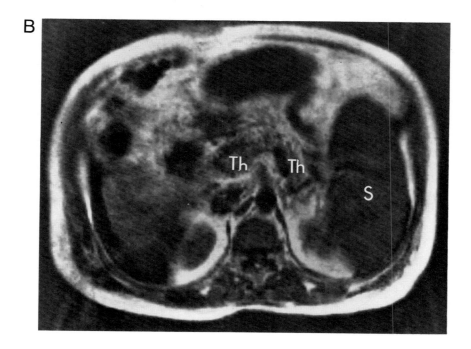

B, T$_1$-weighted axial scan (TR, 0.5 sec; TE, 35 msec): Blood flowing at normal intracorporeal velocity generates no MRI signal and thus a region of low signal intensity. This can be observed in the aortic lumen in this case. In comparison, note the midrange signal intensity of the intraluminal thrombus *(Th)* in the splenic vein. Splenic enlargement is also present (*S*, spleen).

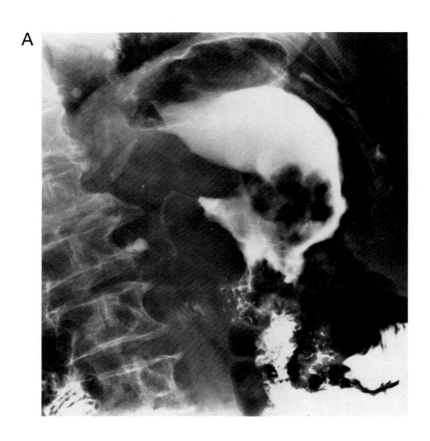

FIG 12–17.
Gastric adenocarcinoma. This 56-year-old patient with history of Billroth II surgery for peptic ulcer disease developed weight loss.

A, upper gastrointestinal series: An infiltrating and fungating process involves the gastric remnant. At surgery, gastric adenocarcinoma was proven.

B, enhanced CT image: Note thickening of the anterior gastric wall by neoplasm (*Ca,* gastric adenocarcinoma).

C, T₁-weighted axial scan (TR, 0.5 sec; TE, 35 msec): Infiltrating gastric neoplasm can be delineated with MRI. Intraluminal margins of tumor will be delineated by gastric gas, with serosal extension marginated by peritoneal fat with its high signal intensity. Note that because of the anterior location of the tumor (*Ca,* gastric adenocarcinoma) in this case, stomach gas is in a relatively posterior position. There is no evidence of exogastric extension and the fat plane *(F)* separating stomach from the anterior portion of pancreas *(P)* is well defined on this study. There is no evidence of perigastric adenopathy (*SV,* splenic vein).

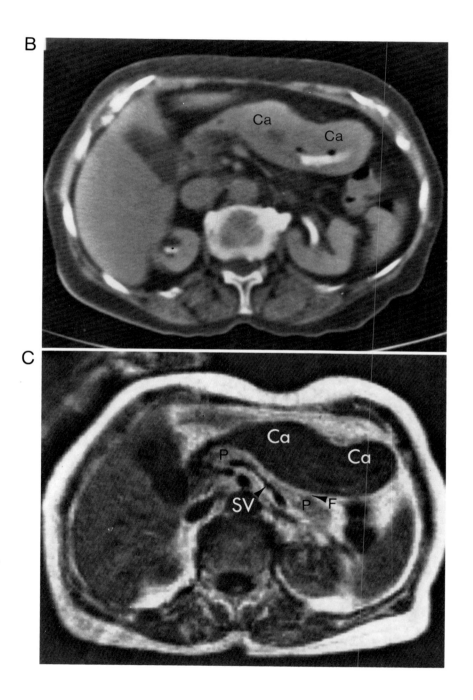

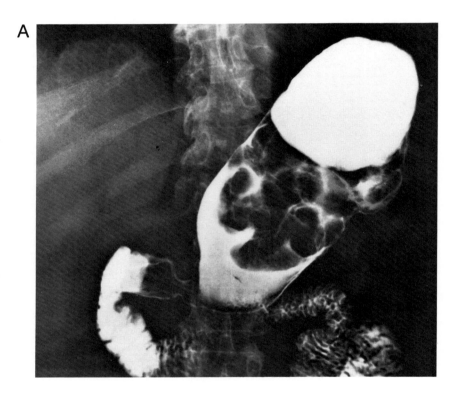

FIG 12–18.
Gastric leiomyosarcoma. A 53-year-old man presented with a rapidly enlarging left upper quadrant mass.

A, upper gastrointestinal series: A bulky gastric leiomyosarcoma fills the gastric fundus.

B, unenhanced CT section: A submucosal gastric leiomyosarcoma *(LE)* with a bulky intraluminal extension is well demonstrated on this CT scan after oral contrast medium administration. There is no evidence of exogastric exten-sion, celiac adenopathy, or usurpation of peripancreatic fat plane.

C, T_1-weighted axial scan (TR, 0.7 sec; TE, 35 msec): In this case, note the similar appearance of the tumor *(LE, gastric leiomyosarcoma)* on the MRI scan and the CT study due to stomach gas, whereas the lack of exogastric exten-sion, pancreatic invasion, or perigastric adenopathy is demonstrated without oral or intravenous contrast medium administration.

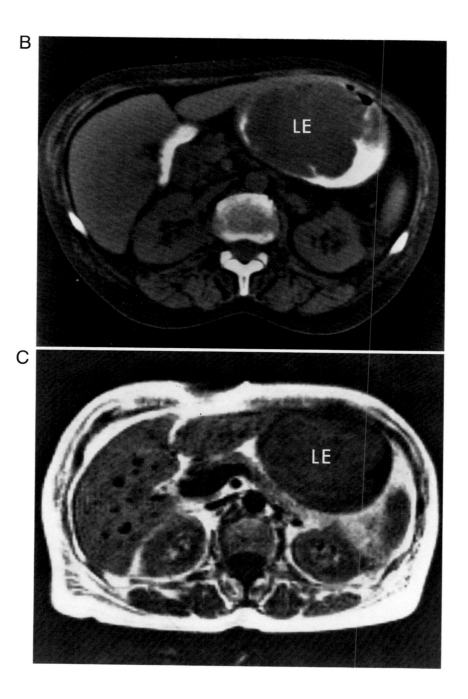

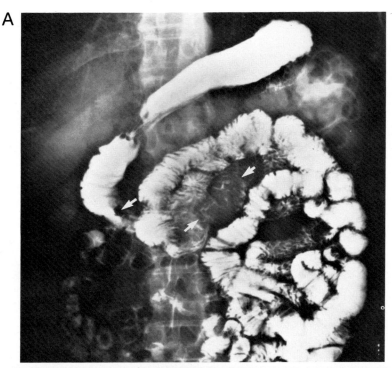

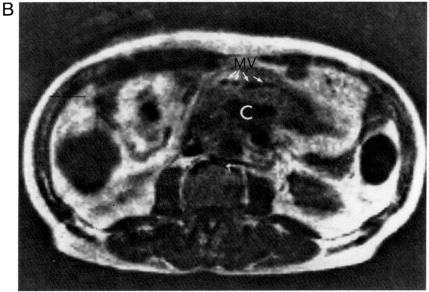

FIG 12–19.
Duodenal adenocarcinoma. This is a 42-year-old man with a history of inflammatory bowel disease.

A, upper gastrointestinal study: A mucosal and submucosal process narrows and distorts the distal second and entire third portions of the duodenum *(arrows)*.

B, T_1-weighted axial scan (TR, 0.5 sec; TE, 35 msec): Magnetic resonance imaging can be used to demonstrate the extent of gastrointestinal primary tumors, particularly in terms of mesenteric involvement, as the low or intermediate signal intensity of the tumor contrasts sharply with the adjacent high signal intensity of the mesenteric fat on T_1 scans. In this case, note the sharp definition of primary duodenal neoplasm that has extended into the root of the mesentery and encases the superior mesenteric artery (*MV,* mesenteric vessels; *C,* cavity).

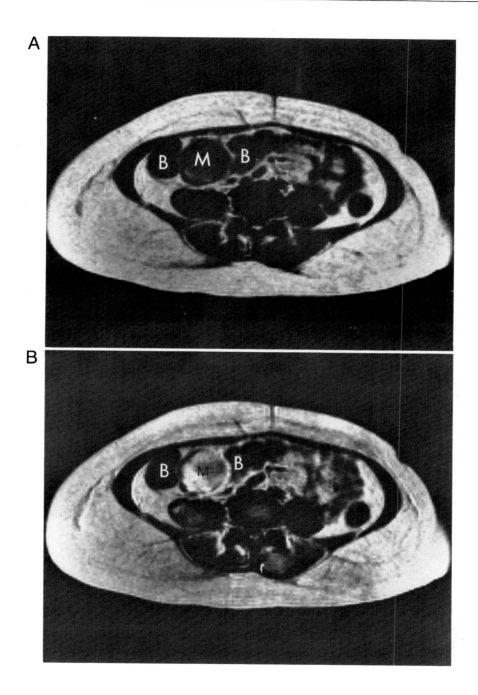

FIG 12–20.
Mesenteric metastasis from malignant melanoma. A 68-year-old man with a three-year history of malignant melanoma complained of recent-onset abdominal pain.

A, T$_1$-weighted axial scan (TR, 0.5 sec; TE, 35 msec): On MRI, air-filled loops of bowel *(B)* contrast only slightly with the large mesenteric metastatic deposit *(M)* in the right midabdomen. The mass does contrast sharply with adjacent mesenteric fat.

B, T$_2$-weighted axial scan (TR, 2.1 sec; TE, 70 msec): The signal intensity for the metastatic lesion has markedly increased between T$_1$- and T$_2$-weighted scans, which allows separation of the mass *(M)* from adjacent air-filled bowel loops *(B)*. The lesion remains separable from adjacent fat.

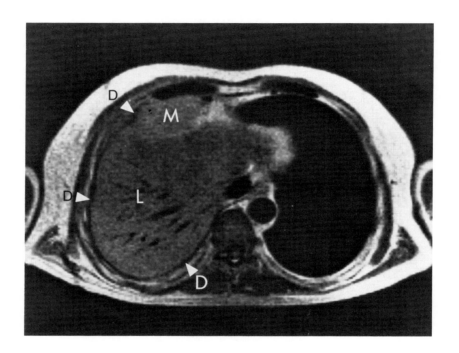

FIG 12–21.
Diaphragmatic metastasis from breast carcinoma. T₁-weighted axial scan (TR, 0.7 sec; TE, 35 msec): Magnetic resonance imaging is useful in demonstrating neoplastic abnormalities of the diaphragm. In this 49-year-old woman with a four-year history of breast carcinoma and new right thoracic pain, a metastatic deposit *(M)* from the breast was located in the anterior right hemidiaphragm *(D)*. A T₁ sequence was utilized to provide significant contrast between the metastatic lesion and the adjacent liver *(L)*. A coronal image is probably more helpful.

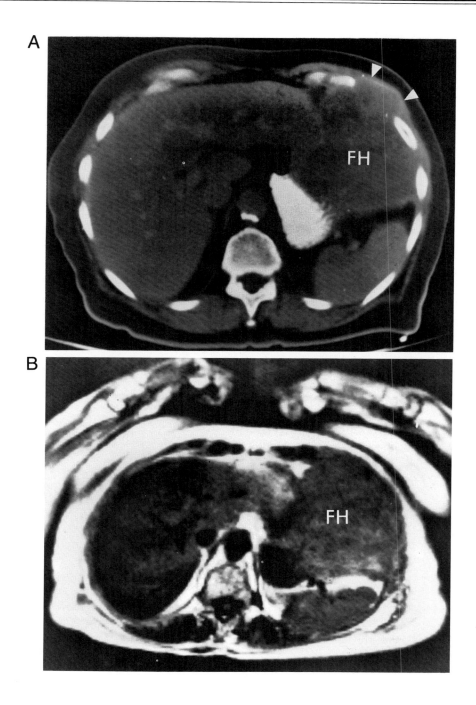

FIG 12–22.

Fibrous histiocytoma with invasion of left hemidiaphragm. A 51-year-old woman presented with a slowly enlarging left upper quadrant mass.

A, enhanced CT scan: A large primary fibrous histiocytoma *(FH)* of the left upper quadrant bulges through several intercostal spaces and directly invades the anterolateral aspect of the left hemidiaphragm. Biopsy proved fibrous histiocytoma *(arrowheads* indicate intercostal bulging).

B, T₁-weighted axial section (TR, 0.7 sec; TE, 35 msec): Fibrous histiocytoma demonstrates a midrange signal intensity on T₁-weighted scans *(FH,* fibrous histiocytoma).

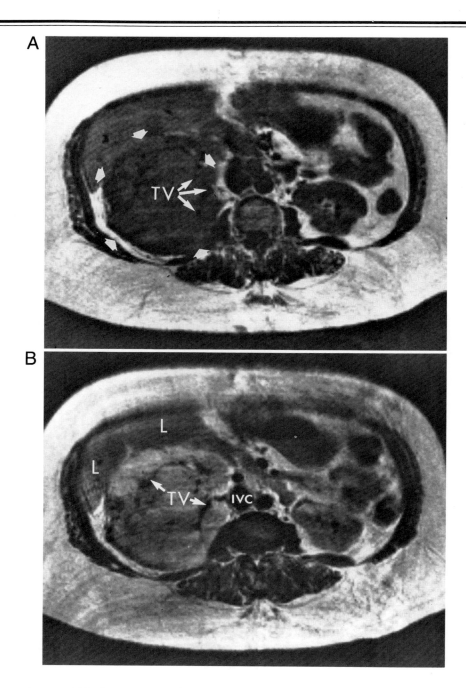

FIG 12–23.

Solid right hypernephroma. This is a 50-year-old woman with gross hematuria and right flank pain.

A, T$_1$-weighted axial scan (TR, 0.5 sec; TE, 35 msec): Magnetic resonance imaging is useful in the diagnosis and staging workup of hypernephroma. On T$_1$ scans, solid hypernephroma demonstrates a midrange signal intensity similar to normal renal parenchyma. Note the marked enlargement of the right kidney *(fat arrows)* with loss of normal anatomical detail. Fat planes adjacent to the liver and psoas have been usurped. Regions of very low intensity in the mass represent tumor vessels *(TV)*.

B, T$_2$-weighted axial scan (TR, 2.1 sec; TE, 35 msec): The signal intensity of hypernephroma increases when going from T$_1$ to T$_2$ scans, as does the signal of normal renal parenchyma (as noted in the left kidney). Tumor vessels are better identified on T$_2$ scans. Contrast differentiation between tumor and liver is better on T$_2$ scans. Note that the inferior vena cava *(IVC)* is free of thrombus and there is no evidence of retroperitoneal adenopathy in this case *(TV,* tumor vessels; *L,* liver).

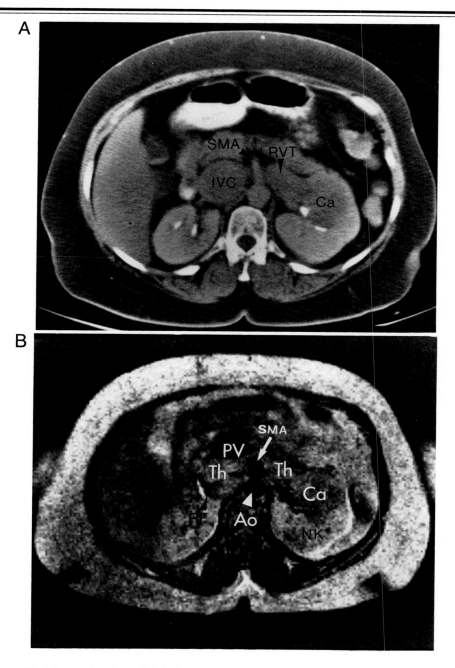

FIG 12–24.
Left hypernephroma with left renal vein and inferior vena cava tumor thrombus. A 49-year-old woman presented with recurrent pulmonary emboli. Venography revealed no evidence of deep leg vein thrombosis.

A, enhanced CT scan: This scan demonstrates a low-attenuation mass *(Ca)*, representing a hypernephroma, in the anterior midpole of the left kidney. Note marked enlargement of the left renal vein and also enlargement of the inferior vena cava due to thrombus (compare with aorta). There is no separation of caval lumen and thrombus on this study. Retroperitoneum is free of adenopathy (*LRVT*, left renal vein tumor thrombus; *IVC*, inferior vena cava; *SMA*, superior mesenteric artery).

B, T_2-weighted axial scan (TR, 2.1 sec; TE, 120 msec): This heavily T_2-weighted scan demonstrates the extension of tumor thrombus *(Th)* within the left renal vein and inferior vena cava. The thrombus is slightly less intense than adjacent normal renal parenchyma. Flow-void phenomenon identifies the superior mesenteric artery *(SMA)*, aorta *(Ao)*, and portal vein *(PV)*. A small amount of flow *(RF)* is identified in the right lateral aspect of the vena cava and at the vena cava–left renal vein junction, information not available with CT (*RF*, residual blood flow in inferior vena cava; *Ca*, left hypernephroma; *NK*, normal kidney). *(Continued.).*

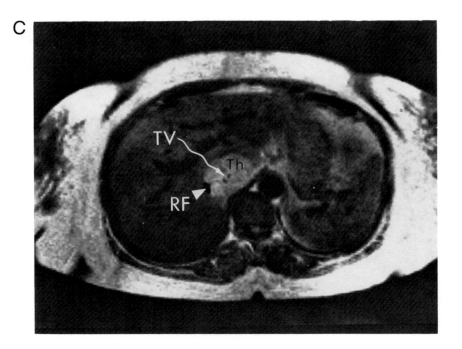

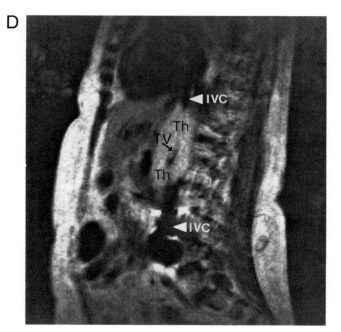

FIG 12–24 (cont.).

C, T$_2$-weighted axial scan (TR, 2.1 sec; TE, 120 msec): This section through the intrahepatic portion of the inferior vena cava depicts the marked enlargement of the vessel by tumor thrombus, the thrombus *(Th)* demonstrated by a high signal intensity. The finding was not well visualized on CT. Note residual blood flow *(RF)* along the right lateral caval lumen and two small low-intensity regions within the center of the thrombus that represent tumor vascularity *(TV)*. Note the contrast differentiation between clot and adjacent nor-mal liver.

D, T$_2$ sagittal scan (TR, 2.1 sec; TE, 35 msec): Sagittal sections are extremely useful in evaluating the inferior vena cava in the presence of renal neoplasm. Note the area of high signal intensity that is markedly expanding the lumen of the vena cava *(IVC)* and that represents tumor thrombus *(Th)*. Note the normal signal intensity in the lower and upper, uninvolved portions of the vessel. Tumor vascularity *(TV)* within the thrombus is demonstrated.

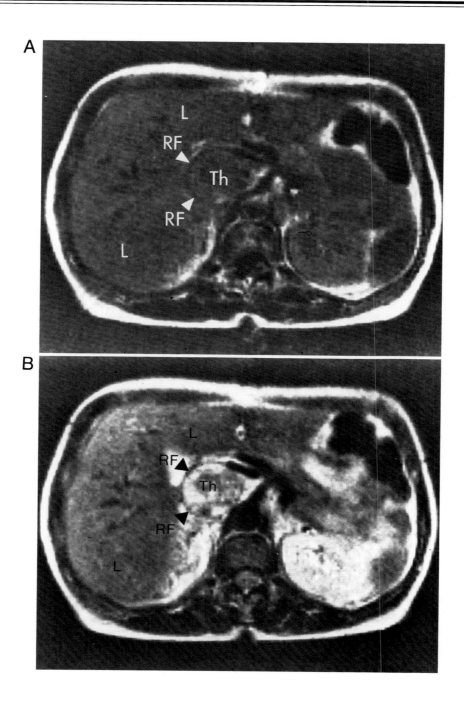

FIG 12–25.

Inferior vena cava tumor thrombus from right hyperne-phroma. This is a 52-year-old woman with known inferior vena cava thrombus due to right renal carcinoma.

A, T₁-weighted axial scan (TR, 0.5 sec; TE, 35 msec): Note the isointensity of the thrombus *(Th)* and adjacent liver *(L)* with only a thin rim of blood flow *(RF)* in the caval lumen separating normal liver from tumor thrombus.

B, T₂-weighted axial scan (TR, 2.1 sec; TE, 70 msec): Note improved visualization of the intrahepatic caval tumor thrombus *(Th)* because of the relatively higher signal inten-sity of the thrombus in comparison with adjacent liver *(L)*. Residual intracaval blood flow *(RF)* is again noted on the periphery of the thrombus.

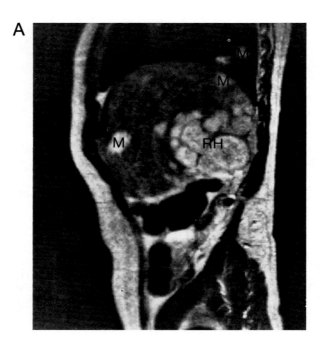

FIG 12–26.
Recurrent hypernephroma with hepatic metastatic disease. This is a 64-year-old man with history of right nephrectomy for renal cell carcinoma.

A, T$_2$ sagittal scan (TR, 2.1 sec; TE, 70 msec): Note the multiseptated recurrent renal mass posterior to the liver (*RH,* recurrent hypernephroma), along with multiple high-intensity regions within the liver and lung that indicate metastatic disease *(M).*

B, T$_2$ sagittal scan (TR, 2.1 sec; TE, 35 msec): Many believe that sagittal MRI sections are the procedure of choice when studying the inferior vena cava. In this case, note the anteriorly displaced but patent inferior vena cava *(IVC)* in the presence of a large retrocaval recurrent hypernephroma *(RH)* (*M,* metastasis).

C, T$_1$ axial scan (TR, 0.5 sec; TE, 35 msec): Note the poorer visual separation of recurrent hypernephroma *(RH)* from liver on this T$_1$ scan.

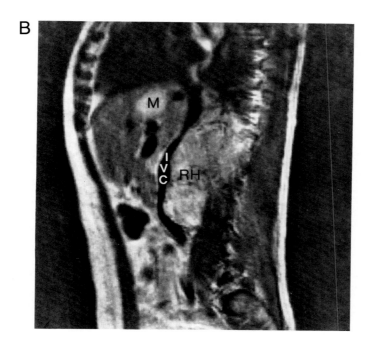

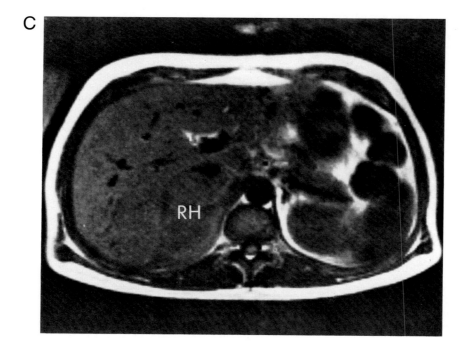

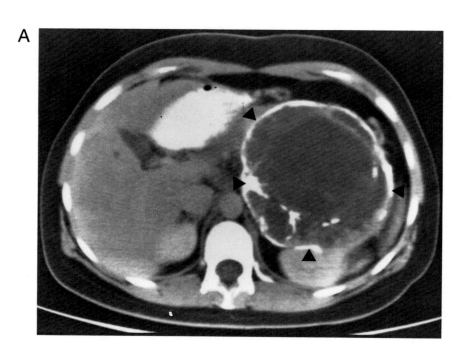

FIG 12–27.
Cystic left hypernephroma with rim calcification. This is a 40-year-old man with left upper quadrant mass.

A, enhanced CT scan: A massive cystic left hypernephroma is demonstrated with rim calcifications *(arrowheads).*

B, T_1-weighted axial scan (TR, 0.5 sec; TE, 35 msec): Low-density concentric bands are defined on the periphery and within the tumor on this T_1 study. The bands indicate areas of calcification and fibrous tumor septa. The mass is nonhomogeneous on the T_1 study, with a low-intensity center implying a fluid nature. Note the sharp interface with the posteriorly compressed part of the left kidney that demonstrates significant corticomedullary differentiation, a finding available mainly on T_1-weighted MRI scans *(arrowheads* indicate calcification; *RC,* renal cortex; *RM,* renal medulla).

C, T_2-weighted axial scan (TR, 2.1 sec; TE, 70 msec): The long T_2 value of this cystic tumor's fluid produces a high signal intensity. A bizarre interior is revealed on this T_2 scan, which also better delineates the rim calcifications *(arrowheads).* The inferior vena cava and retroperitoneum are free of abnormality *(LK,* left kidney).

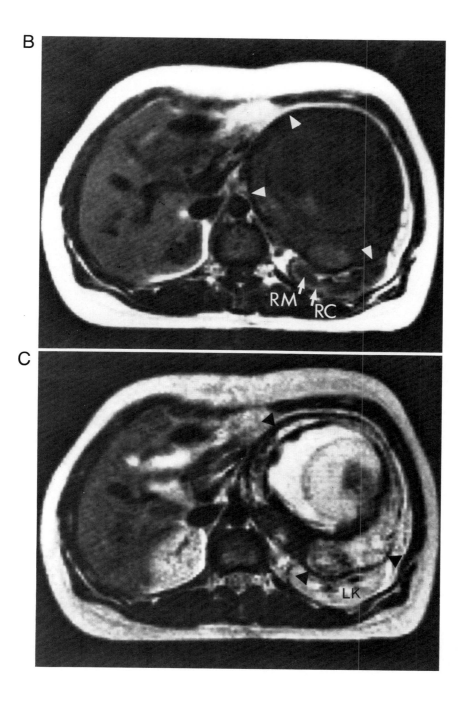

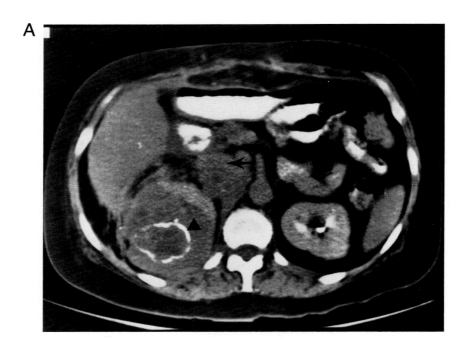

A

FIG 12–28.
Calcified right hypernephroma with retroperitoneal adenopathy. This is a 47-year-old man with right flank pain.

A, enhanced CT study: A centrally calcified *(arrowhead)* right hypernephroma is noted to markedly enlarge the right kidney and compress remaining normal renal parenchyma anteromedially. There is an ill-defined soft tissue density behind the inferior vena cava *(arrow)*. The possibility of retroperitoneal adenopathy or caval thrombus cannot be excluded on this study.

B, T_1 sagittal scan (TR, 0.7 sec; TE, 35 msec): Note the large upper-pole mass *(Ca)* in the right kidney. It has a nonhomogeneous midrange signal intensity, which contrasts with the corticomedullary differentiation that can be noted in the lower pole. Bridging septa *(BS)* of the perirenal compartment are noted. Although calcification within the tumor was suggested by CT, there is no evidence of it here *(RC,* renal cortex; *RM,* renal medulla).

C, T_1 sagittal scan (TR, 0.7 sec; TE, 35 msec): A sagittal scan, 2 cm medial to the image in **B,** demonstrates the entire length of the inferior vena cava *(IVC)* and demonstrates marked anterior displacement of this vessel by retrocaval adenopathy *(N).* This MRI section solves the dilemma raised on CT as to whether the vague density in the pericaval region represented intraluminal thrombus or retroperitoneal adenopathy. The homogeneous low signal intensity of the inferior vena cava excludes the presence of intraluminal thrombus *(RA,* right renal artery).

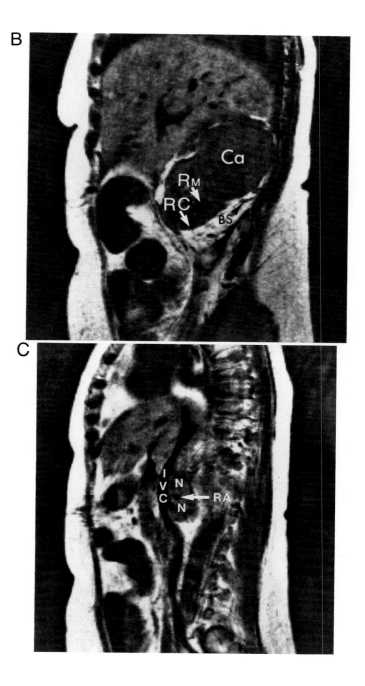

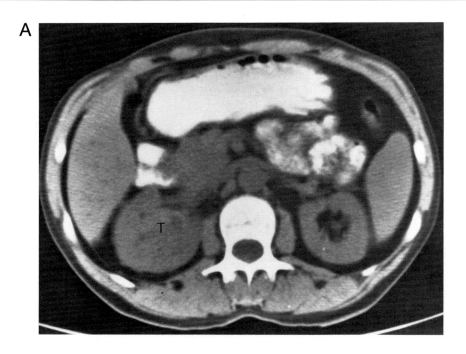

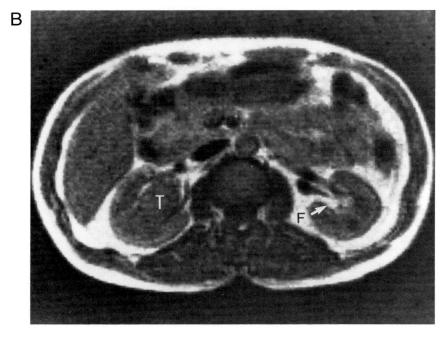

FIG 12–29.
Transitional cell carcinoma of the right kidney. This is a 56-year-old man with hematuria.

A, unenhanced CT section: a vague mass is present in the right renal pelvis (*T,* tumor).

B, T_1-weighted axial scan (TR, 0.5 sec; TE, 35 msec): Transitional cell carcinoma of the kidney is visible on MRI studies when lesions become sizable. Their signal intensity is similar to normal renal medullary signal on T_1- and T_2-weighted studies. Note usurpation of renal sinus fat *(F)* on the right side by the rounded tumor in comparison with the normal left kidney. Biopsy proved transitional cell carcinoma *(T).*

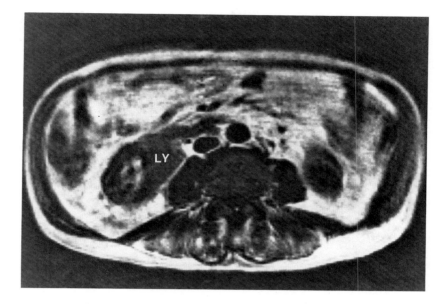

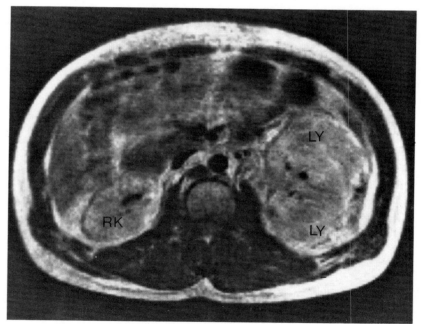

FIG 12–30 (top).
Right renal lymphoma. T₁-weighted axial scan (TR, 0.5 sec; TE, 35 msec): Renal lymphomatous infiltration (*LY,* lymphoma) is demonstrated in the medial lower renal pole in a 40-year-old man with diffuse non-Hodgkin's lymphoma. In our experience, renal lymphoma demonstrates a low signal intensity on T₁-weighted studies that is barely differentiable from normal renal tissue.

FIG 12–31 (bottom).
Left perirenal lymphoma. T₂-weighted axial scan (TR, 2.1 sec; TE, 35 msec): On T₂ scans, renal lymphoma will demonstrate a higher signal intensity than on T₁ scans but will remain similar in intensity to adjacent normal renal tissue, as in this 49-year-old woman with non-Hodgkin's lymphoma. In this case, note the marked expansion of the perirenal space and Gerota's fascia by an infiltrating process that has made the renal border indistinct on the left side. Note the sharp definition of the right kidney *(RK)* in comparison (*LY,* lymphoma).

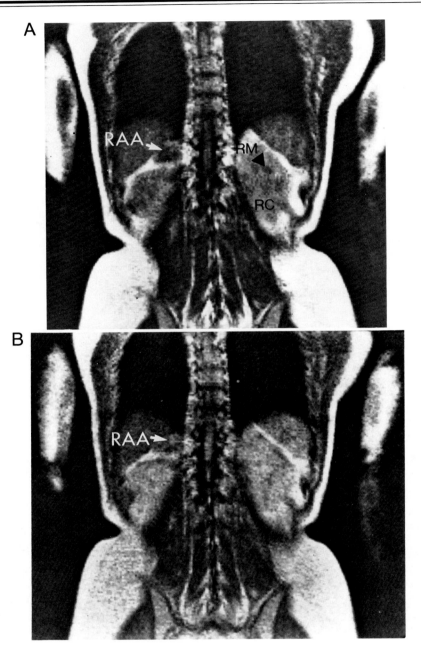

FIG 12–32.
Nonfunctioning right adrenal gland adenoma. This 38-year-old woman was discovered on CT to have an incidental right adrenal nodule.

A, T$_1$ coronal scan (TR, 0.7 sec; TE, 35 msec): It has been suggested by several authors that nonfunctioning adrenal cortical adenomas can be separated from adrenal metastatic lesions on MRI studies. Typically, metastatic lesions (see Fig 7–21) undergo a marked increase in signal intensity on T$_2$-weighted scans, which does not occur in nonfunctioning adenomas. A right adrenal adenoma *(RAA)* demonstrates a lower signal intensity than the adjacent kidney or liver on this T$_1$ scan *(RC,* renal cortex; *RM,* renal medulla).

B, T$_2$ coronal scan (TR, 2.1 sec; TE, 70 msec): Despite utilization of a heavily T$_2$-weighted pulse sequence, the signal intensity of the right adrenal adenoma *(RAA)* remains in the midrange and does not demonstrate the marked increase in intensity that is usually observed in metastatic lesions. This may become a useful indicator for screening the increasing number of nonfunctioning adrenal cortical adenomas encountered in the daily practice of radiology.

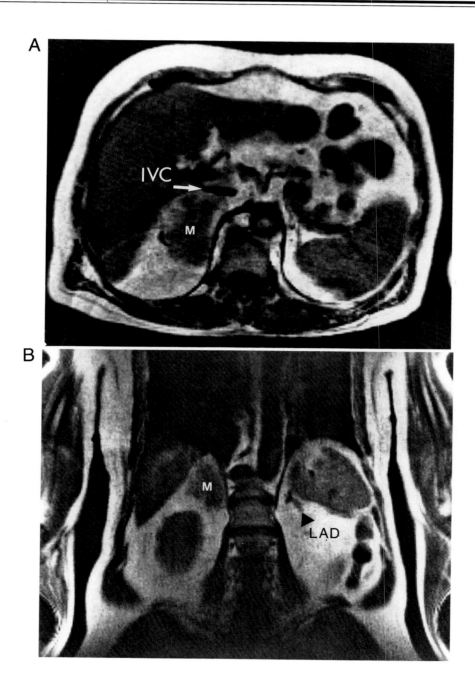

FIG 12–33.

Right adrenal gland metastasis from lung carcinoma. This is a 58-year-old man with small cell lung carcinoma.

A, T₁-weighted axial scan (TR, 0.7 sec; TE, 35 msec): In detecting enlargement of the adrenal glands, MRI is at least as effective as CT. A metastatic deposit *(M)* demonstrates a midrange signal intensity on this T₁-weighted scan. Note sharp definition of the inferior vena cava *(IVC)* anterior to the lesion.

B, T₁ coronal scan (TR, 0.7 sec; TE, 35 msec): In this case, a coronal scan is useful in classifying the retroperitoneal mass as being of adrenal origin. Note the fat plane separating the adrenal mass *(M)* from the right kidney on this section. The normal left adrenal gland *(LAD)* is also demonstrated on this study.

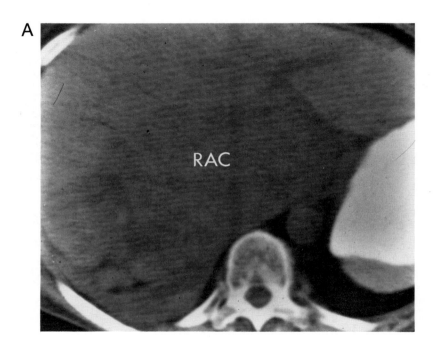

A

RAC

FIG 12–34.
Primary adrenal carcinoma. This is a 50-year-old woman with palpable abdominal mass.

A, unenhanced CT scan: A large right upper quadrant mass is demonstrated. The mass is centered in the right adrenal bed. Its size suggests a primary neoplasm, and extension into the right hemithorax is likely. Precise localization of the inferior vena cava was not obtainable with CT (*RAC,* right adrenal carcinoma).

B, T$_1$-weighted axial scan (TR, 0.5 sec; TE, 35 msec):

The extent of the lesion is as well defined by this axial MRI section as by CT. Note the area of high signal intensity within the lesion, indicating hemorrhage *(H).* The inferior vena cava *(IVC)* is displaced anteriorly by the tumor mass, information not available with CT study.

C, T$_1$ sagittal scan (TR, 0.5 sec; TE, 35 msec): The precise course of the anteriorly displaced inferior vena cava *(IVC)* is noted on this sagittal scan. Note the superb delineation of the cephalocaudal dimension of the tumor with an area of hemorrhage *(H).*

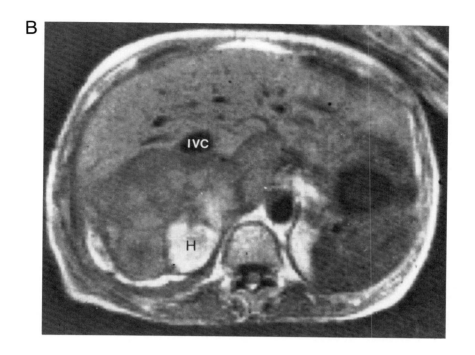

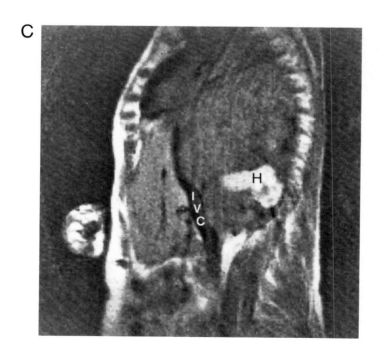

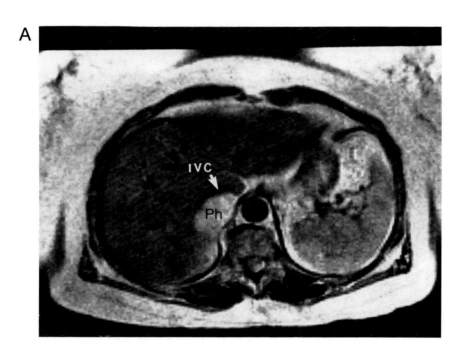

FIG 12–35.
Malignant pheochromocytoma. A 32-year-old woman presented with episodic hypertension.

A, T$_2$-weighted axial scan (TR, 2.1 sec; TE, 35 msec): An oval-shaped mass in the retrocaval region demonstrates a higher signal intensity than adjacent liver. This was found to represent a malignant pheochromocytoma (IVC, inferior vena cava; *Ph,* pheochromocytoma).

B, T$_2$-weighted axial scan (TR, 2.1 sec; TE, 35 msec): This axial section at the inferior border of the tumor (*Ph,*

pheochromocytoma) demonstrates a rounded metastatic deposit *(M)* posterolateral to the triangular primary neoplasm.

C, T$_1$ sagittal scan (TR, 0.5 sec; TE, 35 msec): Sagittal MRI elegantly displays the relationship of the malignant right adrenal pheochromocytoma *(Ph)* to the inferior vena cava *(IVC),* which is posteriorly indented by the lesion but not occluded. Note the lower intensity of the lesion compared with normal liver. There is no evidence of tumor thrombus.

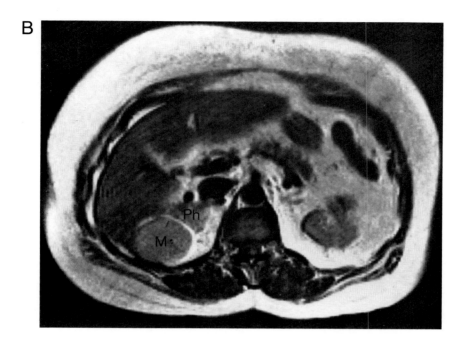

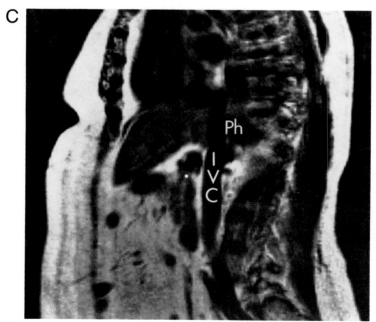

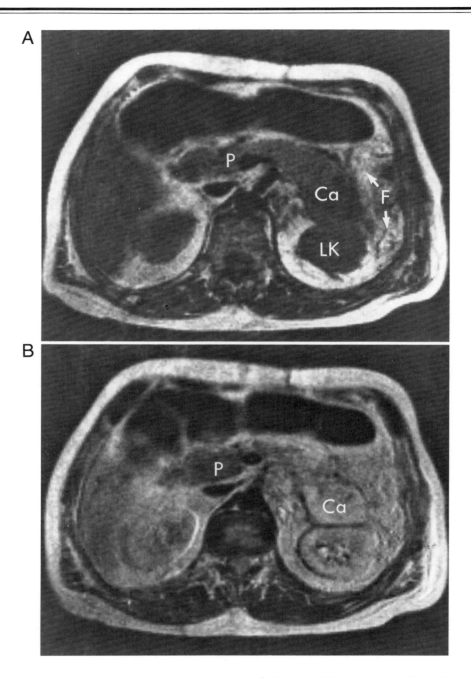

FIG 12–36.
Pancreatic adenocarcinoma. This is a 52-year-old man with abdominal pain.

A, T₁-weighted axial scan (TR, 0.5 sec; TE, 35 msec): Magnetic resonance imaging can delineate pancreatic neoplasm in the tail, although the lack of an oral MRI contrast medium has limited the modality's applications in this area. In this case, the tumor (*Ca,* pancreatic carcinoma) has usurped the fat plane anterior to the left kidney *(LK).* This study delineates changes in the left upper quadrant fascia that may relate to pancreatitis or tumor spread. The signal intensity of the tumor is equal to that of the normal pancreas *(P)* on this T₁ scan (*F,* fascial changes).

B, T₂-weighted axial scan (TR, 2.1 sec; TE, 70 msec): The relatively long T₂ relaxation time of most neoplasms is also typical of pancreatic tumors. In this case, it allows separation of the more intense neoplastic mass (*Ca,* pancreatic carcinoma) from the lower signal intensity of the remaining normal pancreas *(P).* This separation was not available on the T₁ scan.

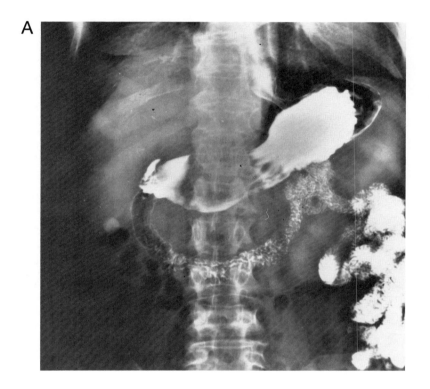

FIG 12–37.
Benign cystadenoma of the pancreas. A 49-year-old woman presented with a slowly enlarging right upper quadrant mass.

A, upper gastrointestinal study: Generalized widening of the duodenal sweep and effacement of the inferior aspect of the gastric antrum is caused by a mass in the region of the head of the pancreas. *(Continued.)*

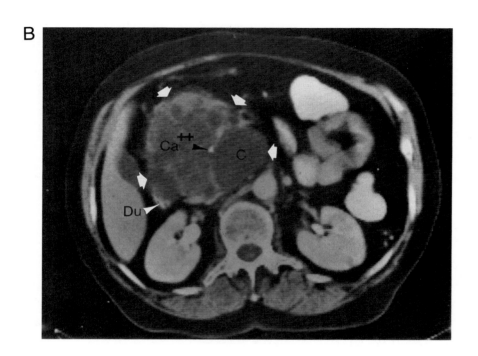

FIG 12–37 (cont.).

B, enhanced CT study: A dynamic CT study demonstrates a mass in the region of the head of the pancreas. Note the large low-attenuation regions *(white arrows)* defining the cystic portion of the mass. A markedly enhancing tumor portion is separated from the cystic region *(C)* by punctate calcification *(Ca⁺⁺)*. The second portion of the duodenum *(Du)* is displaced posterolaterally.

C, T_1-weighted axial scan (TR, 0.5 sec; TE, 35 msec): Note the regions of different signal intensity within the cystadenoma *(arrows)* on this T_1 scan. The cystic region demonstrates a slightly higher signal intensity compared with the remaining, more lateral portion of the tumor because of the complex nature of the cyst fluid. Tumor vascularity is present at the junction of these regions in the posterior portion of the tumor and is defined by flow-void phenomenon *(TV,* tumor vessels; *C,* cyst).

D, T_2-weighted axial scan (TR, 2.1 sec; TE, 70 msec): On the T_2 scan, the cystic portion *(C)* of the tumor *(arrows)* undergoes a marked increase in signal intensity, remaining relatively higher in signal intensity than the more lateral, solid aspect of the tumor. (Neither T_1- nor T_2-weighted studies demonstrated the focal calcification within the tumor that was noted on CT. Failure to visualize calcification is one deficiency of the MRI technique.)

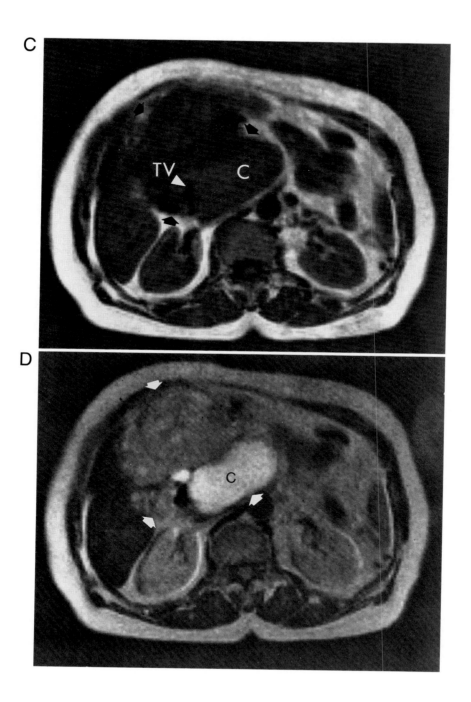

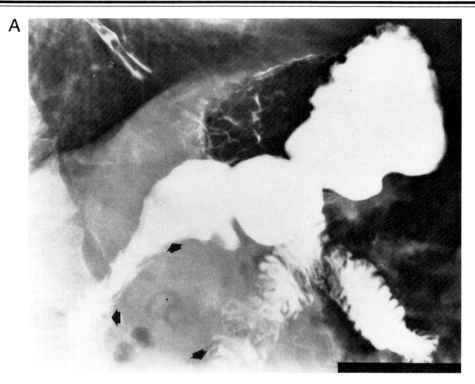

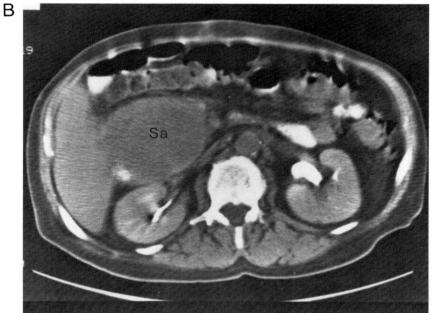

FIG 12–38.

Giant cell sarcoma of the pancreas.

A, upper gastrointestinal series: Note widening of duodenal sweep by mass in region of pancreatic head *(arrows).*

B, enhanced CT section: Note relatively nonenhancing mass in pancreatic head due to giant cell pancreatic sarcoma *(Sa).*

C, T$_1$-weighted axial scan (TR, 0.5 sec; TE, 35 msec):

Note the relatively low signal intensity observed in this mass *(Sa,* giant cell sarcoma) on this T$_1$ scan. A well-defined fat plane is noted around the tumor. Note the marked atrophy *(arrowhead)* of the body of the pancreas.

D, T$_1$ sagittal scan (TR, 0.7 sec; TE, 70 msec): A sagittal scan delineates the borders of the sarcoma and demonstrates the intact fat plane separating the posterior aspect of the mass *(Sa)* from the right kidney *(K).*

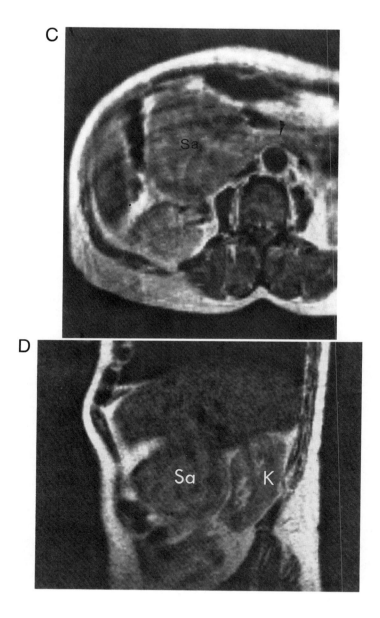

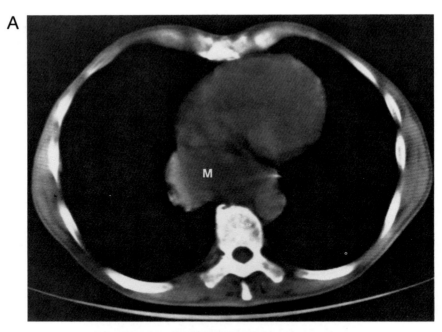

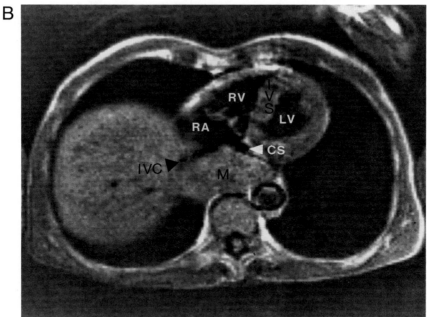

FIG 12–39.
Impingement of inferior vena cava by retrocrural metastatic deposit. This is a 52-year-old man with lower leg edema and a history of carcinoma of the ampulla of Vater.

A, unenhanced CT scan: A nondescript retrocrural mass *(M)* is demonstrated.

B, T$_1$-weighted axial scan (TR, 0.5 sec; TE, 35 msec): Magnetic resonance imaging demonstrates a mass *(M)* of midrange signal intensity in the retrocrural space but in addition demonstrates the anterior displacement and narrowing of the inferior vena cava *(IVC)* at its junction with the right atrium *(RA)*. Gating of the MRI signal acquisition at the systolic phase of the cardiac cycle was utilized to improve definition of pericardiac anatomy (*CS,* coronal sinus; *LV,* left ventricle; *IVS,* interventricular septum; *RV,* right ventricle).

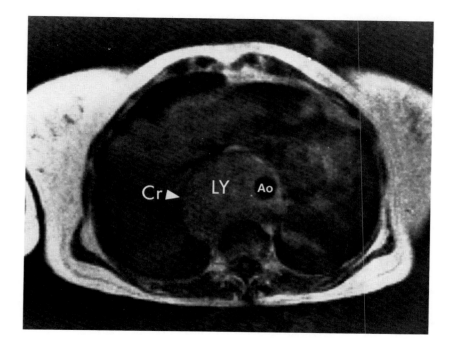

FIG 12–40.

Lymphoma in the retrocrural space. T_1-weighted axial scan (TR, 0.5 sec; TE, 35 msec): Magnetic resonance imaging provides detailed information on the status of the retrocrural space. In this 43-year-old woman with Hodgkin's disease, the diaphragmatic crura *(Cr)* are markedly laterally displaced by a large mass *(LY,* lymphoma) that encases the aorta *(Ao)* and that displays a midrange signal intensity.

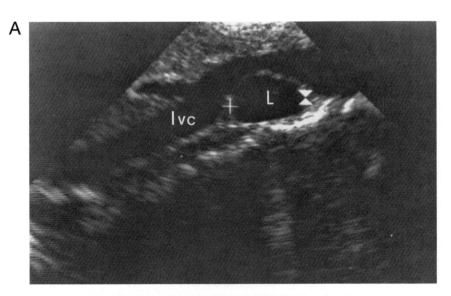

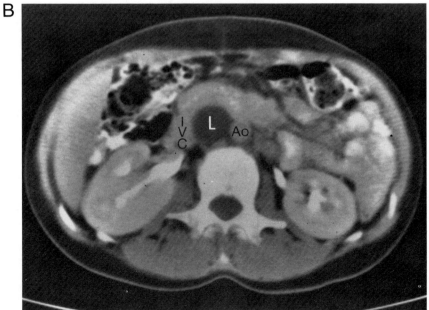

FIG 12–41.
Benign retroperitoneal lymphangioma.

A, real-time ultrasound: Our chief ultrasound technician was scanning her abdomen while evaluating a new real-time ultrasound transducer and discovered a cystic mass (*L,* lymphangioma) lying in a retrocaval location (*IVC,* inferior vena cava). The mass was found to represent a benign cystic lymphangioma of the retroperitoneum.

B, enhanced CT scan: This scan demonstrates a thin-walled cystic lesion *(L)* lying between the aorta *(Ao)* and inferior vena cava *(IVC).*

C, T₁-weighted axial scan (TR, 0.5 sec; TE, 35 msec): As would be expected with a simple cystic lesion, a low signal intensity can be noted within the retroperitoneal lymphangioma *(L)* because of the relatively long T_1 relaxation time of the cyst fluid. Bowel gas in the gut structures and flow-void phenomenon within the aorta and the inferior vena cava delineate the lesion.

D, T₂-weighted axial scan (TR, 2.1 sec; TE, 70 msec): Simple fluid (as present in this lymphangioma) demonstrates a relatively long T_2 relaxation time and will be expected to demonstrate the high signal intensity noted on this T₂ scan *(Ao,* aorta; *IVC,* inferior vena cava; *L,* lymphangioma).

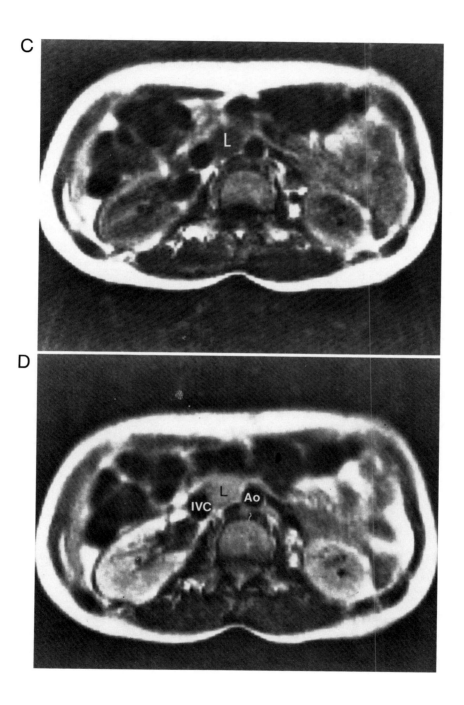

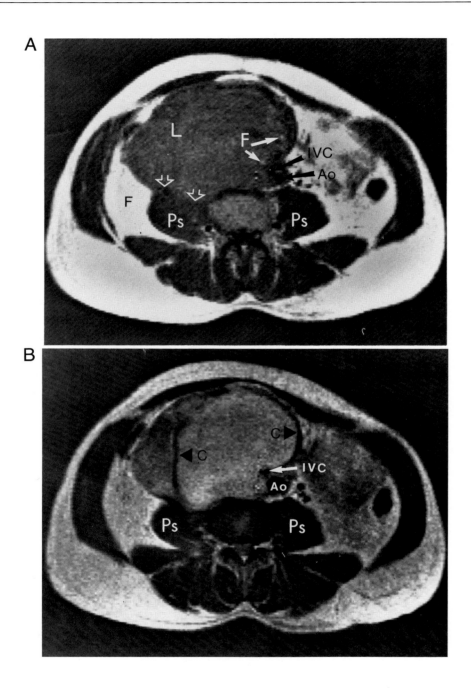

FIG 12–42.
Retroperitoneal liposarcoma. On routine physical examination, a 48-year-old man without symptoms was found to have a large abdominal mass.

A, T_1-weighted axial scan (TR, 0.7 sec; TE, 30 msec): A T_1-weighted MRI study reveals a large lobulated retroperitoneal mass (*L,* liposarcoma). The mass demonstrates a midrange signal intensity and has usurped the fat plane anterior to the right psoas muscle. The inferior vena cava is displaced to the left along the posterolateral aspect of the tumor. There are several punctate high-signal regions that are consistent with fat deposits *(F)* or hemorrhage within the tumor. Biopsy proved liposarcoma (*IVC,* inferior vena cava; *Ps,* psoas muscles; *open arrows* indicate invasion of the right psoas muscle; *Ao,* aorta).

B, T_2-weighted axial scan (TR, 1.4 sec; TE, 70 msec):

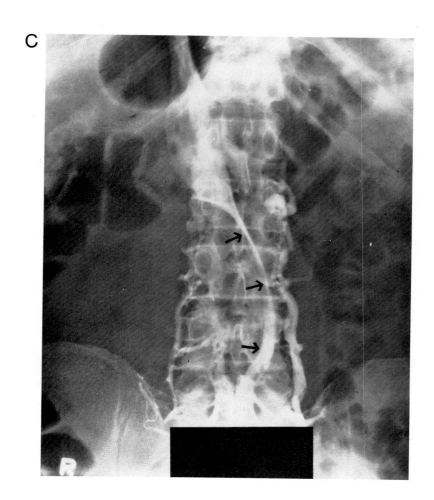

C

The neoplasm demonstrates areas of varying signal intensity. The left two thirds of the lesion demonstrates a very high signal intensity, and there is evidence of a capsule *(C)* separating it from the right portion of the tumor and other retroperitoneal structures. The inferior vena cava *(IVC)* and aorta *(Ao)* are on the left posterolateral aspect of the lesion.

Better visual separation from the right psoas muscle *(Ps)* is available with this pulse sequence.

C, inferior venacavogram: Inferior cavography shows the marked caval narrowing and leftward displacement *(arrows)* demonstrated by the MRI study. The inferior venacavogram roughly approximates the left border of the tumor.

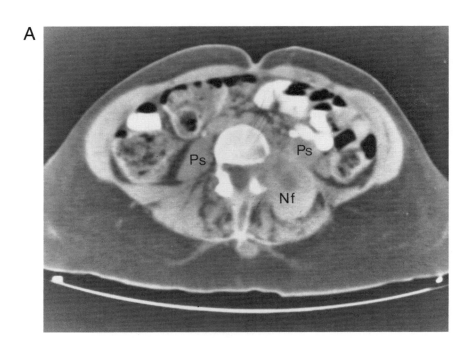

FIG 12–43.
Retroperitoneal malignant neurofibrosarcoma. This 32-year-old woman presented with low back pain.

A, enhanced CT scan: The CT study was performed to assess the cause of pain. It demonstrates a large, lobulated mass *(Nf)* in the left lateral and posterior paraspinal region and slight uplifting of the left psoas muscle *(Ps)*. Biopsy proved neurofibrosarcoma.

B, T$_2$-weighted axial scan (TR, 2.1 sec; TE, 35 msec): Magnetic resonance imaging is extremely valuable in the preoperative workup of paraspinal neurogenic tumors for detecting subtle intraspinal extensions and bony abnormalities not noted on CT or conventional radiography. In this case, note extension of the mass into the left L-4 neural foramen *(arrow)* and actual destruction of the left postero-lateral aspect of the L-4 vertebral body, information not well provided by CT (*Nf,* neurofibrosarcoma).

C, T$_2$ coronal scan (TR, 2.1 sec; TE, 70 msec): A direct coronal image displays high signal intensity within the left paraspinal neurofibrosarcoma *(Nf)* and uplifting of the left psoas muscle *(Ps)*.

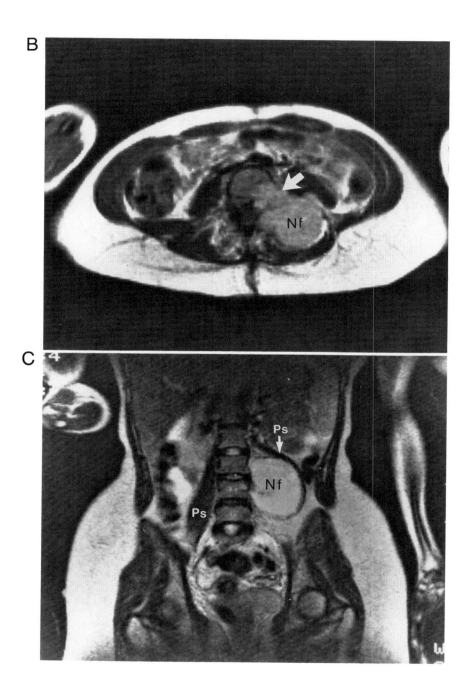

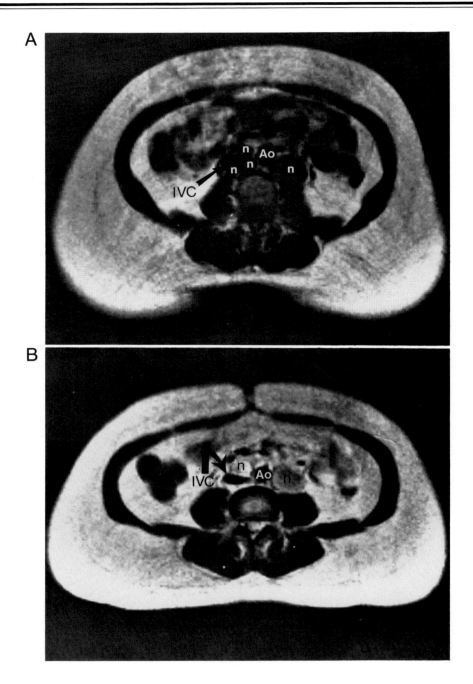

FIG 12–44.
Retroperitoneal adenopathy. This is a 44-year-old woman with non-Hodgkin's lymphoma.

A, T_1-weighted axial scan (TR, 0.5 sec; TE, 35 msec): Note the midrange signal intensity displayed by the enlarged retroperitoneal lymph nodes *(n)*. In demonstrating the presence or absence of retroperitoneal adenopathy, MRI may be as useful and effective as CT. The paraspinal area is relatively fixed; therefore, the MR image in this region is relatively free of respiratory artifact. Flow-void phenomenon within the aorta *(Ao)* and inferior vena cava *(IVC)* allows separation of these structures from adjacent lymph nodes without the need for intravenous contrast administration.

B, T_2-weighted axial scan (TR, 2.1 sec; TE, 70 msec): Retroperitoneal adenopathy undergoes a relative increase in signal intensity on T_2-weighted scans, although in most cases the nodes remain less intense than retroperitoneal fat *(n,* adenopathy; *IVC,* inferior vena cava; *Ao,* aorta).

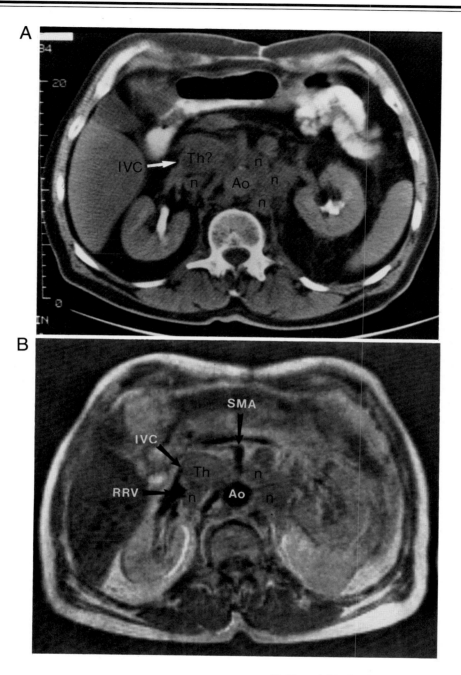

FIG 12–45.
Invasion of inferior vena cava by metastatic adenopathy. This is a 51-year-old man with diffuse retroperitoneal adenopathy secondary to colon carcinoma.

A, enhanced CT scan: It is difficult in this scan, despite the fact that contrast medium was intravenously administered, to separate enlarged retroperitoneal lymph nodes *(n)* from adjacent vascular structures *(Ao,* aorta). There is a suggestion of intraluminal inferior vena cava thrombus *(Th?)* by this scan *(IVC,* inferior vena cava).

B, T$_2$-weighted axial scan (TR, 2.1 sec; TE, 35 msec): Magnetic resonance imaging provides a much better assessment of the pertinent anatomy in this case. Flow-void phenomenon allows separation of the aorta *(Ao)* and the superior mesenteric artery *(SMA)* from adjacent retroperitoneal adenopathy *(n).* The right renal vein *(RRV)* can be identified and traced to the inferior vena cava *(IVC),* which, indeed, is thrombus-laden *(Th).* The intraluminal thrombus demonstrates a midrange signal intensity similar to that of adjacent lymph nodes.

A

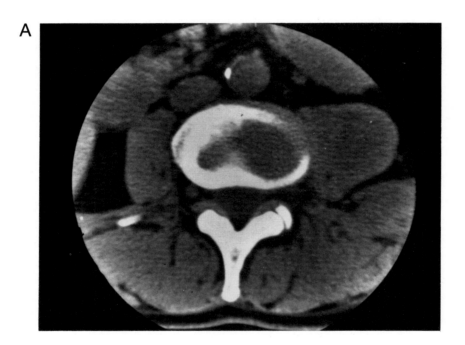

FIG 12–46.
Left psoas metastasis. This is a 70-year-old man with a history of colon carcinoma and left leg pain.

A, unenhanced CT scan: Note enlargement of the left psoas muscle and a subtle low-attenuation region. Intravenous contrast medium could not be used on account of patient allergy.

B, T_1 coronal scan (TR, 0.7 sec; TE, 35 msec) in prone position: An elongated mass *(M)* yielding midrange signal intensity is noted in the left psoas muscle *(Ps)*. Compare this with the lower signal intensity and normal contour of the right psoas muscle. (The patient was prone during this study because of mild claustrophobic reaction.)

C, T_2 coronal scan (TR, 2.1 sec; TE, 70 msec) in prone position: Better contrast definition of the metastatic lesion is available on this T_2-weighted scan, which sharply delineates the border between the mass *(M)* and the normal left psoas muscle *(Ps)*.

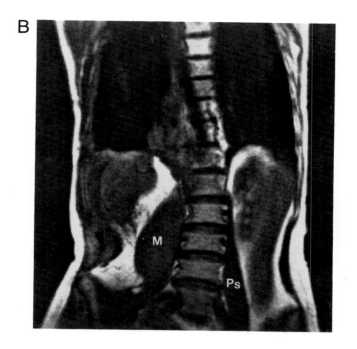

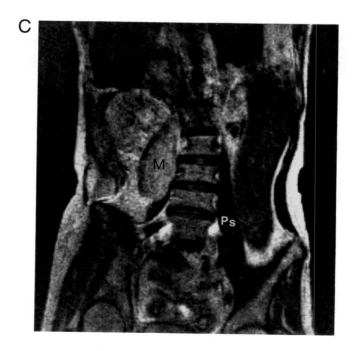

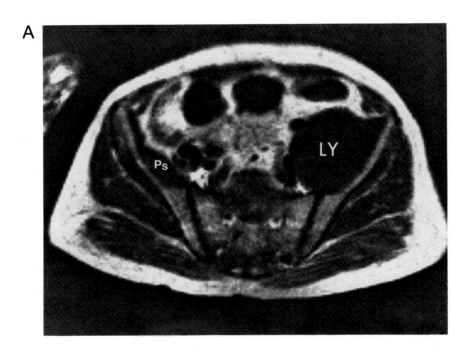

FIG 12–47.
Malignant cystic lymphangioma of the left psoas muscle. This patient is a 49-year-old woman who had a history of colon carcinoma.

A, T_1-weighted axial scan (TR, 0.5 sec; TE, 35 msec): This T_1 section demonstrates a low signal intensity within a cystic lymphangioma *(LY)* of the left psoas muscle. Compare the size of the left psoas muscle to the normal right psoas muscle *(Ps)* on this axial scan.

B, T_2-weighted axial scan (TR, 2.1 sec; TE, 35 msec): There is better contrast definition available on the T_2 scan, which delineates the border of the cystic lymphangioma *(LY)* and the remaining normal left psoas muscle *(Ps)*. Note the common iliac vessels *(V)* along the medial aspect of the lymphangioma.

C, T_1 sagittal scan (TR, 0.5 sec; TE, 35 msec): This format displays the cephalocaudal dimension of the cystic lymphangioma *(LY)*, which demonstrates a low signal intensity.

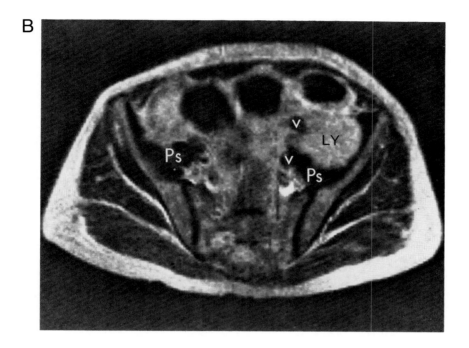

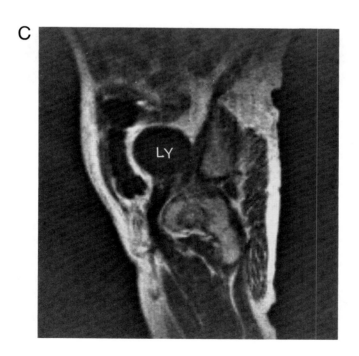

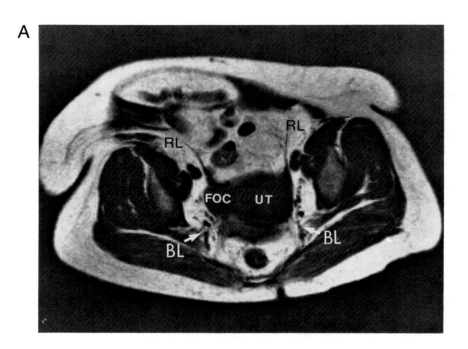

FIG 12–48.

Normal uterus; functional right ovarian cyst.

A, T_1 axial section (TR, 0.5 sec; TE, 35 msec): On T_1-weighted studies, the uterus *(UT)* displays a homogeneous midrange signal intensity. Note the low signal intensity of a small functional right ovarian cyst *(FOC)*. The fibrous nature of the round *(RL)* and broad *(BL)* ligaments is responsible for their low signal intensity.

B, T_2-weighted axial scan (TR, 2.1 sec; TE, 70 msec): Because of differences in their T_2 relaxation times, the various uterine layers can be differentiated with T_2-weighted pulse sequences. The endometrium *(long arrow)* will demonstrate a high signal intensity, contrasting sharply with the adjacent low signal intensity of the stratum basale *(SB)* of endometrium. The myometrium *(M)* demonstrates a midrange signal intensity. Note the marked increase in signal intensity of the functional right ovarian cyst *(FOC)* in comparison with **A.** The thin wall of the cyst is revealed *(BL,* broad ligaments; *RL,* round ligaments).

C, T_2 sagittal section (TR, 2.1 sec; TE, 35 msec): The uterus, cervix, and vagina are best visualized in the sagittal plane. Note the high signal intensity of the endometrial cavity *(EC)* and the lower signal intensity of the stratum basale *(SB)* of endometrium. The myometrium *(M)* demonstrates a relatively midrange signal intensity. The anterior and posterior cervical lips *(CL)* demonstrate a lower signal intensity than the uterus; this allows their precise definition (*B,* urinary bladder).

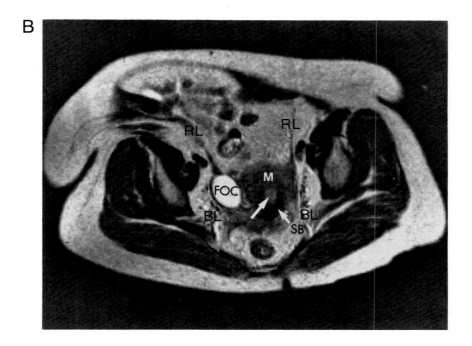

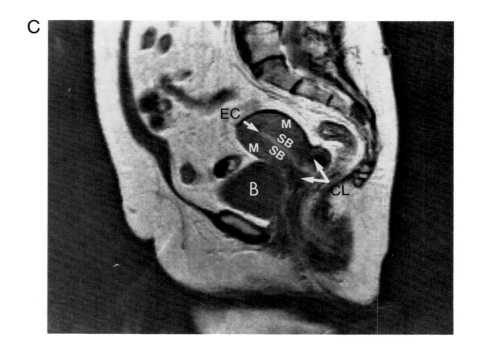

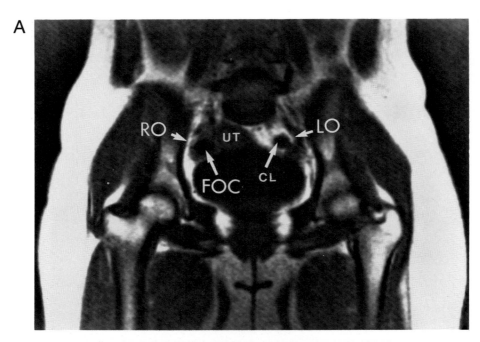

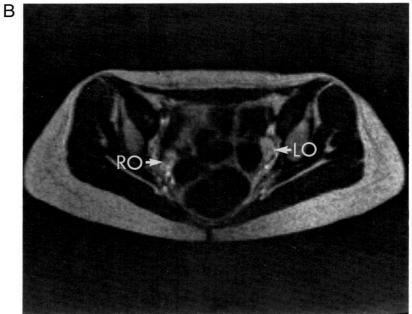

FIG 12–49.
Normal ovaries.

A, T$_1$ coronal scan (TR, 0.7 sec; TE, 30 msec): On T$_1$-weighted scans, the normal ovary demonstrates a signal of midrange intensity. Note, in the left ovary *(LO)* in this case, two punctate high-signal regions that indicate follicle formation. The right ovary *(RO)* in this case demonstrates a large low-signal region, indicating functional ovarian cyst formation *(CL,* corpus luteum; *FOC,* functional ovarian cyst; *UT,* uterus).

B, T$_2$-weighted axial scan (TR, 2.1 sec; TE, 70 msec): The ovaries undergo a homogeneous increase in signal intensity when T$_2$- rather than T$_1$-weighted scans are used. Note the relatively high signal intensity of the ovaries here *(LO,* left ovary; *RO,* right ovary).

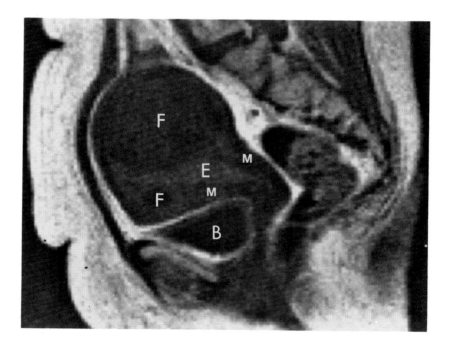

FIG 12–50.
Fibroid uterus. T_1 sagittal scan (TR, 0.5 sec; TE, 35 msec): Magnetic resonance imaging is a useful technique for evaluating uterine masses. Uterine fibroids, in most cases, demonstrate a low signal intensity on T_1- and T_2-weighted images because of their smooth muscle content and the frequent presence of calcification. Their serosal, submucosal, or mucosal origin can be determined with sagittal scans. In this 39-year-old woman, note the large superior/fundal fibroid *(F)* and the smaller, totally submucosal lesion that both demonstrate lower signal intensity than adjacent myometrium or endometrium. In the MRI literature, high signal intensity within uterine fibroid has been attributed to areas of degeneration (*F,* fibroids; *E,* endometrium; *M,* myometrium; *B,* bladder).

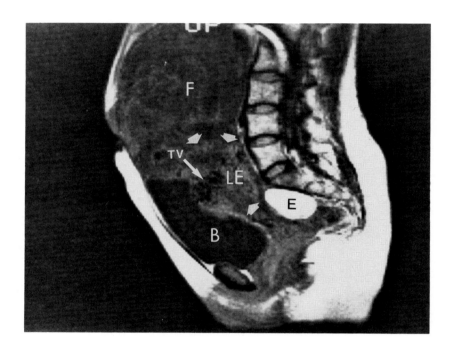

FIG 12–51.

Uterine leiomyosarcoma and endometrioma. A 50-year-old woman presented with an enlarging pelvic mass and was first examined with MRI. T_1 sagittal scan (TR, 0.5 sec; TE, 35 msec): The large size of this uterine mass and the presence of tumor vessels *(TV)* within it suggested that a leiomyosarcoma was present. A slightly higher intensity was noted surrounding the tumor vessels in the area of sarcomatous degeneration. The upper portion of the mass at surgery represented fibroid *(F)* only.

An area of high signal intensity in the presacral zone at surgery represented an endometrioma *(E)* (*LE* and *arrows,* leiomyosarcoma; *B,* bladder).

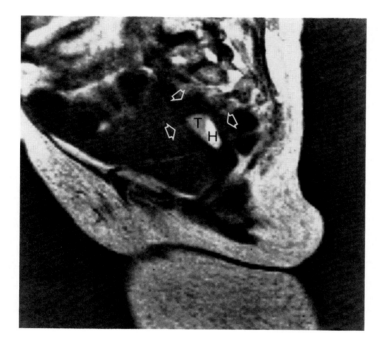

FIG 12–52.

Endometrial carcinoma with hematometra. T_1 sagittal scan (TR, 0.5 sec; TE, 70 msec): Magnetic resonance imaging can play an important role in the diagnosis and staging of endometrial carcinoma. In this 71-year-old woman with uterine bleeding, note the signal level formed by hematometra *(H)* lying atop a shelf of tumor *(T)*. The uterus *(arrows)* is not enlarged, and there is no evidence of tumor outside of the uterine body.

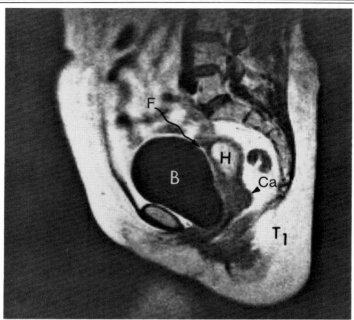

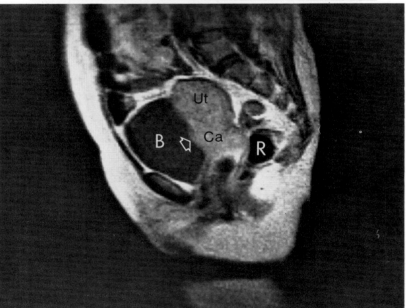

FIG 12–53 (top).
Stage I cervical carcinoma with hematometra. T_1 sagittal scan (TR, 0.6 sec; TE, 35 msec): Stage I lesions confined to the cervix rarely cause abnormal areas of signal intensity but may induce slightly bulbous enlargement of the cervix, as in this 38-year-old woman. Hematometra *(H)* has resulted from obstruction of the cervical canal by the tumor *(Ca);* it demonstrates a high signal intensity within the endometrial canal. Note the intact fat plane *(F, arrow)* separating the uterus and cervix from the urinary bladder *(B),* indicating lack of invasion of the latter structure. The bulbous portion of the cervical tumor is also surrounded by fat posteriorly.

FIG 12–54 (bottom).
Stage II cervical carcinoma, with uterine invasion. T_2 sagittal scan (TR, 1.5 sec; TE, 35 msec): On T_2 sagittal scans, the three layers of uterine tissue should be exhibited. In this 40-year-old woman, the normal pattern of uterine signal intensity has been replaced by a homogeneous high signal intensity that indicates extension of cervical carcinoma *(Ca)* into the uterine body *(Ut).* This pattern indicates a stage II lesion. Note nodular indentation of the posterior bladder wall *(arrow)* but lack of invasion of the bladder *(B)* or of the adjacent rectum *(R).*

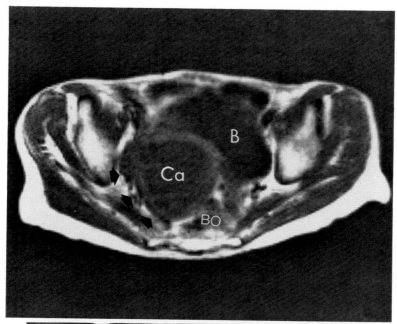

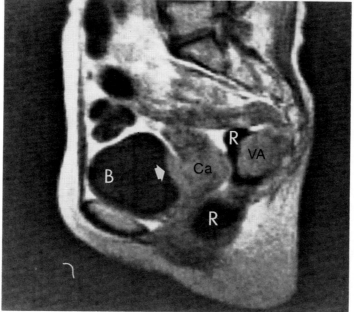

FIG 12–55 (top).
Stage III cervical carcinoma, with right pelvic sidewall invasion. T₁-weighted axial scan (TR, 0.5 sec; TE, 35 msec): The more advanced forms of cervical carcinoma are accurately evaluated with MRI. In this 40-year-old woman, an extensive right parametrial and pelvic sidewall extension *(arrows)* demonstrated as areas of low-intensity signals indicates a stage III lesion *(Ca,* cervical carcinoma; *BO,* bowel; *B,* urinary bladder).

FIG 12–56 (bottom).
Stage IV cervical carcinoma, with invasion of urinary bladder and rectum. T₁ sagittal scan (TR, 1.0 sec; TE, 30 msec): In this 41-year-old woman, the cervical carcinoma *(Ca)* has extended beyond the boundaries of the cervix and has invaded the posterior aspect of the urinary bladder. Note the sessile extension of tumor along the posterior urinary bladder wall *(arrows)*. The tumor extends superiorly, and it appears to be separate from the uterus. The mass has also extended posteriorly into the anterior wall of the rectum *(R),* which contains a villous adenoma *(VA)* in its posterior wall.

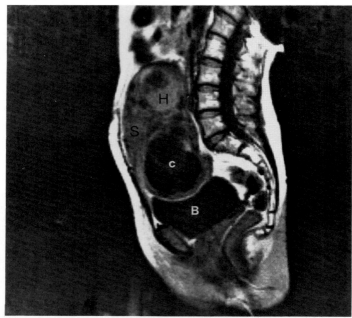

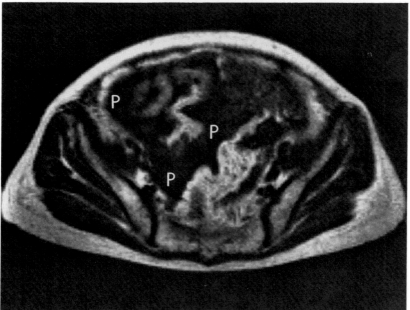

FIG 12–57 (top).
Serous ovarian adenocarcinoma. T_1-weighted sagittal scan (TR, 0.7 sec; TE, 35 msec): Ovarian malignancies made up of solid and cystic elements will demonstrate a complex signal intensity on T_1-weighted scans, with cystic areas *(C)* demonstrating relatively low signal intensity, hemorrhagic areas *(H)* demonstrating a relatively higher signal intensity, and stromatous areas *(S)* showing a midrange signal intensity. A large pelviabdominal serous adenocarcinoma of the ovary is demonstrated in this 52-year-old woman. Note the intact fat plane separating the lesion from the urinary bladder *(B),* which is compressed by the lesion.

FIG 12–58 (bottom).
Pseudomyxoma peritonei. T_1-weighted axial scan (TR, 0.7 sec; TE, 35 msec): A 53-year-old woman with known pseudomyxoma peritonei from ovarian carcinoma was examined with MRI. Malignant ascites and pseudomyxoma peritonei *(P)* both demonstrate a low signal intensity and fill all available peritoneal recesses.

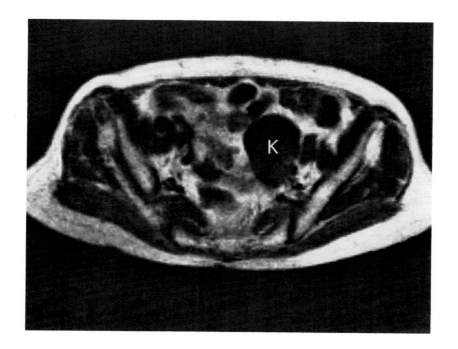

FIG 12–59.
Krukenberg's tumor of the left ovary. T_1-weighted axial scan (TR, 0.5 sec; TE, 35 msec): A relatively low signal intensity is observed in a left ovarian mass in this 65-year-old woman. The mass was found at surgery to be a metastatic deposit from gastric carcinoma, or Krukenberg's tumor *(K).* The appearance of mass with cystic and solid components is not characteristic on MRI and mimics a variety of other lesions.

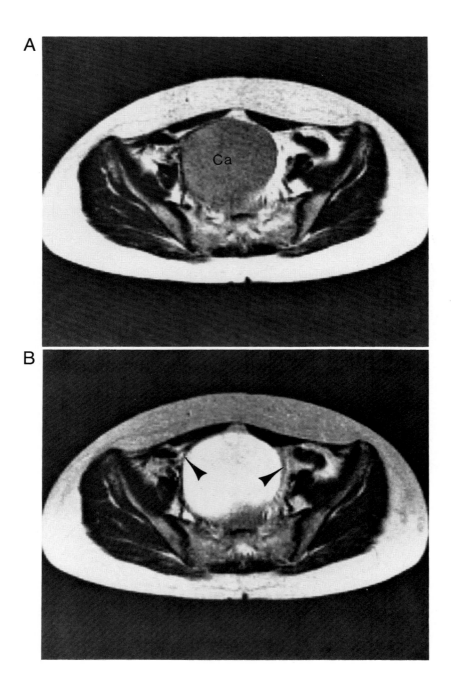

FIG 12–60.
Mucinous ovarian adenocarcinoma. This is a 49-year-old woman with pelvic mass.

A, T$_1$-weighted axial scan (TR, 0.7 sec; TE, 35 msec): Cystic ovarian neoplasms will demonstrate a homogeneous low signal intensity on T$_1$-weighted images. Note sharp definition from adjacent fat, muscle, and bowel structures (*Ca,*

carcinoma).

B, T$_2$-weighted axial scan (TR, 2.1 sec; TE, 35 msec): In totally cystic malignant ovarian lesions, a striking increase in signal intensity will be observed on T$_2$ scans because of the prolonged T$_2$ relaxation time of the fluid within the tumor cyst. The wall of the cyst *(arrowheads)* is frequently visible on the T$_2$ scans.

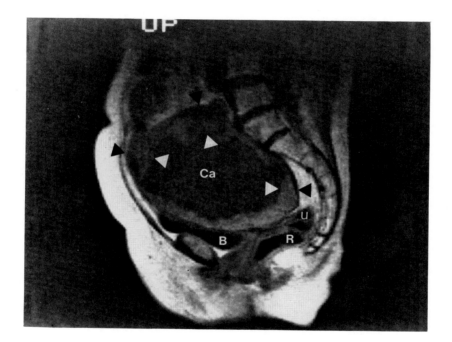

FIG 12–61.
Serous ovarian carcinoma. T_1 sagittal scan (TR, 0.7 sec; TE, 35 msec): Magnetic resonance imaging is useful in defining the origin of masses in the pelvis. In this 50-year-old woman, a thick-walled ovarian carcinoma *(Ca)* is noted to displace the uterus *(U)* posteriorly, but the outer wall of the lesion is definitely separate from the uterus, suggesting an ovarian origin. Note marked compression of the urinary bladder *(B)* (*arrowheads* indicate tumor wall; *R,* rectum).

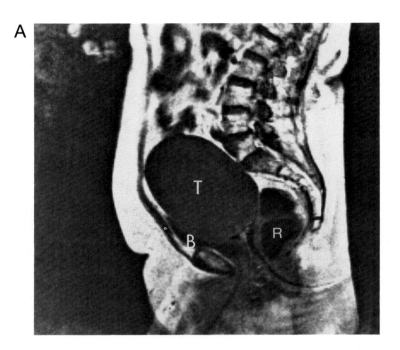

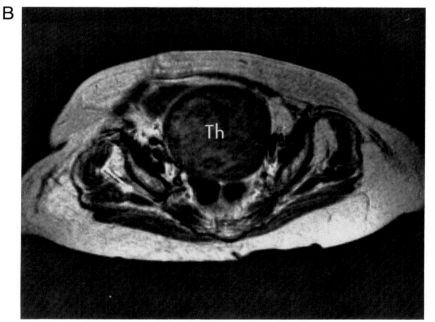

FIG 12–62.
Ovarian thecoma. This is a 39-year-old woman with palpable pelvic mass.

A, T₁ sagittal scan (TR, 0.5 sec; TE, 35 msec): Ovarian thecoma *(T)* presents an appearance similar to ovarian fibroma. The scan demonstrates a homogeneous mass of low signal intensity. The mass was discovered on routine gynecologic examination (*R,* rectum; *B,* urinary bladder).

B, T₂-weighted axial scan (TR, 2.1 sec; TE, 35 msec): Note that the major portion of this tumor does not increase significantly in signal intensity, although some areas in the right half of the tumor are slightly more intense than the left. The lesion is well circumscribed, and there are well-defined adjacent fat planes (*Th,* thecoma).

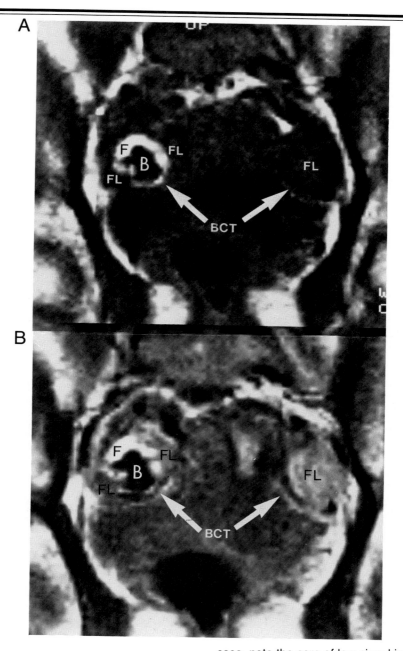

FIG 12–63.
Bilateral benign cystic teratoma.

A, T₁ coronal scan (TR, 0.5 sec; TE, 35 msec): In benign cystic teratoma, MRI can usually provide a specific diagnosis. Characteristic triple signal intensity changes are seen within the lesions in the pelvis of this 29-year-old woman. When a benign cystic teratoma containing bone, fluid, and fat is present, the bone will demonstrate a low signal intensity, the fat a high signal intensity, and, on T₁-weighted scans, the fluid a low signal intensity. When there is a shift to a T₂-weighted scan, the bone and fat intensity will remain the same, whereas the fluid signal intensity will markedly increase. This sequence of intensity changes forms a pattern that allows the specific diagnosis. In this case, note the core of low signal intensity in the right lesion: a bone fragment *(B)* is surrounded by high-signal fat *(F)* and only a small amount of fluid. The left lesion contains mainly fluid and demonstrates a low signal intensity on this T₁-weighted scan *(arrows* indicate the benign cystic teratoma, *BCT).*

B, T₂ coronal scan (TR, 2.1 sec; TE, 70 msec): As stated in **A,** only the fluid element of a benign cystic teratoma will significantly change in signal intensity when there is a shift from T₁ to T₂ scans. Note the high signal intensity now present diffusely in the left lesion, indicating a fluid nature *(FL).* There has been little change in the appearance of the right lesion, which is mainly composed of fat and bone.

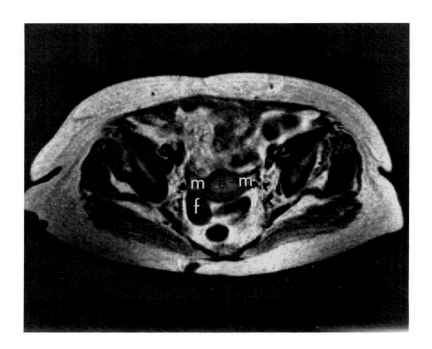

FIG 12–64.
Right ovarian fibroma. T_2-weighted axial scan (TR, 2.1 sec; TE, 70 msec): Magnetic resonance imaging is useful in the diagnosis and staging of benign and malignant ovarian neoplasms, with a narrow differential diagnosis obtainable in most cases. In this 35-year-old woman, note the low signal intensity in a right adnexal mass *(f)* which at surgery was found to be a right ovarian fibroma. These lesions, because of their fibrous nature, typically demonstrate a low signal intensity on T_1- and T_2-weighted studies. Also note the separation of the various uterine layers by signal intensity on this T_2-weighted scan (*e,* endometrium; *m,* myometrium).

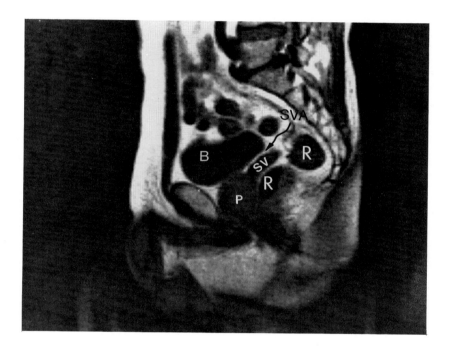

FIG 12–65.
Sagittal view of normal male pelvis. T$_1$-weighted axial scan (TR, 0.5 sec; TE, 35 msec): The midline sagittal MRI scan of the male pelvis is useful in demonstrating the prostate gland and its relationship to the urinary bladder. The normal prostate *(P)* is seen here and demonstrates a midrange homogeneous signal intensity. The medial aspects of the seminal vesicle *(SV)* and the seminal vesicle angle *(SVA)* are visualized. The rectum *(R)* is defined posteriorly and anteriorly by adjacent fat *(B,* urinary bladder).

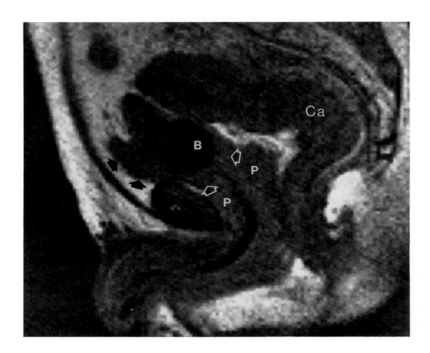

FIG 12–66.
Prostate carcinoma with urinary bladder invasion. T_1 sagittal scan (TR, 0.5 sec; TE, 35 msec): In this 68-year-old man, notice the extension of prostate tumor *(P)* around the anterior aspect of the urinary bladder *(arrows)*, indicating direct invasion of this structure. A Foley catheter has been in-serted, outlining the prostatic urethra through the tumor. The seminal vesicle angles are well maintained.

Also present in this patient is an extensive carcinoma of the rectosigmoid colon (*B,* urinary bladder; *Ca,* rectal car-cinoma).

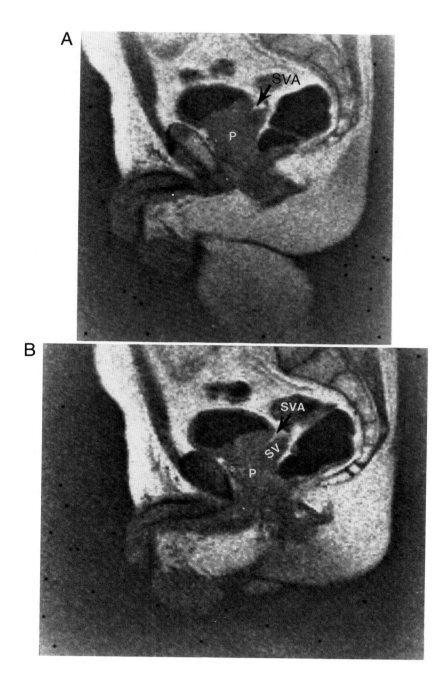

FIG 12–67.

Prostatic carcinoma. This is a 77-year-old man with an enlarged prostate.

A, T_1 sagittal scan (TR, 0.5 sec; TE, 35 msec): Note enlargement of the prostate gland *(P)* and, on this section, the usurpation of the seminal vesicle angle *(SVA),* indicating extension of tumor into this region.

B, T_1 sagittal scan (TR, 0.5 sec; TE, 35 msec): A sagittal scan through the opposite seminal vesicle *(SV)* demonstrates that this angle is intact (*P,* prostate; *SVA,* seminal vesicle angle).

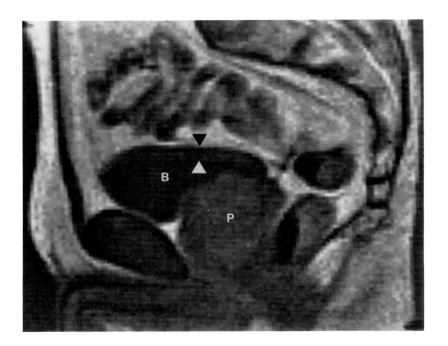

FIG 12–68.
Benign prostatic hypertrophy. T_1 sagittal scan (TR, 0.5 sec; TE, 35 msec): Benign prostatic hypertrophy *(P)* is demonstrated by MRI as generalized enlargement of the gland with a nodular border. There is never evidence of invasion of adjacent structures. Frequently, the urinary bladder wall will be thickened *(arrowheads)* because of hypertrophy from bladder neck obstruction, as in this case. The signal intensity of benign prostatic enlargement may be homogeneous or nonhomogeneous (*B,* urinary bladder).

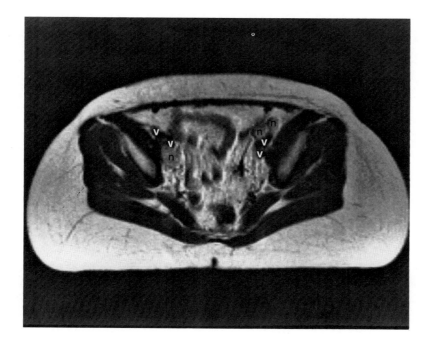

FIG 12–69.
Pelvic adenopathy. T_2-weighted axial scan (TR, 2.1 sec; TE, 70 msec): Metastatic adenopathy in the pelvis and retroperitoneum will demonstrate a relatively low signal intensity on T_1-weighted images and increase to a midrange signal intensity on T_2-weighted images, as in this 50-year-old man with non-Hodgkin's lymphoma. The intensity remains below that of pelvic fat on this T_2-weighted sequence. Note the enlarged right obturator and left external iliac lymph nodes *(n)*, sharply demarcated by pelvic fat and adjacent blood vessels *(v)*.

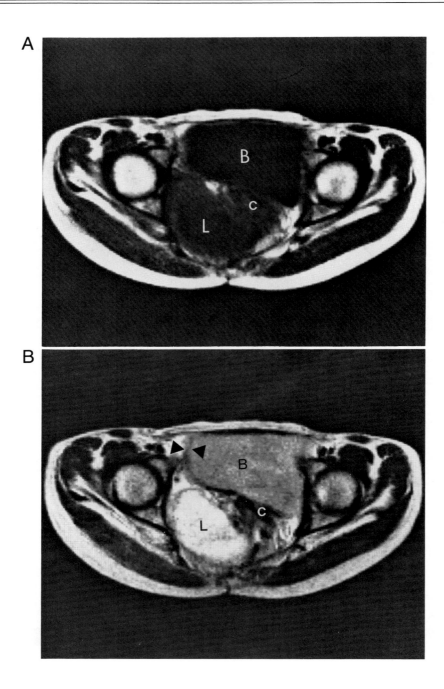

FIG 12–70.
Malignant cystic lymphangioma. This is a 43-year-old woman with metastatic cervical carcinoma and lymphatic obstruction.

A, T_1-weighted axial scan (TR, 0.5 sec; TE, 35 msec): A large cystic lymphangioma *(L)* in the presacral region. As with most simple fluid collections, the intensity is low on the T_1-weighted scan and markedly increases on the T_2-weighted scan (*C,* cervix; *B,* urinary bladder).

B, T_2-weighted axial scan (TR, 2.1 sec; TE, 70 msec): Note marked increase in signal intensity of the interior of the presacral cystic lymphangioma, as would be expected with a cystic fluid collection. Also note the definition of the urinary bladder wall *(arrowheads)* on this T_2-weighted scan (*L,* cystic lymphangioma; *B,* urinary bladder; *C,* cervix).

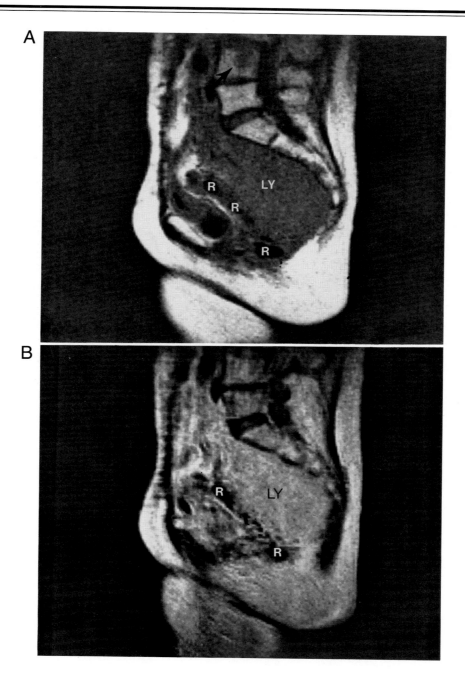

FIG 12–71.
Presacral lymphoma. This is a 50-year-old man with lymphoma.

A, T₁ sagittal scan (TR, 0.5 sec; TE, 35 msec): Lymphoma will demonstrate a midrange signal intensity on T₁-weighted images and markedly increase in signal intensity on T₂-weighted images. On this T₁-weighted scan, note the midrange signal intensity observed in the large presacral lymphomatous mass *(LY)* that is displacing the air-filled rectum *(R)* anteriorly. Note sharp definition of lymphoma borders by pelvic fat. Also note the rounded low-intensity region at the L-4 vertebral body *(arrow)*, indicating a lymphomatous bony infiltrate.

B, T₂ sagittal scan (TR, 2.1 sec; TE, 35 msec): An MRI pitfall in studying lymphoma is that on T2-weighted scans the intensity of lymphoma may equal that of adjacent fatty structures and thus render the borders of the mass invisible. The mass *(LY,* lymphoma) in this case can still be detected by the anterior displacement of the air-filled rectum *(R).*

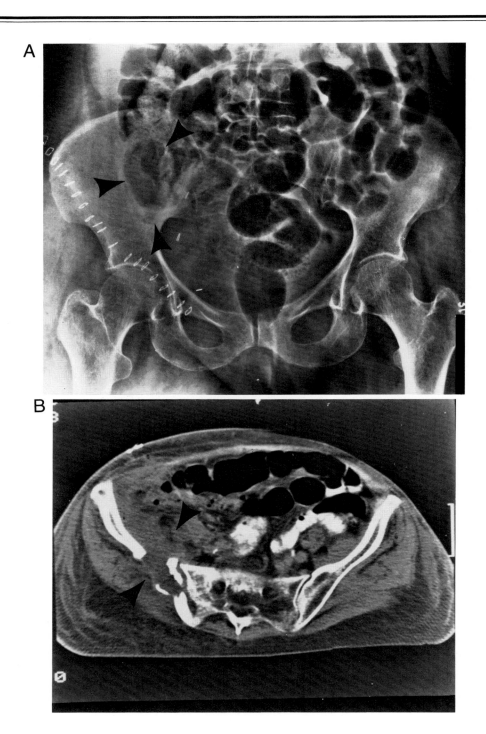

FIG 12–72.
Lymphoma of the right iliac wing. A 72-year-old woman presented with right buttock pain.

A, this view of the pelvis shows a large lytic region in the right iliac wing surrounded by bony sclerosis *(arrowheads)*. Lymphoma was proved by CT-guided biopsy.

B, enhanced CT section: This image defines soft tissue mass *(arrowheads)* adjacent to the defect in the right iliac wing and extending anteriorly into the right iliacus muscle and posteriorly into the right buttock. The right sacroiliac joint is widened on this study.

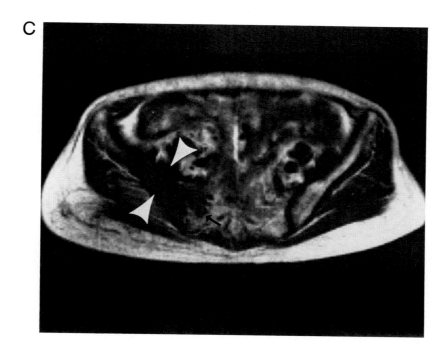

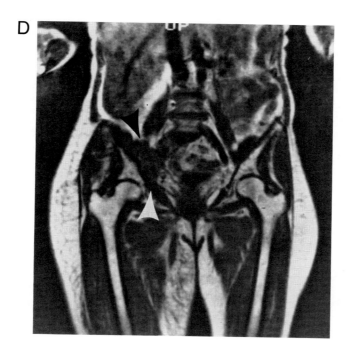

C, T$_1$ axial image (TR, 0.5 sec; TE, 35 msec): The mass demonstrates a low signal intensity on this T$_1$-weighted scan; lymphomatous tissue *(arrowheads)* fills the defect in the right iliac wing and the normal intensity of bone marrow is lost. Bony cortex demonstrates a very low signal intensity on MR images. There is decreased signal intensity *(arrow)* present in the right sacral ala, indicating bony involvement in this region, information not available with CT.

D, T$_1$ coronal scan (TR, 0.7 sec; TE, 35 msec): Coronal MRI demonstrates the extension of tumor in the iliac region, where a large mass of low signal intensity is noted *(arrowheads)*.

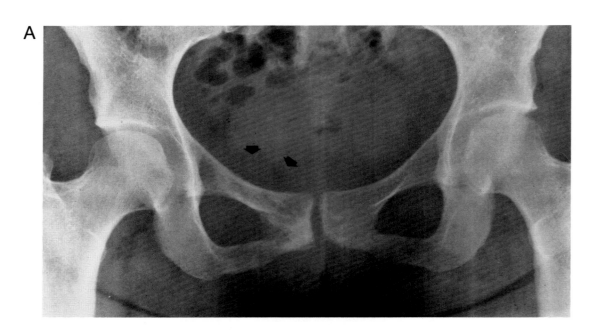

FIG 12–73.
Ewing's sarcoma of right ischium. A 17-year-old girl presented with right-sided pelvic pain.

A, anteroposterior pelvic radiography: This radiograph demonstrates a permeative pattern of bone destruction in the perisymphyseal portion of the right ischiopubic ramus complex. There is a suggestion of elevation of the right obturator fat plane by an associated soft tissue mass *(arrows)*.

B, T$_2$-weighted axial scan (TR, 2.1 sec; TE, 35 msec):

Note the expansion and increased signal intensity of the right pubic bone due to the presence of Ewing's tumor *(E)*. Also there are adjacent soft tissue masses *(arrows)* that extend into the anterior right ischiorectal fat pad *(IR)* and into the space anterior to the vagina *(v)*.

C, T$_2$ coronal scan (TR, 2.1 sec; TE, 70 msec): Coronal MRI demonstrates the elevation of the urinary bladder by the pelvic floor mass *(E,* Ewing's sarcoma).

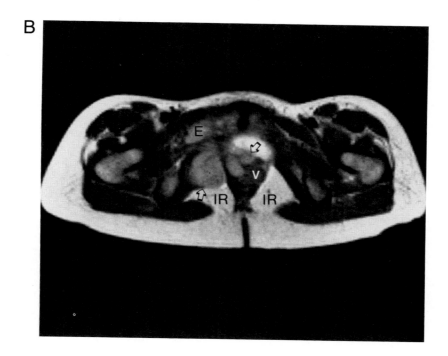

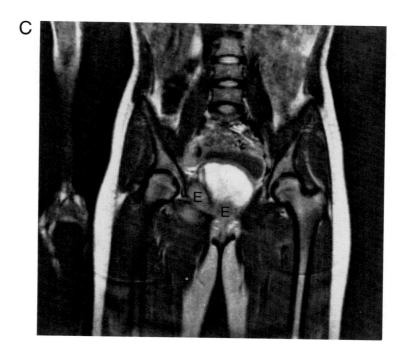

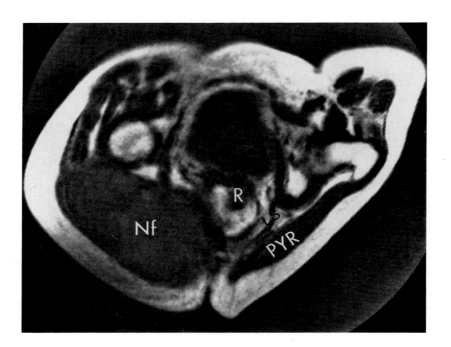

FIG 12–74.

Right pelvic neurofibrosarcoma. T$_1$-weighted axial scan (TR, 0.7 sec; TE, 35 msec): An 80-year-old woman with a history of endometrial carcinoma presented with right-sided sciatica. A large soft tissue mass arising in the region of the right lumbosacral plexus and right piriform muscle was re- vealed by MRI. The mass (*Nf,* neurofibrosarcoma) extends into the posterior pelvis and displaces the rectum *(R)* to the left while also extending laterally around the right acetabulum. A CT-guided biopsy indicated malignant neurofibrosarcoma. Note the normal left piriform muscle *(PYR)* and lumbosacral plexus region *(LS).*

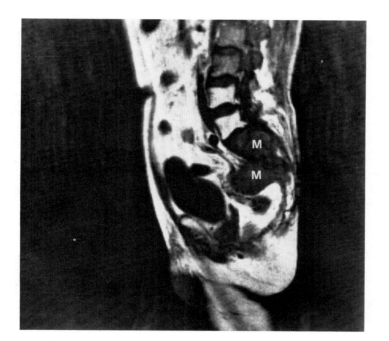

FIG 12–75.

Sacral myeloma. T_1 sagittal scan (TR, 0.5 sec; TE, 35 msec): The sacral and coccygeal structures are best defined on sagittal MRI scans. In this 60-year-old man with sacral pain, notice the large soft tissue mass *(M)* destroying portions of the sacrum and coccyx. The solitary mass was shown by biopsy to be a plasmacytoma. Note the sharp definition of the anterior aspect of the mass by the retrorectal fat.

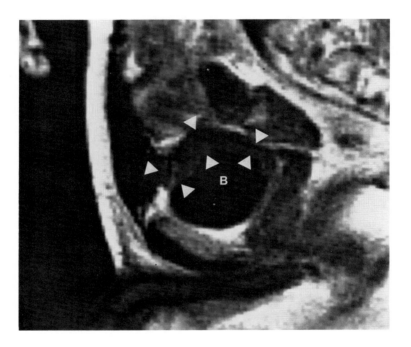

FIG 12–76.
Carcinoma of the urinary bladder. T$_2$ sagittal scan (TR, 2.1 sec; TE, 35 msec): Magnetic resonance imaging is useful in the diagnosis and staging of primary carcinomas of the urinary bladder. Note the marked thickening of the anterosuperior wall of the urinary bladder in this 58-year-old man with a proved adenocarcinoma of the urinary bladder (*arrowheads* indicate the bladder tumor).

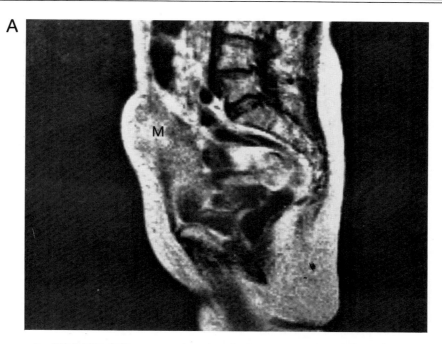

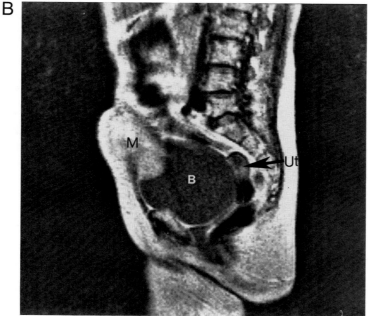

FIG 12–77.

Carcinoma of the urachus. A 32-year-old woman complained of umbilical crusting and a periumbilical mass.

A, T_2 sagittal scan (TR, 2.1 sec; TE, 35 msec): On this sagittal MRI scan, there is a vague area of midrange signal intensity in the space of Retzius that is causing a bulge along the periumbilical portion of the anterior abdominal wall. The urinary bladder is not filled, and the definition of the mass *(M)* in relation to the urinary bladder is poor.

B, T_2 sagittal scan (TR, 2.1 sec; TE, 35 msec): Note the marked improvement in the definition of the urachal carcinoma with the urinary bladder now filled. The mass *(M)* in the space of Retzius is noted to indent the anterosuperior aspect of the urinary bladder *(B)* in a manner characteristic of urachal carcinoma. Carcinoma of the urachus is a rare primary tumor that usually presents as a soft tissue mass in the space of Retzius (*Ut,* uterus).

13

Advances in Nuclear Imaging of Abdominal and Pelvic Malignancies

Donald A. Podoloff, M.D.

Lamk M. Lamki, M.D.

Nuclear medicine imaging since its inception has been closely allied with oncology, beginning in the 1940s with the introduction of iodine 131 for the diagnosis and treatment of thyroid cancer and its detection with stationary uptake probes.[1] This connection[2–6] progressed from Cassen's development in the 1950s of a scanning instrument using isotopes of mercury (used in brain tumors)[2] and the development of a stationary gamma camera for imaging brain tumors, liver, and spleen[3] to clinical application of radioimmunoassay[4] in the 1960s. During the 1960s and 1970s, the development of technetium 99m labeled compounds allowed nuclear physicians to examine the liver and spleen, cardiac blood pool, and osseous structures.[5–7]

Also in the 1970s, the first commercial availability of computer software for nuclear medicine and the almost simultaneous recognition that red cells could be successfully labeled with technetium 99m pertechnetate (in the presence of the reducing agent stannous ion) led to extensive evaluation of the cardiovascular system. Doxorubicin, a drug long used in the therapy of cancer patients, has significant cardiovascular toxicity when used in doses large enough to be tumoricidal. The ability to serially follow cardiac function over time has greatly enhanced the effectiveness of this agent in a wide variety of malignancies.[8–10] In fact, at many institutions where patients with cancer are treated, 15% to 20% of the work done in nuclear medicine is concerned with evaluation of the cardiovascular system by noninvasive techniques.

More recently, the development of positron-emission tomography (PET) has suggested that the ability to examine the metabolic effects of various tumor and tumorlike agents is at hand, but this ability, although feasible in principle, has yet to be evaluated in very many clinical centers.[11] Single photon-emission computed tomography (SPECT) has enabled us to use analogues labeled with ^{99m}Tc to demonstrate the three-dimensional distribution of various radioactive agents employed in the diagnosis of malignancies. The wide availability of gamma cameras and the low cost of SPECT imaging relative to either computed tomography (CT) or PET suggest that this technology represents another leap forward in the continuing battle with cancer.[12] Further, the nuclear medicine physician stands on the threshold of an entirely new era because the development of specific monoclonal antibodies (MoAbs), which can specifically target tumor tissue, offers promise in both immunodetection and immunotherapy. This technology is already being applied in melanoma, lymphoma, and colorectal cancer.[13–17]

Nevertheless, it must be recognized that the application of more conventional radionuclides in the evaluation of abdominal and pelvic malignancies has undergone rather fundamental changes recently. The number of liver-spleen scintigraphic studies performed in most institutions has decreased rather precipitously in response to the failure of these studies to successfully compete with such diagnostic modalities as CT and sonography. Although the sensitivities of liver scintigraphy, CT, and ultrasound are fairly close, CT and ultrasound are much superior because of the information they provide about disease sites adjacent to the liver and spleen.[18]

However, new techniques that assure nuclear imaging a place in the future in the management of neoplasms of the abdomen and pelvis have recently been introduced. The list includes gastrointestinal bleeding scintigraphy, biliary scintigraphy, hepatic and splenic catheter placement and perfusion studies, adrenocortical and medullary scintigraphy, and scintigraphy of the genitourinary tract to evaluate the presence and extent of outflow obstruction and differential renal function.[19–22] Catheter studies at other sites in the abdomen and pelvis have been introduced and are used prior to chemotherapy since they provide a method of determining the distribution of microspheres and presumably of tumoricidal drugs downstream from a particular arterial site.[23] Finally, as previously mentioned, imaging utilizing MoAbs is a rapidly growing area that promises a great deal.

It is the purpose of this chapter to demonstrate the usefulness of modern techniques available in nuclear medicine to the evaluation of malignancies of the abdomen and pelvis. We will discuss in general terms planar and tomographic imaging in the evaluation of such malignancies, and we will demonstrate the use of newer, more specific radiopharmaceuticals in the diagnosis of these malignancies.

As more tissue-specific agents become available, nuclear imaging will be able to take advantage of their ability to image physiologic events rather than anatomical structures. To some degree, this is already happening in the field of MoAbs, where tumor-specific antigens are targets of specific antibodies. The specific monoclonal antibodies are labeled with ^{131}I, ^{111}In, or, more recently, ^{99m}Tc for diagnosis of various malignancies of the abdomen and pelvis. However, when the same MoAbs are tagged with large doses of ^{131}I or beta-emitting yttrium 90, therapeutic potential exists. It should be noted that this particular endeavor is being pursued vigorously by several workers, including commercial manufacturers.[24–26]

Additional examples of tissue specificity are the use of (1) ^{99m}Tc-labeled neoglycolic acid derivatives to image hepatic protein-binding sites and (2) antiferritin antibodies tagged with ^{131}I in the diagnosis and therapy of hepatomas.[27]

IMAGING WITH MONOCLONAL ANTIBODIES

Immunoscintigraphy in oncology is gradually moving to the clinic from the laboratory[28–32] as more clinically useful antibodies become available. Progress has been fairly slow because of the magnitude of the problems involved: (1) finding a highly immunoreactive monoclonal antibody (MoAb) that has high specificity for a given type of tumor and low reactivity with other tissue antigens and (2) selecting the appropriate radioisotope. However, enough progress can be claimed to justify the optimism associated with the current clinical trials. Several MoAbs are now on trial in abdominal and pelvic cancers. In most cases, the antibodies are produced by fusion of myeloma cells with mouse lymphocytes (splenocytes) sensitized to a specific antigen of the tumor of interest (e.g., carcinoembryonic antigen [CEA] of colon cancer). The two cells fuse while in culture with the help of polyethylene glycol. The resultant hybrid cells, which have properties of the lymphocyte and of myeloma cells, produce antibodies while they grow as "hybridomas" in the peritoneal cavities of other mice. The ascitic fluid produced contains the desired MoAb. Several trial and separation procedures are often necessary before the desired clone emerges. Monoclonal antibodies produced in this way are then labeled with a gamma-emitting radioisotope such as ^{131}I, ^{123}I, or ^{111}In. When injected intravenously, the labeled antibody will localize in tumors that contain the antigens against which the antibodies are directed. Unfortunately, some normal tissues may have that antigen (e.g., CEA is found in many tissues other than colon cancer). Some nonspecific localization of the labeled antibody also takes place (e.g., in the liver).

At M. D. Anderson Hospital, we have evaluated ZCE-025, which is an anti-CEA MoAb for the detection of metastatic colon cancer. It is an IgG1 immunoglobulin that reacts with a specific site (epitope) on the CEA molecule. We have also used it for the detection of occult colon malignancies in patients who have rising levels of serum CEA but no obvious recurrent disease by such other investigations as CT, ultrasound, and barium studies. Labeled with ^{111}In, ZCE-025 can detect approximately 80% of the known colon metastases.[32] Like several other ^{111}In-labeled MoAbs, ^{111}In-ZCE-025 localizes normally in several normal tissues, specifically the liver (Fig 13–1), an effect that lowers the target:background ratio. To block the normal liver uptake, we infused unlabeled ZCE-025 in varying doses mixed with ^{111}In-labeled ZCE-025. We found that the best mixture to infuse was 1 mg of the ^{111}In-labeled and 40 mg of the unlabeled ZCE-025 antibody.[33]

We are currently studying fragments of the anti-CEA antibody. Monoclonal antibodies are usually IgGs that can be digested by the enzyme papain to give an Fc fragment (constant-end fragment) and two Fab fragments (antibody-binding fragments). Treatment of the IgG molecule with pepsin results in a double F(ab')$_2$ fragment and an incomplete Fc fragment. The fragments can also be labeled with appropriate radioisotope (e.g., ^{131}I or ^{111}In) and they have certain advantages over the whole antibody for imaging metastases. The Fab and F(ab')$_2$ retain the antigen-binding capacity but not the Fc fragment. Compared with the whole antibody, each has a shorter half-life in the blood pool and localizes less in the liver, resulting in a better target:background ratio. We have used the F(ab')$_2$ fragment and labeled it with ^{111}In-chloride. Indium 111 has certain advantages over [131]I.[34] We have found the fragments to result in a lower liver uptake and greater sensitivity for detecting metastases (Fig 13–2). Other workers are currently studying other MoAbs directed against colon cancer antigens besides CEA (e.g., the MoAb 17-1A and its F(ab')$_2$ fragment).[35] Overall, immunoimaging of colon cancer and its metastases has come a long way since the initial work with radiolabeled polyclonal antibodies.[36]

The other MoAb that we have studied is the anti–prostatic acid phosphatase (anti-PAP) PAY-276, labeled with 5 mCi of ^{111}In-chloride. The highest detection rate of metastases (sensitivity) was achieved when 1 mg of labeled MoAb was mixed and co-infused with 80 mg of unlabeled PAY-276. As we increased the amount of unlabeled antibody co-infused with the 1 mg of ^{111}In-labeled MoAb, the metastatic detection rate improved until the 80-mg dose was reached.[31] Similar findings were observed with other ^{111}In-labeled MoAbs, although the dose for peak sensitivity varied. The unlabeled MoAbs appear to block the liver uptake of the ^{111}In-labeled antibody, allowing more to localize in metastatic lesions and other tissues. Sensitivity was highest for

bony metastases (Fig 13–3), but the soft tissue lesions, including the prostate primary, could occasionally be seen.

We have had fairly extensive experience in assessing for abdominopelvic metastatic disease in patients with melanoma. We have used two ^{111}In-labeled murine MoAbs: the first is the 96.5,[29] which is an IgG2a directed against the melanoma surface antigen P97, and the other is ZME-018,[30] also an IgG2a but directed against the high molecular weight antigen (HMWA) of melanoma. One milligram of each MoAb was labeled with 5 mCi of ^{111}In and mixed with the respective unlabeled MoAb, the mixture then infused into the patient. The detection rate was between 75% and 81% of known metastatic lesions (Fig 13–4). We are at present evaluating the anti-p97 MoAb using the "chase-pulse" method of administration rather than the co-infusion method. In this study, rather than infusing the labeled mixed with the unlabeled MoAb, we inject the unlabeled antibody intravenously (chase) prior to injecting the labeled antibody (pulse); the interval between the two is either 1 or 24 hr. This method may improve the sensitivity for metastatic detection; there are indications so far that this is the case.

To improve on the target:background ratio, we are now trying a Fab fragment of a melanoma antibody instead of the whole antibody, namely, NRX-118.07.03, which is a Fab fragment of the IgG MoAb NR-ML-05 directed against a 250-kilodalton glycoprotein antigen of melanoma. To increase the photon flux, and hence the imaging characteristic, we are now trying the ^{99m}Tc label instead of ^{111}In-chloride. Technetium 99m–labeled MoAbs and their Fab fragments have the advantage of same-day imaging, compared with the 72-hr delay necessary when ^{111}In-labeled MoAbs are used.[34] Technetium 99m also gives better images than ^{111}In, but it is too early to comment on sensitivity and specificity. Other investigators have used ^{131}I for labeling various MoAbs, but one has to sacrifice image quality when using this high-energy (364-KeV) photon and also there is the dose-limiting property of the beta emissions of [131]I. In Europe, an antibody to human milk fat globule (HMFG$_2$) antigen has been labeled with ^{131}I and used to identify ovarian cancer; this technique is not yet widely used in the United States. The place of immunoscintigraphy is not established as yet in the diagnostic algorithm of abdominal and pelvic oncology. However, this place should be better defined as antibody purification techniques are improved and higher specificity achieved. Also, the availability of human MoAbs in the future will eliminate the problems inherent in the use of murine antibodies. An isotope label combining all the desirable features of ^{99m}Tc, ^{111}In, and ^{131}I has yet to be found for diagnostic radioimmunoimaging. Progress in immunotherapy is partly dependent on the previously described advancements needed in diagnostic imaging, but some therapeutic success is already evident with large doses of ^{131}I-labeled MoAbs,[17, 28] and other workers are experimenting with ^{90}Y-labeled MoAbs, an approach that relies on the high flux of beta emissions of the ^{90}Y for radiation effect.

SCINTIGRAPHY OF THE BILIARY SYSTEM AND IN GASTROINTESTINAL BLEEDING

Since patients who harbor malignancies can, of course, also fall victim to the same diseases as others, imaging of the gallbladder and biliary tree has been of significant value in the evaluation of cancer patients with acute cholecystitis, chemical cholecystitis, diffuse hepatocellular disease, and hepatic biliary obstruction (Fig 13–5).[22]

In recent years, radionuclide techniques for the evaluation of gastrointestinal hemorrhage have become first-line and paramount. It is common practice to perform a radionuclide study to evaluate the site of gastrointestinal bleeding before angiography.[37, 38]

SINGLE PHOTON–EMISSION COMPUTED TOMOGRAPHY IN ABDOMINAL AND PELVIC MALIGNANCIES

Patients with hematologic and myeloproliferative disorders have been followed in the past by liver-spleen studies for evaluation of the size of these organs as chemotherapy progresses. More recently, the ability to better quantitate size in these organs has been provided by SPECT (Figs 13–6 and 13–7). One can more accurately and more objectively assess organ response to a variety of therapeutic interventions (Fig 13–8). Moreover, SPECT imaging has demonstrated significant improvement in sensitivity with respect to the evaluation of diffuse hepatocellular disease, whether it is due to chemotherapeutic effect or to miliary metastases (Fig 13–9).[39]

The ability to quantitate lesion response to various chemotherapeutic interventions in the liver and spleen, and elsewhere in the abdomen and pelvis, is being vigorously explored now that SPECT is a routine technology. Early experimental findings and clinical work have demonstrated an excellent correlation between lesion size as measured by SPECT and actual-volume measurements.[40]

MOTILITY STUDIES

Evaluation of therapeutic response in patients with carcinoma of the esophagus has been facilitated by radionuclide evaluation of esophageal motility. Similarly, patients with obstructing lesions of the stomach can undergo a noninvasive radionuclide gastric-emptying study to check progress after surgical or chemotherapeutic interventions (Fig 13–10).[41]

CATHETER PLACEMENT STUDIES

With the introduction of advanced subselective catheterization techniques in the abdomen and pelvis, radionuclide perfusion imaging has proved to be the mainstay in the noninvasive evaluation of these radiologic interventions. Tumors of mesenchymal origin and fibrosarcomas and sarcomas of the abdomen and pelvis have been evaluated by these perfusion techniques. The patient's clinical course and his or her response to chemotherapy can be followed serially (Figs 13–11 to 13–16).[42, 43]

LYMPHOSCINTIGRAPHY

Lymphoscintigraphy has proved valuable in the evaluation of patterns of lymph node drainage in patients with melanoma. Additionally, specific radionuclide antimelanoma antibodies have been used with the lymphoscintigraphy technique to provide better preoperative evaluation in patients with melanoma.[44] After intradermal injection of ^{99m}Tc-labeled colloid compounds around the lesion, visualization of regional lymph nodes is possible and indicative of the lymphatic drainage of the area of the lesion (Fig 13–17). Although it is not possible generally to determine whether or not these lymph nodes are pathologic, the fact that the radiocolloid drains into them suggests that tumor cells can behave in a similar fashion and thus lymph node dissection would seem to be indicated.[44] If one uses a MoAb specific to melanoma antigen, the possibility of having a more tissue-specific lymphoscintigraphy exists. Work in this area is under way in many centers throughout the country, including a study at M. D. Anderson Hospital. Early results are quite encouraging.

RENAL AND HEPATIC FUNCTION STUDIES

In the evaluation of pelvic and genitourinary neoplasms that can cause urinary tract obstruction, the diuretic renal study has been of inestimable value. It is possible to noninvasively quantitate differential renal function and to objectively follow the response to various therapeutic interventions (Fig 13–18).[45]

Specific protein-binding substances tagged with ^{99m}Tc can be used to assess hepatocyte-binding function. It is possible in patients with severe liver disease secondary to malignancy to better depict the distribution of normal and abnormal hepatocytes by using this technique.[46, 47]

ENDOCRINE STUDIES

The entire field of radiopharmaceutical specificity is under review at present. The potential for nuclear imaging techniques to be of value in endocrinology is being pursued by numerous investigators. The introduction of iodocholesterol for the detection of adrenal cortical lesions was rapidly followed by the introduction of *meta*-iodobenzyl-guanidine (MIBG) for the evaluation and therapy of adrenal medullary and extraadrenal medullary tumors throughout the abdomen and pelvis (Fig 13–19).[19, 20, 48]

VENOUS FLOW STUDIES

The management of patients with malignancies has been enhanced by the use of nuclear medicine techniques that have rather general applicability. Included in this area are flow studies to evaluate the vascularity of lesions (Fig 13–20) and venous obstruction of the upper and lower extremities (Figs 13–21 and 13–22).

GALLIUM STUDIES

Gallium 67 citrate has long been a valuable clinical tumor seeker. It has served the medical community well in the diagnosis of malignancies in the abdomen and pelvis (Figs 13–23 to 13–26). Additionally, it has been one of the few tumor-seeking agents that have been routinely available to the general nuclear medicine practitioner. Lately, ^{67}Ga imaging has to some extent been replaced by CT. However, it continues to be valuable in patients with lymphoma who have demonstrated iodine sensitivity and who thus are not candidates for lymphangiography, and it is of extreme value in following pulmonary effects of bleomycin therapy.[49, 50] Cobalt 57 has been tried unsuccessfully for clinical use.[51]

THE FUTURE

The use of serial bone scans to assess a given patient's response to various chemotherapeutic interventions is well accepted and continues to account for nearly half the work in most oncological nuclear medicine departments.[52] This approach will likely continue to be an important diagnostic tool for the oncologist. At present, planar imaging and tomographic scanning of the liver and spleen appear to be playing significant roles in the evaluation of therapeutic response in various lymphomas and leukemias. What contribution SPECT imaging is to make is now being evaluated.[53]

Additionally, standard ventilation-perfusion studies, abscess localization with ^{111}In-labeled white blood cells, and colloid bone marrow scintigraphy have been shown to be valuable in the management of patients with malignancies (Fig 13–27).

Newer technologies, in particular PET and MRI, promise to become important in the management of patients with a variety of pelvic and abdominal malignancies.[54, 55]

REFERENCES

1. Allen H.C. Jr., Risser J.R., Greene J.A.: Improvements in outlining of thyroid and localization of brain tumors by the application of sodium iodine gamma-ray spectrometry techniques, in *Proceedings of the Second Oxford Radioisotope Conference*. New York, Academic Press, 1954, vol. 1, pp. 76–96.
2. Cassen B., Curtis L., Reed C., et al.: Instrumentation of ^{131}I used in medical studies. *Nucleonics* 9:46, 1951.
3. Anger H.O., Van Dyke D.C., Gottschalk A., et al.: The scintillation camera in diagnosis and research. *Nucleonics* 23:57, 1965.
4. Berson S.A., Yalow R.S.: Quantitative aspects of the reaction between insulin and insulin-binding antibody. *J. Clin. Invest.* 38:1996–2016, 1959.

5. Moreno J.B., Deland F.H.: Brain scanning in the diagnosis of astrocytomas of the brain. *J. Nucl. Med.* 12:107–111, 1975.

6. Citrin D.L., Bessent R.G., Grieg W.R.: A comparison of the sensitivity and accuracy of the ^{99m}Tc-phosphate bone scan and skeletal radiograph in the diagnosis of bone metastases. *Clin. Radiol.* 28:107–117, 1977.

7. Bitran J.D., Bekerman C., Desser R.K.: The predictive value of serial bone scans in assessing response to chemotherapy in advanced breast cancer. *Cancer* 45:1562–1568, 1980.

8. Blum R.M., Carter S.K.: Adriamycin: a new anticancer drug with significant clinical activity. *Ann. Intern. Med.* 80:249–259, 1974.

9. Minow R.A., Benjamin R.S., Lee E.T.: Adriamycin cardiomyopathy—risk factors. *Cancer* 39:1397–1402, 1977.

10. Alexander J., Dainiak N., Berger H.J., et al.: Serial assessment of doxorubicin cardiotoxicity with quantitative radionuclide angiocardiography. *N. Engl. J. Med.* 300:278–283, 1979.

11. Larson S.M., Grunbaum Z., Rasey J.S.: Positron imaging feasibility studies: selective tumor concentration of ^{3}H-thymidine, ^{3}H-uridine and ^{14}C-2-deoxyglucose. *Radiology* 134:771–773, 1980.

12. Cowan R.J., Watson N.E.: Special characteristics and potential of single photon emission computed tomography in the brain. *Semin. Nucl. Med.* 10:335–344, 1980.

13. Goldenberg D.M., Kim E.E., Bennett S.J., et al.: Carcinoembryonic antigen radioimmunodetection in the evaluation of colorectal cancer and in the detection of occult neoplasms. *Gastroenterology* 84:524–532, 1983.

14. Larson S.M., Carrasquillo J.A.: Nuclear oncology 1984. *Semin. Nucl. Med.* 14:268–276, 1984.

15. Berche C., Mach J.P., Lumbroso J.D., et al.: Tomoscintigraphy for detecting gastrointestinal and medullary thyroid cancers: first clinical results using radio-labelled monoclonal antibodies against carcinoembryonic antigen. *Br. Med. J. (Clin. Res.)* 285:1447–1451, 1982.

16. Halpern S.E., Dillman R.O., Witztum K.F., et al.: Radioimmunodetection of melanoma utilizing ^{111}In 96.5 monoclonal antibody: a preliminary report. *Radiology* 155:493–499, 1985.

17. Carrasquillo J.A., Krohn K.A., Beaumier P., et al.: Diagnosis and therapy of solid tumors with radiolabeled Fab. *Cancer Treat. Rep.* 68:317–328, 1984.

18. Harbert J.C.: Efficacy of bone and liver scanning in malignant diseases: facts and opinions, in Freeman L.M., Weissmann H.S. (eds): *Nuclear Medicine Annual 1982.* New York, Raven Press, 1982, pp. 373–401.

19. McEwan A.J., Shapiro B., Sisson J.C., et al.: Radioiodobenzylguanidine for the scintigraphic location and therapy of adrenergic tumors. *Semin. Nucl. Med.* 15:132–151, 1985.

20. Munkner T.: ^{131}I-*meta*-iodobenzylguanidine scintigraphy of neuroblastomas. *Semin. Nucl. Med.* 15:154–160, 1985.

21. Carrasco C.H., Freeny P.C., Chuang V.P., et al.: Chemical cholecystitis associated with hepatic artery infusion chemotherapy. *AJR* 141:703–706, 1983.

22. Weissmann H.S., Berkowitz D., Fox M.S., et al.: The role of technetium-99m IDA cholescintigraphy in acute acalculous cholecystitis. *Radiology* 146:177–180, 1983.

23. Bledin A.G., Kim E.E., Harle T.S., et al.: Technetium-99m-labeled macroaggregated albumin arteriography for detection of abnormally positioned arterial catheters during infusion chemotherapy. *Cancer* 53:858–862, 1984.

24. Mitchell M.S., Oettgen H.F. (eds): *Hybridomas in Cancer Diagnosis and Treatment.* Progress in Cancer Research and Therapy. New York, Raven Press, vol. 21, 1982.

25. Gold P., Freedman S.O.: Demonstration of tumor-specific antigens in human colonic carcinomata by immunological tolerance and absorption techniques. *J. Exp. Med.* 121:439–462, 1965.

26. Solter D., Ballou B., Feilan J., et al.: Radioimmunodetection of tumors using monoclonal antibodies, in Mitchell M.S., Oettgen H.F. (eds): *Hybridomas in Cancer Diagnosis and Treatment.* Progress in Cancer Research and Therapy. New York, Raven Press, 1982, vol. 21, pp. 241–244.

27. Order S.E., Klein J.L., Ettinger D., et al.: Use of isotopic immunoglobulin in therapy. *Cancer Res.* 40:3001–3007, 1980.

28. Keenan A.M., Harbert J.C., Larson S.M.: Monoclonal antibodies in nuclear medicine. *J. Nucl. Med.* 26:531–537, 1985.

29. Murray J.L., Rosenblum M.B., Sobol R.E., et al.: Radioimmunoimaging in malignant melanoma with ^{111}In-labeled monoclonal antibody 96.5. *Cancer Res.* 45:2376–2381, 1985.

30. Murray J.L., Rosenblum M.G., Lamki L., et al.: Clinical parameters related to optimal tumor localization of indium-111-labeled mouse antimelanoma monoclonal antibody ZME-018. *J. Nucl. Med.* 28:25–33, 1987.

31. Babaian R.J., Murray J.L., Lamki L., et al.: Radioimmunoimaging of metastatic prostatic cancer using ^{111}In-labeled monoclonal antibody PAY-276. *J. Urol.* 137:439–443, 1987.

32. Lamki L.M., Patt Y.Z., Murray J.L., et al.: Scintigraphic findings of colonic cancer using indium-111-labeled anti-CEA monoclonal antibody (ZCE-025) combined with unlabeled antibody [abstract 593]. *J. Nucl. Med.* 27:1021, 1986.

33. Lamki L., Murray J.L., Rosenblum M., et al.: Effect of unlabeled monoclonal antibody (MoAb) on biodistribution of indium-111 labelled MoAb. *Nucl. Med. Commun.* (in press).

34. Fairweather D.S., Bradwell A.M., Dykes P.W., et al.: Improved tumour localisation using indium-111-la-

belled antibodies. *Br. Med. J. (Clin. Res.)* 287:167–170, 1983.

35. Moldofsky P.J., Powe, J., Hammond N.D.: Monoclonal antibodies for radioimmunoimaging: current perspectives, in Freeman L.M., Weissmann H.S. (eds.): *Nuclear Medicine Annual 1986.* New York, Raven Press, 1986, pp. 57–103.

36. Goldenberg D.M., Deland F., Kim E., et al.: Use of radiolabeled antibodies to carcinoembryonic antigen for the detection and localization of diverse cancers by external photoscanning. *N. Engl. J. Med.* 298: 1384–1386, 1978.

37. Alavi A., Dann R.W., Baum S., et al.: Scintigraphic detection of acute gastrointestinal bleeding. *Radiology* 124:753–756, 1977.

38. Bunker S.R., Brown J.M., McAuley R.J., et al.: Detection of gastrointestinal bleeding sites: use of in vitro Tc-99m-labeled RBCs. *JAMA* 12:789–792, 1982.

39. Ell P.J., Khan O.: Emission computerized tomography: clinical applications. *Semin. Nucl. Med.* 11:50–60, 1981.

40. Mansfield C.M., Park C.H.: Contribution of radionuclide imaging to radiation oncology. *Semin. Nucl. Med.* 15:28–44, 1985.

41. Malmud L.S., Fisher R.S., Knight L.C., et al.: Scintigraphic evaluation of gastric emptying. *Semin. Nucl. Med.* 12:116–125, 1982.

42. Kim E.E., Bledin A.G., Kavanagh J., et al.: Chemotherapy of cervical carcinoma: use of Tc-99m MAA infusion to predict drug distribution. *Radiology* 150:677–681, 1984.

43. Chuang V.P., Wallace S.: Arterial infusion and occlusion in cancer patients. *Semin. Roentgenol.* 16:13–25, 1981.

44. Sugarbaker E.V., McBride C.M.: Melanoma of the trunk: the results of surgical excision and anatomic guidelines for predicting nodal metastasis. *Surgery* 80:22–30, 1976.

45. Thrall J.H., Koff S.A., Keyes J.W.: Diuretic radionuclide renography in the differential diagnosis of hydroureteronephrosis. *Semin. Nucl. Med.* 11:89–104, 1981.

46. Fritzberg A.R., Klingensmith W.C. III, Whitney W.P., et al.: Chemical and biological studies of ^{99m}Tc-N, N'-bis(mercaptoacetamido)-ethylenediamine: a potential replacement for ^{131}I-iodohippurate. *J. Nucl. Med.* 22:258–263, 1981.

47. Stadalnik R.D., Vera D.R., Woodle E.S., et al.: Technetium-99m NGA functional hepatic imaging: preliminary clinical experience. *J. Nucl. Med.* 26:1233–1242, 1985.

48. Schteingart D.E., Seabold J.E., Gross M.D., et al.: Iodocholesterol adrenal tissue uptake and imaging adrenal neoplasms. *J. Clin. Endocrinol. Metab.* 52:1156–1161, 1981.

49. Fonkalsrud E.W., Pederson B.M., Murphy J., et al.: Reduction of infusion thrombophlebitis with buffered glucose solutions. *Surgery* 63:280–284, 1968.

50. Richman D.S., Levenson S.M., Bunn P.A., et al.: ^{67}Ga accumulation in pulmonary lesions associated with bleomycin. *Cancer* 36:1966–1972, 1975.

51. Nouel J.P., Ranault H., Robert J., et al.: Lableomycin marquee au Co-57. *Nouvelle Presse Medicale* 2:95–98, 1972.

52. McNeil B.J.: Value of bone scanning in neoplastic diseases. *Semin. Nucl. Med.* 14:277–286, 1984.

53. Tumeh S.S., Rosenthal D.S., Kaplan W.D., et al.: Lymphoma: evaluation with Ga-67 SPECT. *Radiology* 164:111–114, 1987.

54. Decertaines J., Harry J.Y., Lancien G., et al.: Evaluation of human thyroid tumors by proton nuclear magnetic resonance. *J. Nucl. Med.* 23:48–51, 1982.

55. Bovee W.M., Getreuer K.W., Schmidt J., et al.: Nuclear magnetic resonance and detection of human breast tumor. *JNCI* 67:53–55, 1978.

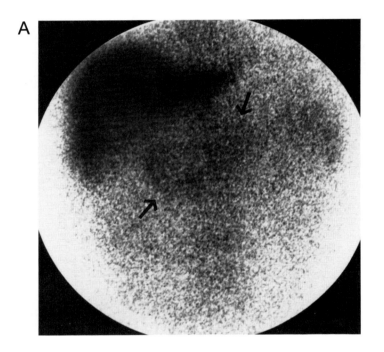

FIG 13–1.
Metastatic colon carcinoma (two examples of monoclonal antibody study).

A and **B,** five years after a colon cancer resection, this man presented with biopsy evidence of recurrent disease in several areas of the body. A ^{111}In-labeled anti-CEA MoAb (^{111}In-ZCE-025) study was undertaken.

This anterior abdomen image **(A)** was taken 72 hr after intravenous infusion of 1 mg of anti-CEA MoAb labeled with 5 mCi of ^{111}In and mixed with 20 mg of unlabeled anti-CEA MoAb in 100 mL of saline solution. Note the abnormal accumulation in the epigastrium *(arrows),* which represents a metastatic lesion from colon cancer.

A CT scan **(B)** shows the retroperitoneal adenopathy of the metastatic colon cancer, corresponding to the area of increased ^{111}In-MoAb uptake in **A.**

C, this is an anti-CEA MoAb study in another patient with metastatic colon cancer to the liver. This is a typical study showing the intense liver uptake of the ^{111}In-labeled anti-CEA. The normal liver concentrates more MoAb than do the metastases, which appear photon deficient and therefore "cold" relative to surrounding liver. This disadvantage can often be overcome by increasing the dosage of unlabeled anti-CEA MoAb to 40 mg, in which case the metastatic lesions appear "hot" because normal liver uptake is diminished (blocked) by the unlabeled MoAb.

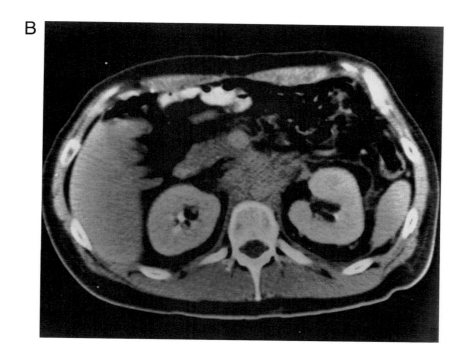

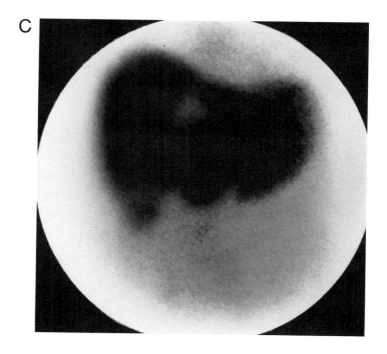

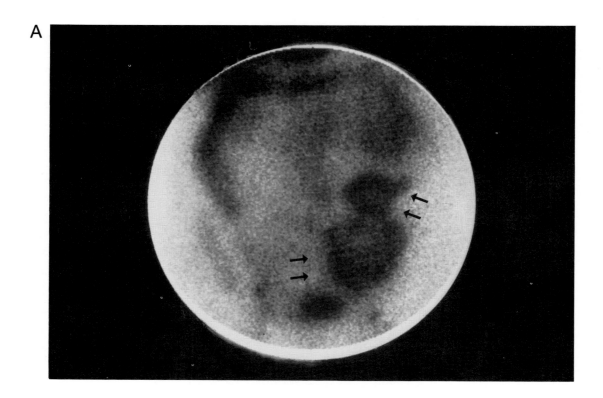

FIG 13–2.

Recurrent and metastatic colon carcinoma (two cases with monoclonal antibody study). These two patients, each with a history of colon carcinoma, underwent study with ^{111}In-labeled $F(ab')_2$ fragments of the anti-CEA MoAb ZCE-025 (**A,** patient 1; **B,** patient 2). The MoAb studies were part of reinvestigation for recurrence of the disease. In patient 1, surgical exploration following the MoAb study confirmed two tumor masses (*arrows* in **A**) in the left pelvis (recurrent colorectal carcinoma). In patient 2, surgery disclosed a metastatic lesion above the left kidney (*arrows* in **B**). Note the high uptake of the ^{111}In-labeled $F(ab')_2$ fragments in the kidneys and reduced uptake in the liver compared with the whole-antibody study in **C.**

For comparison, we show a typical scan **(C)** after intravenous injection of ^{111}In-labeled whole-antibody ZCE-025. In contrast to **A** and **B,** a significant amount of MoAb has been distributed to the liver, spleen, bones, and, to a much lesser extent, kidneys. Colon activity was seen in both whole-antibody and $F(ab')_2$-fragment studies. Note that the antibody would move in the bowel lumen with time (e.g., if we reimaged the area at 72 and 96 hr, the distribution would be different).

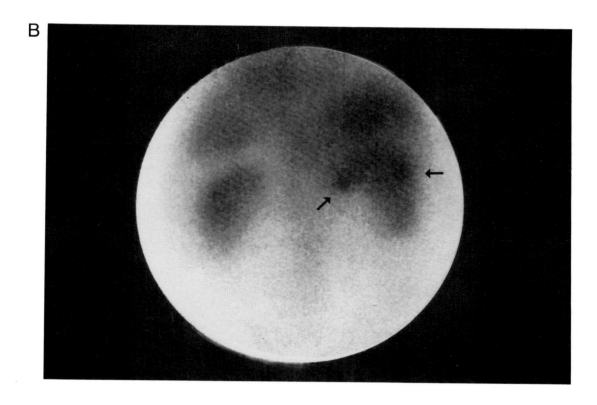

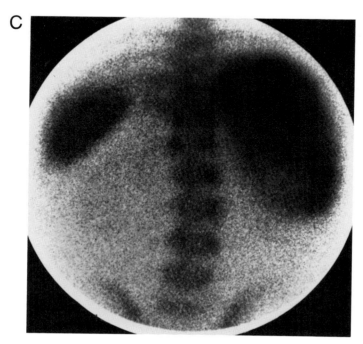

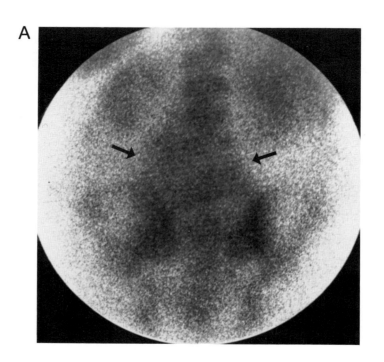

FIG 13–3.
Metastatic carcinoma of the prostate (two cases with monoclonal antibody study).

A and **B,** this patient had been operated on several years earlier for prostatic cancer. He now had known metastasis to the lumbar spine. He underwent study with ^{111}In-labeled anti-PAP MoAb PAY-276.

Image **A** was made at 144 hr following intravenous infusion of a mixture of 1 mg ^{111}In-PAY-276 mixed with 40 mg of unlabeled PAY-276. The metastatic lesion extended to the extraosseous tissues *(arrows).*

A bone scan **(B)** utilizing ^{99m}Tc-labeled methylene diphosphonate (^{99m}Tc-MDP) shows abnormal uptake of ^{99m}Tc-MDP by the calcified metastatic lesion *(arrows)*, confirming the abnormal MoAb uptake in the lumbar spine and surrounding tissues. Plain radiographs further supported these findings.

C, this second patient with a history of prostatic carcinoma underwent imaging with a smaller dosage of unlabeled PAY-276 (5 mg co-infused with 1 mg of ^{111}In-PAY-276). All the activity was localized in the liver, with none in other tissues. Compare this image with **A,** where 40 mg of unlabeled PAY-276 was used (with the labeled 1 mg). In that case **(A)**, the spleen, bones, and kidneys are well visualized. Metastases can be detected better when the preferential liver uptake of labeled MoAb is blocked by the higher dosage of unlabeled MoAb. Five milligrams was not enough to block the liver uptake in **C.**

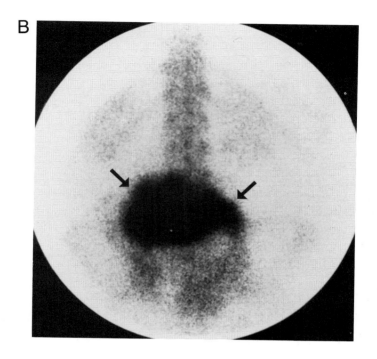

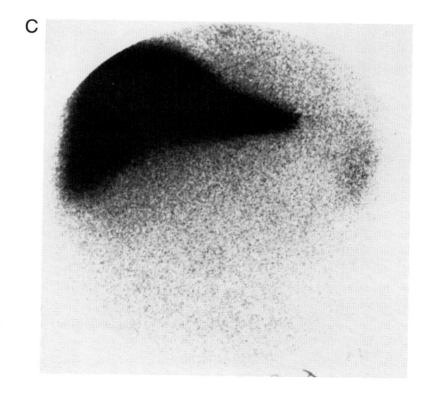

A
B

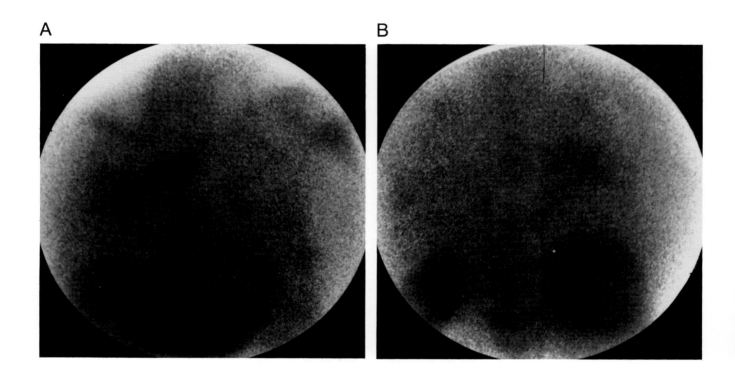

FIG 13–4.
Metastatic melanoma (three cases with monoclonal antibody study).

A and **B**, this patient with metastatic melanoma underwent imaging with ^{111}In-labeled antimelanoma ZME-018. Areas of abnormal uptake in the upper sternal region *(arrow)* and right chest wall were biopsy-proved to be metastatic lesions. Normal soft tissue background activity and liver uptake were also noted. The anterior chest image **(A)** was taken at 72 hr following intravenous infusion of 1 mg of labeled MoAb and 20 mg of unlabeled MoAb. A posterior image **(B)** of the same patient shows the right lesion even better. Clinical examination revealed the lesion to be wrapped around the chest wall and to originate in the right axilla.

C, another patient, with melanoma in the buttock area

and metastases to the pelvis, underwent imaging with ^{111}In-labeled antimelanoma 96.5 MoAb (anti-P97). The metastatic lesions *(arrows)* are seen to take up the antibody quite intensely. The nontumor distribution of ^{111}In-labeled 96.5 MoAb was somewhat similar to that of ^{111}In-ZME-018: namely, it localized in the liver, spleen, and bone marrow, with some to the kidneys and testes, but less spleen and testes uptake compared with ZME localization.

D, this scan is from another melanoma patient who also underwent study with ^{111}In-labeled anti-P97 MoAb. The image is a tomographic section of the body taken 72 hr after infusion. In the left proximal thigh, note the metastatic lesion *(arrows)* concentrating the labeled MoAb. Also note the normal liver, spleen, and bone marrow nonspecific uptake.

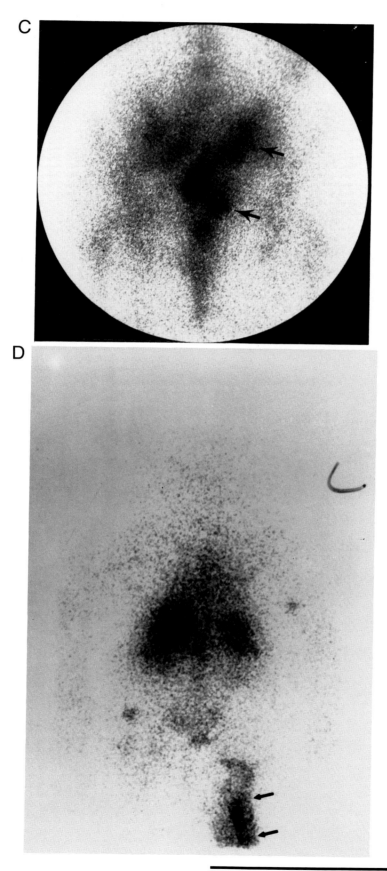

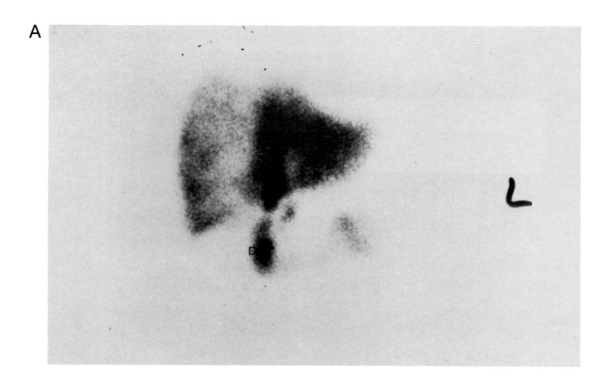

FIG 13–5.
Biliary scintigraphy in hepatoma. This 40-year-old patient with hepatocellular carcinoma presented with right upper quadrant pain, fever, and chills. Ultrasound showed non-homogeneous liver, distended gallbladder with thick wall, and ascites.

A and **B,** cholecystography demonstrates prompt visu-

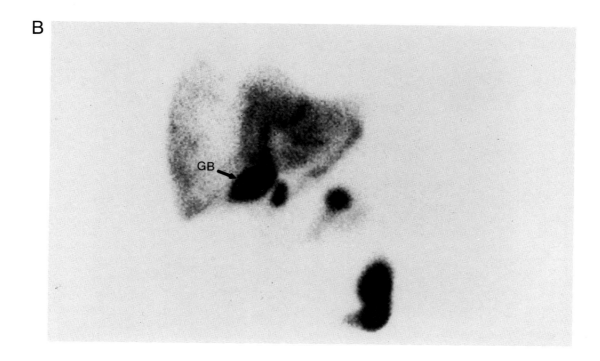

B

alization of the duodenum *(D)*, gallbladder *(GB)*, and intra-hepatic bile ducts. There is distinct preference of uptake in the left lobe of the liver because the tumor occupies large portions of the right lobe. This study helped to exclude acute cholecystitis as a diagnostic consideration in this patient.

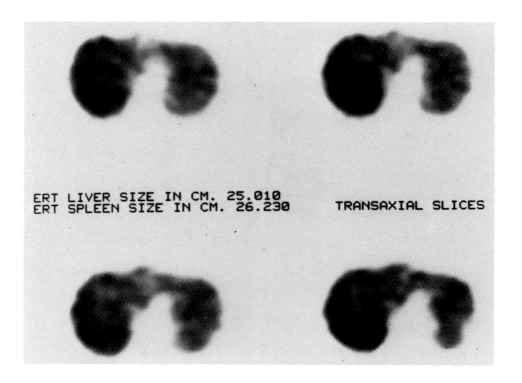

FIG 13–6.
Leukemic infiltration of the liver and spleen (SPECT evaluation). This patient is a 54-year-old woman with chronic lymphocytic leukemia. On this admission, she presented with left upper quadrant pain. Liver-spleen imaging demonstrated significant hepatosplenomegaly and multiple focal defects throughout both the liver and spleen, all better appreciated on this SPECT image. Note that vertical height of the liver and spleen is reported in centimeters.

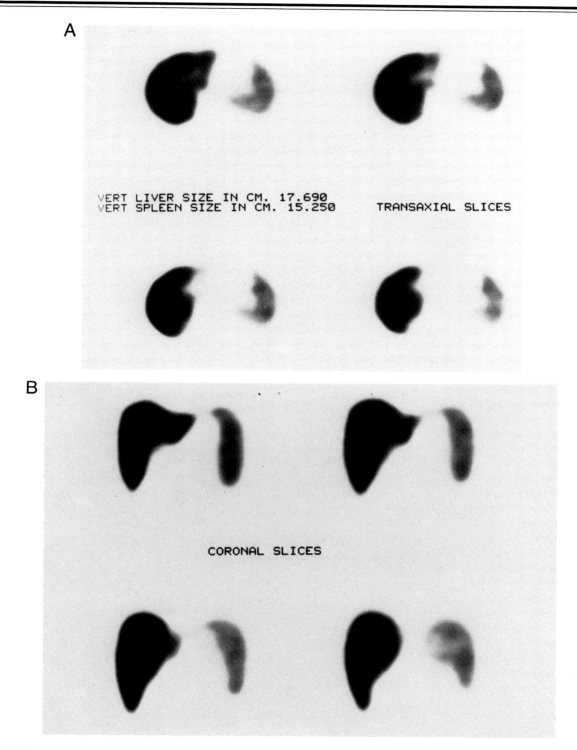

A

VERT LIVER SIZE IN CM. 17.690
VERT SPLEEN SIZE IN CM. 15.250   TRANSAXIAL SLICES

B

CORONAL SLICES

FIG 13–7.
Lymphomatous involvement of the spleen (SPECT evaluation). This patient is a 27-year-old woman with small cell lymphoma who has been receiving chemotherapy for several years.

A and **B,** the first SPECT liver study in axial **(A)** and coronal **(B)** views demonstrates an enlarged spleen with diminished activity due to lymphomatous infiltration. (*Continued.*)

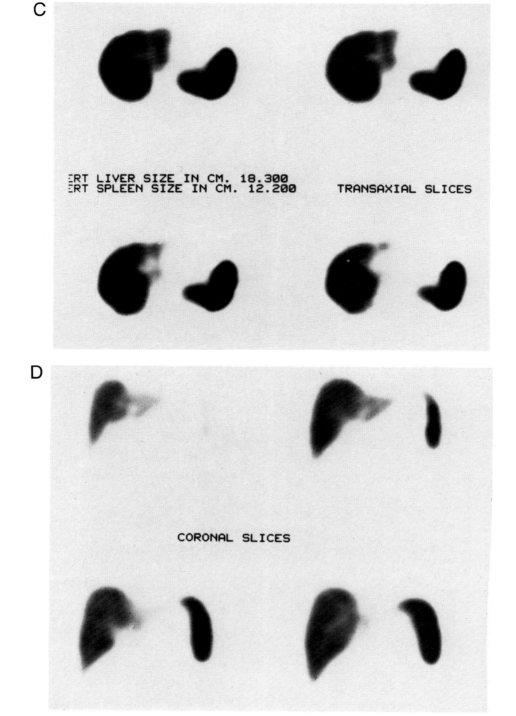

C

RT LIVER SIZE IN CM. 18.300
RT SPLEEN SIZE IN CM. 12.200   TRANSAXIAL SLICES

D

CORONAL SLICES

FIG 13–7 (cont.).
C and **D,** the corresponding second study, after treatment, demonstrates an enlarged spleen with reversal of the normal liver:spleen ratio so that the spleen is now scintigraphically more active than the liver. This increased activity in the spleen is a nonspecific finding and has been associated with a variety of hepatocellular dysfunctions and the presence of neoplasm elsewhere in the body. Note the decrease in vertical height measurement of the spleen between the two studies. Imaging by SPECT enables objective serial measurements to be made more easily than with standard planar techniques.

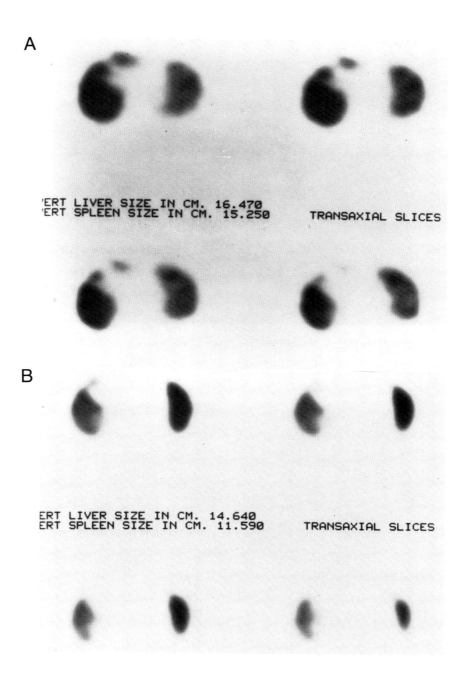

A

'ERT LIVER SIZE IN CM. 16.470
'ERT SPLEEN SIZE IN CM. 15.250   TRANSAXIAL SLICES

B

ERT LIVER SIZE IN CM. 14.640
ERT SPLEEN SIZE IN CM. 11.590   TRANSAXIAL SLICES

FIG 13–8.
Leukemic infiltration of the spleen. This patient is a 43-year-old woman with chronic lymphocytic leukemia.

A, on a SPECT study of the liver and spleen, prior to therapy, splenomegaly and multiple areas of diminished activity throughout the spleen are seen. The overall concentration of the radiopharmaceutical in the spleen, compared with the liver, is significantly diminished.

B, after therapy, a repeat liver-spleen study reveals a significant increase in splenic uptake of radiopharmaceutical and the absence of any photopenic areas. These axial SPECT images on the two studies were taken from approximately the same level in the liver and spleen and demonstrate significant shrinkage in the spleen as well as the disappearance of the previously noted abnormalities.

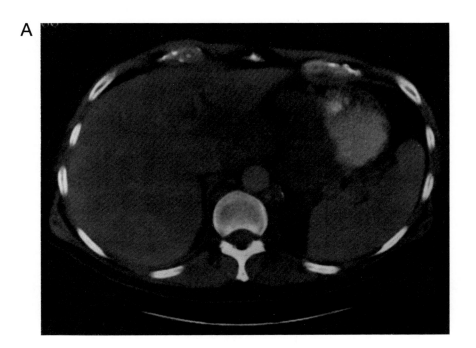

FIG 13–9.
Hodgkin's disease in the liver and spleen (SPECT evaluation). The patient is a 58-year-old man with a history of known Hodgkin's disease.

A, this CT study shows adenopathy in the gastrohepatic ligament and in the retrocrural region. The liver and spleen appear normal.

B, the static planar liver-spleen image is likewise unremarkable.

C, imaging by SPECT demonstrates multiple focal defects involving the liver and spleen.

Liver biopsy revealed a histologic pattern consistent with Hodgkin's disease.

B

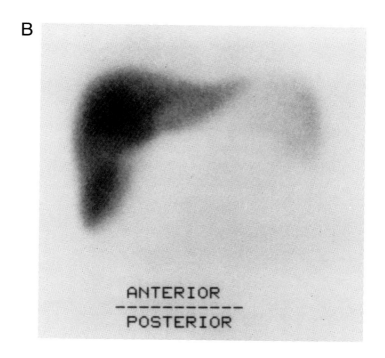

ANTERIOR

POSTERIOR

C

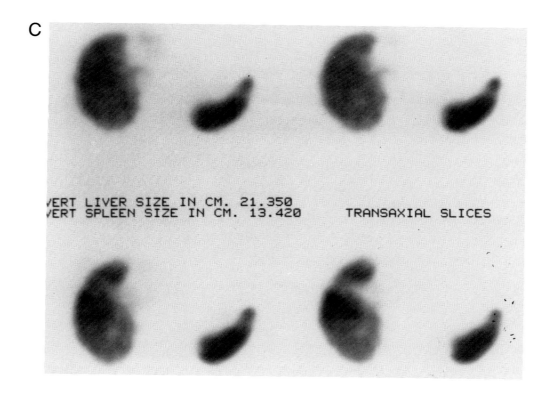

VERT LIVER SIZE IN CM. 21.350
VERT SPLEEN SIZE IN CM. 13.420   TRANSAXIAL SLICES

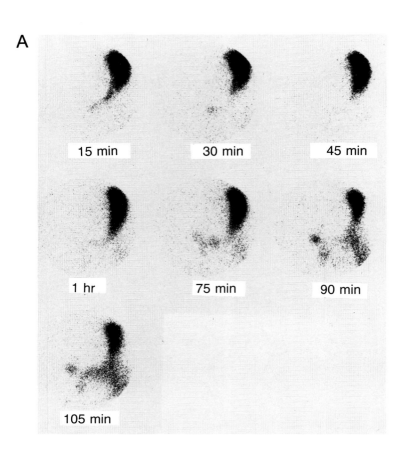

A

15 min   30 min   45 min

1 hr   75 min   90 min

105 min

FIG 13–10.
Delayed gastric emptying in a cancer patient. A 55-year-old woman with synovial cell sarcoma of the right ilium and known metastasis to L-4 presented because of recent episodes of persistent vomiting without obvious cause. An upper gastrointestinal barium examination performed during this admission was reported normal.

A, gastric emptying was studied using ^{99m}Tc-labeled sulfur colloid, some of which was scrambled with eggs and another portion of which was mixed in a glass of apple juice. Examination revealed abnormal delay in gastric emptying of solids but not of liquids. Anterior views of the stomach from

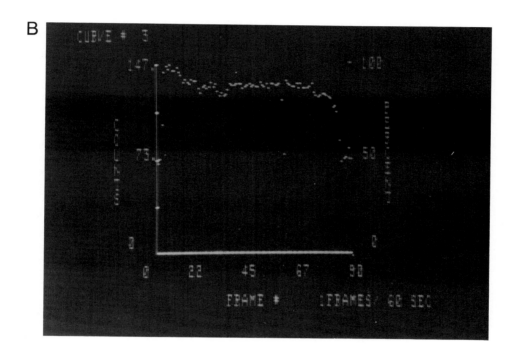

15 to 105 min show significant retention of radiolabeled gastric contents. Only about 10% of the solid meal emptied from the stomach during 1 hr (normal ≥ 50% of solid meal in 1 hr). However, 50% emptying did occur by 90 min. Such patterns have been seen as a consequence of diabetes mellitus and in other cases of gastric autonomic nervous system abnormality. This particular patient was not known to be diabetic. She did, however, have a peripheral neuropathy thought secondary to a toxic effect of chemotherapy or a primary consequence of the malignancy.

B, plot of activity as a function of time demonstrates less than 50% emptying at 1 hr.

A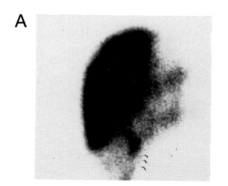

B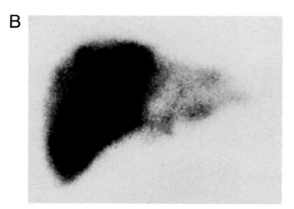

FIG 13–11.

Liver metastases (catheter diversion). The patient is a 41-year-old man with a known history of metastatic disease to the right and left lobes of the liver.

A, on the first flow study, activity is seen in the liver, predominantly in the superior lateral portion of the right lobe.

B, after therapy and after occlusion of the left hepatic artery by placement of an internal stent, there is preferential distribution of particles to the medial and inferior portions of the right lobe of the liver. This technique has been used successfully to selectively divert chemotherapy to specific tumor-bearing portions of the liver, sparing more normal areas from exposure to potentially toxic agents.

A

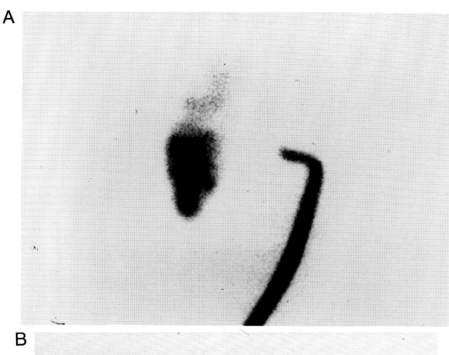

B

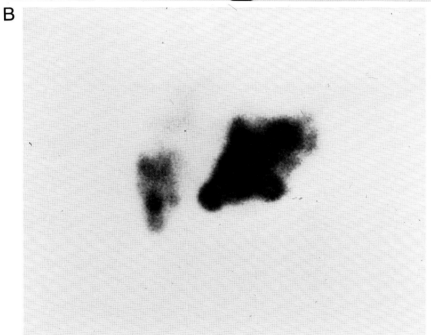

FIG 13–12.
Liver metastasis (continuous vs. pulsatile flow). This 46-year-old woman with carcinoma of the ovary metastatic to the liver was being evaluated for intraarterial chemotherapy.

A, radionuclide catheter study shows a marked difference in distribution of radioactive particles under conditions of continuous and pulsatile flow. Continuous flow to the liver goes mainly to the inferior aspect of the right lobe of the liver.

B, pulsatile flow delivers radiopharmaceutical mainly to the medial segment of the left lobe of the liver. Depending on the site and extent of lesions, a properly chosen dynamic delivery system can be used to successfully divert chemotherapy in a manner analogous to the way the particles are diverted.

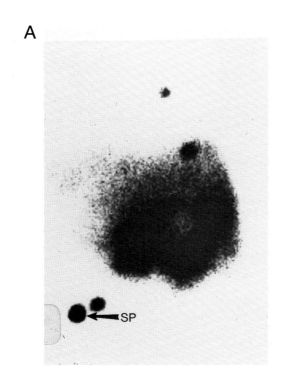

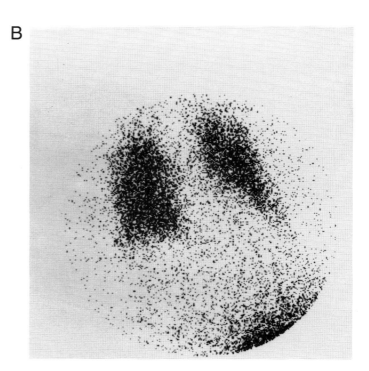

FIG 13–13.
Pelvic leiomyosarcoma (catheter placement for chemotherapy). The patient is a 55-year-old woman with a leiomyosarcoma of the left iliac fossa.

A, catheter approach via right femoral artery with tip of the catheter in the left gluteal artery demonstrates good per-fusion of the tumor mass. Most of the tumor is to the left of the midline (*SP,* symphysis pubis).

B, there is some tumor arteriovenous shunting to the lungs, resulting in significant bilateral pulmonary accumulation of radioactivity.

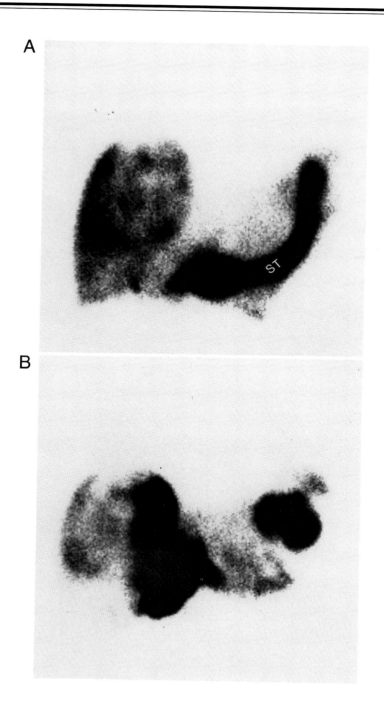

FIG 13–14.

Primary and metastatic adenocarcinoma of the liver (two cases of catheter malposition).

A and **B,** this patient is a 56-year-old man with differentiated adenocarcinoma of the liver who was to undergo regional hepatic arterial chemotherapy.

Prior to the intraarterial therapy, a radionuclide catheter placement study was done. The anterior view **(A)** reveals a large amount of activity outlining the stomach *(ST)*.

Repositioning the catheter the following day **(B)** shows activity mainly in the medial and in a portion of the lateral segment of the left lobe of the liver, with some filling of the right lobe of the liver and no gastric activity. The sequence reveals the utility of this study for checking catheter position prior to chemotherapy. (*Continued*.)

C

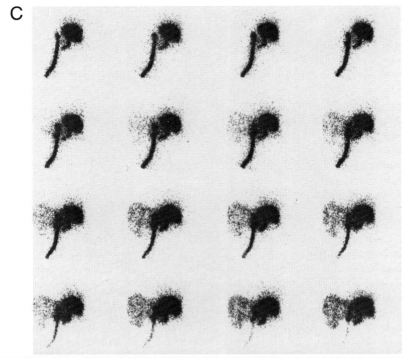

D

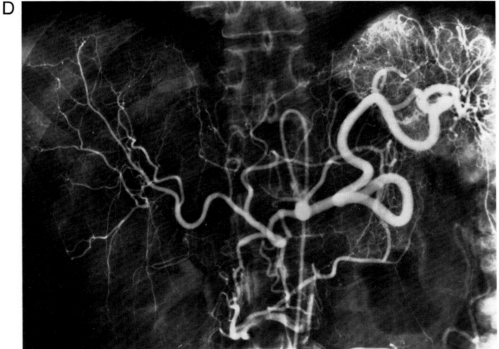

FIG 13–14 (cont.).
C through **F,** this patient is a 62-year-old woman with metastatic colon carcinoma to the liver who was a candidate for intraarterial chemotherapy.

After the catheter was angiographically positioned in the hepatic artery, the flow study **(C)** shows activity to the left upper quadrant in the region of the spleen. Repeat angiography **(D)** proved return of the tip of catheter from the hepatic artery into the celiac axis, with filling of a large, tortuous splenic artery.

By performing angiography **(E),** the catheter was secured in the hepatic artery and repeat nuclear flow study **(F)** shows activity mostly to the left lobe of the liver, with some activity to the right lobe. The catheter was then used for intraarterial chemotherapy.

E
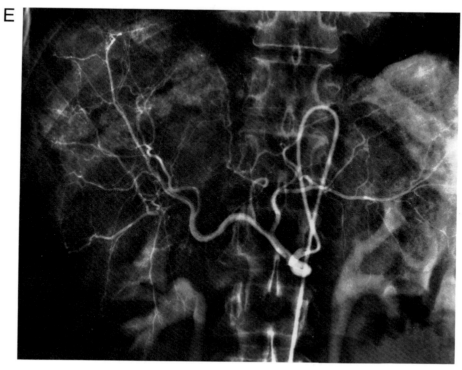

F
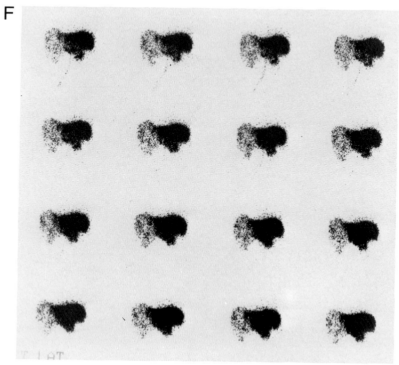

A

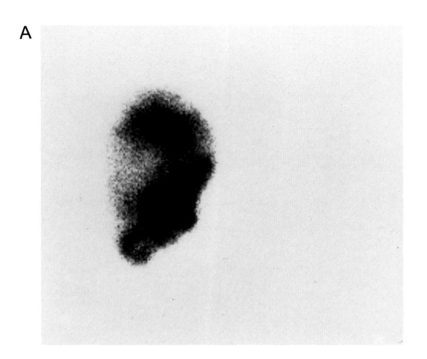

FIG 13–15.
Liver metastases (continuous vs. pulsatile flow). The patient is a 56-year-old man with colon carcinoma metastatic to the liver. Prior to infusion of regional chemotherapy, the patient underwent catheter placement study, and a marked difference in the distribution of particles under conditions of continuous or pulsatile flow was demonstrated.

A, continuous-flow study demonstrates only a small amount of perfusion to the posterior segment of the right lobe of the liver.

B, pulsatile-flow study demonstrates increased distribution of particles to the posterior segment of the right lobe of the liver.

C, eight days later, reimaging was done, and now a large amount of activity is seen in the stomach. These findings were confirmed at contrast angiography, and the catheter was repositioned.

B

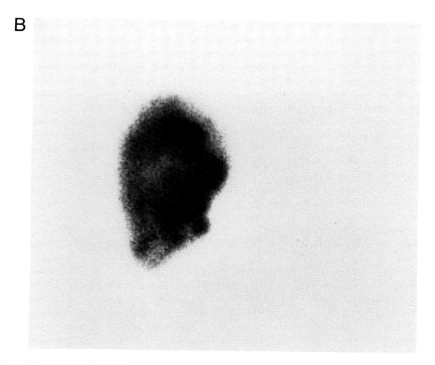

C

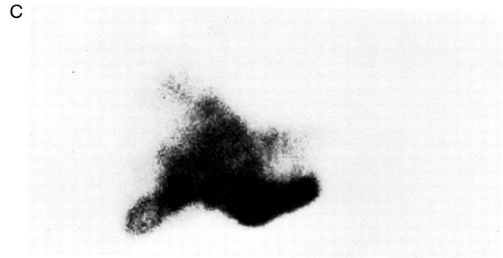

A

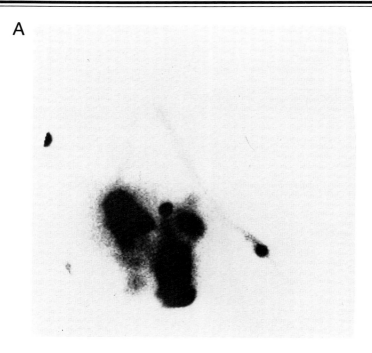

B

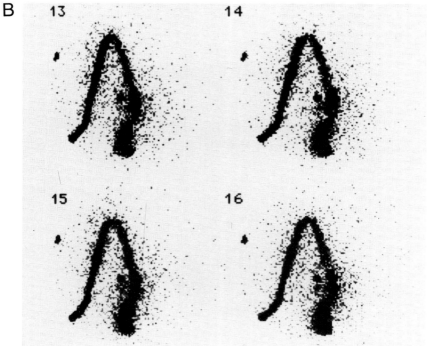

FIG 13–16.
Rhabdomyosarcoma of the perineum (catheter malposition). The patient is a 20-year-old man with a history of rhabdomyosarcoma of the perineum.

A, initial study shows a large amount of activity directed to the shaft of the penis and both sides of the pelvis.

B, repeat flow study after repositioning of the catheter shows activity in the right side of the pelvis and no activity in the penile shaft.

C and **D,** flow studies demonstrate striking difference in distribution over time. These studies prior to chemotherapy allowed recognition of the fact that a large amount of chemotherapy would have been directed to the genitalia rather than the primary tumor (*CR,* iliac crest).

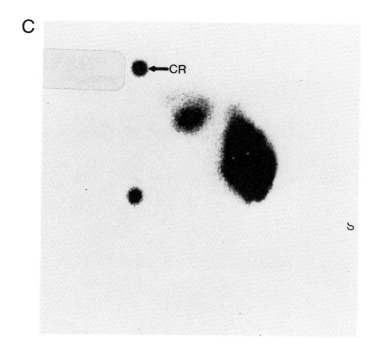

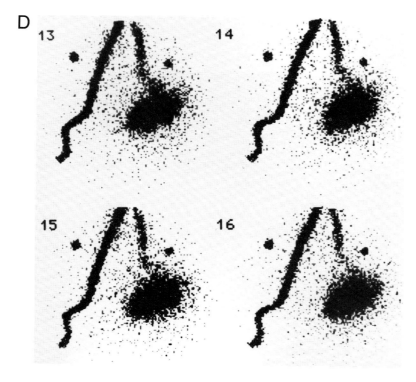

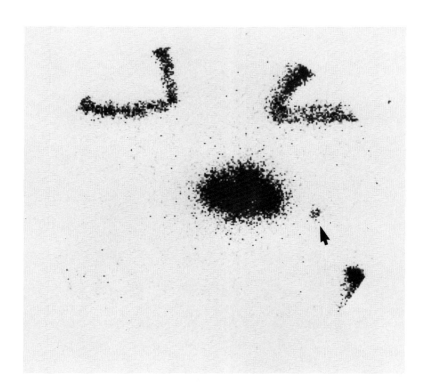

FIG 13–17.
Lymphoscintigraphy in melanoma (lymph node drainage pattern). This patient is a 45-year-old woman with a melanoma of the right back. Lymphoscintigraphy was performed, and the scan demonstrates drainage from the lesion to the right axilla. This study is used to determine lymph node drainage patterns and to assist the surgeon in determining which drainage site should be removed at surgery. Surgical examination of the specimen revealed no evidence of melanoma in the excised lymph nodes.

In this posterior view of the patient's back, the large, dark area in the middle is the injection site, and the small focal area *(arrow)* is the drainage pattern to the right axilla. Radioactive markers are placed on the neck, shoulders, and right side.

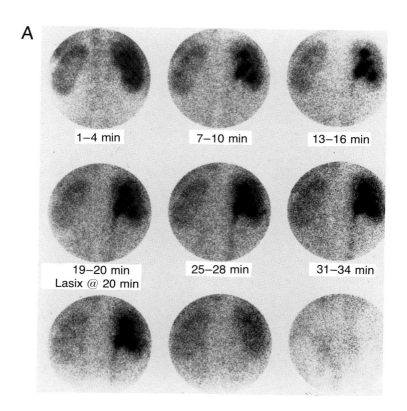

FIG 13–18.
Carcinoma of the prostate, obstructive uropathy, and renal abscess. This patient is a 65-year-old man with a history of carcinoma of the prostate. Interventional diuretic posterior renal study revealed significant decrease in the overall function of the left kidney and moderately severe calicectasis of the right kidney. The right kidney failed to respond to an intravenously administered diuretic agent (furosemide at 40 mg).

A, sequential dynamic ^{99m}Tc-labeled diethylenetriamine pentaacetic acid (^{99m}Tc-DTPA) renal study demonstrates obstruction of the outflow tract of the right kidney.

Note that at 20 min into the study, the patient was given furosemide intravenously and that there was a very delayed response to the intravenous diuretic, indicating almost total obstruction. (*Continued.*)

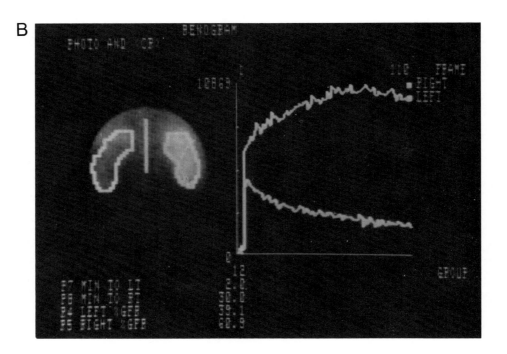

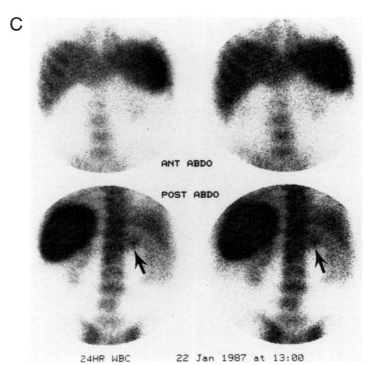

FIG 13–18 (cont.).
B, regions of interest (ROI) and time activity curve of diuretic renogram shows almost complete absence of response of the right kidney to the diuretic.

C, because of intermittent fever, study was done after labeling the patient's white blood cells with [111]In. Posterior view of this study demonstrates a focal area of abnormal accumulation in the superior pole of the right kidney *(arrows).* After intervention and CT-guided aspiration and placement of a nephrostomy tube, the kidney lesion was shown to be an abscess. Note also the abnormal localization of ^{111}In-labeled white blood cells in the lumbar spine at the sites of known blastic metastases.

A

B

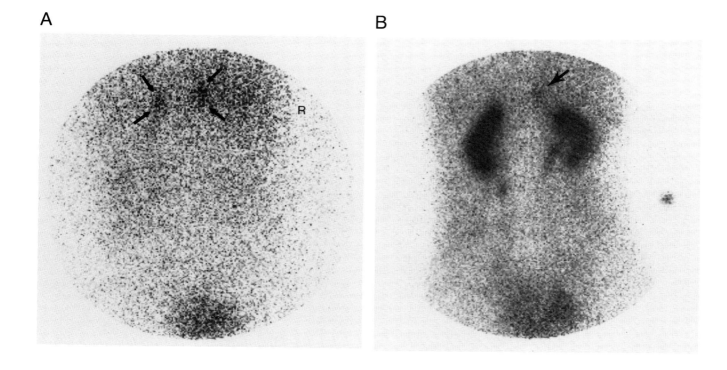

FIG 13–19.
Bilateral adrenal hyperplasia (¹³¹I-MIBG study). The patient is a 24-year-old woman with type IIB multiple endocrine neoplasia syndrome with medullary carcinoma of the thyroid.

A, the ¹³¹I-MIBG study is abnormal; this posterior view shows bilateral adrenal accumulation of the radiopharmaceutical *(arrows).* Activity is somewhat greater on the right

(R) than on the left. The findings are consistent with bilateral adrenal medullary hyperplasia or bilateral pheochromocytoma.

B, a subsequent injection of ^{99m}Tc-labeled DTPA partially obliterates the activity, indicating that the lesions are in fact in the area of the adrenal glands. The right adrenal *(arrow)* is still seen. The relationship of the adrenal lesions and the kidneys is demonstrated.

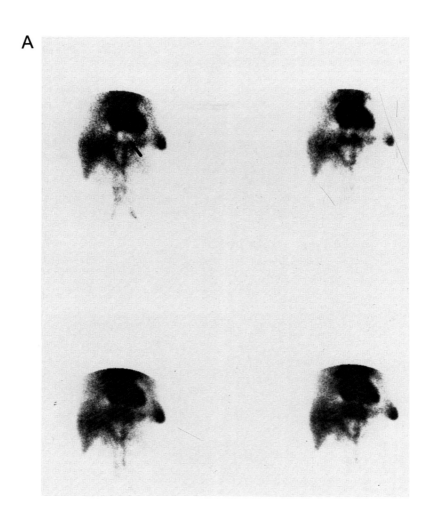

FIG 13–20.

Hemangioma of the liver (blood-pool study). The patient is a 37-year-old woman with breast cancer. A ^{99m}Tc-labeled sulfur-colloid liver scan showed a large focal defect involving the left lobe of the liver. The patient then had a blood-pool study, which was accomplished after red blood cells were labeled in part in vivo and in part vitro ("in vivtro").

A, the first anterior-view blood-pool image shows an area of diminished vascular flow *(arrow)* in the superior aspect of the left lobe of the liver. The area immediately fills in.

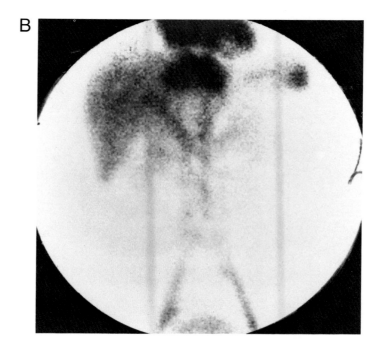

B, over the next hour, anterior view shows an intense localization of the activity in an area involving almost the entire medial segment of the left lobe of the liver (this is the so-called sequestration pattern of hemangioma). Note a small area of diminished activity just superior and lateral to the portal vein; this area was shown by CT and ultrasound to represent a small hepatic cyst. The left lobe lesion was shown to be contrast-enhancing during the same CT examination, consistent with a diagnosis of hemangioma.

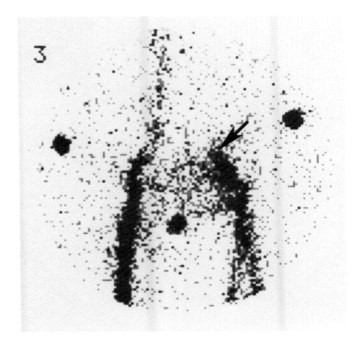

FIG 13–21.
Prostatic carcinoma with pelvic venous obstruction (radionuclide venogram). This 78-year-old man with a history of prostate cancer presented with significant swelling and pain involving the left lower extremity. The radionuclide venogram demonstrates occlusion of the left common iliac vein *(arrow)* with extensive collaterals across the midline.

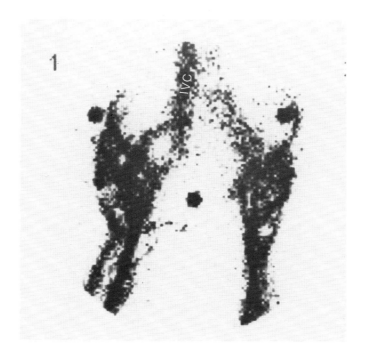

FIG 13–22.

Cervical carcinoma with pelvic venous obstruction (radionuclide venogram). This patient is a 33-year-old woman with a history of carcinoma of the cervix with pelvic metastases. She presented with swelling of the right calf.

Radionuclide venogram demonstrates bilateral iliac vein obstruction with extensive collateral vessels. The patient had undergone rather extensive radiotherapy to the pelvis. Anterior view of the pelvis after bipedal intravenous administration of ^{99m}Tc-labeled macroaggregated albumin (^{99m}Tc-MAA) shows occlusion of iliac vessels and presence of extensive collaterals filling the inferior vena cava *(IVC)*.

A

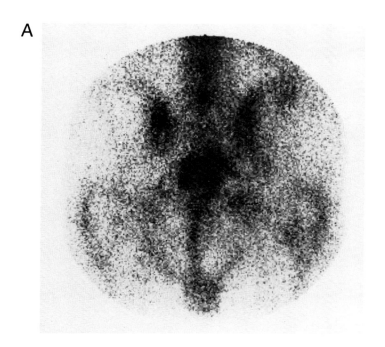

FIG 13–23.
Bladder lymphoma (gallium study). The patient is a 77-year-old man who underwent gallium imaging for staging of lym-

phoma.

A and **B,** there is a large accumulation of gallium in the

B

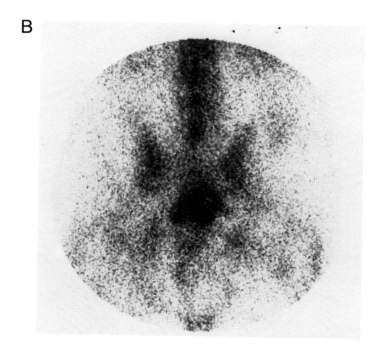

pelvis **(A)**, which fails to change after a bowel movement **(B)**. It was suggested that the patient had lymphomatous involvement in his pelvis. Computed tomography proved that the bladder was the site of the lymphoma.

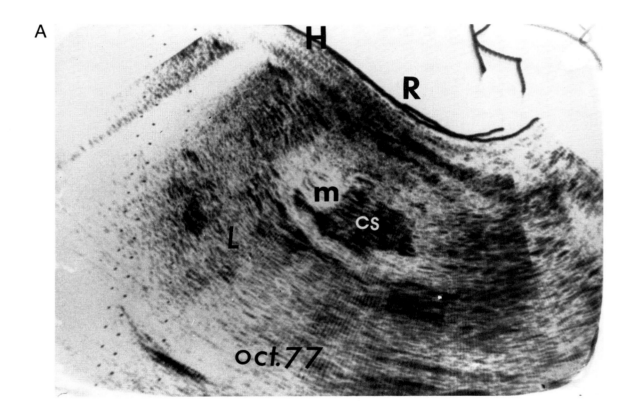

FIG 13–24.
Renal lymphoma (gallium study). This 75-year-old man with a history of poorly differentiated lymphocytic lymphoma originating in the chest underwent diagnostic reevaluation. Excretory urography showed fairly radiolucent renal masses, which were thought to represent cysts.

A and **B,** longitudinal sonography of the right **(A)** and

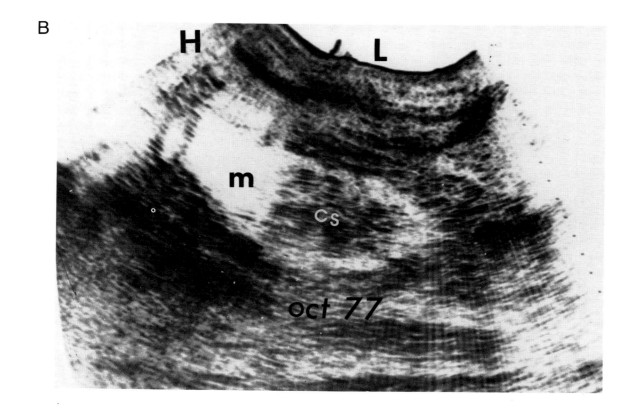

left **(B)** kidneys, made with the patient prone, shows that each organ contains a mass *(m)* in its upper pole, the right mass poorly defined and weakly echogenic, the left large, poorly defined, sonolucent, and with increased through-transmission (*CS,* collecting system; *H,* toward the head; *L,* left; *R,* right). (*Continued.*)

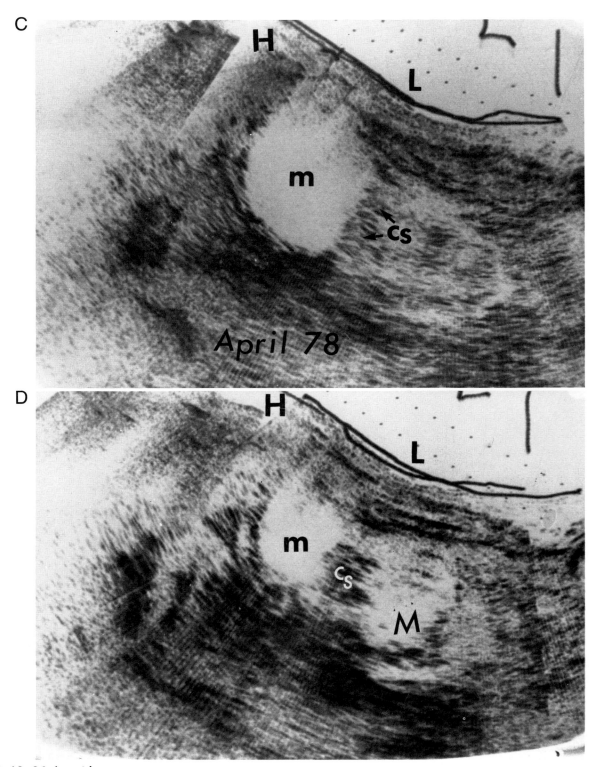

FIG 13–24 (cont.).
C and **D**, these longitudinal sonograms of the left kidney made six months later, again with the patient prone, show that the upper-pole mass *(m)* has grown larger **(C)** and that a new, weakly echogenic mass *(M),* not previously seen, has appeared in the lower portion of the organ **(D)**. In **D,** only part of the superior mass is visible (scale is 1 cm between the dots at the top of each scan; *CS,* collecting system; *H,* toward the head; *L,* left).

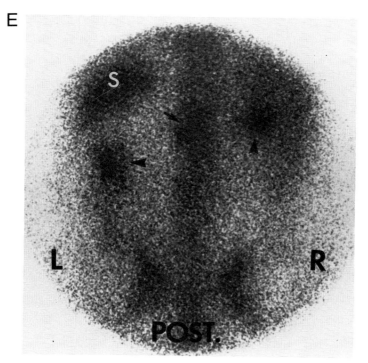

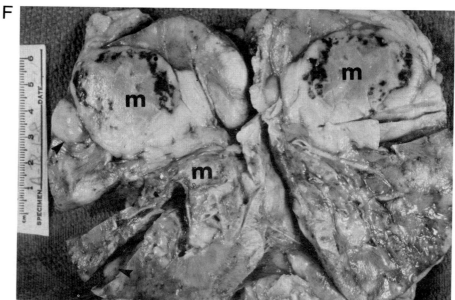

E, a total-body gallium scan (posterior view) made at this time shows multiple areas of increased uptake of radiopharmaceutical within the kidneys *(arrowheads),* corresponding to the renal masses demonstrated on ultrasound. Also note abnormal uptake in the paraspinal nodes *(arrow).* The scan was made 96 hr after injection (*L,* left; *R,* right; *S,* spleen).

F, the patient died within one month, and the autopsy specimen shows lymphomatous masses *(m)* in the left kidney. (From Shirkhoda A., Staab E.B., Mittelstaedt C.A.: Renal lymphoma imaged by ultrasound and gallium-67. *Radiology* 137:175–180, 1980. Reproduced with permission.)

A

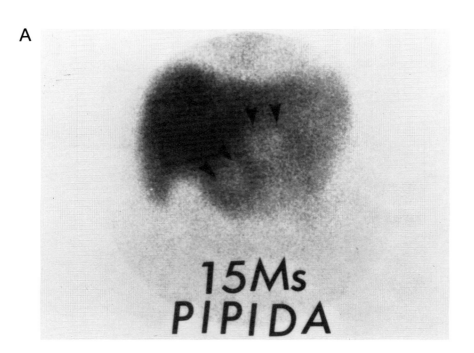

15Ms
PIPIDA

FIG 13–25.
Hepatocellular carcinoma (PIPIDA and gallium studies). This patient has a biopsy-proved diagnosis of hepatocellular carcinoma.

A, on PIPIDA (paraisopropyl immunodiacetic acid) imaging, two well-circumscribed focal photopenic areas *(arrowheads)* involving the left lobe of the liver are demonstrated.

B, a transverse sonogram reveals hypoechoic lesions *(arrows)* in the left lobe of the liver.

C, anterior and right lateral gallium imaging demonstrates filling in of the photopenic areas, which correspond in location to the abnormalities seen on PIPIDA study and sonography. These combined findings suggest a neoplastic or infectious etiology for the lesions. Biopsy proved hepatocellular carcinoma.

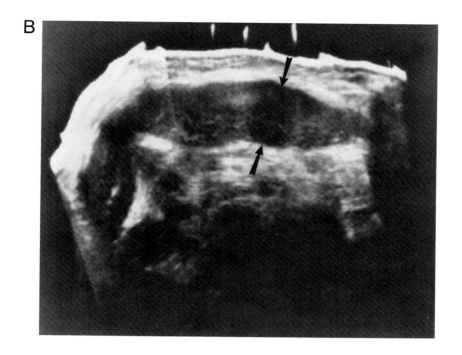

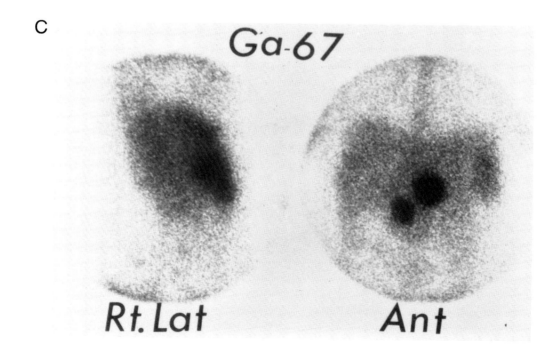

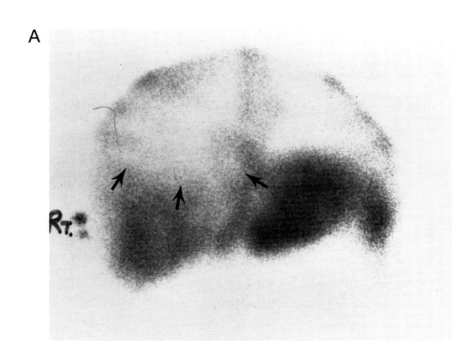

FIG 13–26.
Hepatocellular carcinoma (gallium study). This 67-year-old man presented with weight loss and evidence of ascites.

A, anterior view of ^{99m}Tc–sulfur colloid scan shows an irregular photopenic area in the right and probably the medial segment of the left lobe of the liver *(arrows)*. There is evidence of diversion of colloid to the bone marrow.

B, gallium imaging (48 hr after injection) demonstrates filling in of the photopenic areas seen in **A,** suggesting either inflammation or tumor.

C, an arteriogram demonstrates significant tumor staining. Hepatocellular carcinoma was proved at biopsy.

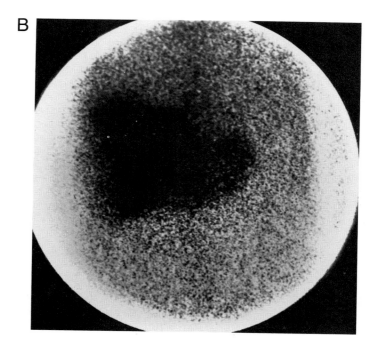

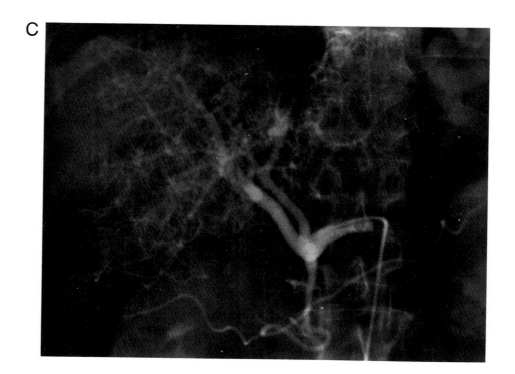

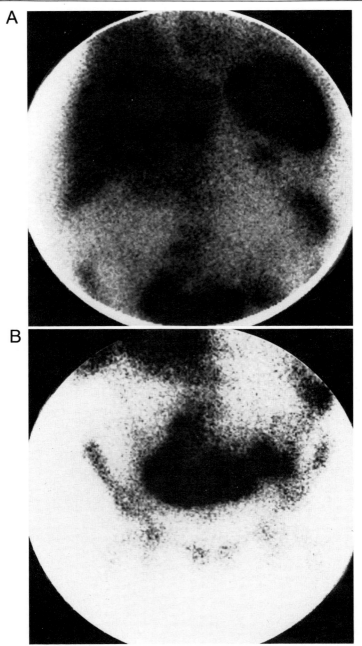

FIG 13–27.
Pelvic abscess following resection of colon carcinoma (¹¹¹In-labeled white blood cell study). This 73-year-old woman with a known history of carcinoma of the colon underwent surgical resection for liver metastases and postoperatively developed sepsis. She also developed a cardiac murmur and was thought to have endocarditis.

The patient's blood cells were labeled with ¹¹¹In and studies were made at 4 hr (**A** and **B**) and 24 hr (**C** and **D**) and demonstrated a large accumulation of radioactivity in the pelvis and in the left upper and lower quadrants. She was treated conservatively and improved without further surgery.

The indium–white blood cell study was helpful in excluding abnormality in the liver and in demonstrating abnormality in the pelvis and left abdomen.

A, anterior view of the abdomen 4 hr after injection of autologous white blood cells labeled with ¹¹¹In-oxine shows abnormal activity in the lower abdomen.

B, anterior view of the pelvis 4 hr after injection of autologous white blood cells labeled with ¹¹¹In-oxine shows a small lesion in the left lower quadrant and a large midline lesion.

C and **D,** these images show the abdomen at 24 hr.

C

D

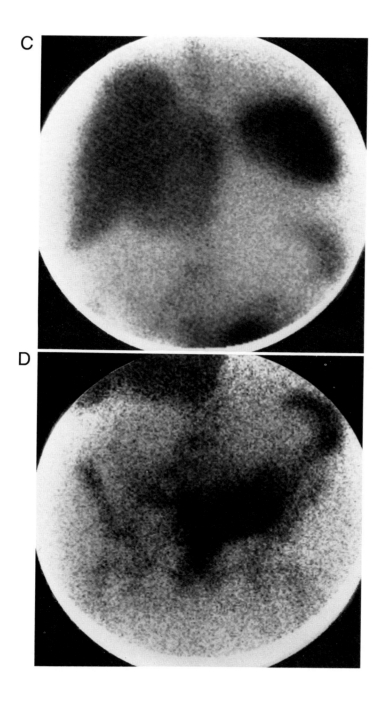

14

Pitfalls in Computed Tomography of the Abdomen and Pelvis

Ali Shirkhoda, M.D.

In this era of sophisticated imaging technology, awareness of conditions that can generate diagnostic confusion is of utmost importance. The emphasis in this atlas has been the application of the most appropriate diagnostic modality for reaching a particular conclusion. But though computed tomography (CT), angiography, ultrasonography, magnetic resonance imaging (MRI), and interventional procedures each have special places, they also each entail pitfalls that can lead to their misinterpretation. Most of the problems arise from incomplete radiologic technique or misreading of a normal anatomical structure, artifact, or (in an oncological context) benign condition. And most can easily be avoided through knowledge of their existence and of appropriate and adequate imaging technique.

Computed tomography has revolutionized the practice of medicine, making such a significant contribution that nowadays this practice would be incomplete without its use. Scanning by CT is increasingly used for diagnosis and management decision making in oncological patients.[1, 2] In many institutions, it has become the primary investigative modality in patients with suspected malignancy in the abdomen or pelvis, both areas whose cross-sectional anatomy it accurately portrays. When an abdominal or pelvic mass is found on palpation, CT can localize the mass with a sensitivity of 99% and a specificity of 97%; it can define the nature of the mass in 88%

of patients and organ of origin in 93%.[3] In staging neoplasms of the kidney and bladder, CT can achieve 90% accuracy.[1] Given this very wide spectrum of CT applications, it is appropriate to discuss the modality's most common pitfalls.

This chapter focuses on those pitfalls when CT is used to image the abdomen or pelvis mostly in an oncological context. Suggestions are made as to how misinterpretation of a normal variant or benign condition as cancer can be avoided.

Knowledge of CT pitfalls in the abdomen and pelvis is of prime importance to the radiologist since these pitfalls can lead to major interpretative errors and thus to erroneous decisions about the patient's management. The limitations inherent in the procedure itself, poor radiologic technique, and observer's errors contribute to most of the inaccurate interpretations of CT images, with the last a significant factor regardless of the radiologist's recognition of limitations and the sophistication of technique.[4] The chance for error is further complicated by the number of decisions that the radiologist must make in obtaining an abdominal or pelvic scan, among them (1) the area to be studied, (2) the slice thickness and the interval between the scans, (3) the use of contrast material (oral, rectal, or intravenous; drip, bolus, or dynamic), and (4) the patient's position and how to assure the patient's immobility.

The improper planning of CT study is one of the

most common problems. The easiest decision would be to administer oral and rectal contrast material and obtain contiguous 5- or 10-mm scans of the entire abdomen and pelvis before and after intravenous contrast in all patients with suspected abdominopelvic pathology. Yet this would probably be a waste of expensive resources and also would deliver unnecessary radiation to the patient. Above all, it would probably be impractical at many institutions because of either an inadequate number of scanners or a large number of patients.

In general, the study should be tailored to a particular area of the body based on the clinical information. Frequently, the study will be limited to the pelvis or the abdomen using a 10-mm slice thickness and equal increments. However, if a small organ such as an adrenal gland is studied, 4-mm sections should be used and the contiguous slices overlapped.

The most common error in body CT scanning is oral and rectal contrast inadequate for the optimal opacification of the gastrointestinal tract. This is particularly the case in patients who are evaluated for a pancreatic mass, lymphoma, retroperitoneal metastases, abscesses, gynecologic tumors, or, sometimes, renal or adrenal masses. An unopacified fluid-filled loop of small or large bowel can simulate a primary tumor or adenopathy. Also, fluid-filled or inadequately distended stomach can mimic neoplasm or even abscess in the upper left quadrant.

The intravenous administration of contrast material should be selectively used not only to differentiate between normal and pathologic situations but also to be more certain about the presence or absence of certain conditions and their specific natures. The most important organs in the abdomen that require the use of intravenous contrast are the liver, kidneys, spleen, and major blood vessels. As important as the type of contrast material is how it is administered: slow drip, fast drip, bolus, or by injector, for example. In many instances, precontrast imaging will increase CT's sensitivity in detecting a lesion.

Care must be taken to assure that the patient is immobile and placed symmetrically within the scanning circle. Even slight asymmetry or motion can create a major problem. In addition, when any part of the patient's body is outside the scanning circle, the CT unit scale will be inaccurate. Sedation is necessary in pediatric patients[5, 6] and might be needed in adults who cannot hold still because of pain.

The following is a brief discussion of the commonly, and some of the uncommonly, encountered pitfalls with CT in four major anatomical areas of the abdomen and pelvis. Case presentations and illustrations of the pitfalls will follow.

GENERAL ABDOMEN AND GASTROINTESTINAL TRACT

Cardiac motion in the upper abdomen often generates artifactual problems in the subdiaphragmatic portion of the liver and in the left upper quadrant. However, this problem is encountered less often when a fast scanner is used.

An inverted dome of the diaphragm, especially on the right side and when associated with pleural effusions, can simulate a cystic liver mass (Fig 14–1). The diaphragm itself may display areas of invagination, which can mimic tumor nodules[7] or metastatic implants (Fig 14–2).

In the upper abdomen, azygos and hemiazygos veins are located behind the crura of the diaphragm and posterior to the aorta. On axial view, particularly when they are engorged, these vessels can mimic lymphadenopathy. Bolus intravenous contrast injection would lead to a correct diagnosis. Noninvasively, these vessels may be identified by MRI studies because the blood flow reads as an area of no signal (Fig 14–3).

Interposition of the colon between the liver and the diaphragm or an unusual shape of the liver and thus the liver's unusual relationship with the colon (Fig 14–4) can yield an image that could be mistaken for a subphrenic abscess.[8] Evaluation of the plain film and use of a contrast enema during CT study will preclude this erroneous diagnosis.

A sliding hiatal hernia may simulate a mass in the gastric fundus[9] or mimic a preaortic node. Suspecting this possibility and repeating the CT study at that level with more oral contrast will solve the problem (Fig 14–5). Occasionally, it is necessary to fluoroscopically examine the esophagus to prevent such a misdiagnosis.

About one third of patients who have CT scans of the upper abdomen show focal thickening in the region of the esophagogastric junction, or what appears to be a mass there.[10] This finding is related to the transverse anatomical plane of section through the esophagogastric junction and carina and should not be interpreted as a neoplasm (Fig 14–6). It has been reported that this finding is seen more often on the same plane as the fissure that separates the caudate lobe from the lateral segment of the liver.[11] Rescanning with additional contrast and with the patient placed in the left posterior or prone position will help differentiate this pseudotumor from a neoplasm.

The esophagus itself can mimic a node in the gastrohepatic ligament, and it may be necessary to perform a repeat scan to rule out adenopathy (Fig 14–7).

Transabdominal fundoplication (Nissen's procedure) can lead to a CT image that simulates a mass at the distal esophagus (Fig 14–8) or at the esophagogastric junction. Thickening of the posterior gastric wall or even an abscess may be mimicked.[10] This procedure is an antireflux operation done for hiatal hernia and involves wrapping part of the fundus completely around the lower 4 to 6 cm of the esophagus.

Retention of food in or inadequate distension of the stomach can potentially give rise to false-positive diagnosis of a gastric wall mass (Fig 14–9), a pancreatic mass invading the stomach, or even an abscess in the left upper quadrant (Fig 14–10).[12] Also, inadequate density of contrast in the stomach can mimic a mass in the liver (Fig 14–11) or in the upper abdomen. Previous history of gastrojejunostomy (Billroth II) can be associated with herniation of jejunal mucosa through the area of anastomosis, so that a gastric tumor is mimicked on scanning.

Giving more oral contrast material to the patient just prior to the beginning of scanning will prevent these misinterpretations. Occasionally, under these circumstances and also when the spleen or an enlarged left lobe of the liver encroaches on the stomach, positional studies (i.e., decubitus or prone) may be necessary.[13]

A prominent papilla in the medial wall of the duodenum can mimic a tumor. This occurs very infrequently and may necessitate other studies such as cholangiography (Fig 14–12) or endoscopic retrograde cholangiopancreatography.

One of the most frequent causes of false-positive results in the abdomen is the presence of fluid-filled bowel loops. A solid mass, an abscess, or mesenteric nodal enlargement may be simulated (Fig 14–13). In cases of cavitating metastases communicating with the small bowel, the contrast-filled tumor on CT may be misread as normal small bowel.[14] It is essential that adequate oral contrast material be administered before the study and that it be continued until the beginning of the CT examination. The transit time of dilute oral contrast material varies, but in most patients the entire small bowel will be opacified within 1 hr.

LIVER, BILIARY SYSTEM, AND SPLEEN

The porta hepatis and hepatoduodenal ligament region are both areas in which there is a likelihood of CT misinterpretation.[15] There are many normal structures at this location, including lymph nodes, fat, and the portal vein, common bile duct, hepatic artery, gallbladder, and caudate lobe and its papillary process. To discriminate the vascular and biliary compartments, it is necessary to use intravenous contrast (Fig 14–14). Posterior to this region is the inferior vena cava, which because of variation in its size may simulate a mass. Occasionally, it may become necessary to inject contrast material into a foot vein for direct opacification of inferior vena cava. The papillary process of the caudate lobe of the liver (Fig 14–15) and replaced right hepatic artery (see Fig 14–47), both of which are located anterior to the inferior vena cava, should not be mistaken for a node. Inferiorly, the caudate lobe is divided into the caudate process laterally and the papillary process medially.[16] A normal or large papillary process may mimic a node at the porta hepatis or a mass in the pancreas. The inferior part of the papillary process can extend medially behind the gastric antrum (Fig 14–15,B) and is separated from the liver on at least one CT scan in 20% of patients.[16]

Normal intrahepatic venous channels are frequently seen on unenhanced liver CT and will disappear or be enhanced upon the intravenous administration of contrast material (Fig 14–16). They should not be mistaken for dilatation in the biliary system or for small hepatic lesions.[17]

The inferior vena cava in its distal segment runs into the liver before reaching the right atrium and produces a well-circumscribed low-density area that can resemble a hepatic lesion.

The rare entity of an intrahepatic gallbladder should not be mistaken for a liver lesion. In this case, ultrasound might become necessary to see the common bile duct and its relationship with the gallbladder, and visualization of the gallbladder itself could be easily achieved by biliary scintigraphy.

The CT diagnosis of hepatic cysts may be difficult (Fig 14–17), primarily because the attenuation values of a simple cyst (particularly when it is small and inflamed) and a neoplastic lesion of the liver can be similar.[18] Aspiration or excision biopsy may prove to be necessary.

In severe cirrhosis, the right and left lobes of the liver shrink and the caudate lobe becomes enlarged.[19] This enlarged lobe should not be mistaken for an intraabdominal or hepatic tumor (Fig 14–18). In patients with malignancy treated by chemotherapy, the liver might undergo fatty infiltration. In these cases, there occasionally remains a focus or several foci of relatively high density within the diffuse fatty liver (Fig 14–19); such foci might represent normal liver tissue and should not be assumed to be metastases.[20] Rarely, the fatty infiltration surrounds islands of normal liver and simulates ductal dilatation or metastases (Fig 14–20).

When surgical clips from previous surgery such as cholecystectomy cause artifact in the liver, the CT diagnosis of metastases might become difficult. In these circumstances, one can place the gantry at such an angle that clips will not be in the x-ray beam and then continue to scan with a thinner slice until the clips are again seen (Fig 14–21). By this technique, most of the area covered by artifacts can be studied.

A normal-variant elongated left lobe of the liver can have the same density as the spleen and on CT simulate splenomegaly. Bolus contrast and the proper setting of windows are needed for diagnosis (Fig 14–22). In the early phase of bolus contrast injection, the spleen may be enhanced very nonhomogeneously, mimicking other conditions such as tumor infiltration (Fig 14–23). This is probably due to variable rates of blood flow through the splenic red pulp.[21] In these cases, repeat CT imaging at the end of the study or sonography is indicated to rule out tumor infiltrate. Also in the spleen, the normal splenic cleft[22] should not be mistaken for laceration (Fig 14–24).

Splenectomy alters the anatomical integrity of the lesser peritoneal cavity, so assessment of abnormal masses or fluid collection there should await opacification of all bowel loops in the area. Accessory splenic tissue may become hypertrophic after splenectomy and measure up to 5 cm in diameter; this hypertrophy should not be mistaken for an enlarged node.[23] Under these circumstances, a scintiscan of the liver and spleen may help decide the necessity of biopsy.

After partial hepatectomy, the gallbladder is in some cases displaced so that a duplication cyst or a gastric diverticulum is mimicked (Figs 14–25 and 14–26). There will also be normal anatomical changes of the remaining hepatic lobe, along with displacement of the major vasculature.[24] Also regarding the gallbladder, opacification of bile within this organ is not unusual after a large dosage of iodinated contrast material injection. Strax et al. reported that abdominal CT 12 to 48 hr after angiography showed enhancement of the gallbladder content in those patients with normal renal and hepatic function who had received more than 37 g of iodine during angiography.[25] This observation on CT (Fig 14–27) should not be mistaken for such conditions as milk of calcium or dense sludge.

RETROPERITONEUM

The crura of the diaphragm, which are ligamentous bands representing extension of the psoas muscles, form the hiatus of the diaphragm through which the abdominal aorta, lymphatic channels, and other neurovascular structures pass.[15] They are tendinous at their origin and blend with the ventral longitudinal ligament along the anterior aspect of the vertebral column. The right crus is larger, longer, and often more lobular than the left crus. Computed tomographic images obtained near the diaphragm demonstrate the crura as their fibers pass from the vertebral bodies anteriorly to meet across the aorta. However, the more caudal images may only demonstrate a portion of the crus, making correct anatomical identification more difficult. Thickened areas of the crus are common, particularly on the right side, and can easily be misinterpreted as diseased nodes (Fig 14–28). Also, certain structures adjacent to the crura, including enlarged nodes and the inferior vena cava, right renal artery, and right adrenal gland, might be mistaken for the crura.[26]

One of the retroperitoneal organs that is often evaluated by CT is the pancreas. On cross-sectional anatomy, it is located posterior to the stomach and anterior to the splenic vessels, left kidney, and aorta. Its head is just medial to the duodenal loop and anterior to the inferior vena cava. The uncinate process can be prominent and simulate a mass. It extends behind the superior mesenteric vein and its characteristic hook contour helps to identify this normal structure.

The pancreas can be extensively replaced by fat, particularly in elderly patients.[27] A layer of fat that is normally present between the splenic vein and the pancreas (Fig 14–29) may simulate a dilated pancreatic duct.[28] In addition, the size of the pancreas may be overestimated because of addition of the spleen (Fig 14–30) or the width of the splenic vein in the absence of intervening fat.[15] In these circumstances, intravenous contrast, preferably in the form of a bolus injection, is necessary for opacification of normal vasculature.

Also in the pancreas, artifact as the result of barium in adjacent bowel or stomach can generate a pseudomass with low density (Fig 14–31); the corresponding CT scan should be repeated in these patients.

The unopacified duodenum or inferior vena cava can cause apparent enlargement of the pancreatic head, and an unopacified duodenal diverticulum may simulate a retroperitoneal or pancreatic mass.[29, 30]

The common bile duct and ampullary region may appear as a prominent lobulation to the posterior lateral aspect of the head of the pancreas and should not be mistaken for a small tumor.

In patients who have had a gastrojejunostomy, obstruction can cause the afferent duodenal loop to become dilated, so that a large cystic mass or cystic masses may be simulated in the upper abdomen because of retained bile and pancreatic juice. Since the serum amylase value is often elevated in these cases, an erroneous diagnosis of pancreatic pseudocyst might be made. In one report, the cause of this apparent cystic mass was proved by intravenous CT cholangiography.[31]

A lobulated kidney, a column of Bertin, and nodular compensatory hypertrophy[32] can each simulate masses on CT and even on ultrasound (Fig 14–32). Since the normal kidney will demonstrate homogeneous contrast enhancement, the CT study should be performed with and without contrast if a mass is suspected. Occasionally, scintigraphy might be necessary (see Fig 14–32,C), using renal cortical agent to differentiate a tumor from a pseudotumor.[33] High-density contrast in the renal collecting system causes streak artifacts secondary to beam hardening. This can lead to lucent and dense bands in the renal parenchyma and should be differentiated from the striations seen in renal inflammatory disease.

In cases of small cysts of the renal cortex, routine CT scanning using a 10-mm slice thickness can show low-density lesion with a high CT number that is beyond what is accepted as cystic fluid. This is due to the presence of high-density contrast-enhanced renal parenchyma within the same voxels shared by the cyst.[34] To overcome this pitfall, the CT scan should be repeated in the area using a thin slice thickness, targeted preferably at 1.5 mm (Fig 14–33).

Organs adjacent to the kidney, such as the duodenum and spleen, can be located more posteriorly than is normal and cause displacement of (Fig 14–34) or pseudomass in (Fig 14–35) the kidney. Also,

because of volume averaging on routine scanning, a splenic lesion can simulate a renal mass. Thinner slices at smaller increments of the table should be used to overcome this pitfall (Fig 14–36).

The pancreatic tail is very close to the anterior surface of the kidney and in thin patients can simulate a left renal mass. Repeat CT with the patient prone will usually separate these two structures (Fig 14–37).

Motion artifact, which can result from breathing, might be misinterpreted as renal subcapsular hematoma and around the liver can simulate ascites (Fig 14–38). That the findings are not seen on adjacent or repeat images suggests motion artifact.

In a patient with a history of nephrectomy, the vascular pedicle may simulate a mass or abnormal node. Also, if the patient had a previous hip replacement and a contralateral nephrectomy, asymmetry of the psoas muscles due to atrophy in the side with normal kidney can represent a major pitfall (Fig 14–39). In fact, ipsilateral thickening of the psoas muscle, which is one of the CT signs of recurrent tumor, can be simulated.

Adhesions and displacement of the bowel loops into the renal fossa postnephrectomy may mimic tumor on CT (Fig 14–40), but reevaluation of the area after the administration of more oral contrast will usually solve the problem. Usually the liver fills the empty renal fossa, although occasionally the gallbladder so shifts. Because of multiple surgical clips, it may be difficult to differentiate normal hepatic parenchyma from locally recurrent tumor (Fig 14–41). In the case of the gallbladder at this site, differentiation from a cystic mass such as lymphocele or abscess may be difficult (Fig 14–42).

Computed tomography is the best procedure for imaging the adrenals. Anatomical variability does exist in these glands' position and shape, particularly with the left adrenal. The relation of the left adrenal to the left kidney depends on the amount and distribution of perirenal fat. As a result, this gland can be intimately related to the esophagogastric junction, the posteromedial aspect of the fundus of the stomach, the superomedial aspect of the spleen, the pancreas, a tortuous splenic artery, the left renal artery and vein confluence, or the fourth portion of the duodenum. Confusion between tortuous splenic vasculature and left adrenal gland nodule (Fig 14–43) occurs most often in elderly patients.[15] Similarly, vascular bundle consisting of the renal artery and vein or a tortuous renal artery can mimic an adrenal mass (Fig 14–44). This condition is most troublesome in patients being evaluated for pheochromocytoma, a disease in which extraadrenal tumors of the renal hilus are not rare. With bolus intravenous contrast injection and properly timed CT scanning, this normal anatomy will be visualized.

A small cyst of the upper-pole renal cortex might project into the adrenal fossa, and it is not unusual for this to be mistaken for an adrenal nodule (Fig 14–45). In these cases, thin-section CT images should be obtained to prove the contiguity of the apparent nodule with the renal cyst.

An accessory spleen also may mimic a left adrenal mass,[35] and in some cases it may be necessary to obtain a liver-spleen scintiscan.

A portion of the stomach can project so that it is in the proximity of the left adrenal and mimic an adrenal mass (Fig 14–46). A diverticulum arising from the gastric cardia can extend into the adrenal fossa and simulate a cystic or solid adrenal mass.[36, 37] Repeat CT imaging with more oral contrast will solve this problem.

One of the common pitfalls in evaluating the adrenals is not to include or recognize the entire gland. Occasionally the nodule will be at the extremity of one of the cross-sectional limbs of the adrenal.

The crura of diaphragm (Fig 14–47), a double or left-sided inferior vena cava (Fig 14–48), tortuous renal arteries (Fig 14–49), retroaortic left renal vein (Fig 14–50), and presence of collateral venous channels in a patient with an occluded inferior vena cava can all be misinterpreted as retroperitoneal nodes.[38–40] By enhancing the vascular structures through intravenous contrast injection (in particular, via a foot vein), proper differentiation will be achieved.

Other abnormalities, such as varices, aneurysms, localized bleeding, and extramedullary hematopoiesis, can mimic retroperitoneal nodes,[41] as can such normal structures as unopacified bowel loops (particularly in thin patients) (Fig 14–51) and psoas minor muscle (Fig 14–52). The psoas minor, which is often absent, is a long, slender muscle that originates from the sides of the 12th thoracic and first lumbar vertebrae and that is ventral to the psoas major. Especially when it exists unilaterally, it can mimic nodes.

PELVIS

The most frequent source of misinterpretation in pelvic CT scans is nonopacified loops of small and large bowel. An adequate volume of dilute oral contrast given 1 to 2 hr prior to the examination is required for opacification of the entire small intestine. Just before beginning the pelvic CT, contrast material should be administered, always via the rectum or a colostomy, to identify the colon.

Mixture of feces and air in the bowel, especially in the colon, occasionally mimics a pelvic abscess. A redundant sigmoid and ascending colon may not completely fill with rectal contrast and may thus mimic the appearance of an adnexal tumor or abscess (Fig 14–53). In these cases, delayed CT scanning to provide time for opacification of the colon from the oral contrast or barium enema is helpful. Occasionally, if the patient has left the CT department, it may become necessary to solve the problem by using water enema during real-time ultrasound examination at a later date (Fig 14–54).

Using a tampon helps to delineate the normal anatomy of the vagina and to prevent a misreading of the normal vagina as a primary or recurrent malignant tumor, for example. Tampon use is also helpful in identifying the uterus and occasionally in recognizing the positions of the ovaries, which could be mistaken for pelvic tumor. However, normal ovaries may become a source of pitfall in the pelvis (Fig 14–55).

If the patient has had a supracervical hysterectomy, one should not mistake the remaining cervix for recurrent mass (Fig 14–56).

A bladder diverticulum may mimic a fluid-filled mass or abscess in the pelvis. It may be necessary to use intravenous contrast and to place the patient in a prone or lateral decubitus position to fill a large diverticulum, or to opacify the entire bladder.[42]

The pelvic vessels are usually symmetric, but sometimes a tortuous vessel or an aneurysm can be misinterpreted as a node. Obviously, bolus intravenous contrast injection is mandatory before contemplating biopsy.

Asymmetry of the piriform or iliopsoas muscles, which may be either developmental or postsurgical (e.g., subsequent to poliomyelitis or amputation of one extremity), can generate confusion (Fig 14–57). Usually, it is the normal or hypertrophic side that simulates a mass or adenopathy.

In patients who had resection of the rectum, displacement of the seminal vesicles or uterus (Fig 14–58) may mimic nodes or locally recurrent neoplasm.

Omentum is sometimes surgically dispatched into the pelvis after rectosigmoid resection or pelvic exenteration (Fig 14–59). The omental lid is formed into a pedicle flap based on either the left or the right gastroepiploic artery, and it is usually swung down to the left paracolic gutter to cover the denuded pelvic walls. This predominantly adipose tissue serves both as a vascular bed to absorb the serous drainage and as a barrier against the intestines.[43] The CT appearance of the lid should not be mistaken for a fatty tumor in the pelvis.

If pelvic CT is performed shortly after percutaneous biopsy (e.g., transperineal prostatic biopsy), the changes in the fascial planes may mimic nodes or tumor infiltration (Fig 14–60). In patients who have undergone transurethral resection of the prostate, thickening of perirectal fascia is seen as a temporary phenomenon.[44]

REFERENCES

1. Husband J.E.: Role of the CT scanner in the management of cancer. *Br. Med. J. (Clin. Res.)* 290:527–530, 1985.
2. Fineberg H.V., Wittenberg J., Ferrucci J.T. Jr., et al.: The clinical value of body computed tomography over time and technologic change. *AJR* 141:1067–1072, 1983.
3. Williams M.P., Scott I.H.K., Dixon A.K.: Computed tomography in 101 patients with a palpable abdominal mass. *Clin. Radiol.* 35:293–296, 1984.
4. Hunter T.B.: Pitfalls of computed tomography of the abdomen and pelvis. *Contemp. Diagn. Radiol.* 6:1–6, 1983.
5. Thompson J.R., Schneider S., Ashwal S., et al.: The choice of sedation for computed tomography in children: a prospective evaluation. *Radiology* 143:475–479, 1982.
6. Strain J.D., Harvey L.A., Foley L.C., et al.: Intravenously administered pentobarbital sodium for sedation in pediatric CT. *Radiology* 161:105–108, 1986.
7. Rosen A., Auk Y.H., Rubenstein W.K., et al.: CT appearance of diaphragmatic pseudotumor. *J. Comput. Assist. Tomogr.* 7:995–999, 1983.
8. Newmark H. III, Burrow R., Silberman E.L., et al.: A pitfall in the diagnosis of a subphrenic abscess seen on computerized tomography. *Computerized Tomography* 4:115–157, 1980.
9. Pupols A., Ruzicka F.F.: Hiatal hernia causing a cardiac pseudomass on computed tomography. *J. Comput. Assist. Tomogr.* 8:699–700, 1984.
10. Thompson W.M., Holvorsen R.A., Wilford M.E., et al.: Computed tomography of the gastroesophageal junction. *RadioGraphics* 2:179–193, 1982.
11. Marks W.M., Callen P.W., Moss A.A.: Gastroesophageal region: source of confusion on CT. *AJR* 136:359–362, 1981.
12. Kaye M.D., Young S.W., Hayward R.: Gastric pseudotumor on CT scanning. *AJR* 135:190–192, 1980.
13. Dixon A.K., Stringer D.A., Hallett M.G., et al.: The use of the right decubitus position in computed tomography of the liver and pancreas. *Clin. Radiol.* 32:113–116, 1981.
14. DuBrow R.A., Rubin J.M.: Intraabdominal metastatic carcinoma: unusual presentation and potential pitfall in CT evaluation. *J. Comput. Assist. Tomogr.* 6:966–968, 1982.
15. Sample W.F., Sarti D.A.: Computed body tomography and gray scale ultrasonography: anatomic correlations and pitfalls in the upper abdomen. *Gastrointest. Radiol.* 3:243–249, 1978.
16. Auh Y.H., Rosen A., Rubenstein W.A., et al.: CT of the papillary process of the caudate lobe of the liver. *AJR* 142:535–538, 1984.
17. Kressel H.Y., Korobkin M., Goldberg H.I., et al.: The portal venous tree simulating dilated biliary ducts on computed tomography of the liver. *J. Comput. Assist. Tomogr.* 1:169–179, 1977.
18. Barnes P.A., Thomas J.L., Bernardino M.E.: Pitfalls in the diagnosis of hepatic cysts by computed tomography. *Radiology* 141:129–133, 1981.
19. Goldberg H.I.: CT scanning of diffuse parenchymal liver disease, in Moss A.A., Goldberg H.I. (eds.): *Computed Tomography, Ultrasound and X-Ray: An Integrated Approach.* New York, Academic Press, 1980, pp. 177–187.
20. Lewis E., Bernardino M.E., Barnes P.A., et al.: The fatty liver: pitfalls in the CT and angiographic evaluation of metastatic disease. *J. Comput. Assist. Tomogr.* 7:235–241, 1983.
21. Glazer G.M., Axel L., Goldberg H.I., et al.: Dynamic CT of the normal spleen. *AJR* 137:343–346, 1981.
22. Jeffrey R.B., Laing F.C., Federle M.A., et al.: Computed tomography in splenic trauma. *Radiology* 141:729–732, 1981.
23. Beahrs J.R., Stephans D.H.: Enlarged accessory spleens: CT appearance in postsplenectomy patients. *AJR* 135:483–486, 1980.
24. Couanet D., Shirkhoda A., Wallace S.: Computed tomography after partial hepatectomy. *J. Comput. Assist. Tomogr.* 8:453–457, 1984.
25. Strax R., Toombs B.D., Kam J., et al.: Gallbladder enhancement following angiography: a normal CT finding. *J. Comput. Assist. Tomogr.* 6:766–768, 1982.
26. Callen P.W., Filly R.A., Korobkin M.: CT evaluation of the diaphragmatic crura. *Radiology* 126:413–416, 1978.
27. Patel S., Bellon E.M., Haaga J., et al.: Fat replacement of the exocrine pancreas. *AJR* 135:843–845, 1980.
28. Seidelmann F.E., Cohen W.N., Bryan P.J., et al.: CT demonstration of the splenic vein—pancreatic relationship: the pseudodilated pancreatic duct. *AJR* 129:17–21, 1977.
29. Marks W.M., Goldberg H.I., Moss A.A., et al.: Intestinal pseudotumors: a problem in abdominal computed tomography solved by direct techniques. *Gastrointest. Radiol.* 5:155–160, 1980.

30. Ginaldi S., Zornoza J.: Large duodenal diverticulum simulating pancreatic mass by computed tomography. *Computerized Tomography* 4:169–172, 1980.

31. Kuwabara Y., Nishitani H., Numaguchi Y., et al.: Case report: afferent loop syndrome. *J. Comput. Assist. Tomogr.* 4:687–689, 1980.

32. Wespes E., Van Gansbeke D., Schulman C.C.: Renal pseudotumors. *World J. Urol.* 2:89–91, 1984.

33. Daly M.J., Henry R.E.: Defining renal anatomy and function with technetium dimercaptosuccinic acid: clinical and renographic correlation. *J. Urol.* 127:712–714, 1982.

34. Goodenough D., Weaver K., Davis D.O., et al.: Volume averaging limitations of computed tomography. *AJR* 138:313–316, 1982.

35. Stiris M.G.: Accessory spleen versus left adrenal tumor: computed tomographic and abdominal angiographic evaluation. *J. Comput. Assist. Tomogr.* 4:543–544, 1980.

36. Schwartz A.N., Goiney R.C., Graney D.O.: Gastric diverticulum simulating an adrenal mass: CT appearance and embryogenesis. *AJR* 146:553–554, 1986.

37. Silverman P.M.: Gastric diverticulum mimicking adrenal mass: CT demonstration. *J. Comput. Assist. Tomogr.* 10:709–711, 1986.

38. Mayo J., Gray R., St. Louis E., et al.: Anomalies of the inferior vena cava [review]. *AJR* 140:339–345, 1983.

39. Royal S.A., Callen P.W.: CT evaluation of the inferior vena cava and left renal vein. *AJR* 132:759–763, 1979.

40. Klimberg I., Wajsman Z.: Duplicated inferior vena cava simulating retroperitoneal lymphadenopathy in a patient with embryonal cell carcinoma of the testicle. *J. Urol.* 136:678–679, 1986.

41. Koehler P.R., Mancuso A.A.: Pitfalls in the diagnosis of retroperitoneal adenopathy. *J. Can. Assoc. Radiol.* 33:197–201, 1982.

42. Newmark H.: A distended bladder simulating a neoplastic or cystic mass on computed tomography. *Computerized Tomography* 4:173–175, 1980.

43. Rutledge R.N., Smith J.P., Wharton J.T., et al.: Pelvic exenteration: analysis of 296 patients. *Am. J. Obstet. Gynecol.* 129:881–892, 1977.

44. Parienty R.A., Vallancien G., Pradel J., et al.: CT features of perirectal fascia thickening after transurethral resection of prostatic adenoma. *J. Comput. Assist. Tomogr.* 11:92–95, 1987.

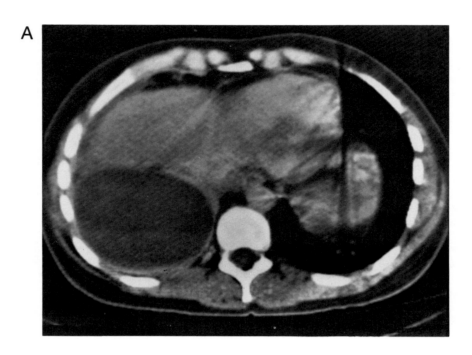

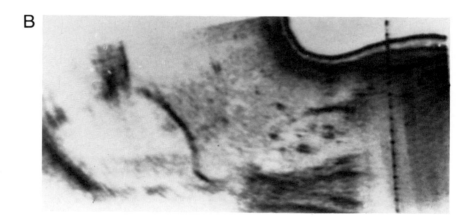

FIG 14–1.

Cystic hepatic mass? A 62-year-old patient with broncho-genic carcinoma of the right upper lobe. The patient had right pleural effusion on chest radiography.

A, the upper abdomen CT image shows a large cystic mass in the posterior aspect of the liver. Based on CT, it could not be determined whether the mass represented hepatic cyst, necrotic hepatic neoplasm, or abscess or if the mass was related to the pleural effusion.

B, a sagittal sonogram of the right upper quadrant clearly shows the inverted right hemidiaphragm and loculated right pleural effusion. The liver is normal.

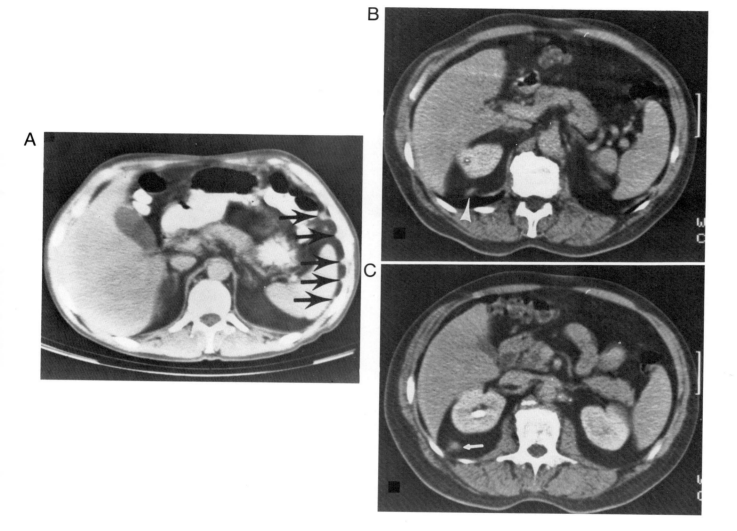

FIG 14–2.
Diaphragmatic implants? (Multiple cases.) Abdominal CT was used to search for metastases in these two patients with malignant melanoma.

A, on this scan of the upper abdomen, nodular densities *(arrows)* in the region of the diaphragm are seen both anteriorly and laterally. These are so-called diaphragmatic pseudotumors and are related to the diaphragmatic fibrous tissue's localized invagination into the adjacent fat.

B and **C,** occasionally, this invagination occurs in the posterior and inferior aspect, adjacent to the perirenal fat, so that perirenal metastasis can be mimicked *(arrow in C)*. Thin slices and demonstration of the area of invagination *(arrowhead in B)* will prove the normal variation. (**B** from Shirkhoda A.: Computed tomography of perirenal metastases. *J. Comput. Assist. Tomogr.* 10:435–438, 1986. Reproduced with permission.)

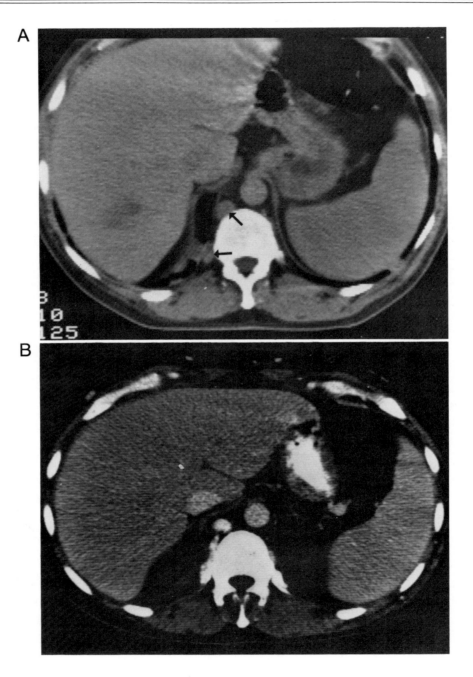

FIG 14–3.
Retrocrural adenopathy? (Multiple cases.)

A, this patient had a thoracic CT scan for evaluation of the extent of bronchogenic carcinoma. On the unenhanced CT of the lower thorax, at least two separate nodules *(arrows)* are seen behind the right crus of diaphragm.

B, scanning was repeated in this patient on the following day, with bolus intravenous contrast. It is seen that both nodules represent vessels. This is a common pitfall in unenhanced CT scans, on which structures such as azygos and hemiazygos veins can mimic lymphadenopathy. Occasionally the vein is not dilated throughout its entire course, which generates more confusion.

C and **D,** another patient with a similar condition was evaluated for metastases, and CT showed a right retrocrural soft tissue density **(C).** Incidentally, notice that a gastric pseudotumor in the adrenal fossa mimics a mass *(m).* The T_1-weighted (TR/TE, 800/25) MR image **(D)** proves the signal-void vascular nature (azygos vein) of the retrocrural densities *(arrowhead).*

C

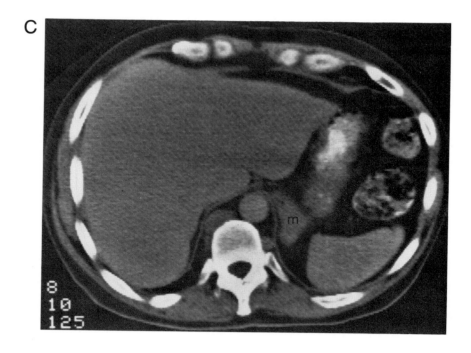

D

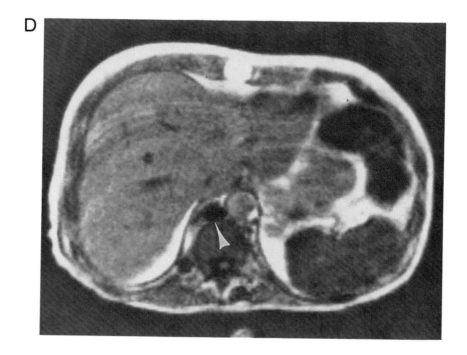

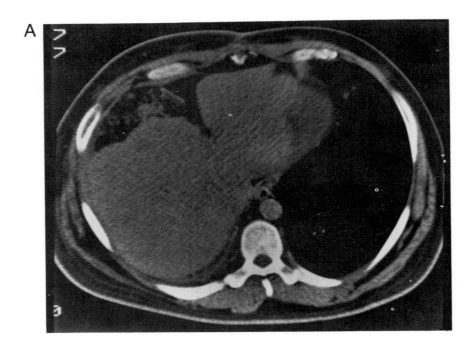

FIG 14–4.
Subphrenic abscess? (Multiple cases.) Computed tomography was used to rule out subphrenic abscess in these two patients, both of whom had recently undergone abdominal surgery.

A, adjacent to the upper portion of the liver and lateral to the falciform ligament, the appearance of the soft tissue with multiple air bubbles could be mistaken for a subphrenic abscess. This results from the very high location of the hepatic flexure of the colon. This patient also has a small right pleural effusion.

B and **C,** in the second patient, the hepatic flexure of the colon is anterior to the right lobe of the liver. Because of this appearance and even questionable extraluminal gas, the possibility of a liver or subphrenic abscess was raised during CT study of the chest.

A scan at a lower level **(C)** shows contiguity of the suspected abnormality with the normal colon.

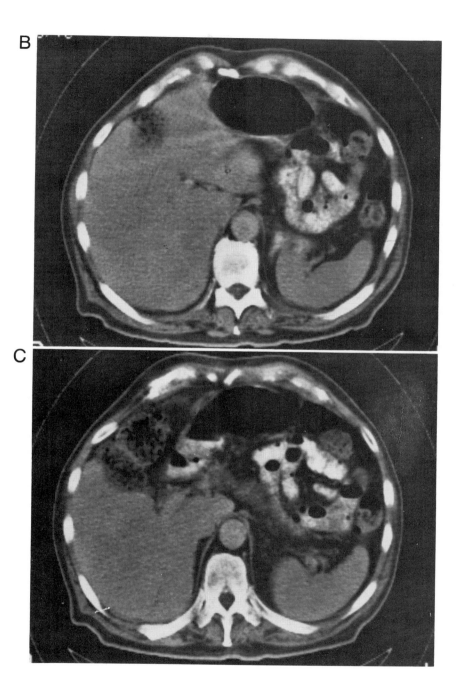

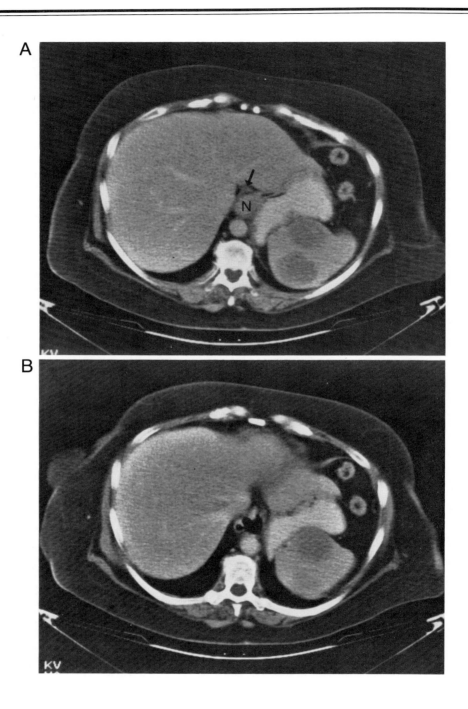

FIG 14–5.
Retroesophageal node? This patient with known lymphoma had an abdominal CT scan for the evaluation of the extent of disease.

A, on this upper abdomen CT image, the spleen is obviously involved by areas of lower attenuation. There seems to be a large node *(N)* behind the esophagus *(arrow),* displacing the esophagus anteriorly.

B, a repeat CT image at the same level following oral administration of a small amount of contrast material demonstrates the esophagus with a probable small sliding hiatal hernia filled with air. There is no evidence of adenopathy.

This is an anatomical area offering many pitfalls. Anytime there is a questionable mass in this region, repeat CT at the same level with more oral contrast is recommended.

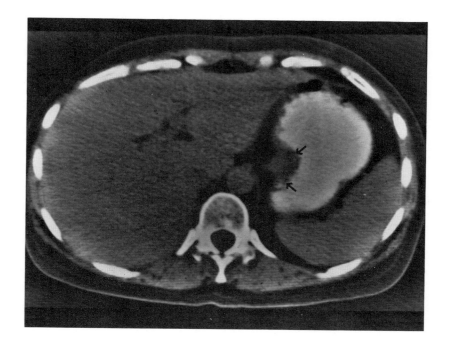

FIG 14–6.
Esophagogastric mass? This patient, who underwent abdominal CT because of possible pancreatic tumor, was found to have a prominent soft tissue mass at the esophagogastric junction *(arrows)*. A double-contrast upper gastrointestinal barium study yielded normal findings.

Such a finding at the esophagogastric junction is seen in more than one third of patients undergoing abdominal CT scan. It is related to the transverse anatomical plane of section through the normal junction and cardia. Variations in gastric distension may affect this prominent soft tissue density.

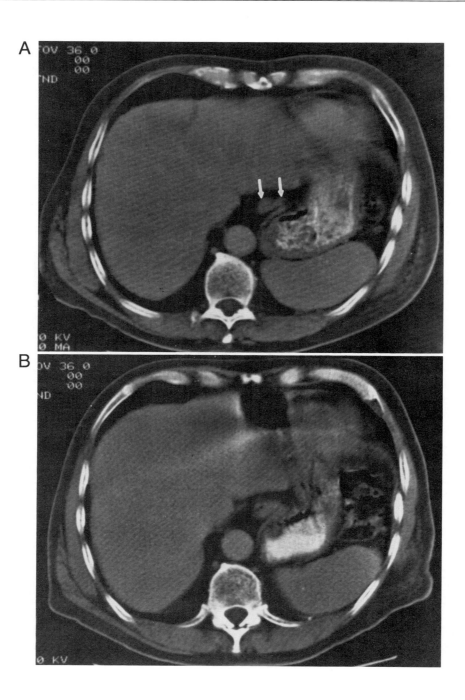

FIG 14–7.
Lymph node in the gastrohepatic ligament? Abdominal CT was used in this patient to assess for metastases from melanoma of the lower extremity.

A, on this upper abdomen image, the only abnormality seen is nodular soft tissue densities in the upper portion of the gastrohepatic ligament *(arrows).* Initially, it was thought that these might represent lymph nodes.

B, on the repeat CT, with more oral contrast, a small amount of air is seen within this soft tissue density, proving the verdict of normal esophagus being imaged just before the esophagogastric junction.

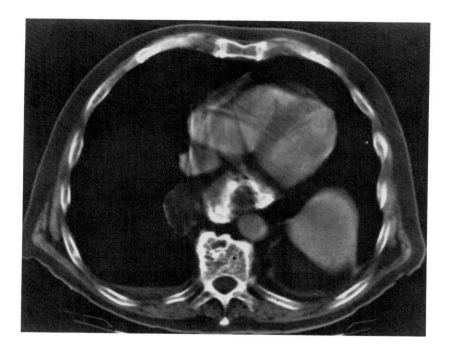

FIG 14–8.
Hiatal hernia with mass? This patient, who had a transabdominal fundoplication as an antireflux operation for hiatal hernia, underwent CT examination because of consistent upper abdominal pain.

A soft tissue mass is seen anterior to the aorta and is surrounded by the oral contrast material. This is a result of the surgery, which involved wrapping part of the fundus around the lower esophagus. It should not be mistaken for a tumor in the esophagus or stomach. Proper knowledge of the type of surgery is essential in such cases.

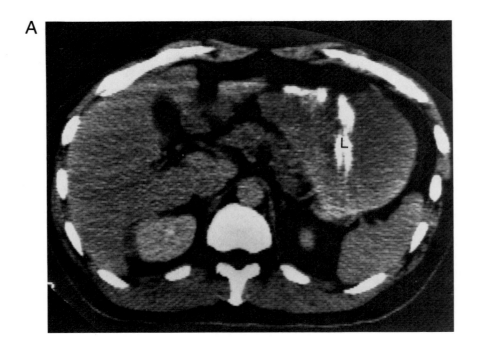

FIG 14–9.
Gastric tumor? (Multiple cases.)

　　A and **B,** CT was used in this lymphoma patient to evaluate response to chemotherapy.

The upper abdomen CT image **(A)** shows marked thickening of the gastric wall, whose density is similar to that of the spleen or liver. A small amount of oral contrast material is seen in the lumen *(L).*

B

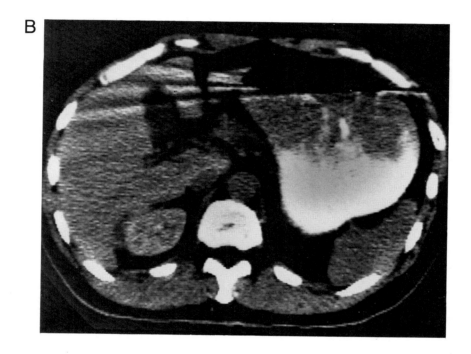

Since the patient was clinically free of symptoms, upper abdomen CT was repeated **(B)** following the administration of more oral contrast. In this image, the pseudomass nature of the gastric wall is obviously due to inadequate distension of the stomach. (*Continued.*)

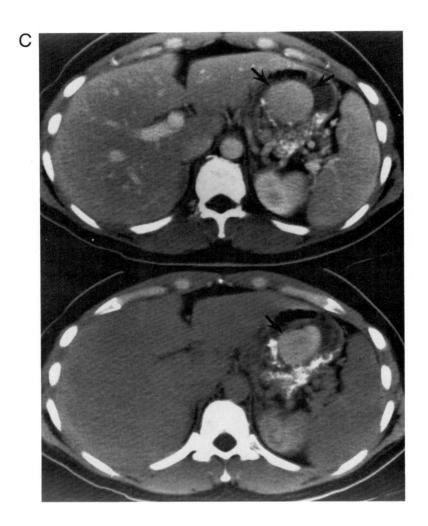

FIG 14–9 (cont.).
C through **E,** CT in this patient with lung carcinoma shows a soft tissue density (*arrows* in **C**), thought to represent a leiomyoma, within the gastric lumen. Fifteen minutes later and at the completion of abdominal study, the images were repeated with more oral contrast. These sequential images **(D)** show the apparent mass in **C** becoming enhanced with barium. A double-contrast gastric study **(E)** proved lack of any abnormality.

D

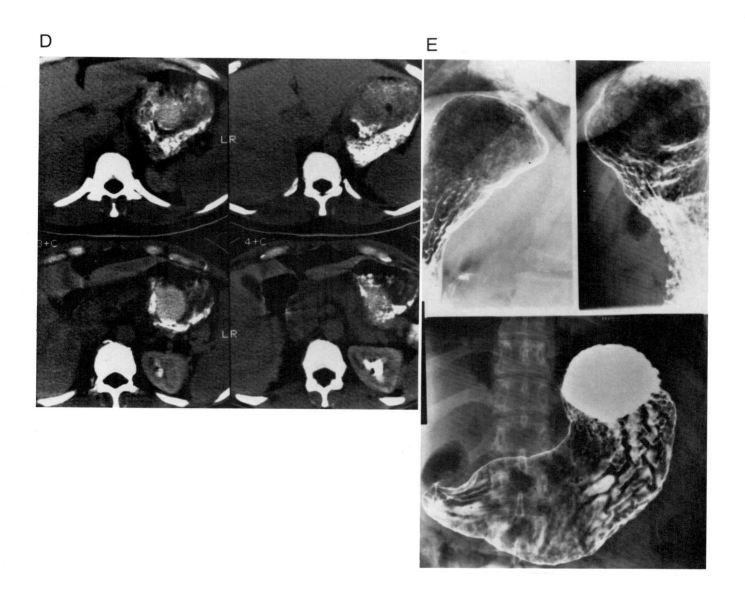

E

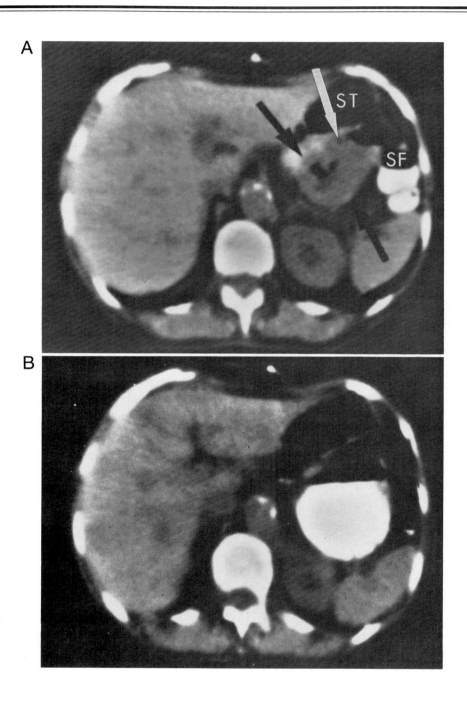

FIG 14–10.
Left upper quadrant abscess? This youngster with a history of abdominal surgery presented with fever, and a CT scan was done to rule out intraabdominal abscess.

A, on this upper abdomen CT image, a soft tissue mass with central air *(arrows)* is seen behind the stomach *(ST)* and medial to the splenic flexure of the colon *(SF).* The ini-tial thought was an abscess or hematoma.

B, before any treatment, CT was repeated with more oral contrast. This proved the common pitfall of the inade-quately contrast-filled stomach, mimicking an abscess in the left upper quadrant. No other abnormalities were discov-ered.

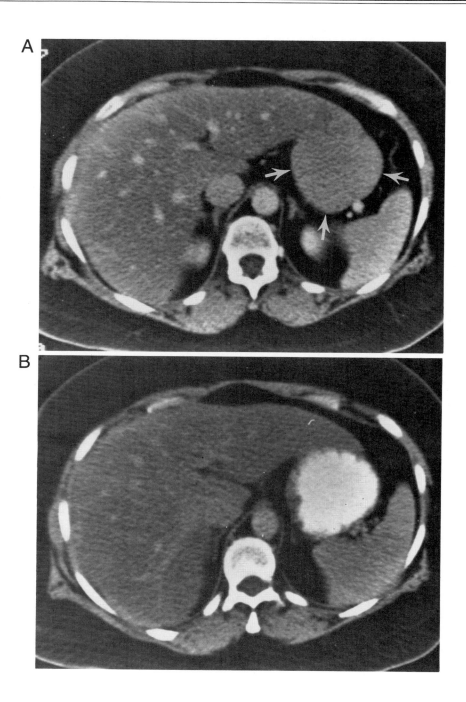

FIG 14–11.
Liver mass? This woman with known breast carcinoma showed abnormal levels of liver enzymes. A CT scan was done to rule out metastases.

A, on this image, a large, relatively enhancing mass contiguous with the left lobe of the liver is seen *(arrows).*

Although the probability of unopacified stomach was raised in this instance, one could conceivably mistake this finding for a large, bulging mass in the liver.

B, CT was repeated with more oral contrast. This image indeed proves the nature of the mass to be inadequately opacified stomach.

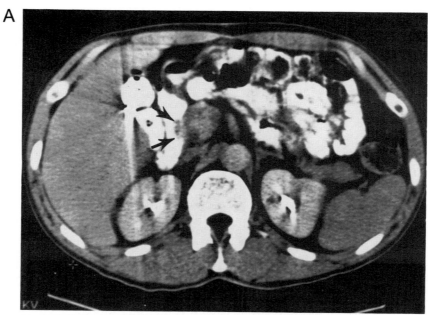

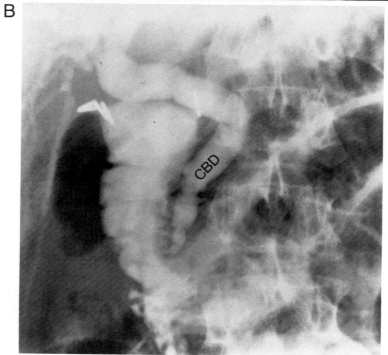

FIG 14–12.
Duodenal lesion? This patient, who had had a cholecystectomy but no history of malignancy, experienced mild abdominal pain.

A, on this upper abdomen CT image, there is a promi-nent soft tissue density *(arrows)* in the medial wall of the descending duodenum.

B, a cholangiogram shows a normal common bile duct *(CBD)* with a normal-variant prominent papilla.

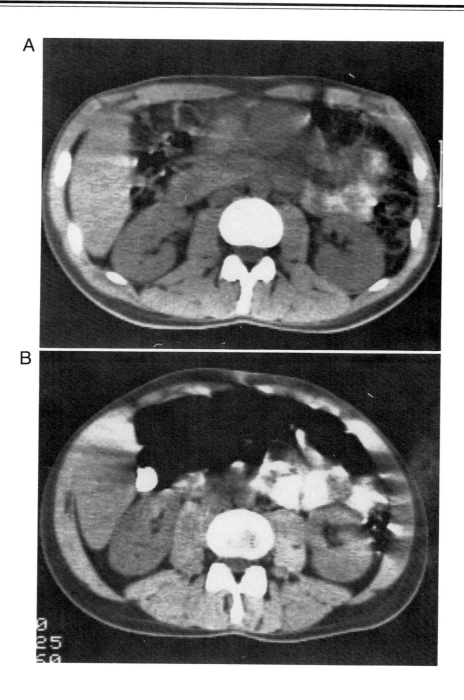

FIG 14–13.
Retroperitoneal, mesenteric adenopathy? (Multiple cases.)

A and **B,** this young man with malignant seminoma had abdominal CT to rule out metastases. The abdominal CT study was performed without intravenous contrast because of a history of allergy to iodine; however, the patient received oral contrast. On image **A,** multiple soft tissue densities are seen in the paraaortic and mesenteric regions. No mass was clinically palpable.

Computed tomography was repeated following the administration of more oral contrast. Image **B** shows that a large amount of gas has moved from the stomach to the small bowel and that most of the pseudotumors are now opacified with oral contrast. No retroperitoneal adenopathy is seen. This is a very frequent source of pitfall in the mesentery and retroperitoneum. The bowel loops can simulate masses, abscesses, and lymph nodes. *(Continued.)*

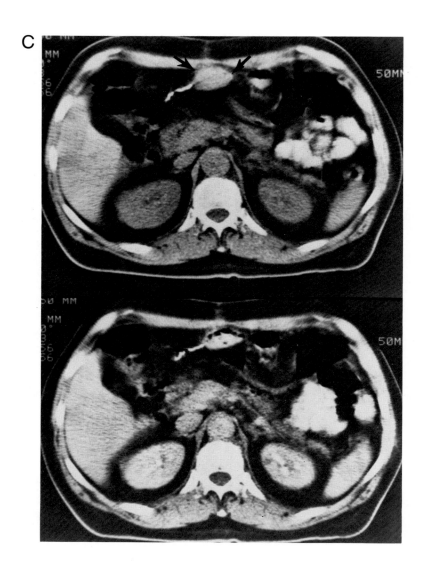

FIG 14–13. (cont.).

C, this different patient with gastric carcinoma had prior gastrectomy and gastroduodenostomy. The one-year follow-up CT scan shows a soft tissue density adjacent to the surgical suture line (*arrows* in *top*), thought to represent recurrence at the anastomotic site. Repeat study with intravenous contrast and more oral contrast *(bottom)* proved the presence of unopacified bowel loop adjacent to the suture line.

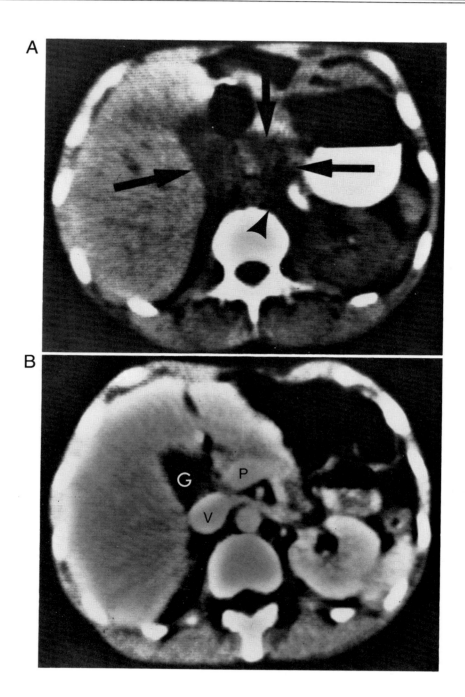

FIG 14–14.
Mass in the porta hepatis? This young girl with a primary rhabdomyosarcoma in the pelvis underwent CT for evaluation of the extent of disease.

A, on the unenhanced CT, fullness in the porta hepatis and celiac axis suggests mass *(arrows)* and nodes in the paraaortic region *(arrowhead).*

B, a repeat CT image made during bolus intravenous contrast shows normal portal vein *(P)*, inferior vena cava *(V)*, gallbladder *(G)*, and renal pedicle. No mass or adenopathy is present.

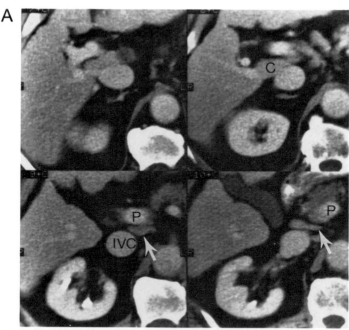

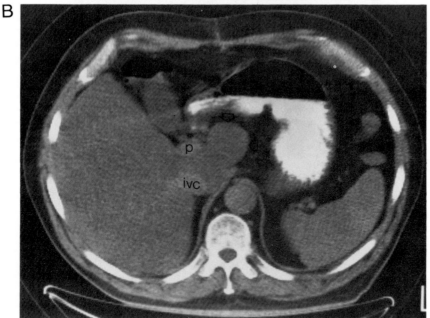

FIG 14–15.
Precaval node? (Multiple cases.)

A, on these four sequential images (left to right), which were obtained at 10-mm intervals, there is a soft tissue density *(arrows)* behind the portal vein *(P)* and anterior to the inferior vena cava *(IVC)*. The connection of this soft tissue density with the caudate lobe *(C)* can be appreciated on sequential images. However, in the third and fourth images, this density, which represents the normal papillary process of the caudate lobe of the liver, could be misread as a small precaval lymph node.

B, in this upper abdomen CT image from another patient, the papillary process of the caudate lobe *(arrows)* is markedly enlarged and is anteriorly outlined by the portal vein *(p)* and posteriorly outlined by the inferior vena cava *(ivc)*.

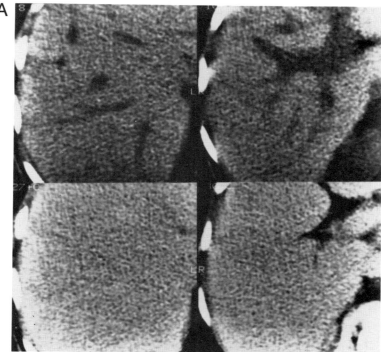

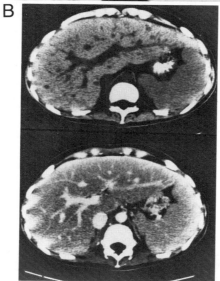

FIG 14–16.
Biliary dilatation?

A, this patient with lymphoma and mildly elevated levels of liver enzymes had liver CT scan to rule out biliary obstruction or metastases.

Top row on the unenhanced CT scan, there are linear areas of low density throughout the liver that simulate intrahepatic ductal dilatation. There are also some small, rounded low-density areas that suggest metastases.

Bottom row, upon repeat CT scans made with drip intravenous contrast, these low densities become isodense to the liver, which proves the structures to be unopacified venous channels. In patients with allergy to iodine, it might be necessary to use ultrasound to prove the nature of the pseudoducts seen on unenhanced CT.

B, in another patient, a bolus contrast causes the low density areas (*top*) to enhance (*bottom*), proving their vascular nature.

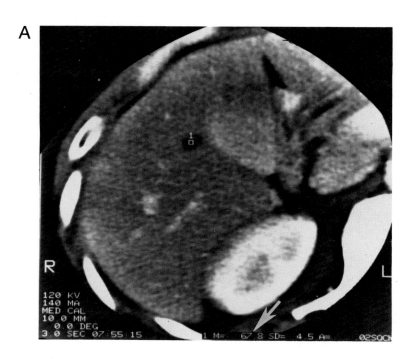

FIG 14–17.

Liver metastasis? This patient with cutaneous malignant melanoma had CT to rule out intraabdominal metastases.

A, a single lesion is seen on enhanced liver CT using 10-mm slice thickness and equal increment. Its attenuation value *(arrow)* is in the soft tissue range (67.8 Hounsfield units).

B, a repeat CT scan was done of the same area but using a 1.5-mm slice thickness. The image shows the same lesion to have the attenuation value *(arrow)* of fluid (−2.8 Hounsfield units). This lesion represented a simple liver cyst and did not change in eight months' CT follow-up. Notice the necessity to change the milliampere setting from 140 to

170 when using a slice thickness of 1.5 mm.

C, the drawings illustrate that a lesion is often only partially imaged when the lesion's dimension and the slice thickness are the same *(1)*. In this example, the attenuation values of the lesion and adjacent liver are additive. The lesion's attenuation value would also be incorrect if the slice thickness exceeded the lesion's width *(2)*. The ideal relationship would have the slice cover the lesion from edge to edge *(3)*. However, to ensure accurate sampling of this small lesion, it will be best to narrow the slice thickness *(4)*, as was done in **B**.

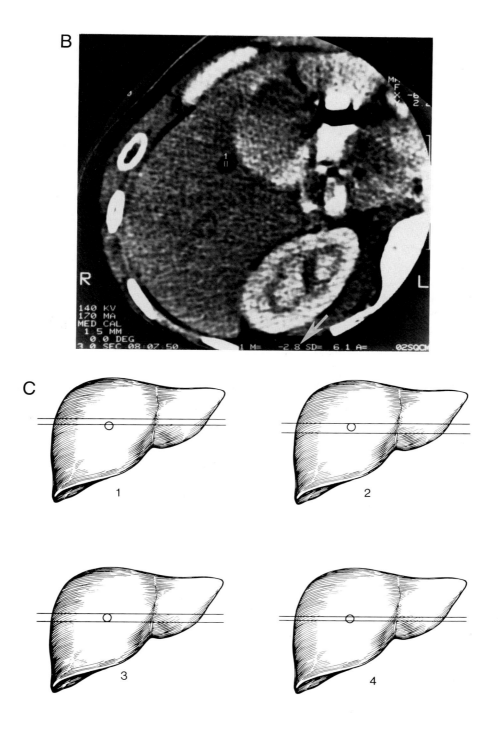

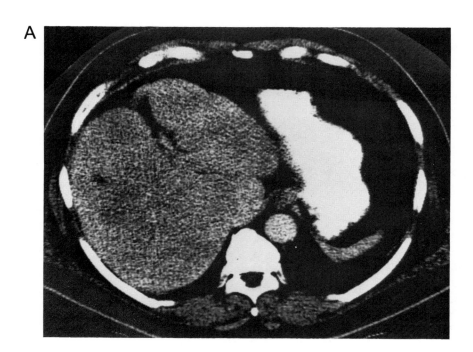

FIG 14–18.

Hepatic mass? The patient had a history of alcohol abuse and weight loss and was evaluated for the possibility of any malignancy.

A, the liver is rather small and shows irregularly outlined low-density areas proved by a biopsy to represent fatty infiltration.

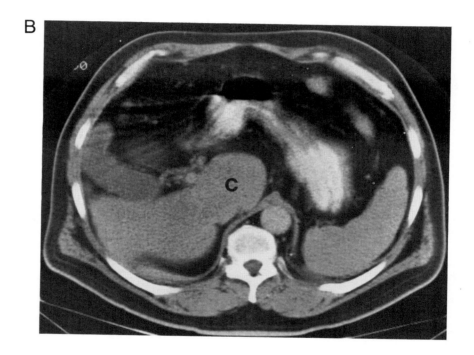

B, on this image, which is 3 cm below **A,** the caudate lobe of the liver *(C)* is hypertrophic and bulbous. This appearance, which is commonly seen in cirrhotic liver, should not be mistaken for a primary hepatic neoplasm. There is a particular risk of mistaking fatty infiltration in the caudate lobe for necrotic tumor.

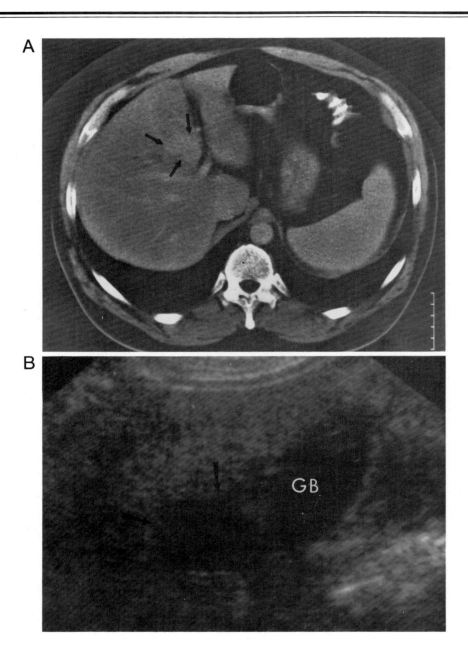

FIG 14–19.

Liver metastasis? (Multiple cases.) Two women, both with known carcinoma of the breast, underwent CT examination to rule out liver metastasis. Each was receiving chemotherapy.

A and **B,** a contrast-enhanced CT scan **(A)** shows diffuse decreased attenuation throughout the liver, this due to fatty metamorphosis. However, there is a well-defined area of high density *(arrows)* in the liver, adjacent to the porta hepatis. This area was thought to represent a focus of metastasis.

A parasagittal sonogram **(B)** through the area in **A** shows the abnormality to be hypoechoic. The gallbladder

(GB) is seen. Percutaneous biopsy proved this area to be normal liver parenchyma not infiltrated by fat. In fact, the sonographic echogenicity of the rest of the liver in this case is coarse because of fatty change. That fatty change probably resulted from chemotherapy.

C and **D,** in the second patient, a contrast-enhanced CT scan **(C)** shows a similar abnormality. A focal area of high density *(arrows),* which was thought to represent enhanced metastasis, is seen in the left lobe.

The transverse sonogram **(D)** in this patient shows a corresponding hypoechoic area *(arrows),* proved by biopsy to represent normal liver.

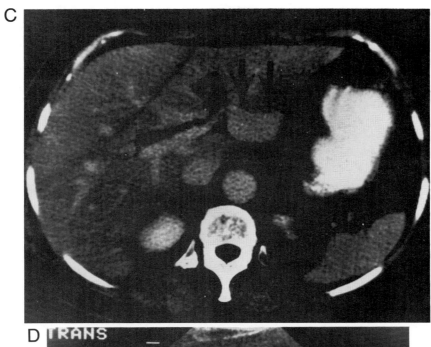

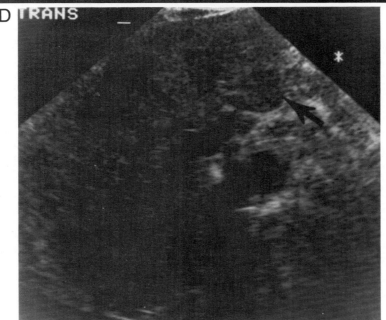

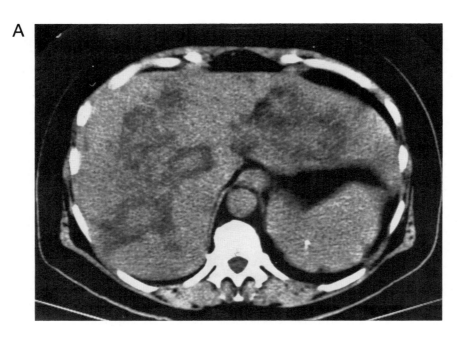

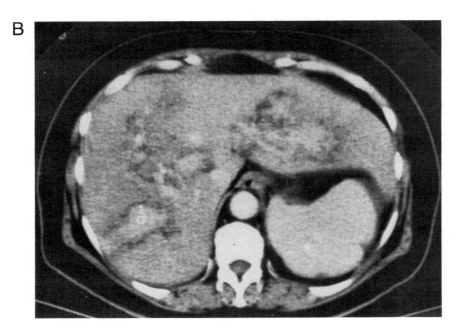

FIG 14–20.

Liver metastasis or biliary ductal dilatation? This woman with hepatomegaly was evaluated by CT as part of the diagnostic workup.

A, the unenhanced CT of the liver shows linear and circular areas of low attenuation in both lobes. The possibility of metastasis or biliary ductal dilatation was raised.

B, a contrast-enhanced CT image of the liver shows normal enhancement of the hepatic parenchyma. Even those islands that are surrounded by the circular and linear low densities enhance.

Percutaneous ultrasound-guided biopsy disclosed hepatic fatty infiltration.

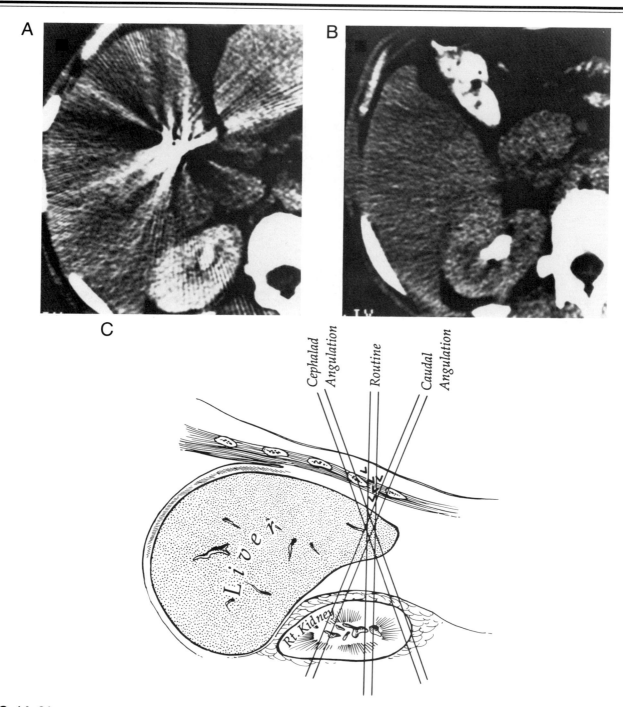

FIG 14–21.
Liver metastasis? This woman with breast carcinoma was evaluated for possible liver metastasis. She had a history of cholecystectomy.

On image **A,** because of artifacts from multiple surgical clips, the right lobe of the liver cannot be evaluated for metastasis. One way to overcome this problem is to angle the gantry in a direction so that the x-ray beam will not interact with the clips. In image **B,** the result of caudad angulation of the gantry is an artifact-free image. At this angle, as seen in the sagital schematic drawing **(C),** one may continue to scan at smaller increments until the clips are seen, so a major portion of the right lobe can be clearly scanned. Routine position of the gantry in **C** shows interaction with clips.

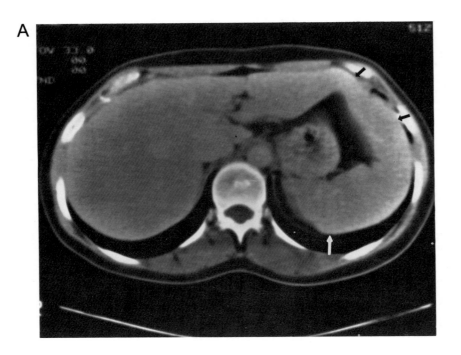

FIG 14–22.
Splenomegaly? In this patient, the normal-variant elongated hepatic left lobe, which extends anterior and lateral to the spleen, can be added to the spleen by CT, mimicking splenomegaly.

A, on this image obtained using a soft tissue window, it was thought that the entire structure *(arrows)* in the left upper quadrant represented a large spleen.

B, on the narrow window, the normal-sized spleen *(S)* is seen, with the enhanced left lobe of the liver *(L)* wrapped in the lateral aspect.

C, in this CT image on the lower level, again the narrow tongue of the left hepatic lobe is seen to wrap around the spleen and to extend to the posterior aspect *(open arrows)*. Incidentally, the lobulated appearance of the spleen generates a pseudomass *(m)* between the spleen and the left kidney on this image.

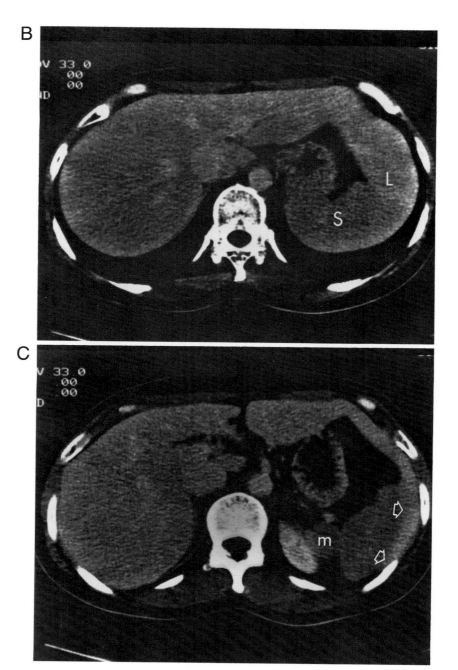

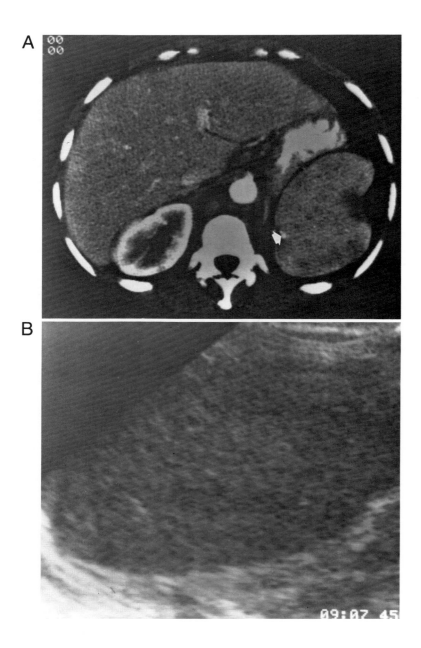

FIG 14–23.
Splenic metastasis? (Multiple cases.)

A and **B,** this patient had been treated for non-Hodgkin's lymphoma and was considered disease free. A CT scan was done as a follow-up study.

The upper abdomen CT image **(A)** was obtained following bolus intravenous injection of contrast material. High-density contrast is seen in the aorta, and cortical blush is seen in the right kidney. The large spleen displays areas of low density, an effect thought to be due to lymphomatous involvement. Incidentally, a granuloma is visible in the spleen *(arrow).*

Because CT showed no other evidence of disease, a splenic sonogram **(B)** was obtained to confirm the abnormality. The sonogram shows homogeneous echo pattern throughout the spleen, with no focal abnormality.

The apparent low-density areas of the spleen seen on bolus CT study were due to the difference of contrast distribution through the splenic red pulp in the early arterial phase.

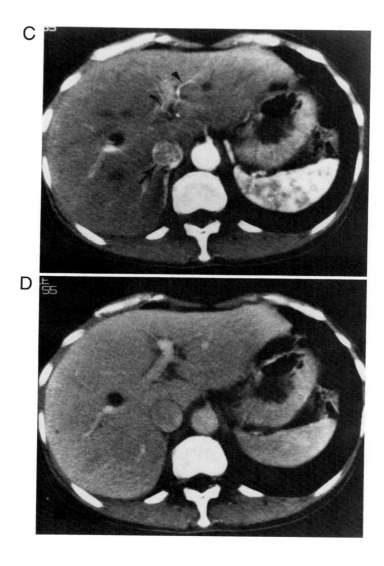

C and D, early arterial-phase CT as a part of workup for metastasis in another patient shows nonhomogeneous splenic enhancement (C). Notice enhancement of hepatic arteries within the liver *(arrowheads)*. Also the mixture of enhanced and unenhanced blood in the vena cava *(arrow)* can mimic clot. Repeat CT, in the equilibrium phase, shows normal spleen and cava. (C and D courtesy of K. Takayasu, M.D., Department of Radiology, National Cancer Center, Tokyo.)

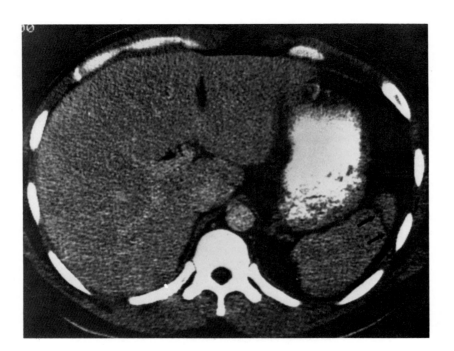

FIG 14–24.
Splenic laceration? An 18-year-old college athlete with a diagnosis of Hodgkin's disease was followed by abdominal CT scan. He had suffered blunt abdominal trauma while playing soccer.

On this upper abdomen CT image, there is a lucent line *(arrows)* in the anterior aspect of the spleen. Because the patient is athletic, one might think of splenic laceration. In fact, the finding represents a congenital cleft of the spleen, which generates so-called pseudosplenic laceration.

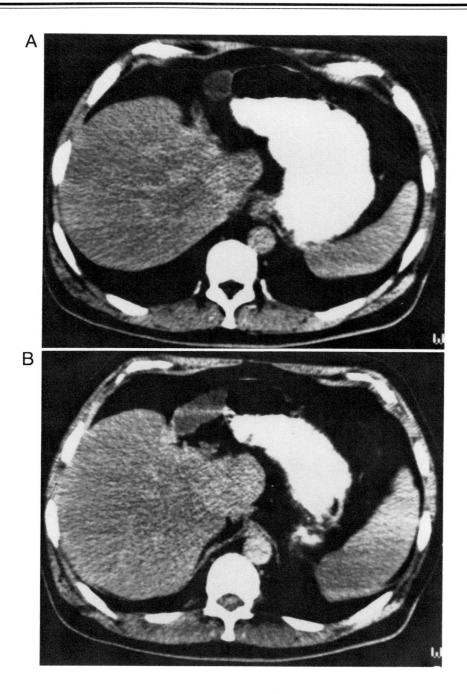

FIG 14–25.

Post-hepatic lobectomy gallbladder/tumor? This patient had a history of left hepatic lobectomy for removal of a single metastasis of colon carcinoma. A repeat CT scan was done because of a rising carcinoembryonic antigen (CEA) titer.

  A and **B,** no evidence of metastasis is seen in the liver. The right lobe is somewhat globular, not an unusual appearance after removal of a lobe. However, there is a small cystic structure adjacent to the fundus of the stomach, anterior and medial to the right lobe of the liver. This structure did not fill with more oral contrast or after rescanning with the patient in different positions. It was evaluated by ultrasound and was proven to represent a displaced gallbladder. Initially, abnormalities such as cystic metastases to the gastrohepatic ligament or a small duplication cyst were considered.

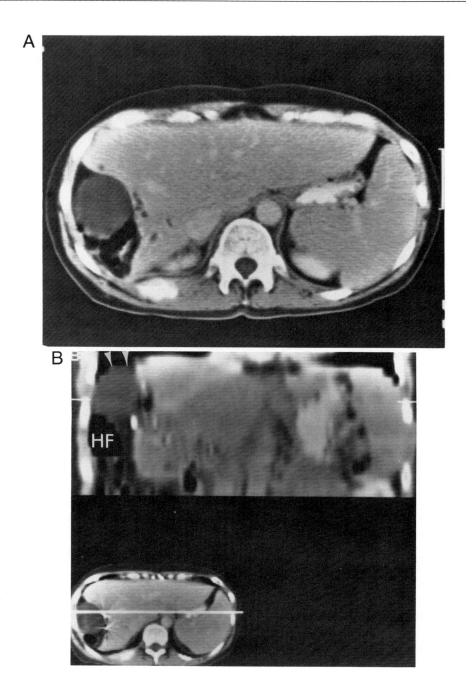

FIG 14–26.
Cystic mass? This patient, who had undergone partial right hepatic lobectomy, was evaluated by CT because of continual tenderness in the right upper quadrant.

A, on this axial CT scan, a well-defined cystic structure is seen lateral to the liver. Posterior to this is the hepatic flexure of the colon. Since the gallbladder could not be localized in its normal location, and since it was not removed at the time of lobectomy, the cystic structure undoubtedly represents this organ displaced.

B, a coronal reconstruction image shows the lateral position of the gallbladder under the diaphragm *(arrowheads)* and above the hepatic flexure of the colon *(HF).*

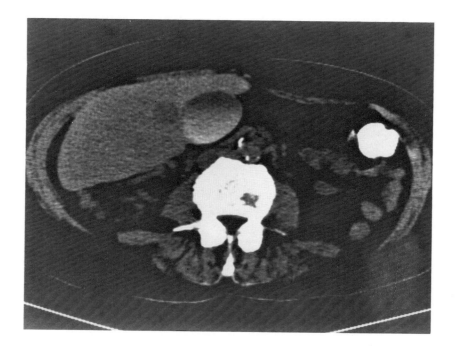

FIG 14–27.
Gallbladder sludge? This patient with renal cell carcinoma had undergone angiographic workup about 20 hr before this CT scan.

There is high-density material within the lumen of the gallbladder. This is iodine from the recent angiography. Such a finding is not uncommon at this location shortly after administration of a large dosage of contrast medium, and it should not be mistaken for milk of calcium, sludge, or hemorrhage within the gallbladder lumen.

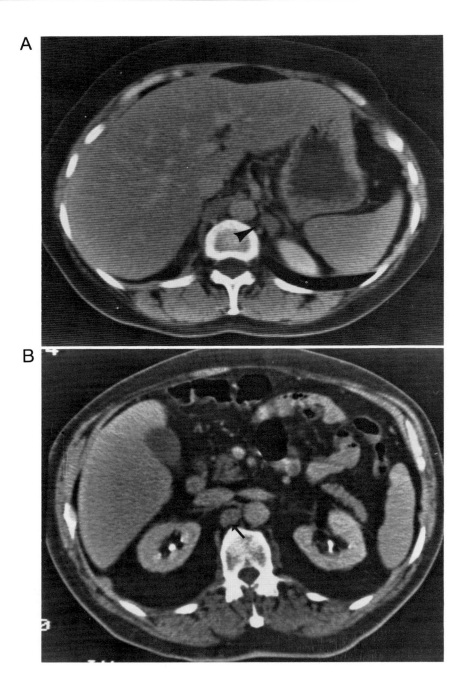

FIG 14–28.
Adenopathy? This patient with Hodgkin's disease in the mediastinum had abdominal CT for evaluation of possible lymphadenopathy.

A, nodular densities are seen adjacent to the aorta and vena cava in both sides of the retroperitoneum. The density in the left side can be mistaken for a node or enlarged adre-

nal gland *(arrowhead)*.

B, the retroperitoneal nodular soft tissue densities are seen in multiple images and represent the tendinous diaphragmatic crura in both sides. Generally, the right crus *(arrow)* is larger, longer, and often more lobular than the left crus. It is potentially a source of misinterpretation as retroperitoneal adenopathy.

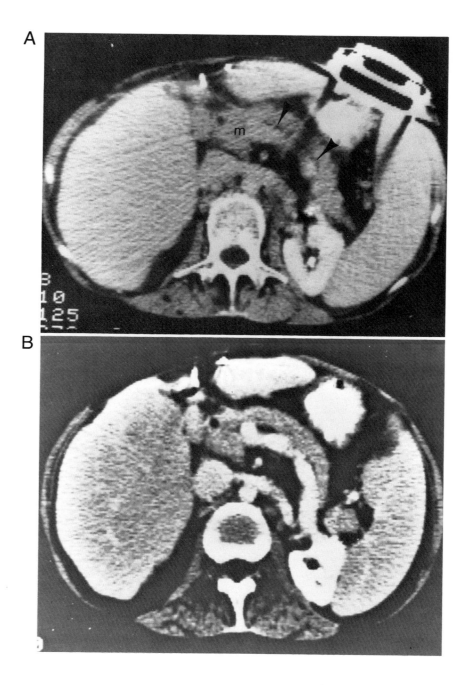

FIG 14–29.

Large pancreas with dilated duct? A 46-year-old woman had abdominal CT to rule out pancreatic abnormality.

A, on this CT image, which was done about 12 hr after intravenous pyelography, the pancreas appears to be enlarged and to have a prominent duct *(arrowheads).* There is a possible mass *(m)* in the pancreatic head.

B, repeat scan on bolus contrast injection proves that there is pseudoenlargement of the pancreas because of added thickness of the unenhanced splenic vein. The apparent dilated duct, or pseudoduct, is attributable to the fat between the pancreas and the splenic vein. The head of the pancreas is normal.

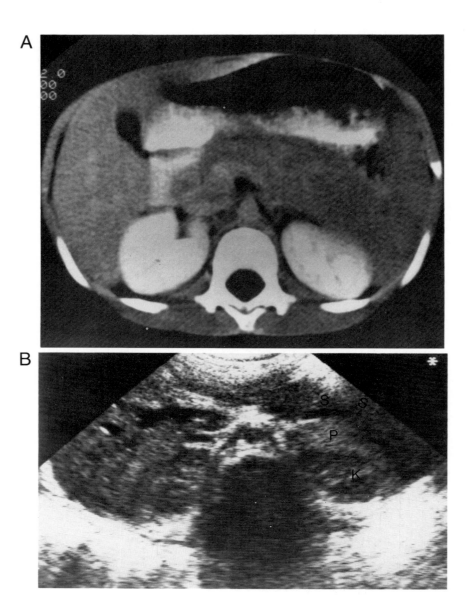

FIG 14–30.
Pancreatic enlargement? On development of fever of unknown origin, this six-year-old leukemia patient had CT to
rule out intraabdominal abscess.

A, the upper abdomen CT image shows a very large
pancreas with loss of fat planes between the pancreas and
the spleen. Such possibilities as pancreatitis, leukemic infiltration of the pancreas, and massive peripancreatic adenopathy were raised.

B, an abdominal sonogram reveals a normal pancreas
(P) with no adenopathy or abnormal fluid collection. However, the spleen *(S)* appears to have a very elongated medial process that extends anterior to the pancreas. The left
kidney *(K)* is seen on this image.

In children and cachectic individuals, because of inadequate retroperitoneal fat, the proximity of the organs can
cause an additive effect that mimics organomegaly.

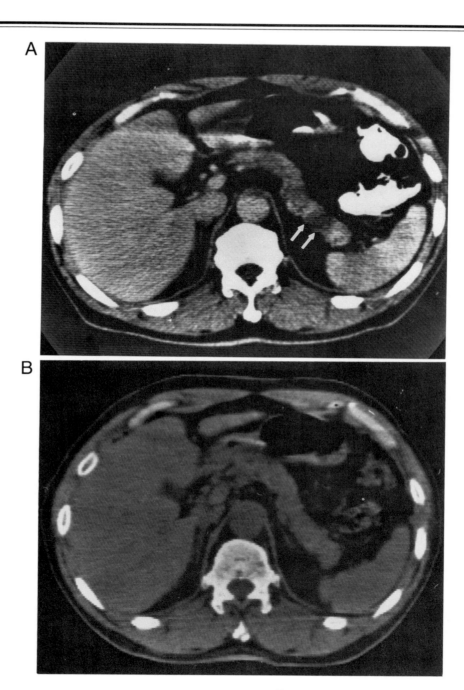

FIG 14–31.
Pancreatic mass? This elderly patient was evaluated because of weight loss and loss of appetite.

A, the upper abdomen CT scan, which was done one day after upper gastrointestinal barium study, demonstrates an area of low density *(arrows)* in the distal end of the body of the pancreas.

Because of the high-density barium in the adjacent splenic flexure of the colon and the possibility of artifact, the decision was made to repeat this image later.

B, this scan was obtained 4 hr after **A** and demonstrates a normal pancreas. The barium has been cleared from the colon by this time.

Artifacts from high-density barium within the gastrointestinal tract or from a metallic device can generate pseudolesions in the liver, pancreas, spleen, and kidneys. Under these circumstances, the study should be repeated after the barium has moved from the area of interest. In cases of artifact from a metallic device, sonography or MRI might be necessary.

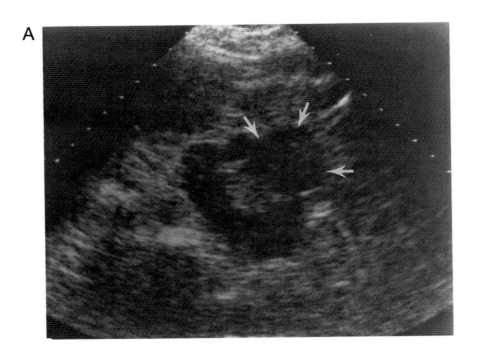

FIG 14–32.
Renal mass? Ultrasonography in this patient with vague abdominal pain showed a probable left renal mass.

A, the sonogram shows a left renal mass *(arrows)* that has the same degree of echogenicity as the renal cortex. There is minimal mass effect on the adjacent renal collecting system. The diagnosis of a primary renal neoplasm could not be ruled out.

B, on this CT image, there appears to be a mass projecting laterally *(arrows)* from the midportion of the left kidney. The mass enhances almost to the same degree as the

renal parenchyma. The possibility of a normal fetal lobulation was raised.

Under these circumstances, the kidney can be evaluated noninvasively by using renal scintigraphic agents that concentrate in the cortex. The favorite agent in this situation is ^{99m}Tc-labeled dimercaptosuccinic acid (^{99m}Tc-DMSA).

C, on this posterior scintiscan, the agent concentrated in the renal cortex and in the normal lobulated region *(arrows),* resulting in a normal scan. Otherwise, there would be a "cold" area in the renal parenchyma. Scintigraphy cannot help to differentiate between cystic and solid masses.

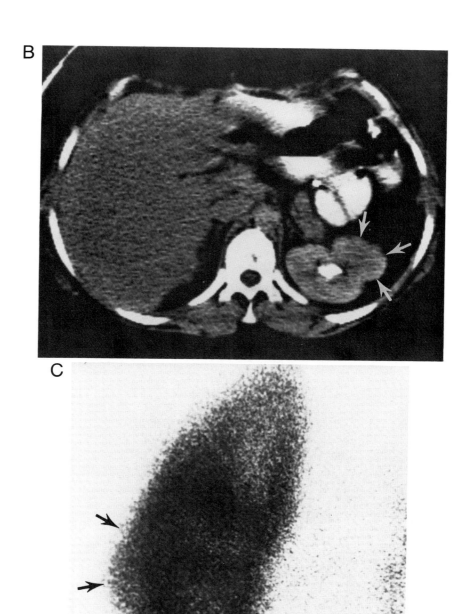

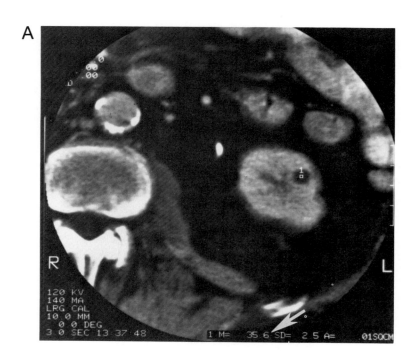

FIG 14–33.
Renal metastasis? This patient with carcinoma of the lung had CT of the abdomen to rule out metastasis.

 A, a single left renal lesion was discovered on routine abdominal CT using 10-mm slice thickness and equal increment. It has an attenuation value of 35.6 Hounsfield units *(arrow),* atypical for a simple cyst.

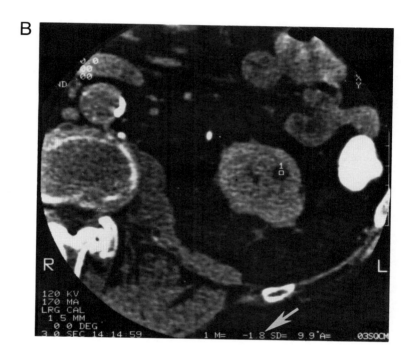

B

B, repeat CT of the same area using a 1.5-mm slice thickness shows the same lesion with an attenuation value of −1.8 Hounsfield units *(arrow)*. A follow-up CT scan in five months showed no change, proving simple renal cyst.

Here also, as in the case of liver (see Fig 14–17), the milliampere setting has to be increased from 140 to 170 when decreasing the slice thickness from 10 to 1.5 mm.

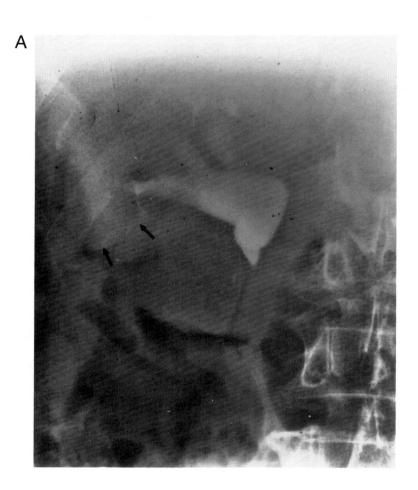

FIG 14–34.

Perirenal mass or abscess? This woman with a gynecologic malignancy underwent intravenous pyelography as a part of the tumor staging procedures.

A, the pyelogram demonstrates lateral displacement of the lower pole of the right kidney *(arrows)* and attenuation of the ureteropelvic junction. The possibility of a mass in the area was raised, and abdominal CT was ordered.

B, the CT image at the corresponding level shows a contrast- and air-filled structure *(D)* infiltrating between the right kidney *(K)* and the proximal ureter *(open arrows)*.

C, the image was repeated a few minutes later. It shows that the contrast has left this portion of the bowel, presumably the duodenum *(D* in image **B**). The renal pelvis and proximal right ureter are seen *(open arrows)*.

Occasionally, if the bowel is not filled with contrast medium, the air-filled structures in the above region can be mistaken for a small abscess in the proximity of the kidney. Under these circumstances, the imaging should always be repeated, with more oral contrast or at a later time.

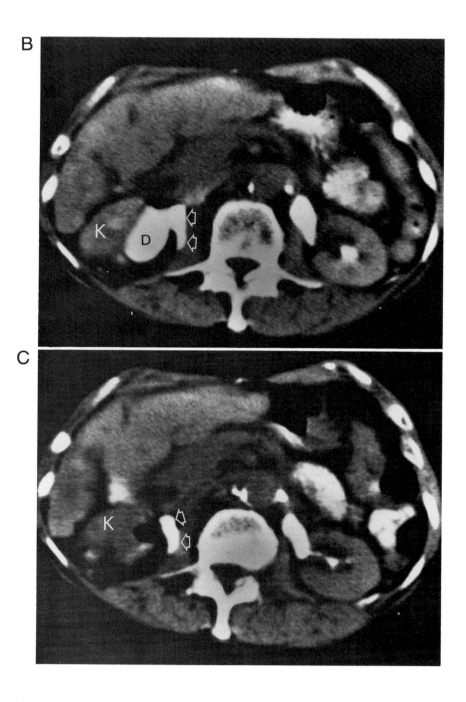

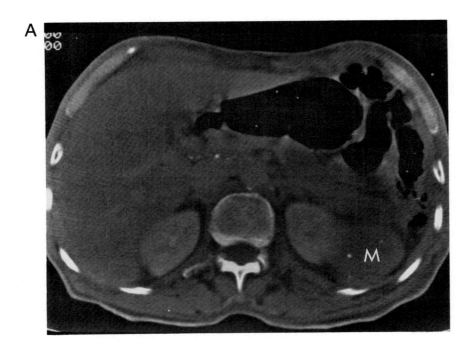

FIG 14–35.
Renal mass? This patient with a primary bladder tumor underwent a workup for possible metastasis.

A, on this midabdominal CT image, there appears to be a mass *(M)* with punctate calcifications blending into the lateral aspect of the left kidney.

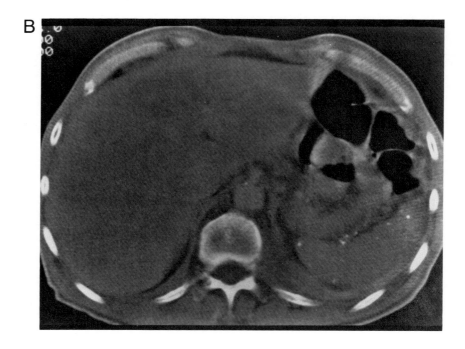

B, because similar calcifications in the spleen are seen on the higher image, it was thought that the apparent left renal mass could be related to lobulated spleen. An ultrasound examination was done (not shown) and confirmed the normal appearance of the left kidney.

Occasionally, this situation can be solved on the CT table by placing the patient in a prone or lateral decubitus position and obtaining images in different phases of respiration. One might attempt to obtain a thin-slice image, which can sometimes show the plane between the spleen and kidney in better detail.

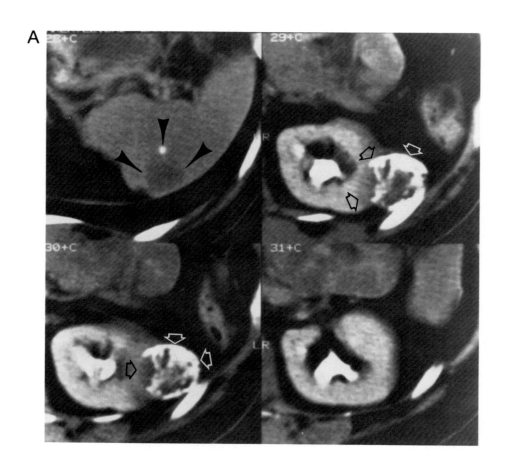

FIG 14–36.
Calcified renal tumor? This 41-year-old woman with known lymphoma underwent CT as follow-up in the abdomen.

A, these four sequential images were made using a 10-mm slice thickness. On the highest image, one can see an area of low density with a flake of calcium *(arrowheads)* in the spleen. The two middle images show what appears to be a calcified left renal mass *(arrows),* and on the lowest image the left kidney is normal.

B, the repeat images, made using a 5-mm slice thickness, show a thick-walled calcified splenic cyst in the lower pole of the spleen, adjacent to the kidney. There is clearly a fat plane between the splenic cyst and the normal left renal cortex.

C, the coronal reconstructed CT image displays the splenorenal relationship, which in this case resulted in a pitfall for renal mass. In **A,** in fact, the middle and the very bottom of the calcified cyst were scanned, but a major part of the cyst was skipped because of the 10-mm slice thickness and probably because of a different phase of respiration.

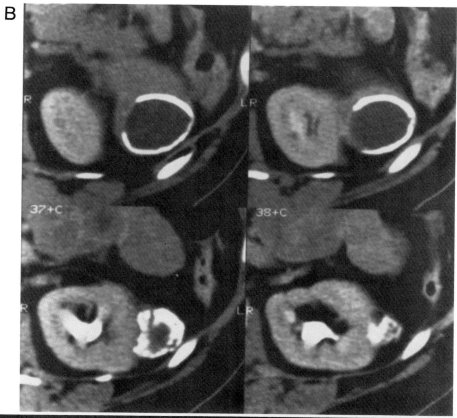

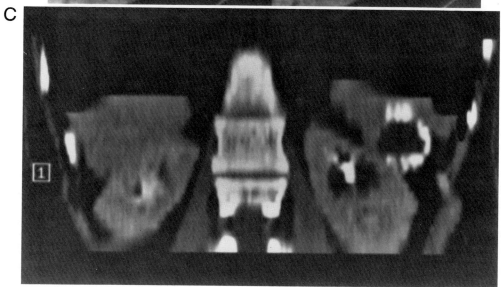

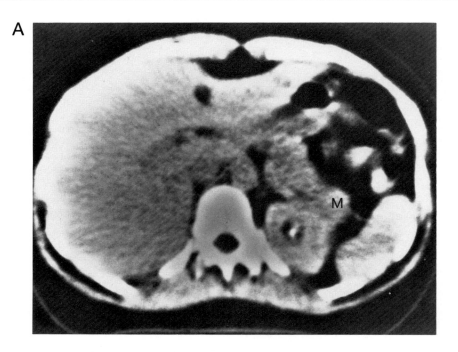

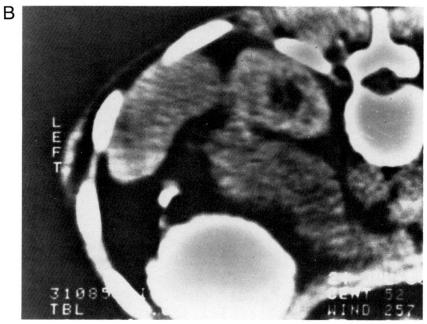

FIG 14–37.
Renal mass? Intravenous pyelography employed to determine the cause of microscopic hematuria in this 34-year-old woman suggested a mass in the left kidney.

A, the CT scan shows a solid mass *(M)* in the lateral and upper pole of the left kidney.

B, the possibility of mass effect from the tail of the pancreas was raised, and the image was repeated at the same level but with the patient in a prone position. Clearly, the pancreas and kidney are separated from each other, and the left kidney is normal.

This case represents the pseudomass effect of the pancreas on the normal left kidney in a patient with little retroperitoneal fat.

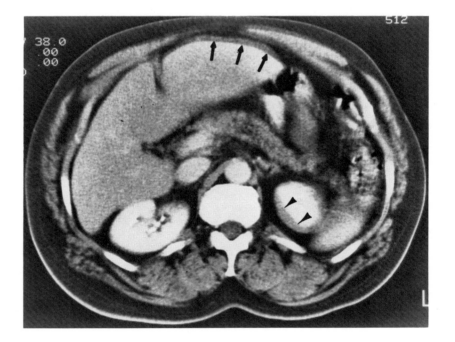

FIG 14–38.
Subcapsular hematoma, ascites? In this 38-year-old woman with melanoma, CT was performed to rule out metastasis.

On this upper abdomen image, there is a crescent-shaped low-density area *(arrowheads)* in the posterior and medial aspect of the left kidney, simulating subcapsular he-matoma. A similar finding *(arrows)* is seen anterior to the left lobe of the liver. The latter simulates ascites.

These apparent abnormalities are artifactual and result from brief internal motion during the exposure time of the CT scan. Shallow breathing, which can minimally displace the liver and kidneys, is usually at fault.

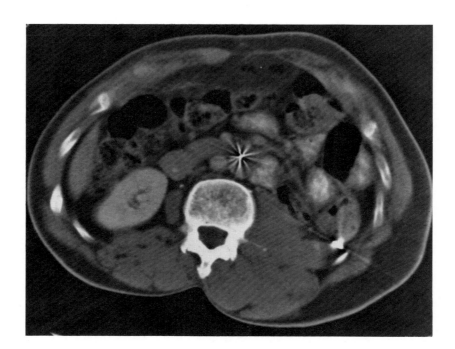

FIG 14–39.
Recurrent renal tumor? This patient had a history of left nephrectomy and right hip replacement. A CT scan was done to rule out the possibility of recurrent tumor.

There appears to be a large soft tissue density blending into the left psoas and left quadratus lumborum muscles. However, given this patient's history, one would suspect atrophy of the right paraspinal and right psoas muscles and avoid reading the normal left psoas muscle as tumor infiltration.

Asymmetry of the paraspinal, psoas, and iliacus muscles is commonly seen in patients with a history of such disabilities as poliomyelitis, previous amputation, and hip or knee prosthesis. Atrophy on one side and hypertrophic or normal anatomical parameters on the other side should not be mistaken for tumor or lymphadenopathy.

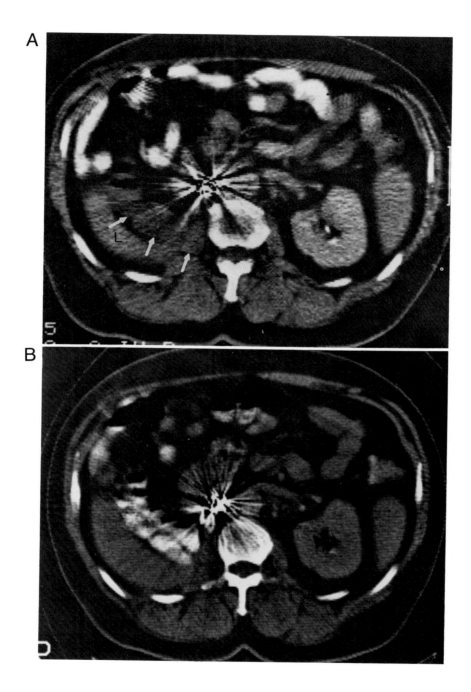

FIG 14–40.
Postnephrectomy recurrent tumor?

A, the CT scan was obtained one year after right nephrectomy and shows soft tissue density *(arrows)* in the renal fossa. Notice that a portion of the enhanced right lobe of the liver *(L)* is also seen behind the soft tissue density.

The question of locally recurrent tumor was raised.

B, the image was repeated at the same level about 30 min later. It shows that the unopacified bowel loops are now opacified, and there is no evidence of locally recurrent tumor.

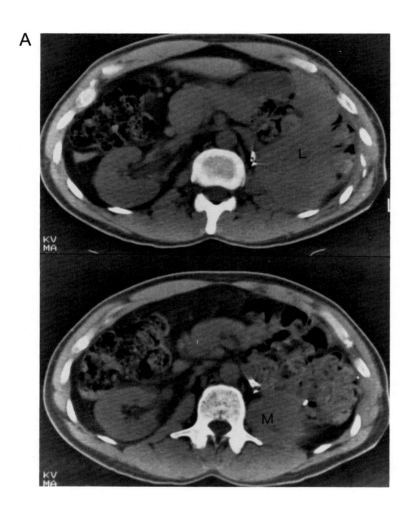

FIG 14–41.
Postnephrectomy recurrent tumor? This patient with situs inversus viscerum had a left nephrectomy for renal cell carcinoma. A CT study was done as follow-up to rule out local disease recurrence.

A, two CT images at 1.6-mm intervals show presence of liver *(L)* in the left side of the abdomen seen on the top image. Notice normal psoas muscles. However, in the bottom image a soft tissue density *(M)* obliterating the left psoas outline is seen in the left renal fossa. From CT, it could not be determined whether the soft tissue density *(m)* represented normal liver or tumor recurrence.

B, sequential axial T_1-weighted magnetic resonance images (TR/TE, 800/25) clearly show the soft tissue *(L)* to have the same signal intensity as the liver. The left psoas muscle *(P)* is clearly seen. No locally recurrent tumor is apparent.

C, the coronal T_1-weighted magnetic resonance image (TR/TE, 800/25) shows the normal outline of the left psoas muscle and absence of any abnormal tissue in the vicinity.

B

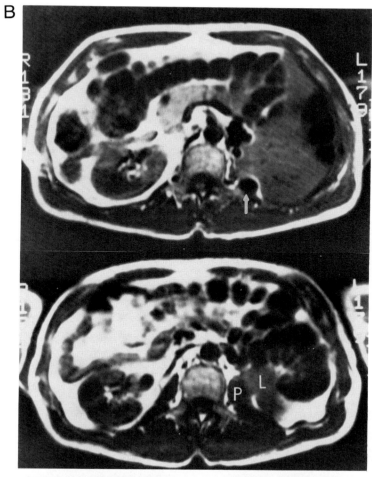

C

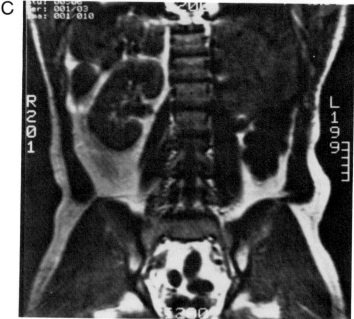

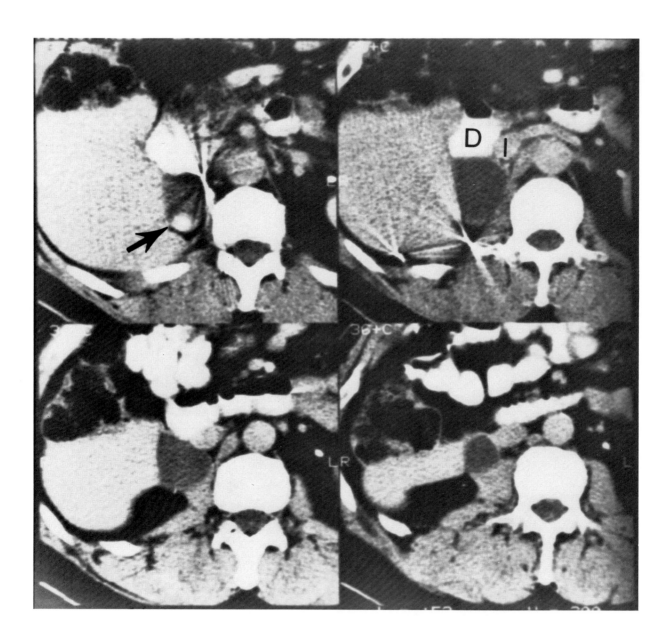

FIG 14–42.
Postnephrectomy hematoma/lymphocele? This patient had a nephrectomy three months previously. Abdominal CT was now used to assess for tumor recurrence or metastasis.

Sequential CT images demonstrate a well-defined cystic structure medial to the right lobe of the liver and behind the inferior vena cava *(I)* and duodenum *(D).* The gallbladder could not be identified, and there was evidence of a stone *(arrow)* within the lumen of the structure, proving displaced gallbladder with cholelithiasis.

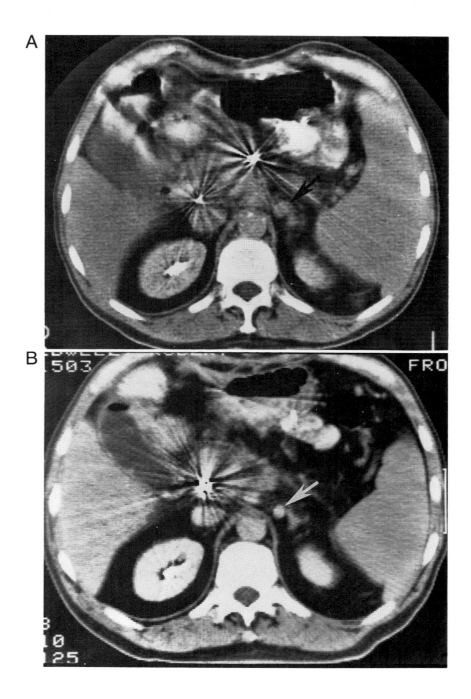

FIG 14–43.
Left adrenal nodule? (Multiple cases.)

A and B, this patient had previously undergone operation for retroperitoneal sarcoma. The present evaluation was for possible tumor recurrence. On this enhanced CT of the upper abdomen **(A)**, a nodular density *(arrow)* is seen in the left adrenal gland.

The repeat CT study at the same level **(B)** made during bolus intravenous contrast injection shows significant enhancement of this apparent nodular density *(arrow)*, which now appears to be adjacent to the left adrenal gland. (*Continued.*)

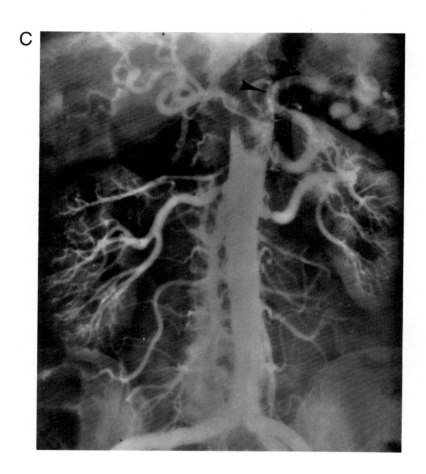

FIG 14–43 (cont.).
C, CT showed similar findings in this different patient (see reference that follows). An angiogram demonstrates the course of a tortuous splenic artery, which crosses the region of the left adrenal gland *(arrowheads).* On axial images made without bolus contrast, such an artery can easily mimic a left adrenal nodule, as was the case in this patient. (**C** from Shirkhoda A.: Current diagnostic approach to adrenal abnormalities. *J. Comput. Tomogr.* 8:277–285, 1984. Reproduced with permission.)

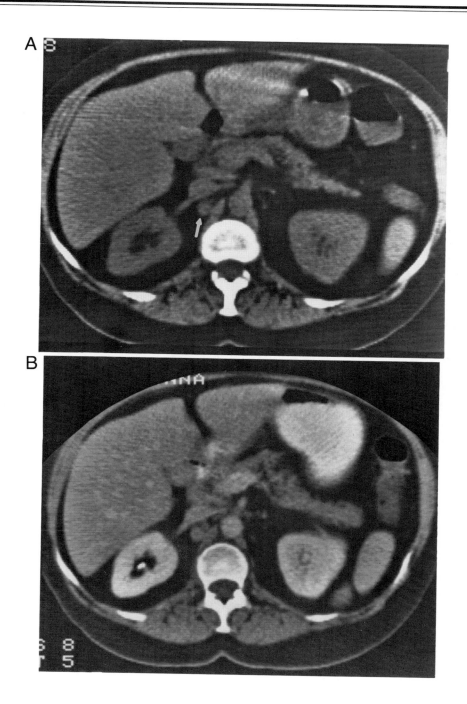

FIG 14–44.
Right adrenal nodule or retrocaval node? This 46-year-old woman with breast carcinoma underwent abdominal CT to rule out metastatic disease.

A, on this unenhanced CT scan, a small nodular density *(arrow)* is seen behind the inferior vena cava and lateral to the right crus of diaphragm.

B, the enhanced CT was obtained on bolus intravenous contrast injection. It shows the nodule to enhance almost to the same density as the aorta.

A tortuous renal artery is a common pitfall in and around the crus of diaphragm and simulates a node or a small adrenal nodule. As in the case of tortuous splenic artery, bolus contrast injection should be used for verification.

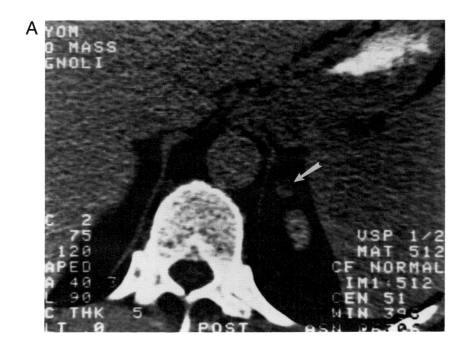

FIG 14–45.
Left adrenal nodule? A small nodule was discovered in the left adrenal gland during upper abdomen CT examination of this 45-year-old man with lung carcinoma.

A, on this CT image, which was obtained using a 5-mm slice thickness, a small nodule is seen *(arrow)* superior and medial to the left kidney in the adrenal fossa.

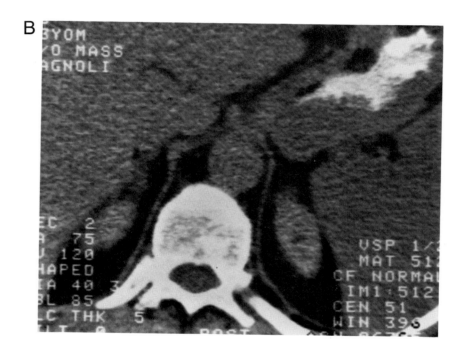

B, in a scan made 5 mm below image **A,** the continuity of this apparent nodule with the upper pole of the left kidney is seen. This suggests that a small renal cortical cyst of the left upper pole is projecting into the adrenal fossa.

On the original scan, the images were made using a 10-mm interval. In image **A,** only the nodule was seen; 10 mm below that, the continuity of the nodule with the upper-pole renal cyst could not be appreciated. This is not an uncommon pitfall.

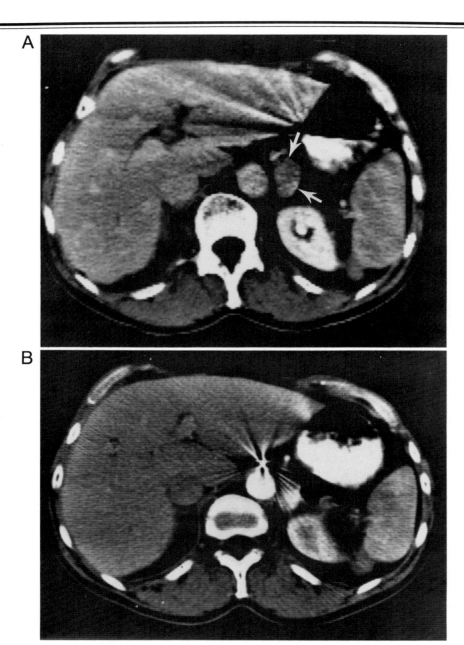

FIG 14–46.
Left adrenal mass? (Multiple cases.)

A and **B,** a 52-year-old woman with a history of hiatal hernia repair was found to have a right renal mass, proved to be carcinoma.

On initial CT assessment, the renal mass (not shown) was confined to the right kidney, and there was no evidence of metastasis. However, in this scan **(A),** a mass is seen in the left adrenal fossa *(arrows).* The mass was thought to displace the partially contrast-filled stomach anteriorly. The focal areas of high density within the mass were thought to be due to artifacts from the barium in the stomach and also from the surgical clips. Similar artifact is also seen in the spleen and liver.

A percutaneous aspiration biopsy was scheduled, and the patient was brought back on a different date and scanning done on a different machine using bolus intravenous contrast and oral contrast **(B).** The previously described mass is seen to be due to a portion of the stomach that is projecting into the proximity of the left adrenal gland. The adrenal gland could not be well seen because of the artifacts from the metallic clips. No adrenal mass was seen at the time of nephrectomy.

C and **D,** a different patient with abdominal pain was reported to have a left adrenal mass *(arrows* in **C**). Double-contrast upper gastrointestinal study **(D)** shows a diverticulum off the gastric fundus projecting posteriorly into the adrenal fossa. A repeat CT scan showed barium enhancement of the mass seen in **C.**

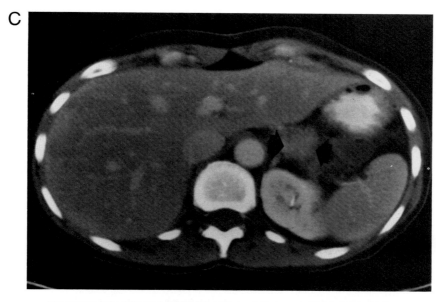

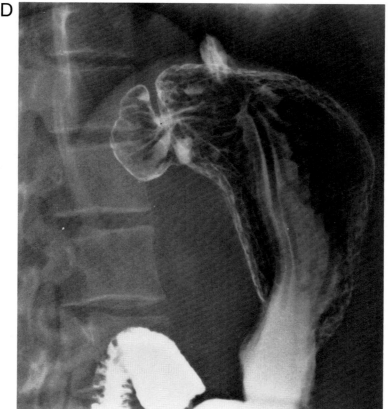

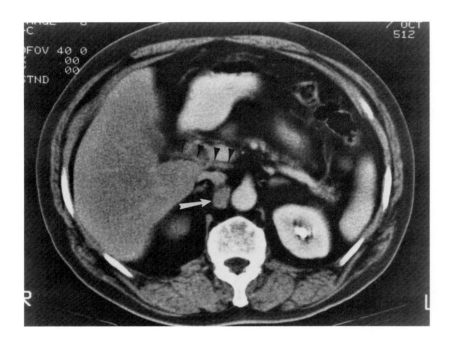

FIG 14–47.

Paraaortic node? This 58-year-old man had undergone colon resection for adenocarcinoma and now had a CT scan as follow-up.

There is a nodular density *(arrow)* lateral to the aorta and behind the inferior vena cava. This is a very common pitfall on the right side because of thickened right crus of

diaphragm. The right crus is often thicker and longer than the left, and its more proximal portion in the upper abdomen can often mimic retroperitoneal adenopathy.

On this image, notice the replaced right hepatic artery *(arrowheads)* that is anterior to the inferior vena cava and behind the portal vein. This also should not be mistaken for a lymph node.

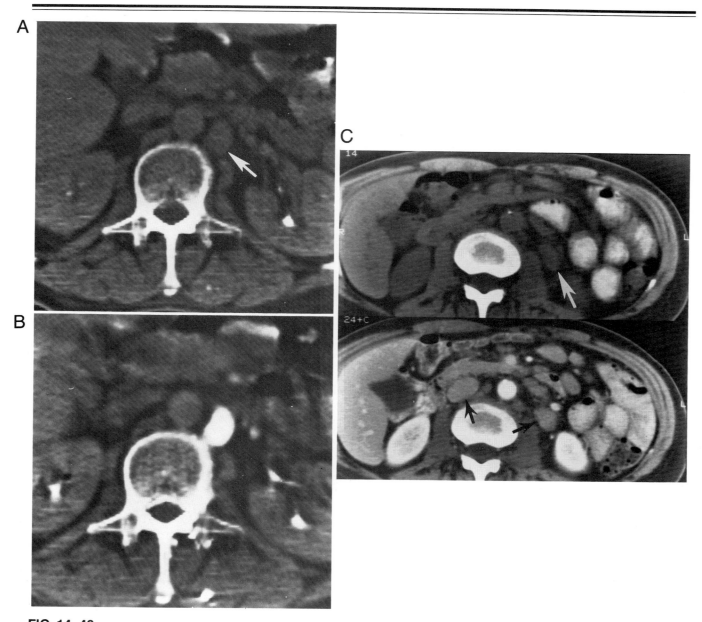

FIG 14–48.

Retroperitoneal adenopathy? (Multiple cases.)

A and **B,** these first two CT scans were part of the evaluation of primary lung carcinoma. A nodular density *(arrow)* is seen to the left of the aorta in the upper abdomen scan **(A).** Additional images obtained at the same time on lower levels suggested a possibly vascular nature of the soft tissue mass.

The upper abdomen study was repeated **(B)** during direct injection of contrast into a vein of the dorsal aspect of a foot. The intense opacification of the structure in question proves a left-sided inferior vena cava.

This uncommon anomaly usually crosses the midline at the level of the kidneys and becomes a right-sided vena cava or drains into the left renal vein. When the CT is strictly done in the upper abdomen as a part of chest study, one might see the very upper portion of the left inferior vena cava and mistake that for a retroperitoneal node. Bolus intravenous contrast, preferably in a foot vein, will demonstrate the vascular nature of this pitfall.

C, in a different patient, the normal right-sided inferior vena cava is seen on the unenhanced *(top)* and enhanced *(bottom)* studies. However, on the unenhanced CT, there is a nodular density *(white arrow)* lateral to the left psoas muscle; this density is obviously a vascular structure since it enhances along with the vena cava *(black arrows).* Such duplication of the inferior vena cava can also be confused with adenopathy.

A

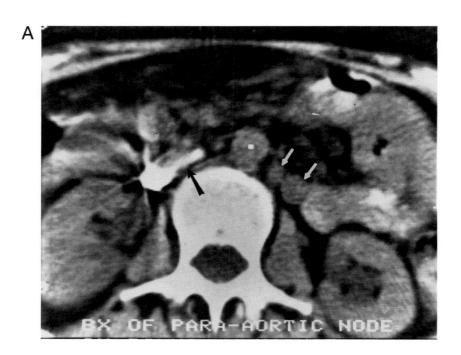

BX OF PARA-AORTIC NODE

FIG 14–49.

Retroperitoneal lymphadenopathy? (Multiple cases.)

A, this 60-year-old man with known prostate cancer was referred for biopsy of a CT-discovered paraaortic node. A CT scan was obtained during hand injection of contrast in a foot vein and shows the opacified inferior vena cava *(black arrow)* in the right and nodular densities *(white arrows)* in the left paraaortic region.

B, the CT image was repeated at the same level during large-bolus injection in the antecubital vein. There is simul-

taneous enhancement of the nodular densities and the aorta, confirming the vascular and probably arterial nature of the densities. The most likely etiology for this finding is tortuous left renal artery.

C, a similar finding in a different patient with extensive arteriosclerosis involves tortuous bilateral renal arteries. Notice the origin of the right renal artery from the aorta *(arrow).* Small low-density areas within the walls of vessels probably represent clots.

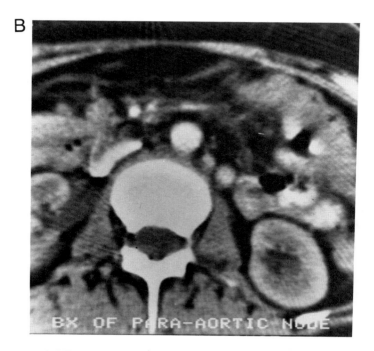

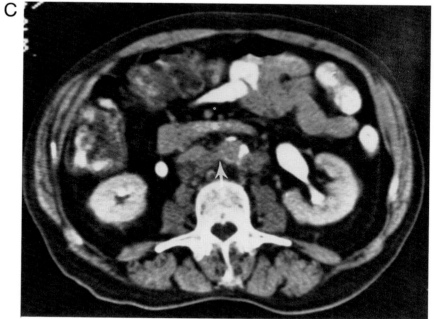

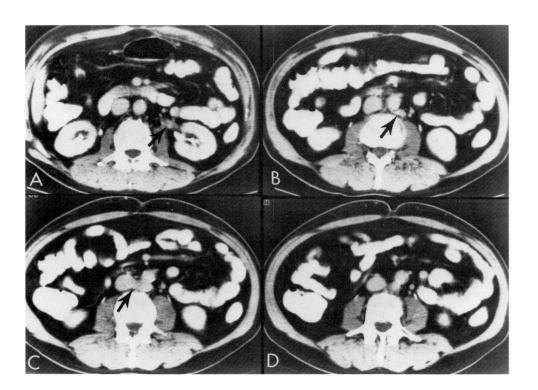

FIG 14–50.
Retroaortic adenopathy? A 38-year-old woman with melanoma of the lower extremity underwent CT scanning at an outside institution and was referred to M. D. Anderson Hospital for percutaneous aspiration biopsy of a retroaortic lymph node.

An enlarged lymph node was suspected from images **C** and **D.** However, the **A** to **D** sequence of four 10-mm slices belies that suspicion. In fact, the left renal vein originates (*arrow* in **A**) in the left kidney and goes behind the aorta in an oblique fashion (*arrow* in **B**), then merging with the inferior vena cava (*arrow* in **C**). In **D,** the lower border of the vein has been imaged because of volume averaging.

A retroaortic left renal vein is not uncommon, but usually it crosses the midline transversely. However, when the renal vein enters the vena cava at a level lower than that at which it originates in the kidney, there is the potential for confusion on CT.

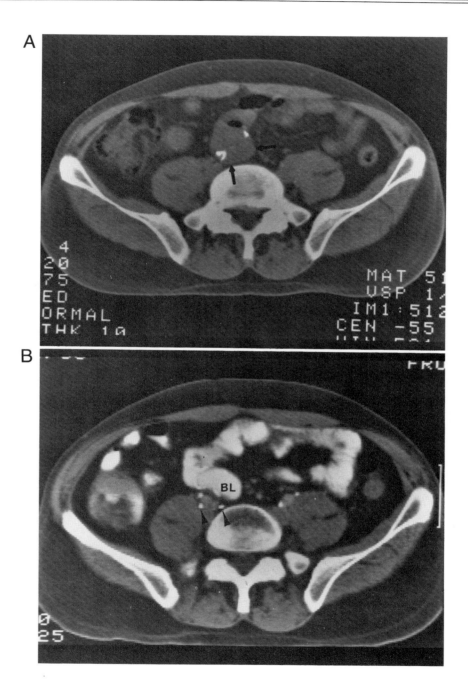

FIG 14–51.
Retroperitoneal adenopathy? A 44-year-old woman had previously undergone lymphangiography for lymphoma and now two years later underwent follow-up CT for the post-chemotherapy evaluation of nodes.

A, the CT scan shows a soft tissue mass *(arrows)* anterior to the proximal right main iliac vessels. The mass was presumed to represent adenopathy. So that the entire nodal system could be evaluated, lymphangiography was repeated. Normal lymphangiographic findings were reported.

B, this CT scan shows the previously described soft tissue density to be due to unopacified bowel loop *(BL)*. Notice residual contrast material *(arrowheads)* in the normal lymph nodes around the enhanced main iliac vessels.

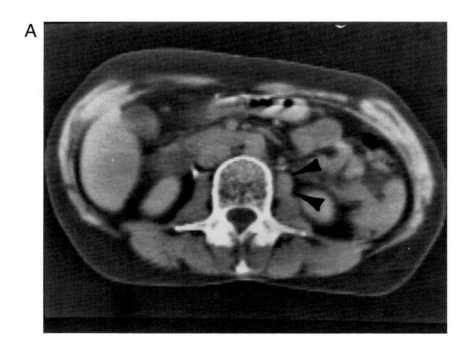

FIG 14–52.
Adenopathy? (Multiple cases.) These abdominal CT scans are from two patients, both evaluated to rule out metastatic disease in the retroperitoneum.

A, unilateral soft tissue density *(arrowheads)* is seen anterior to the left psoas muscle.

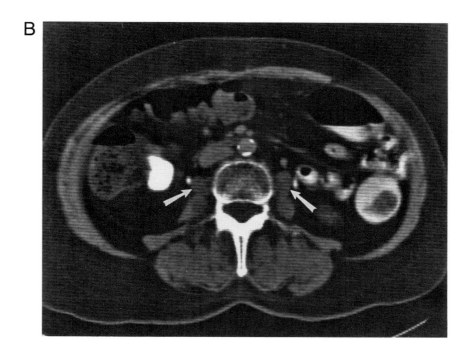

B, there are bilateral soft tissue densities *(arrows)* anterior to the psoas muscles. Both of the ureters, which are opacified, appear to be displaced.

In both of these patients, the psoas minor muscle is being imaged. This muscle, which is often absent, can be unilateral or bilateral and generally extends anterior to the psoas major muscle, particularly when it is unilaterally present. It should not be mistaken for an enlarged lymph node.

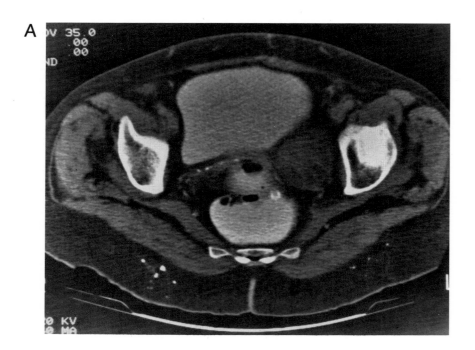

FIG 14–53.

Pelvic abscess, mass? (Multiple cases.)

A through **C,** a 39-year-old woman presented with abdominal pain and irregular vaginal bleeding.

The CT images of the lower pelvis (**A** and **B**) demonstrate a large soft tissue mass *(M)* with multiple irregular densities, in the left side of the pelvis. The patient had received oral and rectal contrast, and it appears that the opacified rectosigmoid colon *(CO)* is draped over the soft tissue

mass **(B).** A barium enema examination was recommended.

A double-contrast barium enema **(C)** demonstrates extensive diverticulosis of the colon. The colon is somehow redundant with the sigmoid and distal descending colon, folding over within the pelvis. This area obviously did not fill with rectal contrast, so that a pelvic mass was mimicked. The finding was originally thought to represent ovarian tumor. Vaginal examination was normal. (*Continued.*)

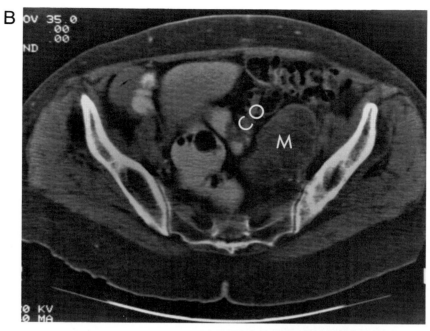

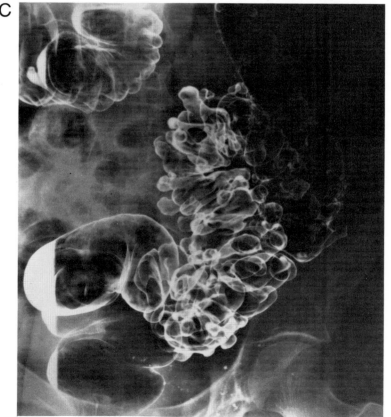

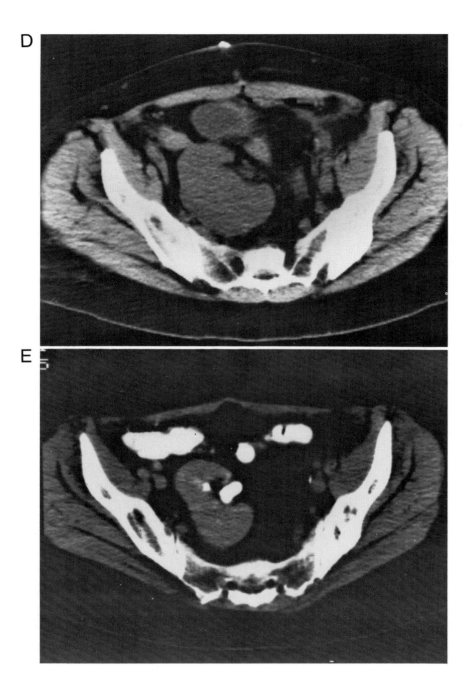

FIG 14–53 (cont.).
D and **E,** in this 76-year-old woman who had hysterectomy at the age of 35, a pelvic mass was palpated. Unen-hanced pelvic CT **(D)** shows a well-defined mass in the right side. Repeat CT with intravenous contrast **(E)** proved a nor-mal pelvic kidney.

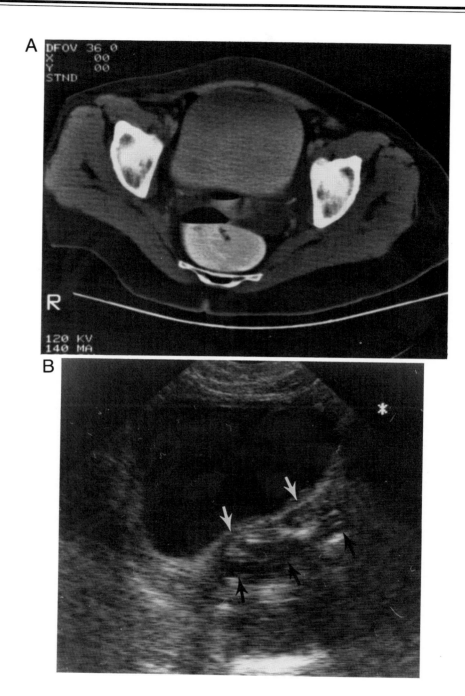

FIG 14–54.

Adnexal mass? Abdominal and pelvic CT examinations were done in this 34-year-old woman with known melanoma.

A, there is a low-density mass in the region of the left, and probably the right, adnexa. The normal uterus was seen on the other CT images. This patient was considered as otherwise having no evidence of disease, and this CT finding warranted additional evaluation for possible biopsy.

B, real-time examination failed to show any definite mass. This examination was done during water enema and shows normal peristalsis in the area of the rectosigmoid colon *(arrows)*. No abnormal adnexal mass was seen.

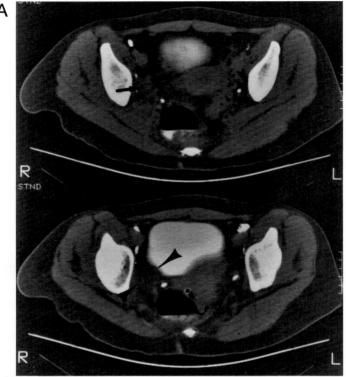

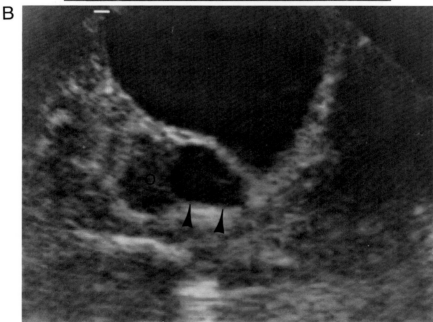

FIG 14–55.
Pelvic adenopathy? A 33-year-old woman with newly diagnosed carcinoma of the cervix had abdominal and pelvic CT as part of the staging procedures. The lymphangiographic findings were normal.

A, there is a soft tissue density *(arrows)* in the right side of the pelvis, adjacent to the internal obturator muscle. This density was also seen on another CT scan. Pelvic adenopathy was strongly suspected. A cystic right adnexal mass *(arrowheads),* presumed to represent an ovarian cyst, is seen in the adjacent image.

B, ultrasonography was done to further evaluate the adnexa. The parasagittal sonogram of the right side of the pelvis shows that the normal right ovary *(O)* contains a cyst *(arrowheads)* in its lower portion.

Occasionally, in this orientation of benign ovarian cyst, axial imaging of the cyst on one image and the solid ovary on another generates the pitfall of adenopathy from the normal ovary.

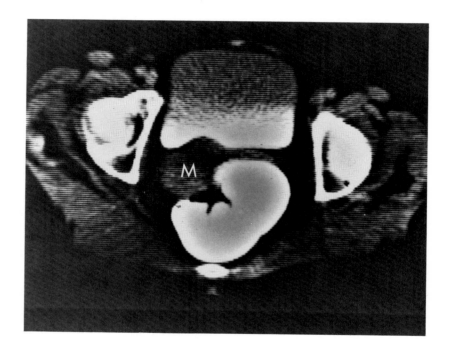

FIG 14–56.

Pelvic mass? A 59-year-old woman with a history of hysterectomy for dysfunctional bleeding presented with lower abdominal pain. On this CT image, there is a soft tissue density behind the bladder and anterior to the rectum. This was thought to represent an adnexal mass, but review of the history revealed that the hysterectomy had been a supracervical one, so that the soft tissue would represent the remaining cervix.

As seen here, this type of hysterectomy, which is not commonly done, can lead to a pitfall in future pelvic imaging.

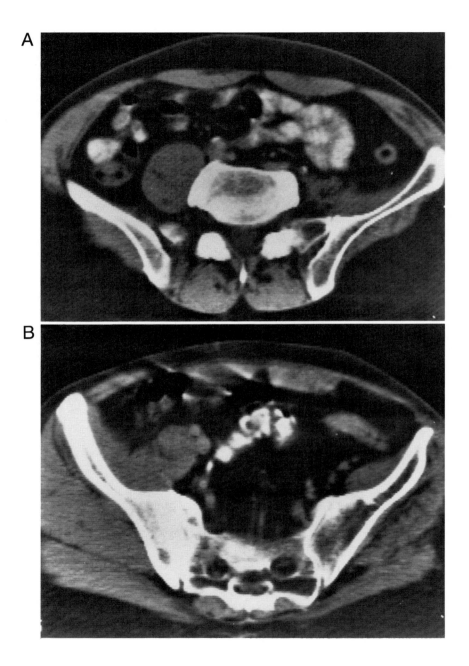

FIG 14–57.
Right iliac mass? This CT scan was made to assess for local disease recurrence or metastasis in a 17-year-old boy who had two years previously undergone hip disarticulation for osteosarcoma of the proximal left femur.

A and **B,** significant atrophy of the left psoas muscle is seen in both images. Normal muscles in the right should not be confused with a pathologic mass in the iliac fossa.

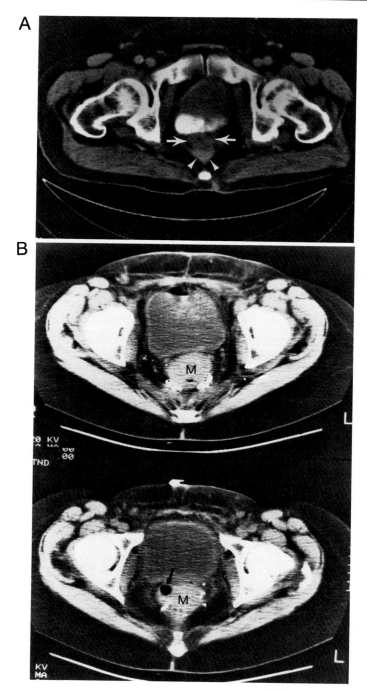

FIG 14–58.
Recurrent rectal carcinoma? (Multiple cases.) From different patients, both of these CT scans were made approximately one year after the treatment of rectal carcinoma by anterior peritoneal resection.

A, in this 61-year-old man, postoperative changes are seen anterior to the coccyx *(arrowheads)*. In addition, there are two nodular densities *(arrows)* behind the bladder and adjacent to the postsurgical scar.

B, in addition to postsurgical changes in this 57-year-old woman, there is a large mass *(M)* in the midline anterior to the coccyx and lower sacrum. Notice the tampon *(arrow)* within the vagina.

After anterior peritoneal resection, changes related to posterior and inferior displacement of the seminal vesicles **(A)** or uterus **(B)** are commonly observed and should not be mistaken for locally recurrent tumor.

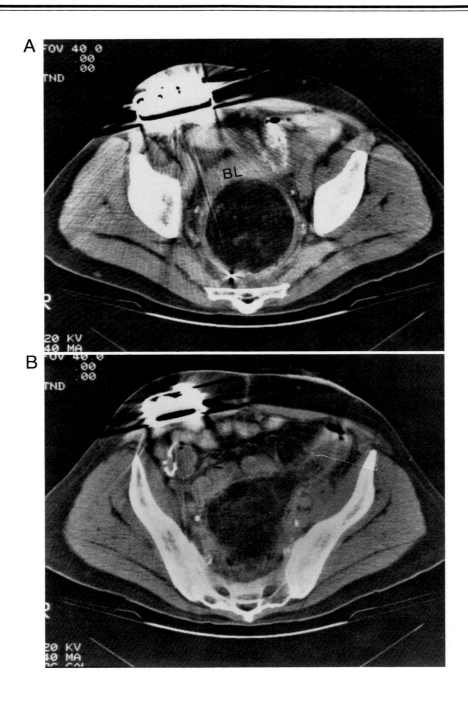

FIG 14–59.
Pelvic fatty tumor? A CT examination was done on this 44-year-old woman who had a history of sigmoid colostomy, followed by radiation therapy for rectal carcinoma.

A, on this lower pelvic CT, there is a well-rounded fatty mass deep within the true pelvis. A small portion of the bladder *(BL)* is seen anterior to the mass. The injection pump for administration of chemotherapy to the liver metas-

tases is seen in the right lower abdomen.

B, the CT image obtained at the midpelvis shows continuity of the fatty mass with the peritoneum. The further history revealed that this mass represents omental fat, which had been surgically dispatched into the pelvis to displace the small bowel upward so that the rectal area could be irradiated.

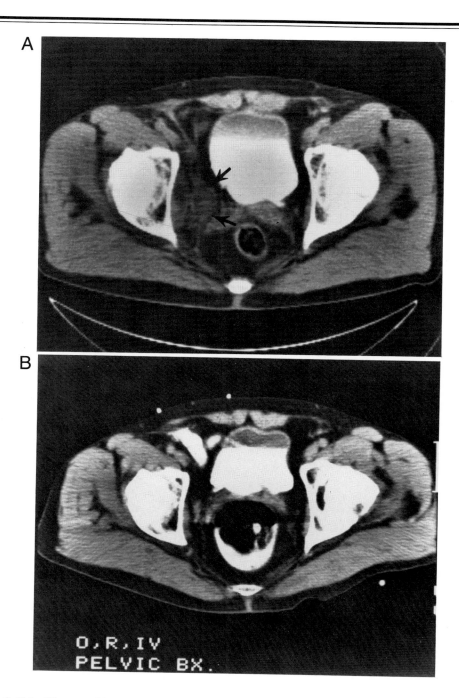

FIG 14–60.

Pelvic adenopathy? This 69-year-old man was referred to M. D. Anderson Hospital shortly after a transperineal biopsy of the prostate that established adenocarcinoma.

A, the CT scan of the pelvis demonstrates a soft tissue mass *(arrows)* in the right side, adjacent to the right internal obturator muscle. The obturator muscle itself also appears to be slightly prominent. With the probable diagnosis of pelvic adenopathy, the patient was scheduled to undergo a CT-guided biopsy.

B, the CT examination was repeated in one week for localization of the soft tissue mass and as a guide for biopsy procedure. As this scan shows, the previously noted abnormality was not seen.

The CT findings at the time of admission were most likely attributable to hematoma following transperineal biopsy. Indeed, lack of adenopathy changed the staging of the prostatic carcinoma and saved the patient an unnecessary biopsy.

Index